FAMILY MEDICAL ADVISOR

FAMILY MEDICAL ADVISOR

The Complete Guide to Alternative & Conventional Treatments

BY THE EDITORS OF TIME-LIFE BOOKS
ALEXANDRIA, VIRGINIA

CONSULTANTS

NEIL BAUM, MD
teaches at Tulane Medical School and serves on the staff of Touro Infirmary and Memorial Medical Center in New Orleans. He is a board-certified urologist with expertise in male sexual dysfunction, urinary incontinence, and male infertility; he has written extensively in these areas. Dr. Baum is the author of *Impotence—It's Reversible.*

HERBERT BENSON, MD
teaches at Harvard Medical School and is chief of the Division of Behavioral Medicine at the Deaconess Hospital. He is also founding president of the Mind/Body Medical Institute, which specializes in the treatment of stress-related illnesses. Dr. Benson has helped draw attention to the field of mind/body medicine through his pioneering work on the relaxation response.

ZOË BRENNER, LAc, Dipl Ac, Dipl Ch (NCCAOM), FNAAOM
has practiced acupuncture since 1977 and Chinese herbal medicine since 1984. She teaches oriental medicine and the history and philosophy of Chinese medicine at the Traditional Acupuncture Institute in Bethesda, Maryland.

DWIGHT C. BYERS
is a leading authority in reflexology. He began teaching with his late aunt, Eunice Ingham, who pioneered and developed the original Ingham method of reflexology. Byers travels throughout the world to teach reflexology, and he serves as president of the International Institute of Reflexology in St. Petersburg, Florida.

BARRIE R. CASSILETH, PhD
is chief of the Integrative Medicine Service at Memorial Sloan-Kettering Cancer Center in New York. She was a member of the founding council of the Office of Alternative Medicine at the National Institutes of Health, and she is now a board member of the American Cancer Society.

EFFIE CHOW, PhD, RN, CA
is president of the East West Academy of Healing Arts in San Francisco. A registered nurse, certified acupuncturist, and qigong master, Dr. Chow has practiced and taught qigong for more than 30 years.

JOHN G. COLLINS, ND, DHANP
teaches homeopathy at the National College of Naturopathic Medicine in Portland, Oregon. He also has a private practice in Portland, Oregon.

STEPHANIE S. COVINGTON, PhD, LCSW
is a psychotherapist and codirector of the Institute for Relational Development in La Jolla, California. She has taught at the California School of Professional Psychology and has written extensively on the subject of addiction. Two of Dr. Covington's recent publications include *A Woman's Way Through the Twelve Steps* and *Helping Women Recover: A Program for Treatment Addiction.* She formerly chaired the Women's Committee of the International Council on Alcoholism and Addiction.

KYLE H. CRONIN, ND
specializes in women's healthcare in her medical practice in Phoenix. Dr. Cronin is a cofounder and former academic dean and currently dean of Curricular Development at Southwest College of Naturopathic Medicine and Health Sciences.

TIMOTHY B. DEERING, MD
is a board-certified internist and gastroenterologist who practices with Asheville Gastroenterology Associates in North Carolina.

PALI C. DELEVITT, PhD
consults on alternative therapies at the cancer center of the University of Virginia, where she also teaches in the School of Medicine. Dr. Delevitt has consulted on curriculum development for the medical schools of Columbia University, Emory University, and Indiana University.

JAMES A. DUKE, PhD
was an economic botanist with the Agriculture Research Service, United States Department of Agriculture, in Beltsville, Maryland, for much of his career. Dr. Duke advises many organizations, including Nature's Herbs and allherb.com.

KATHLEEN FRY, MD, MD(H)
is a board-certified gynecologist specializing in holistic healthcare for women. She is a licensed classical homeopath and current president of the American Holistic Medical Association. Dr. Fry has a private medical practice at Alternatives for Women in Scottsdale, Arizona.

ADRIANE FUGH-BERMAN, MD
is Assistant Clinical Professor in the Department of Health Care Sciences at George Washington School of Medicine. She is editor of the newsletter *Alternative Therapies in Women's Health* and the author of *Alternative Medicine: What Works.* Her articles have appeared in numerous medical and consumer publications. She is on the executive board of the National Women's Health Network. Dr. Fugh-Berman was formerly with the National Institutes of Health, at the Contraception and Reproductive Health Branch and at the Office of Alternative Medicine.

ALAN R. GABY, MD
is past president of the American Holistic Medical Association. He is professor of therapeutic nutrition at Bastyr University in Kenmore, Washington, and the author of *The Patient's Book of Natural Healing.*

DAVID E. GOLAN, MD, PhD
is an attending physician at Brigham and Women's Hospital in Boston and an associate professor of biological chemistry and molecular pharmacology at Harvard Medical School. A board-certified internist and hematologist, Dr. Golan directs research on blood cell membranes. He has also created a computer-learning program for pharmacology.

CONSTANCE GRAUDS, RPh
is founder and president of the Association of Natural Medicine Pharmacists. She is assistant clinical pharmacy professor at the University of California, San Francisco. Grauds is the natural medicine editor for *Pharmacy Times* and the author of *Kava and Anxiety.* As a trained specialist in the field of natural medicines, she is also a consultant to the pharmaceutical and natural medicine industries.

ELLIOT GREENE, MA
is a past president of the American Massage Therapy Association and currently serves on the regulatory Massage Therapy Advisory Committee for the State of Maryland. Nationally certified in massage therapy by the National Certification Board for Therapeutic Massage and Bodywork, he has more than 27 years of experience in the field. Mr. Greene maintains a private practice in Silver Spring, Maryland.

KEITH S. HECHTMAN, MD, FAAOS, FAOSSM
is a board-certified orthopedic surgeon who is fellowship-trained in sports medicine. He is an associate professor in the Department of Orthopaedics and Sports Medicine at the University of Miami in Florida. Dr. Hechtman trains medical students, residents, and fellows in the specialty of sports medicine. He is the team physician for Florida International University and the University of Miami. He is also Medical Director of Athletics of Miami-Dade County High Schools.

VICTOR HERBERT, MD, JD, MACP
teaches medicine at the Mount Sinai-New York University Health System, where he also chairs the Committee to Strengthen Nutrition. A former president of the American Society for Clinical Nutrition, Dr. Herbert consults in the field of nutrition for many organizations, including the World Health Organization.

DAVID HOFFMANN, MNIMH
is a member of the British National Institute of Medical Herbalists and founding president of the American Herbalist Guild. His writings on therapeutic herbalism were a valuable resource during the preparation of this volume.

MAURITA HOLLAND, MALS
is an associate professor of information and library science at the University of Michigan in Ann Arbor. Some of her students provided research for this book and are listed individually in the acknowledgments section.

TORI HUDSON, ND
is a professor at the National College of Naturopathic Medicine and is medical director of A Woman's Time clinic for women in Portland, Oregon. Dr. Hudson specializes in women's healthcare; in 1990, she received a national award for her research and in 1999 she was named Naturopathic Physician of the Year.

GRACE BROOKE HUFFMAN, MD
serves as a primary care physician at two offices in Maryland and teaches at Georgetown University School of Medicine in Washington, D.C. A board-certified family practitioner, she has additional certification in geriatrics.

STEVEN IDELL, MD, PhD, FACP, FACCP
is chief of the pulmonary division and chairman of the Department of Specialty Care Services at the University of Texas Health Center at Tyler. His research in pulmonary diseases is sponsored by the National Institutes of Health.

JENNIFER JACOBS, MD, MPH
specializes in homeopathic medicine and has a private practice in family medicine in Edmonds, Washington. She conducts research in the use of homeopathic medicines in primary care at the University of Washington. Dr. Jacobs is the coauthor of *Healing with Homeopathy.*

JOSEPH J. JACOBS, MD, MBA
began his medical career as a pediatrician with the Indian Health Service in Gallup, New Mexico, and has continued working with American Indians throughout his career. Dr. Jacobs was director of the Office of Alternative Medicine at the National Institutes of Health from 1992 to 1994 and is a former president of the Association of American Indian Physicians.

JONATHAN M. KAGAN, MD
is clinical assistant professor of ophthalmology at New York Medical College and a fellow of the American Academy of Ophthalmology. Dr. Kagan maintains a private practice in New York City. He conducts clinical trials of new drugs for ophthalmic use, and he is among the first surgeons to perform laser vision correction.

STEVEN W. KAIRYS, MD, MPH, FAAP
is associate chair of pediatrics at the Dartmouth-Hitchcock Medical Center, where he directs primary care activities and the Children at Risk Program. He is founder and president of the New Hampshire Alliance for Children and Youth in Concord, New Hampshire.

J. DANIEL KANOFSKY, MD, MPH
teaches psychiatry, epidemiology, and social medicine at the Albert Einstein College of Medicine and at the Bronx Psychiatric Center, both in New York City. A board-certified psychiatrist, Dr. Kanofsky is also a fellow of the American College of Nutrition.

TED KAPTCHUK, OMD, CA
is a research associate at Beth Israel Hospital. As a doctor of Oriental Medicine, Dr. Kaptchuk practices both Chinese herbal medicine and acupuncture. He is the author of *The Web That Has No Weaver.*

ROBERT B. KLEIN, MD, FAAP, FAAAI
is chairman of pediatrics at the University of Texas Health Center at Tyler. His other specialties include allergy, pulmonology, and immunology. Dr. Klein also consults on childhood tuberculosis and asthma in Croatia for the U.S. State Department.

ROBERT KOTLER, MD, FACS
practices facial plastic surgery in Beverly Hills, California. Dr. Kotler is a former commissioner and regional consultant to the Medical Board of California. He also teaches at UCLA Center for the Health Sciences.

JOSEPH J. LAMB, MD
is a board-certified internist and a senior clinician with American WholeHealth, Inc. in Alexandria, Virginia, where he practices integrative medicine. Dr. Lamb is the school physician at Episcopal High School in Alexandria. He is on the clinical faculty at George Washington School of Medicine.

JESSE M. KRAMER, MD
is a dermatologist practicing in Santa Rosa, California. He teaches family medicine physicians through the University of California in San Francisco.

DAVID B. LARSON, MD, MSPH
is a psychiatrist; his particular interest is the influence of religious commitment on physical and mental health. Currently the president of the National Institute for Healthcare Research, Dr. Larson has worked for the National Institutes of Health and the U.S. Department of Health and Human Services. He serves as an adjunct faculty member for several universities, including Duke and Northwestern University Medical Centers.

DANA J. LAWRENCE, DC, FICC
is dean of Postgraduate and Continuing Education, director of Publications and Editorial Review, and a professor in the Department of Chiropractic Practice at the National College of Chiropractic in Lombard, Illinois. He is editor of the school's *Journal of Manipulative and Physiological Therapeutics.*

KAREN SUE LEVENTHAL, RPh
is a registered pharmacist in Maryland, Pennsylvania, and Washington, D.C. She is currently working for Rite Aid Corporation in Washington, D.C, where she is a pharmacy manager. She received her Bachelor of Science in Pharmacy from the University of Pittsburgh School of Pharmacy.

NORMAN S. LEVY, MD, PhD, FAAO, FACS
practices ophthalmology in Gainesville, Florida, specializing in glaucoma. He conducts research at the University of Florida. Dr. Levy is a former professor and chief of ophthalmology at the Veterans Administration hospitals in Gainesville and Lake City, Florida.

PHILIP LEVY, MD, FACE
practices at the Phoenix Endocrinology Clinic, Ltd., and is a clinical professor of medicine at the University of Arizona in Tucson. He is an active member of the American Diabetes Association, the Endocrine Society, and the American Association of Clinical Endocrinologists.

JOHN E. LONSTEIN, MD
is a board-certified orthopedic surgeon and past president of the Scoliosis Research Society. Dr. Lonstein teaches at the University of Minnesota and practices with Twin Cities Spine Surgeons, Ltd. He is also chief of Spine Service and Cerebral Palsy Spine Service at Gillette Children's Hospital in Minnesota.

DAVE MANNINO, MD, FACCP
works at the Centers for Disease Control and Prevention at the National Center for Environmental Health in Atlanta. He teaches at the Emory School of Public Health.

ROY J. MATHEW, MD
teaches at Duke University Medical Center in Durham, North Carolina. He is also director of the Alcoholism and Addictions program, which provides treatment for people with alcoholism and drug addiction and offers consultation services for other medical specialists regarding addictions. Dr. Mathew's research focuses largely on the effects of alcohol and drugs on the brain and behavior.

ALEXANDER MAUSKOP, MD, FAAN
is director of the New York Headache Center and the not-for-profit New York Headache Foundation. He also teaches clinical neurology at the State University of New York, where he conducts research on the role of magnesium in headaches.

JEFFREY MIGDOW, MD
directs prana yoga-teacher training through the Open Center in New York City. He began his yoga training more than 20 years ago at Kripalu Center in Lenox, Massachusetts. In his medical practice, Dr. Migdow counsels patients on lifestyle and recommends a wide variety of homeopathic, nutritional, and other therapies. He is the coauthor of *Breathe In, Breathe Out.*

JOHN R. MOFFETT, PhD
is a former research scientist in the Biology Department at Georgetown University in Washington, D.C. His specific areas of research are neurotransmitters in the visual system and toxins released by immune cells.

ANNE MOORE, MD
teaches clinical medicine at Weill Medical College of Cornell University and chairs the New York Hospital breast cancer tumor board. Board certified in internal medicine with subspecialties in hematology and oncology, Dr. Moore is also on the staff of the New York Presbyterian Hospital-Cornell Medical Center.

LEN OCHS, PhD
is a social psychologist who has spent 20 years developing computerized biofeedback instrumentation. Dr. Ochs is past president of the Biofeedback Society of New York. He is currently researching energy field neurofeedback systems to treat fibromyalgia and traumatic brain surgery.

STEPHEN OLMSTEAD, MD
practices internal medicine and cardiology in Seattle, where he also teaches at the University of Washington.

ELSA RAMSDEN, EdD, PT
is a licensed physical therapist and certified medical psychologist. She is *emerita* professor at the University of Pennsylvania and an adjunct professor at Widener University. She has taught overseas at the University of Queensland in Brisbane, Australia, and the University of Uppsala, Sweden, and she was a Fulbright senior scholar to Australia.

JOHN C. REED, MD, MD(H)
is a board-certified family physician who is the National Medical Director for American WholeHealth, Inc. and WholeHealthMD.com. Dr. Reed has integrated acupuncture, homeopathy, and osteopathic medicine into his medical practice. He has consulted for the Office of Alternative Medicine at the National Institutes of Health and was coeditor of that office's report, *Alternative Medicine: Expanding Medical Horizons.* He currently consults with American WholeHealth's integrative medicine practices in the Washington, D.C., metropolitan area.

NORMAN E. ROSENTHAL, MD
is clinical professor of psychiatry at Georgetown University Medical School and a guest researcher at the National Institutes of Health. Dr. Rosenthal is a former president of the Society for Light Therapy and Biological Rhythms.

BEVERLY RUBIK, PhD
is founding director of the Center for Frontier Sciences at Temple University in Philadelphia. Her particular interests in the field of alternative medicine include spiritual healing, acupuncture, and homeopathy.

MILDRED SEELIG, MD, MPH
teaches nutrition at the University of North Carolina, Chapel Hill, and preventive medicine at Emory University in Atlanta. Dr. Seelig is editor emeritus of the Journal of the American College of Nutrition.

WINIFRED SEWELL, MS, DSc
is a fellow of the Medical Library Association. She has taught at the University of Maryland School of Pharmacy as well as the College of Library and Information Services.

SCOTT SHANNON, MD
practices integrative psychiatry, holistic medicine, and medical acupuncture in Fort Collins, Colorado. Board certified in two specialties, he consults with large hospital systems and major corporations on the integration of alternative therapies with conventional treatments. An officer of the American Holistic Medical Association, Dr. Shannon teaches other physicians nationally about holistic medicine.

JILL M. SIEGFRIED, PhD
is professor and vicechairman of the Department of Pharmacology at the University of Pittsburgh School of Medicine. She specializes in cancer pharmacology and conducts research in lung cancer. Dr. Siegfried is director of the Lung Cancer Basic Science Program at the University of Pittsburgh Cancer Institute.

J. JAMISON STARBUCK, JD, ND
practices family medicine in Missoula, Montana. She is a regular feature writer and monthly columnist for two national health magazines, a freelance writer, and an editor. Dr. Starbuck is a past president of the American Association of Naturopathic Physicians.

JAMES P. SWYERS, MA
is a science writer and editor who formerly served as managing editor of *Alternative Medicine: Expanding Medical Horizons,* a report published by the Office of Alternative Medicine at the National Institutes of Health. Before turning to journalism, he worked as a research biochemist and molecular biologist.

MICHAEL A. TANSEY, PhD
is an EEG neurofeedback clinician and researcher. He is a past president of the Society for the Study of Neuronal Regulation.

DICK W. THOM, DDS, ND
is an associate professor at the National College of Naturopathic Medicine in Portland, Oregon, where he teaches clinical and physical diagnosis, neurology, endocrinology, and therapeutic drainage. Dr. Thom is also a clinic supervisor at Natural Health Centers. He maintains a private practice at Natural Choices Health Clinic in Beaverton, Oregon.

ALEX A. TIBERI, OMD, LAc
is chairman of the Department of Oriental Medicine at the Pacific College of Oriental Medicine in San Diego. At his private practice at the Pacific Center of Health, he specializes in acupuncture for sports medicine. Dr. Tiberi has also served as a national examiner for the National Commission for the Certification of Acupuncturists.

ANDREW J. VICKERS
directs the information service at the Research Council for Complementary Medicine in the United Kingdom. He also teaches research methodology at the University of Westminster and the London School of Acupuncture.

ROBERT C. WARD, DO, FAAO
teaches biomechanics and family medicine at Michigan State University's College of Osteopathic Medicine. He was in private family practice for 12 years prior to teaching.

CAROLINE WELLBERY, MD, PhD
is assistant professor of Family Medicine at Georgetown University in Washington, D.C. She practices medicine at Unity Health Care.

FAMILY MEDICAL ADVISOR

FAMILY MEDICAL ADVISOR

Project Manager
Anna Burgard

Technical Specialist
Monika Lynde

Production Manager
Carolyn Bounds

Quality Assurance
Jim King, Stacy L. Eddy

Special Contributors
Susan C. Ashton, Celia Beattie, Yvonne Beran, Judy Lyon Davis, Stephanie Summers Henke, Kathleen Mallow

PROJECT EDITOR
Robert Somerville

Senior Art Director: Fatima Taylor

Deputy Editors:
Kristin Baker Hanneman, Tina S. McDowell

Administrative Editor: Judith W. Shanks

EDITORIAL STAFF
Text Editors: Glen Ruh, Jim Watson

Associate Editors / Research and Writing:
Nancy Blodgett, Kristin Dittman, Stephanie Summers Henke, Jennifer I. Vermillion

Technical Art Assistant: Dana R. Magsumbol

Copyeditors:
Mary Beth Oelkers-Keegan (principal), Claudia S. Bedwell, Donna D. Carey

Editorial Assistant: Katrina Barnes Johnson
Picture Coordinator: Paige Henke

SPECIAL CONTRIBUTORS
Alan H. Anderson, Charlotte Anker, Adrianne Appel, Jamie Baylis, Angela Burbage, Nancy Cardwell, Leslie Carper, Lisa Ann Clark, Mary E. Collins, George Constable, Margery A. duMond, Juli Duncan, Phyllis A. Friedemann, Ruth Goldberg, Debra S. Greinke, Peter Gwynne, Harriet Harvey, Lydia Preston Hicks, Silvia Hines, Donald E. Holmes, Judith Klein, Sarah Labouisse, Jeffrey Laign, Amy McGoldrick, Elizabeth Moore, Narisara Murray, Ann Perry, Susan Perry, Barbara Fairchild Quarmby, Eugenia S. Scharf, Jacqueline L. Shaffer, Colette Stockum, Janet Barnes Syring, Michael Tenneson, Monika Thayer, Susan Gregory Thomas, Victoria Valentine, Mary Weideman, Jayne Rohrich Wood

John Drummond, Robert Herndon (design), Barbara L. Klein (index)

CORRESPONDENTS
Maria Vincenza Aloisi (Paris), Christine Hinze (London), Christina Lieberman (New York)

Pre-Press Services, Time-Life Imaging Center
Printed in U.S.A.
10 9 8 7 6 5 4 3 2 1

CIP data available upon application:
Time-Life Books
2000 Duke Street
Alexandria, VA 22314

The textual and visual descriptions of medical conditions and treatment options in this book should be considered as a reference source only; they are not intended to substitute for a health-care practitioner's diagnosis, advice, and treatment. Always consult your physician or a qualified practitioner for proper medical care.

Before using any drug or natural medicine mentioned in this book, be sure to check the Index of Conventional and Natural Medicines, beginning on page 882, for any warnings or cautions. You should keep in mind that herbal remedies are not as strictly regulated as drugs.

CONTENTS

Introduction **12**
How to Use This Book 14

Dictionary of Conventional Medicine and Alternative Therapies **16**

General Guidelines to Health **30**
Children's Health 32
Adult Health 37
Women's Health 38
Men's Health 42
Growing Older 44

Emergencies/First Aid **46**
Your Medicine Chest 78

Ailments and Options **80**

Index of Conventional and Natural Medicines **882**
About Herbal and Homeopathic Remedies 1025

Eating for Health **1028**
The Food Guide Pyramid 1031
Essential Vitamins and Minerals 1032

A Visual Diagnostic Guide **1042**

Atlas of the Body **1052**

Appendix **1068**
Abbreviations, Professional Titles 1070
Health Associations and Organizations 1071
Gallery of Acupressure and Yoga Positions 1076

Glossary 1094 ◆ Bibliography 1100 ◆ Index 1118 ◆ Picture Credits / Acknowledgments 1152

INTRODUCTION

When you or someone you love is ill or suffering even a minor ailment, you want to know you are making the best choices about treatment. On the eve of the 21st century, those choices are more plentiful than ever. Even as healthcare practitioners embrace the technological advances and the research breakthroughs occurring in modern medicine, they are turning with new interest to the alternative, or natural, therapies from medicine's foundations. Venerable healing practices, from acupressure and herbal remedies to yoga and meditation, are increasingly taking their place alongside modern forms of treatment such as immunotherapy and laser surgery.

In the context of the many options available, these pages offer clear, concise information on hundreds of health problems, ranging from relatively benign conditions to the most serious diseases. For any given ailment, conventional therapeutic approaches represent the best of modern medical science and mainstream medical practices. Alternative therapies also stand on extensive evidence of their benefits—even if those benefits sometimes defy scientific understanding.

In the end, the best decision will be the one you make in conjunction with your healthcare practitioner. The goal of this volume is to provide a solid base of knowledge to help in that process, so you can make informed—and thus more confident—choices about healthcare.

HOW TO USE THIS BOOK

The main section of this book consists of some 300 entries and charts covering several hundred ailments. You may want to begin by turning to a symptoms chart *(see example below)*, which will name several related problems and help you decide which ailment entry to look up based on your symptoms. Ailment entries *(example opposite)* provide a more complete list of symptoms, plus guidelines to discern whether the condition is potentially serious or requires your doctor's attention.

After explaining what causes the ailment, each entry describes conventional and alternative treatment options; for more information about types of therapies, turn to the ***Dictionary of Conventional Medicine and Alternative Therapies,*** beginning on page 18. If specific acupressure techniques or yoga positions are listed as treatment options but not illustrated, check the appendix for the galleries of acupressure points and yoga positions. These are sets of illustrations and capsule descriptions of most of the pressure points and positions described throughout the book.

While reading an ailment entry, you may be referred to other entries or to the ***Emergencies/First Aid*** section. Bold italic type indicates cross references to other ailment entries or to medicines or herbs described more fully in the ***Index of Conventional and Natural Medicines*** *(example opposite)* beginning on page 882. Plain bold type is used to emphasize a concept, or to indicate a therapeutic technique or a subcategory of the main ailment.

Other sections are useful as references or to supplement information in the ailment entries. For an overview of health concerns specific to women, men, children, and the elderly, consult the ***General Guidelines to Health*** starting on page 30. ***Your Medicine Chest*** on page 78 describes the various herbs, homeopathic remedies, and over-the-counter drugs you should have at hand in your home. Use the ***Visual Diagnostic Guide*** to identify problems you can see, such as skin rashes, eye infections, and canker sores. The ***Atlas of the Body*** contains detailed illustrations of the different bodily systems and the five senses. Technical medical terms and procedures mentioned in the book are defined in the ***Glossary,*** beginning on page 1094.

If you can't find the ailment or medicine you're looking for, check the general index at the end of the book to see if it's listed by an alternate name. For example, "pinkeye" is not in the ailments section, but you will find it in the index with page numbers for the ailment entry "conjunctivitis," another name for this eye infection. The index makes it easier to find medicines also, by listing the generic names, top brand names, and drug classes of conventional drugs, plus the common and Latin names of herbs.

If you want more information about one of the ailments or treatment options presented in the book, contact any of the groups listed in the appendix under ***Health Associations and Organizations.***

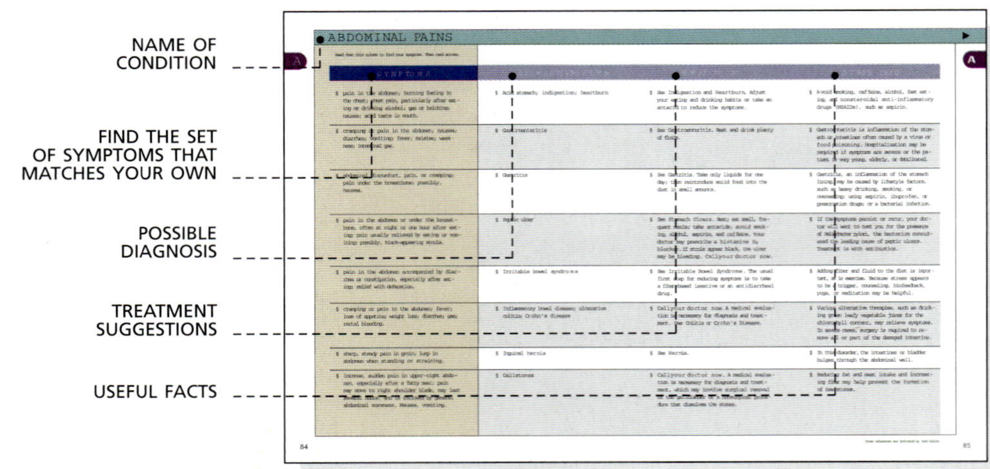

SYMPTOMS CHARTS

Some symptoms, such as abdominal pains, can be caused by any of several different ailments. Charts are a convenient way to identify an ailment by your symptoms and to locate the appropriate ailment entry. To use these charts, start in the far left column and read down until you find the set of symptoms that corresponds most nearly to your own. Read across to find the name of an ailment you can look up for a description and information about causes, treatment, and prevention. Symptoms charts are listed alphabetically with ailment entries.

AILMENT ENTRIES

Each of the nearly 300 ailment entries in this book follows a consistent format. Symptoms and information about when you need to call your doctor are listed first. Each entry describes the ailment and how it affects your body. Next, the entry outlines the underlying causes of the ailment and the tests and procedures your doctor may use to confirm a diagnosis. The treatment segment presents conventional and alternative recommendations for curing the problem or alleviating the symptoms. Be sure to refer to the ***Index of Conventional and Natural Medicines*** for important information about medicines printed in bold italics; always check for possible side effects and adverse interactions with other medicines or foods. Most ailment entries conclude with advice on preventive measures you can use to stay healthy.

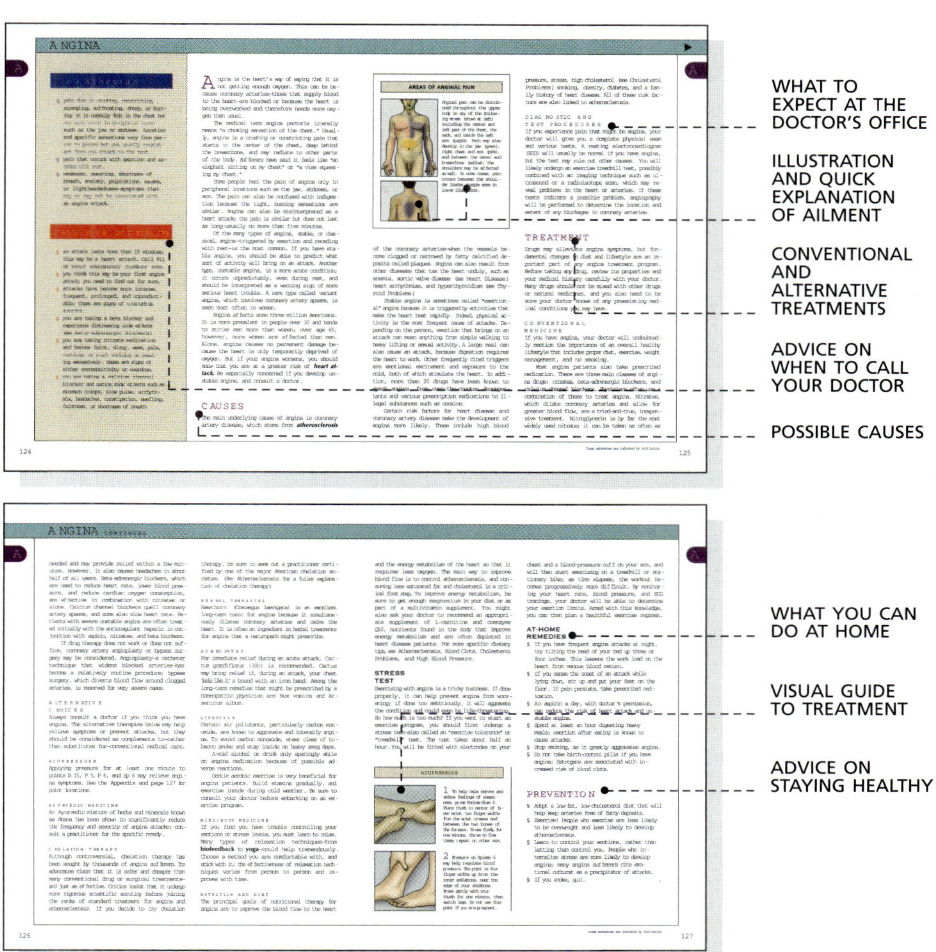

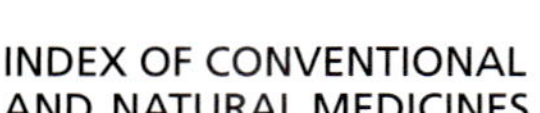

INDEX OF CONVENTIONAL AND NATURAL MEDICINES

This section lists in alphabetical order the most commonly used medicines and herbal remedies; icons identify each entry as a prescription or over-the-counter drug, Chinese or Western herb, or homeopathic remedy. Every entry starts with a general description and specifies the target ailments. Side effects are categorized as either not serious or serious, with guidance on when you should call your doctor about a reaction to medication. Any special information or particular cautions are also listed, as are possible interactions with foods and other drugs. Herb and homeopathic entries also include information on the different types of preparations available for the given remedy.

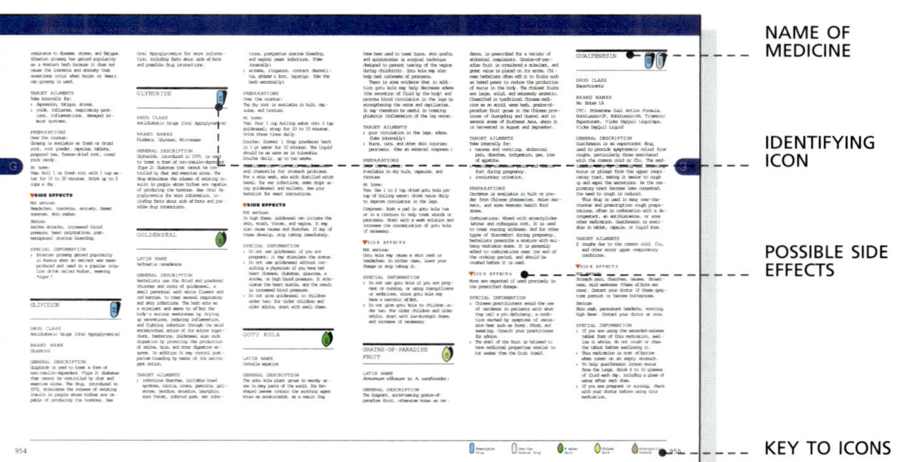

DICTIONARY OF CONVENTIONAL MEDICINE AND ALTERNATIVE THERAPIES

The world of medicine can seem bafflingly complex, with numerous fields of specialization apportioned between two broad sectors, generally called conventional and alternative. The definitions and explanations on the following pages offer a map of the terrain, one that covers all of the medical disciplines and therapeutic options cited in this book. (Note: Ailments that appear in boldface italics are discussed in detail in the alphabetically organized section of the book that begins on page 80.)

The distinction between conventional and alternative approaches to medicine is best understood in terms of basic perceptions of health. Conventional medicine, also called biomedicine, typically views health as an absence of disease. The main causes of illness are considered to be pathogens—bacteria or viruses—or biochemical imbalances. Scientific tests are often used in diagnosis, and drugs, surgery, and radiation are among the key tools for dealing with the problems. Alternative medicine, by contrast, tends to view health as a balance of body systems—mental, emotional, and spiritual, as well as physical. All aspects of a person are seen as interrelated—a principle called holism, meaning "state of wholeness." Any disharmony is thought to stress the body and perhaps lead to sickness. To fight disease, alternative medicine uses a wide range of therapies to bolster the body's own defenses and restore balance.

For suggestions on finding and working with a doctor or an alternative practitioner, see page 29.

CONVENTIONAL MEDICINE: MEDICAL SPECIALTIES

ALLERGY AND IMMUNOLOGY

Allergy is a subspecialty of immunology, the study of the workings of the immune system. Allergists treat such conditions as ***asthma, eczema,*** and ***hay fever***—immune responses brought on by artificial or naturally occurring allergens in water, food, or the air.

ANESTHESIOLOGY

Anesthesiologists chemically induce unconsciousness in patients undergoing surgery, and they treat any heart or respiratory complications that may arise at that time. They may also provide and monitor various types of pain relief during other types of medical procedures, such as childbirth.

DENTISTRY

This field includes numerous specialties relating to the care of the teeth, gums, and jaws. **Dental surgeons** hold four-year dental degrees and emphasize family practice. **Orthodontists** have two additional years of specialized training in positioning teeth. **Oral surgeons,** with three years of added training, perform surgery for such conditions as ***temporomandibular joint syndrome*** and jaw reconstruction.

DERMATOLOGY

Dermatologists treat problems of the skin, mouth, hair, and nails—conditions such as ***acne, psoriasis,*** allergies, and ***skin cancer.***

EPIDEMIOLOGY

Epidemiology is the statistical study of disease among populations or groups of people. Once dedicated to infectious diseases and epidemics, this specialty has expanded to cover noninfectious diseases such as ***cancer*** and ***heart disease.***

FAMILY PRACTICE

Family practice physicians are generalists. Most of them provide a wide range of care, and they usually place special emphasis on looking after the medical, psychological, and social needs of families on a continuing basis. They will refer complicated problems to specialists.

INTERNAL MEDICINE

Internists focus on adult care and are experts on the workings of the internal organs and body systems. They treat a broad spectrum of problems, ranging from common complaints to severe diseases. Subspecialties of internal medicine include **cardiology,** which addresses disorders of the heart, lungs, and blood vessels (***angina*** or ***atherosclerosis,*** for example); **endocrinology,** which covers disorders of the endocrine glands (***diabetes*** or ***thyroid problems,*** for example); **gastroenterology,** targeting diseases of the digestive system, including ***stomach ulcers*** or ***colitis;*** **hematology,** which treats diseases of the blood, spleen, and lymph nodes (***anemia*** or ***leukemia,*** for example); **infectious diseases,** focused on bacterial and viral diseases such as ***AIDS*** or ***meningitis;*** **nephrology,** dealing with problems of the kidneys; **oncology,** which is concerned with all forms of ***cancer;*** **pulmonology,** which treats the lungs and airways in conditions such as ***pneumonia, pleurisy,*** or ***emphysema;*** and **rheumatology,** which addresses diseases of the joints, muscles, bones, and tendons (***arthritis,*** for example).

MEDICAL GENETICS

Medical geneticists counsel potential parents on the risks of passing on hereditary disorders, and diagnose such disorders in children after they're born.

NEUROLOGY

Neurologists focus on dysfunctions of the brain, spinal cord, peripheral nerves, and other parts of the nervous system. They frequently act as consultants to other physicians in determining the cause of such symptoms as dizziness or headaches, and they treat disorders ranging from ***Alzheimer's disease*** to ***multiple sclerosis.***

NUCLEAR MEDICINE

Specialists in nuclear medicine administer radioactive materials internally to identify and treat disorders in body tissues and organs. Thyroid cancer, for example, can be detected and attacked with radioactive iodine, which is absorbed by thyroid cells.

OBSTETRICS AND GYNECOLOGY (OB-GYN)

Obstetrician-gynecologists care for women during pregnancy and childbirth. They also deal with female reproductive tract disorders, such as ***endometriosis,*** as well as conditions caused by imbalances in hormone production. They perform surgery, including Cesarean sections, tubal ligations, and hysterectomies.

OPHTHALMOLOGY

Ophthalmologists treat eye and vision problems, such as ***glaucoma*** or ***cataracts,*** often with drugs or surgery. They have medical degrees, unlike optometrists, who are licensed only to diagnose vision problems and prescribe glasses and contact lenses.

OTOLARYNGOLOGY (EAR, NOSE, AND THROAT)

Otolaryngologists deal with disorders of the ear, the nose, the throat, and related areas of the head and the neck. They are experts in assessing and treating ***hearing problems*** and sinus conditions as well as many other problems, and all are surgeons, trained to perform operations for such conditions as ***tonsillitis*** and deviated septum.

PATHOLOGY

Pathologists are trained to recognize the causes, the effects, and the characteristics of disease. They conduct their work primarily through laboratory analysis of tissue samples and body fluids. They perform autopsies, and they also examine biopsies, often in order to determine the presence of ***cancer;*** they routinely serve as consultants to other physicians.

PEDIATRICS

Pediatricians specialize in the medical problems of children, from birth through adolescence, treating such ailments as ***asthma, diaper rash, chickenpox,*** abnormal growth and development, and sports-related injuries.

PHYSICAL MEDICINE AND REHABILITATION

Physiatrists work with patients who are injured or physically disabled, especially if the problem is musculoskeletal, neurological, or cardiovascular. They provide pain relief and help the patient regain or achieve a higher level of psychological and physical functioning.

HOW SPECIALISTS ARE CERTIFIED

Medical doctors in every state are required by law to have a license to practice; it is issued by a state licensing board upon their graduation from an accredited medical school and upon passage of a licensure exam. Many then continue their training in order to become specialists, and at the end of the process, they typically seek certification by a board of experts. In most cases, the board will be one that operates under the authority of a national oversight group, the American Board of Medical Specialties (ABMS).

To be certified by an ABMS-recognized board, doctors must complete a residency program lasting from three to seven years, depending upon the specialty, and pass an examination prepared and scored by the board's members. Some specialty boards allow doctors to apply for certification upon completing their residency; others—mostly surgical boards—require doctors to practice for a certain number of years and complete a set number of medical procedures before they can take the exam.

Specialists may go on to become subspecialists, which usually involves additional training and perhaps several years of practice, then passing an additional subspecialty exam administered by their primary specialty board. These boards sometimes require doctors to pass exams every 7 to 10 years in order to keep their certification.

The American Board of Medical Specialties, by far the best-known and most widely accepted certification authority, oversees 37 areas of specialization and 75 subspecialties. It does not have the certification field to itself, however. Certificates are also issued by self-designated boards—some entirely reputable, some not. These self-designated boards may not require that a specialist get extra training or pass an exam; in the most dubious cases, they may offer an impressive-looking diploma after a doctor merely attends a weekend course—or for no more than the payment of a fee.

With the growth of managed care programs, board certification has become a benchmark for doctors' qualifications, and most hospitals insist that a doctor be certified by one of the 24 member boards of the ABMS to have admitting privileges. Nonetheless, many doctors who are not board certified provide quality care—and it should be remembered that a certificate is never a measure of a doctor's personality or compassion. ■

PREVENTIVE MEDICINE

Preventive medicine specialists develop regimens to help at-risk groups learn healthful habits and avoid disease and injury. Their recommendations may address diet, behavior, occupational or environmental factors, and public awareness about healthcare.

PSYCHIATRY

Psychiatrists are physicians specializing in the treatment of mental, emotional, or addictive illnesses—among them, ***depression*** and ***anorexia nervosa.*** Like psychologists and clinical social workers, they use psychotherapy, but only psychiatrists have medical degrees and can prescribe drugs.

RADIOLOGY

Radiologists use external radiant energy in many forms to diagnose and treat diseases. Among their procedures are x-rays (including mammography), computed tomography (CT), positron emission tomography (PET), magnetic resonance imaging (MRI), and angiography.

SURGERY

General surgeons perform a wide range of operations involving many parts of the body. In addition, they are trained to recognize problems that should be referred to more highly specialized surgeons who must go through additional training and certification by their own surgical boards. These specialized categories include **colorectal,** to treat the lower digestive tract; **neurosurgery,** which deals with peripheral nerves as well as the brain and spinal cord; **orthopedic,** for problems in the musculoskeletal system; **otolaryngologic,** dealing with the head and neck; **plastic surgery,** to reconstruct, repair, or improve the appearance and function of any part of the body; and **cardio/thoracic,** focusing on the chest, especially the heart and lungs.

UROLOGY

Urologists specialize in genital and urinary tract disorders. Among the conditions they treat—by surgery, if necessary—are ***kidney stones,*** chronic ***bladder infections,*** and ***prostate problems.*** ■

ALTERNATIVE THERAPIES

ACUPRESSURE

This therapy involves pressing points on the body with fingers or hands to alter the internal flow of a supposed vital force or energy called chi (pronounced "chee"), strengthening it, calming it, or removing a blockage of the flow. Acupressure is one of a number of treatment methods regularly used in traditional Chinese medicine, or TCM, a system of healthcare that originated in China thousands of years ago and is still widely practiced in Asian countries today.

According to TCM, acupressure points are aligned along 14 bodily meridians, or pathways *(illustration, pages 22-23).* Twelve of the meridians are bilateral; that is, identical versions of them (with the same sets of points) exist on both sides of the body. The other two are unilateral, running along the midline of the body. The 14 meridians do not correspond to any known physiological processes or anatomical structures in the body, such as nerves or blood vessels. Nevertheless, some well-controlled studies suggest that acupressure can be effective for a number of health problems, including ***nausea,*** pain, and ***stroke***-related weakness. A single point may be pressed for relief from a particular symptom or condition; or to promote overall well-being of the body, a series of points can be worked on in a specific order.

Acupressure can be administered by someone trained in the technique or it may be practiced at home. The force used on different points varies, but in general, most points call for a steady, downward pressure lasting one to two minutes. If you are applying pressure to a point several times in succession, complete this process on one side of the body before switching to the other side.

The risks of acupressure are minimal, provided certain cautions are observed. During pregnancy, the points designated Spleen 6 and Large Intestine 4 should never be used; avoid the abdominal area entirely, if possible. Never apply pressure to open wounds, varicose veins, tumors, inflamed or infected skin, sites of recent surgery, or areas where a broken bone is suspected.

ACUPUNCTURE

Acupuncture, like acupressure, is based on the traditional Chinese theory of meridians—energy pathways that are believed to run through the body, carrying the vital force or energy called chi. In this therapy, the flow of chi is controlled by the insertion of hair-thin needles at specific points—the same meridian-aligned ones used in acupressure *(illustration, pages 22-23).* Unlike acupressure, acupuncture must be performed by a trained practitioner.

An average treatment involves the insertion of 5 to 15 fine needles. They may penetrate as little as a fraction of an inch (on the fingertips, for example) or as much as three or four inches (where a thick layer of fat or muscle exists). The procedure usually causes little pain, although often there may be a tingling or heavy sensation. In addition to (or sometimes instead of) inserting needles, acupuncturists may opt for a treatment called moxibustion. This consists of applying heat directly above acupuncture points by means of small bundles of smoldering herbs, usually ***mugwort leaf.***

The ability of acupuncture to relieve pain in many patients is well documented, and the physical basis of the pain relief has been demonstrated through laboratory tests on animals; acupuncture can trigger the release of endorphins and other forms of neurotransmitters that serve as the body's natural painkillers. However, researchers remain unclear as to how acupuncture is able to provide long-lasting pain relief. Along with its pain-controlling benefits, acupuncture has been found effective in stroke rehabilitation, in providing relief from ***nausea,*** and as treatment for ***asthma.*** It has also been recommended as a treatment for drug addiction. The practice of acupuncture is licensed in 37 states and the District of Columbia.

AROMATHERAPY

In aromatherapy, the essential oils of plants are used to promote relaxation and help relieve the symptoms of certain ailments. Essential oils are extremely concentrated fragrant extracts, cold-pressed or steam-distilled from blossoms, leaves, or roots. The oils often are diluted with so-called carrier oils, such as almond or soy, and can be applied through massage, mixed with water and used as compresses on the skin, added to a bath, or diffused into the air and inhaled. Essential oils should never be ingested; one drop of oil can be equivalent to an ounce or more of a whole plant. Taken internally, the oils of such plants as thuja, wormwood, ***mugwort leaf,*** tansy, ***hyssop,*** and ***sage*** are toxic, and they can even be lethal.

Aromatherapists believe that the fragrance of the oils has a healing effect on the brain's limbic system, which is involved in memory, emotion, and hormone control. Some practitioners also theorize that the oils are absorbed through the skin and work directly in the body. However, critics of aromatherapy suggest that the relaxation attributed to the oils may actually be due to their application by massage, hot baths, and other pleasant methods.

AYURVEDIC MEDICINE

Ayurvedic medicine is a system of diagnosis and treatment that has been practiced in India for more than 5,000 years. The term Ayurveda comes from the Sanskrit roots *āyur,* which means "life," and *veda,* meaning "knowledge." Ayurvedic theory holds that all diseases of the body arise from stresses in the awareness, or consciousness, of the individual; the stresses lead to unhealthy lifestyles, producing a cycle of ill health. Physical manifestations of disease are attributed to the imbalance of three basic physiological principles, called *doshas.* The *vata* dosha represents the kinetic energy of the body; vata makes the heart beat, causes blood to flow, and stimulates brain and nerve functions. The *kapha* dosha is potential energy, responsible for physical strength and the lubrication of tissues. The *pitta* dosha, considered a mediator between vata and kapha, governs the metabolic processes of the body, from digestion to cell operation. If these three principles cease to operate in harmony, sickness ensues. Evaluation of the doshas is performed by a technique called *nadi vigyan,* which involves taking the pulse at the wrist; this assessment determines the precise form treatment will take.

Ayurvedic practitioners prescribe a variety of precise body postures, all derived from the age-old discipline of yoga, along with breathing exercises and meditative techniques *(see **Mind/Body Medicine: Yoga,** page 27)*. In addition, practitioners use herbs, emetics and enemas, oil massage, and dosha-specific diets toward a goal of helping detoxify the system and bring it back into balance.

Some Ayurvedic herbal mixtures have been found to contain high levels of lead and can be toxic. Be sure to thoroughly investigate the ingredients of any remedy before using it; don't hesitate to ask the practitioner about this.

BODY WORK

Body work is an umbrella term for the many techniques, both ancient and modern, that promote relaxation and treat ailments (especially those of the musculoskeletal system) through lessons in proper movement, postural reeducation, exercise, massage, and various other forms of bodily manipulation. Some types of body work—including massage, qigong, reflexology, shiatsu, and t'ai chi—can be practiced at home. Others may require the guidance of a trained professional. Forms of body work include the following:

- **The Alexander technique** focuses on correcting habitual posture and movement patterns that are believed to damage or impair the body's functioning.
- **Aston-Patterning** is a technique that tailors guided movement and postural retraining to the particular characteristics of each client's body.
- **The Feldenkrais method** features individual sessions during which verbally directed exercises, touch, and movement are used to teach new patterns in order to improve posture, movement, and breathing.
- **Hellerwork,** an offshoot of **Rolfing** (Structural Integration), combines touch and movement retraining to teach stress-free methods for performing everyday activities.

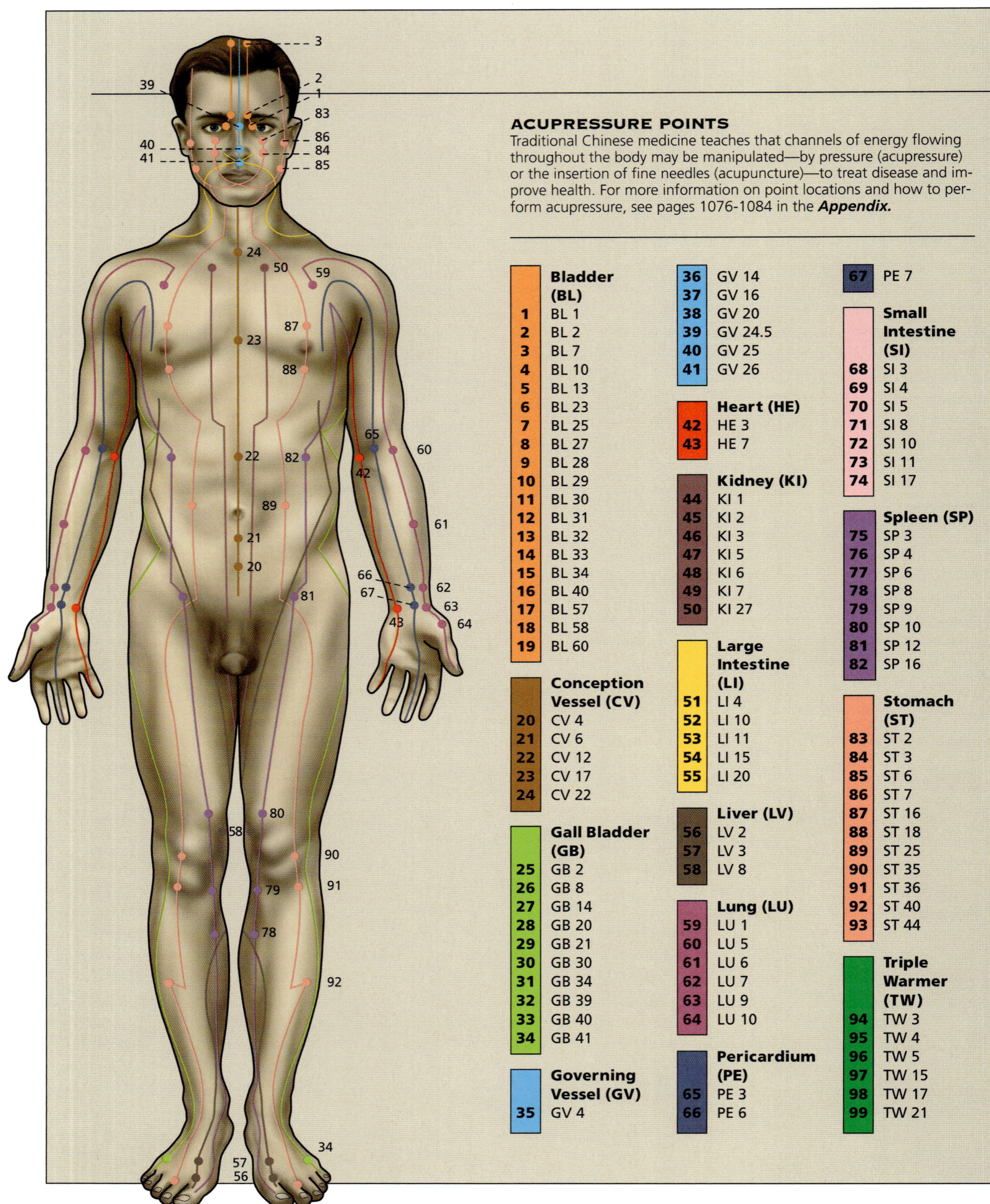
ACUPRESSURE POINTS
Traditional Chinese medicine teaches that channels of energy flowing throughout the body may be manipulated—by pressure (acupressure) or the insertion of fine needles (acupuncture)—to treat disease and improve health. For more information on point locations and how to perform acupressure, see pages 1076-1084 in the Appendix.
Bladder (BL)
1 BL 1
2 BL 2
3 BL 7
4 BL 10
5 BL 13
6 BL 23
7 BL 25
8 BL 27
9 BL 28
10 BL 29
11 BL 30
12 BL 31
13 BL 32
14 BL 33
15 BL 34
16 BL 40
17 BL 57
18 BL 58
19 BL 60
Conception Vessel (CV)
20 CV 4
21 CV 6
22 CV 12
23 CV 17
24 CV 22
Gall Bladder (GB)
25 GB 2
26 GB 8
27 GB 14
28 GB 20
29 GB 21
30 GB 30
31 GB 34
32 GB 39
33 GB 40
34 GB 41
Governing Vessel (GV)
35 GV 4
36 GV 14
37 GV 16
38 GV 20
39 GV 24.5
40 GV 25
41 GV 26
Heart (HE)
42 HE 3
43 HE 7
Kidney (KI)
44 KI 1
45 KI 2
46 KI 3
47 KI 5
48 KI 6
49 KI 7
50 KI 27
Large Intestine (LI)
51 LI 4
52 LI 10
53 LI 11
54 LI 15
55 LI 20
Liver (LV)
56 LV 2
57 LV 3
58 LV 8
Lung (LU)
59 LU 1
60 LU 5
61 LU 6
62 LU 7
63 LU 9
64 LU 10
Pericardium (PE)
65 PE 3
66 PE 6
67 PE 7
Small Intestine (SI)
68 SI 3
69 SI 4
70 SI 5
71 SI 8
72 SI 10
73 SI 11
74 SI 17
Spleen (SP)
75 SP 3
76 SP 4
77 SP 6
78 SP 8
79 SP 9
80 SP 10
81 SP 12
82 SP 16
Stomach (ST)
83 ST 2
84 ST 3
85 ST 6
86 ST 7
87 ST 16
88 ST 18
89 ST 25
90 ST 35
91 ST 36
92 ST 40
93 ST 44
Triple Warmer (TW)
94 TW 3
95 TW 4
96 TW 5
97 TW 15
98 TW 17
99 TW 21

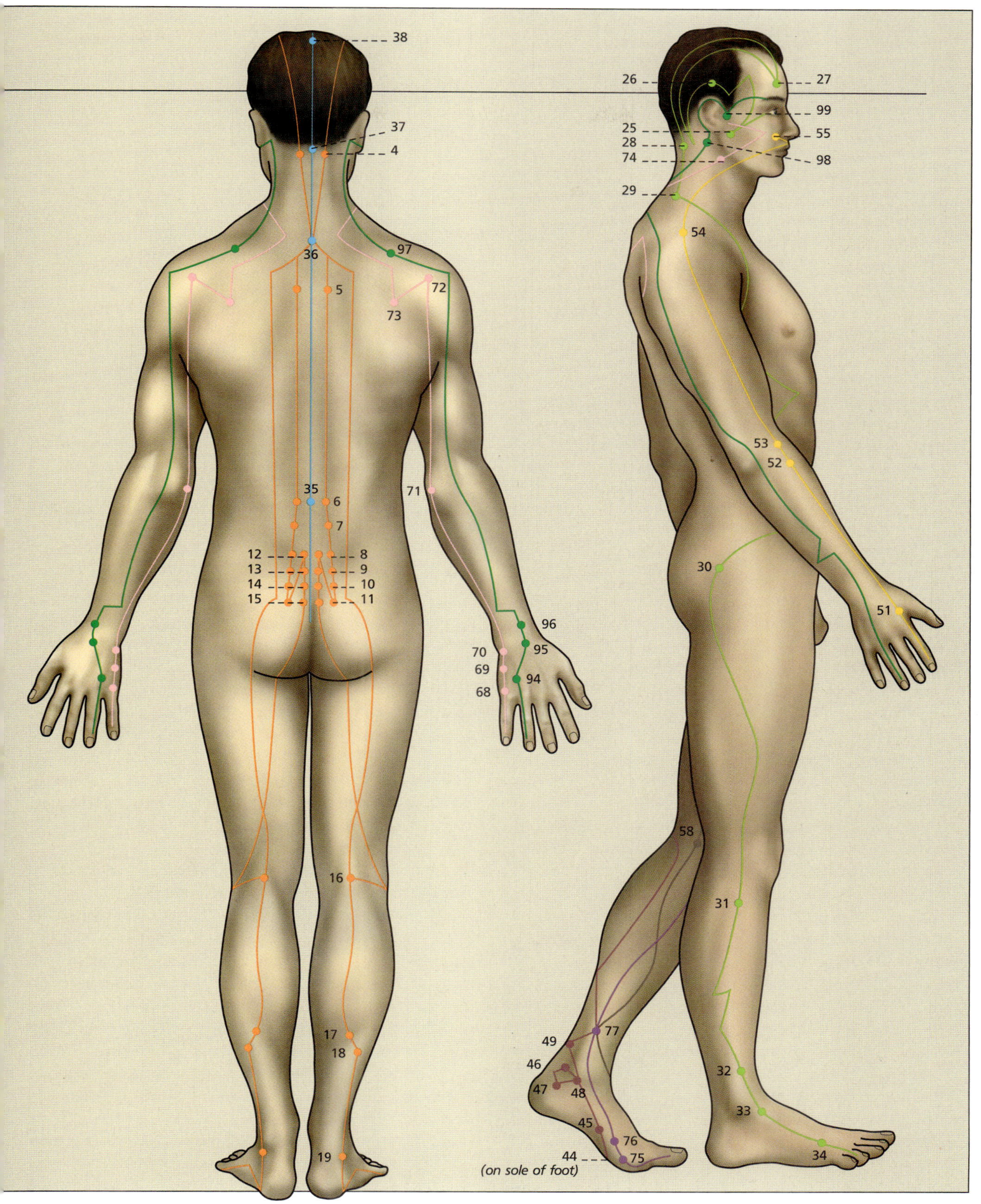

Cross references are indicated by ***bold italics.***

- **Massage** includes an assortment of manual therapies that manipulate the soft tissues of the body in order to reduce tension and stress, increase circulation, aid the healing of muscle and other soft-tissue injuries, control pain, and promote overall well-being.
- **Myotherapy** is a form of deep massage used to reduce tension and pain originating in specific points in the muscle layers of the body.
- **Qigong** ("chee-goong"), an ancient Chinese discipline, emphasizes breathing, meditation, and stationary and moving exercises to enhance the flow of energy or chi (sometimes also spelled "qi") through the body.
- **Reflexology** involves the manipulation of specific areas on the feet—and sometimes the hands—with the goal of bringing the body into homeostasis, or balance. According to reflexologists, distinct regions of the feet *(illustration, page 25)* correspond to particular organs or body systems, and the stimulation of the appropriate region is intended to eliminate energy blockages thought to produce pain or disease in the associated structures. The arrangement of reflexology areas on the feet mirrors the organization of the body to the extent that organs on the right side of the body are represented on the right foot, and so with the left.

  Reflexology features a few basic techniques that can be performed either by yourself or by a partner. The basic thumb technique uses the inside edge of the thumb pad (the side away from the fingers) to "walk" along reflex areas; walking consists of a forward, creeping movement, with the first joint of the thumb bending and unbending slightly as the digit inches ahead. The finger technique uses the same walking motion but with the edge of the index finger closest to the thumb. When working a specific area, one hand should work and the other should hold the foot in a comfortable position with the sole flat and toes straight.

  Practitioners of reflexology claim that it can relieve a wide variety of ailments. Critics say that treatments are no more than glorified foot massages.
- **Rolfing,** also called Structural Integration, is based on the belief that proper alignment of the various parts of the body is necessary for physical and emotional health. The method uses deep massage and movement exercises to loosen or release adhesions in the fascia—the connective tissue covering muscles—in an effort to bring the body back into correct alignment.
- **Shiatsu,** a Japanese technique similar to acupressure, uses finger and thumb pressure on precise body points to encourage the proper flow of chi—or ki, as the Japanese call it—a vital force or energy believed to circulate through the body.
- **T'ai chi,** one style of qigong, is a martial art involving meditation and slow, flowing self-guided movements that follow set forms. It is intended to affect the flow of chi (energy) and bring about physical self-awareness.
- **Therapeutic Touch** does not involve actual physical contact, despite its name. The practitioner's hands move in slow, rhythmic motions two to six inches above the patient in an effort to detect what are said to be blockages in the body's energy field that may cause or contribute to illness. The technique was devised a few decades ago as a contemporary version of various ancient practices in which a healer consciously strives to direct and focus energy to the receiver to balance and unblock energy flows. Sessions typically last about 20 minutes and are said to produce a sense of relaxed well-being as well as relief from pain and other symptoms.
- **Trager Psychophysical Integration** (Trager approach) features gentle touch and rhythmic rocking and shaking movement, along with a series of directed body exercises intended to help identify and correct chronic tension patterns that affect posture and movement. Research suggests that it is beneficial for people with severe neuromuscular problems produced by injury or such diseases as ***multiple sclerosis*** or muscular dystrophy.

CHINESE HERBS

The use of herbs, along with acupuncture and acupressure, is a major component of the system of traditional Chinese medicine, or TCM. Doctors of traditional Chinese medicine usually practice under the title "licensed," or "certified," acupuncturist, and they recommend herbal combinations according to complex rules of diagnosis, which are intended to help the body correct imbalances of energies. In TCM, ailments are believed to be caused by disturbances in the bodily flow of a type of energy called chi, or by a lack of balance in the complementary states of yin (which is characterized by darkness and quiet) and yang (which is characterized by light and activity).

Chinese herbs, like other TCM remedies (such as minerals and animal products, like hide and bone), can be prepared in numerous ways: steeped in hot water to make a tea or infusion; boiled to produce a stronger solution called a decoction; used to make powders, pills, or syrups that may all be taken internally; and fashioned into plasters or poultices that are applied to the skin. Treatments should be prescribed and monitored by a trained practitioner, because some Chinese herbs can be toxic in large doses; others, such as ***safflower flowers,*** should be used with caution during pregnancy. Complex mixtures should be formulated only by a trained practitioner.

In recent years, Chinese herbal medicine has been sub-

REFLEXOLOGY AREAS

Manually working specific areas on the feet is thought by proponents of reflexology to improve the function of corresponding organs and body parts. For more information, see page 24.

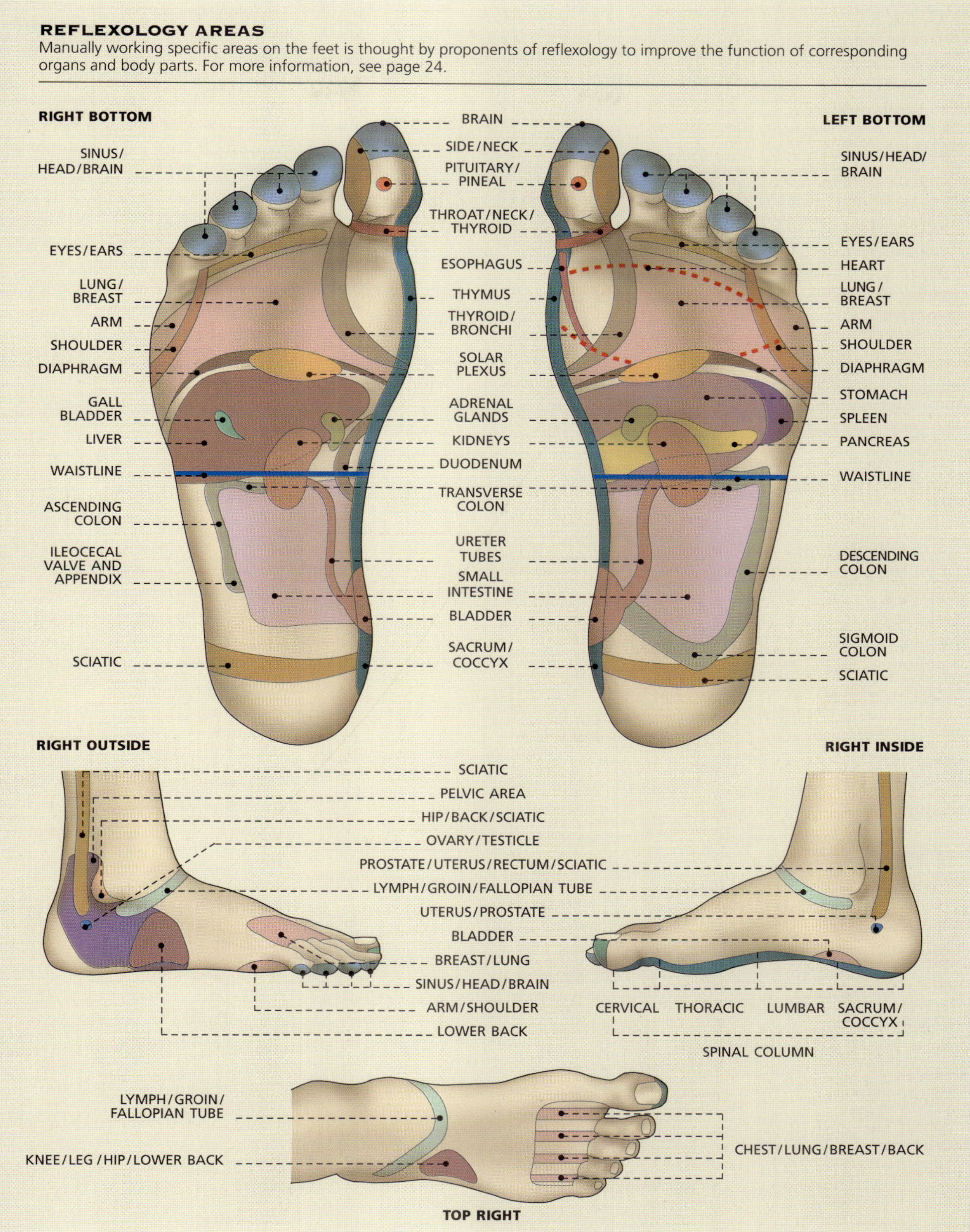

jected to increasingly rigorous study in China, the United States, and elsewhere. The evidence indicates that although some remedies do not perform as claimed, others are effective. In China today, herbal remedies are often prescribed along with modern biomedical treatments.

CHIROPRACTIC

Chiropractic, a system of healing taught in five-year chiropractic colleges and licensed in all 50 states according to standards set by the Council of Chiropractic Education and the Federation of Chiropractic Licensing Boards, is based on the idea that the human body has an innate self-healing ability and seeks homeostasis, or balance. According to chiropractic theory, the nervous system plays a significant role in maintaining homeostasis—and hence health. But problems in the joints, called subluxations, are believed to interfere with proper functioning of the nervous system, and as a result, the body's ability to maintain optimal health is diminished. Chiropractors seek to bring the body back into balance through manual manipulation of the spine and other joints and muscles, allowing the neuromusculoskeletal system to function smoothly.

Today, chiropractors are divided into two major camps. One, traditionalist in stance, sees subluxations as the cause of most ailments. The other, considered progressive, aims at establishing chiropractors as providers of primary care, emphasizing the treatment of back pain and musculoskeletal problems, along with manipulation.

Although chiropractic is categorized as alternative medicine, it has gained a degree of acceptance, in part because of a number of recent studies that have shown it to be quite effective in treating problems such as acute lower-back pain. The services of chiropractors are covered by Medicare and, in many states, by Medicaid and most major private plans.

HERBAL THERAPIES

Herbal medicines are prepared from a variety of plant materials—leaves, stems, roots, bark, and so on. They usually contain many biologically active ingredients and are used primarily for treating mild or chronic ailments. (At least a quarter of all conventional pharmaceuticals include some of the same ingredients, although generally in purified form.) Herbs can be prepared at home in many ways, using either fresh or dried ingredients. Herbal teas and infusions can be steeped to varying strengths. Roots, bark, or other plant parts can be boiled into strong solutions called decoctions. Honey or sugar can be added to infusions and decoctions to make syrups. In stores, herbal remedies can also be purchased in the form of pills, capsules, or powders, or in more concentrated liquid forms called extracts and tinctures. They can be applied topically in creams or ointments, soaked into cloths and used as compresses, or applied directly to the skin as poultices.

In the United States today, herbal remedies are not regulated and come in unpredictable strengths; the amount of the active ingredients varies greatly, depending on whether more than one species of the herb is used and how and when the herb is gathered and prepared. Because some herbs can be toxic or carcinogenic, all herbs should be used under the guidance of a healthcare practitioner familiar with herbal medicine.

Across the spectrum of alternative medicine, the use of herbs is varied: Naturopathic medicine, traditional Chinese medicine, and Ayurvedic medicine all differ in how diseases are diagnosed and what herbal remedies are prescribed. For more information on herbal medicines, see ***About Herbal Preparations*** *(pages 1025-1026).*

HOMEOPATHY

Homeopathy, founded by a German physician named Samuel Hahnemann in the 1790s, is based on the idea that "like cures like"; that is, substances that cause certain symptoms in a healthy person can also cure those same symptoms in someone who is sick. This so-called law of similars gives homeopathy its name: "homeo" for similar, "pathy" designating disease. In his experiments, Hahnemann developed a method of "potentizing" homeopathic remedies by diluting them in a water-alcohol solution and then vigorously shaking (or succussing) the mixtures. The results convinced him that a high degree of dilution not only minimizes the side effects of the remedies but also simultaneously enhances their medical efficacy.

Modern homeopaths usually prescribe doses at dilution ratios ranging from 1x (1 part substance to 9 parts dilution medium) to 200c (200 repetitions of diluting 1 part substance with 99 parts dilution medium); higher ratios are indicated with an "m," for a 1 to 999 ratio. *(See also **About Homeopathic Remedies,** page 1027.)* Critics of homeopathy argue that, in the more extreme dilution ratios (which are considered higher potencies), the remedies may not contain even a single molecule of the original healing substance. Nonetheless, studies have shown that homeopathic remedies may be effective for certain disorders, such as childhood ***diarrhea, hay fever, asthma,*** and the ***flu.*** Further research is now being conducted under the auspices of the National Institutes of Health.

Most homeopathic remedies have undergone "provings," or medical observations in which healthy individuals are given doses of undiluted homeopathic substances. Mental, emotional, and physical changes brought on during these tests help provide homeopathic physicians with a better understanding of which remedy will best suit a particular set of symptoms. Over the past 200 years, provings for almost 2,000 substances have been conducted.

The majority of homeopaths practice "constitutional" homeopathy, based on the idea that each person's constitution—or mental, physical, and emotional makeup—may need to be treated along with any specific ailments. Classically, only one homeopathic medicine is used at a time. An extensive patient history is taken and the patient's physical and psychological symptoms are observed, then an initial prescription is made. If the medication does not have the desired effect or if the symptoms persist, a second analysis is done and a second prescription is given. This process continues until the correct medication for the underlying ailment is found. Constitutional treatment is generally used for chronic problems; acute, or short-term, ailments and injuries are usually treated with remedies specific to the illness.

Recently, over-the-counter combination homeopathic remedies have become available for a wide variety of common ailments. These products contain several of the most common remedies for a particular problem and can be useful for self-treatment of minor conditions. For prolonged or serious illness, a professional homeopath can prescribe specific single remedies.

Homeopathic practitioners usually have prior medical training, such as a degree in medicine, osteopathy, or naturopathic medicine. The pharmaceuticals they prescribe are recognized and regulated by the FDA, and may be purchased over the counter at specialty drugstores.

HYDROTHERAPY

Hydrotherapy literally means water therapy, in the form of ice, liquid, and steam, to relieve the symptoms of numerous types of ***infections,*** acute and chronic pain, ***circulatory problems,*** and more. Treatments include wraps, sprays, and douches, as well as steam rooms and saunas, and both hot and cold baths—among them, whirlpool baths, hand or foot baths, and sitz baths, which involve immersion of only the pelvic area. The aim is to stimulate an immune response or to detoxify the body by changing body temperature. Hydrotherapy is often used by naturopaths.

MIND/BODY MEDICINE

This umbrella term covers activities and therapies that focus on the interrelationship of mind and body; the goal in all forms of mind/body medicine is to address particular disorders and promote overall health by combining both mental and physical approaches. Yoga, for example, involves both physical movement and a meditative state of mind, and may serve the dual purpose of improving a person's physical condition and combating emotional problems such as ***depression*** and ***anxiety.*** As noted below, the two-way connection between mind and body is exploited in many ways to influence the hormonal, nervous, and immune systems.

- **Biofeedback** uses computerized machines to measure and display body functions and states such as heart rate, skin temperature, muscle tension, and brain activity. By monitoring these functions through stages of rest and activity, patients are able to see how and why they change, and eventually can learn to control them.
- **Guided imagery** teaches patients to imagine scenarios that may help influence certain physiological conditions. A cancer patient, for example, may imagine a tumor dissolving under an attack by immune system "bullets." While there are no conclusive studies on imagery, patients often report physical and psychological benefits.
- **Hypnotherapy,** administered by a professional, uses a relaxed, focused state of awareness to help change physiological and psychological reactions to pain, illness, or anxiety. Self-hypnosis may be learned and applied to certain conditions as well.
- **Meditation** includes a number of different Asian and Western practices. All share the basic characteristics of sitting or resting quietly, usually with the eyes closed, and performing mental exercises designed to relax the body and focus concentration.
- The **relaxation response** is a state of psychological and physiological rest characterized by lowered oxygen consumption and reduced heart rate. It can be induced by many different techniques, including **meditation, yoga, t'ai chi, qigong,** and **hypnotherapy.** This deep relaxation can relieve ***stress*** and its many symptoms.
- **Spirituality** is a source of relaxation and comfort for many people, whether it involves practicing a particular religion or contemplating spiritual values outside of a religious context.
- **Support groups** bring together people, and family members, who are suffering from the same disease or similar types of trauma. Within the group, they can share experiences and feelings, which may yield great psychological benefits and perhaps improve the functioning of their natural bodily defenses as well.
- **Yoga** is a series of body positions and movements developed over thousands of years to calm the mind, relax the body, and ease the spirit *(see also **Ayurvedic Medicine,** page 21).* Meditation and breathing exercises lead into cycles of stretches and poses that may vary from session to session. Yoga can be learned in a class and practiced at home; however, modified movements may be required during pregnancy or if a person has a condition such as heart disease. A yoga specialist can recommend the appropriate adjustments.

NATUROPATHIC MEDICINE

Naturopathic medicine provides holistic, or whole body, healthcare by taking advantage of resources drawn from numerous traditional healing systems. Dating back to the late part of the 19th century, naturopathy is organized around three fundamental principles: The physician should strive to aid the body's natural healing abilities; the root cause of an illness should be addressed rather than its symptoms; and above all, only therapies that cause no harm should be used (which means that toxic drugs and surgery are avoided whenever possible).

A naturopathic doctor, or ND, may pay considerable attention to a patient's lifestyle, since naturopathic theory holds that physical, psychological, and even spiritual elements can all contribute to disease. In treating patients, the naturopathic practitioner may use a number of therapies, including homeopathy, herbal remedies, traditional Chinese medicine, spinal manipulation, nutrition, hydrotherapy, massage, counseling, and exercise.

Doctors of naturopathy train at accredited four-year naturopathic medical schools. The first two years include many of the same core science classes as conventional medical schools, as well as classes in naturopathic medical philosophy; while the final two years focus on training in natural healing techniques. At present, naturopathic doctors are licensed to practice in eleven states and in Puerto Rico; most other states allow naturopathic doctors to practice in limited ways. Many private insurance plans cover naturopathic care.

NUTRITION AND DIET

Conventional and alternative practitioners alike acknowledge the importance of a healthful diet. Alternative practitioners, however, place more emphasis on dietary intervention in some conditions where conventional medicine would resort first to drugs or even surgery. Treatment of ***atherosclerosis,*** for example, may take the form of an extremely low-fat diet along with a program of meditation, exercise, and support-group therapy.

Some diets, such as traditional Japanese and Mediterranean ones, contain small amounts of animal fat. Because they are low in saturated fats, these diets appear to protect against ***heart disease*** and some forms of ***cancer.*** Vegetarian diets have been shown to lower blood pressure, decrease arthritic pain, and reduce the risk of cardiovascular disease and some cancers. Particular foods may be beneficial: ***Garlic,*** for example, is said to reduce the levels of cholesterol in the bloodstream and protect against some forms of cancer.

Vitamins and mineral supplements figure in the dietary recommendations of many therapies. Although some vitamins, such as ***A*** and ***D,*** are fat-soluble and can reach toxic levels in the body if not carefully monitored, others, like ***vitamin C,*** are water-soluble and are not stored; any bodily excess is usually excreted. Generally, vitamins and minerals are recommended for daily use as a preventive measure. They often come in tablet form, and doses are measured by weight in milligrams (mg), or thousandths of a gram; in micrograms (mcg), or millionths of a gram; or in a universal standard known as international units (IU). Orthomolecular medicine, a form of nutrient therapy, uses combinations of vitamins, minerals, and amino acids normally found in the body to treat specific conditions, such as ***asthma, heart disease, depression,*** and ***schizophrenia.*** Such therapy can also be used to maintain general good health.

OSTEOPATHY

Osteopathy focuses on correcting structural problems in the musculoskeletal system to improve overall bodily functioning. To restore structural balance and thus help a patient regain health, an osteopathic physician will combine manipulation of the joints, physical therapy, and instruction in proper posture. Because osteopathic care is holistic, or targeted at the whole body, the doctor also considers psychological factors, lifestyle, and diet in addressing an illness and maintaining health.

Ever since it was founded by an American doctor named Andrew Taylor Still in the late 19th century, osteopathy has blended all aspects of conventional medicine with its central tenets of the importance of the body's structure and its predisposition toward health over illness. Doctors of osteopathy, or DOs, train at their own four-year medical colleges and can enter either MD or DO residency programs. They are licensed to practice in all 50 states, and can prescribe drugs, perform surgery, and further specialize in any of the medical subspecialties, such as cardiology, neurology, or obstetrics and gynecology.

Apart from the emphasis they place on musculoskeletal function and alignment (an emphasis that can vary from doctor to doctor), most osteopathic physicians practice much like conventional medical doctors. ■

HOW TO CHOOSE A HEALTHCARE PRACTITIONER

Becoming a patient means becoming a consumer, with the same options and rights as a purchaser of any other service or product. To ensure satisfaction in the medical marketplace, you need to know how to find or change doctors, what sort of relationship to expect, and when to seek a second opinion.

CONVENTIONAL MEDICINE

For a doctor who will oversee your general health (and also suggest specialists when necessary), a good choice within conventional medicine is a family physician with an emphasis on long-term primary care. When looking for candidates, ask for names and recommendations from a regional hospital or medical school, or try a local pharmacist. You may find that family and friends can provide valuable opinions based on their experience with particular doctors. In your search, don't hesitate to act on personal considerations such as a preference for a male or female doctor, or an older or younger one. If you have beliefs or philosophies that play a major role in your healthcare, be sure that you choose a doctor who will respect your views. If board certification is important to you, medical directories—such as the *Directory of Medical Specialists,* published for the American Board of Medical Specialties—can provide the necessary information; these directories can usually be found at a local library. *(For more information on board certification, see page 19.)*

The doctor-patient relationship is built on mutual respect, trust, and communication; you should keep this in mind as you evaluate someone you are considering as your regular physician. Your doctor should take time to explain procedures to you and discuss optional treatment plans—all the while avoiding confusing medical jargon and allowing you to ask questions and add observations of your own. Although bedside manner is not a gauge of skill, a physician should be friendly and approachable. But keep up your end of the doctor-patient commitment by being on time for your appointments, following through on all treatment plans, and reporting any new symptoms or adverse drug responses immediately.

If you are ever given a diagnosis that requires surgery, involves a debilitating or fatal disease, or calls for very complex or costly treatment, you should seek a second opinion. You have an absolute right to one; moreover, some insurance plans actually require a second opinion before approving certain medical procedures. Your doctor should readily provide you with a referral upon request and also should be prepared to share your medical records with other physicians. If you are reluctant to ask for a referral, call a local hospital or medical school to get one, or consult medical directories in your local library.

ALTERNATIVE MEDICINE

When searching for an alternative practitioner, you may want to begin with a recommendation from a conventional doctor. Illness-related self-help groups, books on alternative healing, and organizations listed in ***Health Associations and Organizations*** *(pages 1071-1075)* may be good sources for names. You should fully investigate any alternative practitioner's background and experience and be aware of any licensing requirements in your state or district. Be extremely suspicious of anyone who expresses hostility or derision toward mainstream medicine or makes grandiose claims for a cure. Get explicit information about the treatment you will receive, and remember that *you* are in charge of the entire treatment process. Above all, trust your own instincts and judgment. ■

GENERAL GUIDELINES TO HEALTH

This section is a brief summary of basic health issues related to different stages of life—beginning with infancy, moving into childhood and adolescence, and continuing through maturity and old age. Understanding normal human development and the potential problems males and females face throughout life is one of the keys to establishing a personal plan for healthful living. By adopting good habits and making sensible lifestyle choices at an early age, you can help ensure full, healthy lives for yourself and other family members.

CONTENTS

Children's Health 32
The Healthy Adult 37
Women's Health 38
Men's Health 42
Growing Older 44

CHILDREN'S HEALTH

A new baby is probably the most exciting and challenging event a family experiences. A good prenatal program will see that you and your partner are well prepared to care for the new family member. Most babies are born with everything they need to grow into healthy adults, but it's never too early to start preventive healthcare practices to ensure your child's long-term health and well-being.

Every child should have regular medical checkups, learn to practice good hygiene and nutrition, and get plenty of rest and exercise. For the first several years, a family doctor or pediatrician should monitor your baby's development and be on call when the inevitable childhood ailments come along. A baby gets a ***hepatitis*** shot shortly after birth and should have a complete course of inoculations before the age of two. Your state or locality will require inoculations against certain infectious childhood diseases, and no child should start school without them. *(See the **Immunization Schedule,** opposite.)*

Most children develop in size, stature, and motor skills at roughly the same age, but don't be overly concerned if your child's milestones are slightly different from those of other children in the family or the neighborhood. If your child's development differs significantly or consistently from that of peers, you may want to consult your pediatrician. In addition to your child's physical health, mental and emotional well-being needs to be developed and nurtured. Affection and support from family and friends help encourage self-confidence, and interacting with children of a similar age cultivates important socialization skills.

INFANCY (BIRTH TO 1 YEAR)

Even though an infant seems helpless, the first year of life is a period of remarkable growth and development. Care for your child's health during this period begins with a complete physical examination at birth, during which your baby's heart rate, breathing, and reflexes will be checked. The remains of the umbilical cord usually fall off within the first two weeks. Until then, clean the stump every day with alcohol and keep it dry. If your baby boy has been circumcised, keep his penis dry and cover it at each diaper change with a gauze pad moistened with petroleum jelly until healing is complete.

A newborn's head has two soft spots, or fontanels, where the skull plates have not yet fused together. The smaller spot on the back of the head usually closes 8 to 12 weeks after birth; the larger spot in the front generally closes between 6 and 18 months. Even though the brain is covered by a tough membrane, these soft spots should be safeguarded from injury. The fontanels will rise and fall as the baby breathes or cries. If you notice an unusually bulging or sunken soft spot, however, notify your doctor.

Usually for the first six months, a baby's nutritional needs are satisfied by either breast milk or infant formula; breast-feeding is also often supplemented by the occasional bottle. A big advantage of breast-feeding is that breast milk helps the baby's immune system fight off ***infections*** and may help protect against ***allergies*** in the future. At about six months your infant may be ready to start eating soft foods; drinking from a cup typically comes a few months later. Your pediatrician can advise you about weaning your child completely from the breast or the bottle. Most children triple their birthweight during this first year. *(See **Growth Charts,** pages 34-35.)*

Spitting up a small amount of milk or food soon after eating is normal for an infant, as he gets rid of swallowed air and gas. If he vomits frequently and has a ***fever*** or ***diarrhea,*** or if you see blood or green bile in the vomit, however, call your pediatrician. In newborns, stools are greenish black or mustard-colored and may be very watery; breast-fed babies usually have more bowel movements than those fed on formula. To prevent ***diaper rash,*** change diapers before or after each feeding, after each bowel movement, and every time the baby wakes from a sleep. Wash and dry the diaper area at each change; if you see signs of irritation, apply a mild skin ointment or barrier cream.

The baby's first vocal response is crying, which usually stops when he is held or fed. *(See **Colic.**)* At one to two weeks your baby will start following your eyes with his own, and at four to six weeks he may smile at a nearby face; what looks like a smile before this age is probably just a reaction to intestinal gas. By about 12 weeks you can expect to hear his first laugh. Sometime between 5 and 10 months, most babies get their first teeth, and some babies have as many as eight teeth by their first birthday.

At the age of about three to four months, many babies are able to raise their head and shoulders when lying on their stomach. By six months, an infant may be able to sit up with some help. Most children learn to crawl at about eight months, and about the time of their first birthday they take their first independent steps. Children of this age may also point with their fingers and speak a few intelligible words, including "mama" and "dada."

Some babies have patches of discolored skin, or birthmarks, on their face or body. Most birthmarks are harmless and fade away as the child ages, although tan, brown, or purplish red birthmarks may be permanent. Because some skin marks are disfiguring, and in rare cases carry a risk of ***cancer,*** ask your doctor about treatment options.

Children are naturally inquisitive and need to be protected from accidentally hurting themselves. Before your child starts to crawl, take steps to childproof your home. You can, for example, install safety gates at the top and bottom of stairs and put childproof latches on doors and cabinets; you may also want to put protective covers over electrical outlets. If your child injures himself, refer to the ***Emergencies/First Aid*** section for appropriate care. Infants may also have minor health problems, including ***anal fissures, croup, diarrhea, constipation, eczema, gastroenteritis,*** and ***jaundice.***

A baby should sleep on a firm mattress. Some experts recommend that to prevent your baby from being smothered in bed, you should not cover him with a fluffy comforter or blanket, and should keep all pillows or stuffed animals out of the crib during the first year. Sudden infant death syndrome (SIDS), or crib death, happens to some babies in their sleep without apparent cause. SIDS strikes about 1 out of 2,000 babies in the first year, affects more boys than girls, and occurs more frequently in colder months. Placing the baby on his back or side to sleep is believed to reduce the risk of SIDS.

YOUR PRESCHOOL CHILD (AGES 1 TO 5)

The next few years are a period of rapid development. Your child's individuality becomes more apparent, especially as language skills improve. At 18 months she can stack blocks, throw a ball, and push toys around the room. She will soon be able to run, walk up and down stairs without help, and feed herself with a spoon.

Some children use simple words at about one year, but long before they start putting words together as statements, they understand and respond with actions to much of what you say. During the second year a child may be easily frus-

IMMUNIZATION SCHEDULE

DISEASE	Birth	2 Months	4 Months	6 Months	6-18 Months	12-15 Months	12-18 Months	4-6 Years	11-12 Years	14-16 Years
Hepatitis B			△							▲
Diphtheria										■
Tetanus										■
Pertussis (whooping cough)										
Hemophilus influenzae B				●						
Polio										
Measles									□	
Mumps									□	
Rubella (German measles)									□	
Chickenpox							○			

Immunization against contagious diseases is one of the most important aspects of preventive healthcare, protecting not only individuals but the general public. Because certain types of immunization are effective only for limited periods, booster shots are required to maintain immunity. The inoculations listed above are recommended for all children by the Advisory Committee on Immunization Practices. State and local health authorities may recommend or require specific inoculations before a child can attend public school. From time to time, other inoculations may be recommended or required to prevent or control the spread of communicable diseases.

Key

- △ If not given at birth.
- □ If not given at 4-6 years.
- ○ If your child is older and has not yet had chickenpox, this vaccine may be given at any time.
- ▲ If your child was not inoculated as an infant, this shot should be given before leaving high school.
- ■ Booster needed every 10 years.
- ● Depending on the vaccine used, may not be required.

trated and throw temper tantrums. Learning to disregard such outbursts, while praising your child's positive behavior, is a parent's best course of action.

Two-year-olds are able to run well and are beginning to dress and undress themselves. Most children are toilet-trained by the end of this year and stay dry all day, although some, particularly boys, may not stay dry all night until age five or six. Their vocabularies expand dramatically, and by her third birthday, your child will probably be speaking short sentences. She will crave your affection and approval, and will understand your disapproval. Between 18 months and three years, a child becomes more responsive—and sometimes deliberately unresponsive—to parental guidance. During this period, sometimes called the terrible twos, children are developing a sense of independence as well as responsibility. As much as children enjoy praise for things they do well, don't be surprised when they occasionally answer "no" to your requests.

Three-year-olds learn to use simple sentences, get dressed and undressed with help, and use the toilet on their own. They will play with more complicated toys, such as swings, slides, and tricycles. They are now more interested in interacting with playmates, rather than just playing alongside them as one- and two-year-olds do. At this age, signs of sibling rivalry and jealousy are not unusual. If your child hasn't done so already, he is likely to stop sucking his thumb or finger during this year.

By the age of four, children are using more complex sentences. A sense of imagination may make your child fear the dark or imaginary monsters; such fears are normal and usually disappear in a year or two. Five-year-olds have the motor skills to hop on one foot and skip. Physical independence and curiosity make young children particularly accident prone. Most scrapes and bruises heal quickly, but some injuries may require medical attention. You and your family should be alert for hazards to children—such as fires or unfenced pools—that could cause severe injuries.

The preschool child may contract such illnesses as the ***common cold, flu,*** or ***strep throat,*** especially when exposed to other children in group activities. Many childhood ill-

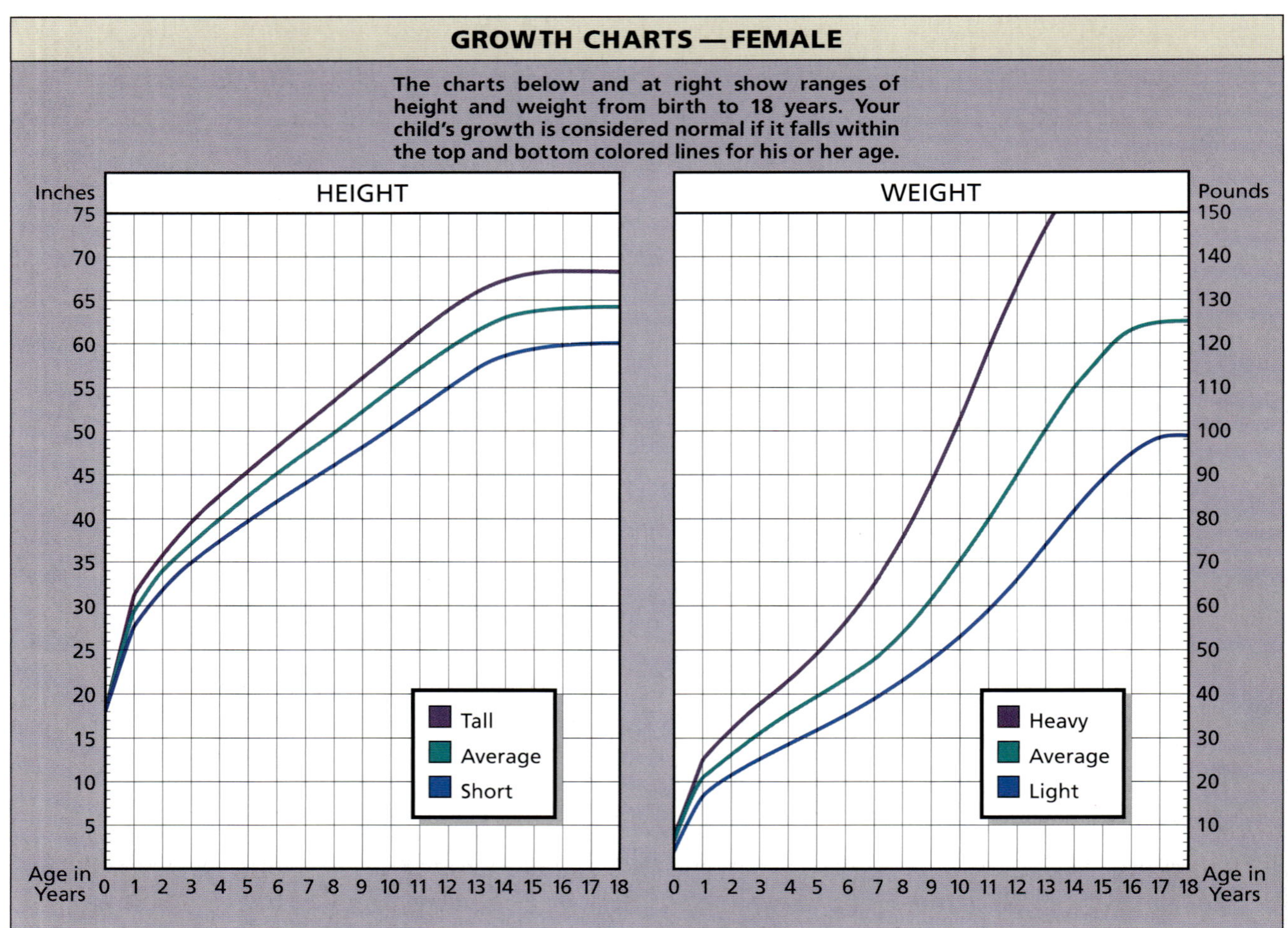

nesses are accompanied by ***fever.*** Unlike an adult, a child under the age of eight may suffer no ill effects from a temperature as high as 106°F (41.1°C), although a child between one and three years with a fever over 101°F (38.3°C) may suffer febrile seizures. Such seizures are frightening to a parent but are rarely life-threatening to the child. *(See **Emergencies/First Aid: Seizures.**)*

YOUR SCHOOL-AGE CHILD (AGES 6 TO 12)

By age six, most children enter elementary school, where the relaxed atmosphere of preschool and kindergarten is replaced with more structure and regimentation. In the classroom and in organized sports, the school-age child is presented with opportunities for intellectual, physical, and psychological growth. Many children develop close friendships, usually with children of the same sex. Your child will begin learning to read and write; those who experience unusual difficulty with schoolwork can be tested for developmental problems, such as ***attention deficit disorder,*** or specific learning disabilities, such as dyslexia.

Once a child starts school, she is likely to be exposed to ***chickenpox*** and other infectious illnesses. Baby teeth begin to fall out, usually painlessly. Except for wisdom teeth, the permanent teeth are usually in place by the early teens. Your child should have dental examinations every six months, and if the teeth do not come in straight, you may want to consult an orthodontist about corrective work.

Some children between the ages of three and nine experience severe, recurring "growing pains" in the arms and legs. In most cases these pains occur in the evening and last a few hours but are not a serious health problem. Children may also complain about recurring ***headaches*** or stomachaches. As your child becomes more independent and adventurous, the likelihood of accidental injury also increases. To minimize the risks, teach your child how to cross streets and ride a bicycle safely, how to swim, and how to use a seat belt when riding in a car. Instruct your child that knives, guns, and tools are not toys and are not to be used without parental guidance.

You should also explain to your child the hazards of

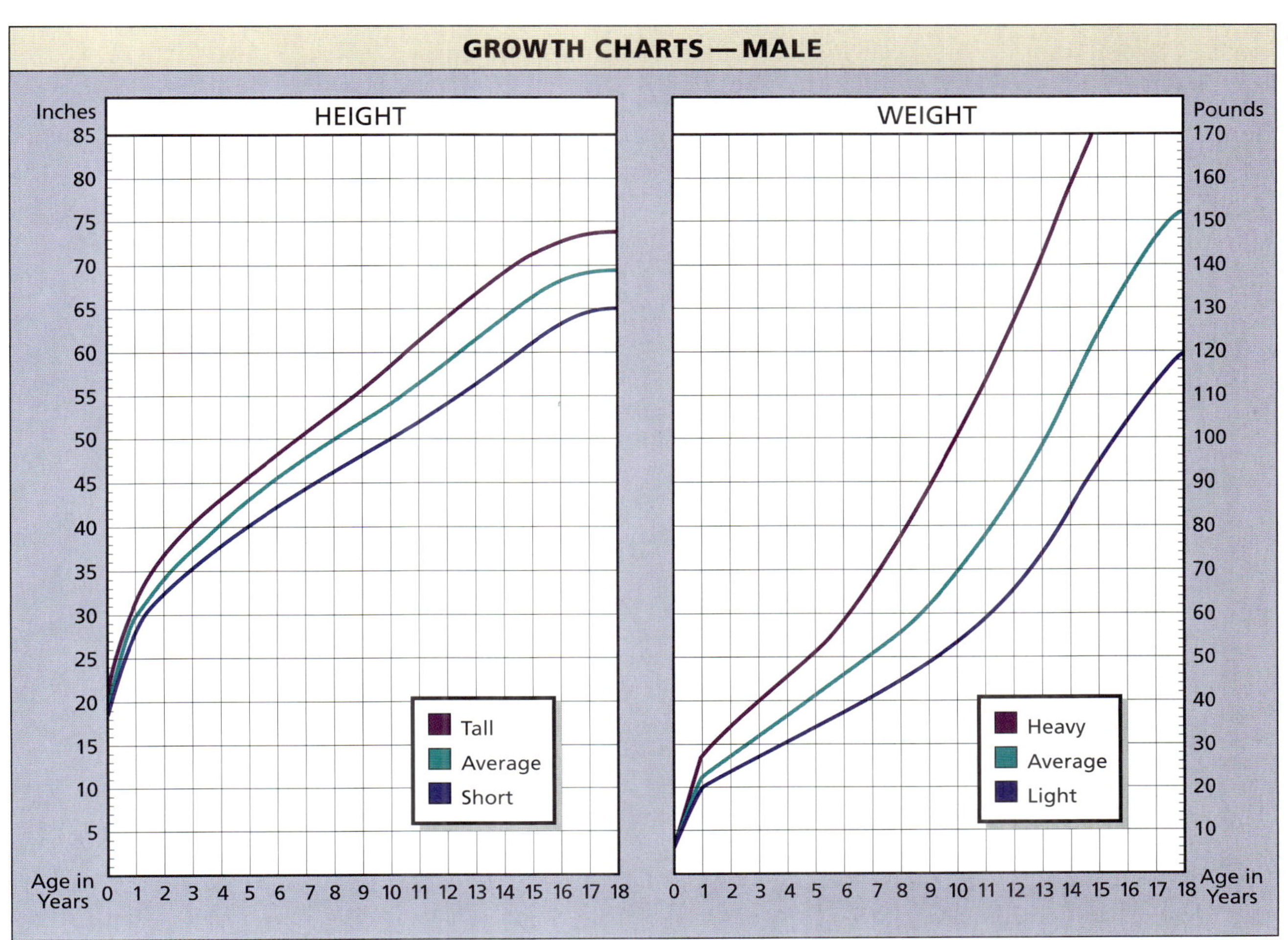

contact with strangers, the difference between "good" and "uncomfortable" touching, when to say "no," and other precautions against potential child abuse.

For most girls, puberty begins sometime after the 10th birthday, for boys sometime after the 11th. Early signs of puberty in girls include growth of pubic hair, breast development, and a noticeable increase in physical size. Early signs of puberty in boys include enlargement of the testicles and penis and the emergence of pubic hair. A year or two later, boys begin to grow rapidly in weight and stature. If your child shows signs of puberty before the age of eight, you should speak with your doctor. Although the underlying cause of premature, or precocious, puberty may simply be an early-maturing endocrine system, it is wise to check for other potential disorders. In any case, remember that preadolescent children who are beginning to mature physically are still children mentally and emotionally and need to be treated as such.

ADOLESCENCE (AGES 13 TO 18)

During the teenage years, or adolescence, your child becomes more independent and socially mature, and takes on many adult physical attributes. In girls, menstruation typically begins between 11 and 14. Pubic hair, breasts, and all sweat glands are usually developed by age 14. The growth spurt that began at 10 or 11 usually slows down after the first menstrual period. It is not unusual for adolescent girls to suffer from painful menstruation; they may not establish regular menstrual patterns until about 17. If your daughter is 15 and has had no significant physical growth, or by 17 has not begun to menstruate, discuss delayed puberty with your doctor. If she has severe ***menstrual problems,*** she may need a pelvic exam by a pediatrician-gynecologist; in any case, girls should have a pelvic exam by their 18th birthday, and earlier if they are sexually active.

At 13 or 14 your son's voice box begins to grow and his voice begins to change. Underarm and facial hair, as well as sweat glands, begin to develop between 13 and 15, and most boys are able to ejaculate seminal fluid by this age. The growth spurt that began between 13 and 15 usually ends at around 17 or 18. If your son is 15 and has had no significant physical growth, or if his voice has not begun to change by 16, discuss delayed puberty with your doctor.

It is natural for adolescents to explore and experiment with their own sexuality, often through masturbation. They start to develop relationships with members of the opposite sex, and some may experiment with homosexual relationships, although few will ultimately become gay or lesbian. As your child enters puberty, you should explain the changes your child is experiencing, the differences between sex and love, homosexuality, and the potential consequences of unprotected sex—including pregnancy and ***sexually transmitted diseases.***

Rapid physical and hormonal growth may cause other changes, such as ***vision problems,*** iron deficiency ***anemia,*** and ***acne.*** A common infectious disease that affects children of all ages, but especially adolescents, is ***mononucleosis.*** Eating disorders, including ***anorexia nervosa*** and ***bulimia,*** sometimes affect teenage girls and young women; the warning signs are extreme weight loss, fluctuating weight, or binge-and-purge eating. Some adolescents, especially girls, are susceptible to migraine ***headaches.*** More girls than boys are subject to ***scoliosis,*** a sideways curvature of the spine; many schools routinely screen children for this condition.

The physical, intellectual, and psychological development that occurs during adolescence may be associated with emotional or behavioral instability: It is not uncommon for teenagers to suffer ***depression, anxiety,*** and ***panic attacks.*** Out of curiosity, in response to depression or other trauma, or as a result of peer pressure, many adolescents experiment with drugs, alcohol, and tobacco. You should discuss with your child the potential health hazards, as well as the social and legal repercussions, of smoking, drinking, and ***drug abuse.*** ■

THE HEALTHY ADULT

Early adulthood is, for most people, a period of good health. A young adult is more likely to have an accidental injury than a systemic disorder, but a few ailments, such as ***testicular cancer*** and ***multiple sclerosis,*** tend to strike young and middle-aged people rather than the elderly.

GOOD HEALTH HABITS

To keep your body in top shape, you should exercise regularly, eat a balanced diet, keep your weight within sensible limits, drink alcoholic beverages only in moderation, avoid abuse of legal or illegal drugs, and not smoke.

If you have a chronic ailment or condition, or if you think you have a hereditary predisposition to a certain disorder, advise your family doctor and educate yourself to recognize the likely symptoms. For example, if you are overweight or have a family history of ***diabetes,*** you are at some risk of developing Type 2 (noninsulin-dependent) diabetes as you approach middle age. Early detection of the disease is critical; even though there is no cure, it can be effectively controlled.

HEALTHCARE OPTIONS

Choosing a family doctor or other healthcare provider and carrying adequate health insurance give you protection against unexpected disease or injury. Most employers offer basic health programs to ensure productivity in the workplace. At the very minimum, look into a low-cost major medical policy that covers the potentially devastating expense of a catastrophic medical situation.

Periodic checkups may help detect health problems in their early stages, when treatment is likely to be most effective. Even if you received childhood inoculations against tetanus and diphtheria, your immunizations should be renewed every 10 years. A dental examination every six months will help detect tooth and ***gum problems,*** and if necessary an annual checkup by an ophthalmologist will monitor any ***vision problems.*** *(See* ***Women's Health*** *and* ***Men's Health,*** *on the following pages.)*

EMOTIONAL WELL-BEING

In addition to maintaining physical health, it is important to keep your mental and emotional health under control. Learning to cope with the changes and personal crises of life can have a direct effect on your physical well-being, while ***stress*** and ***anxiety*** place you at greater risk for a variety of health problems. Sometime after the age of 40, some people experience a so-called midlife crisis, as they reflect on their own aging and accomplishments. If you find yourself overwhelmed by self-examination or ***depression*** at any stage of your life, you should seek professional counseling. ■

HEIGHT AND WEIGHT GOALS

WOMEN			
Height	Small Frame	Medium Frame	Large Frame
4′10″	102-111 lbs.	109-121 lbs.	118-131 lbs.
4′11″	103-113	111-123	120-134
5′0″	104-115	113-126	122-137
5′1″	106-118	115-129	125-140
5′2″	108-121	118-132	128-143
5′3″	111-124	121-135	131-147
5′4″	114-127	124-138	134-151
5′5″	117-130	127-141	137-155
5′6″	120-133	130-144	140-159
5′7″	123-136	133-147	143-163
5′8″	126-139	136-150	146-167
5′9″	129-142	139-153	149-170
5′10″	132-145	142-156	152-173
5′11″	135-148	145-159	155-176
6′0″	138-151	148-162	158-179
MEN			
5′2″	128-134 lbs.	131-141 lbs.	138-150 lbs.
5′3″	130-136	133-143	140-153
5′4″	132-138	135-145	142-156
5′5″	134-140	137-148	144-160
5′6″	136-142	139-151	146-164
5′7″	138-145	142-154	149-168
5′8″	140-148	145-157	152-172
5′9″	142-151	148-160	155-176
5′10″	144-154	151-163	158-180
5′11″	146-157	154-166	161-184
6′0″	149-160	157-170	164-188
6′1″	152-164	160-174	168-192
6′2″	155-168	164-178	172-197
6′3″	158-172	167-182	176-202
6′4″	162-176	171-187	181-207

By keeping your weight within these ranges, you join those people identified by the Metropolitan Life Insurance Company as having fewer illnesses and longer lives than the general population.

WOMEN'S HEALTH

All women should have a periodic checkup by a family doctor, a women's health specialist, or another licensed healthcare provider. The checkup should include appropriate blood, urine, and stool tests; a pelvic examination to check the health of the reproductive organs; and a Pap smear and breast examination to detect early signs of ***cervical cancer*** and ***breast cancer.*** If you are over 50 or have entered menopause, you should have an annual breast x-ray, or mammogram, which can detect tumors before they can be felt. (When to begin annual mammograms is a controversial issue, with some doctors suggesting that they begin as early as the age of 35.) If a lump appears—or if you detect a lump through your own breast self-examination—your doctor will follow up with appropriate tests, even though most breast lumps are benign. *(See **Breast Cancer, Breast Problems, Cervical Problems, Ovary Problems, Uterine Problems, Vaginal Problems.**)*

THE REPRODUCTIVE PROCESS

During fetal development of a female baby, millions of egg cells are created and stored in her two ovaries. When puberty begins, the ovaries start releasing eggs in the process called ovulation. Normally, ovulation alternates between the two ovaries, with one egg being released about every 28 days. The egg then travels toward the uterus through the fallopian tube. If sexual intercourse has occurred within 72 hours before or 24 hours after ovulation, millions of male sperm cells are swimming toward the egg. If a single sperm penetrates the egg, fertilization occurs. Normally, the fertilized egg implants itself in the lining of the uterus, or endometrium, where it will develop into an embryo. If the egg is not fertilized, it and the blood-filled endometrium are expelled from the uterus during menstruation.

If two eggs are released by the ovaries and fertilized by separate sperm cells, the eggs develop into fraternal twins. If the fertilized egg splits in two early in its development, identical twins occur. In rare cases, three or more fertilized eggs develop; such multiple conceptions can be either identical or fraternal, or a combination of the two.

MENSTRUATION

The menstrual cycle varies from individual to individual. On average, a menstrual period begins every 28 days and lasts 4 days, although periods from 23 to 35 days apart and lasting from 2 to 7 days are still considered normal. Most women use either vaginal tampons or sanitary pads to absorb the flow of blood. A tampon should not be left in the vagina for longer than eight hours, because extended use of a single tampon has been linked to ***toxic shock syndrome,*** especially in women under the age of 30.

Unusual stress or long-distance travel may upset your regular menstrual cycle. Irregular periods are also common in young women who have just begun to menstruate and in older women nearing menopause. Absence of a period typically indicates pregnancy but may be due to ***stress,*** excessive exercise or athletic activity, ***obesity, anorexia nervosa,*** or other illnesses. During their menstrual periods some women experience abdominal pain, cramps, or low-back pain. Hormonal changes can cause unusually heavy periods—those that last more than seven days—and irregular menstrual cycles. If, after years of relatively pain-free periods, you start having menstrual pain or heavier-than-usual menstrual flow, you should notify your doctor. The unusual pain or the heavy flow may be caused by a tumor in the uterus, ***endometriosis,*** or ***pelvic inflammatory disease.***

Premenstrual syndrome (PMS) strikes some women with varying degrees of severity about a week before a period begins. Hormonal imbalances may cause temporary breast tenderness, swelling, water retention, weight gain, food cravings, or mood swings. If menstruation has not begun by the time a young woman turns 17, she should see her doctor to determine if she has a disorder in her reproductive or endocrine system.

PREGNANCY

One of the first indications of pregnancy is the absence of a menstrual period. Other early signs are tender or swollen breasts, frequent urination, and perhaps nausea or vomiting. Pregnancy test kits available at most drugstores test your urine for a hormone that is present only when you are pregnant, but at-home tests are not always accurate, especially in the early days of a pregnancy. As soon as you think you might be pregnant, you should see a doctor or visit a healthcare center for more accurate testing.

On average, babies are born 266 days—or 38 weeks—after fertilization. Even if you can't tell exactly when fertilization occurred, you can estimate the baby's due date with reasonable accuracy, especially if your periods are regular: From the first day of your previous menstrual period, add 40 weeks, or 280 days. As a convenient benchmark, doctors commonly divide pregnancy into three trimesters of 13 weeks. In terms of the baby's development, the first trimester is perhaps the most important; the microscopic embryo grows to a fetus about three inches long, and all its major organs are formed. The baby is enclosed in amniotic fluid and is connected to the mother's circulatory system by the umbilical cord. During the second and third trimesters, the baby's organs and limbs continue to develop. Although birth size and weight can vary considerably, a typical full-term baby is about 20 inches long and weighs about 7½ pounds.

Babies born between the 20th and 35th week of pregnancy are considered premature; some do not survive the birthing process and are stillborn. In general, a baby's chance of survival increases the longer it stays in the womb.

Even though 1 in 4 pregnancies ends in miscarriage before the 13th week of pregnancy, the majority of these happen early—often before a woman even knows she is pregnant. Such spontaneous abortions occur because of genetic abnormalities or developmental defects in the baby. Miscarriages due to falls, injury, or stress are very rare. *(See **Pregnancy Problems.**)*

PRENATAL CARE

Proper prenatal care should begin as soon as you know you are pregnant. Your doctor will warn you that using tobacco, alcohol, and drugs—whether they are prescription or over-the-counter, legal or illegal—is potentially hazardous to your baby's development. Proper nutrition is very important, and the quality of the food you eat is more important than quantity. A good diet during pregnancy will be high in fresh fruits and vegetables but low in sugar and salt, with a sensible balance of vitamins, minerals, proteins, and fats. Taking a prenatal multivitamin supplement helps ensure that you and your baby receive the necessary vitamins.

Most pregnant women gain between 20 and 30 pounds before delivery. Of this weight, 6 to 9 pounds will be the baby; the rest is due to breast and uterus enlargement, increased blood supply, amniotic fluid, and the placenta.

During pregnancy you may develop ***varicose veins, hemorrhoids, backaches, anemia, constipation,*** or ***heartburn;*** if you are over 35 you are at a slightly greater risk of developing ***diabetes*** or ***high blood pressure.*** These problems usually subside or disappear soon after the baby is born. If your nipples are inverted, you can place plastic or rubber inserts inside your bra after the 15th week of pregnancy; the suction of these inserts will draw out the nipples by the time your baby is born so you can breast-feed successfully.

Children born to women over the age of 35 are at slightly greater risk of having chromosomal abnormalities, such as Down syndrome. If one or both sides of the family have a history of any chromosomal disorders, you may want to have genetic counseling to determine the likelihood of your child's inheriting a given problem. Prenatal tests such as amniocentesis and ultrasound imaging may help detect such disorders early in the pregnancy.

If you should contract either toxoplasmosis or ***German measles*** (rubella) during your pregnancy—especially in the first trimester—your baby is at risk of a major congenital defect. Blood tests before you get pregnant can determine whether you are immune to either disease. Rubella is entirely preventable by vaccination, and all women should be protected against it. If you are not already immune, you should be vaccinated against it and then wait three months before you start trying to get pregnant. The parasite that causes toxoplasmosis is carried by raw meat and cat feces. If you are not immune to toxoplasmosis, your doctor can suggest ways to guard against infection.

A relatively rare, though preventable, disease occurs when the mother's blood is incompatible with the baby's blood because of the so-called Rh factor. Although the mother is unaffected, the incompatibility can cause the baby serious blood disorders that could result in ***anemia*** or even death. Your doctor can determine if your child is at risk of developing Rh disease and can recommend preventive treatment—usually inoculation with the drug Rh immunoglobulin early in the third trimester and again after the birth to protect the next child. For other potential complications, see ***Pregnancy Problems.***

LABOR AND DELIVERY

Before the baby is due, you should consider your birthing options. Your doctor or prenatal clinic can provide information about various natural-childbirth approaches, as well as the pros and cons of using drugs or anesthetics to relieve pain during delivery. An injected epidural anesthetic alleviates the pain while still allowing you to remain awake and aware of the birth, and it tends to have fewer potential side effects than a general anesthetic.

The need for surgical procedures depends on a number of circumstances, and you may want to discuss the various options with your obstetrician. During normal delivery, the vaginal opening can be surgically enlarged in a procedure called episiotomy. In a Cesarean section, the baby is surgically removed from the womb. A C-section delivery may be elective or may be used in an emergency when the life of the mother or child is at risk.

The first signs of labor may be difficult to detect. Some women have so-called Braxton Hicks contractions for a few weeks before the due date; they occur irregularly, will not increase in intensity, and do not indicate the beginning of labor. For most women, the start of active labor is indicated when "the water breaks." This release of the amniotic fluid that protects the baby can be anything from a trickle to a gush of fluid from the vagina. Other signs can include a light discharge of blood-tinged mucus or uterine contractions at regular intervals.

Labor is divided into three stages. During the first and longest stage, uterine contractions cause the cervix to open so the baby can leave the uterus; this may take 12 hours or more for first-time mothers. During the second stage, uterine contractions actually push the baby out of the uterus; for first-time mothers, this may last several hours, although a child is sometimes delivered after only a few minutes. The final stage of labor consists of expelling the placenta, a quick and relatively painless process. After a woman's first delivery, labor is usually shorter, on average between 4 and 8 hours, because the uterus and vaginal muscles are more flexible. If you should go into delivery sooner than expected and you are not with your obstetrician, midwife, or family doctor, follow the guidelines in ***Emergencies/First Aid:*** **Emergency Childbirth.**

BREAST-FEEDING AND AFTER

Although breast-feeding is an entirely natural process, both you and your new baby not only must learn how to do it but also must establish a comfortable routine. This may take several days, so don't be frustrated if you have difficulty at first; your doctor, nurse, or midwife will offer advice as needed. For the first two to three days of nursing, the baby receives colostrum, a thin, sticky fluid rich in protective antibodies; but colostrum is soon replaced by actual milk. Many authorities recommend breast-feeding for the first year, though some women may wean their baby to a bottle (and formula) after only a few weeks. In any event, after several months you can introduce your baby to bottled water and juice, and later to solid foods. You and your baby will know when she is ready to be weaned from the breast or bottle.

Some women who breast-feed their babies develop engorged breasts or cracked nipples; if this happens, ask your healthcare practitioner for appropriate treatment. A new mother may feel varying degrees of postpartum depression for a few weeks after the baby is born, a condition generally attributable to fatigue, hormonal recovery, and emotional changes. If you feel overwhelmed by these "baby blues," you should discuss the situation with your doctor.

INFERTILITY

If you have been trying to get pregnant for a year or more without success, you and your partner should investigate possible causes of ***infertility.*** In women, causes may include the failure of an ovary to release an egg, a blockage or other abnormality in the fallopian tubes, a disorder of the uterus or cervix, or a ***sexually transmitted disease*** (STD). While many cases of infertility can be resolved successfully, the alternatives include artificial insemination, surrogate fertilization, and adoption. *(For information about male infertility, see **Men's Health,** pages 42-43.)*

Fertility is definitely affected by age. In both men and women, fertility peaks sometime in the twenties. After the age of 37, a woman's fertility begins to decline significantly. Whereas men produce sperm most of their lives, a woman cannot conceive a child after menopause.

FAMILY PLANNING

Every woman should consider the consequences of becoming sexually active: It takes only one act of sexual intercourse to become pregnant. There are a number of ways to be sexually active and prevent conception.

Natural family planning is the practice of determining the fertile and infertile days of a woman's menstrual cycle to predict when she is likely to ovulate and therefore likely to conceive. Coordinating intercourse with ovulation can be helpful in becoming pregnant; conversely, abstaining from sexual intercourse during the time near ovulation can serve as a form of contraception.

Modern natural family planning originates from the rhythm method, first introduced in the 1930s, in which a woman predicts ovulation based on the timing of her previous menstrual cycle. This method is not particularly effective and is no longer recommended. Modern forms of natural family planning include a method that relies both on observations of cervical mucus and on basal—or resting—temperature readings to determine a two- to three-day window during which ovulation will occur. Advocates of modern forms of natural family planning suggest that preventing pregnancy usually involves 10 to 14 days of abstinence from intercourse each month.

Preventing sperm from reaching an unfertilized egg is called barrier contraception. Methods include a man's use of a condom and a woman's use of a diaphragm, female condom, or cervical cap. All barrier methods are more effective in combination with spermicidal cream or gel that destroys sperm on contact. An intrauterine device (IUD) inserted in the uterus prevents a fertilized egg from becoming implanted in the uterine wall; although IUDs can be highly effective, some women who use them experience uncomfortable and occasionally serious side effects. Women under the age of 30 who use internal contraception devices are also at somewhat elevated risk of developing ***toxic shock syndrome.***

Hormone-based birth control—using either oral pills or timed-release capsules implanted under the skin—is among the most effective means of contraception. The synthetic hormones temporarily suppress the release of eggs from the ovaries while allowing menstruation to continue. Contraceptive pills or capsules must be prescribed by a physician, who will advise about the most appropriate type, their potential side effects, and other complications, which these days are rare. After discontinuing birth-control pills, most women resume normal ovarian function and can conceive successfully.

Sterilization is a permanent form of contraception. Treatment for some diseases, such as ***cervical*** or ***uterine cancer,*** requires a hysterectomy—the surgical removal of the uterus and often the ovaries, fallopian tubes, and cervix. After bearing one or more children, some women elect to have their tubes surgically severed or tied, effectively preventing contact between eggs and sperm.

On rare occasions, an egg will be fertilized and implanted outside the uterus in the fallopian tube. This is called an ectopic pregnancy—a painful and potentially life-threatening condition for the mother, requiring the fetus to be surgically aborted. Elective abortions are generally performed during the first trimester of pregnancy, typically by a method known as dilation and curettage (D and C) of the uterus.

OTHER SEXUAL CONCERNS

An active sex life that includes multiple partners raises concerns about ***sexually transmitted disease*** (STD), or venereal disease (VD). Direct body contact and exchange of fluids during intercourse and oral sex leave partners open to such highly contagious diseases as ***syphilis, gonorrhea, genital herpes,*** and ***genital warts,*** as well as to transmission of the human immunodeficiency virus (HIV), the cause of ***AIDS*** (acquired immune deficiency syndrome). While bacterial STDs can usually be cured, viral STDs generally cannot, which can mean lifelong consequences for affected people; AIDS is eventually fatal.

Male condoms, properly used, can prevent some STDs but should not be considered 100 percent effective. If any symptoms of an STD appear, both partners should be checked by a doctor immediately, and any person with a known STD should avoid sexual contact entirely. Every woman has the right to know whether her partner has ever had an STD, and should not be afraid to ask.

SEXUAL DYSFUNCTION

A woman's sexual desire, or libido, naturally fluctuates; there may be times when she is not interested in having sex at all. This may be due to illness, the side effects of certain medications, ***stress, depression,*** or problems in the relationship. If your sexual desires are diminished for an extended period of time, if sexual intercourse is consistently uncomfortable, or if you are unable to have an orgasm, you may wish to discuss the problem with your doctor. *(See* ***Sexual Dysfunction.****)*

MENOPAUSE

Sometime between the ages of 40 and 55, most women's supply of eggs becomes depleted, and the ovaries no longer produce the quantities of estrogen—the primary female hormone—needed for the menstrual cycle to continue. For a period of several years the interval between menstrual periods becomes longer. Eventually, ovulation ceases, menstruation stops altogether, and pregnancy is no longer possible. This is menopause, the natural endpoint of a woman's reproductive years.

Other symptoms of menopause may include hot flashes, felt predominantly in the upper body; drying and thinning of the vaginal walls, which may cause painful intercourse; and various emotional complications. Elderly women and women who have had many children may lose strength in the pelvic muscles that hold the uterus or cervix in place. These conditions are usually minor, but treatment may be necessary if the symptoms cause undue discomfort. *(See* ***Uterine Problems, Cervical Problems.****)* The threat of ***osteoporosis*** is a serious concern for postmenopausal women, as decreasing amounts of estrogen just after menopause speed up depletion of calcium in the bones. To help counter some of the effects of menopause, ask your doctor about the pros and cons of hormone replacement therapy (HRT). *(See* ***Menopausal Problems.****)*

OTHER HEALTH CONCERNS

Among treatable ailments that tend to afflict women are urinary tract infections (including ***bladder infections***), ***irritable bowel syndrome,*** and ***yeast infections.*** Some women are predisposed to chronic ailments such as ***arthritis, diabetes, obesity,*** and the eating disorders ***bulimia*** and ***anorexia nervosa.***

Of all the health issues that concern women, probably the most significant is ***cancer.*** While the disease strikes a relatively small percentage of women, the incidence of various types of cancer is rising as other ailments are brought under control. Every woman should be alert to the warning signs of cancer in any part of the body and should see a doctor at once if a suspected symptom appears. If symptoms persist, or if you feel unsure, get a second opinion. If a tumor is discovered, whether it is benign or malignant, discuss treatment options with a specialist to be sure that you get the most appropriate treatment possible. *(See* ***Cancer.****)* ■

MEN'S HEALTH

Every man should establish basic habits that will help ensure decades of continuing good health. First and foremost is a balanced diet that provides proper nutrition and keeps your body weight within recommended limits for your height and build. It is a good idea to start exercising at an early age, through either active sports or a regular fitness program. The importance of physical fitness continues into a man's middle years and beyond. An active lifestyle that includes regular exercise can help prevent ***obesity*** and can also be an important aspect of your mental and emotional well-being, especially as a means of relieving ***stress.***

A regular physical checkup by a family physician or health service monitors your heart, lungs, and circulation, and includes analysis of your blood, urine, and stool for such things as blood sugar, cholesterol, and signs of systemic diseases. After the age of 50, your physical is likely to include a digital check of your prostate gland. Depending on your overall health and family history of specific ailments, you may need other tests, such as an electrocardiogram (ECG) to check heart function, a sigmoidoscopy to check for ***colorectal cancer,*** or a stress test to check your cardiovascular system.

It is always important to report any apparent symptoms of disease or physical disorders to your doctor without delay, and to ask about any unusual conditions, changes in your body, or reduced physical ability. The essential keys to keeping diseases and disorders at bay are prevention, early detection, and prompt, professional treatment.

THE REPRODUCTIVE SYSTEM

After puberty, a man's testicles manufacture sperm cells and the male sex hormone testosterone continuously into old age. Sperm and fluids from the seminal vesicles and the prostate gland combine to create semen, which is ejaculated through the urethra during orgasm. If semen is not ejaculated in a few days, the sperm cells are reabsorbed and replaced. In a typical ejaculation about 500 million sperm cells are expelled, even though only one is needed to fertilize an egg cell. Since sperm can live in a woman's reproductive tract for up to 72 hours, fertilization can occur up to three days after sexual intercourse.

SEXUAL DYSFUNCTION

Impotence—not being able to have an erection or to maintain it long enough to reach orgasm—afflicts most men at some time or other. Temporary impotence can occur if you drink too much alcohol, when you are overly excited, or during an emotional crisis. Premature ejaculation occurs under some of the same circumstances and can be frustrating to both you and your partner. Both problems tend to disappear when the underlying cause goes away. If either problem occurs regularly or persists in spite of your best efforts, you should see a doctor or a sex therapist to discuss treatment options. *(See **Sexual Dysfunction.**)*

Various disorders of the sexual organs can complicate or prevent normal sexual activity. You should visually examine your penis and testicles on a regular basis, and report any abnormalities to your doctor. *(See **Penile Pain, Testicle Problems, Testicular Cancer.**)*

INFERTILITY

Most men have no problem fathering children, but there is perhaps nothing more upsetting to a couple than finding out that one person is infertile. Two of the most common causes of ***infertility*** in men are low sperm count and poor sperm motility. Other men have difficulty controlling the timing of their ejaculations, or they may ejaculate little or no semen. Various other genital disorders can cause infertility, among them varicocele, or enlarged veins in the scrotum, and inflammation of the testicles, sometimes caused by ***mumps.*** Fortunately most such conditions can be remedied with proper treatment.

SEXUAL RESPONSIBILITY

A man has an obligation to father children in a responsible fashion and to share with a woman the decision to let pregnancy begin. Withdrawing the penis during intercourse prior to ejaculation is not an effective way to prevent fertilization. A more reliable preventive method is to use a condom, which physically blocks sperm from entering the vagina; condoms are even more effective if the woman also uses a spermicidal cream.

Sterilization is a reliable, but usually permanent, form of male contraception, which some men choose after having children. In a surgical procedure called vasectomy the vas deferens is severed and tied off, preventing sperm from reaching the urethra and being ejaculated. A vasectomy does not affect a man's ability to have erections and orgasms. In theory, vasectomies can be surgically reversed, but in practice, reversal is fully successful in only about 30 percent of cases. *(See **Women's Health,** pages 38-41, for more information about fertilization and contraception.)*

Condoms are also an effective means of preventing ***sexually transmitted diseases*** (STDs), which can result from either heterosexual or homosexual contact. STDs are by definition highly contagious, and men with active sex lives and multiple partners should be alert to the possibility of being infected and of transmitting disease. At the first symptom of an apparent STD, see a doctor and have a thorough physical checkup. If you know or suspect you are carrying an STD, avoid any sexual contact until you get a complete diagnosis and medical treatment if necessary.

SYSTEMIC DISORDERS

Numerous ailments can strike men at any time in their adult lives. Men are somewhat more likely than women to suffer cardiovascular ailments, such as ***atherosclerosis*** and ***heart attacks.*** They are also at somewhat greater risk for ***lung cancer*** and gastrointestinal problems, although those tendencies may be changing as people become more conscious of the importance of good diet and the hazards of smoking.

You should discuss with your doctor any discoloration, sores, or lumps that appear anywhere on your body. The same is true for difficulties with urination, ***sexual dysfunction,*** or any other apparent physical symptoms. It is important to understand any disorders that may have been passed on from one generation of your family to another, whether they are benign conditions like ***hair loss*** or potentially fatal diseases like ***diabetes*** or ***cancer.*** Being conscious of such inherited tendencies and alert to their warning signs can make the difference between a healthy life and early disability. If you have a family history of a systemic ailment, or recognize the potential symptoms of some other disorder, consult a doctor and discuss preventive measures. A change in lifestyle at an early age may be the key to long-term health.

OTHER MALE CONCERNS

Poor hygiene is associated with urinary tract infections and cancer of the penis, and more uncircumcised than circumcised men develop these problems. Uncircumcised men should wash under the foreskin daily. *(See* ***Penile Pain.****)* You should also carefully self-examine your testicles for lumps or enlargement once a month. ***Testicular cancer,*** although rare, is most likely to strike men under the age of 40. If you experience any pain or swelling in the testicles or scrotum that is not readily explained, see your physician. *(See* ***Testicle Problems.****)*

Bladder and prostate problems develop gradually over a period of years, which is why many men accept difficulty in urination and ejaculation as normal consequences of aging. The prostate is a walnut-sized gland that partially surrounds the urethra—the tube that takes urine out of the bladder. Over time the prostate can swell, constricting the urethra and causing frequent, painful urination. *(See* ***Bladder Infections, Prostate Problems, Urinary Problems.****)*

An unrelated disorder, ***prostate cancer*** is the most common type of cancer in men, especially those over 50. As with all cancers, early detection is critical for successful treatment; therefore it is important to have regular physical checkups and to be examined if symptoms appear. Although medical intervention remains somewhat controversial, you should discuss any apparent difficulties with your doctor, who can inform you about the latest research findings and recommend appropriate treatment.

MENTAL HEALTH

Men and women alike can be challenged by emotional and psychological difficulties, often in times of personal crisis but sometimes as a recurring or lifelong problem. If you tend to react to ***stress*** in your life with anger or ***depression,*** or if you have difficulty coping with enforced or accidental changes—such as the breakup of a relationship, the loss of a job, or the death of a family member or friend—you may benefit from professional counseling or therapy, with or without medication.

Some people are considered Type A personalities, given to aggressive attitudes and stressful patterns of behavior. Although women can have such traits too, men seem to be particularly disposed. Some studies associate aggressive behavior and a stressful lifestyle with such ailments as ***high blood pressure,*** gastrointestinal problems, and some forms of ***cancer.*** Authorities believe that learning to control such tendencies can have a beneficial effect on overall health.

Emotional well-being is as important as physical fitness, and your emotional and mental state can have a profound effect on your physical health. This is particularly true when disease strikes. A positive, realistic attitude—as well as a clear understanding of the ailment—can be an important contribution to a successful recovery. ■

GROWING OLDER

Thanks to monumental advances in medical science and the healing arts, most people today can look forward to longer, more productive lives than their grandparents might have imagined. Men born in the second half of the 20th century can expect to live an average of more than 70 years; for women the average life span is more than 75 years.

Adequate exercise, proper nutrition, and appropriate medical care when needed can help keep you in good physical and mental health through your middle years—between 40 and 65—and well into old age. On the other hand, poor nutrition, obesity, systemic diseases, and excessive use of tobacco, alcohol, and drugs tend to accelerate the inevitable process of aging.

THE AGING PROCESS

Physical fitness and mental productivity generally peak in the mid-twenties and stay stable for many years. Eventually, however, all body systems begin to become less efficient. You may not start to notice changes until you are in your forties or fifties, but sometimes the effects of aging come on without warning. For many people, the first sign of aging is loss or graying of hair. ***Hair loss*** that begins while you are still in your twenties is usually hereditary, but whenever it occurs, it is nearly impossible to prevent.

Accumulation and redistribution of body fat may also contribute to a changing appearance. In middle age, a man's excess fat tends to settle at the abdomen; in women, fat gravitates to the breasts, abdomen, and hips. Bones reach their maximum density between the ages of 25 and 35, and their slow erosion to ***osteoporosis*** may result in losing several inches of height by the late seventies, while also contributing to lower body weight. Bones may also develop calcification and lose protective cartilage at the joints, or may develop other symptoms of ***arthritis.***

Over the years your skin slowly thins, loses elasticity, and begins to wrinkle, especially on the face and hands. Age spots or patches that appear on the backs of the hands and elsewhere are usually harmless and may actually disappear over time. The best thing you can do for your skin is to avoid overexposing it to the sun. What was once considered a healthy tan—or even one severe ***sunburn*** at an early age—is now considered a potential risk factor for ***skin cancer.*** Itchy, reddened skin and other forms of ***dermatitis*** may also be associated with aging. Cosmetic surgery may tighten areas of loose skin and eliminate existing wrinkles for a time, but the skin and underlying fat layers will continue to grow thinner and new wrinkles will eventually appear.

Disorders of the joints and the skeletal system may become apparent as people get older, making arthritic conditions some of the more widespread ailments of the elderly. *(See **Arthritis, Joint Pain.**)* The combination of slower reflexes and a deterioration in the sense of balance makes older people prone to falls and other accidents. Brittle bones, weaker muscles, and thinner skin mean that such accidents may also have more serious consequences. The healing process is much slower in older adults than in younger people, so relatively minor injuries can become serious, even life-threatening.

Exercise and good nutrition can help keep your body limber and strong, although muscles, too, will atrophy naturally over time. Shrinking gum tissue can cause teeth to become loose and susceptible to decay, so regular dental checkups and corrective dental work are important for good oral health. If tooth and gum deterioration interferes with eating, or if you begin to lose your teeth, you should speak with your dentist about being fitted for dentures. *(See **Gum Problems, Toothache.**)*

SENSORY CHANGES

Each of the physical senses tends to degenerate as you age, at varying rates for different people. When you first detect changes in your vision, see an ophthalmologist about glasses or contact lenses to correct near- or farsightedness. Adults over 60 may be susceptible to ***glaucoma, cataracts,*** and ***macular degeneration;*** these conditions, if left untreated, can eventually lead to partial or total blindness. Because eyesight tends to deteriorate slowly, you may not be aware of progressive vision loss, so you should schedule an annual vision exam to check your eyes for these disorders. *(See **Vision Problems.**)*

Hearing loss is usually a gradual process that may be noticeable after age 40; some people may notice significant loss over time while others may notice little change. *(See **Hearing Problems, Tinnitus.**)* Your senses of smell and taste will also become less acute, but the gradual loss is usually a problem only if it adversely affects your appetite. Older people are more susceptible to **hypothermia, heatstroke,** and **heat exhaustion** than are younger people *(see these entries in **Emergencies/First Aid**)*. Temperature sensitivity may be affected by ***circulatory problems*** or a ***thyroid problem.***

SYSTEMIC CHANGES

All your internal systems become less efficient as you age. The muscles of your heart and blood vessels lose some of their elasticity, making it harder for blood to circulate through your body. Cardiovascular deterioration eventually makes physical exertion very tiring. Because your heart has to work harder to do its job, a slight increase in blood pressure is normal; a significant increase may mean you are at risk for having a ***heart attack*** or ***stroke;*** adults who smoke are at markedly greater risk of stroke. Regular physical exercise—walking, swimming, golf, or tennis—will help keep your cardiovascular system healthy, but consult your doctor before you start any new exercise programs.

Urinary tract infections such as ***kidney*** and ***bladder infections*** become more common with increasing age and can lead to more serious repercussions. Older adults are also susceptible to gastrointestinal problems, such as ***irritable bowel syndrome*** and ***diverticulitis.*** Poor diet may cause ***anemia*** to develop in older adults. Elderly adults are also prone to suffer from ***incontinence*** and ***constipation.***

Your body's immune system is also likely to become less effective with age. You may find yourself more susceptible to common illnesses, and whenever you get them you may take longer to recover than you did in the past. Many doctors recommend that adults over 65 get an annual ***flu*** shot to protect against active strains of the influenza virus. Some older people may need a pneumococcal shot to prevent ***pneumonia.***

For various reasons, your risk of developing ***cancer*** becomes more likely after the age of 50. You should advise your doctor of any family history of a particular form of cancer and educate yourself about its possible warning signs. Women should be particularly alert to signs of ***breast cancer, uterine cancer, cervical cancer,*** and ***ovarian cancer.*** Men should be aware of the warning signs of ***prostate*** and ***testicular cancer,*** and should understand that they are statistically at somewhat higher risk than women for ***lung*** and ***colorectal cancer.***

Aging also affects the brain and the nervous system. Mild tremors in the hand or head are common in older adults; for many people this is harmless, but it may be a symptom of ***Parkinson's disease.*** Forgetfulness, partial memory loss, and progressively increasing confusion have many causes, ranging from minor infections or sleep deprivation to ***stroke*** or ***Alzheimer's disease.*** If you notice such symptoms in yourself or in another adult family member, arrange a medical examination to determine the cause.

MAKING ADJUSTMENTS

Physical changes related to aging will be accompanied by changes in your personal life. Retirement and adopting a slower-paced lifestyle may have a substantial psychological effect that some people find difficult to accept. Finding new outlets—travel, volunteer work, or pursuing a lifelong interest—can ease the adjustment to a different role in your family and community.

Around the house, a modest investment in safety—grab rails in the bathtub or shower, reinforced stair banisters, and securely fastened floor coverings, for example—can help prevent accidents. If balance or mobility becomes a problem, using a cane or a walker may be a wise decision. At some point, because of declining vision and physical reflexes, most older adults find it prudent to stop driving a car.

Retirement communities offer many benefits for older adults, but the decision to change one's lifestyle in a major way should be made with a clear understanding of the financial and social consequences, and the possibility of some initial emotional trauma. The death of friends or a spouse will inevitably cause grief and perhaps ***anxiety*** about changes in your own life. If you feel overwhelmed by your feelings, or if you or others around you sense you are suffering from ***depression,*** you should seek help from your healthcare practitioner or a counselor.

CARING FOR THE ELDERLY

The time-honored concept of younger family members caring for an older generation is still valid, but for many people today it is unrealistic or impossible. If you choose to be a primary caregiver, you may find that enrolling an older person in a day-care program eases the mental and physical strain associated with such care over the long term. If caring for a chronically ill or bedridden person at home yourself is not feasible or acceptable, you can consider home care by a trained nurse or other provider, on either a part- or full-time basis.

The time may come when you need to place an elderly spouse or parent in a nursing home or similar facility. This is not an easy decision, but it may be the best solution, especially when the person is ill, family members are far away, or at-home facilities are inadequate or unsuitable. With careful research and planning, a suitable and caring environment for any elderly person can be found. ■

EMERGENCIES/ FIRST AID

CONTENTS

Emergency First Steps 47
Bleeding 48
Burns 49
Cardiac and
  Respiratory Arrest 50
Choking 54
Drowning or Near-Drowning 57
Ear Emergencies 58
Electric Shock 59
Emergency Childbirth 60
Eye Emergencies 62
Fractures and Dislocations 64
Head, Neck, and Back Injuries 66
Heart Attack 67
Heatstroke and
  Heat Exhaustion 68
Hypothermia and Frostbite 69
Internal Bleeding 70
Loss of Consciousness 71
Nose Emergencies 72
Poisoning 73
Seizures 74
Shock 75
  Anaphylactic Shock 75
Snakebites 76

See also *Ailments and Options* for:

Abdominal Pains 84
Breathing Problems 212
Diabetes 316
Fainting 364
Insect and Spider Bites 508
Nausea 616
Stroke 788
Vomiting 868

What to Do in an Emergency

1 Call 911 or your emergency number, or tell someone nearby to do so.

2 Check the victim's ABCs *(right).*

3 Stop any severe bleeding *(page 48).*

4 Prevent shock *(page 75).*

5 **Try to determine what happened.** Look around the scene for any clues, such as a Medic Alert tag on the victim or an open container of a poisonous chemical.

The Recovery Position

Placing an unconscious victim who is breathing in the recovery position will keep the airway open. CAUTION: Do not place the victim in this position if you suspect a neck or back injury.

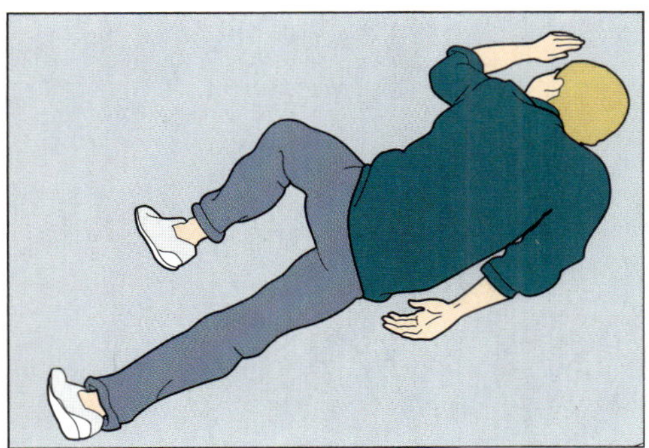

Support the victim's head and roll him onto his stomach. Bend the victim's arm and knee that are closest to you. Carefully tilt back the head so the airway remains open.

Checking the ABCs:

AIRWAY, BREATHING, CIRCULATION

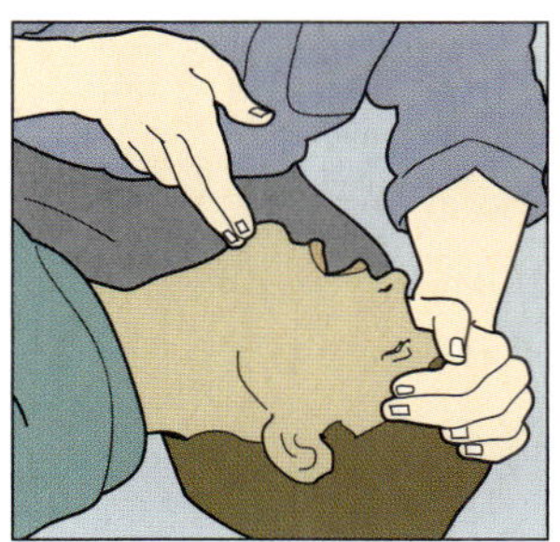

A

OPENING THE VICTIM'S AIRWAY. Gently tilt back the victim's head and lift the chin. CAUTION: If you suspect a head, neck, or back injury, just lift the chin.

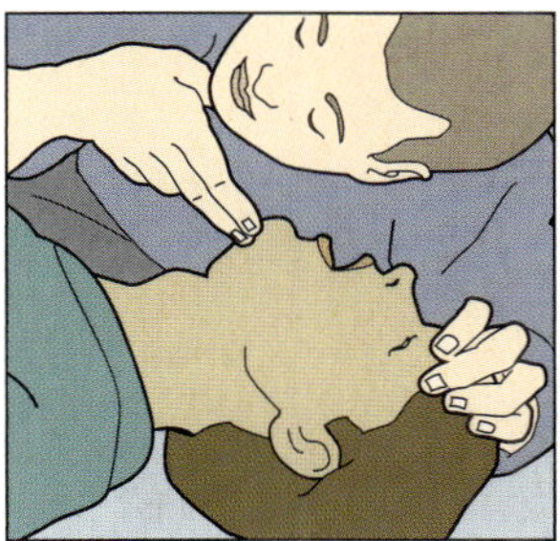

B

LOOKING, LISTENING, AND FEELING FOR BREATHING. Look for the victim's chest to rise. Put your ear to the victim's mouth, and listen and feel for exhaled air; chest movement alone might not mean breathing.

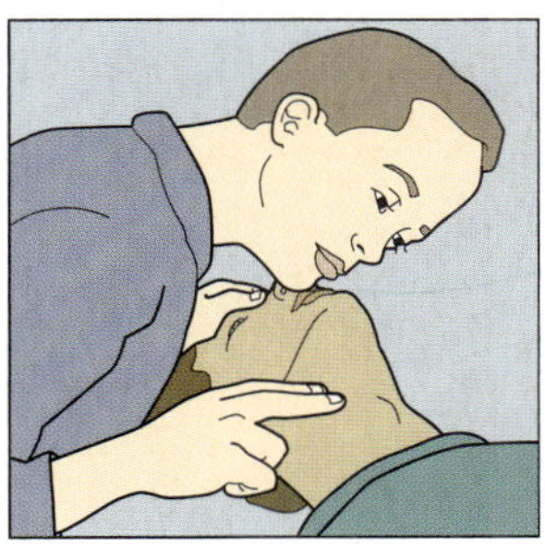

C

CHECKING FOR A PULSE. Gently press two fingers, not your thumb, in the depression on the side of the victim's neck, next to the Adam's apple, and feel for a pulse.

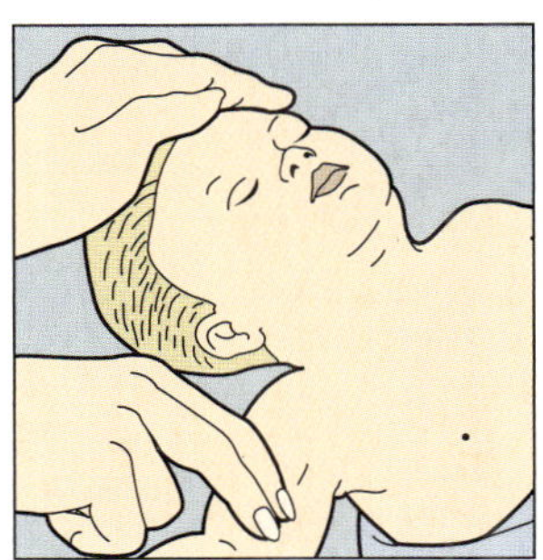

CHECKING FOR AN INFANT'S PULSE (UP TO 1 YEAR OLD). Gently press two fingers, not your thumb, on the inside of the infant's arm between the elbow and shoulder, and feel for a pulse. If you do not feel a pulse, listen for a heartbeat.

BLEEDING

IMPORTANT!

- If the bleeding is severe, call 911 or your emergency number.
- For specific bleeding sites, see also Ear Emergencies *(page 58)*, Eye Emergencies *(page 62)*, or Nose Emergencies *(page 72)*.

CAUTION: If you suspect a head, neck, or back injury, see page 66.

1 Lay the victim flat on his back. Raise the victim's feet several inches. If possible, elevate the wound above heart level.

2 Check the victim's ABCs *(page 47)*. **If the victim is not breathing or does not have a pulse or heartbeat, begin CPR** *(pages 50-53).*

3 Remove any visible objects from the wound. CAUTION: Do not remove any object or pull on any clothing that is stuck in the wound. Do not probe the wound or disturb it in any way.

4 Apply direct pressure to the wound with a clean cloth or your hand. If blood seeps through the cloth, do not remove it; put another cloth on top and keep pressing. You may need to apply firmer pressure if blood continues to seep through. For an embedded object, put pressure around the wound, not on the object.

5 If the bleeding does not stop, apply pressure to an arterial pressure point. Keep direct pressure on the wound as you press the arterial point. Do not apply pressure to arteries leading to the head or neck unless bright red blood is spurting from an injured neck artery.

6 When the bleeding stops, apply a bandage. Do not remove any cloths placed on the wound to help stop the bleeding; place a clean cloth over the wound. If there is an object embedded in the wound, bandage around it to support it.

7 Keep the victim calm and still.

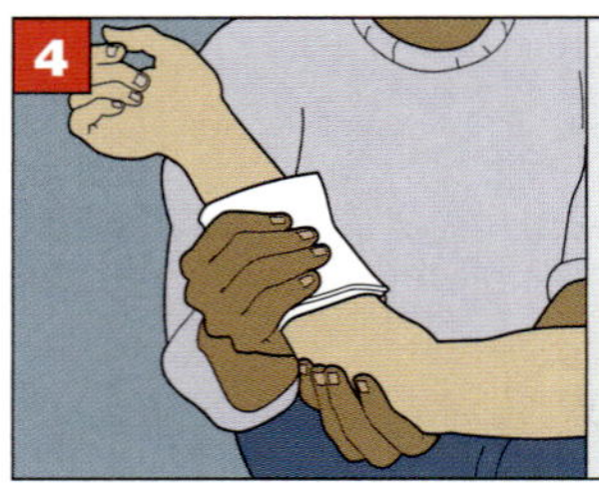

Applying direct pressure. Use a clean cloth, or your hand alone if necessary, to put pressure directly on the wound. Hold the edges of flesh together.

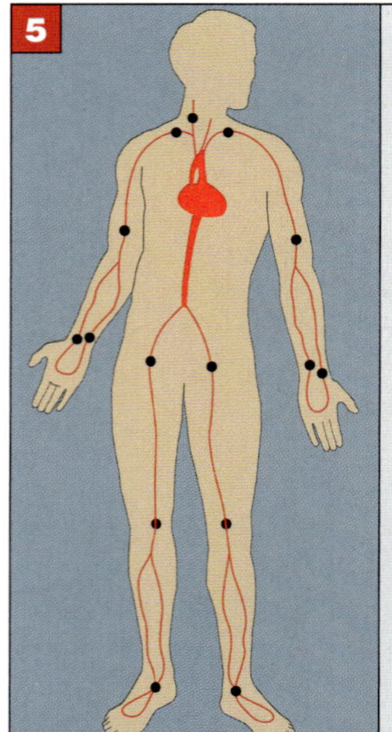

Applying pressure to an arterial pressure point. Apply pressure with your fingers held flat against the arterial pressure point that is closest to the wound, between it and the heart.

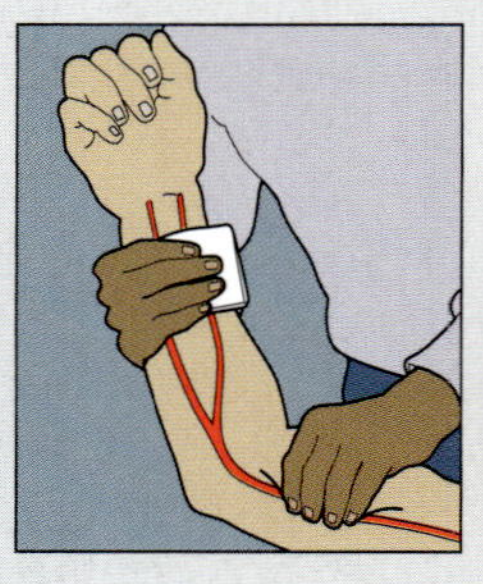

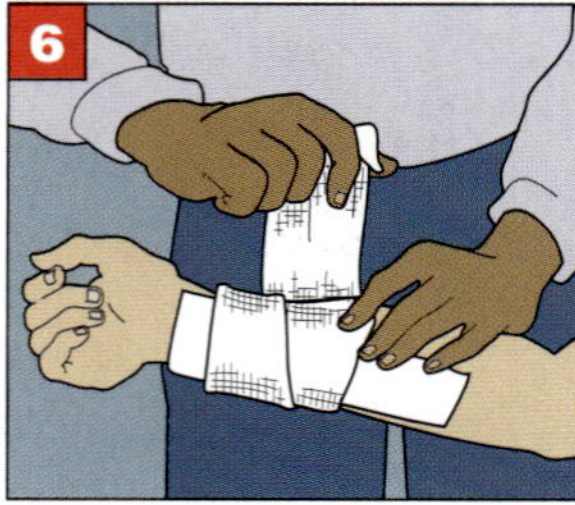

Bandaging a wound. Wrap a bandage or a clean cloth around the wound; tie it in place.

BURNS

IMPORTANT!

- Call 911 or your emergency number if the burns involve more than one body part or the face, neck, hands, feet, or genitals, or if the victim has trouble breathing. Call if the victim is a child or is elderly.
- Call 911 or your emergency number if the burns are caused by chemicals. See the box below.
- If you suspect that the victim has been electrocuted, see Electric Shock *(page 59).*
- If the victim has a chemical burn in the eye, see Eye Emergencies *(page 62).*
- If the victim spilled a chemical that caused the skin to freeze, give first aid for chemical burns, then give first aid for frostbite *(page 69).*
- If the victim spilled a chemical that was absorbed through the skin without burning it, see Poisoning *(page 73).*

CAUTION: If you suspect a head, neck, or back injury, see page 66.

1 Remove the victim from the cause of the burns.

2 Remove any clothing or jewelry from the burned area. CAUTION: Do not remove any hot or smoldering clothing that is dry or is stuck to the burned skin. Do not breathe or cough on the burned skin.

3 Cover small burns with wet cloths. If the burned area is smaller than the size of the victim's chest, loosely cover it with a sheet or towel that has been soaked in cold water, or hold the burned skin under cold running water. CAUTION: Do not place ice on the burned skin. Do not break any blisters. If the burned area is larger than the size of the victim's chest, do not apply water or cover the burn.

4 Separate burned fingers or toes. If fingers or toes have been burned, gently place dry cloth dressings between them. CAUTION: Do not use cotton or any adhesive bandages.

5 Loosely cover the burned skin with a clean, dry cloth. If fluid oozes through the cloth, place another cloth over it. CAUTION: Do not spread any ointments, lotions, butter, baking soda, or ice on the burn.

6 Elevate a burned arm or leg above the level of the victim's heart.

DEEP BURNS

For deep burns (indicated by charred or white skin), you should also check the victim's ABCs *(page 47).*

CLOTHING ON FIRE

1 Lay the person on the ground so the burning clothing is on top.
2 Smother the flames with a blanket, coat, or any other cloth that is nearby and handy. Direct the flames away from the person's face, or **tell the victim to roll over slowly.**

CHEMICAL BURNS

SYMPTOMS

- Burn marks
- Headache
- Breathing problems
- Seizures
- Blisters
- Dizziness
- Abdominal pain
- Unconsciousness

1 Remove the victim from the chemical.
2 Flush the burn with water and remove contaminated clothing. Place the burned area under running water for at least 15 minutes to dilute the chemical. As you flush the burn, remove any jewelry or clothing that may have come in contact with the chemical. CAUTION: For a dry chemical, such as lime, brush off any particles before flushing with water.
3 Check the victim's ABCs *(page 47).*
4 If the victim is not breathing or does not have a pulse or heartbeat, begin CPR *(pages 50-53).*
5 Cover the burn with a clean, dry cloth.

CARDIAC AND RESPIRATORY ARREST

IMPORTANT!

- If the victim is not breathing and does not appear to be choking, call 911 or your emergency number, or tell someone nearby to do so; then begin CPR *(below)*. If the victim is an infant or a child younger than eight years old, see also pages 52-53. If you suspect choking, see pages 54-56.
- If victim has trouble breathing, see page 212.
- If you suspect that the victim is having a heart attack, see page 67.

SYMPTOMS

- Pale or bluish face
- Chest does not rise or fall
- No heartbeat or pulse
- Unconsciousness
- No exhaled breath

CPR

Treatment for cardiac or respiratory arrest is called cardiopulmonary resuscitation (CPR). The goals of CPR are to open the airway, reestablish breathing, and reestablish circulation. It is best to give CPR only if you have been trained in the procedure.

CAUTION: If you suspect a head, neck, or back injury, see page 66.

1 **Lay the victim flat on his back.**

2 **Sweep the victim's mouth.** CAUTION: If you see an object lodged in the victim's throat, do not try to retrieve it, as this might force the object farther down the airway; give first aid for choking *(page 54).*

3 **Open the victim's airway.** Gently tilt back the victim's head and lift the chin.

4 **Look, listen, and feel for breathing.** Be sure to put your ear to the victim's mouth; chest movement alone might not mean breathing.

5 **If the victim is not breathing, give breaths.** Watch for the chest to rise with each breath; let the chest fall before you give the second breath. If the victim's chest does not rise, gently tilt his head farther back and try again to give two slow breaths. If the chest still does not rise, give first aid for choking *(page 54).* CAUTION: If the head is tilted too far or not far enough, you may not successfully open the airway.

6 **Check for a pulse.**

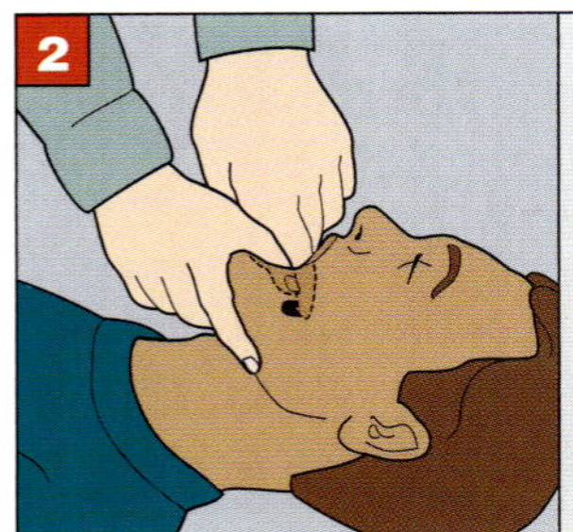

Finger sweep, adult. Hold the victim's tongue and lift the chin. Slide your index finger down the inside of the cheek and sweep out any loose objects.

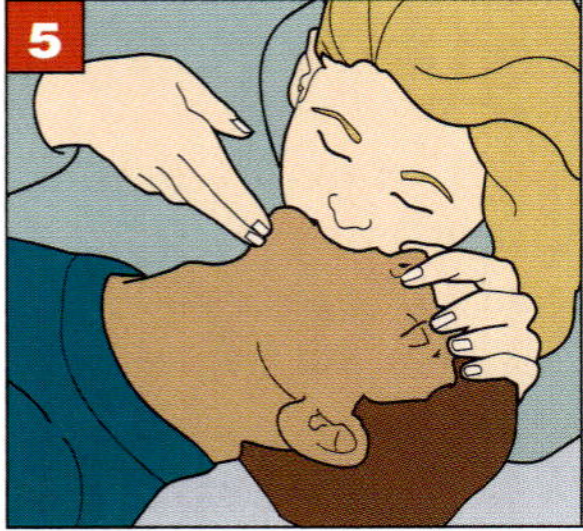

Giving breaths, adult. Pinch the nose shut and seal your lips tightly around the mouth. Give two slow breaths; remove your mouth between breaths.

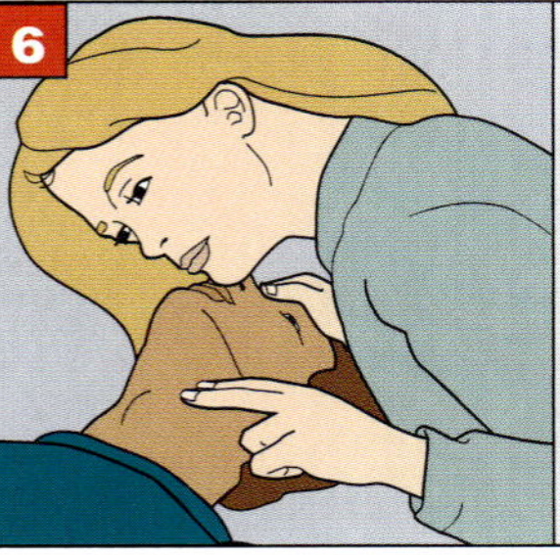

Checking the pulse, adult. Gently press two fingers, not your thumb, in the depression on the side of the victim's neck, next to the Adam's apple; feel for a pulse.

7 If you feel no pulse, give chest compressions. See the illustrations at right and on pages 52-53.

8 Repeat steps 3, 4, and 5. If the victim is an infant or a child younger than eight years old, give only one breath.

9 Give chest compressions, breaths, and recheck for a pulse. For an adult or child over eight years old, repeat a series of 15 chest compressions, followed by two breaths, 4 times; then recheck for a pulse. For an infant or a child younger than eight years old, repeat a series of 5 chest compressions, followed by one breath, 10 times; then recheck for a pulse. Repeat the series of chest compressions, breaths, and pulse checking until the victim has a pulse or begins to breathe on his own, or until medical help arrives.

10 If the victim is not breathing but has a pulse, give breaths. For an adult or child over eight years old, give 1 breath every five seconds. Check the pulse every 12 breaths. For a child between one and eight years old, give 1 breath every four seconds; check the pulse every 15 breaths. For an infant, give 1 breath every three seconds; check for a pulse or heartbeat every 20 breaths. Continue until help arrives.

7

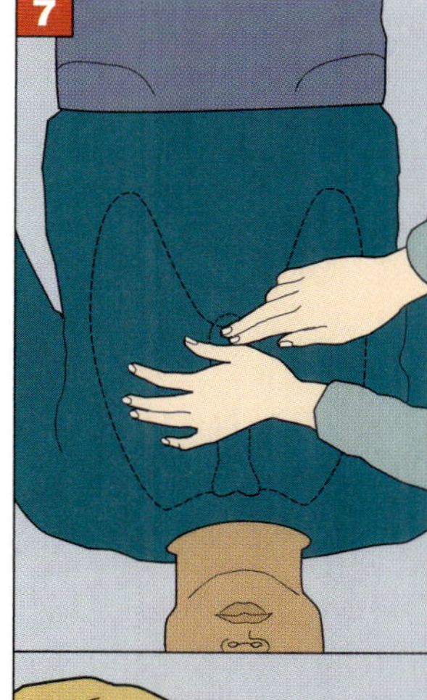

Placing your hands, adult. Place your middle finger in the notch where the ribs meet the bottom of the breastbone. Put your index finger next to and above your middle finger. Place the heel of your other hand next to and above your index finger. Remove your fingers and place that hand over your other hand; interlace your fingers and keep them up, off the chest.

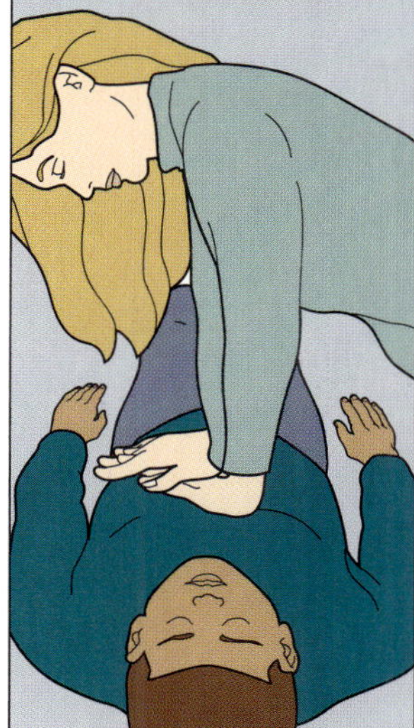

Giving chest compressions, adult. Position yourself so that your shoulders are directly over your hands; keep your arms straight. Press down forcefully to depress the victim's breastbone 1½ to 2 inches. Release the pressure, but don't lift your hands off the chest. Give 15 chest compressions, at the count of "one and two and three and...." CAUTION: Do not rock back and forth.

CONTINUED ▶

INFANT (UP TO 1 YEAR OLD)

SWEEP, BREATHS, PULSE

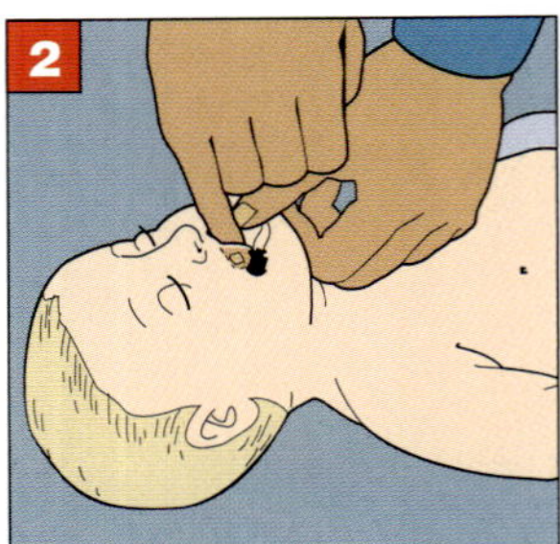

Finger sweep. Hold the tongue and lift the chin. Look in the mouth; if you can see an object and think you can easily remove it, slide your little finger down the inside of the cheek and sweep out the object.

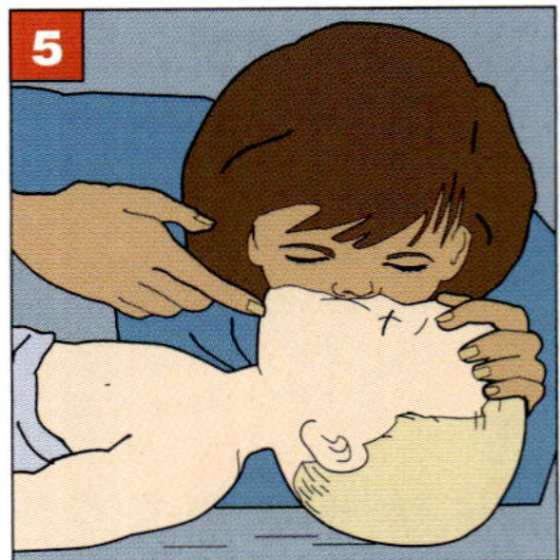

Giving breaths. Keep the chin lifted with one hand and seal your lips over the nose and mouth. First give two breaths, then one thereafter. Remove your mouth between breaths. Breathe forcefully but not so hard that air goes into the stomach.

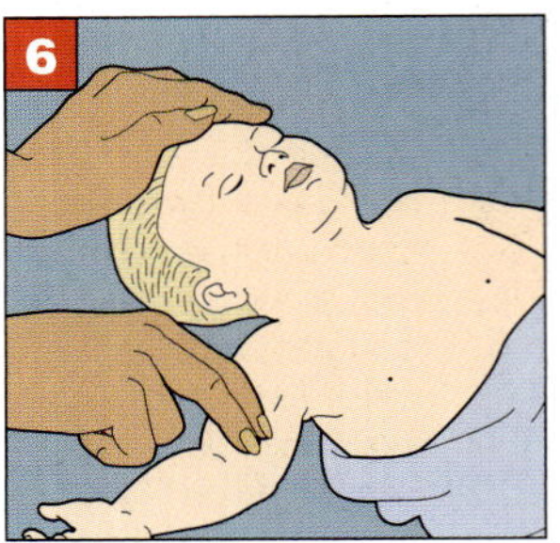

Checking the pulse. Gently press two fingers, not your thumb, on the inside of the infant's arm between the elbow and shoulder. If you do not feel a pulse, listen for a heartbeat.

CHEST COMPRESSIONS

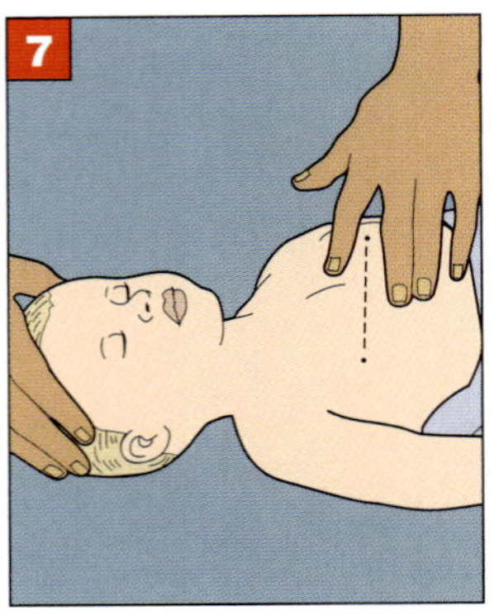

Placing your hands. Place your index finger just below an imaginary line between the nipples, in the center of the chest, on the breastbone. Place your two middle fingers next to and below your index finger, then lift your index finger. Use your free hand to help keep the infant's head tilted back.

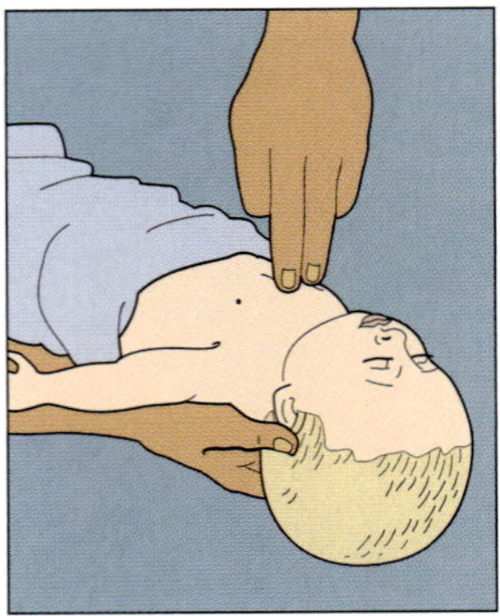

Giving chest compressions. Bend your elbow slightly and press straight down on your fingers, depressing the infant's breastbone $1/2$ to 1 inch. Release the pressure, but don't lift your fingers. Give five chest compressions, at the count of "one two three...." CAUTION: Do not rock back and forth.

See pages 50-51 for complete instructions.

CHILD (BETWEEN 1 AND 8 YEARS OLD)

SWEEP, BREATHS, PULSE

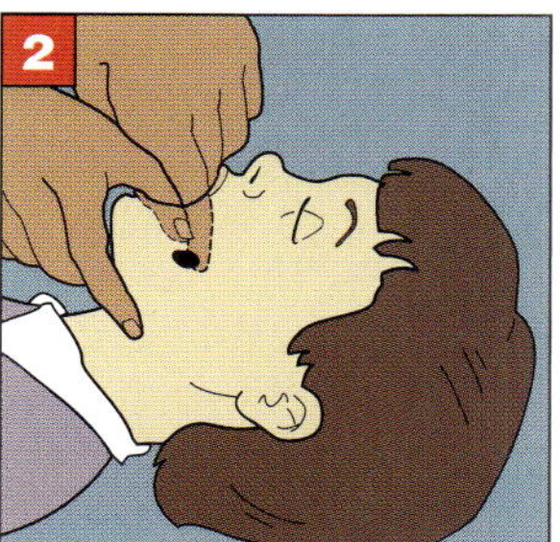

Finger sweep. Hold the victim's tongue and lift the chin. Slide your index finger down the inside of the cheek and sweep out any loose objects.

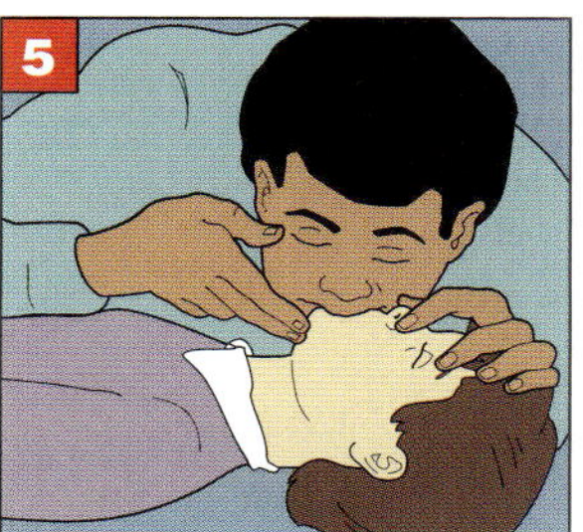

Giving breaths. Pinch the nose shut and seal your lips tightly around the mouth. Give two slow breaths initially; give one breath thereafter. Remove your mouth between breaths.

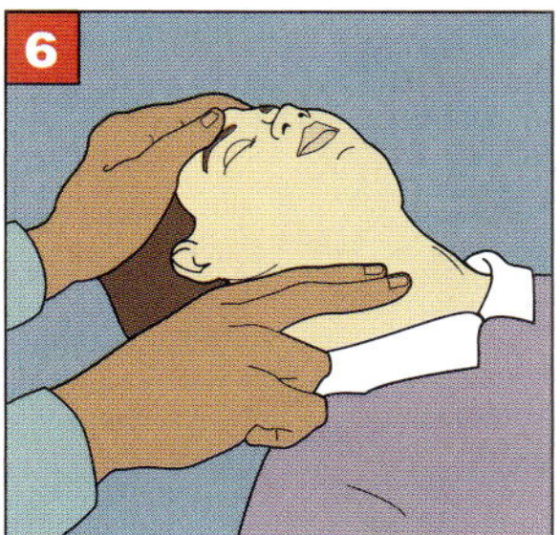

Checking the pulse. Gently press two fingers, not your thumb, in the depression on the side of the victim's neck, next to the Adam's apple, and feel for a pulse.

CHEST COMPRESSIONS

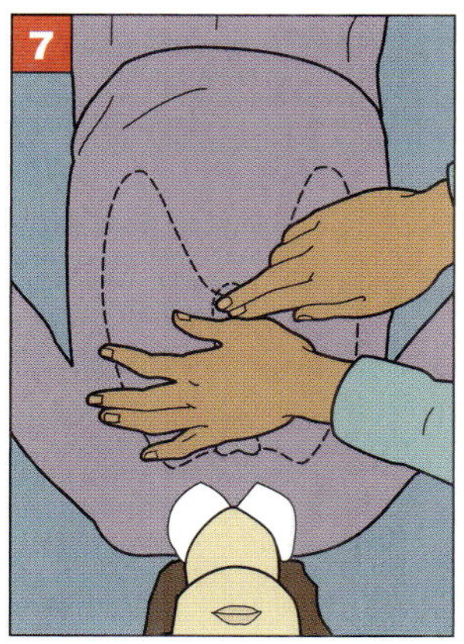

Placing your hands. Place two fingers of your right hand in the notch where the ribs meet the bottom of the breastbone. Place the heel of your left hand next to your right index finger, keeping your fingers off the child's chest. Now remove your left hand and put the heel of your right hand where the left hand was. Use your left hand to keep the child's head tilted back *(below)*.

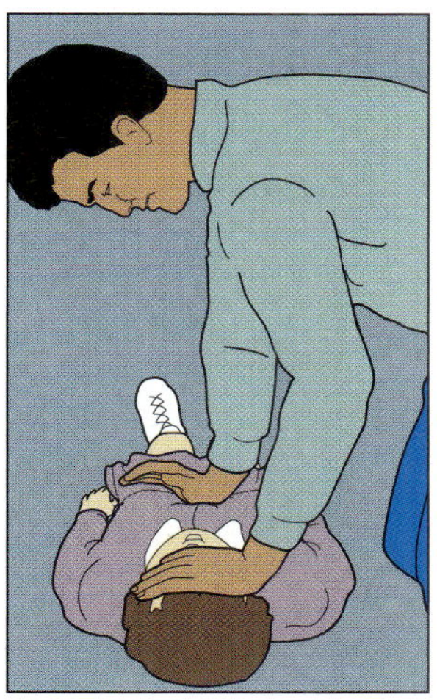

Giving chest compressions. Position yourself so that your shoulders are directly over the child's chest; keep your arm straight. Press down forcefully on your hand to depress the child's breastbone 1 to 1½ inches. Release the pressure, but don't lift your hand. Give five chest compressions, at the count of "one and two and three and...." CAUTION: Do not rock back and forth.

See pages 50-51 for complete instructions.

CHOKING

IMPORTANT!

- If you suspect that an object is caught in a victim's throat and he cannot cough, breathe, speak, or cry, call 911 or tell someone nearby to do so. Begin first-aid treatment for choking *(below)*. If you are the victim, see the box below, right. If the victim is an infant (up to one year old), see the box on page 56.
- If you suspect that an object is caught in a victim's throat but he is able to cough, breathe, talk, or cry, do not intervene. But be prepared to act if the situation worsens.

CAUTION: If you suspect a head, neck, or back injury, see page 66.

1 **Do not try to retrieve an object lodged in the victim's throat.** This might force the object farther down the airway.

2 **Give abdominal thrusts (the Heimlich maneuver).** Continue giving abdominal thrusts until the object is dislodged or until the victim loses consciousness. CAUTION: If the victim is pregnant or obese, place your fist on the middle of the victim's breastbone; do not place your hands on the ribs or on the lower edge of the breastbone.

3 **If the victim loses consciousness, lay him flat on his back.**

4 **Sweep the victim's mouth.** CAUTION: Remember, do not try to retrieve an object lodged in the victim's throat.

5 **Open the victim's airway.** Gently tilt back the victim's head and lift the chin.

6 **Look, listen, and feel for breathing.** Be sure to put your ear to the victim's mouth; chest movement alone might not mean breathing. If the victim is breathing, give first aid for unconsciousness *(page 71)*.

7 **Breathe twice into the victim's mouth.** Watch for the victim's chest to rise with each breath; let the chest fall before you give the next breath. If the victim's chest does not rise with each breath, gently tilt the head farther back and try again to give two slow breaths.

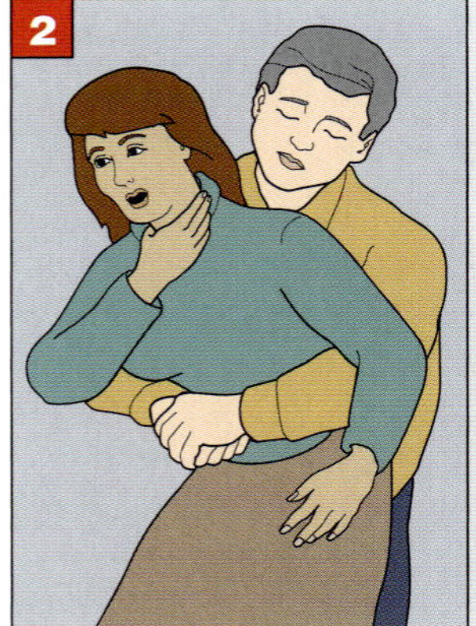

2 **Abdominal thrust.** Place your arms around the victim's waist. Make a fist with one hand and place it in the middle of the victim's abdomen, just above the navel and below the ribs. Hold your fist with your other hand. Give quick, repeated thrusts, pushing inward and upward.

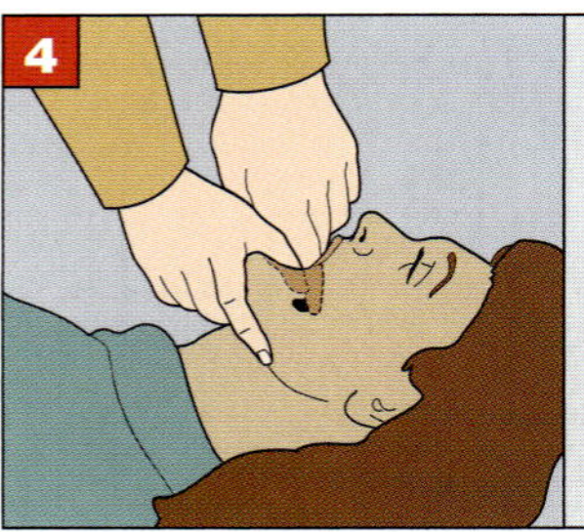

4 **Finger sweep.** Hold the victim's tongue and lift the chin. Slide your index finger down the inside of the cheek and sweep out any loose objects.

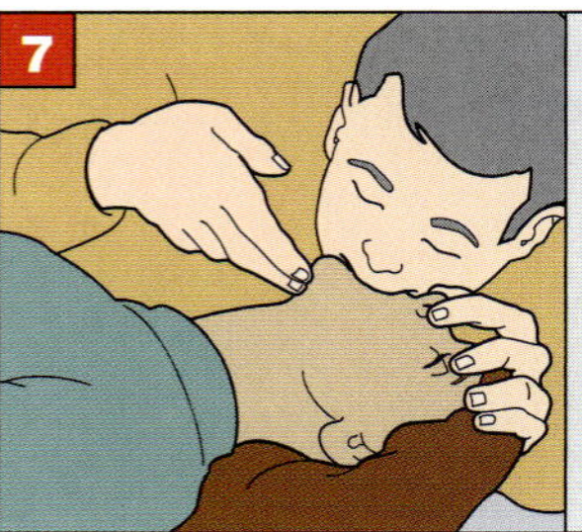

7 **Breathe into the victim's mouth.** Pinch the victim's nose shut and seal your lips tightly around the mouth. Give two slow breaths; remove your mouth between breaths.

8 **If the victim's chest still does not rise, give five abdominal thrusts.** CAUTION: Do not press to either side as you thrust.

9 **Sweep the victim's mouth, make sure the airway is open, and breathe twice again into the victim's mouth.**

10 **If the victim's chest still does not rise, give abdominal thrusts, sweep the mouth, and give breaths.** Give five abdominal thrusts. Sweep the victim's mouth, and give two slow breaths. Repeat this sequence of abdominal thrusts, sweeps of the mouth, and slow breaths until the object is dislodged or until medical help arrives.

11 **If the object is dislodged but the victim is not breathing, begin CPR** *(pages 50-53)*.

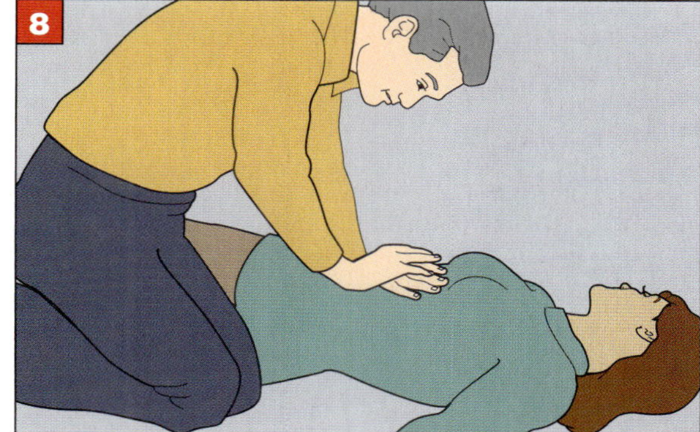

Abdominal thrust. Position the heel of one of your hands against the middle of the victim's abdomen, just above the navel and below the ribs. Place your other hand on top of the first. Give quick thrusts, pressing your hands inward and upward.

SELF

Give yourself abdominal thrusts until the object is dislodged. Get medical help to check for complications arising from either the choking episode or the first aid. CAUTION: If you feel or see an object lodged in your throat, do not try to retrieve it, as this might force the object farther down your airway.

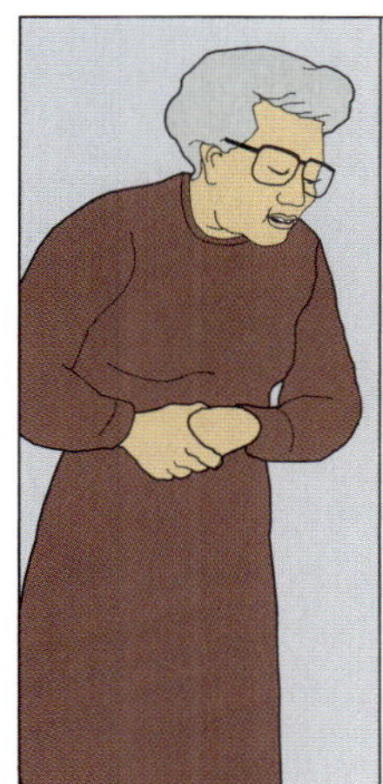

Abdominal thrust. Make a fist with one hand and place it in the middle of your abdomen, just above the navel and below the ribs. Hold your fist with your other hand. Keeping your elbows out, press your fist with a quick, upward thrust into your abdomen.

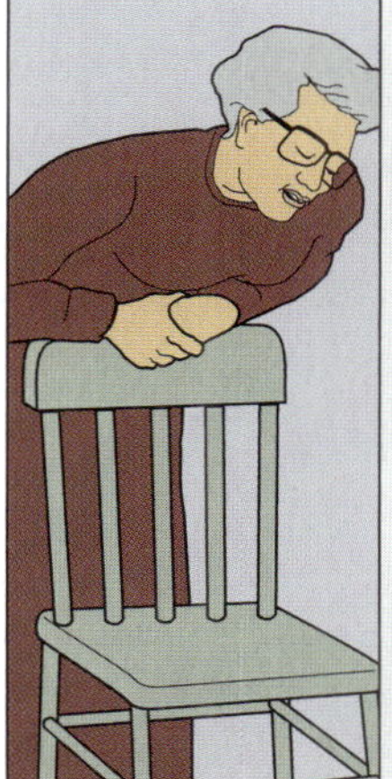

Abdominal thrust with the help of an object. Make a fist with one hand and place it in the middle of your abdomen, just above the navel and below the ribs. Bend over the back of a chair, a countertop, or some other firm, hard object and forcefully press it against your fist.

CONTINUED ▶

INFANT (UP TO 1 YEAR OLD)

1 Give back blows and chest thrusts. Give four back blows. If the object is not dislodged, give four chest thrusts. Repeat sets of four back blows and four chest thrusts until the object is dislodged or the infant loses consciousness.

2 If the infant loses consciousness, sweep the infant's mouth with your little finger. CAUTION: Do not try to retrieve an object lodged in the infant's throat.

3 Give breaths. If the infant isn't breathing, give two breaths into the mouth and nose. If the infant's chest does not rise with each breath, gently tilt the head farther back and try again to give two breaths.

4 If the infant's chest does not rise with breaths, continue giving breaths, back blows, and chest thrusts and sweeps of the mouth. Repeat a sequence of two breaths, four back blows, four chest thrusts, and a sweep of the mouth until the object is dislodged or until medical help arrives.

5 If the object is dislodged but the infant is not breathing, begin CPR *(page 52)*.

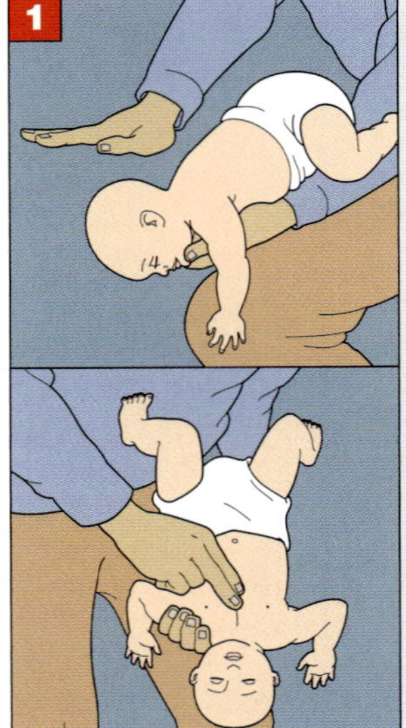

Back blow. Lay the infant facedown on your lower arm, supporting the head with your hand. Hold the chin between your index finger and thumb. Strike the back between the shoulder blades with the heel of your other hand.

Chest thrust. Turn the infant onto his back, with his head lower than the rest of his body. Place your index and middle fingers on the breastbone just below the nipples. Give quick thrusts.

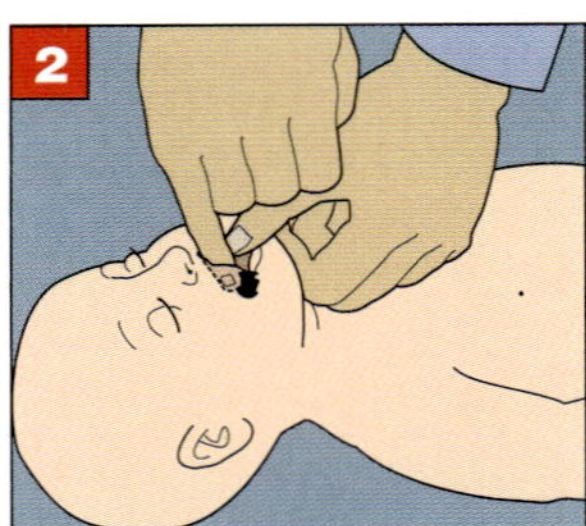

Finger sweep. Hold the infant's tongue and lift the chin. If you see an object and believe that you can easily remove it, slide your little finger down the inside of the cheek and sweep the object out.

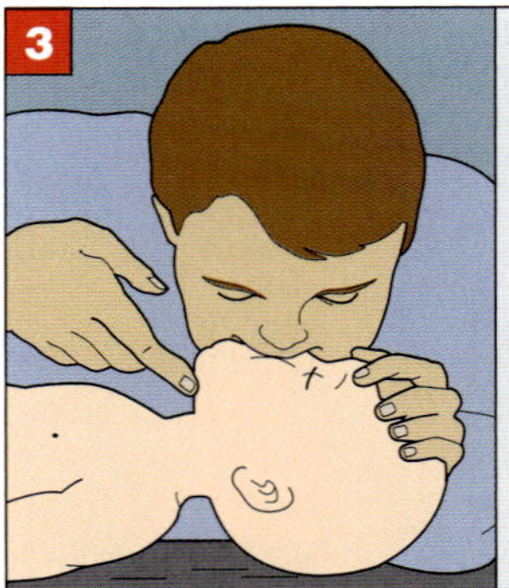

Breathe into the infant's mouth. Keep the head tilted with one hand and the chin lifted with your other. Tightly seal your lips around the mouth and nose. Give two breaths; remove your mouth between breaths. Breathe forcefully but not so hard that air goes into the infant's stomach.

DROWNING OR NEAR-DROWNING

IMPORTANT!

- If a victim is floating facedown in the water or is having difficulty swimming, call 911 or your emergency number, or tell someone nearby to do so; begin the first-aid steps described here.

SYMPTOMS

- Cold, pale skin
- Blue face
- Unconsciousness
- No exhaled breath

CAUTION: If you suspect a head, neck, or back injury, see page 66.

1 Pull the victim to safety. CAUTION: Be careful if you stretch out your arm or leg to the victim; the victim may inadvertently pull you into the water. Try to keep the victim's head, neck, and back aligned as you pull him to shore; if possible, slip a board under his back to tow him or to carry him out of the water.

2 Check the victim's ABCs *(page 47).* **If the victim is not breathing or does not have a pulse or heartbeat, begin CPR** *(pages 50-53).*

3 Place the victim in the recovery position *(page 47).* CAUTION: Do not place the victim in the recovery position if you suspect a neck or back injury, perhaps caused by a diving accident.

4 Remove any wet clothing and cover the victim with a coat, blanket, or dry clothing.

5 Keep the victim still and quiet while you wait for medical help to arrive.

WATER RESCUE

Unconscious victim. If possible, wade out and tow the victim faceup to shore; be careful of strong currents. If the water is too deep for wading, look for a boat to use to get to the victim. If there is no boat nearby and you are a strong swimmer, swim out to the victim and tow him faceup to shore. Otherwise, get help.

Conscious victim. Pull the drowning victim to safety with the help of a stick, oar, rope and life ring, towel, or nearby boat. If necessary, wade toward the victim, but be careful of strong currents. CAUTION: Do not swim out to the victim, unless you have been trained in water rescues.

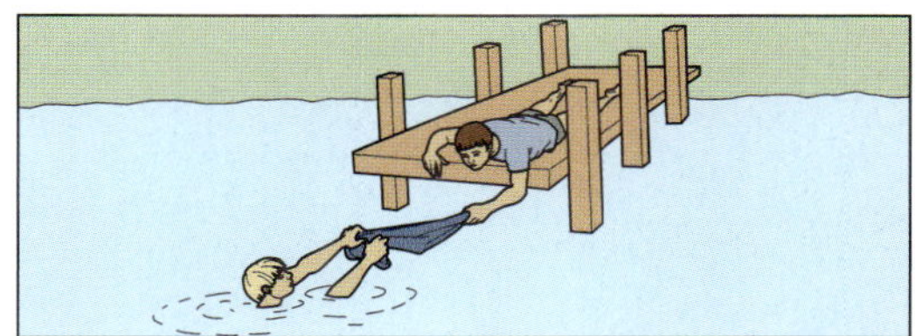

ICE RESCUE

Unconscious victim. If you can't reach the victim, tie a rope to a tree and then around your waist; slide on your belly to the victim. Otherwise, form a human chain with rescuers lying flat on the ice, and pull the victim to shore. CAUTION: Stay as far away as possible from the break in the ice.

Conscious victim. Tell the victim not to climb out but to hang on to the edge of the ice. Pull the victim out with the help of a big stick, rope, or ladder. Or form a human chain with rescuers lying flat on the ice.

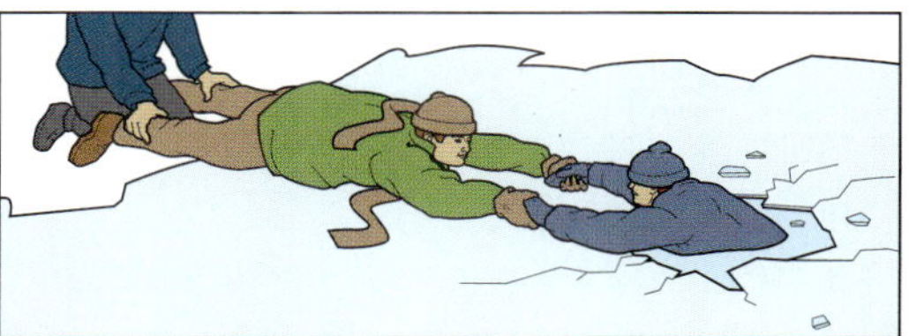

EAR EMERGENCIES

IMPORTANT!

- If you suspect a head injury or if blood or other fluids are draining from the ear after trauma to the head, call 911 or your emergency number.

SYMPTOMS

- Earache
- Difficulty hearing
- Swelling, redness of ear
- Bleeding
- Dizziness
- Nausea or vomiting

Foreign Objects

1 Shake the object out. Tilt the victim's head so that the affected ear is near the ground. Ask the victim to shake his head, or shake it for him. CAUTION: Do not hit the victim's head to try to free the object.

2 Pick the object out. If the object does not fall out, look into the ear. If you can see the object and it is pliable but is not a live insect, try to remove it with tweezers. CAUTION: Never poke at an object. Do not try to pick out a hard object such as a bean or a bead.

3 If there is a live insect inside the ear, kill the insect by pouring a small amount of oil, vinegar, or alcohol onto it. This will help alleviate pain. Then float the insect out with warm, not hot, oil.

4 If the object is securely lodged in the ear, take the victim to the nearest hospital.

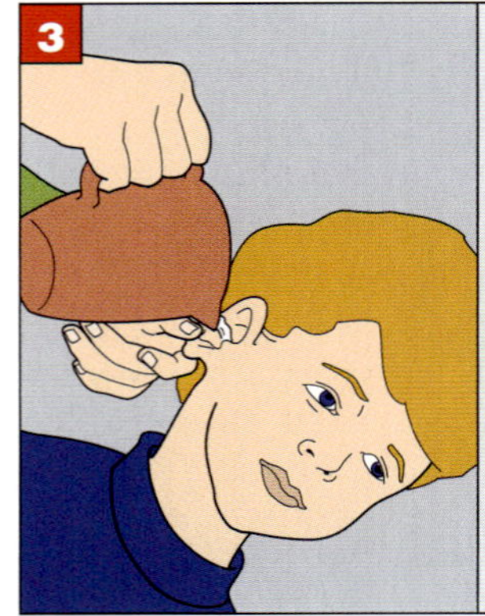

Floating an insect out of the ear. Tilt the victim's head so that the affected ear is toward the sky. Gently pull the victim's earlobe backward and upward, and pour a little warm mineral, olive, or baby oil into the ear. This should float the insect out of the ear.

Blood or Other Fluids from inside the Ear

1 Loosely cover the ear with a clean cloth and tape the cloth in place. CAUTION: Do not try to stop the drainage. Do not try to clean the ear.

2 Lay the victim flat on his back. CAUTION: If you suspect a head, neck, or back injury, see page 66.

ELECTRIC SHOCK

IMPORTANT!

- If a victim is near a high-voltage current, stay at least 20 feet away. If the victim is inside a car, tell him to stay there; however, if the car is burning, tell him to jump out and away from the car. Call the power company to have the power turned off; then call 911 or your emergency number. Once the power is off, begin the first-aid steps described here.
- If a victim is touching a live household electrical wire or you otherwise suspect that he has been electrocuted by household current, call 911 or your emergency number and begin the first-aid steps described here. Do not touch the victim if he is still in contact with a live current.
- If you suspect that a victim has been struck by lightning, call 911 or your emergency number. You may immediately touch the victim and begin the first-aid steps described here.

SYMPTOMS

- Burn marks on mouth or skin
- Tingling sensation
- Dizziness
- Feeling a severe jolt
- Muscle pains
- Bleeding
- Headache
- Unconsciousness

CAUTION: If you suspect a head, neck, or back injury, see page 66.

1 Stop the flow of electricity. Unplug the electrical appliance or turn off the house's main power switch. If you are not able to do this, separate the victim from the live current. CAUTION: Do not touch the victim's skin while he is still touching the live current. Do not touch the electrical wire.

2 Check the victim's ABCs *(page 47).* **If the victim is not breathing or does not have a pulse or heartbeat, begin CPR** *(pages 50-53).*

3 Check for and treat any other serious injury. Treat any entry and exit burns *(page 49).*

4 Make the victim comfortable. Cover the victim with a coat or blanket. Do not place a pillow under the head; this might cause the airway to become blocked.

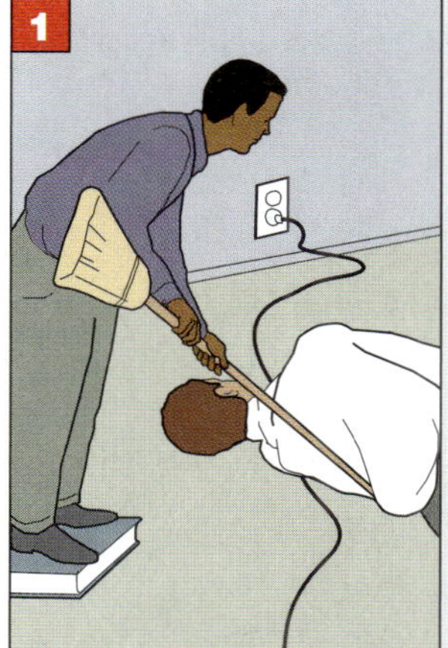

1 **Separating the victim from the current.** Stand on a pile of clothes, a book, or a piece of wood; make sure you are not standing in a pool of water. Use a dry, nonconductive material such as a wooden broom handle or a chair to separate the victim from the live current.

EMERGENCY CHILDBIRTH

IMPORTANT!

- If labor is proceeding faster than expected (the mother may feel an overwhelming urge to push or she may feel the baby's head between her legs), call 911 or your emergency number; then begin the first-aid steps described here. It is imperative to get medical help as soon as possible, because there may be complications that could endanger the life of the mother and baby.
- If uterine contractions are regular and occurring three to five minutes apart, take the mother to the hospital.
- If there is a liquid discharge from the mother's vagina, call her physician.
- Childbirth is a natural process, so interfere only when needed. Do not try to delay delivery. Do not let the mother cross her legs, and do not try to push the baby back into the mother's vagina.

Preparing the Mother

1 Make the mother comfortable. Place her on a large, flat area with pillows or other comfortable, supportive materials. Put a clean sheet or newspapers under her. Make sure she is warm. Help her remove any clothing below her belly.

2 Keep the mother calm. The mother may be in great pain; tell her to take deep, slow breaths.

3 Wash your hands with soap and water. Scrub under your fingernails with soap and water, and remove all of your jewelry.

The Delivery

1 Bloodstained fluid will appear. It is normal for there to be some bloodstained fluid; do not be alarmed. CAUTION: Get immediate medical help if the mother bleeds more than 1 to 2 cups of blood before, during, or after delivery.

2 Support the baby as he emerges. The baby will be slippery; you may want to use a clean, dry towel to hold him. CAUTION: Do not pull on the baby.

3 Make sure the umbilical cord is not around the baby's neck. If the umbilical cord is wrapped around the baby's neck, hook your finger underneath it and gently slip it over the baby's head.

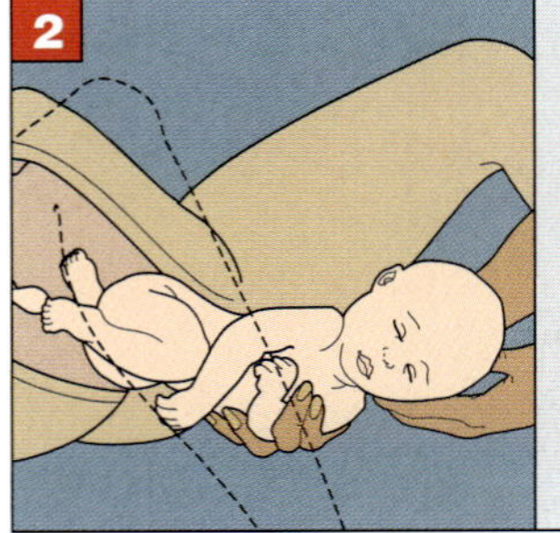

Support the baby. Most babies emerge headfirst. Support his head, and the rest of his body, as he emerges. He will naturally turn to one side and the rest of his body will follow.

4 The baby's shoulder may get stuck. If a shoulder seems stuck, gently press just above the mother's pubic hair or raise her legs up; tell her to push hard.

5 The baby may still be in the amniotic sac. If this is the case, tear the sac open.

6 The baby's head may not emerge first. If this happens, gently press just above the mother's pubic hair. Note the time. Support the baby's body as he emerges. If the head is not delivered within three minutes, lift the baby's body to expose his face so he can breathe. Tell the mother to keep pushing. CAUTION: Do not pull the baby out of the vagina.

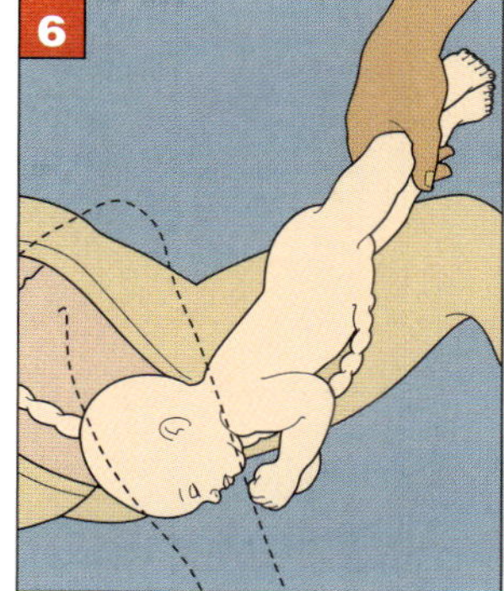

6 **Let a breech baby breathe.** Lift the baby's body upward until you can see his face. Clean the baby's mouth and nose with a clean, dry towel.

After the Birth

1 Help the baby begin to breathe. Hold the baby so fluids drain from his mouth and nose. Clean his mouth and nose with a clean, dry towel. If he is not breathing, hold him so his head is lower than his feet and tap his soles. Immediately rub his back. If this doesn't work, begin CPR *(pages 50-53)*.

2 Dry and wrap the baby. Use a clean, dry towel; do not wash off any white material on his body. Wrap him in a clean, dry towel.

3 Tie a string around the umbilical cord.

4 Save the placenta. The mother will usually expel the placenta within 30 minutes. Place it in a container to give to medical personnel. If it is not entirely expelled within 30 minutes, get immediate medical help. Do not pull on the umbilical cord or try to get the placenta out.

5 Massage the mother's lower abdomen. After the placenta is expelled, rub the mother's lower abdomen to help control any bleeding.

6 Keep the mother and baby warm until medical help arrives.

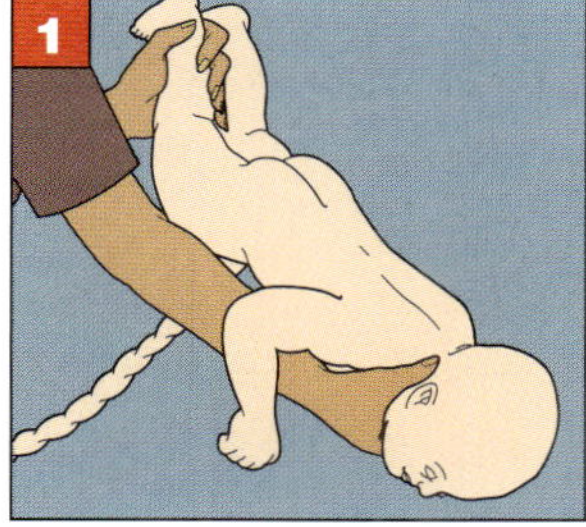

1 **Drain the baby's fluids.** Hold the baby so his head is lower than his feet and turn his head sideways.

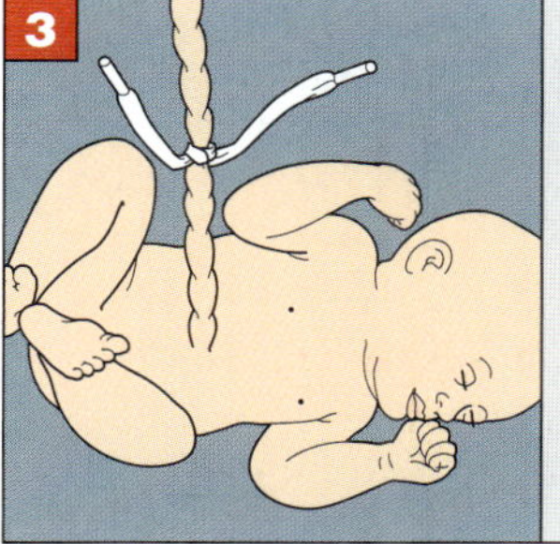

3 **Tie off the umbilical cord.** Use a string or shoelace and tie it tightly around the umbilical cord at least four inches from the baby's navel. CAUTION: Do not use thread to tie the umbilical cord.

EYE EMERGENCIES

IMPORTANT!

- If you suspect a head injury, an object is embedded in the eye, or a chemical was spilled in the eye, call 911 or your emergency number.
- If there is a pool of blood inside the eye, cover both eyes with a clean cloth and take the victim to the nearest hospital.
- If there is bleeding from inside the eye, elevate the victim's head above his heart, cover both eyes with a clean cloth, and take the victim to the nearest hospital. CAUTION: If you suspect a head, neck, or back injury, do not reposition or move the victim; call 911 or your emergency number.

SYMPTOMS

- Cut or bruise on eye
- Pain in or around eye
- Bloodshot eye
- Dry or itchy eye
- Tears
- Rapid blinking
- Inability to keep eye open
- Sensitivity to light
- Impaired vision
- Headache
- Unequally sized pupils

Foreign Objects

CAUTION: Do not touch or attempt to remove anything embedded in the eye. If the object is large, such as a pen, place a paper cup over the eye so that it supports the object; you may need to punch a hole in the cup. Tape the cup in place. Cover the victim's other eye with a clean cloth to help keep the injured eye from moving. If the object is small, cover both eyes with a clean cloth and loosely tie it in place.

1 Wash your hands with soap and water.

2 Look for the object. Ask the victim to slowly roll his eyes as you look for the object. CAUTION: Do not let the victim rub his eye.

3 Cause tears to form in the eye. If you see the object, gently pull the upper eyelid down over the lower eyelid. This will cause tears, which may wash the object out.

4 Remove a visible object. If the object does not wash out with tears, flush it out with running water or lift it off with a clean, damp cloth. Alternatively, the victim can open his eyes underwater in a bowl of fresh tap water. Once the object is out, the victim should take out any contact lenses. CAUTION: Do not use tissue or cotton to lift off the object. Do not lift off an object that is on the victim's iris or pupil.

5 Remove an object from the lower eyelid. If you see the object on the lower eyelid, flush it out with water or lift it off with a clean, damp cloth. Once the object is out, the victim should take out any contact lenses.

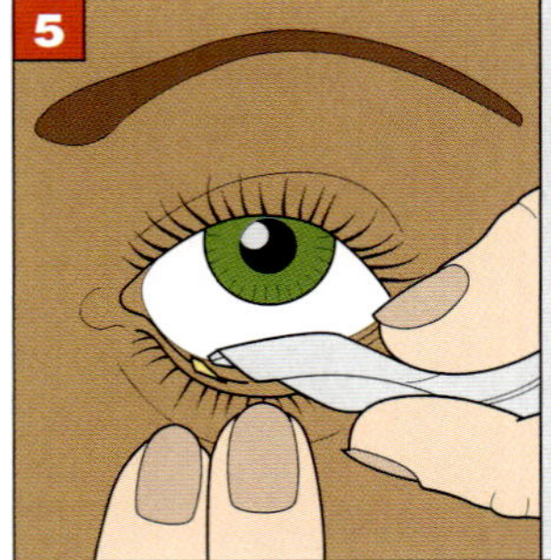

Lifting an object off the lower eyelid. Tell the victim to look up, and gently pull down the lower eyelid. Lift the object off the eye with a clean, damp cloth. CAUTION: Do not use tissue or cotton to lift off the object.

6 Remove an object off the upper eyelid. If you do not see the object on the eye or inside the lower eyelid, lift the victim's upper eyelid. If you see the object on the upper eyelid, flush it out with water or lift it off with a clean, damp cloth. Once the object is out of the eye, flip the upper eyelid back into place. The victim should now take out any contact lenses. CAUTION: Do not use tissue or cotton to lift off the object.

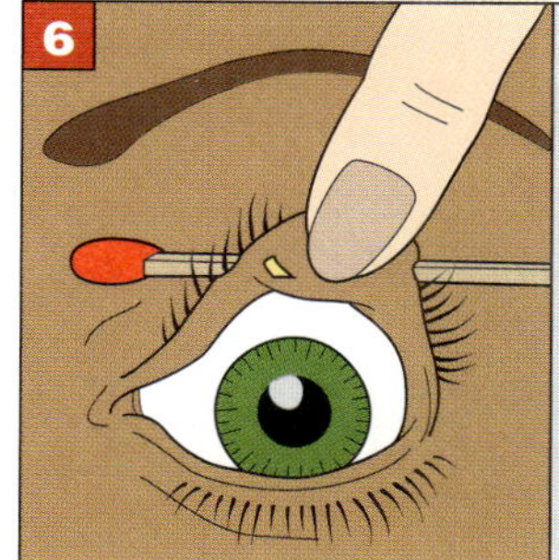

Raising the upper eyelid. Tell the victim to look down. Place a cotton swab, matchstick, or coffee stirrer across the upper eyelid. Hold the victim's upper eyelashes and eyelid, and fold the upper eyelid over the matchstick.

7 If necessary, cover both eyes and get medical help. If you cannot find or remove the object, or if the victim is in pain or has difficulty seeing after you've removed the object, cover both eyes with a clean cloth and tie it in place. Take the victim to the nearest hospital.

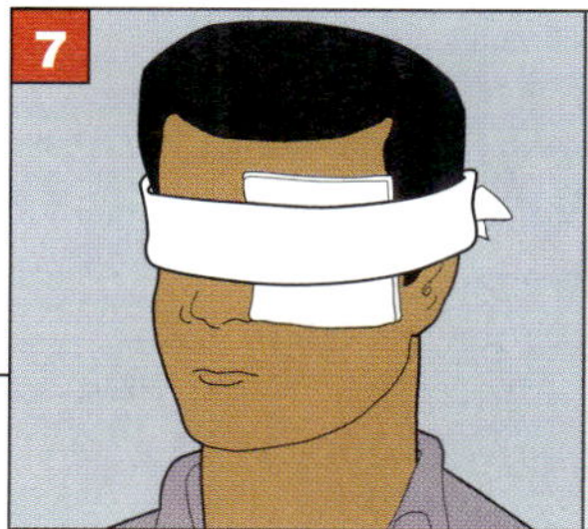

Covering both eyes. Place a clean cloth over the injured eye. Wrap another clean cloth around the victim's head so that it covers both eyes; tie it in place.

Chemical in the Eye

CAUTION: Do not waste any time to begin flushing the eye, and make sure that water is getting underneath both eyelids. Do not put anything other than water in the eye. Do not let the victim rub his eye.

1 Flush the eye with water. See the illustration at right. If you cannot get the victim to a faucet, keep flushing the eye with glasses of water for 15 minutes, making sure that the water flows across the eye away from the inner corner.

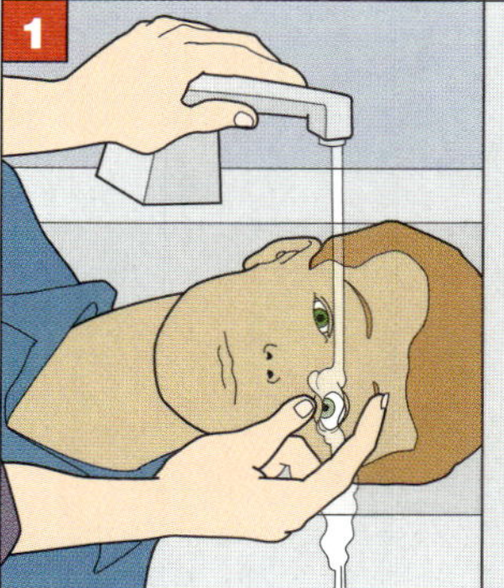

Flushing the eye. Hold the person's open eye under running water from a faucet for at least 15 minutes. The water should run from the inside of the eye to the outside. If both eyes are affected, let the water run over both eyes.

2 Ask the victim to remove his contact lenses, if he is wearing any.

3 Cover the eye. After flushing the eye, cover it with a clean cotton cloth. Then tie a bandage over both eyes; this will help inhibit movement of the affected eye.

4 Identify, if you can, the chemical that caused the burn. At a minimum, be prepared to tell emergency medical personnel whether the chemical was wet or dry.

FRACTURES AND DISLOCATIONS

IMPORTANT!

- Call 911 or your emergency number.
- If you suspect that the victim has broken his neck or back, see Head, Neck, and Back Injuries *(page 66).*
- If you suspect that the victim has broken his nose, see Nose Emergencies *(page 72).*

SYMPTOMS

- Pain
- Misshapen body part
- Bruising
- Discoloration of skin
- Swelling
- Visible bone
- Numbness in limb
- Loss of function of joint, limb, or digit

CAUTION: If you suspect a head, neck, or back injury, see page 66.

1 Check the victim's ABCs *(page 47).* **If the victim is not breathing or does not have a pulse or heartbeat, begin CPR** *(pages 50-53).*

2 Do not move the victim. CAUTION: Do not move someone with an injured hip, pelvis, or upper leg unless it is absolutely necessary. If you must move him to safety, immobilize the victim's head between your arms, grab his clothes at his shoulders, and drag him.

3 Check for and treat any other serious injuries. CAUTION: If the victim is bleeding around or near a broken bone, do not wash or probe the wound. Place a clean cloth over the wound and tie a bandage over it.

4 Immobilize the injured bone or joint. If a finger or toe is broken, apply a cold compress to it and elevate it above the level of the victim's heart. Place a small cloth or piece of cotton between the injured digit and an uninjured one, and then tape them together. See the illustrations opposite for instructions on how to immobilize an injured leg or arm. CAUTION: Do not attempt to straighten or change the position of any misshapen bone or joint. When applying a sling or splint, do not cut off blood circulation to the injured limb. Do not tie the splint in place over the break.

IMMOBILIZING AN INJURED ARM

LOWER ARM, WRIST, OR HAND

STABILIZE THE INJURED ARM

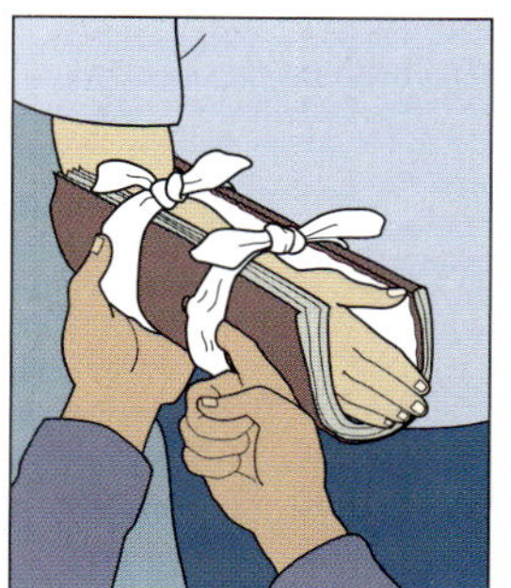

Stabilizing the arm. Support the injured bone or wrist with your hands, and place the lower arm at a right angle over the victim's chest. The victim's thumb should be pointing upward. Place the arm and wrist on a magazine or newspaper padded with a towel or pillow, and tie the magazine in place.

PLACE THE ARM IN A SLING

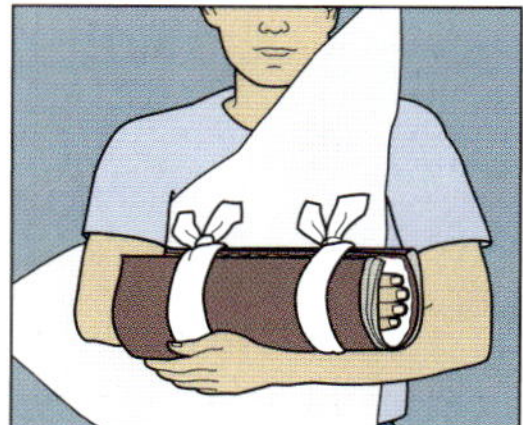

1 Position a cloth to be used as a sling. Locate a large piece of cloth or a long-sleeved shirt or sweater; fold the cloth in half, so it forms a triangle. Slide the cloth or shirt between the victim's arm and body, so the long side of the cloth or the shirt's top is closest to the uninjured arm.

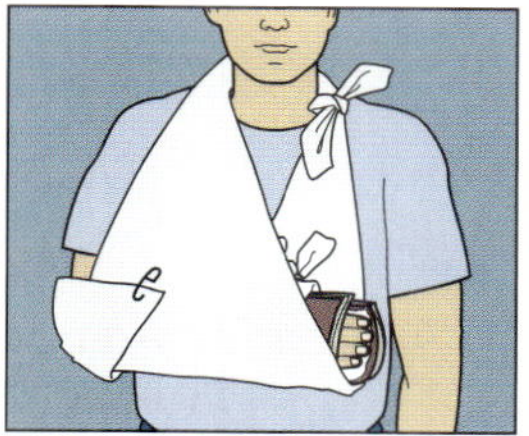

2 Tie the cloth in place. Pull one end of the cloth behind the victim's neck; place the other half over the injured arm. Tie the sling over the shoulder of the uninjured side; fold over any extra material that is behind the elbow and pin it in place. Make sure the sling is snug but not tight.

UPPER ARM, SHOULDER, OR COLLARBONE

STABILIZE THE INJURED SHOULDER OR COLLARBONE

1 Support the injured bone or joint with your hands. Position the injured arm across the chest, thumb pointing up, and place it in a sling *(above)*.

2 Secure the sling in place. Tie a piece of cloth around the sling and the victim's chest and arm.

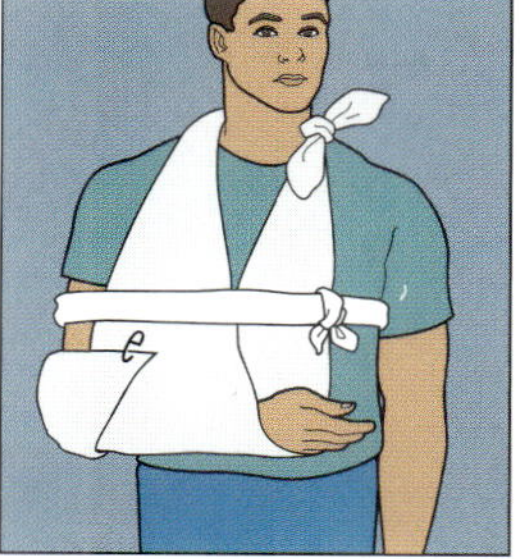

IMMOBILIZING AN INJURED LEG

LOWER LEG

SPLINT THE LOWER LEG

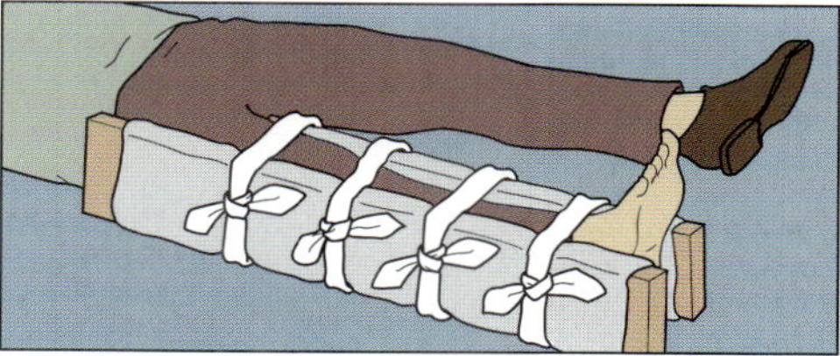

Using boards as a splint. Locate two long boards; one should extend from the victim's hip to the heel, and the second should stretch from the groin to the heel. Pad the boards with blankets or pillows, then place the boards so the padded side touches the injured leg. Tie the boards in place at the groin, thigh, knee, and ankle.

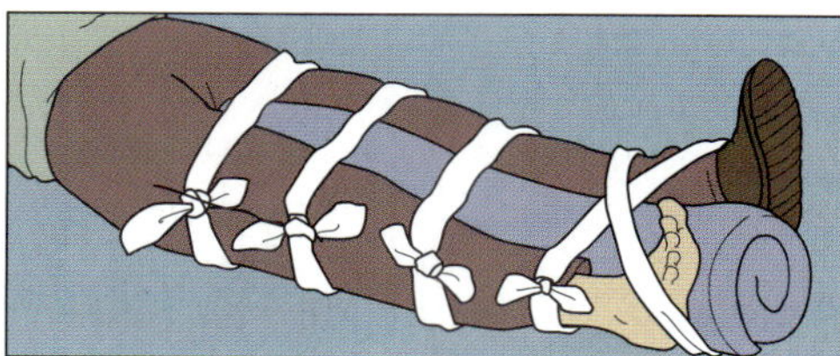

Using a blanket as a splint. If boards are unavailable, roll up a blanket, place it between the victim's legs, and tie the victim's legs together at the groin, thighs, knees, and ankles.

UPPER LEG OR HIP

SPLINT THE UPPER LEG OR HIP

CAUTION: Do not splint an injured upper leg or hip unless you have to move the victim. Do not tie the splint in place over the break.

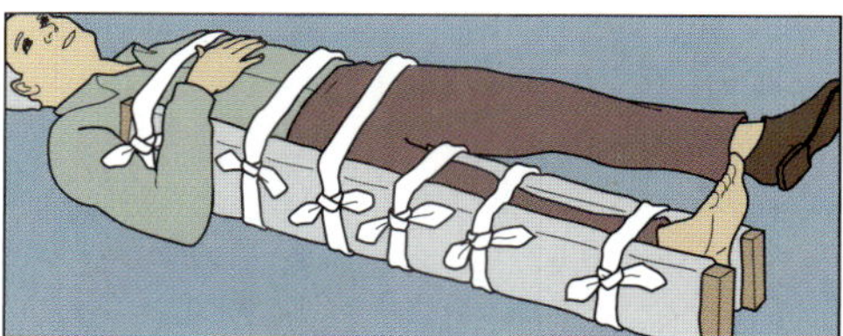

Using boards as a splint. Locate two long boards: one to extend from the victim's armpit to the heel, and the other from the groin to the heel. Pad the boards with blankets or pillows, then place the boards padded side in. Tie the boards in place at the chest, waist, groin, thigh, knee, and ankle.

HEAD, NECK, AND BACK INJURIES

CAUTION: Do not move the injured person unless it is absolutely necessary.

1 Keep the victim calm and completely still.

2 Check the victim's ABCs *(page 47).* **If the victim is not breathing or does not have a pulse or heartbeat, begin CPR** *(pages 50-53).* CAUTION: When opening the victim's airway, just lift the chin. If you need to place the victim on his back, support his head, neck, and back together and carefully roll him onto his back; make sure you keep the head, neck, and back aligned as you roll him. It is best to have at least one other person help you do this.

3 Treat obvious injuries.

4 Make the victim comfortable. Keep the victim warm, with a blanket or coat, until medical help arrives. CAUTION: Do not put a pillow under the head, as this might cause the airway to become blocked. Do not give him anything to eat or drink.

5 Keep the airway open. If the victim begins to choke or vomit or becomes unconscious, support his head, neck, and back together and carefully roll him onto his side. It is best to have someone else help you do this. CAUTION: Make sure that the victim's head and neck move with his body.

IMPORTANT!

- Call 911 or your emergency number.
- If you suspect the victim has suffered a head injury and he is bleeding from his ear, eye, or nose, give first aid as described below and then give first aid for ear emergencies *(page 58),* eye emergencies *(page 62),* or nose emergencies *(page 72).*
- If you can, find out how the victim was injured. A head, neck, or back injury is particularly likely if the victim was in an accident involving sudden acceleration or deceleration (as in car accidents) or from jumping or diving, or if there are gunshot wounds to the head or chest. Multiple wounds and unconsciousness after physical trauma are other possible indicators.

SYMPTOMS

Head Injuries

- Head wound
- Bruise or lump on scalp
- Bleeding from ear, nose, or mouth that is not due to injury to those areas
- Fluid draining from ear or nose
- Black eyes
- Bruise behind ear
- Headache, nausea, or vomiting
- Altered mental state
- Vision changes
- Slurred speech
- Irregular pulse
- Unconsciousness

Neck or Back Injuries

- Pain in back or neck
- Tingling sensation in arms or legs
- Loss of movement in arms or legs
- Loss of bladder or bowel control
- Odd position of head, neck, or back
- Unconsciousness

HEART ATTACK

IMPORTANT!

- Call 911 or your emergency number.

SYMPTOMS

- Crushing or spreading chest pain that may radiate to one or both arms or to the neck or jaw
- Irregular heartbeat
- Difficulty breathing
- Fear or anxiety
- Dizziness
- Heavy sweating
- Nausea or vomiting
- Pale or bluish lips or fingernails
- Pale, bluish, or clammy skin
- Unconsciousness

CAUTION: If you suspect a head, neck, or back injury, see page 66.

1 Check the victim's ABCs *(page 47).* **If the victim is not breathing or does not have a pulse or heartbeat, begin CPR** *(pages 50-53).*

2 Make the victim comfortable and keep him calm. Loosen any tight clothing, especially around the victim's neck, chest, and waist. If the victim is unconscious, place him in the recovery position *(page 47).* Keep the victim warm; if necessary, cover him with a blanket or additional clothing. Stroke the victim's forehead with a cool, wet cloth. CAUTION: Do not try to revive an unconscious victim by slapping or shaking him or throwing cold water on him. Do not give the victim anything to eat or drink.

3 Continue to monitor the victim's breathing and pulse, and if necessary, begin CPR.

HEATSTROKE AND HEAT EXHAUSTION

Heatstroke

Cool the victim. Quickly move the victim to a cooler site. Place cool, wet cloths on the forehead and torso, or wrap the victim in wet towels or sheets. Fan him with an electric fan, a hair dryer set on cold, or your hand. CAUTION: Do not use an alcohol rub to cool the victim; do not give him anything to eat or drink.

Heat Exhaustion

1 **Move the victim to a cooler site.**

2 **Have the victim lie or sit down, and elevate his feet.**

3 **Cool the victim.** Place cool, wet cloths on the forehead and torso, or wrap the victim in wet towels or sheets. Fan the victim with an electric fan, a hair dryer set on cold, or your hand. CAUTION: Do not use an alcohol rub to cool the victim.

4 **Give the conscious victim a cool drink.** If the victim is conscious and is able to swallow and breathe without difficulty, give him salt water (1 tsp salt mixed with 1 qt water) to sip. CAUTION: Do not force the victim to drink; do not give him anything that is alcoholic or caffeinated.

5 **If the victim's condition does not improve, call 911 or your emergency number.**

IMPORTANT!

- If you suspect that the victim is suffering from heatstroke, call 911 or your emergency number.
- Untreated heat exhaustion may progress to become heatstroke.

SYMPTOMS

Heatstroke

- Body temperature above 102°F
- Flushed, dry, hot skin
- Constricted pupils
- Confusion
- Rapid pulse
- Seizures
- Unconsciousness

Heat Exhaustion

- Cool, clammy skin
- Excessive perspiration
- Dilated pupils
- Rapid pulse
- Headache
- Nausea or vomiting
- Abdominal or limb cramps
- Dizziness
- Unconsciousness

HYPOTHERMIA AND FROSTBITE

IMPORTANT!

- Call 911 or your emergency number.
- If the victim has symptoms of both hypothermia and frostbite, treat for hypothermia first.

SYMPTOMS

Hypothermia

- Shivering
- Uncoordinated movements
- Drowsiness, weakness
- Unconsciousness
- Cardiac arrest

Frostbite

- Numb, cold skin
- Pink skin that becomes pale, and then later becomes blackened or hard and frozen
- Blisters

Hypothermia

CAUTION: If you suspect a head, neck, or back injury, see page 66.

1 Check the victim's ABCs *(page 47)*. **If the victim is not breathing or does not have a pulse or heartbeat, begin CPR** *(pages 50-53)*. CAUTION: Hypothermic victims often have very slow and weak pulses; therefore, take a little extra time and care to check for the pulse.

2 Gently take or lead the victim to shelter. Change the victim into dry clothing.

3 If medical help is unavailable, slowly rewarm the victim. Cover the head and neck. Use your own body heat, blankets, or aluminum foil to slowly warm the victim. Place warm compresses to the neck, chest, and groin. If the victim is conscious and can swallow, give warm, sweetened, nonalcoholic beverages to sip. CAUTION: Do not use any form of direct heat, such as an electric blanket, to warm the victim.

Frostbite

CAUTION: If there is any chance of the skin refreezing, do not thaw it. Move the victim out of the cold and wait for emergency help.

1 Move the victim to a nearby shelter. Remove any tight clothing or jewelry.

2 If you can keep the frostbitten skin warm and help will not arrive soon, slowly thaw the skin. Place frostbitten hands or feet in a bowl of warm, not hot, water for at least 30 minutes. Gently stir the water, and add warm water as it cools. Or soak a cotton cloth in warm water; resoak the cloth to keep it warm. If water is not available, use your own skin, blankets, or newspaper to warm the skin. CAUTION: Frostbitten skin may be permanently damaged if warmed too quickly; do not use direct heat, such as an electric blanket. Do not massage the skin.

3 Dry the thawed skin and keep it warm. Once the damaged skin is soft and sensation returns, place a clean, dry cloth over the skin; place clean, dry cloths between frostbitten toes and fingers. Wrap the skin with dry cloths in order to keep it warm.

4 Do not let the victim smoke or drink alcohol while you wait for medical help.

INTERNAL BLEEDING

IMPORTANT!

- Call 911 or your emergency number.

SYMPTOMS

- Bruises
- Coughing or vomiting blood
- Rectal bleeding
- Vaginal (but not menstrual) bleeding
- Blood in urine
- Bleeding from the nose or ear
- Skull, chest, or abdominal wounds
- Dizziness
- Fainting
- Weak pulse
- Shortness of breath
- Shallow breathing
- Dilated pupils
- Pale, clammy skin

CAUTION: If you suspect a head, neck, or back injury, see page 66.

1 **Check the victim's ABCs** *(page 47)*. **If the victim is not breathing or does not have a pulse or heartbeat, begin CPR** *(pages 50-53)*. While you wait for medical help, periodically recheck the victim's ABCs.

2 **Keep the victim calm and still. Do not give him anything to eat or drink.**

3 **If the victim's arm or leg is swollen or misshapen, immobilize it** *(page 65)*.

4 **Begin treatment for shock** *(page 75)* **while you wait for medical help.**

LOSS OF CONSCIOUSNESS

IMPORTANT!

- Call 911 or your emergency number.

CAUTION: If you suspect a head, neck, or back injury, see page 66.

1 Check the victim's ABCs *(page 47).* **If the victim is not breathing or does not have a pulse or heartbeat, begin CPR** *(pages 50-53).*

2 Remove the victim from an injurious site.

3 Loosen any tight clothing, especially around the victim's neck.

4 Place the victim in the recovery position *(page 47).*

5 Keep the victim warm, with a blanket or coat, until medical help arrives. Stroke the victim's forehead with a cool, wet cloth. CAUTION: Do not try to revive the victim by slapping or shaking him or throwing cold water on him. Do not place a pillow under the head, as this might cause the airway to become blocked.

NOSE EMERGENCIES

IMPORTANT!

- If a nosebleed does not stop after 15 minutes, clear or bloody fluid is draining from the nose after an injury, or you suspect a head or neck injury, call 911 or your emergency number.

SYMPTOMS

Foreign Objects

- Irritation
- Difficulty breathing through nostril
- Foul-smelling discharge from nostril
- Bleeding from nostril

Nosebleed

- Bleeding from nostril
- Bleeding in the back of the throat
- Gagging
- Choking

Foreign Objects

CAUTION: Do not use tweezers or other tools to try to remove the object. Do not ask the victim to inhale sharply.

1 Ask the victim to try to blow out the object. Press the unaffected nostril with one finger; ask the victim to blow his nose. If the object is not dislodged, ask the victim to sniff some pepper to help him sneeze and blow the object out.

2 If the object is still not dislodged, take the victim to the nearest hospital.

Nosebleed

CAUTION: If your nose is misshapen or misaligned, or you have swelling, pain, or bruises around your eyes, your nose may be broken. Sit down and press a cold cloth against your nose. Ask someone to take you to the nearest hospital.

1 Sit down.

2 If there are clots of blood in your nose, try to blow them out, once.

3 Pinch your nose shut. Hold both nostrils, below the bridge, between your thumb and index finger for 10 minutes. Breathe through your mouth.

4 If the bleeding does not stop, place a cloth packing in the bleeding nostril. Roll a small, clean cloth and place it in the bleeding nostril; hold both nostrils between your thumb and index finger. CAUTION: Do not push the cloth too far into the nose; make sure that you will be able to pull it out.

5 Once the bleeding stops, place a cold cloth over your nose and face.

6 Remove the cloth packing in your nostril after 30 to 60 minutes. It is best to dampen the cloth before removing it. Do not blow or pick your nose, strain yourself, or bend over for 24 hours. Rub petroleum jelly inside the nostril to help prevent further bleeding or drying.

POISONING

CAUTION: If you suspect a head, neck, or back injury, see page 66.

1 Check the victim's ABCs *(page 47).* **If the victim is not breathing or does not have a pulse or heartbeat, begin CPR** *(pages 50-53).*

2 Try to identify the poison. If possible, ask the victim what he swallowed or inhaled. Otherwise, look around for any open or nearby containers of chemicals or for any plants or household items that the victim may have swallowed; sniff the air for unusual odors.

3 Call your local poison control center or 911. Tell emergency personnel what chemical, plant, or household item the victim swallowed. Wait for instructions as to how to proceed.

4 Follow the instructions given by the poison control center or by 911 personnel. Depending on the poison, you may be instructed to induce vomiting by giving the victim syrup of ipecac, to give milk or water to drink, or to give activated charcoal. CAUTION: Do not try to induce vomiting unless told to do so; do not induce vomiting if it has been more than one hour since the victim ingested the poison. Do not give the victim anything to eat or drink unless told to do so. Do not rely on poisoning instructions given on container labels.

5 Place the victim in the recovery position *(page 47).*

6 Save any vomit for medical personnel.

IMPORTANT!

- If chemicals have splashed or spilled into the victim's eyes, see Eye Emergencies *(page 62).*
- If chemicals have splashed or spilled onto the victim's skin, see Burns *(page 49).*
- If the victim inhaled poisonous gas, take him to fresh air and then begin the first-aid steps for poisoning described here.
- Since a poisoning victim may exhibit few symptoms or symptoms that are not listed below, it is very important to examine the scene for clues.

SYMPTOMS

- Headache
- Dizziness
- Fever
- Abdominal pain
- Vision problems
- Seizures
- Unusual breath odor
- Chills
- Drowsiness
- Burns on skin
- Nausea or vomiting
- Breathing problems
- Unconsciousness

POISONOUS HOUSEHOLD ITEMS

In addition to this list of poisonous household items, many cleansers, detergents, deodorizers, and disinfectants are poisonous. Drugs, medications, herbal remedies, and vitamins, whether prescription or over the counter, may be poisonous if mixed together, mixed with alcohol, or taken in large quantities; see the ***Index of Conventional and Natural Medicines.*** Call your local poison control center about specific items.

- Alcohol
- Antifreeze
- Fuels
- Herbicides
- Insecticides
- Iron pills
- Lye
- Mothballs
- Paint
- Pesticides
- Polishes
- Solvents
- Tobacco products
- Turpentine
- Windshield fluid

POISONOUS PLANTS

There are hundreds of potentially poisonous plants in the U.S. Many plant parts, including seeds, berries, nuts, and bulbs, are potentially poisonous. If you have a question about a plant, call your local poison control center. Some of the most poisonous plants are:

- Castor bean
- Dieffenbachia
- Foxglove
- Jimson weed
- Oleander
- Philodendron
- Poison hemlock
- Pokeweed
- Pothos
- Water hemlock

SEIZURES

IMPORTANT!

- If this is the first time the victim has had a seizure, if the victim has more than one seizure per hour, or if the seizure lasts more than two minutes, call 911 or your emergency number.
- Seizures, while frightening, are usually not life-threatening. You should be more concerned about the seizure's cause, so be sure to determine if the victim is wearing a Medic Alert tag or if he is suffering from another injury.

SYMPTOMS

- Tingling sensation
- Twitching, muscle spasms
- Body stiffening
- Drooling
- Loss of bladder or bowel control
- Temporary respiratory arrest
- Unconsciousness

CAUTION: If you suspect a head, neck, or back injury, see page 66.

1 If the victim suspects that he is going to have a seizure or if he begins to lose his balance, help him to the ground.

2 Lay the victim on his side to prevent any vomit from entering his lungs. CAUTION: Do not put your hands in or near the victim's mouth during the seizure.

3 Loosen any tight clothing on the victim.

4 Prevent the victim from injuring himself. Remove eyeglasses. Push away any objects or furniture that might injure the victim if he collides with it. CAUTION: Do not try to restrict his movements, unless he is going to hurt himself.

5 When the seizure has ended, help the victim into a comfortable position on his side. The victim is likely to be tired and confused; he may fall asleep.

6 Check the victim's ABCs *(page 47).* **If the victim is not breathing or does not have a pulse or heartbeat, begin CPR** *(pages 50-53).*

FEBRILE SEIZURES

Seizures in young children or infants are often caused by sudden high fevers. If the child has such a fever, take off his clothes and sponge his body with lukewarm, not cold, water. Call your doctor for further advice. CAUTION: Do not give the child a bath.

SHOCK

IMPORTANT!

- Call 911 or your emergency number.

SYMPTOMS

- Restlessness or anxiety
- Weak, rapid pulse
- Cold, clammy, pale skin
- Shaking chills
- Chest pain
- Rapid, shallow breathing
- Dizziness or general weakness
- Nausea or vomiting
- Unconsciousness

CAUTION: If you suspect a head, neck, or back injury, see page 66.

1 Check the victim's ABCs *(page 47)*. **If the victim is not breathing or does not have a pulse or heartbeat, begin CPR** *(pages 50-53)*.

2 Position the victim so he is comfortable. Unless the victim is more comfortable sitting up, lay him on his back, with his head lower than the rest of his body. If you do not suspect any broken leg bones, elevate the legs 8 to 12 inches. Recheck the victim's airway.

3 Try to determine the cause of shock and perform first aid for the appropriate emergency.

4 Make the victim warm and comfortable. Loosen any tight clothing and cover the victim with a blanket or additional clothing. Do not use an electric blanket or any other form of direct heat. If the victim is lying down, do not place a pillow under the head, as this might cause the airway to become blocked.

5 Keep the airway open. If the victim begins to choke or vomit, turn his head to one side so that the vomit will not block his airway.

6 If medical help is more than an hour away, give the conscious victim a clean cloth soaked in water to suck on.

ANAPHYLACTIC SHOCK

IMPORTANT!

- If you suspect a severe allergic reaction, the victim may be in anaphylactic shock.

SYMPTOMS

- Itching
- Flushed face
- Dizziness
- Nausea or vomiting
- Wheezing
- Unconsciousness
- Hives
- Warm skin
- Swollen face or tongue
- Abdominal cramps
- Difficulty breathing

In addition to treating the victim as you would for shock, perform these steps:

- **Try to keep the victim calm.**
- **Determine if the victim was stung by an insect.** If so, carefully scrape the stinger off the victim's skin. CAUTION: Do not use tweezers; this may push more venom into the skin.
- **Administer medicine, if available.** Some people are prone to anaphylactic shock and may have emergency supplies on hand. If this is the case, help the victim with his medicine. This may include giving the victim a shot of epinephrine; follow the instructions on the medication.

SNAKEBITES

IMPORTANT!

- If you aren't sure that the bite was by a poisonous snake, assume it was and begin the first-aid steps described here.

SYMPTOMS

Rattlesnake, Copperhead, and Cottonmouth Bites

- Increasing pain at bite site
- Rapid swelling and skin discoloration at bite site
- Twitching skin
- Dizziness
- Nausea
- Sweating
- Numbness around mouth

Coral Snake Bites

- Pain at bite site
- Drowsiness
- Slurred speech
- Double vision
- Sweating
- Nausea
- Delirium
- Seizures

1 **Keep the victim calm and still, and if possible, place the bite below the level of the victim's heart.**

2 **Identify the snake, if you can.** If you have to kill the snake, do not damage its head. CAUTION: Do not endanger yourself by getting too close to the snake.

3 **Call 911 or your emergency number and report what kind of snake bit the victim.**

4 **Check the victim's ABCs** *(page 47).* **If the victim is not breathing or does not have a pulse or heartbeat, begin CPR** *(pages 50-53).*

5 **If the bite is on the victim's arm or leg, tie a band above it.** Loosen the band for a minute or two every 15 to 30 minutes. If swelling extends to the band, move it a few inches higher. CAUTION: Do not apply a band if you suspect that the victim was bitten by a coral snake.

6 **If you are sure that the snake was poisonous, the bite occurred within 5 minutes, and it will take more than 30 minutes to get medical help, cut into the bite and suck out the venom.** With a sterile razor blade, cut just through the skin and through the bite mark. With a suction cup or your mouth, suck out the venom. CAUTION: Cut along the length of a limb, not across it. Do not make any cuts on the victim's head, neck, or torso. Do not swallow the venom; spit it out. Do not suck the venom if you have open sores in or on your mouth. Do not make any cuts if the victim was bitten by a coral snake.

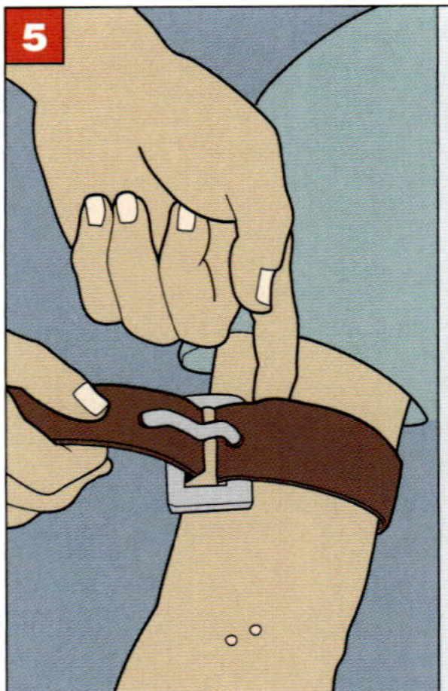

Tie a band above the bite. Use either a belt or scarf to tie a band two to four inches above the bite; the band should be between the bite and the victim's heart. Make sure you can slip your finger between the band and the victim's skin and that you can feel a pulse below the band. If you cannot do this, loosen the band until you can.

7 **Gently wash the bite with soap and water.** Pat, don't rub, it dry.

8 **Remove any constricting jewelry or clothing near the bite.**

9 **Place a clean cloth bandage over the bite.**

10 **Watch for signs of a severe allergic reaction.** See Anaphylactic Shock *(page 75)*.

11 **If the victim needs to move, do not let him walk; carry him.**

HEAD SHAPES AND BITE MARKS

NONPOISONOUS SNAKE

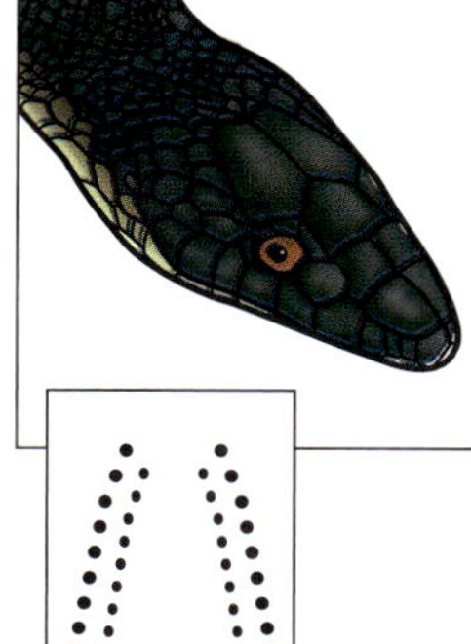

Nonpoisonous snakes tend to leave a bite pattern similar to that shown above, with double rows of bite marks.

POISONOUS SNAKE

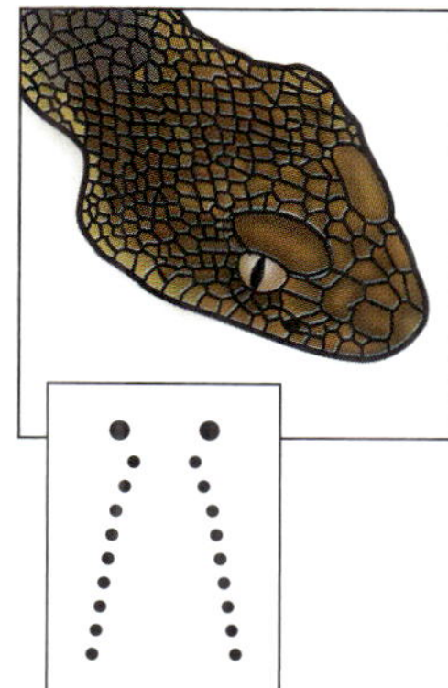

Poisonous snakes (except the coral) have a distinctive triangular head; the bite usually includes two fang puncture wounds.

POISONOUS SNAKES IN THE U.S.

There are four types of poisonous snakes in the United States: rattlesnakes, copperheads, cottonmouths (also called water moccasins), and coral snakes (also called harlequin or bead snakes). It is important to be able to recognize the snake that bit the victim so that the proper antivenin can be administered at the hospital.

Rattlesnakes, copperheads, and cottonmouths have triangular heads, slitlike eyes, long fangs, and a similar bite pattern. Rattlesnakes and copperheads shake their tails when disturbed, but only rattlesnakes have rattles on the end of their tails. Cottonmouths can be recognized by the white lining of their mouths.

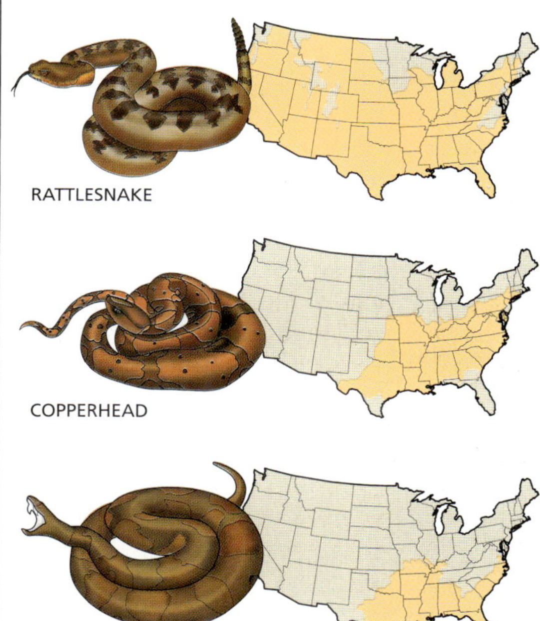

RATTLESNAKE

COPPERHEAD

COTTONMOUTH

Coral snakes have red, black, and yellow or white bands and a black snout. They can be distinguished from similarly colored nonpoisonous snakes with the help of this rhyme: "Red next to yellow will kill a fellow; red next to black won't hurt Jack."

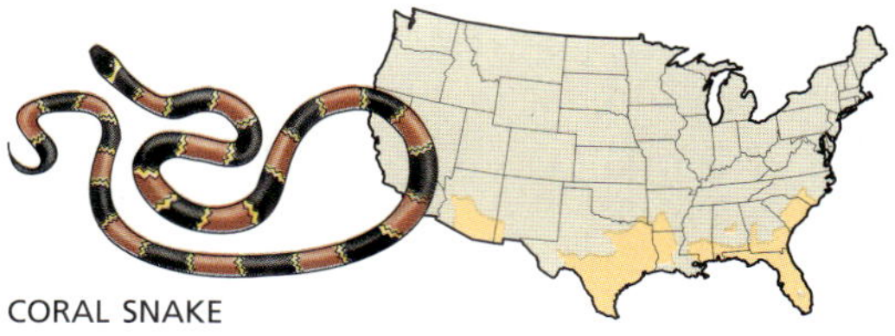

CORAL SNAKE

YOUR MEDICINE CHEST

CONVENTIONAL

It is helpful to have some medications for common ailments on hand in your home so that when the occasional cold or flu strikes you'll be prepared. All of the items below are available over the counter (OTC) at most drugstores and supermarkets. When it comes to brand names among OTC classes, most preparations have the same active ingredients and differ only in packaging. Keep in mind that OTC products are still drugs and can have potentially dangerous side effects if misused; for more information on a specific medication see the ***Index of Conventional and Natural Medicines,*** beginning on page 882.

All of these substances should be stored away from light, humidity, and the reach of children. Check expiration dates on all your medications periodically; many of these preparations have a limited shelf life.

Members of your family may have other, specific needs, such as epinephrine for bee allergies. These should also be included in your home medicine chest.

FIRST-AID SUPPLIES

In addition to your home pharmacy, you should also keep a supply of bandages and first-aid materials on hand for emergencies. These items should be stored in clean, airtight containers.

- Adhesive bandages, assorted sizes
- Adhesive tape
- Antiseptic wipes
- Butterfly bandages
- Cold packs (disposable)
- Cotton, both roll and balls
- Cotton-tipped swabs
- Elastic bandage
- First-aid manual
- Gauze bandages, various sizes, in pads and rolls
- Hand wipes (disposable)
- Insect repellent
- Latex gloves
- Safety pins
- Scissors (kept solely for this purpose)
- Sling (triangular bandage)
- Soap
- Sterile nonstick dressings
- Thermometer (if there are children under age five in the household, be sure to include a rectal or ear thermometer)
- Tissues
- Tongue depressors (for finger splints)
- Tweezers

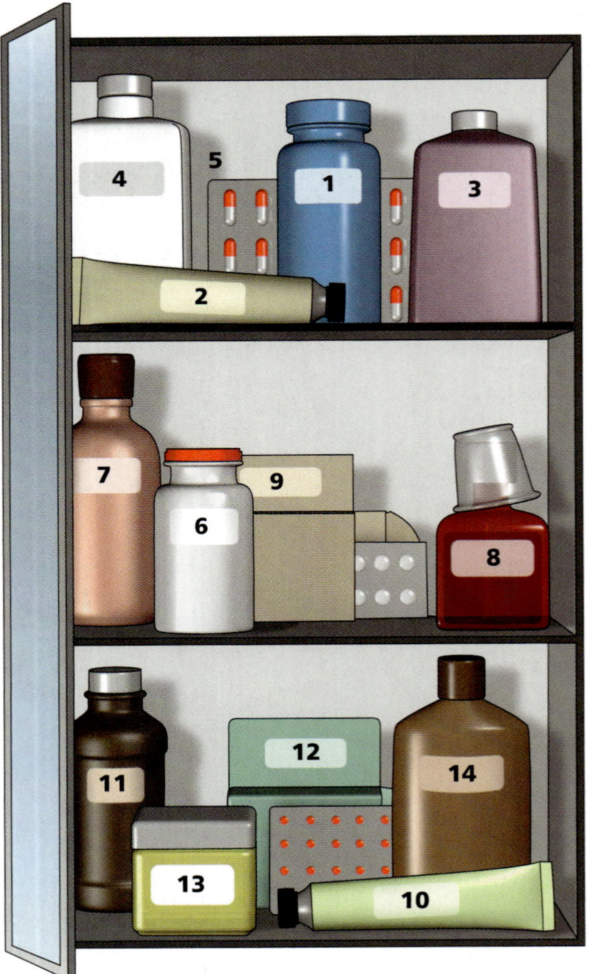

CONVENTIONAL

1 Antacid indigestion
2 Antibiotic cream cuts, scratches
3 Antidiarrheal medication
4 Antifungal medication athlete's foot or jock itch
5 Antihistamine capsules allergies
6 Aspirin or **acetaminophen** pain such as headaches or muscle cramps
7 Calamine lotion itching of skin rashes and insect bites
8 Cough/cold/flu medicine
9 Dimenhydrinate tablets motion sickness
10 Hydrocortisone cream skin rashes and insect bites
11 Hydrogen peroxide antiseptic for cuts and scratches
12 Laxative constipation
13 Petroleum jelly chafing
14 Sunscreen

ALTERNATIVE

Natural preparations can be used for many common ailments. These herbs, oils, and homeopathic medications can usually be found at health food stores or specialized pharmacies. Oils and homeopathic pharmaceuticals are commonly prepackaged, but herbs may be purchased loose and combined at home to create specific preparations. Don't forget that herbs, like OTC drugs, are powerful substances and should be used with care. Preparation and dosage directions for natural medicaments can be found in the ***Index of Conventional and Natural Medicines,*** beginning on page 882.

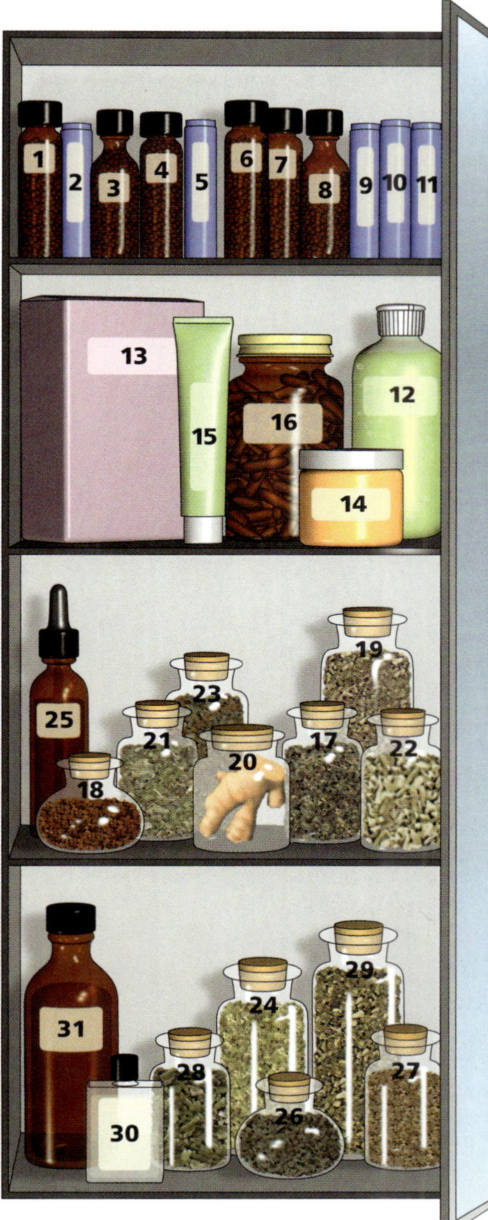

HOMEOPATHIC

1 ***Aconite*** colds, croup, fever, shock
2 ***Apis*** bites and stings, hives
3 ***Arnica*** bruises, dislocated joints, shock, surgery
4 ***Arsenicum album*** colds, food poisoning, influenza
5 ***Belladonna*** earache, high fever, headache, infection, heatstroke
6 ***Bryonia*** back pain, fever, headaches, influenza
7 ***Gelsemium*** fever and influenza
8 ***Hepar sulphuris*** abscesses, boils, croup, sore throat
9 ***Hypericum*** injury to nerves, insect bites
10 ***Pulsatilla*** childhood infections, colds, fever, sinus problems, teething
11 ***Rhus toxicodendron*** back pain, chickenpox, influenza, poison ivy, sprains, strains

HERBAL

12 Aloe *(Aloe barbadensis)* apply gel externally for bee stings, sunburn
13 Chamomile *(Matricaria recutita)* tea for indigestion
14 Chickweed *(Stellaria media)* cream for relief of skin irritation
15 Comfrey *(Symphytum officinale)* leaf ointment for cuts but not puncture wounds
16 Dandelion *(Taraxacum officinale)* root decoction as a secretory laxative
17 Elder *(Sambucus nigra)* flower, **peppermint** *(Mentha piperita),* and **yarrow** *(Achillea millefolium)* hot infusion of equal parts three times daily to relieve sinus pain
18 Flaxseed bulk laxative
19 Gentian *(Gentiana lutea)* hot tea to relieve indigestion
20 Ginger *(Zingiber officinale)* hot infusion of root as needed to relieve nausea, coughs
21 Horehound *(Marrubium vulgare)* hot infusion as needed for coughs
22 Marsh mallow *(Althaea officinalis)* hot infusion as needed for wet coughs
23 Meadowsweet *(Filipendula ulmaria),* **wild cranesbill** *(Geranium maculatum),* and **peppermint** *(Mentha piperita)* infusion of equal parts to relieve symptoms of diarrhea
24 Mullein *(Verbascum thapsus)* hot infusion three times daily for coughs; good for children
25 Osha *(Ligusticum porterii)* root for sore throat relief, viral infections
26 Peppermint *(Mentha piperita)* tea or infusion to relieve indigestion, diarrhea, migraines
27 Psyllium *(Plantago psyllium)* bulk laxative
28 Calendula *(Calendula officinalis)* gargle infusion for sore throat
29 Sourdock *(Rumex crispus)* decoction three times daily as secretory laxative
30 Tea tree oil (*Melaleuca* spp.) externally for athlete's foot
31 Witch hazel *(Hamamelis virginiana)* distilled, use externally for relief of itching ■

AILMENTS AND OPTIONS

Before using any drug or natural medicine mentioned in the following ailment entries, be sure to check the Index of Conventional and Natural Medicines, starting on page 882, for any warnings or cautions. You should keep in mind that herbal remedies are not as strictly regulated as drugs.

CONTENTS

A

Abdominal Pains 84
Aches and Pains 88
Acne 90
Adenoid Problems 94
AIDS 96
Alcohol Abuse 102
Allergies 106
Alzheimer's Disease 110
Anal Bleeding 114
Anal Fissure 116
Anemia 118
Aneurysm 122
Angina 124
Ankles, Painful 128
Ankles, Swollen 130
Anorexia Nervosa 132
Anxiety 134
Appendicitis 138
Arm Pain 140
Arthritis 142
Asthma 148
Atherosclerosis 152
Athlete's Foot 156
Athletic Injuries 158
Attention Deficit
Disorder 162

B

Backache 164
Back Problems 166
Bad Breath 170
Bedsores 172
Bedwetting 174
Bee and Wasp Stings 176
Black Eye 178
Bladder Cancer 180
Bladder Infections 182
Blisters 186
Blood Clots 188
Blood Poisoning 190
Body Odor 192
Boils 194
Bone Cancer 196
Bone Spurs 198
Bowel Movement
Abnormalities 200
Brain Cancer 202
Breast Cancer 204
Breast Problems 208
Breathing Problems 212
Bronchitis 214
Bulimia 218
Bunion 220
Burns 222
Bursitis 224

C

Cancer 226
Canker Sores 232
Carpal Tunnel Syndrome . . 234
Cataracts 238
Celiac Disease 240
Cervical Cancer 242
Cervical Problems 244
Chest Pain 248
Chickenpox 250
Chlamydia 252
Cholesterol Problems 254
Chronic Fatigue
Syndrome 258
Circulatory Problems 262
Cirrhosis 266
Cold Sores 270
Colic 272
Colitis 274
Colorectal Cancer 276
Common Cold 280
Congestion 284
Conjunctivitis 286
Constipation 288
Corns and Calluses 292
Cough 294
Crohn's Disease 298
Croup 302
Cuts, Scratches,
and Wounds 304

D

Dandruff 306
Depression 308
Dermatitis 312
Diabetes 316
Diaper Rash 322
Diarrhea 324
Disk Problems 326
Diverticulitis 330
Dizziness 334
Drug Abuse 336

E

Earache 340
Eczema 342
Emphysema 346
Endometriosis 350
Environmental Poisoning . . 354
Epilepsy 358
Eye Problems 360

F

Facial Pain 362
Fainting 364
Fatigue 366
Feet, Aches and Pains 370
Fever and Chills 372
Flu 374
Fluid Retention 378
Flushed Face 380
Food Poisoning 382

CONTENTS CONTINUED

G
Gallstones 384
Gas and Gas Pains 388
Gastritis. 390
Gastroenteritis 392
Genital Herpes. 394
Genital Warts. 396
German Measles. 398
Glaucoma 400
Goiter 404
Gonorrhea. 406
Gout 408
Graves' Disease 412
Groin Strain. 416
Gum Problems 418

H
Hair Loss 422
Hamstring Injury 426
Hand and Wrist Pain 428
Hangover. 430
Hay Fever 432
Headache 436
Hearing Problems. 442
Heart Arrhythmias 448
Heart Attack 452
Heartburn 456
Heart Disease 458
Hemorrhoids 464
Hepatitis 468
Hernia. 472
Hiatal Hernia 474
Hiccups. 476
High Blood Pressure 478
Hives. 482
Hypoglycemia 484

I
Immune Problems 486
Impetigo 490
Impotence 492
Incontinence 494
Indigestion 498
Infections 500
Infertility 502
Inflammation 504
Ingrown Nail 506
Insect and Spider Bites 508
Insomnia 510
Irritability 514
Irritable Bowel Syndrome. 516
Itching Skin 520

J
Jaundice 522
Jock Itch 524
Joint Pain. 526

K
Kidney Cancer 528
Kidney Disease. 530
Kidney Infections 534
Kidney Stones 536
Knee Pain 538

L
Lactose Intolerance 540
Laryngitis. 542
Leg Pain 544
Leukemia. 546
Lice. 550
Liver Cancer 552
Lou Gehrig's Disease 554
Lumps 556
Lung Cancer 558
Lupus 562
Lyme Disease. 564
Lymphoma. 566

M
Macular Degeneration . . . 570
Malaria 572
Manic-Depression. 574
Measles 578
Ménière's Disease. 580
Meningitis 584
Menopausal Problems. . . . 586
Menstrual Problems 588
Mononucleosis 594
Motion Sickness 598
Multiple Sclerosis 600
Mumps 604
Muscle Cramps 606
Muscle Pain 608
Muscle Weakness 610

N
Nail Problems 612
Nasal Polyps 614
Nausea 616
Neck Pain 620
Neuralgia. 622
Nicotine Withdrawal 624
Numbness and Tingling. . . 626

O
Obesity 628
Obsessive-Compulsive Disorder 632
Oral Cancer. 634
Osteoporosis 636

Otitis Media. 640
Ovarian Cancer 644
Ovary Problems 646

P

Pain, Chronic. 648
Pancreatic Cancer 654
Pancreatic Problems 656
Panic Attack 658
Parkinson's Disease 660
Pelvic Inflammatory Disease 664
Penile Pain. 666
Phlebitis 668
Phobias 670
Pinched Nerve 672
Plantar Warts. 674
Pleurisy 676
Pneumonia. 678
Poison Ivy 682
Postnasal Drip 684
Posttraumatic Stress Disorder 686
Pregnancy Problems 688
Premenstrual Syndrome . . 694
Prostate Cancer 698
Prostate Problems. 702
Psoriasis 706
Pupil Dilation. 710

R

Rabies 712
Rashes. 714
Raynaud's Syndrome. 718
Respiratory Problems 720
Restless Leg Syndrome . . . 722
Rheumatic Fever 724
Rocky Mountain Spotted Fever 726

S

Scabies 728
Scarlet Fever 730
Schizophrenia 732
Sciatica 734
Scoliosis 736
Seasonal Affective Disorder 738
Sexual Dysfunction. 740
Sexually Transmitted Diseases. 744
Shingles. 746
Shin Splints 748
Shoulder Pain. 750
Sickle Cell Anemia 752
Sinusitis. 754
Skin Cancer 758
Sneezing 762
Snoring 764
Sore Throat 766
Sprains and Strains 770
Staph Infections 772
Stomach Cancer 776
Stomach Ulcers 778
Strep Throat. 782
Stress 784
Stroke 788
Sty 792
Sunburn. 794
Swallowing Difficulty 796
Sweating, Excessive 798
Swimmer's Ear 800
Syphilis 802

T

Teething Problems 804
Temporomandibular Joint Syndrome. 806
Tendonitis 810
Tennis Elbow 812
Testicle Problems 816
Testicular Cancer 818
Tetanus 820
Throat Cancer 822
Thyroid Problems 824
Tics and Twitches 828
Tinnitus 830
Tonsillitis 834
Toothache 836
Toxic Shock Syndrome . . . 838
Trembling 840
Trichomoniasis 842
Tuberculosis. 844

U

Urinary Problems 846
Uterine Cancer 848
Uterine Problems 850

V

Vaginal Problems 854
Varicose Veins 858
Vision Problems 862
Vitiligo 866
Vomiting 868

W

Warts 872
Wheezing 874
Whooping Cough 876
Worms 878

Y

Yeast Infections 880

ABDOMINAL PAINS

A

Read down this column to find your symptoms. Then read across.

SYMPTOMS	AILMENT/PROBLEM
◆ pain in the abdomen; burning feeling in the chest; chest pain, particularly after eating or drinking alcohol; gas or belching; nausea; acid taste in mouth.	◆ Acid stomach; ***indigestion; heartburn***
◆ cramping or pain in the abdomen; nausea; diarrhea; vomiting; fever; malaise; weakness; intestinal gas.	◆ ***Gastroenteritis***
◆ abdominal discomfort, pain, or cramping; pain under the breastbone; possibly, nausea.	◆ ***Gastritis***
◆ pain in the abdomen or under the breastbone, often at night or one hour after eating; pain usually relieved by eating or vomiting; possibly, black-appearing stools.	◆ Peptic ulcer
◆ pain in the abdomen accompanied by diarrhea or constipation, especially after eating; relief with defecation.	◆ ***Irritable bowel syndrome***
◆ cramping or pain in the abdomen; fever; loss of appetite; weight loss; diarrhea; gas; rectal bleeding.	◆ Inflammatory bowel disease; ulcerative ***colitis; Crohn's disease***
◆ sharp, steady pain in groin; lump in abdomen when standing or straining.	◆ Inguinal ***hernia***
◆ intense, sudden pain in upper-right abdomen, especially after a fatty meal; pain may move to right shoulder blade, may last several hours, and is followed by general abdominal soreness. Nausea, vomiting.	◆ ***Gallstones***

A

WHAT TO DO	OTHER INFO
◆ See ***Indigestion*** and ***Heartburn.*** Adjust your eating and drinking habits or take an ***antacid*** to reduce the symptoms.	◆ Avoid smoking, caffeine, alcohol, fast eating, and ***nonsteroidal anti-inflammatory drugs (NSAIDs),*** such as ***aspirin.***
◆ See ***Gastroenteritis.*** Rest and drink plenty of fluids.	◆ Gastroenteritis is inflammation of the stomach or intestines often caused by a virus or ***food poisoning.*** Hospitalization may be required if symptoms are severe or the patient is very young, elderly, or debilitated.
◆ See ***Gastritis.*** Take only liquids for one day; then reintroduce solid food into the diet in small amounts.	◆ Gastritis, an inflammation of the stomach lining, may be caused by lifestyle factors, such as heavy drinking, smoking, or overeating; using ***aspirin, ibuprofen,*** or prescription drugs; or a bacterial infection.
◆ See ***Stomach Ulcers.*** Rest; eat small, frequent meals; take ***antacids;*** avoid smoking, alcohol, ***aspirin,*** and caffeine. Your doctor may prescribe a ***histamine H_2 blocker.*** If stools appear black, the ulcer may be bleeding. **Call your doctor now.**	◆ If the symptoms persist or recur, your doctor will want to test you for the presence of *Helicobacter pylori,* the bacterium considered the leading cause of peptic ulcers. Treatment is with ***antibiotics.***
◆ See ***Irritable Bowel Syndrome.*** The usual first step for reducing symptoms is to take a fiber-based ***laxative*** or an ***antidiarrheal drug.***	◆ Adding fiber and fluid to the diet is important, as is exercise. Because stress appears to be a trigger, counseling, acupuncture, biofeedback, yoga, or meditation may be helpful.
◆ **Call your doctor now.** A medical evaluation is necessary for diagnosis and treatment. See ***Colitis*** or ***Crohn's Disease.***	◆ Various alternative therapies, such as drinking green leafy vegetable juices for the chlorophyll content, may relieve symptoms. In severe cases, surgery is required to remove all or part of the damaged intestine.
◆ See ***Hernia.***	◆ In this disorder, the intestines or bladder bulges through the abdominal wall.
◆ **Call your doctor now**. A medical evaluation is necessary for diagnosis and treatment, which may involve surgical removal of the gallbladder or a nonsurgical procedure that dissolves the stones.	◆ Reducing fat and meat intake and increasing fiber may help prevent the formation of new stones.

Cross references are indicated by ***bold italics.***

SYMPTOMS	AILMENT/PROBLEM
◆ acute, constant abdominal pain radiating to the back and chest; fever; nausea; vomiting; abdominal distention; clammy skin.	◆ Pancreatitis
◆ severe cramping pain that is usually worse on the left side of the abdomen; chills; fever; nausea; history of constipation.	◆ ***Diverticulitis***
◆ sharp pain in the side that moves toward the groin and/or abdomen; frequent urge to urinate; blocked flow of urine; painful urination; cloudy or foul-smelling urine; blood in urine; fever and chills; nausea and vomiting; profuse sweating.	◆ ***Kidney stones***
◆ pain low in the abdomen that is accompanied by painful and frequent urination; constant urge to urinate; possibly, blood in urine.	◆ Urinary tract infection
◆ pain radiating from below the breastbone into the neck and arms; heartburn; vomiting; belching; bloating; difficulty swallowing.	◆ ***Hiatal hernia***
◆ crampy pain in the pelvic area during menstruation.	◆ Menstrual cramps
◆ extremely severe abdominal pain with or without other acute symptoms.	◆ **Emergency conditions:** intestinal obstruction, peritonitis, ***appendicitis,*** ileus, ***pelvic inflammatory disease, heart attack,*** abdominal aortic ***aneurysm,*** ischemic bowel, ruptured ectopic pregnancy, ruptured ovarian cyst, perforated peptic ulcer, anaphylactic shock, chemical burn, diabetic emergency, poisoning.

WHAT TO DO	OTHER INFO
◆ **Call your doctor now** to avoid possible life-threatening complications. See ***Pancreatic Problems.***	◆ The cause is usually heavy drinking or gallbladder disease. To control chronic pancreatitis, avoid alcohol and fatty foods.
◆ **Call your doctor now.** Severe cases may require hospitalization and surgery. Treatment for milder cases usually involves bed rest, stool softeners, a liquid diet, ***antibiotics,*** and possibly, ***antispasmodic drugs.***	◆ Although you should eat low-bulk foods during the inflammatory period, a high-fiber diet may be preventive.
◆ **Call your doctor now.** A medical evaluation is necessary for diagnosis and treatment. Commonly, the first step is to drink plenty of water and take a pain reliever until the stone passes.	◆ Infection, blockage, or large stones may make surgery necessary. A new treatment method uses high-energy shock waves to break up the stones without surgery.
◆ If you also have fever, chills, back pain, and possibly, nausea and vomiting, you may have a ***kidney infection.*** **Call your doctor now.** See ***Bladder Infections*** and ***Kidney Infections.***	◆ Pregnant women, people with ***diabetes,*** and nursing-home patients are at greatest risk for serious complications of a urinary tract infection.
◆ See ***Hiatal Hernia.***	◆ Lifestyle changes that may alleviate symptoms include avoiding smoking and alcohol, and eating smaller meals, none within two hours of going to bed.
◆ See ***Menstrual Problems.*** Take a pain reliever such as ***aspirin*** or ***ibuprofen*** or the homeopathic remedies *Magnesium phosphate* or *Colocythis.*	◆ Chiropractic, acupuncture, Chinese herbs, or ***magnesium*** supplements may help. For severe cramps, your doctor may recommend a prescription anti-inflammatory drug. See also ***Ovary Problems.***
◆ **Call your doctor, 911, or your emergency number now. Follow instructions to obtain immediate medical care.**	

Cross references are indicated by ***bold italics.***

ACHES AND PAINS

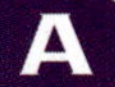

Read down this column to find your symptoms. Then read across.

SYMPTOMS	AILMENT/PROBLEM
◆ pain and swelling of muscles and joints in an active person; possibly, headache.	◆ Overexertion
◆ achiness with runny nose, sneezing, and cough; possibly, sore throat, headache.	◆ ***Common cold***
◆ achiness with runny nose, sneezing, cough, headache, sore throat, weakness, chills, and fever; possibly, vomiting and/or diarrhea.	◆ ***Flu***
◆ achiness with fever, chills, and chest pain; cough that produces sputum.	◆ ***Pneumonia***
◆ joints painful, red, warm, stiff, and/or swollen; pain worse in the morning.	◆ Inflammatory ***arthritis***
◆ chronic, widespread muscle pain and stiffness, especially in the morning; sleep disturbance and chronic fatigue.	◆ Fibromyalgia
◆ muscle or joint pain with headache, fatigue, malaise, and fever; months before, a circular or oval red rash up to eight inches or more in diameter with a white center may have appeared on the skin, from a tick bite that may or may not have been noticed.	◆ Lyme arthritis, a later stage of ***Lyme disease***

A

WHAT TO DO	OTHER INFO
◆ Consider anti-inflammatory drugs, heat rubs or massage, a cream containing ***aspirin,*** or the homeopathic remedy ***Arnica.*** Also, set limits to exercise; pay attention to your body's early signals of overexertion.	◆ The achiness may not be felt until two to three days after the overexertion. People who exercise to maintain a mood uplift need to be especially cautious.
◆ See ***Common Cold.*** Rest, drink plenty of fluids, and if needed, take a ***decongestant.***	◆ ***Vitamin C*** is widely believed to lessen the severity of colds. The herb **echinacea** (*Echinacea* spp.) may also help.
◆ See ***Flu.*** Rest, drink plenty of fluids, and if needed, take an anti-inflammatory drug to reduce fever and achiness. For prevention, eat a healthful diet to improve your immune defenses. The herb osha *(Ligusticum porteri)* can help your immune system fight the virus.	◆ Flu shots are often recommended for people over 65 and for those with chronic diseases. Children under 18 who may have a viral infection should not take ***aspirin*** or aspirin-containing products, which have been linked in young people with the neurological disorder Reye's syndrome. Children under 12 should not take aspirin when ill.
◆ **Call your doctor now.** A medical evaluation is needed for diagnosis and treatment, which may involve ***antibiotics.*** If you are elderly, have another serious illness, or fail to improve with treatment, you may need to be hospitalized. See ***Pneumonia.***	◆ Muscle aches are more likely to be caused by an "atypical" pneumonia, which comes on more slowly and is caused by a virus or other microorganism rather than by a bacterium.
◆ See ***Arthritis.*** Take an anti-inflammatory drug for pain relief.	◆ The condition may be helped by acupuncture, homeopathy, herbal medicine, yoga, and nutritional changes. Aching in joints also may be caused by a noninflammatory arthritis, such as osteoarthritis, in which redness, warmth, and swelling do not occur.
◆ Treatment frequently involves ***analgesics,*** a low-dose ***antidepressant,*** and/or injection of a local ***anesthetic,*** possibly with a ***corticosteroid,*** into aching points of the body.	◆ Fibromyalgia was previously believed to be psychogenic but is now recognized as a syndrome with uniform signs and symptoms. Aerobic exercise, stress management, massages, and acupuncture may be helpful.
◆ **Call your doctor now.** The usual treatment is ***antibiotics.*** See ***Lyme Disease.***	◆ Lyme arthritis, which is characterized by back and joint pain, can occur months, or even years, after the bite of a deer tick, the cause of ***Lyme disease.***

ACNE

A

SYMPTOMS

- persistent, recurrent red spots or swellings on the skin, generally known as pimples; they may become inflamed or pus-filled, and typically appear on the face, chest, shoulders, neck, or upper portion of the back, particularly in adolescents.
- Dark spots with open pores at the center are **blackheads.**
- Spots that bulge under the skin and have no opening are **whiteheads.**
- Red swellings or lumps, sometimes visibly filled with pus, are **pustules,** which develop from blackheads or whiteheads.
- Inflamed, fluid-filled lumps under the skin, which may become as large as an inch across, are **nodules,** or **cysts.**
- Abnormally flushed cheeks and nose are a sign of **rosacea,** an acnelike disorder that affects adults—mostly women—over 30 years of age.

CALL YOUR DOCTOR IF:

- your acne doesn't respond in two to three months to over-the-counter remedies; you may need medical treatment.
- you have severe acne, which may produce cysts under the skin and persistent pimples that may become infected. A dermatologist may recommend prescription drugs to control the condition and prevent permanent scars.
- your skin becomes abnormally flushed around your cheeks and nose. You may have **rosacea,** which can be controlled with appropriate antibiotic medication.

Nearly everyone suffers from outbreaks of pimples at some point in life, making acne one of the most common skin disorders. It starts when tiny hair follicles become plugged with oily secretions from the skin's sebaceous glands. **Blackheads** appear as small, usually flat spots with centers darkened by exposure to air; **whiteheads** are similar lesions without the color. Both types of pimples can develop into swollen, tender inflammations. **Cysts,** or **nodules,** associated with severe cases of acne, are firm swellings below the skin's surface that become inflamed and sometimes infected.

Although acne remains largely a curse of adolescence, about 20 percent of all cases occur in adults. Acne commonly arises during puberty and tends to be worse in people with oily skin. It occurs in both sexes, although teenage boys tend to have the most severe cases. Women are more likely than men to have mild to moderate forms into their thirties and beyond, and are somewhat more susceptible to **rosacea.**

Myths about harmful diets and uncontrolled sex drives causing acne have been replaced by the simple truth that heredity and hormones are behind most forms. Swearing off chocolate or scrubbing your face 10 times a day won't change your predisposition to this unsightly, sometimes painful, and often embarrassing skin disorder.

CAUSES

The cause of acne is not fully understood. While poor hygiene, poor diet, and stress can aggravate acne, they clearly do not cause it. Common **acne vulgaris** in teenagers starts with an increase in hormone production. During puberty, both boys and girls produce high levels of androgens—male sex hormones that include testosterone. Androgens can in turn step up production of sebum, the substance that lubricates the skin and helps it retain moisture, and keratin, a primary constituent of hair. Tiny hair follicles, especially those on the face, neck, chest, and back, can become plugged with sebum and keratin. As the follicles fill up and bacteria multiply, **blackheads** or **whiteheads** form on the skin's surface, a condition called

noninflammatory acne. If the follicle wall ruptures under pressure and sebum leaks into nearby tissue, the result is a **pustule,** or **inflammatory acne.** If pustules become infected, matters are further complicated: The infection can penetrate deep into the skin and create **cysts,** which can rupture and leave temporary or permanent scars.

Various factors appear to make certain people prone to developing acne, such as family history of the condition, ***stress,*** and using contraceptives or ***corticosteroids.*** Taking oral contraceptives may trigger acne in some women but actually suppress it in others, depending on the type of pill taken. Anabolic steroids taken by some bodybuilders can also lead to severe outbreaks.

Acne has many subtypes. Some forms—**acne neonatorum** and **acne infantum**—occasionally affect newborns and infants, usually boys. A pimply rash appears on the face but usually clears within weeks with no lasting effect. Adults, usually women, who escape their teen years almost pimple free may develop persistent **adult-onset acne** as they get older. In some cases the outbreaks are allergic reactions to cosmetics or foods, while others are linked to menstruation. Both **premenstrual** and **postmenopausal acne** tend to be relatively milder than cosmetic-related flareups.

Despite the normal increase in androgen levels during puberty, some researchers believe that flareups of acne have less to do with an individual's androgen levels than with how that person's skin responds to an increase in the production of sebum. The bacteria *Propionibacterium acnes* and *Staphylococcus epidermidis* occur naturally in healthy hair follicles. If too many of them accumulate in plugged follicles, they may secrete enzymes that break down sebum, promoting localized inflammation. Some people are simply more sensitive than others to this reaction, so that sebum levels that might cause a pimple or two in one person may result in widespread outbreaks, or **acute cystic acne,** in another person.

Rosacea

W. C. Fields, with his bulbous nose and flushed complexion, may be the best-known victim of rosacea, but fair-skinned women over 30 are actually the most prone to the condition. Rosacea starts with a persistent, abnormal blush on the cheeks and nose, which is made more obvious by consuming spicy foods, hot drinks, or alcohol. The inflammation tends to spread, and a few rosacea patients, usually men, develop a severe form in which the nose becomes red, thickened, and tender.

To control mild cases, your doctor will probably prescribe an oral ***antibiotic*** *such as metronidazole or a topical* ***corticosteroid.*** *Lotions or gels containing sulfur as an active ingredient may be prescribed or purchased over the counter. Because many rosacea patients also suffer from migraine* ***headaches,*** *some researchers suspect that an intolerance to certain types of food may be a factor. Some cases respond particularly well to large doses of* ***B vitamins,*** *especially* ***vitamin*** B_2 *(riboflavin). In severe cases of rosacea, surgery or laser treatments may reverse the inflammation and swelling.*

TREATMENT

The occasional pimple or two need no treatment. Over-the-counter cover-up creams and cosmetics, if used at all, should be water based and hypoallergenic. Even if outbreaks of acne cannot be eliminated, conventional and alternative treatment can provide relief. Conventional medicine favors drug therapies that inhibit sebum and keratin production, limit bacterial growth, or encourage shedding of skin cells to unclog pores. Because many therapies can have potent side effects, any patient with a skin problem should proceed with caution when trying a new treatment.

People with severe, persistent cases need the care of a dermatologist.

CONVENTIONAL MEDICINE

To treat mild acne, your doctor may recommend a topical over-the-counter medication containing benzoyl peroxide or prescribe the antiacne drugs azelaic acid or ***tretinoin*** (retinoic acid), a ***vitamin A*** derivative. Before applying the medication, wash the affected area with a mild oil- and scent-free soap. When pus-filled pimples are ready to break, applying a hot towel for a few minutes may encourage the process. Infected pimples should be opened only by a nurse or doctor using surgical instruments and following antiseptic practices. Squeezing pimples yourself may lead to further infection and the possibility of permanent scars.

For moderate to severe cases, a mainstay of treatment is ***tetracycline,*** an ***antibiotic*** that is usually taken orally, sometimes in combination with topically applied tretinoin. Other useful antibiotics are oral ***erythromycin*** and clindamycin.

For chronically inflamed **cysts,** a doctor may prescribe the drug isotretinoin, but because of its potentially severe side effects, the treatment must be monitored carefully, especially in women of childbearing age. A less common treatment option is to inject ***triamcinolone,*** a type of ***corticosteroid,*** directly into the cysts. This treatment may leave some patients' skin temporarily darkened around the lesion. Because many acne sufferers are relieved by summer sun, a dermatologist may also recommend controlled exposure to ultraviolet light to keep outbreaks in check.

Patients taking ***antiacne drugs*** should be alert to possible side effects and interactions. The drugs tretinoin and benzoyl peroxide can leave skin reddened, dry, and sensitive to sunlight. Benzoyl peroxide may inhibit the healing effects of tretinoin, so never apply them at the same time. Taking antibiotics for more than a few weeks may leave women susceptible to ***yeast infections.***

Some adults carry scars or pitted skin from cysts or deep pimples that were scratched or severely infected. Two relatively aggressive surgical procedures can improve the skin's appearance: dermabrasion, in which a dermatologist essentially sandpapers frozen skin, and chemical peeling. Both procedures remove the scarred surface and expose unblemished skin layers. Before considering such treatment, however, discuss the procedures, necessary precautions, and likely results with at least two dermatologists.

ACUPRESSURE

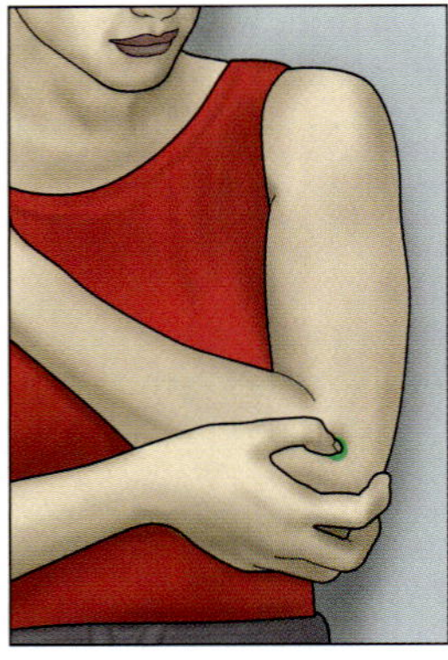

1 Acupressure may help to ease inflammation, hormonal imbalances, and emotional distress associated with acne. Apply firm pressure with your thumb to Large Intestine 11, at the outer end of the elbow crease. Hold for one minute, and repeat on the other arm.

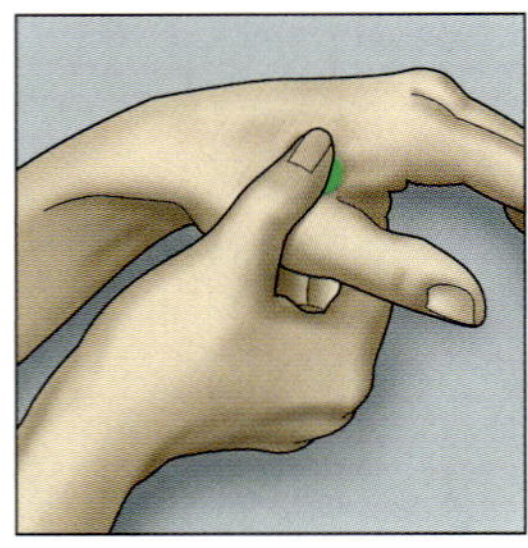

2 To help ease skin irritation, press your right thumb into Large Intestine 4, between the thumb and index finger of your left hand, pushing against the bone above your index finger. Hold for one minute, then repeat on the other hand. Do not use this point if you are pregnant.

ALTERNATIVE CHOICES

Some alternative therapies for acne attempt to reduce inflammation and fight infection. Other approaches use herbal or dietary measures to control factors that may promote acne, such as stress. For mild or moderate acne, these approaches may make sense, but **acne vulgaris** and **rosacea** respond much more slowly than most other ailments to any therapy. Be patient: Many acne treatments take up to a year to produce results.

CHINESE HERBS

Chinese herbal medicine for acne seeks to rid the

skin of dampness and heat, which are believed to be causative factors. Preparations commonly used for the purpose include ***cnidium seed*** *(Cnidium monnieri)* and ***honeysuckle flower*** *(Lonicera japonica).* Consult a practitioner of Chinese medicine for specific formulations and dosages.

HERBAL THERAPIES

Many herbs are used to help heal the skin and soothe inflammation and itching. Among those a trained herbalist may recommend are ***calendula*** *(Calendula officinalis),* ***tea tree oil*** (*Melaleuca* spp.), ***goldenseal*** *(Hydrastis canadensis),* and Oregon grape *(Mahonia aquifolium)* root. Drinking tea made with a combination of ***nettles*** *(Urtica dioica)* and cleavers (*Galium* spp.) tincture may be effective. CAUTION: Never use any herbal preparation on newborns without consulting your doctor.

If stress may be contributing to your acne, try relaxing with a cup of tea made from ***lavender*** *(Lavandula officinalis)* or ***chamomile*** *(Matricaria recutita).* A facial sauna two to three times a week with either of these herbs may also help.

HOMEOPATHY

For minor outbreaks of acne, ***Hepar sulphuris*** or ***Silica,*** in 6x potency tablets taken three times a day for up to a week, may help speed healing.

NUTRITION AND DIET

Most doctors now believe that acne is not a food-related problem and rarely ask patients to change their diets as a means of reducing outbreaks. Some alternative therapists, however, make a change in diet the basis of treatment. While experts in both camps concede that chocolate, fats, and other suspect foods don't cause acne, debate continues over whether they can aggravate the condition.

Among vitamin and mineral supplements, nutritionists generally suggest ***zinc,*** which plays a part in how the body processes hormones. A 30- to 50-mg zinc supplement daily may contribute to reducing inflammation and healing damaged skin. ***Chromium*** supplements are said to boost the body's ability to break down glucose. Large amounts of ***vitamin A*** may reduce sebum and keratin production, but since large doses can cause headaches, fatigue, muscle and joint pain, and other side effects, taking megasupplements is not advised unless monitored carefully by your doctor or other healthcare practitioner. ***Vitamin E,*** an antioxidant, may also be included in a natural antiacne regimen at doses of 200 to 400 IU a day. ***Vitamin B_6,*** which aids in the metabolism of hormones, can be particularly effective for women suffering from premenstrual acne; 50 mg a day is a typical dosage.

AT-HOME REMEDIES

- Washing your face gently with unscented, oil-free soap—or a medicated or ***calendula*** soap—helps keep your skin clean, but scrubbing already inflamed skin only makes acne worse.
- Resist the urge to pop pimples. Let them break when they're ready, then wash gently.
- For mild to moderate acne, try over-the-counter treatments that contain benzoyl peroxide.
- Expose your acne to sunlight in moderation, but be careful to avoid overexposure.
- Men with moderate to severe acne should use a new razor blade every time they shave to lower the risk of infection. Instead of alcohol-based aftershaves, try herbal alternatives that include essential oils of ***lavender, chamomile,*** or ***tea tree.***

PREVENTION

Because of acne's association with fluctuating hormone levels and possible genetic influences, many doctors believe there is no way to prevent it. Although the accepted wisdom is that neither good hygiene nor diet can prevent outbreaks, the tips in **Nutrition and Diet** *(left)* may be helpful.

Good general hygiene and sensible skin care are especially important during adolescence. The basics include a daily bath or shower, and washing face and hands with unscented or mildly antibacterial soap. Teenage girls are better off not using cosmetics regularly. And despite claims to the contrary, few if any commercial skin medications have any beneficial effect on acne. ■

ADENOID PROBLEMS

A

SYMPTOMS

Adenoid-related problems produce symptoms in the ears, nose, and throat. Any of the following may be indicative of adenoid problems:

- sleep apnea, in which the sleeping child may interrupt a normal breathing pattern with either short periods of not breathing many times through the night, or longer periods of not breathing—up to 20 seconds—once or twice a night.
- mouth breathing (nasal obstruction).
- snoring (obstructed airway).
- nasal voice.
- secretions from the nose during the day combined with a cough at night, caused by sinus drainage.
- recurring ear infections in association with the above symptoms.

CALL YOUR DOCTOR IF:

- your child has intervals of not breathing many times each night; this may indicate sleep apnea syndrome, which can cause behavioral problems in children because of sleep disturbances, or in severe cases can put pressure on the cardiac system.
- you notice your child having difficulty breathing or breathing open-mouthed because of extreme nasal congestion. While these symptoms are not life-threatening, they indicate that your child's adenoids may be obstructing the nasal airway.
- your child has recurrent ear infections that respond poorly to antibiotic treatment; untreated ear infections can cause hearing loss.

The adenoids, masses of lymph tissue located in the top of the throat behind and above the tonsils *(below, right),* play a special role during childhood: By making antibodies, they help the young child's body fight respiratory tract infections. From the time your child is three until around the age of seven, the adenoids grow so that they can give extra protection to the lungs and chest. After about the age of eight, they usually begin to shrink, and by the time your child is an adolescent, they have virtually disappeared.

When the adenoids become infected or irritated they swell, often blocking the airway to the nose and the Eustachian tube to the ear, causing mild to severe discomfort and difficulty breathing or hearing. Left untreated, enlarged adenoids can lead to chronic ***sinusitis,*** and in severe cases, sleep apnea—in which the child stops breathing for seconds at a time during the night.

You may have grown up in an era when removing the adenoids and tonsils was standard practice and may have undergone one of these procedures yourself. But because doctors now understand more clearly the role of the adenoids in fighting infection, the chances of your child's undergoing an adenoidectomy are much more remote—usually limited to the most severe cases.

CAUSES

The primary reason for chronic adenoid problems is structural: The adenoids grow so large that they block the nasal passages. But infection or irritation, perhaps caused by ***allergies,*** can also cause problems by making the adenoids swell.

TREATMENT

Adenoid problems are difficult to diagnose because the symptoms can point to any number of conditions and it is hard to tell even by examination if enlarged adenoids are the cause. Always take your child to a pediatrician or to an alternative practitioner for an examination if he or she has had recurrent ear infections, a blocked nose, or any of the other symptoms listed at left.

CONVENTIONAL MEDICINE

Your child's pediatrician will take a history of your child's ear, nose, and throat problems and probably refer you to either an ear, nose, and throat (ENT) specialist or an allergist for an evaluation of your child's symptoms. The ENT specialist will want to examine your child and may also order x-rays to help determine the size and shape of the adenoids. The allergist will probably test for any sensitivity to airborne allergens (for example, cigarette smoke, dust, pollen, or pet dander).

If allergies are to blame, treatment for the allergies—such as a course of allergy shots to desensitize your child—or elimination of allergens is the appropriate action. If allergies are not the cause, the ENT specialist may recommend surgery to remove the adenoids. Surgery is called for as a first-line defense only in cases of severe sleep apnea, in which the enlarged adenoids can cause chronic pressure on the cardiac system and could possibly lead to heart failure.

THE ADENOIDS

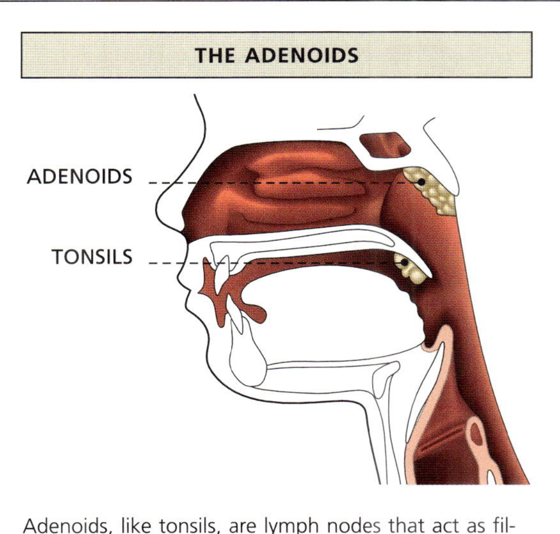

Adenoids, like tonsils, are lymph nodes that act as filters against germs. They are small, pink lumps on the back wall of the throat *(shown here in yellow)*, just above the roof of the mouth. When the adenoids become infected, they may swell and hamper breathing.

ALTERNATIVE CHOICES

Alternative therapists usually seek an allergy-related cause first. Always take your child to a professional for evaluation and treatment; at-home care can only alleviate the symptoms.

HERBAL THERAPIES

Echinacea (*Echinacea* spp.) is believed to help fight infection. Cleavers *(Galium aparine)* may help reduce swelling of lymphatic tissue. Consult a medical herbalist for appropriate dosages.

HOMEOPATHY

Because chronic adenoid problems give rise to other problems, you should consult a homeopathic physician for remedies appropriate to the condition as well as to the individual. The practitioner will monitor your child's progress and change remedies if they do not bring relief in a short time.

OSTEOPATHY

Manipulative treatment of the neck, which is thought to drain the lymphatic system, would be the prescribed course of treatment.

AT-HOME REMEDIES

These remedies may alleviate some symptoms, but they will not clear up the underlying condition. Always seek help from a professional when your child has a chronic problem.

- For children with allergies, reducing or eliminating dietary and environmental irritants can make your child more comfortable. For example, an electrostatic air filter may lower the amount of dust or mold in the house.
- A humidifier may help a child who is congested by preventing the mucus from getting too thick. Use a humidifier with a humidistat to ensure the proper amount of moisture in the air, and clean the humidifier thoroughly before and after use.
- An over-the-counter decongestant may temporarily alleviate stuffiness.
- Chicken soup may also open blocked nasal passages. ■

AIDS

A

SYMPTOMS

The following are among the most common symptoms of AIDS:

- long-term fatigue you can't explain.
- swollen lymph nodes.
- a fever that lasts more than 10 days.
- night sweats.
- unexplained weight loss.
- purplish or discolored lesions on skin or mucous membrane that do not go away.
- persistent, unexplained cough or sore throat.
- shortness of breath.
- persistent colds.
- persistent severe diarrhea.
- ***yeast infections.***
- easy bruising or bleeding that cannot be explained.

CALL YOUR DOCTOR IF:

- you have more than one of the above symptoms; you may not have AIDS, but you do have a condition that requires treatment.

For a person who has contracted the virus that causes AIDS, the long-term outlook is undeniably grim. But a diagnosis of AIDS should not be taken as an immediate death sentence. With proper care the AIDS sufferer can stave off the worst symptoms and live a productive life for many years.

Acquired immune deficiency syndrome (AIDS) is not a single disease in itself. Rather, a severely impaired immune system leaves the AIDS sufferer highly susceptible to a whole host of infections and diseases. AIDS is thought to be caused by the human immunodeficiency virus (HIV), which is spread through infected semen, vaginal fluids, and blood. HIV damages the body's ability to produce adequate numbers of white blood cells called T cells, leaving it unable to fight off invading bacteria or viruses.

Symptoms differ widely from country to country and even from risk group to risk group. In the United States and Europe, AIDS sufferers often develop Kaposi's sarcoma (a rare form of skin cancer), pneumocystis ***pneumonia,*** and ***tuberculosis.*** In Africa, AIDS usually causes sufferers to waste away from fever, diarrhea, and a persistent cough. Developing any of the 28 or so diseases and sets of symptoms associated with AIDS in the United States and testing positive for antibodies to HIV will almost certainly lead to a diagnosis of AIDS.

In most cases AIDS starts with flulike symptoms that resemble ***mononucleosis.*** These may persist for two weeks to a few months after the virus enters the body.

After this first stage, symptoms may disappear for several years. How the AIDS patient takes care of himself or herself during this time is extremely important, because HIV is multiplying in the body, slowly at first and then rapidly. As the virus systematically destroys the cells that fight off infection, the immune system begins to fail and the patient becomes vulnerable to various illnesses and tumors. This stage is sometimes called **ARC,** or **AIDS-related complex.** Full-blown AIDS—the stage in which serious infections begin to develop—may not appear until 5 to 10 years after the onset of HIV infection. Death usually occurs 2 to 3 years later.

Doctors in the United States first recognized AIDS in 1981, but undiagnosed cases had begun showing up in 1979. Before that, AIDS probably existed in Africa and some Caribbean countries.

Although AIDS can strike anyone, it first occurred among homosexual and bisexual men who had many sexual partners. Because many of these men also used recreational drugs such as "poppers" (amyl nitrate), doctors thought at first that the drugs caused the disease. Eventually, research showed that AIDS is transmitted via bodily fluids. That hypothesis was borne out when intravenous-drug users, heterosexuals, and people who got blood transfusions began to contract AIDS.

This most serious health crisis of our time has now reached epidemic levels. Worldwide, more than 22 million people are infected with HIV. In the United States as many as 1 to 2 million people are thought to have the virus, and the number of AIDS cases doubles every year; in many U.S. cities, AIDS is the leading cause of death for adults 25 to 44 years old.

At greatest risk for AIDS are people who engage in sex without using condoms and infants born to AIDS-infected mothers. Also at great risk are male and female intravenous-drug users who share needles, and people who received blood transfusions or clotting factors between 1977 and 1985, prior to the establishment of standard AIDS screening of donated blood. Currently, as AIDS spreads through the heterosexual population, women make up the fastest-growing group of infected people. In the United States, more than 80,000 women between the ages of 15 and 44 have contracted the virus.

The good news is that AIDS is preventable. Provided you are not at risk because of intravenous drug use, you can avoid HIV infection through a monogamous relationship, or reduce the risk of infection by practicing safe sex—which means, first and foremost, using condoms.

According to recent indicators, more people are taking such precautions. The National Health and Social Life Survey, which was published in 1995, found that nearly 3 in 10 American adults say they have dramatically altered their sexual behavior to lower the risk of contracting AIDS. This landmark study of adult sexual behavior investigated the sex habits and attitudes of about 150 million people. Results of the survey include:

- 29 percent reported using condoms more often.
- 26 percent said they were likely to be monogamous.
- 25 percent said they were choosing their partners more carefully or getting to know them better before being intimate.
- 11 percent said they had decided to abstain from sex because they were afraid of contracting AIDS.

CAUSES

Scientists suspect that at least two viruses cause AIDS: **HIV-1** and **HIV-2.** Worldwide, the viruses infect equal numbers of people, but HIV-1 is much more prevalent in North America.

Researchers don't yet know precisely how HIV works, and some are asking whether in fact the virus causes AIDS or merely shows up in conjunction with it. For some reason the immune system can't detect HIV. The virus enters the body through small abrasions or cuts in mucous membranes in the mouth, vagina, or rectum and destroys T cells, so the immune system fails. Patients then develop infections that eventually kill them.

AIDS is not a highly contagious disease. The only way you can get it is to have unprotected vaginal, oral, or anal sex with an infected partner or to share tainted blood, which may occur through IV-drug use or transfusions.

You can't get AIDS from kissing. A protein in human saliva keeps the AIDS virus from infecting white blood cells. The protein attaches itself to white blood cells and protects them from infection. The discovery may lead to new strategies for developing AIDS medicines, such as injecting this protein directly into the bloodstream to keep the virus from attacking blood cells.

You also needn't worry about catching AIDS if you live with someone who has it. HIV cannot be transmitted by toilet seats or objects handled by people who have AIDS. Nor will you get the disease if you share food with someone who is infected, because HIV dies very quickly once it is outside the body.

DIAGNOSTIC AND TEST PROCEDURES

Within a few weeks of infection, your body should be producing antibodies to the virus, which your doctor can detect in blood tests. However, your body may take as long as 35 months to produce a detectable level of antibodies, so if you think you've been infected, particularly if you're in a high-risk group, you should be tested for the disease every 6 months.

The first test you'll be given is the ELISA, or enzyme-linked immunosorbent assay. This test is generally reliable, but a positive result (meaning antibodies have been detected) should always be confirmed; the doctor may follow up with the Western blot, a blood test that almost never gives a false-positive reading.

Before deciding to have an AIDS test, make sure you get advice from a counselor. A positive test result for AIDS may cause you profound psychological distress. The counselor can help you deal with the anxiety, grief, and fear you'll probably experience at first.

If you test positive, make sure your doctor gives you a complete workup to detect other ***sexually transmitted diseases,*** such as ***gonorrhea, genital herpes,*** or ***syphilis***.

It is extremely important that you notify your sexual partners of your diagnosis. They too must be tested and treated.

TREATMENT

Almost everyone who develops full-blown AIDS eventually succumbs to the disease, but ***antibiotic*** and ***antiviral drugs*** can prolong life for several years. In any event, you should never try to treat yourself for this life-threatening illness: Always seek the advice of a qualified practitioner. And beware of claims made for "miracle" cures. They simply don't exist.

Currently there are several hundred human studies to test drugs for the treatment of AIDS and related conditions. These include antiviral drugs, drugs that modify the immune system, anti-infective drugs, and ***anticancer drugs.***

One study by the National Institute of Allergy and Infectious Diseases (NIAID) has found that a naturally produced protein may rebuild AIDS-damaged immune systems. Called interleukin 2, the protein dramatically increased T cell counts in 6 out of 10 people who took it. However, it did not work for people with advanced AIDS, and it also has severe side effects, including rash, nausea, diarrhea, and depression. Further studies on the protein are being conducted.

Another experimental treatment, now in use in France, is **passive immunotherapy.** The therapy does not increase the life span of AIDS sufferers, but it may keep them from getting as sick as they otherwise might. Patients with advanced AIDS are injected with plasma from healthier HIV-infected donors. Researchers hope the injections will bolster the advanced patients' immune systems and help them fight off diseases associated with AIDS. Initial results have been promising.

Although a number of vaccines to prevent AIDS are under investigation, scientists have had difficulty finding one that works. The theory is that injecting someone with a weakened form of the virus would spur that person's immune system to mount a huge attack against HIV and build up a resistance. Doctors are understandably reluctant to inject anyone with HIV, however, fearing that even a weakened virus might cause AIDS.

In related work, a team of researchers from NIAID has developed a vaccine with a "suicide gene" that allows itself to be killed off once its job is done. The weakened HIV carries an extra gene taken from the herpesvirus. Cells that become infected with HIV then can be selectively destroyed with ganciclovir, a herpes medicine. So far the

CAUTION!

Seek help immediately if you think you have AIDS, and don't fail to notify your sexual partners if you test positive for HIV. They too will require testing and possibly treatment. In some states the health department will require that sexual partners be notified. Ask your doctor for advice.

vaccine has been examined only in the test tube. Animal and human trials are being planned.

CONVENTIONAL MEDICINE

The current treatment of choice for AIDS patients is the combination use of several powerful ***antiviral drugs.*** This multi-drug cocktail, while not a cure for AIDS, has lengthened the survival time for AIDS patients. It may help stave off the worst symptoms of the disease for many years.

Zidovudine, known better by the trade name AZT, and other similar drugs, including didanosine and zalcitabine, are reverse transcriptase inhibitors. These drugs are frequently paired with protease inhibitors, including indinavir and ritonavir. Both types of drugs slow down the HIV virus by interfering with the way it goes about propagating itself. These drugs have multiple side effects; close consultation with your physician is critical. There are also many drugs available to fight secondary infections.

Unfortunately, the HIV virus adapts and can become resistant to drugs; this ability has made it difficult not only to control HIV infection but also to create a vaccine.

ALTERNATIVE CHOICES

Combined with medical treatment, many alternative therapies can lengthen and improve the quality of the AIDS patient's life. Studies demonstrate that many AIDS patients respond well to immune-bolstering nutritional programs. Patients also show marked improvement after using stress-reduction techniques. Again, beware of any treatment that claims to be a "miracle" cure.

ACUPRESSURE

Your immune system may function more efficiently if you reduce stress in your life. One acupressure massage that seems to relieve fatigue and tension is known as the Shoulder Well. Press Gall Bladder 21, the highest point of the shoulder muscle midway between the outer tip of the shoulder and the spine. Do this at home several times a day. *(See the **Appendix** for more information on the location of Gall Bladder 21.)*

ACUPUNCTURE

When combined with Chinese herbs, acupuncture seems to boost immune functions and reduce symptoms of AIDS, including night sweats, fatigue, and digestive problems. Acupuncture may also help your body fight off secondary infections and eliminate lesions. Seek the advice of a qualified practitioner.

AROMATHERAPY

You may also reduce stress by inhaling the aromas of various oils, such as ***lavender*** *(Lavandula officinalis).* To heal lesions brought on by AIDS, aromatherapists recommend that you apply the antiviral oils of ***tea tree*** (*Melaleuca* spp.) and ***garlic*** *(Allium sativum).*

BODY WORK

Several studies indicate that moderate exercise substantially increases immune system activity. In one study, aerobic training boosted immune cells in AIDS patients. Too much aerobic exercise can suppress immunity, however, so ask your doctor to recommend an exercise program for you.

CHINESE HERBS

Many Chinese herbs have been effective in treating symptoms of AIDS such as night sweats, fatigue, neuropathy, and diarrhea. Chinese herbs also may relieve the side effects of some conventional drugs.

Tonic herbs to strengthen the system include ***astragalus*** *(Astragalus membranaceus),* ***ganoderma*** *(Ganoderma lucidum),* and ***Asian ginseng*** *(Panax ginseng).* ***Licorice*** *(Glycyrrhiza glabra)* is thought to enhance the immune system and inhibit the herpesvirus.

Trichosanthin, a protein in Chinese cucumber root, has been extracted to form tricosantin, or Compound Q, which seems to purify the blood and ward off a variety of infections.

An extract of ***shiitake*** *(Lentinus edodes)* mushrooms has also been successfully used to treat AIDS symptoms.

To treat your specific symptoms, consult a Chinese herbalist.

HERBAL THERAPIES

Herbalists recommend several plant-based medicines for boosting the immune system and strengthening the body. ***Echinacea*** *(Echinacea* spp.) increases immune system functions by stimulating T cells, but it may not be as effective in treating AIDS because it stimulates HIV as well. Ask your doctor before trying it.

Garlic *(Allium sativum)* has been used by AIDS patients for its antibacterial and antiviral properties, and some studies have indicated that ***hyssop*** *(Hyssopus officinalis)* may be useful in treating Kaposi's sarcoma.

A promising herbal remedy is ***St.-John's-wort*** *(Hypericum perforatum),* which contains hypericin, a chemical that has been shown to inhibit the growth of the virus that causes one form of ***leukemia.*** Researchers hope that hypericin can be used to reduce AIDS symptoms such as fever and swelling of lymph nodes. Hypericin isn't effective if you just drink St.-John's-wort tea; to get the powerful extract, consult your doctor or a qualified herbal practitioner.

HOMEOPATHY

Besides seeking conventional treatments, you may also wish to consult a homeopathic physician, who will take your complete medical, emotional, and genealogical history and then help you make healthful changes in your lifestyle. In addition, many homeopathic remedies have been helpful in treating the symptoms of AIDS. ***Hypericum,*** a homeopathic drug derived from St.-John's-wort, is one remedy a homeopath might prescribe.

HEAT THERAPY

Several studies have shown that HIV is sensitive to heat and becomes increasingly inactive as body temperature is raised above normal for extended periods of time. Raising body temperature stimulates the immune system in general by increasing production of antibodies and interferon, a protein substance produced by virus-invaded cells that prevents reproduction of the virus.

Ask your doctor about the experimental therapy hyperthermia—heat therapy—in which AIDS patients combine hot baths with hot drinks and then wrap themselves in blankets. This should be done only under strict supervision. Heat may elevate your body temperature to dangerous extremes and impair organ functioning.

MIND/BODY MEDICINE

Many doctors and psychologists believe that there is a vital relationship between your emotions and the way your immune system functions. Negative emotions such as guilt, hopelessness, suppressed anger, and fear are common among AIDS patients and may suppress the body's ability to fight off infection. Practitioners of mind/body medicine believe you'll be healthier and live longer if you do everything you can to maintain a positive attitude. Low moments are unavoidable, and you should not chide yourself for having them; but do what you can to avoid dwelling on negative thoughts.

To help, try relaxation techniques such as **biofeedback, yoga,** exercise, and **meditation. Massage** therapy can improve your circulation and give you a greater sense of ease and well-being. The massage should not be too fast or deep, however, or your adrenal system, which releases powerful chemicals in response to real or imagined stress, could become overstimulated and challenge your immune system. Seek the advice of a licensed massage therapist.

Also, try joining a support group to help you deal with the anxiety you may be feeling. Sharing your fears—and also your victories—with others can be of enormous benefit. *(See the **Appendix**.)*

NUTRITION AND DIET

What you put into your body once you're diagnosed with HIV may have a profound effect on how long you live. With proper nutrition you can strengthen your body's ability to fight the virus.

Avoid foods that impair the immune system. For example, there are some indications that 100 grams of simple sugar—such as honey or refined sugar—can significantly decrease the ability of white blood cells to kill bacteria and viruses for up to five hours. The typical American consumes about 150 grams of sugar a day.

Stay away from alcohol and caffeine, which deplete the body of vitamins and minerals. And smoking heavily tends to increase suppressor

A

T cells and decrease helper T cells (two types of immune cells that, in proper proportion, help keep the immune system in balance).

Eat more foods rich in beta carotene *(see **Vitamin A**)*, such as green, leafy vegetables and orange and yellow vegetables. If you develop candidiasis or other infections common with AIDS, you may want to increase consumption of ***garlic,*** which contains the powerful antibiotic allicin.

Take ***vitamin C*** supplements to boost your immune system. Some naturopaths and dietitians recommend taking vitamin C until it causes diarrhea, then cutting back to the highest tolerable level; one approach is to take dosages every two hours. CAUTION: You should check with your doctor before trying this approach. ***Zinc*** also stimulates the immune system and is antiviral.

DIET POINTERS

For AIDS patients, nutritionists recommend in particular that you:

- *reduce your consumption of polyunsaturated and saturated fats and oils.*
- *use monounsaturated oils (such as olive oil) and increase your intake of omega-3 fatty acid, which is found in fish but is also effective when obtained through supplements.*
- *eat small portions throughout the day to optimize absorption of nutrients from foods.*
- *eat a balanced meal—65 percent complex carbohydrates, 15 percent protein, and 20 percent fat.*
- *make sure fruits and vegetables are clean and free of parasites and bacteria by steaming them lightly before eating.*
- *eat a wide variety of foods to help avoid becoming sensitized to specific food families.*

AT-HOME REMEDIES

If you have HIV, you may stave off symptoms of AIDS if you:

- eat nutritious, balanced meals to bolster your immune system.
- take vitamin supplements.
- try acupressure exercises to relax.
- take up meditation or yoga to relieve stress.
- try to maintain a positive attitude.
- don't smoke or drink.
- follow a moderate exercise program approved by your doctor.

If you have AIDS:

- eat nutritious, balanced meals to bolster your immune system.
- take vitamin supplements.
- try acupressure exercises to relax.
- take up meditation or yoga to relieve stress.
- try to maintain a positive attitude.
- follow a moderate exercise program approved by your doctor.
- try inhaling or bathing with oils of tea tree and garlic.

PREVENTION

- Condoms reduce the risk of HIV infection. Use a latex condom with the spermicide nonoxynol-9, which has been shown to kill HIV outside the body. Use a condom for all kinds of sex, including oral, anal, and vaginal. This is not necessary if you and your partner are monogamous and not infected.
- Don't use oil-based lubricants, which can eat through condoms.
- Learn the sexual history of a potential partner and ask about HIV test results.
- Don't have sex with prostitutes.
- Don't share a needle if you use intravenous drugs; bleach needles to clean them.
- When in Third World countries, carry a supply of disposable sterile needles in case you require medical injections.
- Get tested every six months if you're in a high-risk group; your sexual partner should be tested as well. ■

ALCOHOL ABUSE

A

SYMPTOMS

The following symptoms are associated with abuse of alcohol:

- temporary blackouts or memory loss.
- recurrent arguments or fights with family members or friends.
- continuing use of alcohol to relax, to cheer up, to sleep, to deal with problems, or to feel "normal."
- headache, anxiety, insomnia, nausea, or other unpleasant symptoms when you stop drinking.
- flushed skin and broken capillaries on the face; a husky voice; trembling hands; chronic diarrhea; and drinking alone, in the mornings, or in secret. These symptoms are specifically associated with **chronic alcoholism.**

CALL YOUR DOCTOR IF:

- you have any of the symptoms above and are unable to stop drinking on your own. You need medical intervention to treat alcoholism. You may also be susceptible to ailments such as ***cirrhosis,*** alcoholic ***hepatitis,*** and ***heart disease.***
- you drink regularly and experience chronic or periodic ***depression.*** You may be at risk of suicide.
- you have tried to stop drinking and experienced withdrawal symptoms such as headache, anxiety, insomnia, nausea, or delirium tremens. You need medical attention by a physician or a treatment center.

People have been brewing and fermenting alcoholic drinks since the dawn of time. Consumed in moderate amounts, alcoholic beverages are relaxing and in some cases may even have beneficial effects on health *(see* ***Atherosclerosis****).* Consumed in excess, alcohol is poisonous to human systems and is considered a drug. Nearly 100,000 Americans die each year as a result of alcohol abuse, and alcohol is a factor in more than half of the country's homicides, suicides, and traffic accidents. Alcohol abuse also plays a role in many social and domestic problems, from job absenteeism and crimes against property to spousal and child abuse.

The immediate physical effects of drinking alcohol range from mild mood changes to complete loss of coordination, vision, balance, and speech—any of which can be signals of the temporary systemic poisoning known as **acute alcohol intoxication,** or drunkenness. These effects usually wear off in a matter of hours after a person stops drinking *(see* ***Hangover****).* Many law-enforcement agencies regard a .08 percentage of alcohol in the bloodstream as evidence of intoxication. Larger amounts of blood alcohol can impair brain function and eventually cause unconsciousness; an extreme overdose can be fatal.

Chronic alcoholism is a progressive, potentially fatal disease, characterized by an incessant craving for, increased tolerance of, physical dependence upon, and loss of control over drinking alcohol. The physical dependence on alcohol may or may not be obvious to other people. While some chronic alcoholics get very drunk, others exercise enough control to give the appearance of coping with everyday affairs in a near-normal way. However, alcoholism can lead to a number of physical ailments, including ***hypoglycemia, kidney disease,*** brain and heart damage, enlarged blood vessels in the skin, chronic ***gastritis,*** and pancreatitis *(see* ***Pancreatic Problems****).*

Alcoholism can also lead to ***impotence*** in men, damage to the fetus in pregnant women, and an elevated risk of ***cancer*** of the larynx, esophagus, stomach, pancreas, and upper gastrointestinal tract. Because alcoholics seldom have adequate diets, they are likely to have nutritional deficiencies. Heavy drinkers typically have impaired liver function, and at least 1 in 5 develops ***cirrhosis.***

The alcoholic's continual craving for alcohol makes abstinence—an important goal of treatment—extremely difficult. The condition is also complicated by denial: Alcoholics employ a range of psychological maneuvers to blame their problems on something other than drink, creating significant barriers to recovery. Historically, alcoholic behavior was blamed on a character flaw or weakness of will; many authorities now consider chronic alcoholism a disease that can afflict anyone.

Virtually every culture has warned against overuse of alcohol, and some have prohibited it outright, rarely with lasting success. While laws and educational programs in the United States are designed to prevent alcohol abuse, commercial and social pressure continues to put people at risk. Alcoholism is particularly insidious among young people and the elderly, in part because the symptoms are not easily recognized until the affected person becomes truly alcohol dependent.

ALCOHOL AND YOUR BODY

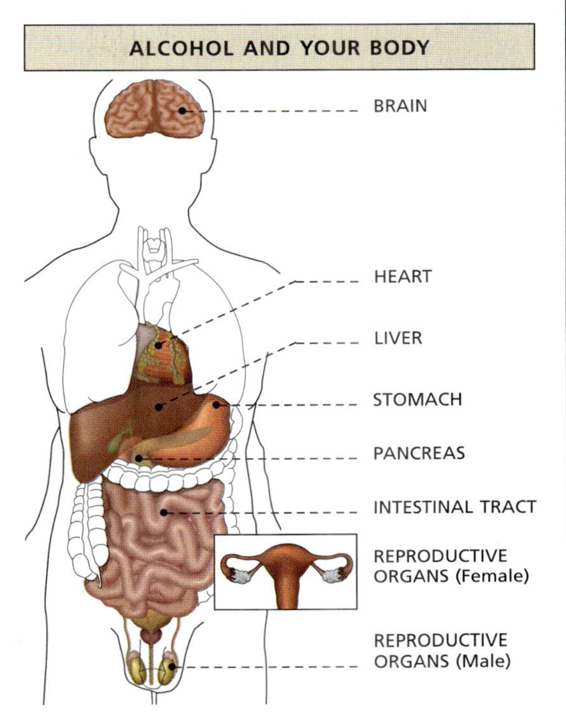

Excessive alcohol intake can have drastic consequences. Heavy drinking can cause acute gastritis and can lead to pancreatitis. Long-term abuse can lead to cardiomyopathy (weakening of the heart), cirrhosis of the liver, and cancer of the upper intestinal tract. Chronic alcoholism is the second leading cause of brain damage and can also impair sexual function.

CAUSES

The cause of alcoholism seems to be a blend of genetic, physical, psychological, environmental, and social factors that vary among individuals. Genetic factors are considered crucial: A given person's risk of becoming an alcoholic is four to five times greater if a parent is alcoholic. Some children of alcohol abusers, however, overcome the hereditary pattern by becoming teetotalers.

TREATMENT

The goal of treatment is abstinence. Among alcoholics with otherwise good health, social support, and motivation, the likelihood of recovery is good: 50 to 60 percent remain abstinent at the end of a year's treatment, and a majority of those stay dry permanently. Those with poor social support, poor motivation, or psychiatric disorders tend to relapse within a few years of treatment. For these people, success is measured by longer periods of abstinence, reduced use of alcohol, better health, and improved social functioning.

CONVENTIONAL MEDICINE

Treatment can begin only when the alcoholic accepts that the problem exists and agrees to stop drinking. He or she must understand that alcoholism is curable and must be motivated to change. Treatment has two stages: withdrawal—sometimes called detoxification—and recovery. Because withdrawal does not stop the craving for alcohol, recovery is often difficult to maintain. For a person in an early stage of alcoholism, withdrawal may bring anxiety and poor sleep. Withdrawal from long-term dependence may bring the uncontrollable shaking, spasms, panic, and hallucinations of delirium tremens (DT). If not treated professionally, people with DT have a mortality rate of more than 10 percent, so withdrawal from late-stage alcoholism should be attempted only at an inpatient center.

Treatment may involve one or more medications. Disulfiram interferes with alcohol metabolism so that drinking a small amount will cause nausea, vomiting, confusion, and breathing difficulty. Naltrexone reduces the craving for alcohol but is recommended only in comprehensive programs that teach patients new coping skills. ***Benzodiazepines*** are antianxiety drugs used to treat withdrawal symptoms such as ***anxiety*** and poor sleep, and to prevent seizures and delirium. They must be used with care, since they may be addictive. ***Tricyclic antidepressants*** may be used to control any resulting anxiety or ***depression,*** but because those symptoms may disappear with abstinence, the medications are usually not started until after detoxification.

Because an alcoholic remains susceptible to becoming dependent again, the key to recovery is total abstinence. Recovery typically takes a broad-based approach, which may include education programs, group therapy, family involvement, and participation in self-help groups.

ALTERNATIVE CHOICES

Once an alcoholic accepts his or her condition and stops using alcohol, a number of alternative therapies can help the recovery process.

ACUPUNCTURE

Treatment by a licensed acupuncturist is often found effective in relieving the symptoms of alcoholic withdrawal and is reported to prevent seizures, to help prevent relapse, and to increase the likelihood of a patient's completing a recovery program.

BODY WORK

Massage, as part of a physical therapy program, can ease recovery by relaxing the body and soothing the anxiety associated with withdrawal.

HERBAL THERAPIES

Ask an herbal therapist about taking ***milk thistle*** *(Silybum marianum)* to protect against, or even reverse, liver damage from alcohol abuse. The product is sold under the name silymarin in 70- to 210-mg capsules at health food stores.

For withdrawal symptoms, try infusing 2 tsp ***skullcap*** *(Scutellaria lateriflora),* ***lavender*** *(Lavandula officinalis),* or motherwort *(Leonurus cardiaca)* in water, and take three times a day. Some treatment centers use a sleep-mix tea made from equal parts ***chamomile*** *(Matricaria recutita),* ***hops*** *(Humulus lupulus),* ***skullcap, peppermint*** *(Mentha piperita),* ***yarrow*** *(Achillea millefolium),* and either ***catnip*** *(Nepeta cataria)* or ***valerian*** *(Valeriana officinalis).*

HYDROTHERAPY

Warm salted baths may be effective in drawing drugs and toxins from the body. Dissolve ½ cup sea salt or epsom salts in a tub of warm water and soak in it 10 to 20 minutes every day.

MIND/BODY MEDICINE

Because alcoholics commonly use alcohol to deal with ***stress,*** various relaxation techniques, such as **massage** and **meditation,** may prove helpful. **Hypnotherapy** may help unlock psychological difficulties that underlie behavioral problems.

NUTRITION AND DIET

Poor nutrition goes with heavy drinking: Because an ounce of alcohol has more than 200 calories but no nutritional value, ingesting large amounts of alcohol tells the body that it doesn't need more food. Alcoholics are often deficient in ***vitamins A, B complex,*** and ***C;*** carnitine; ***magnesium, selenium,*** and ***zinc;*** as well as essential fatty acids and antioxidants. Restoring such nutrients—particularly thiamine ***(vitamin B_1)***—can aid withdrawal and recovery. One study found that recovery programs were twice as effective when nutritional therapy was incorporated.

Some therapists think stabilizing blood sugar levels can help make treatment more successful. Recommendations include eliminating dietary sugar, even fruit juice, which has more sugar than whole fruit; reducing the amounts of simple carbohydrates in the diet, such as those found in white flour and instant potatoes; and increasing vegetable protein and the complex carbohydrates found in whole grains, beans, and vegetables.

AT-HOME REMEDIES

Abstinence is the most crucial—and probably the most difficult—step to recovery. To learn to live without alcohol, you must:

- Avoid people and places that make drinking the norm, and find new, nondrinking friends.
- Join a self-help group *(see* ***Support for Recovery,*** *right).*
- Enlist the help of family and friends.
- Replace your negative dependence on alcohol with positive dependencies such as a new hobby or volunteer work with church or civic groups.
- Start exercising. Exercise releases chemicals in the brain that provide a "natural high." Even a walk after dinner can be tranquilizing.

PREVENTION

Returning to drink is a major problem for recovering alcoholics; preventing this may be difficult, but it can be supported by continued therapy, positive motivation, and strong social support. Other ways to prevent relapse include changing routines, accepting a new sense of values, and avoiding activities or people associated with the drinking habit. For example, 90 percent of alcoholics smoke; alcoholics who stop smoking as well as drinking are more likely to achieve long-term abstinence—to say nothing of the other health benefits.

A SELF-SCREENING TEST

No single symptom defines alcoholism, but honest answers to the following questions will help you decide if you are at risk.

- Has a friend or relative ever suggested that you drink too much?
- Is it hard to stop drinking after you have had one or two drinks?
- Have you ever been unable to remember what you did during a drinking episode?
- Do you ever feel bad about how much you drink?
- Do you get into arguments or physical fights when you've been drinking?
- Have you ever been arrested or hospitalized because of drinking?
- Have you ever thought about getting help to control or stop your drinking?

If you answered yes to one or more questions, you may have a serious alcohol problem. For your own good, it's time to discuss the situation openly with a physician or mental health professional. ■

SUPPORT FOR RECOVERY

Despite the contention that alcoholism is a disease, not a weakness of will, the social stigma still lingers—especially for women. Many alcoholics deny that drinking is a problem, and family and friends who cover up an alcoholic's behavior only help stifle any incentive to reach out for help. It is vital for family and friends to learn about alcoholism and to motivate a loved one to seek help.

Group support helps many alcoholics lead normal, productive lives. About one million Americans are members of Alcoholics Anonymous (AA). For many, the positive peer pressure of AA is crucial to staying sober. Yet opinions differ about certain aspects of AA and similar groups. Some therapists are concerned because AA does not diagnose psychiatric disorders or provide medical evaluation. For those who object to the spiritual emphasis of AA's 12-step program, alternative groups such as Rational Recovery and Women for Sobriety are available.

ALLERGIES

A

SYMPTOMS

- Sneezing, wheezing, nasal congestion, and coughing indicate ***asthma,*** or drug or respiratory allergies.
- Itchy eyes, mouth, and throat are symptoms of respiratory allergies.
- Stomachache, frequent indigestion, and heartburn are signs of food sensitivities.
- Irritated, itchy, reddening, or swelling skin is associated with drug, food, and insect sting allergies.
- Stiffness, pain, and swelling of joints may indicate food or drug allergies.

CALL YOUR DOCTOR IF:

- you have violent stomach cramps, vomiting, bloating, or diarrhea; this could point to a serious food or other allergic reaction or ***food poisoning.***
- breathing becomes extremely difficult or painful; you may be experiencing an ***asthma*** episode, another serious allergic reaction, or a ***heart attack.*** **Get emergency medical treatment.**
- you suddenly develop skin welts, accompanied by intense flushing and itching; your heart may also be beating rapidly. These symptoms may indicate the onset of anaphylactic shock, an extremely serious allergic reaction. **Get emergency medical treatment.** *(See also **Shock** in **Emergencies/First Aid.**)*

The term *allergy* applies to an abnormal reaction by your immune system to a substance that is usually not harmful. Allergies come in a variety of forms and vary in severity from mildly bothersome to life-threatening. An estimated one-fifth of the Western Hemisphere's population suffers from allergies. No one knows why some people develop them, but heredity seems to play a role in their development. Although allergies may flare up and subside throughout your life, people rarely acquire new ones past the age of 40.

The immune system protects the body from foreign substances—known as antigens—by producing antibodies and other chemicals to fight against them. Usually, the immune system ignores benign substances, such as food, and fights only dangerous ones, such as bacteria. A person develops an allergic reaction when the immune system cannot tell the good from the bad and releases a type of chemical called histamine to attack the harmless substance as if it were a threat. Histamine produces many of the symptoms associated with allergies. Substances that may trigger allergic reactions, known as allergens, range from pollen to pet dander to ***penicillin.***

Most allergic reactions are not serious, but some, such as anaphylaxis, can be fatal *(box, page 108).* Only a few allergies can be cured outright, but a variety of conventional and alternative treatments are available to relieve the symptoms. If your allergy is severe, it is vital that you visit a conventional medical doctor and get immediate treatment on an emergency basis.

CAUSES

Allergies come in many distinct forms and are typically grouped in general categories according to the types of substances that cause them or the parts of the body they affect.

Skin allergies: Contact ***dermatitis*** is caused by direct, topical exposure to a specific allergen; atopic dermatitis has no known cause, but it is usually hereditary. ***Hives,*** or urticaria, is an eruption of itchy, swollen, reddened welts that can last for minutes or days. Angioedema is characterized by a deeper swelling around the eyes and lips, and sometimes of the hands and feet as well. Both hives and angioedema stem from the body's adverse reaction to certain foods, pollen, animal dander, drugs, insect stings, cold, heat, light, or even emotional ***stress.***

Respiratory allergies: Some 20 million Americans suffer from ***hay fever*** (allergic rhinitis). Typical symptoms include itchy eyes, nose, and roof of mouth or throat, along with nasal congestion, coughing, and sneezing. If you (or members of your family) have other allergies such as ***dermatitis*** or ***asthma,*** you are more likely to have hay fever. The terms *allergic rhinitis* and *hay fever* apply specifically to reactions caused by the pollens of ragweed, grasses, and other plants whose pollen is spread by the wind. But the same symptoms can be produced by other airborne substances that you inhale. These can include molds, dust, and animal dander. If, for example, you are allergic to pet dander (dead skin scales and saliva), being near a cat will make you sneeze, wheeze, and sniffle. Mold allergies are caused by airborne spores. Outdoor molds—alternaria and hormodendrum—thrive in warm seasons or climates, while indoor molds—penicillium, aspergillus, mucor, and rhizopus—grow year round in damp locations (basements and bathrooms, for example). Dust causes allergies because it harbors offenders such as pollen, mold spores, and microscopic dust mites; it may also contain irritating fibers from fabrics, upholstery, and carpets.

Asthma: Asthma has various causes, but the chief ones are allergies to pollen, mold spores, animal dander, and dust mites. *(See* ***Asthma.****)*

Food allergies: An estimated 70 percent of people with food allergies are under 30; most are children under the age of 6. It is sometimes difficult to pinpoint the specific allergens responsible for a food allergy, because reactions are often delayed or may be caused by food additives or even by eating habits. However, approximately 90 percent of food allergies are caused by proteins in cow's milk, egg whites, peanuts, wheat, or soybeans. Other common food allergens include berries, shellfish, corn, beans, yellow food dye No. 5, and gum arabic (an additive in processed foods). The classic symptoms of food allergies include stomach cramps, diarrhea, and nausea. In more severe cases, there may be vomiting, swelling of the face and tongue, and respiratory congestion, as well as dizziness, sweating, and faintness.

Drug allergies: The most common drug allergy is to drugs in the ***penicillin*** family. Other common drug allergens include sulfas, barbiturates, ***anticonvulsants, insulin,*** local ***anesthetics,*** and dyes injected into blood vessels for x-rays. Almost one million Americans have reactions to ***aspirin;*** these responses are not true allergies but rather "sensitivities."

Insect sting allergies: Some studies speculate that people who have other allergies (food, drug, or respiratory) may be more susceptible to insect sting allergies, which affect about 15 percent of the population. Venom in stings of bees, wasps, hornets, yellow jackets, and fire ants is a common allergen. *(See* ***Insect and Spider Bites.****)*

FOOD ALLERGY OR INTOLERANCE?

Two out of five Americans believe that they are allergic to certain foods, but fewer than 1 percent have genuine allergies; most are unable to tolerate certain foods, often because they lack an enzyme needed for proper digestion.

Some people are sensitive to lactose, a sugar found in milk; in general, however, they can tolerate dairy products such as yogurt, sour cream, and hard cheese. Some children cannot tolerate gluten, found in wheat products. Monosodium glutamate (MSG), a flavor enhancer, can cause flushing, headaches, and numbness. Sulfites, used as a preservative in many foods and wines, can cause sensitivity as well as trigger allergic reactions.

DIAGNOSTIC AND TEST PROCEDURES

After taking a full family and personal medical history, your physician will ask you a series of questions about your exposure and reactions to various allergens to eliminate and identify your allergies' causes. You may be asked to keep track of potential allergens and your allergic reactions for a week to aid in diagnosis. After this, your physician will choose a testing method.

The most common test for respiratory, penicillin, insect sting, skin, and food allergies is a skin test. A small amount of the allergen is placed on, or injected just underneath, the skin, and the physician watches for allergic symptoms. The symptoms—swelling, itchiness, and redness—generally appear within 20 minutes. Skin tests are not completely reliable, because if too much of the allergen is administered, even a nonallergic person may react. Also, extremely sensitive people may go into anaphylactic shock from skin tests. An alternative for respiratory allergies is RAST (for radioallergosorbent test), which measures the levels in the bloodstream of the antibodies associated with allergies.

TREATMENT

The best treatment for allergies is to avoid the substances that trigger them, but this can be difficult. The basic medications for allergies are ***antihistamines,*** which counteract the histamine chemicals that cause the allergic reactions. Prescription ***corticosteroid*** drugs may also be used for severe symptoms. In emergency situations—when anaphylactic shock occurs—injections of ***epinephrine*** are used to dilate bronchial passages. Immunotherapy, or allergy shots, may cure some allergies by introducing small amounts of the offending allergens in order to help the body learn to deal with them.

CONVENTIONAL MEDICINE

If you are extremely allergic and likely to go into anaphylactic shock, you should always carry with you a prescribed emergency kit.

WHAT TRIGGERS ANAPHYLACTIC SHOCK?

The most severe and dangerous of allergic reactions is anaphylaxis, or anaphylactic shock, which begins within minutes after exposure and advances quickly. Although any allergen can trigger anaphylactic shock, the most common are insect stings, certain foods (such as shellfish and nuts), and injections of certain drugs. Standard emergency treatment includes an injection of ***epinephrine*** *to open up the airways and blood vessels; in severe cases, cardiopulmonary resuscitation (CPR) may be necessary. See* ***Shock*** *in* ***Emergencies/First Aid.***

Skin allergies: Atopic and contact ***dermatitis*** can be treated with a variety of ***corticosteroids,*** usually ***hydrocortisone. Hives*** and angioedema often need no medication, but severe cases may require prescription ***antihistamines, terbutaline,*** or oral ***corticosteroids.***

Respiratory allergies: ***Hay fever*** is generally treated with over-the-counter ***antihistamines,*** but your doctor may prescribe other, more powerful drugs—such as ***cromolyn***—if your symptoms are severe. The same treatments apply to other respiratory allergies, but if your symptoms are severe, your physician may prescribe ***corticosteroids,*** in nasal spray or oral form. Immunotherapy has a high success rate, curing 70 percent to 80 percent of people treated for respiratory allergies.

Food allergies: The best treatment for food allergies is avoidance. If your reactions to certain foods are irritating but not life-endangering, your doctor may prescribe ***antihistamines*** or topical creams to help relieve symptoms.

Drug allergies: The only effective treatment for drug allergies is avoidance. Skin rashes associated with drug allergies are generally treated with ***antihistamines;*** occasionally they are treated with ***corticosteroids.***

Insect sting allergies: Avoidance is the best treatment, but immunotherapy may cure insect sting allergies.

ALTERNATIVE CHOICES

Since allergies can be difficult to diagnose, and are in many cases incurable, alternative remedies for them have become quite popular. But if you have a severe allergy, or in case of an emergency, you must see a conventional physician.

ACUPRESSURE

To relieve symptoms associated with respiratory allergies, try Large Intestine 4, the highest spot of the area between the index finger and thumb; rub firmly for one minute, then repeat on the other hand. Do not use this point if you are pregnant. To fortify the immune system, firmly massage Triple Warmer 5, two finger widths from your wrist on the top of your forearm, specifically the area between the two arm bones.

AROMATHERAPY

To relieve nasal congestion, try mixing 1 drop of ***lavender*** *(Lavandula officinalis)* oil and 1 tsp of a carrier oil such as sweet almond or sunflower oil; massage into the skin around your sinuses once a day. ***Eucalyptus*** *(Eucalyptus globulus),* cedarwood, and ***peppermint*** *(Mentha piperita)* oils also act as decongestants; dab on a handkerchief and inhale.

CHINESE HERBS

In acute allergic reactions ***ephedra*** *(Ephedra sinica)* acts like the decongestant ***epinephrine,*** which opens up the lungs' airways when breathing is difficult. But be careful: Large quantities of this herb are equivalent to large quantities of the drug epinephrine and can have serious side effects. Do not use ephedra if you have ***high blood pressure*** or ***heart disease.*** Prepare an infusion by combining 5 grams ephedra, 4 grams ***cinnamon*** *(Cinnamomum cassia)* sticks, 1.5 grams ***licorice*** *(Glycyrrhiza uralensis),* and 5 grams ***apricot seed*** *(Prunus armeniaca);* let steep in cold water, then bring to a boil. Strain and drink hot.

HERBAL THERAPIES

Infusions of ***chamomile*** *(Matricaria recutita),* elder *(Sambucus nigra)* flower, ***eyebright*** *(Euphrasia officinalis),* ***garlic*** *(Allium sativum),* goldenrod *(Solidago virgaurea),* ***nettle*** *(Urtica dioica),* and ***yarrow*** *(Achillea millefolium)* have antimucus and anti-inflammatory effects.

HOMEOPATHY

For a runny nose, itchy throat, and sneezing, a homeopathic practitioner might suggest ***Arsenicum album*** (6c); for chronic thick mucus, ***Pulsatilla*** (6c); for a runny nose, sore upper lip, and itchy eyes, ***Allium cepa*** (6c).

NUTRITION AND DIET

Vitamin C and bioflavonoids (found in the white pith of citrus fruits) act as natural antihistamines, so you should increase your citrus intake or take 500 mg of vitamin C three times daily. ***Vitamins A*** and ***B complex*** are thought to be powerful stimulants to the immune system. Products made with bee pollen and royal jelly may alleviate or eliminate the symptoms of respiratory allergies but should not be taken if you are allergic to bee stings. For food allergies, read labels carefully and make sure you know what foods to avoid.

PREVENTION

Respiratory allergies: Install a high-efficiency air cleaner to help remove pollen and mold spores, and use an air conditioner in your home and car during warm seasons to keep pollen out; regularly clean damp areas with bleach to kill molds. Consider hiring a special cleaning service to rid furniture and upholstery of dust mites. Isolate (or, if you can stand it, get rid of) your pets and keep them outside as much as possible. Regular baths for your pet will help reduce dander.

Food allergies: Instead of dairy products, try tofu-based foods. Always check food labels for additives that are known allergens, such as yellow food dye No. 5 and gum arabic. ■

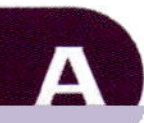

SYMPTOMS

- mood changes: depression, paranoia, agitation, anxiety, selfishness, childish behavior.
- disorientation, confusion, inattention, loss of memory for recent events, inability to retain new information.
- increased tendency to misplace things.
- dizziness or impaired equilibrium.

CALL YOUR DOCTOR IF:

- a family member or friend exhibits signs of Alzheimer's disease over a period of time. Because the person may not be aware of having these problems, it is often up to others to help.

ALZHEIMER'S DISEASE

Alzheimer's disease, a progressive degeneration of brain tissue that primarily strikes people over age 65, is marked by a devastating mental decline. Intellectual functions such as memory, comprehension, and speech deteriorate. Attention tends to stray, simple calculations become impossible, and ordinary daily activities grow increasingly difficult, with bewilderment and frustration worsening at night. Dramatic mood swings occur—outbursts of anger, bouts of fearfulness, periods of deep apathy. The sufferer, increasingly disoriented, may wander off and become lost. Physical problems, such as an odd gait or a loss of coordination, gradually develop. Eventually, the patient may become totally noncommunicative, physically helpless, and incontinent. The disease is invariably fatal.

Alzheimer's can run its course from insidious onset to death in just a few years, or it may play out over a period of as long as 20 years; the average duration, however, is about 7 years. Among American adults, it is the fourth leading cause of death (after heart disease, cancer, and stroke). By the age of 80, about 1 person out of 3 has the disease. Women are twice as susceptible as men, and Caucasians are about four times as susceptible as African Americans.

CAUSES

Although many people develop Alzheimer's as they grow older, the disease is not a natural result of aging; it is an abnormal condition whose causes continue to be investigated.

The gradual loss of brain function that characterizes Alzheimer's disease seems to be due to two main forms of neural damage: Nerve fibers grow tangled, and protein deposits known as plaques build up in the affected tissue. Researchers are not yet sure why or how this tissue degeneration occurs, but some of the most promising recent research points to a normally occurring blood protein called ApoE (for apolipoprotein E), which is required for the transport of fatty substances in the body. As with all proteins, its form is genetically determined, and several different types have been identified—

some of them apparently associated with a higher risk of Alzheimer's. It may be that certain forms of ApoE lead to destruction of nerve cells in the brain. Another possibility is that the protein, perhaps working in combination with other substances, is involved in the formation of the plaques. Whether or not ApoE is part of the causative mechanism of Alzheimer's, genes almost certainly can play a role in the disease: A person with a parent who had Alzheimer's is known to be at higher risk.

Other causes have been proposed. One theory suggests that ingesting tiny particles of aluminum—from cookware, for example—may lead to Alzheimer's. Another proposes a link between plaque formation and free radicals—unstable, free-ranging molecules that can produce destructive chemical reactions. Both theories are controversial and unproved. Indeed, many researchers now consider the link between Alzheimer's and aluminum extremely questionable.

Another controversy centers on zinc. In a 1991 study, Alzheimer's patients were given zinc supplements because other studies suggested that zinc could help improve mental alertness in the elderly (zinc has also been shown to play a role in the functioning of memory). However, after only two days the patients' mental abilities deteriorated so rapidly that the study was considered too harmful for the subjects and was immediately abandoned. Three years later, laboratory tests showed that zinc could cause proteins to form clumps similar to the plaques found in the brains of Alzheimer's victims. But the connection between zinc and Alzheimer's remains unclear. For one thing, scientists remain unsure whether plaques cause Alzheimer's or are themselves a result of the disease; if the latter, zinc's ability to form plaques might be unrelated to what causes Alzheimer's in the first place.

In a minority of cases, trauma may be a contributing factor. About 15 percent of Alzheimer's sufferers have a history of head injury.

DIAGNOSTIC AND TEST PROCEDURES

Diagnosis by a professional is particularly important because a number of other ailments—many of which are treatable—share some symptoms associated with Alzheimer's disease. These include respiratory infections, inadequate nutrition, ***vitamin B12*** deficiency, ***anemia, hypoglycemia, depression,*** and cerebral vascular insufficiency (decreased blood flow to the brain due to constricted arteries). An adverse reaction to prescribed medication, or a harmful combination of medicines, can sometimes cause Alzheimer's-like symptoms. Other diseases and conditions sometimes confused with Alzheimer's are ***Parkinson's disease, stroke, thyroid problems,*** brain tumors, advanced ***syphilis,*** and Huntington's chorea—an inherited degenerative nerve disease.

To check for Alzheimer's, the doctor will probably begin with physical and psychological tests designed to eliminate other possible causes of mental impairment. Verbal tests and interviews of the family are the usual next steps, but they will not produce a definitive diagnosis. Until recently, only a postmortem examination of brain tissue could yield absolute proof of Alzheimer's—the telltale evidence of nerve tangles, protein plaques, and general brain shrinkage from cell death.

Although there is currently no accepted diagnostic test for Alzheimer's, recent studies suggest that genetic testing may prove to be useful.

TREATMENT

Alzheimer's disease is incurable: Nothing can halt or reverse it. However, certain medications seem to slow its general progress to some degree in the early stages, and others can help with mood changes and other specific behavioral problems of the disease.

Caring for an Alzheimer's patient is often stressful for family members; support organizations can help caregivers cope with problems and feelings. Eventually, full-time nursing care will be necessary. Some families are able to provide this full-time care at home, while others turn to professional caregivers.

CONVENTIONAL MEDICINE

- In 1993 tacrine hydrochloride became the first drug approved by the FDA for treatment of Alzheimer's. In tests, it delayed progression of the disease by six months, and it improved mental functioning in cases that were not far advanced. The possible side effect of liver toxicity must be monitored weekly. Newer drugs, including donepezil, are as effective and may have fewer side effects.
- Studies suggest that the experimental drug acetylcarnitine can bring temporary improvements in verbal ability, memory, attention span, and other mental functions among Alzheimer's patients.
- In one test, estrogen replacement therapy helped retard the onset of memory and reasoning deficiencies in 40 percent of female Alzheimer's patients.
- A number of drugs are prescribed for specific symptoms: haloperidol and thioridazine for aggressive behavior and agitation, ***sertraline*** for depression, and ***zolpidem*** and ***diphenhydramine*** for insomnia.

ALTERNATIVE CHOICES

As with conventional medicine, alternative therapies for the treatment of Alzheimer's cannot promise a cure, but in some cases they may help slow the progress of the disease or help address specific symptoms.

ACUPRESSURE

Not surprisingly, Alzheimer's patients easily become depressed and anxious. To help ease these burdens, practitioners suggest the acupressure techniques illustrated at right; they are specifically designed to promote relaxation and to serve as a general health tonic.

ACUPUNCTURE

Acupuncture promotes relaxation, can help improve general health, and can help an Alzheimer's patient be more alert and aware. Consult a qualified practitioner.

ACUPRESSURE

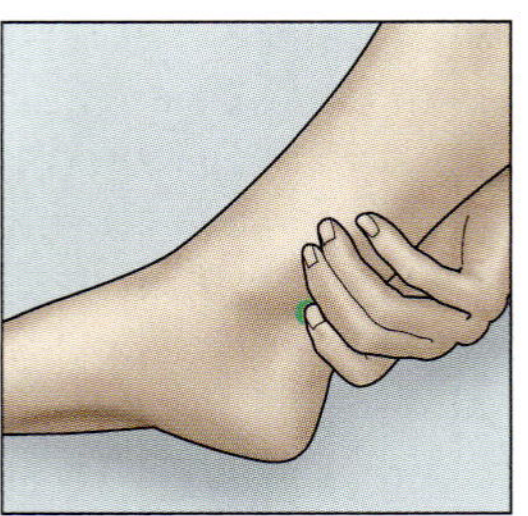

1 Pressing Kidney 3, located on the inside of the ankle between the anklebone and the Achilles tendon, may help stimulate mental activity. Apply firm pressure and hold for one to two minutes, then repeat on the other foot.

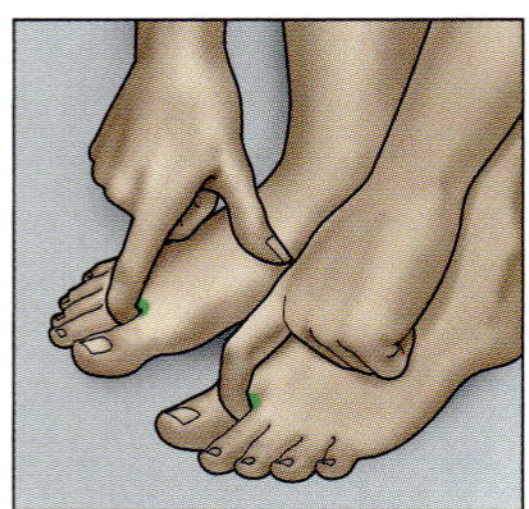

2 Pressing Liver 2—on the top of the foot, in the web between the first and second toes—may help relieve irritability. Press steadily for one minute.

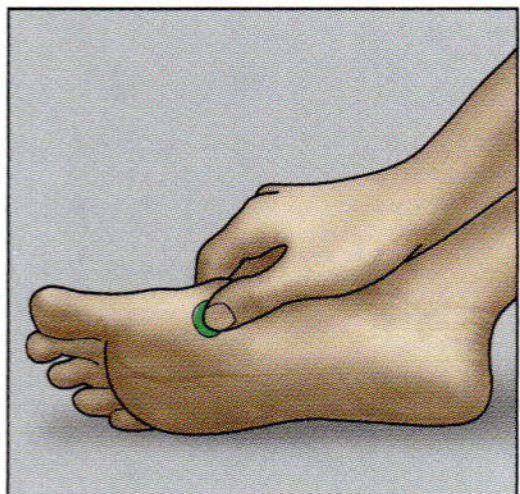

3 Pressing Spleen 3 may aid memory. The point is located on the inside of the foot, just behind the bulge made by the large joint of the big toe. Maintain a steady pressure for one minute, then repeat on the other foot.

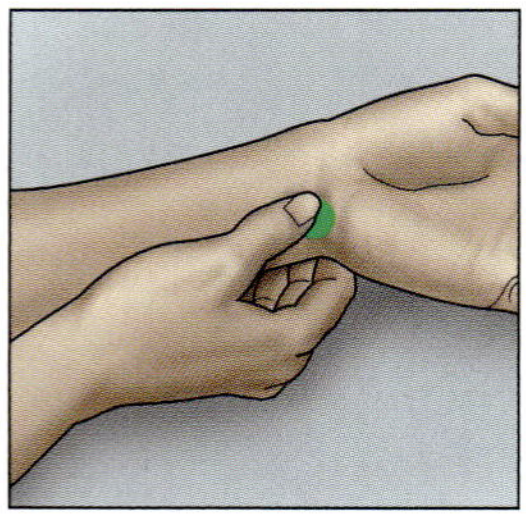

4 Sleeping habits may be improved by pressing Heart 7, located along the crease on the inside of the wrist, directly in line with the little finger. Squeeze firmly between the thumb and index finger for one minute, then repeat on the other hand.

CHELATION THERAPY

Chelation therapy, which involves the nonsurgical removal of accumulated metals in the body, targets aluminum—believed by some researchers to have a causative role in Alzheimer's; it has been suggested that aluminum molecules link with calcium molecules to bind together the deposits called plaque. The chelation technique involves a series of intravenous injections of the amino acid ethylenediaminetetraacetic acid (EDTA), which is thought to loosen the hold of the calcium and capture the aluminum, later releasing it as waste. Studies have suggested that this therapy can slow the progress of the disease. It is controversial and may have potentially dangerous side effects, however. Consult your doctor before undertaking treatment.

HERBAL THERAPIES

Ginkgo biloba extract (GBE), from the ***ginkgo*** tree (*Ginkgo biloba*), is said to alleviate early symptoms of Alzheimer's—among them, deterioration of short-term memory, depression, absentmindedness, anxiety, dizziness, inability to concentrate, confusion, and ringing in the ears. The recommended average dose is 80 to 120 mg, taken three times daily; look for capsules containing 24 percent ginkgo flavoglycosides. According to the proponents of this therapy, positive results are seen after four to six weeks.

HOMEOPATHY

To avoid overmedication with conventional drugs, consult a homeopath for remedies that may help in treating unusual or disruptive behavior; typically, you will see results within a week.

AT-HOME CARE

- ◆ To help an Alzheimer's patient cope with episodes of disorientation and mental lapses, promote a feeling of safety in every way possible: Maintain a stable, familiar living environment; stick to routine; when you must be absent, leave reminder notes and simple directions.
- ◆ Wandering and getting lost is a common problem with Alzheimer's patients; have the patient wear an ID bracelet with a phone number on it.
- ◆ To induce someone with Alzheimer's to talk more, go for a walk. Studies suggest that walking may stimulate areas of the brain linked to speech.
- ◆ To help an Alzheimer's patient develop a more positive outlook on the present, try eliciting reminiscences: Often, long-term memories are not initially impaired, and pleasant recollections can create feelings of happiness and well-being. This can be effectively done in a group. Good nostalgia-promoting materials include old magazines, photo albums, and favorite family stories. Avoid pressuring the patient to remember. A subtle question or two may provide the key to a memory.
- ◆ See the ***Appendix*** for professional associations that may help you and the patient cope.

PREVENTION

No one knows for sure what causes Alzheimer's, so any preventive measures are highly speculative at best. But it's important to remember that even if Alzheimer's runs in your family, you will not necessarily develop it yourself. If you are concerned about the possibility that you might eventually develop Alzheimer's, your best strategy is to maintain a healthful lifestyle: Eat right and exercise regularly to keep your entire body—and especially the nerve cells in your brain—in good shape. In particular, avoid cigarette smoke and air pollution as best you can; this will help you minimize your exposure to free radicals, which some studies have implicated in the formation of nerve plaques.

Although some studies suggest a link between Alzheimer's and zinc, doctors do not recommend that you attempt to limit your daily intake; zinc is an essential mineral, and while you should avoid overdosing on zinc, you would do more harm than good by restricting your intake below the recommended daily allowance (15 mg for men, 12 mg for women). ■

ANAL BLEEDING

A

Read down this column to find your symptoms. Then read across.

SYMPTOMS	AILMENT/PROBLEM
◆ bright red blood on stools or toilet paper; possibly, anal pain.	◆ Bleeding from the lower gastrointestinal tract, perhaps caused by ***hemorrhoids, anal fissure,*** diverticulosis, or vascular ectasia (blood vessels in the colon become distorted, then tangle and bleed)
◆ anal pain and itching; bright red bleeding from the anus; difficult, strained bowel movements but the bowels are never completely emptied.	◆ Anorectal stricture (a narrowing and tightening of the anal canal), caused by inflammation, scarring from a previous surgery, or ***laxative*** abuse
◆ recurrent watery or frequent stools that may contain blood (bleeding may be profuse); lower abdominal pain; weakness; nausea; vomiting; possibly, joint pain, skin sores in the anal region, and/or fever.	◆ ***Colitis, Crohn's disease,*** or ***gastroenteritis***
◆ bright or dark red bleeding from the anus; pain around the navel.	◆ Meckel's diverticulum (a bulging pouch in the small-intestine wall); may lead to peritonitis or intussusception (in which the intestine folds into itself, causing blockage)
◆ frequent or watery stools; bright or dark red bleeding from the anus; rectal fullness; lower abdominal pain; possibly, vomiting.	◆ Rectal prolapse (part of the rectum falls through the anus)
◆ infrequent or hard stools; bright red blood and mucus in stools; rectal fullness; cramping in left abdomen.	◆ Proctitis (inflammation of the rectum), often due to ***infection***
◆ vague abdominal and anal pain; anal itching or discharge; possibly, painless anal bleeding, or bright red stools, mucous anal discharge, and/or a lump near the anus.	◆ Polyps (tissue growths that protrude into the gastrointestinal tract), or ***colorectal cancer***
◆ blood in stools; vomiting with blood; easy bruising; spiderlike blood vessels on the skin; fatigue; yellowish skin or eyes.	◆ ***Cirrhosis***
◆ infant with dark red bloody stools that look like currant jelly; colic; shortness of breath; vomiting that may contain greenish yellow bile.	◆ Infant intussusception (see Meckel's diverticulum, above)

A

WHAT TO DO	OTHER INFO
◆ To help keep stools soft, which minimizes pain and bleeding, change to a high-fiber diet and drink six to eight glasses of water a day.	◆ Warm 15-minute sitz baths three times daily will relieve achiness.
◆ Take over-the-counter ***analgesics*** to alleviate pain; your doctor can dilate or surgically remove the scar tissue and/or the stricture area.	
◆ For ***gastroenteritis,*** fight dehydration (drink 8 to 10 glasses of water daily) and get plenty of rest. For ***colitis*** or ***Crohn's disease,*** avoid stressful situations and foods that disagree with you.	◆ For ***colitis,*** eating 1 clove of raw ***garlic*** *(Allium sativum)* daily may reduce cramping; drinking warm ***chamomile*** *(Matricaria recutita)* tea as often as desired can help the intestinal lining heal.
◆ Call your doctor without delay. You will probably need surgery to remove the diverticulum or any ulcerated area of the intestine.	◆ If your symptoms mimic ***appendicitis,*** you may have surgery to remove the appendix.
◆ Call your doctor without delay. Surgery is sometimes required for rectal prolapse.	
◆ See your doctor. ***Antibiotics*** can cure bacterial proctitis, and you can get symptom relief for the viral form.	◆ Potential causes include ***sexually transmitted diseases*** (especially the ***gonorrhea, chlamydia,*** and ***syphilis*** bacteria, and the herpesvirus), ***laxative*** overuse, rectal injury, ***allergy.***
◆ See your doctor without delay because of the possibility of cancer. Benign polyps may be surgically removed.	◆ Much serious anal bleeding is "occult," or hidden. If you are over 50, see your doctor for a test for occult bleeding every three years.
◆ **Get medical help immediately;** the bleeding can be life-threatening.	◆ Abstain from alcoholic beverages and any unnecessary medications. Sound nutrition is essential to stop the progression of cirrhosis.
◆ **Get medical help immediately** to prevent shock and/or death.	◆ Most cases occur in infants between 4 and 11 months old. Intussusception may recur and is second only to appendicitis in causing abdominal pain in children under age 13.

Cross references are indicated by ***bold italics.***

ANAL FISSURE

A

SYMPTOMS

- drops of bright red blood on bowel movement, toilet tissue, or clothing; occasionally the bleeding is more profuse.
- tearing or burning pain in the anal region during a bowel movement; dull ache may continue for several hours.
- a small piece of skin at the end of the fissure (called a "sentinel pile") that may show outside the anus.
- hard or infrequent stools, usually from deliberately retaining painful bowel movements.

CALL YOUR DOCTOR IF:

- you notice any ***anal bleeding.*** You may have a serious disorder, such as ***colorectal cancer,*** Meckel's diverticulum, or ***cirrhosis.*** Anal bleeding should never be ignored.
- he or she has confirmed you have an anal fissure, but after one month of treatment the fissure has not healed. There may be another reason for the fissure or for the poor healing, such as ***colorectal cancer.***

An anal fissure, also called an anal ulcer, is a single shallow crack in the lining of the anus (the lowest region of your intestines, which also opens to the outside). A fissure begins just inside the anal opening and extends ¼ to ¾ inch along the anal wall.

An anal fissure can be excruciatingly painful. Passing stools irritates it, and the anal sphincter muscles, at the anal opening, may respond by going into spasm. These combined effects cause extreme pain that is made even worse if the stools are either hard or watery. Despite the pain, a fissure is not dangerous and will probably heal with simple treatment. Don't ignore it, however: If a fissure becomes chronic, scar tissue can form and impede bowel movements, and you may need surgery to correct the problem.

CAUSES

Often it isn't clear why an anal fissure has developed. Posterior fissures, along the back anal wall, are probably the result of straining with ***constipation;*** in passing large, hard stools, the anal lining stretches too much and breaks. Anterior fissures, along the front wall, are usually related to scar-tissue buildup from a previous surgery, or to the extreme pressure that the anal region endures during childbirth. Anal fissures can also be a side effect of another condition, such as proctitis (inflammation of the rectum), ***Crohn's disease,*** or ***colorectal cancer.***

DIAGNOSTIC AND TEST PROCEDURES

Because any touch to this sensitive area can cause extreme pain, doctors try to do as little as possible to diagnose anal fissure and rule out serious disorders such as ***colorectal cancer, syphilis, tuberculosis, Crohn's disease,*** and ***AIDS.*** A visual examination—a close look at the anal region—is often all that is needed. Your doctor may insert a lubricated, gloved finger to manually examine the anus, or perhaps insert a small, thin instrument called an anoscope to get a clearer, closer view (using local anesthesia if necessary).

TREATMENT

Practicing good anal hygiene in order to avoid infection and keeping the stools soft to minimize pain and spasm will encourage a fissure to heal itself. Anal fissures, however, often reappear. Surgery is the only treatment known that can break this cycle, and thus it is the best choice of treatment for persistent fissures.

CONVENTIONAL MEDICINE

Anesthetic creams applied directly to the fissure are the first line of defense, along with warm sitz baths and dietary changes to avoid ***constipation.*** This combination is usually successful if the fissure is treated early. If a fissure doesn't respond to these therapies yet is not terribly severe, a physician may apply a local anesthetic and insert a gloved finger into the anus to dilate the anal sphincter. This decreases the pressure inside the anal canal, creating an environment more conducive to healing.

If the anal fissure is extraordinarily painful, resistant to other forms of treatment, or longstanding, surgery is the best option. This involves dividing the lower anal sphincter so it can't tighten and potentially cause fissures. The surgeon may also remove the fissure and the skin just around it, including the sentinel pile if one is present. This 20-minute outpatient procedure is performed under local or spinal anesthetic and is highly effective.

The fissure usually heals, and recurrence is unlikely. More than 90 percent of those who have surgery have no repeat fissure if they maintain a high-fiber diet afterward. It takes three or four days to recover, and you may have trouble controlling flatulence after surgery.

ALTERNATIVE CHOICES

You can often heal an anal fissure by regulating your bowel movements *(see* ***Constipation*** *and* ***Diarrhea****)* and keeping your stress and anxiety levels low. If you can maintain these lifestyle changes, it is unlikely the fissure will return.

HERBAL THERAPY

Slippery elm *(Ulmus fulva)* powder, taken daily, can help keep stools soft. Use up to one tbsp each day, added to oatmeal or applesause.

HOMEOPATHY

For up to seven days, 12c of one of the following, taken four times daily, may help. If one remedy doesn't work, try another. *Aesculus* can help soothe burning anal pain accompanied by lower-back pain and large, dry, hard stools. Try *Graphites* for painful bowel movements with lumps and mucus. For sharp pains during and after constipated bowel movements that feel as if they tear the anus, use *Nitric acid.* When anal fissure pain is sharp and burning as though glass were in the anus, use *Ratanhia.*

AT-HOME REMEDIES

- Apply an over-the-counter cream containing 1 percent ***hydrocortisone*** or ***vitamins A*** and ***D*** just inside the anus. (Small rubber finger covers are available for this purpose.) The hydrocortisone can reduce swelling and pain, and the vitamin cream soothes pain and promotes healing. Suppositories move too far up into the rectum to help.
- Several times a day, sit in a warm sitz bath for 20 minutes. This relaxes the anal sphincter, reducing spasms and their associated pain.
- See ***Hemorrhoids*** for more suggestions.

PREVENTION

Prevention involves avoiding constipation and diarrhea through diet and exercise. Among other benefits, a healthy diet and regular exercise promote good bowel health and offer protection against anal fissures. ■

ANEMIA

A

SYMPTOMS

- weakness, fatigue, and a general feeling of malaise; you may be mildly anemic.
- your lips look bluish, your skin is pasty or yellowish, and your gums, nail beds, eyelid linings, or palm creases are pale; you are almost certainly anemic.
- in addition to feeling weak and tired, you are frequently out of breath, faint, or dizzy; you may have severe anemia.
- your tongue burns; you may have **vitamin B_{12} anemia.**
- your tongue feels unusually slick and you experience movement or balance problems, tingling in the extremities, confusion, depression, or memory loss; you may have **pernicious anemia.**
- other possible symptoms: headaches, insomnia, decreased appetite, poor concentration, and an irregular heartbeat.

CALL YOUR DOCTOR IF:

- you have the symptoms of **pernicious anemia;** this disorder can damage the spinal cord.
- you have been taking iron supplements and experience symptoms such as vomiting, bloody diarrhea, fever, jaundice, lethargy, or seizures; you may be suffering from **iron overload,** which can be life-threatening, especially in children.

To stay healthy, the organs and tissues of the human body need a steady supply of oxygen. Anemia, in which body tissues are deprived of oxygen, is caused by a reduction in the number of circulating red blood cells or by inadequate amounts of an essential protein called hemoglobin. The severity of anemia can range from mild to life-threatening.

Normally, the heart pumps oxygen-depleted blood to the lungs, where hemoglobin in the red blood cells binds to oxygen collected there; oxygen-rich blood then travels through the circulatory system to the rest of the body. Oxygen starvation occurs if the body lacks sufficient numbers of red blood cells, which survive for only about 120 days and must constantly be replaced. Anemia can occur if large amounts of blood are lost or if something interferes with the production of red blood cells or accelerates their destruction. Because hemoglobin is the main component of red blood cells and the carrier for oxygen molecules, anemia also occurs if the hemoglobin supply is insufficient or if the hemoglobin itself is dysfunctional.

In all, more than 400 different forms of anemia have been identified, many of them rare. An anemic person often appears pale and weak and may feel breathless, faint, or unusually aware of a pounding heart. The disorder may arise from a number of underlying conditions, some of which may be hereditary, but in many cases poor diet is to blame. Although some forms of anemia require supervised medical care, those stemming from improper nutrition can typically be treated at home once a physician has determined the cause.

CAUSES

Chronic blood loss, perhaps as a result of ***stomach ulcers, hemorrhoids,*** or gastrointestinal tumors, can bring on anemia, as can chronic alcohol abuse. More often, however, the problem can be traced to dietary deficiencies; indeed, anemia in alcoholics arises largely because they tend to prefer booze to food and often fail to eat properly. Anemia can also result when the digestive system loses its ability to absorb key vitamins and minerals.

A

Iron deficiency anemia, the leading form of anemia worldwide, occurs when the body does not store enough iron, the primary raw material of hemoglobin. Iron deficiency is usually a dietary problem, but in many cases other conditions complicate the picture. For example, women who lose excessive amounts of blood through heavy menstrual flows *(see* ***Menstrual Problems****)* may have a lower-than-average iron level. Women who are pregnant or nursing may also have low iron levels because of loss to the developing fetus or because of milk production. Iron deficiency anemia also afflicts patients who have had surgery to remove part of the stomach, thereby impairing the ability to absorb iron.

Megaloblastic anemias, in which red blood cells become unusually large, occur when the body lacks either ***folic acid*** or ***vitamin*** B_{12}, both critical to cell production.

Hemolytic anemias may arise when red blood cells have genetic defects that cause them to be destroyed prematurely, perhaps by infections. In some cases, the cells are destroyed by the body's own immune system. Some hemolytic anemias are inherited, while others are acquired. **Thalassemia** is an inherited type of hemolytic anemia that stems from the body's inability to produce sufficient amounts of hemoglobin. One kind of thalassemia, common to people of Mediterranean, African, or Middle Eastern origin, is marked by the production of red blood cells that are smaller and more fragile than normal. This type strikes only those people who inherit the responsible gene from both parents.

In ***sickle cell anemia,*** an inherited disease that disproportionately affects people of African and Mediterranean descent, the body produces red blood cells that have a crescent, or sickle, shape rather than the normal oval shape. The deformed cells cannot carry sufficient quantities of hemoglobin, nor can they squeeze easily through tiny blood vessels. Capillaries can become clogged by these abnormal red blood cells, sometimes leading to a life-threatening condition called a sickle cell crisis.

Of the **megaloblastic anemias,** the most common is the type caused by ***folic acid*** deficiency. People with this form of anemia usually aren't getting enough folic acid in their diet. While just one cup of spinach provides enough folic acid to meet the FDA's recommended daily allowance, this vitamin deficiency is still prevalent in the United States and throughout the world. For some people, the problem is caused not by dietary inadequacies but by an inability to absorb sufficient amounts of folic acid. Certain intestinal disorders, such as some inflammatory bowel diseases and ***Crohn's disease,*** as well as some drugs, including sulfasalazine (used to treat ulcerative ***colitis***), can interfere with folic acid metabolism. Heavy consumption of alcohol can also lower blood levels of folic acid by interfering with proper nutrition and by hindering the digestive system's ability to absorb the vitamin.

Because most people, especially those who consume meat and eggs, get plenty of ***vitamin*** B_{12} from their diet, anemia linked to a **vitamin** B_{12} **deficiency** usually signals the body's inability to absorb the vitamin. This type of anemia can occur in people who have had surgery along the digestive tract. However, the most common form of

THE IRON FACTS ABOUT SPINACH

Spinach, long heralded by mothers and Popeye the Sailor as a great source of iron, is in fact an iron-blocker. Technically speaking, the vegetable does contain a significant amount of iron. But, like butter beans, lentils, beet greens, and other leafy vegetables, spinach also contains phytate, a chemical that prevents iron from entering the bloodstream. So if your iron count needs a boost, try eating liver, which is high in available iron. Or garnish your spinach salad with slices of orange, as citrus fruits contain vitamins and acids that counteract the effects of phytate and promote iron absorption.

A

B_{12} deficiency anemia, known as **pernicious anemia,** results when the stomach fails to produce a chemical that normally combines with vitamin B_{12} to aid its absorption in the small intestine. Pernicious anemia is a rare condition that most commonly affects older people.

DIAGNOSTIC AND TEST PROCEDURES

Before beginning a treatment program, you need to find out what kind of anemia you have. The only way to know for sure is to have your doctor run tests on a sample of your blood. The results of these tests will quickly reveal whether your anemia is linked to a nutritional deficiency or to some other cause.

TREATMENT

Conventional remedies for anemia range from simple dietary changes and vitamin supplements to hormone treatments and, in severe cases, surgery. Some alternative practitioners approach the disorder through dietary modifications; others emphasize techniques to improve circulation and digestion.

CONVENTIONAL MEDICINE

Once blood tests reveal the underlying problem, treatment paths are well delineated. For anemia caused by a deficiency in iron or folic acid, your doctor will undoubtedly recommend dietary changes and possibly supplements. Because iron supplements can upset the stomach, you should get ones made from ferrous gluconate, which is easier on the digestive system than ferrous sulfate. In general, liquid solutions are less likely than tablets or pills to cause upset. Avoid enteric-coated supplements, since your body cannot absorb the iron as effectively. WARNING: Iron is extremely toxic in large quantities. Excessive use of supplements can lead to **iron overload**, possibly resulting in abdominal pain, nutritional imbalances, digestive problems, or even death, especially in children. Supplements pose a particular threat to people with the inherited disorder hemochromatosis, in which the digestive tract absorbs higher-than-normal amounts of iron. Be sure to consult your doctor or a professional nutritionist before taking iron supplements.

Since **vitamin B_{12} anemia** is almost always linked to the body's inability to absorb the vitamin through the digestive tract, regular B_{12} injections are the only recourse. Most people learn to self-administer B_{12} injections at home.

In some cases of anemia caused by excessive blood loss, surgery is the only solution. To determine whether surgery is necessary, your doctor will run extensive tests to identify the cause of the bleeding. Some conditions—such as bleeding of the digestive tract, a frequent cause of iron deficiency anemia in men—can be corrected only through an operation. Doctors may also prescribe transfusions of red blood cells or injections of hormones to speed red blood cell production. (Supplements of hormones should be a last resort for women, as the drugs can produce unwanted side effects.) Severe cases of **thalassemia** may require lifetime blood transfusions, and treatment of other **hemolytic anemias** may involve surgery to remove the spleen.

ALTERNATIVE CHOICES

Some remedies treat anemia by promoting better circulation, others by increasing iron absorption, stimulating digestion, or adjusting the diet to include more iron- or vitamin-rich foods.

CHINESE MEDICINE

According to traditional Chinese medicine, anemia is a symptom of a weak spleen. A healthy spleen maintains the integrity of blood vessels and nourishes the blood itself, while a weak spleen produces deficient blood. Treatment would typically involve ways to stimulate the spleen, including **acupuncture** and **herbal therapies.** Research suggests that ***Asian ginseng*** *(Panax ginseng)* is useful as a general tonic to counteract anemia-induced fatigue. ***Dong quai*** *(Angelica sinensis),* another Asian herb used medicinally for thousands of years, might be prescribed for women with heavy menstrual flow. For anemic patients that have a sallow, yellowish complexion, a Chinese herbalist might recommend a combination of dong quai and ***Chinese foxglove root*** *(Rehmannia glutinosa).* For patients that have a stark white complexion, the remedy might be a mixture of ginseng and ***astragalus*** *(Astragalus membranaceus).*

HERBAL THERAPIES

In the history of folk medicine, bitter substances have always been thought to stimulate digestion and thereby promote the absorption of valuable nutrients. The bitter herb ***gentian*** *(Gentiana lutea)* is a popular remedy in Europe for a number of nutritionally based ailments, including anemia. Gentian can be brewed into a tea or ingested in the form of a commercially available alcoholic extract. ***Dandelion*** *(Taraxacum officinale)* is also thought to benefit people with anemia, simply because it is rich in vitamins and minerals. Other iron-rich herbs include ***parsley*** *(Petroselinum crispum)* and ***nettle*** *(Urtica dioica).* While many herbs used to treat anemia have anecdotal support, not all have been studied scientifically. Among those that have been shown to promote digestion are anise *(Pimpinella anisum),* caraway *(Carum carvi),* cumin *(Cuminum cyminum),* and linden (*Tilia* spp.).

HOMEOPATHY

Homeopathy offers a number of remedies that may be helpful in treating anemia. Consult a professional homeopath for an evaluation that will determine which substances are most suitable for your condition.

NUTRITION AND DIET

Adjusting your diet is the easiest, most healthful, and longest-lasting way to combat any anemia linked to nutritional deficiency. A vast array of foods can boost your ***iron*** count, including enriched breads and cereals, rice, potatoes, carrots, broccoli, tomatoes, dried beans, blackstrap molasses, lean red meat, liver, poultry, dried fruits, almonds, and shellfish. Research indicates that iron from animal sources is absorbed more readily than plant iron. Evidence also suggests that ***vitamin C, vitamin B complex,*** and ***copper*** help the body absorb iron, so drink citrus fruit juice with your meals and make sure that your daily multivitamin contains copper. Avoid caffeinated or carbonated beverages, antacids, calcium supplements, and black tea, all of which contain ingredients that interfere with iron absorption. Take calcium supplements away from meals.

If you're low on ***folic acid,*** step up your consumption of citrus fruits, mushrooms, green vegetables, liver, eggs, milk, and bulking agents like wheat germ and brewer's yeast. Also, pumpkin is an excellent source of folate, which is the ***vitamin B complex*** component of folic acid. Keep in mind that folic acid is destroyed by heat and light, so fruits and vegetables should be eaten fresh and cooked as little as possible.

AT-HOME REMEDIES

- Your diet should include foods recommended on these pages. The specific choices should be dictated by the type of anemia you have.
- Keep track of the foods you eat and find out whether they are rich in ***iron, folic acid,*** or ***vitamin*** B_{12}. You might be surprised to learn that some of the foods you eat are preventing the absorption of needed nutrients. *(See "The Iron Facts about Spinach," page 119.)*
- Don't drink caffeinated tea, coffee, or cola with meals; caffeine inhibits iron absorption. The tannin in black tea has the same effect. However, you should drink citrus juices, because they are rich in ***vitamin C,*** which promotes iron absorption.
- Consider taking a daily multivitamin. However, be sure to consult a doctor before taking iron supplements; excess amounts of iron in your system can be harmful.

PREVENTION

- Avoid excessive consumption of alcohol. Chronic drinking can undermine proper nutrition and interfere with the digestive system's ability to absorb folic acid, necessary for the production of red blood cells.
- Take a daily multivitamin to maintain a healthful balance of vitamins and minerals. ■

ANEURYSM

A

SYMPTOMS

Although most aneurysms have no symptoms, in some cases the following symptoms may occur:

- Sudden and severe pain, often described as "ripping or tearing," or an unusual pulsing sensation, pain, or a lump anywhere in your body where blood vessels are located.
- Pain in the abdomen or lower back extending into the groin and legs may indicate an **abdominal aneurysm,** which can sometimes be seen or felt as a throbbing lump and may be accompanied by weight loss or loss of appetite.
- A pain in the chest, hoarseness, persistent coughing, and difficulty swallowing may indicate a **thoracic aneurysm.**
- A throbbing sensation or lump directly behind the knee may indicate a **peripheral aneurysm;** the knee is a common site for this type of aneurysm, especially in smokers.
- A severe headache, like none you've ever had before, accompanied by radiating neck pain, may indicate a **dissecting** or rupturing **berry aneurysm** in the head. Dissecting aneurysms, most commonly characterized by severe pain, can also occur elsewhere in the body and are always an emergency situation.

CALL YOUR DOCTOR IF:

- you suspect you have an aneurysm. Many aneurysms are serious and require a medical evaluation. An aneurysm that ruptures is potentially life-threatening.

An aneurysm is a permanent ballooning in the wall of an artery. The pressure of blood passing through can force part of a weakened artery to bulge outward, forming a thin-skinned blister.

Although any weak blood vessel can be affected, aneurysms usually form in the abdominal or thoracic portions of the aorta, the main blood vessel that carries blood from the heart, or in arteries nourishing the brain. Aneurysms in any of these places are serious, while those in peripheral arteries are often less hazardous.

The gravest threat an aneurysm poses is that it will burst and cause a ***stroke*** or life-threatening hemorrhage. But even if it doesn't rupture, a large aneurysm can impede circulation and promote unwanted blood-clot formation.

Detecting an aneurysm on your own is difficult since symptoms are rare. But certain people are at higher risk of developing aneurysms. Your best strategy is to know if you are at risk *(see **Causes,** below),* to be familiar with the symptoms of an aneurysm, and to take preventive steps.

CAUSES

Any condition that causes arterial walls to weaken or deteriorate can result in an aneurysm. The most common culprits are ***atherosclerosis*** and ***high blood pressure.*** Penetrating wounds and infections can also lead to an aneurysm. Some types, such as **berry aneurysms,** are the result of congenital, or inherited, weakness in artery walls.

TREATMENT

The only way to get rid of an aneurysm is to have it surgically removed—often a risky procedure, but highly effective when successful. Sometimes, however, surgery is impossible, or it may pose more danger than the aneurysm. Careful monitoring and drug therapy may then be the best course.

CONVENTIONAL MEDICINE

Your doctor will probably determine the size, type, and location of an aneurysm using any of various imaging techniques. This information will help determine the best course of treatment.

For inoperable aneurysms, you may be prescribed drugs that lower your blood pressure or reduce the force of your heart's contractions, thereby minimizing the risk of a rupture. But even for an operable aneurysm, your doctor may first try drug therapy and advise a wait-and-see approach, with periodic testing to track the aneurysm's growth. You may need surgery if your doctor finds that the aneurysm has become dangerously swollen.

A surgeon can neutralize an aneurysm by inserting a clip that cuts off blood flow to the affected area. An aneurysm may also be removed and the section of artery replaced with a synthetic graft.

TYPES OF ANEURYSMS

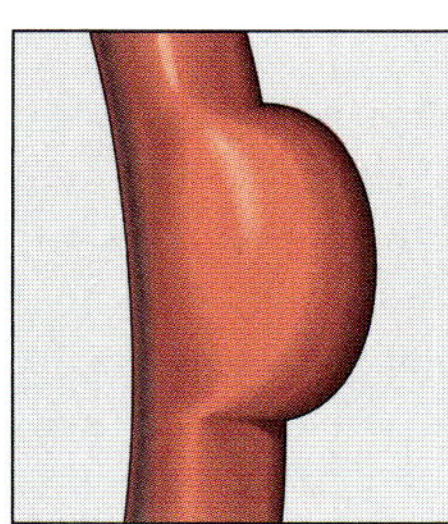

SACCULAR

A saccular aneurysm is a balloonlike bulge in an artery wall. Usually caused by a congenital weakness in the wall's muscular middle layer, this type of aneurysm may contain a blood clot.

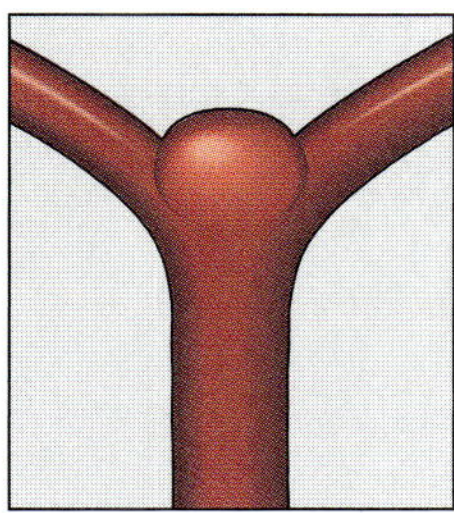

BERRY

Berry aneurysms, a type of saccular aneurysm, are named for their small, round appearance. These bulges most often occur in branching arteries at the base of the brain.

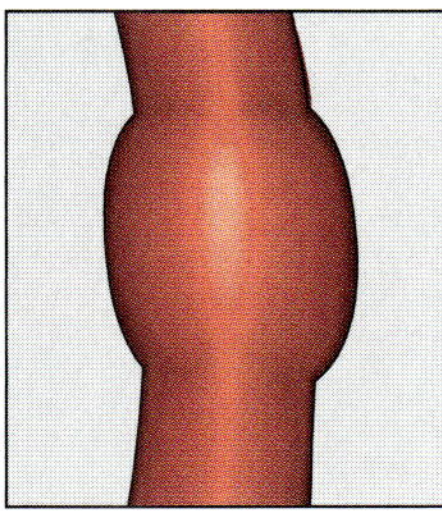

FUSIFORM

Damage to the artery wall's inner and middle layers can cause a sausage-shaped swelling known as a fusiform aneurysm. High blood pressure and atherosclerosis are the primary causes of this type of aneurysm.

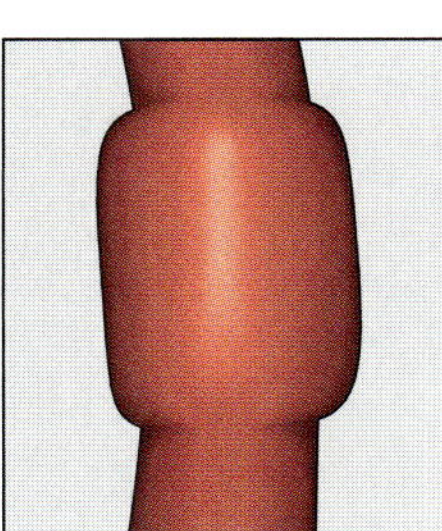

CYLINDROID

A cylindroid, or tubular, aneurysm is an elongated swelling that causes an abrupt change in an artery's normal diameter. Often the result of atherosclerosis or syphilis, a cylindroid aneurysm can develop along a length of artery.

ALTERNATIVE CHOICES

The following treatments—all primarily intended to prevent aneurysms—should be pursued along with, not instead of, your doctor's orders.

HOMEOPATHY

For a small, relatively benign aneurysm or as a preventive remedy for someone at high risk of developing an aneurysm, a professional homeopath might recommend *Baryta carbonica* to tone and strengthen arterial walls.

MIND/BODY MEDICINE

Keeping your mind and body relaxed may prevent an aneurysm from worsening. Try exercises that you can do at home such as **yoga** or **meditation.**

NUTRITION AND DIET

Dietary changes that lower blood pressure and slow atherosclerosis may help prevent an aneurysm from developing. See entries on ***Atherosclerosis, Blood Clots, High Blood Pressure,*** and ***Cholesterol Problems.***

PREVENTION

Know if you are at risk, and take appropriate steps to keep an aneurysm from forming. Especially if you have a family history of ***stroke*** or ***heart disease,*** make changes in your diet and lifestyle to improve your overall health. Exercise regularly, watch what you eat, and if you smoke, stop. ■

ANGINA

A

SYMPTOMS

- pain that is crushing, constricting, strangling, suffocating, sharp, or burning; it is normally felt in the chest but may also occur in peripheral areas such as the jaw or abdomen. Location and specific sensations vary from person to person but are usually consistent from one attack to the next.
- pain that occurs with exertion and recedes with rest.
- weakness, sweating, shortness of breath, anxiety, palpitations, nausea, or lightheadedness—symptoms that may or may not be associated with an angina attack.

CALL YOUR DOCTOR IF:

- an attack lasts more than 15 minutes; this may be a ***heart attack.*** **Call 911 or your emergency number now.**
- you think this may be your first angina attack; you need to find out for sure.
- attacks have become more intense, frequent, prolonged, and unpredictable; these are signs of **unstable angina.**
- you are taking a beta blocker and experience distressing side effects *(see **Beta-Adrenergic Blockers**).*
- you are taking ***nitrate*** medication and become faint, dizzy, weak, pale, restless, or start vomiting or sweating excessively. These are signs of either oversensitivity or overdose.
- you are taking a ***calcium channel blocker*** and notice side effects such as stomach cramps, slow pulse, arrhythmia, headaches, constipation, swelling, faintness, or shortness of breath.

Angina is the heart's way of saying that it is not getting enough oxygen. This can be because coronary arteries—those that supply blood to the heart—are blocked or because the heart is being overworked and therefore needs more oxygen than usual.

The medical term angina pectoris literally means "a choking sensation of the chest." Usually, angina is a crushing or constricting pain that starts in the center of the chest, deep behind the breastbone, and may radiate to other parts of the body. Sufferers have said it feels like "an elephant sitting on my chest" or "a vise squeezing my chest."

Some people feel the pain of angina only in peripheral locations such as the jaw, abdomen, or arm. The pain can also be confused with indigestion because the tight, burning sensations are similar. Angina can also be misinterpreted as a heart attack; the pain is similar but does not last as long—usually no more than five minutes.

Of the many types of angina, **stable,** or **classical, angina**—triggered by exertion and receding with rest—is the most common. If you have stable angina, you should be able to predict what sort of activity will bring on an attack. Another type, **unstable angina,** is a more acute condition; it occurs unpredictably, even during rest, and should be interpreted as a warning sign of more serious heart trouble. A rare type called **variant angina,** which involves coronary artery spasms, is seen most often in women.

Angina affects some three million Americans. It is more prevalent in people over 30 and tends to strike men more than women; over age 65, however, more women are affected than men. Alone, angina causes no permanent damage because the heart is only temporarily deprived of oxygen. But if your angina worsens, you should know that you are at a greater risk of ***heart attack.*** Be especially concerned if you develop **unstable angina,** and consult a doctor.

CAUSES

The main underlying cause of angina is coronary artery disease, which stems from ***atherosclerosis***

A

AREAS OF ANGINAL PAIN

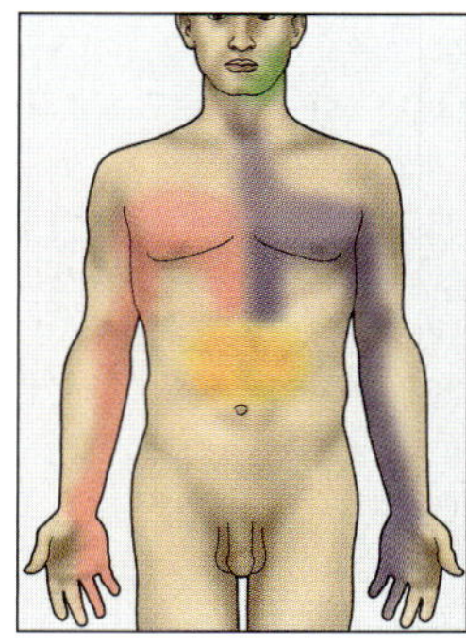

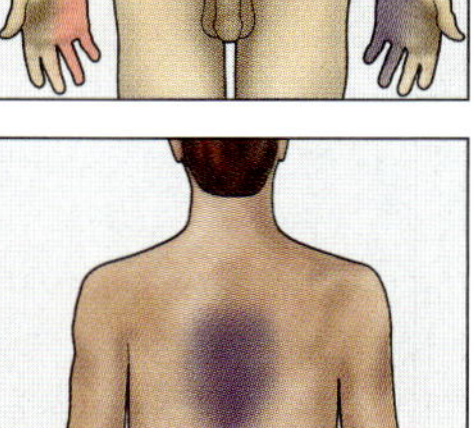

Anginal pain can be distributed throughout the upper body in any of the following areas *(shown at left)* including the center and left part of the chest, the neck, and inside the left arm *(purple)*. Pain may also develop in the jaw *(green)*, right chest and arm *(pink)*, and between the navel and breastbone *(yellow)*; the shoulders may be affected as well. In some cases, pain occurs between the shoulder blades *(purple area in lower illustration)*.

of the coronary arteries—when the vessels become clogged or narrowed by fatty calcified deposits called plaques. Angina can also result from other diseases that tax the heart unduly, such as ***anemia,*** aortic valve disease *(see **Heart Disease**)*, ***heart arrhythmias,*** and hyperthyroidism *(see **Thyroid Problems**)*.

Stable angina is sometimes called "exertional" angina because it is triggered by activities that make the heart beat rapidly. Indeed, physical activity is the most frequent cause of attacks. Depending on the person, exertion that brings on an attack can mean anything from simple walking to heavy lifting or sexual activity. A large meal can also cause an attack, because digestion requires the heart to work. Other frequently cited triggers are emotional excitement and exposure to the cold, both of which stimulate the heart. In addition, more than 20 drugs have been known to spark angina, from over-the-counter decongestants and various prescription medications to illegal substances such as cocaine.

Certain risk factors for ***heart disease*** and coronary artery disease make the development of angina more likely. These include ***high blood pressure, stress,*** high cholesterol *(see **Cholesterol Problems**)*, smoking, ***obesity, diabetes,*** and a family history of heart disease. All of these risk factors are also linked to atherosclerosis.

DIAGNOSTIC AND TEST PROCEDURES

If you experience pain that might be angina, your doctor will give you a complete physical exam and various tests. A resting electrocardiogram (ECG) will usually be normal if you have angina, but the test may rule out other causes. You will likely undergo an exercise treadmill test, possibly combined with an imaging technique such as ultrasound or a radioisotope scan, which may reveal problems in the heart or arteries. If these tests indicate a possible problem, angiography will be performed to determine the location and extent of any blockages in coronary arteries.

TREATMENT

Drugs may alleviate angina symptoms, but fundamental changes in diet and lifestyle are an important part of any angina treatment program. Before taking any drug, review its properties and your medical history carefully with your doctor. Many drugs should not be mixed with other drugs or natural medicines, and you also need to be sure your doctor knows of any preexisting medical conditions you may have.

CONVENTIONAL MEDICINE

If you have angina, your doctor will undoubtedly mention the importance of an overall healthy lifestyle that includes proper diet, exercise, weight management, and no smoking.

Most angina patients also take prescribed medication. There are three main classes of angina drugs: ***nitrates, beta-adrenergic blockers,*** and ***calcium channel blockers.*** Physicians often use a combination of these to treat angina. ***Nitrates,*** which dilate coronary arteries and allow for greater blood flow, are a tried-and-true, inexpensive treatment. ***Nitroglycerin*** is by far the most widely used nitrate; it can be taken as often as needed and may provide relief within a few minutes. However, it also causes headaches in about half of all users. ***Beta-adrenergic blockers,*** which are used to reduce heart rate, lower blood pressure, and reduce cardiac oxygen consumption, are effective in combination with nitrates or alone. ***Calcium channel blockers*** quell coronary artery spasms, and some also slow heart rate. Patients with severe unstable angina are often treated initially with the anticoagulant ***heparin*** in conjunction with ***aspirin,*** nitrates, and beta blockers.

If drug therapy does not work or does not suffice, coronary artery angioplasty or bypass surgery may be considered. Angioplasty—a catheter technique that widens blocked arteries—has become a relatively routine procedure; bypass surgery, which diverts blood flow around clogged arteries, is reserved for very severe cases.

ALTERNATIVE CHOICES

Always consult a doctor if you think you have angina. The alternative therapies below may help relieve symptoms or prevent attacks, but they should be considered as complements to—rather than substitutes for—conventional medical care.

ACUPRESSURE

Applying pressure for at least one minute to points B 15, P 5, P 6, and Sp 6 may relieve angina symptoms. See the ***Appendix*** and page 127 for point locations.

AYURVEDIC MEDICINE

An Ayurvedic mixture of herbs and minerals known as Abana has been shown to significantly reduce the frequency and severity of angina attacks; consult a practitioner for the specific remedy.

CHELATION THERAPY

Although controversial, chelation therapy has been sought by thousands of angina sufferers. Its advocates claim that it is safer and cheaper than many conventional drug or surgical treatments—and just as effective. Critics insist that it undergo more rigorous scientific scrutiny before joining the ranks of standard treatment for angina and atherosclerosis. If you decide to try chelation therapy, be sure to seek out a practitioner certified by one of the major American chelation societies. *(See **Atherosclerosis** for a fuller explanation of chelation therapy.)*

HERBAL THERAPIES

Hawthorn *(Crataegus laevigata)* is an excellent long-term tonic for angina because it simultaneously dilates coronary arteries and calms the heart. It is often an ingredient in herbal treatments for angina that a naturopath might prescribe.

HOMEOPATHY

For immediate relief during an acute attack, *Cactus grandiflorus* (30c) is recommended. Cactus may bring relief if, during an attack, your chest feels like it's bound with an iron band. Among the long-term remedies that might be prescribed by a homeopathic physician are ***Nux vomica*** and ***Arsenicum album.***

LIFESTYLE

Certain air pollutants, particularly carbon monoxide, are known to aggravate and intensify angina. To avoid carbon monoxide, steer clear of tobacco smoke and stay inside on heavy smog days.

Avoid alcohol or drink only sparingly while on angina medication because of possible adverse reactions.

Gentle aerobic exercise is very beneficial for angina patients. Build stamina gradually, and exercise inside during cold weather. Be sure to consult your doctor before embarking on an exercise program.

MIND/BODY MEDICINE

If you find you have trouble controlling your emotions or stress levels, you must learn to relax. Many types of relaxation techniques—from **biofeedback** to **yoga**—could help tremendously. Choose a method you are comfortable with, and stick with it; the effectiveness of relaxation techniques varies from person to person and improves with time.

NUTRITION AND DIET

The principal goals of nutritional therapy for angina are to improve the blood flow to the heart

A

and the energy metabolism of the heart so that it requires less oxygen. The main way to improve blood flow is to control atherosclerosis, and consuming less saturated fat and cholesterol is a critical first step. To improve energy metabolism, be sure to get enough ***magnesium*** in your diet or as part of a multivitamin supplement. You might also ask your doctor to recommend an appropriate supplement of L-carnitine and coenzyme Q10, nutrients found in the body that improve energy metabolism and are often depleted in heart disease patients. For more specific dietary tips, see ***Atherosclerosis, Blood Clots, Cholesterol Problems,*** and ***High Blood Pressure.***

STRESS TEST

Exercising with angina is a tricky business. If done properly, it can help prevent angina from worsening; if done too ambitiously, it will aggravate the condition and could even be life-threatening. So how much is too much? If you want to start an exercise program, you should first undergo a stress test—also called an "exercise tolerance" or "treadmill" test. The test takes about half an hour. You will be fitted with electrodes on your chest and a blood-pressure cuff on your arm, and will then start exercising on a treadmill or stationary bike; as time elapses, the workout becomes progressively more difficult. By monitoring your heart rate, blood pressure, and ECG tracings, your doctor will be able to determine your exertion limits. Armed with this knowledge, you can then plan a healthful exercise regimen.

ACUPRESSURE

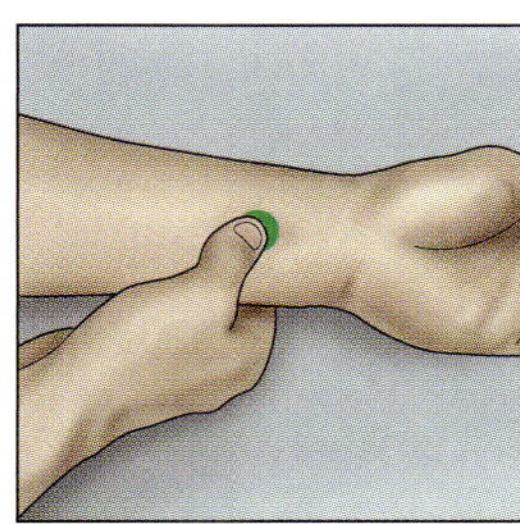

1 To help calm nerves and reduce feelings of uneasiness, press Pericardium 6. Place thumb in center of inner wrist, two finger widths from the wrist crease and between the two bones of the forearm. Press firmly for one minute, three to five times; repeat on other arm.

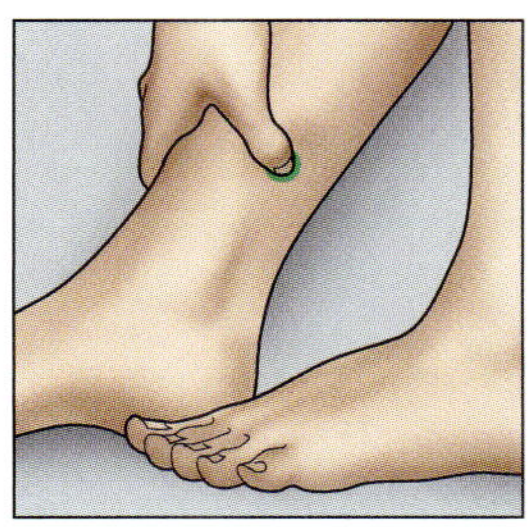

2 Pressure on Spleen 6 may help regulate blood pressure. The point is four finger widths up from the inner anklebone, near the edge of your shinbone. Press gently with your thumb for one minute, then switch legs. Do not use this point if you are pregnant.

AT-HOME REMEDIES

- If you have frequent angina attacks at night, try tilting the head of your bed up three or four inches. This lessens the work load on the heart from venous blood return.
- If you sense the onset of an attack while lying down, sit up and put your feet on the floor. If pain persists, take prescribed medication.
- An ***aspirin*** a day, with doctor's permission, can reduce the risk of heart attack and unstable angina.
- Spend at least an hour digesting heavy meals; exertion after eating is known to cause attacks.
- Stop smoking, as it greatly aggravates angina.
- Do not take birth-control pills if you have angina: Estrogens are associated with increased risk of blood clots.
- Eat green leafy vegetables such as kelp or collard greens. These contain vitamin K, a natural blood thinner.

PREVENTION

- Adopt a low-fat, low-cholesterol diet that will help keep arteries free of fatty deposits.
- Exercise! People who exercise are less likely to be overweight and less likely to develop atherosclerosis.
- Learn to control your emotions, rather than letting them control you. People who internalize stress are more likely to develop angina; many angina sufferers cite emotional outburst as a precipitator of attacks.
- If you smoke, quit. ■

ANKLES, PAINFUL

A

Read down this column to find your symptoms. Then read across.

SYMPTOMS	AILMENT/PROBLEM
◆ pain following injury; ankle is not mis-shapen and can move and bear weight without severe pain.	◆ Soft-tissue injury, such as sprain, strain, or tear
◆ dull ache or pain, ranging from the heel through the back of the ankle and into the lower calf, especially when running or jumping; mild swelling or tenderness.	◆ Achilles ***tendonitis***
◆ spontaneous onset of pain, redness, warmth, and swelling in ankle and/or other joints.	◆ Rheumatoid ***arthritis; bursitis***
◆ spontaneous onset of pain, redness, warmth, and swelling in ankle and/or other joints; recent illness, such as sore throat, rash, or other infection; fever of 100°F or higher.	◆ ***Rheumatic fever;*** infectious ***arthritis***
◆ gradual development of pain and stiffness in ankle, especially when the ankle is moved.	◆ Osteoarthritis
◆ sudden shooting pains in ankle; stiffness and tingling.	◆ ***Bone spur***
◆ chronic pain in feet and legs, especially when walking; feet and legs feel cold.	◆ Poor circulation; peripheral vascular disease
◆ sudden onset of intense, throbbing pain in ankle; ankle swelling; feeling of heat in joint.	◆ ***Gout***

WHAT TO DO	OTHER INFO
◆ See ***Sprains and Strains.*** If you are experiencing intense pain, you may have a severe sprain or a fracture that requires medical attention; call your doctor.	◆ Rest, ice, compression, and elevation—known collectively as RICE—are the initial treatment for most soft-tissue injuries. You may also need rehabilitation exercises.
◆ See ***Tendonitis.*** Rest the ankle, apply ice, and if needed, take pain-relieving medication. Wearing a half-inch lift or pad in the heel of your shoe may aid recovery.	◆ Osteopathy and chiropractic may be helpful. A doctor or physical therapist can prescribe stretching exercises. If the tendon is severed rather than inflamed, surgery is required.
◆ See ***Arthritis*** and ***Bursitis.*** Rest the ankle and apply ice for the first 24 hours, then heat. Take an anti-inflammatory drug for severe pain.	◆ Supplements of fish oil and ***vitamins C***, ***B_6***, and ***E*** may help relieve the pain of arthritis. Bursitis may respond to ***vitamin B_{12}*** injections.
◆ Call your doctor. You will need medical treatment, which is usually ***antibiotics*** and/or anti-inflammatory drugs. See ***Arthritis*** and ***Rheumatic Fever.***	◆ Rheumatic fever is a serious complication of prior streptococcal infection. Infectious arthritis is usually a complication of another illness or injury.
◆ See ***Arthritis.*** Your doctor may prescribe an ***analgesic*** and exercises. Heat treatments, physical or occupational therapy, acupuncture, and yoga may be helpful.	◆ Osteoarthritis involves loss of bone tissue and wearing out of joints, which may be caused by either injury or aging.
◆ See ***Bone Spurs.*** Rest your ankle and take an anti-inflammatory drug. Try padding inside your shoe.	◆ These abnormal growths at the ends of bones are common in older people who have ***disk problems*** and in people who use their muscles extensively, such as athletes or dancers.
◆ Call your doctor to have the underlying cause (***diabetes*** or vascular disease) diagnosed and treated. See ***Circulatory Problems.***	◆ The risk factors associated with poor circulation include aging, ***obesity,*** lack of exercise, and smoking. ***Vitamin E*** and the herb ***ginkgo*** *(Ginkgo biloba)* may be helpful.
◆ See ***Gout.*** Seek medical care. Treatment usually consists of anti-inflammatory medication and the drugs colchicine, allopurinol, or probenecid. Gout attacks may be prevented with a low-purine diet.	◆ Gout is caused by excess uric acid in a joint. ***Vitamin C,*** cherries, and the herb ***devil's claw*** *(Harpagophytum procumbens)* may be helpful.

ANKLES, SWOLLEN

A

Read down this column to find your symptoms. Then read across.

SYMPTOMS	AILMENT/PROBLEM
◆ swelling occurring after injury; ankle is not misshapen and can move and bear weight without severe pain.	◆ Soft-tissue injury, such as sprain, strain, or tear
◆ spontaneous onset of swelling, pain, redness, warmth, and stiffness in ankle and/or other joints.	◆ ***Arthritis***
◆ swelling after periods of standing; aching in lower leg, especially calf, that is worse at the end of the day; swelling and discoloration of veins in legs.	◆ ***Varicose veins***
◆ swelling accompanied by weakness, fatigue, and/or dizziness; shortness of breath that worsens; cough.	◆ Congestive heart failure
◆ swelling in ankle accompanied by a hard, red, cordlike swelling of calf veins on the same leg; pain; redness; tenderness; itching.	◆ ***Phlebitis***
◆ swelling while taking oral contraceptives or ***corticosteroid*** medications.	◆ Drug side effect
◆ swelling in a woman within a few days of her menstrual period; swelling not accompanied by pain.	◆ ***Premenstrual syndrome*** (PMS)
◆ painless swelling of ankles in a woman who is more than three months pregnant; swelling also occurs in face and fingers; weight gain of more than four pounds in the previous week.	◆ ***Pregnancy problem*** or preeclampsia

WHAT TO DO	OTHER INFO
◆ Apply cold compresses until the swelling goes down, then apply warmth. If you are experiencing intense pain, you may have a severe sprain or a fracture that requires medical attention. Call your doctor.	◆ Mild sprains are often compressed with an elastic bandage to reduce swelling. Severe sprains may require a cast or surgery. ◆ Use the homeopathic remedy ***Arnica*** to reduce swelling.
◆ Rest the ankle, apply heat, and take an anti-inflammatory drug.	◆ Hydrotherapy, acupuncture, nutritional therapy, and homeopathy have been found to relieve symptoms in some people.
◆ Rest and elevate your feet. If the leg is significantly swollen or painful, or sores appear on the skin, call your doctor.	◆ Possible treatments include pain medications, elastic stockings, and injections of a drug that causes vein walls to cave in.
◆ **Call your doctor now.** If you are short of breath, **seek emergency medical care.** In addition to various heart medications, treatment usually involves resting with legs raised and wearing anti-embolism stockings. See ***Heart Disease.***	◆ After conventional treatment has been established, nutritional and herbal therapy may be helpful in preventing the underlying heart disease from worsening.
◆ Call your doctor; a medical evaluation is necessary for diagnosis and treatment. Treatment usually involves rest, elevation of the leg, anti-inflammatory drugs, and possibly, ***antibiotics.*** If a blood clot has formed, you may be hospitalized and treated to ensure that the clot does not break off and travel to the lung.	◆ Warm compresses may ease inflammation for superficial phlebitis; elastic stockings or bandages may reduce swelling. Smokers should quit smoking.
◆ Call your doctor to discuss a possible change in medication.	
◆ Implement dietary changes and an exercise regimen.	◆ PMS is believed to be caused by a hormonal imbalance. Dietary changes, nutritional supplements, acupuncture, herbal therapy, and homeopathy may reduce symptoms.
◆ **Call your doctor now.** You could have preeclampsia, a serious condition requiring immediate medical treatment. See ***Pregnancy Problems.***	◆ Avoid standing for long periods, and rest with feet up. For preeclampsia, treatment includes rest, ***diuretics,*** and medication to lower blood pressure. In severe cases, hospitalization may be needed, with delivery of baby by induction or Cesarean section.

ANORЕXIA NERVOSA

A

SYMPTOMS

- significant weight loss.
- fear of becoming fat, even when emaciated.
- excessive dieting and exercising.
- distorted body image.
- abnormal food preoccupations, such as counting all calories or obsessively studying cookbooks.
- constipation.
- dry, sallow skin.
- increase in facial and body hair; loss of some head hair.
- cessation of menstrual periods.
- suppression of sexual desire.
- hands and feet cold at normal room temperature.
- chronic ***insomnia;*** an unexplained increase or decrease in energy level.

CALL YOUR DOCTOR IF:

- your child or teenager is obsessed with dieting and continues to feel fat, usually after a major weight loss.
- your child chronically uses laxatives, diuretics, emetics, or diet pills.
- your child overexercises to lose weight.
- your child is preoccupied with food, calories, and food preparation.

Anorexia nervosa is an eating disorder centered on an overwhelming dread of becoming fat. The result of this unfounded fear is self-starvation and major weight loss; in addition to emaciation, the undernourishment may cause hormonal disturbances, ***anemia,*** irregular heartbeat, brittle bones, and many other problems.

Usually the condition occurs during early adolescence to young adulthood, although it may strike later. Some 90 percent of sufferers are female; about 1 percent of American women are afflicted. Anorexia is dangerous, and professional help should be sought early. Prompt treatment will usually keep the condition from progressing, but some cases are very resistant to treatment and may require hospitalization. As many as 15 percent of anorexics die from complications.

Although its focus is on food, anorexia is an illness of the mind. Often it begins with a relatively normal desire to lose a few pounds. But because dieting only temporarily relieves underlying psychological problems, it soon becomes compulsive; food intake is gradually minimized until eating is almost eliminated. The victim becomes obsessed with her body image and frequently sees herself as fat even though the opposite is true. Ironically, she ritualizes food preparation and consumption. She becomes fascinated with recipes and cooking yet will not eat the food herself, especially in the presence of others. She may intersperse fasting with periodic binging and purging *(see* ***Bulimia****)*, particularly when she is trying to regain normal eating habits. About half of all anorexics become bulimic at some point.

Anorexics tend to come from families that have high standards of achievement, and they are often perfectionists, compulsive in many aspects of their life, especially school. Denial often accompanies their intense focus on remaining thin: Anorexics will typically refuse to admit that anything is wrong, and they become angry or defensive at expressions of concern by others.

CAUSES

While some studies indicate that genes can play a predisposing role in anorexia, most researchers believe that psychological factors are key. Anorexics tend to have low self-esteem and feel undeserving of love. In adolescence, such feelings may be exacerbated by sexual changes, cultural messages that glorify thinness, and pressures or tensions within the family. Extreme fasting may be an anorexic's way of attempting to exert control over her life—not just shaping her appearance but also retarding maturation and sexual development.

DIAGNOSTIC AND TEST PROCEDURES

Although some screening measures—such as the Eating Attitude Test (EAT)—can help identify potential anorexics, the predominant indicator is emaciation for no evident physical reason other than fasting. Blood and urine should be thoroughly tested to rule out other possible causes of weight loss and, more important, to reveal hormonal imbalances and low levels of such important nutrients as ***potassium, zinc,*** and fatty acids. Zinc deficiency—common in anorexics, especially those who are vegetarians—may impair many of the body's biochemical actions, retarding growth and sexual development, and ultimately contributing to the anorexia itself. Because extreme hormonal and nutritional imbalances can lead to death, frequent monitoring is essential.

TREATMENT

Psychotherapy, regular medical monitoring, and nutritional guidance should be part of any treatment program for anorexia. Close cooperation among all health professionals involved is important. All these professionals should be experienced specifically in treating eating disorders.

CONVENTIONAL MEDICINE

Treatment of anorexia will vary, depending on the stage at which it is recognized and the patient's willingness to cooperate. Hospitalization is usually necessary if the patient has lost more than 25 percent of normal body weight.

The primary focus of treatment is individual psychotherapy to uncover emotional problems and interpersonal difficulties that may underlie the disorder. Family therapy is also important if the patient is living at home, and behavior therapy can help change detrimental habits. In addition, a goal of a specific weight range should be set, and ongoing nutritional education and medical monitoring are important.

Supplements of ***zinc*** sulfate will redress any zinc deficiency. Other nutritional supplements, appetite enhancers, ***antidepressants,*** and ***anti-anxiety drugs*** are often prescribed as well.

ALTERNATIVE CHOICES

Alternative therapies may help with some of the symptoms of anorexia, and can serve as useful adjuncts to treatments that address nutrition and the emotional roots of the disorder.

HERBAL THERAPIES

See ***Anxiety*** for herbs that calm. To relax stomach muscles, try ***peppermint*** *(Mentha piperita);* make a tea by pouring boiling water over 1 to 3 tsp of dried herbs or a handful of fresh herbs. Steep for 10 to 15 minutes. Take a small cupful three or four times a day.

MIND/BODY MEDICINE

Yoga, t'ai chi, dance, and swimming are among the exercise or relaxation techniques that can reduce anxiety and increase body awareness.

EEG **biofeedback** can help bring anxiety and eating habits under control. **Hypnotherapy** may also be useful in exploring underlying emotional problems. ■

I M P O R T A N T !

As a parent or friend of someone coping with anorexia, avoid commenting about eating, weight, grooming, or school performance unless you are asked. Show her that you value her and others for their internal qualities, such as thoughtfulness and perceptiveness.

ANXIETY

SYMPTOMS

- heart palpitations.
- sense of impending doom.
- inability to concentrate.
- muscle tension; muscle aches.
- ***diarrhea.***
- ***chest pain.***
- dry mouth.
- excessive ***sweating.***
- undereating or overeating.
- ***insomnia.***
- irritability.
- breathlessness; hyperventilation.
- loss of sex drive. *(See **Impotence.**)*

For school-age children:

- fear of being away from the family.
- refusal to go to school.
- fear of strangers.
- unnecessary worry.

CALL YOUR DOCTOR IF:

- your anxiety seems irrational or more extreme than the situation warrants.
- your anxiety inhibits normal activities.
- low-level anxiety persists for many weeks.
- your symptoms suddenly become severe or uncontrollable. You may be experiencing a ***panic attack.***
- anxiety is accompanied by weight loss and bulging of the eyes; you may have ***thyroid problems.***

Almost everyone feels anxious from time to time. When there is a threat of some kind, anxiety is normal—bound up with the way the body prepares to deal with danger: Adrenaline and cortisone are released in the bloodstream; heart rate quickens; breathing becomes shallow and rapid; muscles tense; sugar is released by the liver; and the mind goes on full alert. But when anxiety is not tied to an identifiable threat or is more severe and long-lasting than warranted, it is a clinical disorder, debilitating and disruptive.

Many different anxiety disorders are recognized. Among them are ***phobias*** (fear of certain situations, such as confining spaces, or of particular things, such as insects); ***panic attacks*** (a sudden onset of extreme fear or tension, for no evident reason); ***obsessive-compulsive disorder*** (persistent, irrational thoughts, such as a dread of infection, or repetitive behavior, such as checking that doors are locked); ***posttraumatic stress disorder*** (prolonged anxiety after a traumatic event); and generalized—or "free-floating"—anxiety (an inexplicable feeling of apprehension that may last for months).

Anxiety disorders can vary greatly in their severity; they may be mild or completely immobilizing. The incidence of the different disorders also varies: Phobias, panic attacks, and obsessive-compulsive disorder, for example, occur less frequently than generalized anxiety (which afflicts twice as many women as men). The disorders usually become noticeable during the teen years or early adulthood and are considerably more common among adults than children.

Some anxieties are very difficult to treat; others respond well to medications, psychotherapy, and alternative therapies. What does not work is self-treatment with alcohol or recreational drugs to alleviate the symptoms. Many sufferers choose this path, but ultimately it will only make the condition worse.

CAUSES

Anxiety can be caused by a recognizable stress—such as an accident, a death in the family, or the loss of a job; in such cases, adjustments to the situation, along with the passage of time, will have an ameliorating effect. In other cases, the stress is invisible—a buried memory of some unhappy or frightening facet of childhood, lurking below the surface of the conscious mind and revealing its presence in anxiety.

Genetic inheritance may predispose some individuals to anxiety: Studies of identical twins show that if one member of an identical pair suffers from anxiety, there is at least a 50 percent chance that the other will, as well. Food sensitivities may also contribute to anxiety, although more research must be done to certify this connection. In addition, anxiety frequently follows a sudden withdrawal from alcohol, tobacco, or other drugs.

DIAGNOSTIC AND TEST PROCEDURES

The first step is to rule out the possibility that the symptoms are being caused by an organic disease. Among the conditions that produce symptoms similar to those of anxiety are hyperthyroidism *(see* ***Thyroid Problems****);* hyper- or hypocalcemia (too much or too little calcium); coronary artery disease *(see* ***Heart Disease****);* tachycardia (rapid heart rate—*see* ***Heart Arrhythmias***); and other heart problems. A thorough evaluation by your doctor will determine if any of these conditions are the cause.

If no organic culprit can be found and the symptoms seem out of proportion to any situation you are facing, the condition will be classified as an anxiety disorder.

TREATMENT

Anxiety can be treated with conventional medications, psychotherapy, and many alternative approaches. A combination of conventional and alternative methods is often effective.

CONVENTIONAL MEDICINE

Psychotherapy and psychoanalysis both aim at identifying conflicts and other stresses—perhaps long buried—that may lie at the roots of anxiety. Behavior modification—a therapy that concentrates on changing patterns of behavior—can help the patient avert anxiety or better cope with it, as can cognitive therapy, which concentrates on changing ways of thinking.

Medication is useful for alleviating the symptoms of anxiety and is often prescribed in conjunction with other therapies. The most prominent of ***antianxiety drugs*** are those known as ***benzodiazepines;*** among them are ***lorazepam, diazepam, alprazolam,*** and ***clonazepam.*** They have drawbacks: Benzodiazepines sometimes cause drowsiness, irritability, dizziness, and dependency. Nonetheless, in recent decades they have largely replaced barbiturates, which not only pose a clear danger of addiction but also can be a threat with suicidal patients. Another antianxiety drug is ***buspirone.*** It has fewer side effects than the benzodiazepines but should not be taken if you have liver or kidney disease; also, check with your doctor before taking it during pregnancy or breast-feeding.

ALTERNATIVE CHOICES

Many alternative practices and treatments can relieve the symptoms of anxiety. **Meditation,** exercise (especially aerobic exercise), and **relaxation** techniques are among the most effective. Their usefulness varies from person to person, however. For example, people with physical symptoms—such as stomachache or sweating—do better with exercise, while those with mental symptoms benefit more from meditation or another form of mental relaxation.

Chinese and **Ayurvedic medicine** use various herbal preparations that can serve as a tonic for the whole system and diminish tension.

A gentle **massage** will help relax almost everyone.

ACUPRESSURE

A number of acupressure points are said to help calm the body and quiet the mind. Two are shown on page 137. For others, consult a practitioner. The effectiveness of particular pressure points is thought to depend on the underlying reasons for the anxiety.

ACUPUNCTURE

Weekly acupuncture treatments—also tailored to the cause of the anxiety—may be beneficial. Consult an acupuncturist experienced in treating mental states.

AROMATHERAPY

Aromatherapy is believed to be very effective with anxiety. Try essential oil of ***lavender,*** jasmine, or blue ***chamomile.*** Put a drop or two on a tissue and inhale it, or include the oils in a steam inhalation or a steamy bath. Or you can rub a drop into your temples.

BACH FLOWER REMEDIES

Developed at the turn of the 20th century by the British bacteriologist and homeopath Edward Bach, these remedies are used to treat a variety of psychological states. In all, there are 38 remedies, each specific to a particular emotional condition. Liquid in form, the remedies are made by soaking flowers on the top of a bowl of water in the sun for several hours; this procedure, according to practitioners, releases the flowers' energy into the water. Bach remedies can be bought at health food stores.

Agrimony and aspen are considered useful for mild to moderate cases of anxiety. Cherry plum used alone is said to be good for severe cases, or it can be used as part of the so-called rescue remedy—a combination of flowers recommended for all manner of anxiety-provoking situations, from a visit to the dentist to the shock felt after a car accident. Put 5 drops into water or 2 drops directly on your tongue. Use as often as needed, up to every hour.

HERBAL THERAPIES

Chamomile *(Matricaria recutita),* lemon balm *(Melissa officinalis),* and linden (*Tilia* spp.) flowers are all considered mild relaxants and tranquilizers. Lemon balm is particularly good for digestive problems linked to anxiety. ***Skullcap*** *(Scutellaria lateriflora)* is somewhat stronger, while ***valerian*** *(Valeriana officinalis),* ***hops*** *(Humulus lupulus),* and ***passionflower*** *(Passiflora incarnata)* all have an even stronger effect on the central nervous system. These three help with ***insomnia*** and can be combined to advantage. However, hops should not be used with marked ***depression,*** and valerian—to be effective—must be used in fairly high dosage (½ to 1 tsp of the tincture). If the anxiety is associated with palpitations, use motherwort *(Leonurus cardiaca).* If it is connected to high blood pressure, use cramp *(Viburnum opulus)* bark and linden blossoms. For all herbs, make an infusion by pouring boiling water over 1 to 3 tsp of the dried herbs or a handful of fresh herbs. Steep for 10 to 15 minutes. Take a small cupful three or four times a day.

You can buy the tincture of any of these herbs in a health food store; follow the directions on the bottle.

HOMEOPATHY

If the anxiety is the result of a sudden fright or shock, try ***Aconite. Ignatia*** is the "grief remedy," said to benefit someone who is upset by a sudden loss. ***Gelsemium*** is recommended for anticipatory and performance anxiety, such as stage fright or agoraphobia (a fear of public places). The homeopathic minerals *Biochemic phosphates* (3x) relieve the physical symptoms of anxiety. If none of these prove effective, seek out a homeopath. A skilled practitioner may be able to prescribe a mixture whose ingredients and strength are better suited to your anxiety.

MIND/BODY MEDICINE

A wide variety of mind/body treatments and practices can relieve anxiety. The key is to find the one or two that you prefer and to use them consistently. Among the useful meditation and relaxation techniques are progressive muscle relaxation, autogenic training, the **relaxation response,** transcendental **meditation** (TM), and Oriental exercise techniques such as **yoga, t'ai chi,** and **qigong.** For best results, meditation and relaxation practices should be undertaken daily or even twice a day.

Since anxiety is almost always accompanied by shallow breathing, deep breathing exercises are very helpful; it is impossible to be anxious when breathing deeply and slowly. Try the following form of **yoga** breathing: Lie on your back in a comfortable place. Breathe in slowly through

ACUPRESSURE

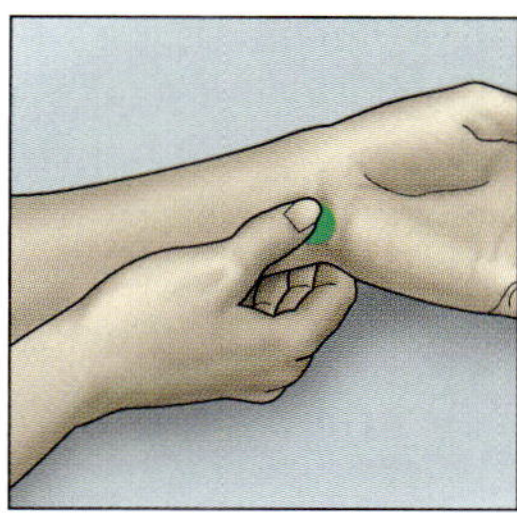

1 Anxiety-induced sleeping problems may be improved by pressing Heart 7, located along the crease on the inside of the wrist, directly in line with the little finger. Squeeze firmly between the thumb and index finger for one minute, then repeat on the other hand.

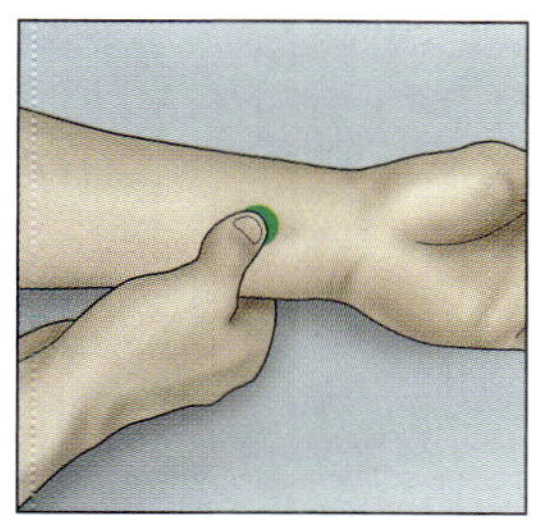

2 To help calm nerves and reduce feelings of uneasiness, press Pericardium 6. Place your thumb in the center of your inner wrist, two finger widths from the wrist crease and between the two bones of the forearm. Press firmly for one minute, three to five times, then repeat on the other arm.

your nose, using your diaphragm to suck air into your lungs while allowing your abdomen to expand. (Put your hand on your abdomen just below the navel to make sure the abdomen is being pushed up and out by the diaphragm.) After the abdomen is expanded, continue to inhale as deeply as possible. Then exhale through your nose, reversing the process: Contract the abdomen while exhaling slowly and completely. Repeat several times.

Therapeutic Touch (which does not involve direct touch) is particularly useful for bedridden patients and those with chronic diseases or injuries too sensitive for direct touch. In addition to relieving anxiety, Therapeutic Touch also diminishes pain. Call your hospital for the name of a nurse who practices it.

EEG **biofeedback,** used to retrain thought patterns, can be especially helpful with conditions that combine both physical and mental symptoms—as is the case with anxiety. In a series of sessions with a therapist, the patient watches his or her own brain-wave patterns on an electroencephalograph and gradually learns to control the waves. Practitioners estimate that after about a dozen sessions, the patient will be able to exert the control over mental activity without the help of the therapist or monitoring instrument.

Hypnotherapy is recommended for specific ***phobias*** such as fear of flying, stage fright, or fear of exams and sports contests. It also helps with general anxiety. Children and adolescents learn self-hypnosis far more quickly than adults, perhaps because they are so accustomed to using their imaginations. Hypnosis is not a magical or sinister process in which you are under the control of the hypnotist; instead, it is a form of concentration. All hypnosis is self-hypnosis; the hypnotist is there simply to teach you how to use the technique to best advantage. Hypnotherapy can frequently be enhanced if used in combination with biofeedback.

AT-HOME REMEDIES

- Daily exercise can be one of the most potent treatments for anxiety symptoms. If you find that exercise works for you, push yourself to go for brisk walks, or undertake an active sport that you enjoy.
- ***Magnesium*** supplements are helpful, especially if you suffer from muscle spasms. Take no more than 300 mg three times a day; too much magnesium can cause diarrhea.
- Avoid alcohol, and reduce or eliminate your consumption of sugar and caffeine.
- Trim a hectic schedule to its most essential items, and do your best to avoid activities you don't find relaxing.
- If you begin to hyperventilate, exhale into a paper bag and inhale the air within the bag. This increases the amount of carbon dioxide you are inhaling, which can reduce the urge to hyperventilate. Inhaling from a bag will help relieve any dizziness or tingling you might feel. ■

APPENDICITIS

A

SYMPTOMS

The classic symptoms of appendicitis include:

- dull pain near the navel or the upper abdomen that becomes sharp as it moves to the lower right abdomen. This is usually the first sign.
- loss of appetite.
- nausea and/or vomiting soon after abdominal pain begins.
- temperature of 99°F to 102°F.
- constipation or diarrhea with gas.

Almost half the time, other symptoms appear, including:

- dull or sharp pain anywhere in the upper or lower abdomen, back, or rectum.
- painful urination.
- vomiting that precedes the abdominal pain.

CALL YOUR DOCTOR IF:

- you have pain that matches the symptoms above. Acute appendicitis is a medical emergency that can be fatal. Prompt surgery is often essential. Do not eat, drink, or use any pain remedies, ***antacids, laxatives,*** or heating pads, which can cause an inflamed appendix to rupture.
- you have symptoms of appendicitis, but your appendix has already been removed. You may have ***pelvic inflammatory disease, colorectal cancer, diverticulitis,*** a tubal pregnancy, ***gastroenteritis,*** or problems with your colon. **Seek medical care immediately.**

Appendicitis is an inflammation of the appendix, a 3½-inch-long tube of tissue that extends from the large intestine. The appendix contains lymphoid tissue and may produce antibodies; however, no one is absolutely certain what its function is. One thing we do know: We can live without it, without apparent consequences.

Appendicitis is a medical emergency that requires prompt surgery to remove the appendix. Left untreated, an inflamed appendix will eventually burst, or perforate, spilling infection into the abdominal cavity. This can lead to peritonitis, a serious ***infection*** of the abdominal cavity's lining (the peritoneum) that can be fatal unless it is treated quickly with strong antibiotics.

Sometimes a pus-filled abscess forms outside the inflamed appendix. Fibrous scar tissue then "walls off" the appendix from the rest of the abdomen, preventing infection from spreading. An abscessed appendix is a less urgent situation, but unfortunately, it can't be identified without surgery. For this reason, all cases of appendicitis are treated as emergencies.

In the United States, 1 in 15 people gets appendicitis. Although it can strike at any age, appendicitis is rare under age 2 and most common between ages 10 and 30.

CAUSES

Appendicitis occurs when the tube-shaped appendix becomes blocked, often by fecal material, a foreign body, or ***cancer.*** Blockage may also be due to infection: Like other lymphoid tissue, the appendix swells in response to any infection in the body. As it expands, its opening gradually closes.

DIAGNOSTIC AND TEST PROCEDURES

Diagnosing appendicitis can be tricky. Time is critical, yet appendicitis symptoms are frequently vague, or extremely similar to other, less urgent ailments (including ***bladder infection, colitis, Crohn's disease, gastritis, gastroenteritis,*** and ***ovary problems***). By gently pressing on your lower right abdomen, your doctor will feel for a hardened, inflamed appendix. Appendicitis can cause

WARNING SIGNS

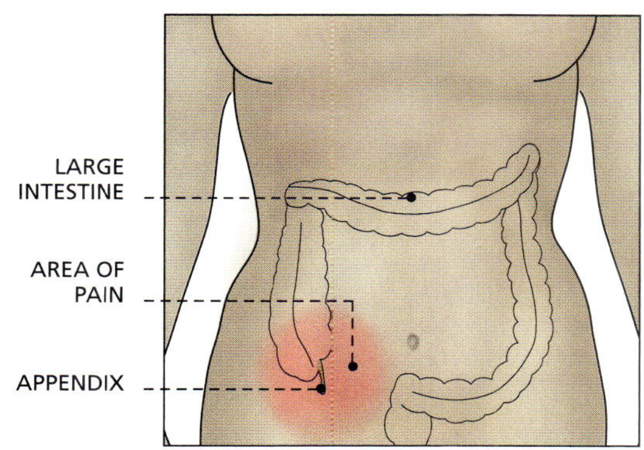

The appendix is a 3½-inch-long extension of the large intestine. If it becomes blocked or its opening to the intestine obstructed in some way, the appendix can become inflamed—the classic symptom of which is a persistent sharp pain in the lower right side of the abdomen *(above).*

rectal pain instead of abdominal pain, so your doctor will also examine your rectum by inserting a lubricated, gloved finger. A blood test will show if your white blood cell count is elevated, meaning your body is fighting infection. CT scans and ultrasound have proved fast and reliable—though not perfect—in revealing appendicitis.

TREATMENT

Surgery to remove the appendix, which is called an appendectomy, is the standard treatment for appendicitis.

CONVENTIONAL MEDICINE

If appendicitis is even suspected, physicians tend to err on the side of safety and quickly remove the appendix to avoid its rupture. If the appendix has formed an abscess, you may have two procedures: one to drain the abscess of pus and fluid, and a later one to remove the appendix.

Antibiotics are given before an appendectomy to fight possible peritonitis. General anesthesia is given, and the appendix is removed through a 4-inch incision. If you have peritonitis, the abdomen is also drained of pus. Within 12 hours of surgery you may get up and move around. You can usually return to normal activities in two or three weeks. If surgery is done with a laparoscope (a thin telescope-like instrument for viewing inside the abdomen), the incision is smaller and recovery is faster.

ALTERNATIVE CHOICES

If you have appendicitis you need a physician's care, but alternative therapies can be helpful in preparing for or recuperating from appendectomy.

ACUPRESSURE

Massaging the following points each day can help to speed your recovery from appendectomy. To improve appetite and intestinal function, massage Stomach 36 and Bladder 25; add Large Intestine 4 to calm pain; Liver 3 to reduce abdominal bloating; and Spleen 6 to promote overall healing. See the ***Appendix*** for information on point locations.

HOMEOPATHY

Taken before surgery, one dose of ***Arnica*** (30c) may minimize pain and swelling; repeat every 2 hours, as needed, until the pain and swelling is gone. One dose of ***Phosphorus*** (30c), also taken before surgery, may help minimize nausea from the anesthesia; if needed, repeat every two hours after surgery until the nausea dissipates. After surgery, applying a solution of ***Hypericum*** and *Calendula* (4 drops of each, added to 1 cup water) three or four times daily can help your incision heal.

AT-HOME CARE

- ◆ Keep your incision clean to promote healing and avoid infection.
- ◆ Once your incision has closed, prick open a ***vitamin E*** capsule and apply the gel directly to your wound to minimize scarring. ■

ARM PAIN

A

Read down this column to find your symptoms. Then read across.

SYMPTOMS	AILMENT/PROBLEM
◆ moderate to severe pain following an injury; arm is not misshapen.	◆ Soft-tissue injury, such as a sprain or strain
◆ radiating pain in elbow or biceps when bending arm.	◆ ***Tendonitis***
◆ gradually worsening pain in elbow, at bony protuberance, that may radiate down forearm into hand; pain follows chronic repetitive movement.	◆ Epicondylitis, commonly known as ***tennis elbow***
◆ pain in arm or hand with weakness, numbness, or tingling; difficulty clenching the fist or grasping small objects.	◆ ***Carpal tunnel syndrome***
◆ spontaneous onset of pain, redness, warmth, and swelling in elbow and/or other joints.	◆ Rheumatoid ***arthritis; gout; bursitis***
◆ spontaneous onset of pain, redness, warmth, and swelling in elbow and/or other joints; fever and general malaise.	◆ Bone or joint infection, such as osteomyelitis or infectious ***arthritis***
◆ arm pain with numbness or tingling; stiff neck; cracking sound when neck is moved.	◆ Cervical osteoarthritis (cervical spondylosis) or other problem involving neck bones
◆ pain accompanied by numbness or tingling that may radiate to the hand; reduced ability to pick up and hold objects with pinched fingers.	◆ ***Neuralgia***
◆ pain that radiates from center of chest down left arm during exercise, then disappears after five minutes of rest.	◆ ***Angina***
◆ persistent severe pain radiating from center of chest down left arm; nausea; shortness of breath.	◆ ***Heart attack***

A

WHAT TO DO	OTHER INFO
◆ See ***Sprains and Strains.***	◆ A homeopathic cream containing ***Arnica*** may be helpful.
◆ Apply ice and stretch the area.	◆ Osteopathy, chiropractic, or acupuncture may be helpful.
◆ Take a pain reliever if needed, rest the arm, and exercise it gently.	◆ Your doctor may advise use of a splint, heat therapy, or physical therapy. Acupuncture or chiropractic may help.
◆ Stop, limit, or modify the activity that brings on the discomfort. A wrist splint may be helpful.	◆ Pain may be temporarily relieved by shaking the hands vigorously or dangling the arms. Acupuncture, osteopathy, or chiropractic may be helpful.
◆ For pain relief, rest the arm; apply ice for the first 24 hours, then heat; and take an anti-inflammatory drug.	◆ ***Vitamins C, B_6,*** and ***E*** may help arthritis. Gout sometimes can be controlled by a low-purine diet but often requires medication to prevent recurrences.
◆ The usual treatment is joint aspiration—surgical cleansing—and ***antibiotics.***	◆ If more than one joint is affected, you should be examined for ***rheumatic fever.***
◆ See ***Arthritis.***	◆ Spinal bones may be putting pressure on nerves in the neck. Chiropractic may help.
◆ See ***Neuralgia.***	◆ The cause may be cervical osteoarthritis. Acupuncture may help relieve pain.
◆ See ***Angina, Heart Attack,*** and ***Heart Disease.*** If you have angina, you will probably be treated with ***nitroglycerin.*** If this is the first time you have had this pain or if the pain does not abate when you stop exerting yourself, **call your doctor, 911, or your emergency number now.**	◆ Angina is a chronic condition. Alternative methods such as acupuncture, chelation therapy, or nutritional therapy may help.
◆ **Call your doctor, 911, or your emergency number now.** See page 67 of ***Emergencies/First Aid*** and ***Heart Attack.***	◆ Medications, exercise, dietary changes, relaxation techniques, herbal therapies, and many other treatments may be used for preventive purposes or after conventional emergency treatment.

ARTHRITIS

A

SYMPTOMS

- Pain and progressive stiffness without noticeable swelling, chills, or fever during normal activities probably indicate the gradual onset of **osteoarthritis.**
- Painful swelling, inflammation, and stiffness in the arms, legs, wrists, or fingers in the same joints on both sides of the body, especially on awakening, may be signs of **rheumatoid arthritis.**
- Fever, joint inflammation, tenderness, and sharp pain, sometimes accompanied by chills and associated with an injury or another illness, may indicate **infectious arthritis.**
- In children, intermittent fever, loss of appetite, weight loss, anemia, or blotchy rash on the arms and legs may signal **juvenile rheumatoid arthritis.**

CALL YOUR DOCTOR IF:

- the pain and stiffness come on quickly, whether from an injury or an unknown cause; you may be experiencing the onset of **rheumatoid arthritis.**
- the pain is accompanied by fever; you may have **infectious arthritis.**
- you notice pain and stiffness in your arms, legs, or back after sitting for short periods or after a night's sleep; you may be developing **osteoarthritis** or another arthritic condition.
- a child develops pain or a rash on armpits, knees, wrists, and ankles, or has fever swings, poor appetite, and weight loss; the child may have **juvenile rheumatoid arthritis.**

American workers lose more time to pain in the joints than to any other type of ailment. To the extent that our jobs and leisure activities become more sedentary, the likelihood of such ailments increases. Fortunately, many of the problems commonly labeled "arthritis" are easily healed or controlled, and the prospects of debilitating complications are far less than they were for our parents and grandparents.

Although the term is applied to a wide variety of disorders, arthritis means the inflammation of a joint, whether as the result of a disease, an infection, a genetic defect, or some other cause. Many people, however, perceive it as any kind of pain or discomfort associated with body movement, including such localized problems as low back pain, ***bursitis, tendonitis,*** and general stiffness or pain in the joints. *(See also **Backache** and **Joint Pain.**)*

For many—although by no means everyone—arthritis seems to be an inevitable part of the aging process, and there are no signs of real cures on the immediate horizon. On the positive side, advances in both conventional medical treatment and alternative therapies make living with arthritis more bearable.

MAJOR TYPES OF ARTHRITIS

Rheumatoid arthritis, sometimes called rheumatism or synovitis, tends to affect people over the age of 40, and women two to three times as frequently as men. It may occur in children, particularly girls from 2 to 5 years of age. It is characterized by inflammation and pain in the hands—especially the knuckles and second joints—as well as in the arms, legs, and feet, and by general fatigue and sleeplessness. It can also cause systemic damage to other parts of the body, including the heart, lungs, eyes, nerves, and muscles. The discomfort of rheumatoid arthritis can develop over weeks or months and tends to be most severe on awakening.

Rheumatoid arthritis in older people may eventually cause the hands and feet to become gnarled and misshapen as muscles weaken, tendons shrink, and the ends of bones become abnormally enlarged.

While there is no complete cure, treatment begun at the onset of the disorder relieves symptoms in most people. Symptoms may endure for five years or more, after which they tend to stabilize or decline. With early treatment, the likelihood of permanent disability is reduced in all but 5 to 10 percent of sufferers.

Juvenile rheumatoid arthritis, or Still's disease, is characterized by chronic fever and anemia. The disease can also have secondary effects on the heart, lungs, eyes, and nervous system. Arthritic episodes in children younger than the age of five can last for several weeks and may recur, although the symptoms tend to be less severe in recurrent attacks. Treatment is essentially the same as for adults, with heavy emphasis on physical therapy and exercise to keep growing bodies active. Permanent damage from juvenile rheumatoid arthritis is now rare, and most affected children recover from the disease fully without experiencing any lasting disabilities.

Infectious arthritis refers to various ailments that affect larger arm and leg joints as well as the fingers or toes. Arthritic infection is usually a complication of an injury or of another disease and is much less common than arthritic conditions that come on with age. Because the symptoms may be masked by the primary injury or illness, however, infectious arthritis may go unnoticed and, if left untreated, can result in permanent disability.

Osteoarthritis, or degenerative joint disease, refers to the pain and inflammation that can result from the systematic loss of bone tissue in the joints. It is the most common form of arthritis, particularly in the elderly. In osteoarthritis, the protective cartilage at the ends of bones in joints—especially in the spine and legs—gradually wears away. The inner bone surfaces become exposed and rub together. In some cases, bony spurs develop on the edges of joints, causing damage to muscles and nerves, pain, deformity, and difficulty in movement. *(See **Bone Spurs.**)*

Although the mechanism of osteoarthritis is unknown, some people appear to have a genetic predisposition to degenerative bone disorders. In rare cases, congenital bone deformation appears at an early age. Misuse of anabolic steroids, which are popular among some athletes, can

JOINT DEGENERATION

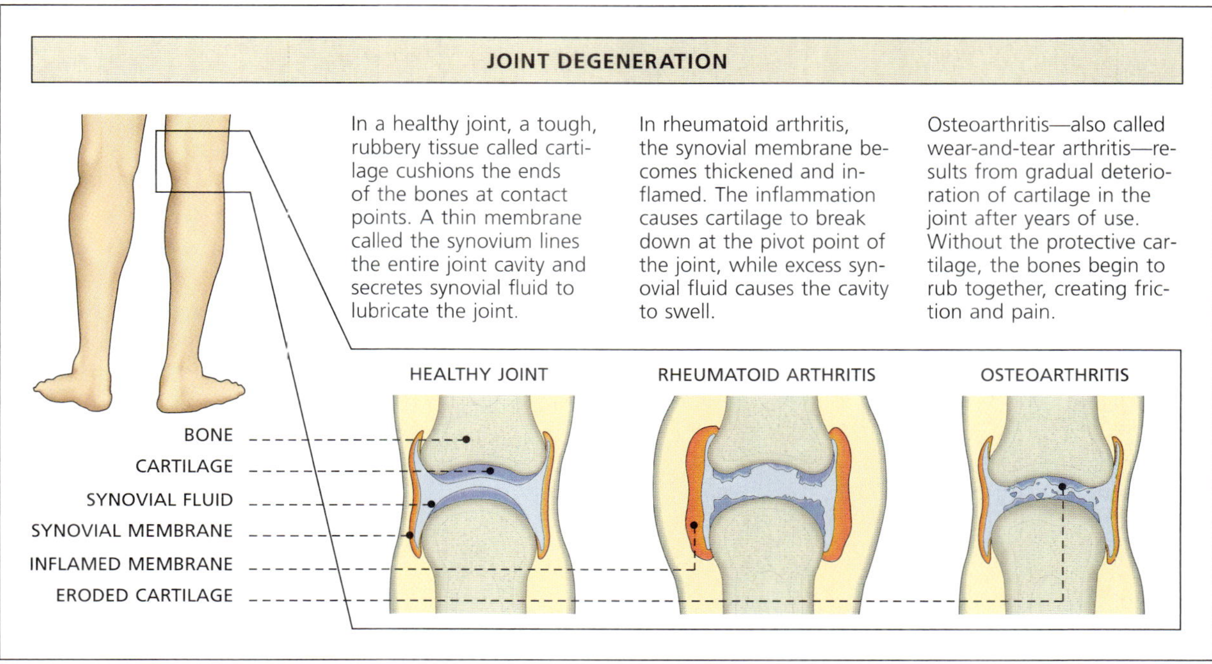

In a healthy joint, a tough, rubbery tissue called cartilage cushions the ends of the bones at contact points. A thin membrane called the synovium lines the entire joint cavity and secretes synovial fluid to lubricate the joint.

In rheumatoid arthritis, the synovial membrane becomes thickened and inflamed. The inflammation causes cartilage to break down at the pivot point of the joint, while excess synovial fluid causes the cavity to swell.

Osteoarthritis—also called wear-and-tear arthritis—results from gradual deterioration of cartilage in the joint after years of use. Without the protective cartilage, the bones begin to rub together, creating friction and pain.

also bring on early osteoarthritic degeneration.

In many people the onset of osteoarthritis is gradual and has no serious debilitating effect, although it can change the shape and size of bones. In other people, bony growths and gnarled joints may cause painful muscle inflammation or nerve damage, along with significant changes in posture and mobility.

Other arthritic conditions include ankylosing spondylitis (arthritis of the spine), ***bone spurs*** (bony growths on the vertebrae or other areas), ***gout*** (crystal arthritis), and systemic ***lupus*** (inflammatory connective-tissue disease). See also ***Back Problems, Bursitis,*** and ***Tendonitis,*** all of which can result from strain, injury, or other irritation.

CAUSES

Each of the three major types of arthritic condition has its own apparent causes:

Rheumatoid arthritis. The cause of rheumatoid arthritis is not fully understood. Some researchers think it may be an autoimmune disorder *(see **Immune Problems**).* Another theory suggests that it is an immune reaction to a viral or bacterial infection somewhere in the body.

Infectious arthritis. This type of arthritis is caused by a bacterial or viral invasion of the joints and typically comes on the heels of another disease, such as ***staph infection, tuberculosis, gonorrhea,*** or ***Lyme disease.***

Osteoarthritis. This common degenerative joint disease is part of the aging process. The condition may be associated with broken bones and can develop in young adults from wear and tear on the body's load-bearing joints, often as a result of intense athletic activity. In cases of osteoarthritis, the cartilage and bone cannot repair themselves sufficiently to keep up with the damage.

DIAGNOSTIC AND TEST PROCEDURES

In addition to symptom analysis, blood tests are commonly used to confirm **rheumatoid arthritis;** the majority of sufferers have antibodies called rheumatoid factors (RF) in their blood, although RF may also be present in other disorders.

X-rays are used to diagnose **osteoarthritis,** typically revealing shrunken joints or calcification at the ends of the bones. If your doctor suspects **infectious arthritis** as a complication of some other disease, testing a sample of fluid from the affected joint will usually confirm the diagnosis.

TREATMENT

Sometimes arthritic damage can be slowed or stopped, but in most cases the damage continues as the disease runs its course, regardless of whether drugs or other therapies are used to relieve the symptoms. Predictably, the duration and intensity of the actual pain and discomfort depend on the type of arthritis and the degree of severity. The process may take a few days in the case of minor joint problems in otherwise healthy adults, while in others it may last months or years. In older people with severe rheumatoid or degenerative conditions, for example, the effects may be lifelong.

CONVENTIONAL MEDICINE

In the case of localized pain, stiffness, and immobility, the typical three-stage therapy consists of medication to relieve pain and inflammation, rest to let injured tissues heal themselves, and exercise to rebuild mobility and strength.

To reduce pain and inflammation in mild cases of **rheumatoid arthritis** and **osteoarthritis,** your doctor may prescribe ***aspirin,*** another ***nonsteroidal anti-inflammatory drug (NSAID)*** such as ***ibuprofen,*** or one of the new ***NSAIDs*** known as the ***COX-2 inhibitors.*** These drugs fight pain and inflammation without causing stomach ulcers. Other drugs, including methotrexate and D-penicillamine, may induce the remission of **rheumatoid arthritis.** Physicians may combine these drugs with regimens of heat, rest and exercise, physical therapy, and physical aids such as canes or walkers. Controlled application of deep heat and ultrasound can also soothe affected joints.

In more advanced cases, your doctor may recommend ***corticosteroid*** injections to ease the pain and stiffness of affected joints. Depending on the individual, results range from temporary relief to long-lasting suppression of symptoms.

Early this century, researchers discovered that certain compounds containing gold, delivered orally or by injection, gave relief to some patients and total remission in others. Note, however, that because the side effects of gold therapy can range from minor skin rash to severe blood and kidney disorders, this therapy should be approached with caution.

WARNING!

BEWARE OF QUACK CURES

Because neither conventional nor alternative medicine can cure rheumatoid arthritis or osteoarthritis, unproven treatments abound. Over the years, arthritis sufferers have reported relief with remedies ranging from copper bracelets to laser treatments. While such therapies claim success in individual cases, you should exercise caution and a degree of skepticism when considering what's right for you.

In general, untested and unproven remedies that aren't injected or swallowed will probably do no harm. Invasive treatments may have dangerous side effects or cause other systemic problems, however. The results, if any, may not justify the money spent. The Arthritis Foundation estimates that people from every income bracket spend more than a billion dollars each year on dubious arthritis treatments.

Your best defense against unscrupulous practices is to know as much as you can about your ailment and the risks and intended benefits of suggested treatments. Understanding the underlying causes of the disease and maintaining a healthy skepticism about claims for quick cures will help you avoid placing your health and your pocketbook at risk.

In cases of arthritic complications from injury or infection, specific therapy will depend on the nature and seriousness of the underlying condition. The major concern is for healing the affected area before more serious complications occur. Treatment of **infectious arthritis** typically involves large intravenous doses of ***antibiotics*** as well as drainage of excess fluid from the joints.

Various forms of surgery may be needed to reduce the discomfort of arthritis or to restore mobility. Synovectomy is the removal of damaged connective tissue lining a joint cavity, and allows the body to regenerate new, healthy tissue in its place. This operation is most common in the knee. In cases of severe arthritic damage to the neck or foot, bones can be surgically removed or fused. Although movement is limited after such surgery, the operations relieve excruciating pain and help prevent further damage to nerves or blood vessels.

If arthritic pain and inflammation become truly unbearable, or arthritic joints simply refuse to function, the answer may lie in surgical replacement. Today, hip and shoulder joints—as well as smaller joints in elbows, knees, and fingers—can be replaced with reliable artificial joints made of stainless steel and plastic.

Because one of the most trying aspects of arthritis is learning to live with pain, many doctors recommend training in pain management, including cognitive therapy. Such programs focus on improving patients' emotional and psychological well-being by teaching them how to relax and conduct their daily activities at a realistic pace. Learning to overcome mental stress and anxiety can be the key to coping with the physical limitations that may accompany chronic rheumatoid arthritis and osteoarthritis. Cognitive therapy may include various techniques for activity scheduling, imaging, relaxation, distraction, and creative problem solving.

ALTERNATIVE CHOICES

Because medical science has not found any full cures for the various kinds of arthritis, many people turn to alternative treatments to ease their pain and disability. While few alternative approaches can definitively be substantiated in controlled studies of their effectiveness, research indicates that some of these methods can play a significant role in treating arthritic ailments. **Meditation,** self-hypnosis, **guided imagery,** and **relaxation** techniques, for example, can have positive effects in controlling chronic arthritis pain. Arthritis sufferers should be extremely cautious, however, about practices that claim to "cure" the disease. Furthermore, what appears to work for one person under a given set of circumstances may not work at all for someone else.

ACUPRESSURE AND ACUPUNCTURE

Some arthritis patients find that these therapies, administered by a trained practitioner, offer effective relief from the pain of **rheumatoid arthritis** or **osteoarthritis** for several weeks or months.

BODY WORK

In combination with other treatments, soft-tissue massage around affected joints or compassionate touching by a physician or other practitioner can have a comforting, reassuring effect on those who suffer from arthritis. Manipulation by a trained therapist constitutes passive exercise for people unable to perform vigorous exercise. In addition to making a patient feel better physically, sympathetically administered touch therapy can help soothe the emotional effects of chronic illness. Studies suggest that relieving stress and tension has a positive influence on the body's hormonal balance.

CHIROPRACTIC

After diagnostic examination, testing, and appropriate conventional therapy, a chiropractor may manipulate the spine and other arthritic joints to relieve pain and help reestablish normal use.

HERBAL THERAPIES

Among the various remedies herbalists recommend to relieve pain is up to 1 tsp of tincture made from 2 parts willow (*Salix* spp.) bark and 1 part each of ***black cohosh*** *(Cimicifuga racemosa)* and ***nettle*** *(Urtica dioica),* taken once a day. To relieve muscle tension, rub a tincture of ***lobelia*** *(Lobelia inflata)* and cramp *(Viburnum opulus)* bark

YOGA TECHNIQUES

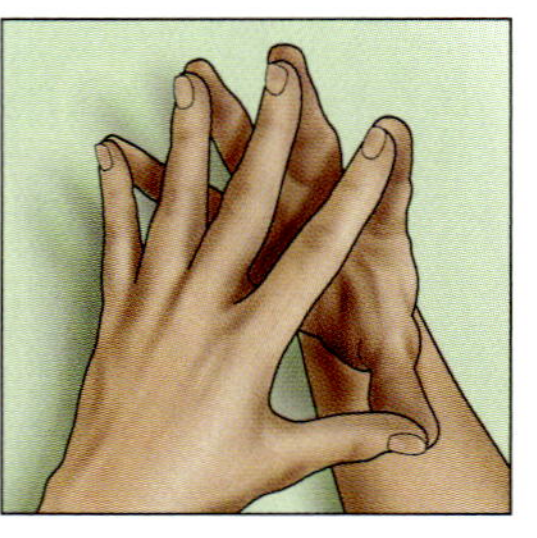

1 To loosen the joints of the hand, use the **Spider Push-Up.** Press your fingertips together firmly, palms two to three inches apart. Push your palms toward each other while keeping your fingertips touching. Do this 20 times.

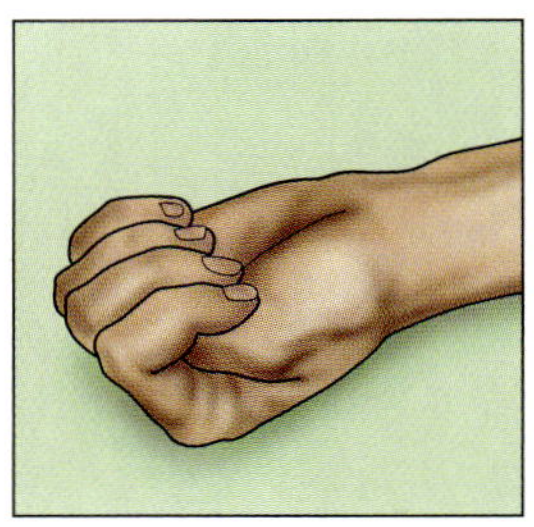

2 To ease stiff finger joints, do the **Thumb Squeezer.** Curl your fingers into a fist around your thumb, gently squeeze, then slowly release. Do this 10 times with each hand.

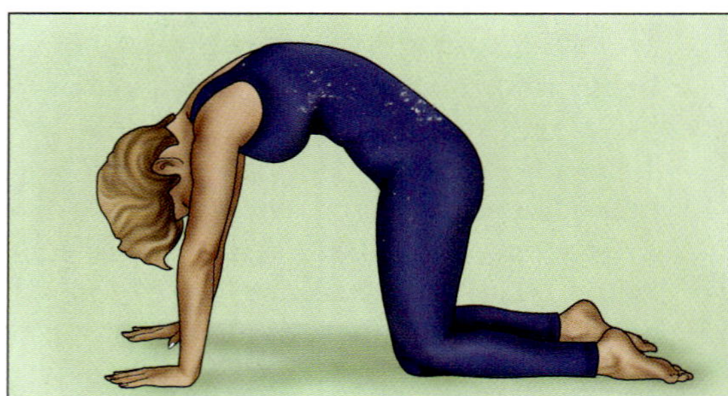

3 The Dog and **Cat** help stretch your hips and back. On your hands and knees in the table position, inhale as you lower your back and lift your head and buttocks (Dog). Then exhale as you arch your back and drop your head and buttocks (Cat). Repeat 10 times.

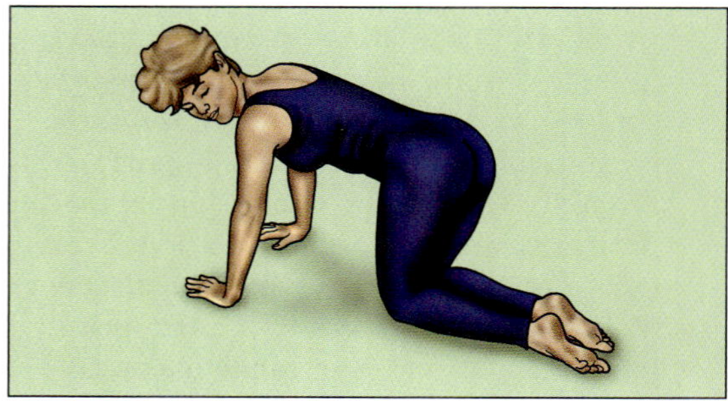

4 Do the **C** exercise on your hands and knees. Exhale and swing your head and buttocks as far to the left as you can. Breathe deeply as you hold this position for 10 seconds; exhale as you slowly straighten your back. Repeat to the right. Do this 10 times.

AN AGE-OLD DISEASE

Arthritis in one form or another has been around for a long time. Some Egyptian mummies show unmistakable symptoms of osteoarthritis, as do the frozen remains of a Copper Age man discovered in 1991 in the Tyrolean Alps. Rheumatoid arthritis, however, has been affecting humans for a relatively short time, according to some authorities. The disease was possibly introduced by a new strain of virus only about two centuries ago.

on the affected area. CAUTION: Lobelia may cause dermatitis in some people.

HOMEOPATHY

For chronic **osteoarthritis** and **rheumatoid arthritis,** constitutional remedies will be prescribed after consultation with a trained homeopathic practitioner. Homeopathic remedies to relieve immediate pain and joint stiffness may include ***Rhus toxicodendron*** or ***Bryonia.***

HYDROTHERAPY

Swimming or other water exercise, preferably in a heated pool, allows arthritis patients to work on movement of affected joints and improve muscle strength; the water helps support the body and reduce the stress of gravity.

NUTRITION AND DIET

Avoiding specific foods can stop arthritic symptoms tied to allergies, especially to grains, nuts, meats, eggs, and dairy products. Use trial and error, preferably under the supervision of a doctor.

Some practitioners recommend cutting out plants in the nightshade family: tomato, potato, eggplant, and pepper. They believe the alkaloids in these foods inhibit formation of the collagen that makes up cartilage.

Low-fat, low-protein vegetarian diets may ease the pain and inflammation of **rheumatoid arthritis.** Positive results are reported from eliminating partially hydrogenated fats and polyunsaturated vegetable oils, and supplementing the diet with flax oil, sardines, and other oily fish as a source of omega-3 fatty acids.

Vitamin therapy may relieve certain arthritic symptoms. Beta carotene *(see **vitamin A**)* has an antioxidant effect on cells, neutralizing destructive molecules called free radicals. ***Vitamins C, B_6,*** and ***E,*** as well as ***zinc,*** are thought to enhance collagen production and the repair of connective tissue. Vitamin C may also be advised for people taking aspirin, which depletes the body's vitamin C balance. ***Niacin*** (vitamin B_3) may also be helpful, although excessive use may aggravate liver problems. Always take vitamin supplements under professional guidance, since overdoses of some vitamin compounds can have side effects or undesirable interactions with drugs.

The nutritional supplement glucosamine sulfate may act to repair cartilage and reduce pain and inflammation; take 1500 mg daily.

YOGA

A number of yoga positions *(opposite)* may have beneficial effects on arthritis.

AT-HOME REMEDIES

Heat and rest—traditional remedies for arthritic pain—are very effective in the short term for most people with the disease. Overweight sufferers should begin weight reduction, especially when arthritis strikes the lower back and legs.

If arthritic pain comes on unexpectedly, supplement an over-the-counter painkiller with dry heat from a heating pad or moist heat in the form of a hot bath or a hot-water bottle wrapped in a towel. Regular exercise is important to keep the joints mobile. People with weakened, badly deformed fingers from **rheumatoid arthritis** benefit from specially designed utensils and door and drawer handles; people suffering weakness in the legs and arms from **osteoarthritis** can use special bathroom fixtures, especially tub rails and elevated toilet seats. ■

ASTHMA

SYMPTOMS

- restlessness or insomnia.
- increasing, but relatively painless, tightness in chest.
- mild to moderate shortness of breath.
- when breathing, a wheezing or whistling sound that can range from faint to clearly audible.
- coughing, sometimes accompanied by phlegm.

CALL YOUR DOCTOR IF:

- you or another person is experiencing an episode of asthma for the first time; asthma is a chronic condition and can be quite serious if not treated properly.
- the prescribed asthma medicine does not work in the time it is supposed to; you need a new prescription, or you may be suffering from a severe episode.
- you or the person with asthma has a suffocating feeling, making it difficult to talk; nostrils flare, the skin between the ribs appears sucked in, and the lips or the skin under the nails looks grayish or bluish. These are all signs of extreme oxygen deprivation. **Get immediate emergency treatment.**

Asthma is a chronic respiratory disease that, like ***bronchitis*** and ***emphysema,*** causes a tightening of the chest and difficulty in breathing. In the case of asthma, however, these symptoms are not always present. They come in episodes set off by various environmental or emotional "triggers," such as pollen, animal dander, tobacco smoke, and stress. Some people with asthma experience only mild and infrequent episodes; for them the condition is an occasional inconvenience. For others, episodes can be frequent and serious, requiring emergency medical treatment. If you have asthma, you should be monitored by a physician regularly, and you must seek immediate medical intervention for a serious episode. By identifying your triggers, you can learn to lessen the intensity and frequency of asthma attacks and perhaps even avoid them completely.

Asthma is not a problem with breathing in, but with breathing out. During an asthma episode, muscle spasms and swelling bronchial tissues narrow the lungs' tiny airways, which then become clogged with excess mucus. Stale air gets trapped in the bottom of the lungs, forcing you to use the top part to gasp for air. Mild and moderate episodes consist of short incidents of breathlessness and wheezing. In severe cases, the lungs' airways become so narrow and clogged that breathing is impossible.

An episode may pass quickly or last more than a day. Sometimes symptoms recur suddenly and with surprising intensity. This "second wave" attack can be more severe and dangerous than the initial episode and may last days or even weeks.

A fairly common disease, asthma affects somewhere between 15 million and 16 million Americans. More prevalent in children than in adults, asthma is the leading cause of school absenteeism and pediatric hospital admission. Although asthma is seldom fatal, it is quite serious. If you have asthma, you should seek the help of a doctor before trying alternative therapies.

CAUSES

Asthma has no single cause; rather, episodes can be brought on by a variety of factors working alone or in combination. ***Allergies*** are the primary offenders. Between 50 percent and 90 percent of people with asthma have allergies. The most common allergens, or allergy-causing substances, are pollen, grass, dust, mold, tobacco smoke, and animal dander. When inhaled, these substances can trigger the release of histamine and other body chemicals, causing an allergic reaction and asthma episodes. Other allergens include chemical fumes; ***aspirin*** or aspirin-like compounds, such as phenylbutazone, indomethacin, ***ibuprofen,*** and other ***nonsteroidal anti-inflammatory drugs (NSAIDs);*** and sulfites, high concentrations of which are found in some foods and liquids *(see* ***Prevention,*** *page 151).* Another factor in allergy-related asthma is heredity: Scientists have discovered a gene that appears to make people susceptible to the disease.

Lung infections can also induce asthma. Bronchiolitis, a viral respiratory infection that usually affects children aged two and younger, is a common cause of childhood asthma. Adults may develop asthma as a result of an upper respiratory infection, such as ***bronchitis.*** Other asthma triggers include exercise, emotional stress, and environmental stresses such as air pollution.

ASTHMATIC AIRWAYS

Air travels down the trachea and into the lungs through branching tubes called bronchioles, which normally are lined with a thin mucous membrane. For people with asthma, certain conditions or inhaled substances can act as "triggers," prompting the release of chemicals that cause the bronchioles to constrict and produce too much mucus. The clogged airways trap air and make breathing difficult.

DIAGNOSTIC AND TEST PROCEDURES

To determine if you have asthma, your doctor will probably administer a pulmonary function test, which measures the strength of your exhalation. Normally, a person without asthma can exhale about 75 to 85 percent of the air in the lungs within a second, emptying them within three seconds. However, it takes a person with asthma six or seven seconds to expel all the air from the lungs. The pulmonary function test used most often is called a peak flow test, which takes readings as you exhale into a device called a peak flow meter. Your doctor can prescribe a peak flow meter for you, so that you can monitor your condition at home.

TREATMENT

If you have asthma, you should see a doctor regularly; for severe episodes, conventional medical treatment is always necessary. However, a number of alternative treatments can be helpful when used in conjunction with conventional therapy.

CONVENTIONAL MEDICINE

Following a diagnosis of asthma, your first step should be to work with your doctor to develop a treatment plan. As part of this plan, the physician might ask you to keep a daily diary, noting environmental and emotional factors that bring on asthma episodes. This not only will help the doctor monitor the disease but will help you recognize and avoid your asthma triggers.

To treat asthma medicinally, doctors generally prescribe ***bronchodilators,*** drugs that help dilate the lungs' constricted airways. These medications are available in two forms: inhaled and oral. Inhaled bronchodilators, which come in aerosol or metered-dose inhaler form, resemble ***epinephrine*** (the synthetic version of the hormone adrenaline produced by the body). Doctors usually prefer inhaled bronchodilators, such as isoproterenol, metaproterenol, isoetharine, and ***albuterol,*** because they are delivered directly to the lungs, and because they use 1,000 times less medicine than oral forms. Generally, one or two "puffs" relieve the wheezing and chest tightness associated with mild to moderate episodes. WARNING: Bronchodilators are potent drugs. If overused, they can cause dangerous side effects, such as ***high blood pressure.***

Oral bronchodilators, which include ***theophylline,*** metaproterenol, ***albuterol,*** and ***terbutaline,*** are available in liquid, tablet, or capsule form. They are frequently prescribed for people who cannot tolerate inhaled medication or who suffer from chronic asthma. In severe cases, ***corticosteroids*** may be prescribed, but a doctor needs to monitor this treatment carefully because of serious side effects. Emergency situations may require an injection or inhaled dose of ***epinephrine*** to help open the lungs' airways.

A new class of asthma medications, known as leukotriene modifiers, can prevent chronic asthma attacks by relaxing airway muscles and reducing airway swelling and inflammation.

If your asthma has been caused by ***allergies*** (especially to pollen or stinging insects), your doctor might suggest immunotherapy. By gradually exposing your body to a certain allergen through a series of injections, immunotherapy can help your immune system build up defenses; over time, your allergic reactions may lessen or disappear entirely.

ALTERNATIVE CHOICES

Many people have reported success with alternative asthma treatments, but even advocates recommend these methods only as complements to conventional therapies. Remember: Once diagnosed, asthma should be monitored by a physician, and serious episodes always require conventional medical attention.

ACUPRESSURE

Applying gentle pressure to certain body points may help relieve some of the discomfort of asthma. Reaching over your left shoulder with your right hand, press firmly on the part of your back in between the left shoulder blade and spine (point BL 13); take five deep breaths, then repeat on the other side. Or put your fists on your chest, thumbs pointing upward, and feel for the sensitive spot next to the breastbone, just underneath the collarbone (point KI 27). Press firmly for two minutes. *(See the **Appendix** for more information about point locations.)*

ACUPUNCTURE

Several medical studies suggest that acupuncture may help alleviate the symptoms of asthma. The procedure should be carried out only by a licensed acupuncturist.

AROMATHERAPY

Essential oils such as ***eucalyptus*** *(Eucalyptus globulus),* ***hyssop*** *(Hyssopus officinalis),* aniseed *(Pimpinella anisum),* ***lavender*** *(Lavandula officinalis),* pine *(Pinus sylvestris),* and ***rosemary*** *(Rosmarinus officinalis)* may help ease breathing and relieve nasal congestion. Inhaled through the nose, a few drops of one of the oils or a mixture of several dabbed on a handkerchief or tissue can help ease breathing during a mild episode of asthma. If you feel congested at other times (not during an episode), mix a few drops of essential oil in a sink full of hot water, cover your head with a towel, and inhale the fragrant steam through your nose.

CHINESE HERBS

The Chinese herb ***ephedra*** *(Ephedra sinica)* is a potent bronchodilator used for acute attacks. CAUTION: Large quantities of this herb can have the same effect as large quantities of ***epinephrine;*** do not use it if you have ***high blood pressure*** or ***heart disease.*** Prepare an infusion by combining 5 grams ephedra, 4 grams ***cinnamon*** sticks *(Cinnamomum cassia),* 1.5 grams ***licorice*** *(Glycyrrhiza uralensis),* and 5 grams ***apricot seed*** *(Prunus armeniaca).* Steep the mixture in cold water, then bring to a boil. Drink it hot.

HERBAL THERAPIES

Elecampane *(Inula helenium),* a root that acts as a soothing expectorant, may help clear the body of excess mucus. To prepare an infusion, shred the root to yield 1 tsp and add a full cup of cold water; let the infusion stand for 10 hours, then strain and drink it hot three times daily. An infusion made from ***mullein*** *(Verbascum thapsus)* is recommended for soothing the mucous membranes, especially during nighttime episodes.

HOMEOPATHY

Homeopaths offer a variety of treatments for asthma symptoms. Following are just a few: To help calm restlessness and anxiety, take ***Arsenicum album*** (30c) as required. For symptoms that worsen at night or during cold weather, or that come on very suddenly, take ***Aconite*** (30c) as required. For symptoms exacerbated by dampness, take *Natrum sulphuricum* (30c) as required. For more remedies, consult a licensed homeopath.

REFLEXOLOGY

Massage the skin between the big toe and second toe on both feet; this area is said to correspond to your throat and lungs. Then, flexing so the toes are spread apart, massage the ball of the foot, the area said to correspond to the lungs and chest.

YOGA

Yoga can help you learn to breathe deeply and to relax, thereby helping you deal more effectively with stress, a common trigger for asthma. *(See **Wheezing** for exercises.)*

PREVENTION

- Learn to identify your triggers: Keep a diary detailing all the environmental and emotional factors that affect you every day over the course of several months. When you have an asthma attack, go back to your diary to see which factor, or combination of factors, might have contributed to it.
- Monitor the shifts in your lung capacity at home using a peak flow meter, a device that your doctor can prescribe for you. Alerted to reductions in your ability to exhale, you can take precautions and lessen the severity of an asthma episode.
- Avoid foods and drinks that have high concentrations of sulfites, such as beer, wine, wine vinegar, instant tea, grape juice, lemon juice, grapes, fresh shrimp, pizza dough, dried fruits (such as apricots and apples), canned vegetables, instant potatoes, corn syrup, fruit topping, and molasses. Some nutritionists recommend that you also steer clear of foods that cause excess mucus production, such as milk.
- A daily dose of ***B-complex vitamins*** (50 to 100 mg) and ***magnesium*** (400 to 600 mg) may help reduce the frequency and severity of asthma episodes.

ASTHMA
MYTHS AND FACTS

MYTH: *Asthmatics shouldn't exercise.*
FACT: *Exercise is as important for people with asthma as it is for anyone else. Equipped with the proper medication, people with asthma can exercise normally. Note: Many doctors recommend swimming for people with asthma, as humidity helps ease breathing. But the chlorine in swimming pools may cause an allergic reaction, triggering an asthma episode.*

MYTH: *You'll grow out of it.*
FACT: *This is both true and false. Although about half of the people who had asthma when they were between the ages of 2 and 10 seem to "outgrow" the disease, in many cases it recurs when they hit their thirties. It's also possible to develop asthma as an adult even if you did not have it as a child.*

MYTH: *Allergic mothers shouldn't breast-feed.*
FACT: *Infants who are breast-fed are less likely to become allergic than those who are not.* ■

ATHEROSCLEROSIS

A

SYMPTOMS

In its early stages, atherosclerosis has no obvious symptoms. Damaged or partially blocked blood vessels may cause one or more of the following:

- dull, crampy pain in your buttock, thigh, and calf muscles during exertion. This may be a sign of atherosclerosis in the pelvic region or leg.
- sudden onset of localized paralysis, tingling, or numbness in a limb; partial vision or speech loss. These symptoms may indicate **cerebral atherosclerosis,** which can lead to ***stroke.***
- ***angina,*** a feeling of tightness or heavy pressure in the chest. This may signal atherosclerosis in the coronary arteries.

CALL YOUR DOCTOR IF:

- you experience ***angina*** pain for the first time, or angina attacks progress from predictable to unstable. Either event is a serious condition that needs immediate medical attention.
- you have discolored, ulcerous skin and sudden sharp pains in the legs or feet when you are at rest. This may indicate severe atherosclerosis and possibly a circulatory blockage that needs treatment to prevent gangrene.
- you notice unexplained loss of balance, coordination, speech, or vision. Any such loss indicates a temporary halt in the flow of blood to the brain, a situation that can result in ***stroke*** if left unattended.

Atherosclerosis—also known as arteriosclerosis or hardening of the arteries—is an inflammatory disease that results in scarring of the artery walls, primarily from long-term buildup of fatty deposits and calcifications. Atherosclerosis is one of the most common cardiovascular diseases and is so prevalent in developed countries that many Americans assume it is a natural consequence of aging. Overwhelming evidence links atherosclerosis closely to diet and lifestyle, suggesting that it can be prevented or slowed, and in some cases, even reversed.

Depending on the location and degree of arterial damage, atherosclerosis can lead to kidney problems, ***high blood pressure, stroke,*** and other life-threatening conditions. Atherosclerosis tends to target the aorta—the body's largest artery, which leads from the heart—and arteries leading to the brain, the lower limbs, and the kidneys. Damage to arteries carrying blood to the legs and feet makes walking painful; severely restricted circulation to the limbs can cause skin ulcers and even gangrene (tissue death). Blockage in the coronary arteries, which feed oxygen-rich blood directly to the heart muscles, is known as **coronary artery disease** or **coronary heart disease.** This disorder and its complications—***angina, heart arrhythmia,*** and ***heart attack***—are the leading causes of death in the U.S. and most of Europe.

CAUSES

Arterial deposits begin as thin, fatty streaks on an arterial wall. In a person with a healthy lifestyle, the streaks may come and go. But if a person's arteries are damaged—typically from ***high blood pressure, stress,*** or smoking—the inner surface of the walls can start to deteriorate. To compensate, the artery grows new tissue that may create tiny bumps or scars. Cholesterol, white blood cells, and other deposits can start to accumulate within these bumps, forming plaque that clogs the arteries. Eventually, calcium deposits and scar tissue surround the soft plaque, making the arteries hard and inelastic. Because atherosclerosis progresses slowly—usually over many years—it is commonly thought of as an affliction of the el-

HARDENING OF THE ARTERIES

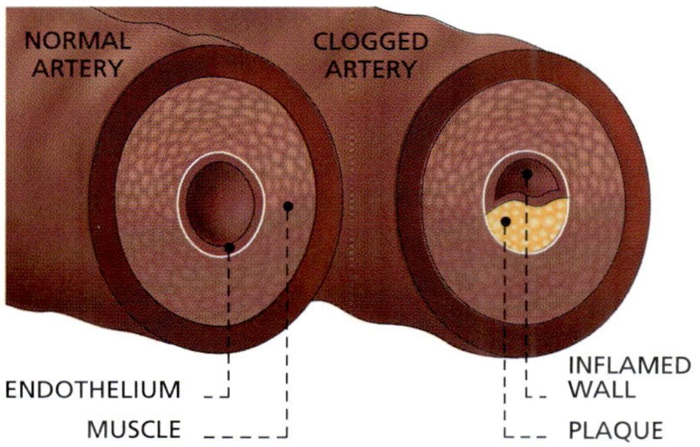

Inside a normal artery, a layer of muscle surrounds the endothelium, the smooth inner lining through which blood flows *(above, left)*. In some people the endothelium can develop streaks or bumps of fat deposits. Over time, continued accumulation of fatty deposits results in inflammation of the artery wall. Eventually, a hard, calcified plaque can develop that may obstruct blood flow *(above, right)*.

derly. However, studies show that arterial deposits can begin in childhood, with significant plaque formation by the time a person is 30.

While the stages of atherosclerosis are well established, the reasons for its development are less clear. People with a high level of blood cholesterol—especially low-density lipoprotein (LDL) cholesterol—are at risk for developing atherosclerosis. LDL cholesterol—the kind that forms arterial plaque—can react with unstable chemical compounds called free radicals in a complicated process that degrades both the transport mechanism for moving cholesterol through the bloodstream and the tissue lining of arterial walls. Nonetheless, most people with high cholesterol do not develop atherosclerosis, and many people with atherosclerosis have normal cholesterol levels. *(See **Cholesterol Problems**.)*

Artery walls can become damaged by high blood pressure, by the carbon monoxide in tobacco smoke, and by stress. For example, one study in a war-torn country found that citizens exposed to ongoing battle had greater plaque buildup than those out of harm's way.

While virtually everyone can expect to develop arterial deposits to some degree over time, other factors influence susceptibility to actual atherosclerosis:

- **Age.** Atherosclerosis tends to affect people over 35, although it can begin much earlier.
- **Gender.** Premenopausal women are less likely than men of the same age to have atherosclerosis, but after menopause the risk is about equal.
- **Heredity.** A family history of atherosclerosis increases the risk of developing the disease.
- **Obesity.** Obese people are more likely to have atherosclerosis, probably because as a group they tend to have high cholesterol and high blood pressure. *(See **Obesity**.)*
- **Lifestyle.** Lack of exercise is associated with atherosclerosis and the eventual onset of coronary ***heart disease.***

DIAGNOSTIC AND TEST PROCEDURES

Doctors usually look for characteristic symptoms of arterial blockage in various parts of the body as indications of atherosclerosis. To determine the precise location and extent of blockage, your doctor may order an angiogram, which highlights arterial plaque on an x-ray.

TREATMENT

After addressing any obvious symptoms, the first step in treating atherosclerosis is to eliminate or reduce risk factors for the disease, for example by lowering the amount of saturated fat in the diet to prevent further plaque buildup. If you have high blood pressure you should take steps to regulate it, such as losing weight, exercising regularly, and reducing stress. People with diabetes must control their blood sugar levels. Smokers should quit.

CONVENTIONAL MEDICINE

No drug treats atherosclerosis directly, although various medications may be prescribed to treat contributing conditions such as ***high blood pressure, blood clots,*** or ***cholesterol problems.*** Sever-

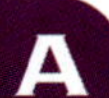

al surgical procedures have been developed to restore damaged arteries: Portions of a diseased artery can be opened and obstructing plaque deposits removed, or a damaged section of artery can be replaced.

One of the more common procedures is bypass surgery, in which blood is rerouted around a blockage using either grafted or synthetic blood vessels. Balloon angioplasty is a nonsurgical technique that opens arteries by splitting and flattening plaques against vessel walls *(right).* Various other techniques use catheterization, lasers, and stents—tiny pieces of woven wire mesh—to restore blocked blood vessels to an acceptably functioning state.

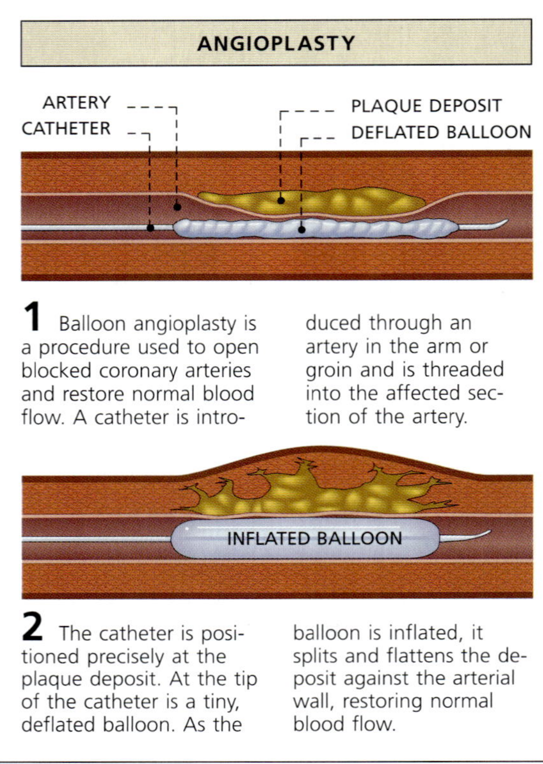

1 Balloon angioplasty is a procedure used to open blocked coronary arteries and restore normal blood flow. A catheter is introduced through an artery in the arm or groin and is threaded into the affected section of the artery.

2 The catheter is positioned precisely at the plaque deposit. At the tip of the catheter is a tiny, deflated balloon. As the balloon is inflated, it splits and flattens the deposit against the arterial wall, restoring normal blood flow.

ALTERNATIVE CHOICES

Since diet and lifestyle are significant factors in both the development and the prevention of atherosclerosis, alternative therapies offer a range of choices to keep the ailment at bay.

AYURVEDIC MEDICINE

Ayurvedic therapy combines diet, herbal remedies, relaxation, and exercise. Consult a specialist for a comprehensive program of treatment.

CHINESE HERBS

Numerous Chinese herbal combinations are recommended for atherosclerosis, including siler *(Ledebouriella divaricata),* platycodon *(Platycodon grandiflorum),* and ***bupleurum*** *(Bupleurum chinense)* in an appropriate combination. Consult a practitioner of Chinese medicine.

HERBAL THERAPIES

Herbal remedies to combat atherosclerosis are typically intended to reduce existing plaques or to improve blood-vessel integrity so plaques are less likely to form. ***Garlic*** *(Allium sativum)* is considered one of the best plaque fighters; ***hawthorne*** *(Crataegus laevigata)* is commonly used to treat atherosclerosis because of its reputation for improving coronary blood flow. For herbs that may provide relief from discomfort associated with atherosclerosis of the lower limbs, see ***Circulatory Problems.***

HOMEOPATHY

Various long-term remedies may be prescribed by a licensed homeopath for treating atherosclerosis. Diagnosis and prescriptions will vary according to the homeopath's evaluation of the patient.

LIFESTYLE

The benefits of lifestyle improvement have been demonstrated in a yearlong program designed for heart disease patients, conducted by Dr. Dean Ornish, that involved strict vegetarianism, exercise, and stress reduction. At the end of the trial, a measurable reversal of plaque buildup in the coronary arteries was reported in 82 percent of participants.

MIND/BODY MEDICINE

Since stress is believed to accelerate the rate at which atherosclerosis develops, therapeutic relaxation techniques may help prevent or retard its progress. A number of approaches can help you relax, including **yoga, meditation, guided imagery,** and **biofeedback.**

NUTRITION AND DIET

Diet and lifestyle changes, if started early and maintained aggressively, may be enough to prevent or even reverse atherosclerosis. First, your diet should be not only low in cholesterol and saturated fat, but high in antioxidants, which neutralize free radicals believed to aggravate tissue damage. The key antioxidants are ***vitamins E*** and ***C,*** beta carotene *(see **vitamin A**),* and ***selenium,*** which can be toxic in high dosages. Be careful about taking any vitamin indiscriminately, however: Too much ***vitamin D,*** for example, may actually accelerate calcification of arterial plaques. To be safe, seek advice from a doctor or nutritionist.

Some evidence suggests that ***garlic*** *(Allium sativum),* eaten in large quantities, deters oxidation of cholesterol. Grape-skin extracts and gugulipid *(Commiphora mukul),* an herb from southern India, are reputed to reduce plaque deposits. ***Alfalfa*** *(Medicago sativa)* and bromelain, a pineapple enzyme, are reported to have done the same in animals and may work on humans.

Numerous studies over the past 30 years have indicated moderate alcohol consumption—a glass or two of wine a day—may protect against atherosclerosis and coronary artery disease. One study suggests that flavonoids in grape skins, which give red wine its color and flavor, inhibit buildup of fatty deposits.

For more nutritional information, see ***Cholesterol Problems*** and ***Blood Clots.***

PREVENTION

Atherosclerosis develops when genetic predispositions meet known risk factors head-on. If you have a family history of atherosclerosis, the prudent course of action is to accept what you cannot change and change what you can.

- Adopt a low-fat, low-salt, high-fiber, natural food diet. Take extra pains to avoid foods high in saturated fat and cholesterol.
- If you smoke, quit.
- Know your blood pressure. If it's high, get it down. *(See **High Blood Pressure.**)*
- Get moderate exercise—a 30-minute walk, swim, or bicycle ride—several times a week, and daily if possible.
- Find a relaxation program that you enjoy, and incorporate it into your daily routine.
- If you have a high-risk family history, be sure to get checked regularly by a cardiologist.

CHELATION THERAPY: THE JURY IS STILL OUT

Every year thousands of people in the U.S. look to chelation therapy for treatment of atherosclerosis—more people than have bypass surgery. Chelation involves injecting a chemical called EDTA into the bloodstream. One theory holds that chelation removes the calcium in arterial plaque; another suggests that EDTA works as an antioxidant.

While chelation therapy has proved beneficial for ailments like lead poisoning, its use as a cardiovascular treatment remains controversial. Advocates tout chelation as a safe, relatively inexpensive, and effective alternative to other treatments. Critics cite the lack of reliable scientific testing and claim that chelation is ineffective or potentially dangerous (early trials sometimes caused kidney damage).

Treatment typically requires from 10 to 40 sessions and may cost thousands of dollars. Until chelation therapy survives at least one rigorous scientific study, physicians will undoubtedly remain divided over its merits. Once science provides answers, chelation therapy will become either a standard recommendation of every cardiologist or a therapeutic relic. ■

ATHLETE'S FOOT

A

SYMPTOMS

- itchy, scaly, red rash that usually starts between the toes; if untreated, develops into cracked, blistered skin that may become infected.
- dry, flaking skin on the soles of the feet.
- unpleasant foot odor.
- yellowish, brittle, flaky toenails.

CALL YOUR DOCTOR IF:

- the rash does not respond to treatment with over-the-counter antifungal medication or other at-home measures in four to six weeks; or if the condition becomes incapacitating. You need a medical diagnosis and prescription medication.
- the rash develops blisters, intense redness, painful swelling, or pus; or if you develop a fever. These are signs of a secondary bacterial infection, which requires treatment with oral antibiotics.
- your toenails become brittle or discolored, usually whitish. This form of athlete's foot is difficult to eradicate and usually requires long-term medical treatment to prevent recurrence.

Athlete's foot is a common fungal ***infection,*** and you don't have to be an athlete to get it. This annoying ailment occurs most often in men and boys, but it is common enough in women and girls, too. Virtually unheard of in ancient Greece and Rome, when people went barefoot or wore sandals, athlete's foot is a by-product of a society that keeps its feet enclosed in shoes most of the time.

CAUSES

The various kinds of fungi that cause athlete's foot belong to a group called dermatophytes, which also cause ***jock itch.*** The fungi thrive in closed, warm, moist environments and feed on keratin, a protein found in hair, nails, and skin. Athlete's foot is mildly contagious; it can be spread through direct contact with the infection and by skin particles left on towels, shoes, and floors of shower stalls and around swimming pools. Although walking barefoot in the shower at the gym or around the pool may increase your chance of contracting athlete's foot, you are more likely to develop the infection from not changing sweaty socks and shoes. The risk of developing athlete's foot can also depend on your susceptibility. For example, people who have taken an ***antibiotic*** for two weeks or longer are at greater risk because the drug not only fights infection but can kill beneficial bacteria that help keep the athlete's foot fungus from spreading. *(See **Yeast Infections.**)*

TREATMENT

You should treat athlete's foot at the first sign of itchy feet or redness between your toes. Most cases of athlete's foot can be cured with over-the-counter antifungal powder and basic good hygiene. Wash and dry your feet thoroughly morning and evening, change your socks or stockings daily, and don't wear the same shoes day after day. Sprinkle antifungal powder on your feet and in your shoes daily.

Make sure your feet get plenty of air. If you can't go barefoot or wear sandals, wear cotton socks and shoes made of a natural, porous material such as leather or fabric, not water-resistant synthetics. If not treated properly and promptly, the infection can be very persistent. Even when treated with ***antifungal drugs,*** the infection may take several weeks to disappear.

CONVENTIONAL MEDICINE

Doctors prescribe oral ***antifungal drugs*** for athlete's foot only when topical remedies fail, since the treatment may have serious side effects, such as liver toxicity. Typical oral medications are ***ketoconazole*** and griseofulvin. The same treatment options apply to athlete's foot affecting the toenails.

ALTERNATIVE CHOICES

AROMATHERAPY

To combat infection, put 5 drops of ***tea tree oil*** (*Melaleuca* spp.) in your bathwater. To relieve itching, try 2 drops of ***peppermint*** *(Mentha piperita)* oil and 4 drops of ***chamomile*** *(Matricaria recutita)* oil in the bathwater.

HERBAL THERAPIES

Soak your feet for half an hour in a solution of 6 tsp ***goldenseal*** *(Hydrastis canadensis)* to a pint of water; you can also powder your feet with goldenseal. Or rub ***tea tree oil*** (*Melaleuca* spp.) on the affected area daily. Try other herbal baths and ointments, following label directions: ***Myrrh*** *(Commiphora molmol)* is said to fight fungus; ***lavender*** *(Lavandula officinalis)* may reduce inflammation; ***calendula*** *(Calendula officinalis)* cream is recommended to heal cracked skin.

HOMEOPATHY

To soothe inflammation, try an over-the-counter preparation containing *Calendula.* A professional homeopath may recommend *Graphites* for a condition with weeping skin.

AT-HOME REMEDIES

Soak your infected feet in warm, salted water (1 tsp salt per cup) for 5 to 10 minutes every day. Dry your feet thoroughly, then apply a baking soda paste between your toes, or dab on an aluminum chloride solution, available from your local pharmacy. You may prefer using an over-the-counter antifungal powder, cream, or spray. The most effective products contain terbinafine, undecylenic acid, or the antifungal drugs ***clotrimazole*** or ***miconazole.*** One percent terbinafine ointment can lead to a complete cure in a week. As long as the area is not blistered or cracked, remove flakes of dead skin with a soft brush before using a topical powder or ointment. Do not tear off flaking skin; you may break nearby healthy skin and spread the infection.

Use the same topical treatment for athlete's foot of the toenails, but don't expect fast action. Keep your nails short, and clean out debris under and around infected nails using a smooth wooden toothpick or matchstick rather than a nail file that might scratch or break the skin.

PREVENTION

Your coach and the school nurse were on the right track when they made you wear shower shoes in the locker room and around the pool. But we now know that susceptibility is as big a factor as actual contact with the fungus. Cut your risk by keeping your feet clean, dry, and powdered with an over-the-counter fungicide. Other sensible steps:

- Wear cotton socks, and shoes that breathe; shoes that keep water out also keep sweat in.
- Never share shoes, socks, or towels.
- If you get athlete's foot, wash your socks and towels in the hottest water possible—or boil them.
- Be doubly cautious of your feet if you take an ***antibiotic*** for two weeks or more. The medication can kill beneficial bacteria that normally control the fungus that causes athlete's foot. Take *Lactobacillus acidophilus* capsules to replenish the beneficial bacteria. ■

ATHLETIC INJURIES

SYMPTOMS

- Pain, discomfort, restricted movement, tenderness, and possible swelling may be indicative of some form of muscle or ligament injury, such as a sprain or strain.
- Pain, swelling, tenderness, and deformity may indicate a **fracture.**
- Pain, restricted movement, misshapen appearance, and swelling in a joint are symptoms of a **dislocation.**
- Localized pain just below the kneecap may be a sign of patellar ***tendonitis.*** In adolescents, the condition may indicate Osgood-Schlatter disease if accompanied by swelling.
- Pain in the elbow, often accompanied by tenderness in the inner or outer portion of the elbow and forearm, and possibly a weak and painful grasp, may indicate **epicondylitis.**

CALL YOUR DOCTOR IF:

- your muscles gradually become weak for no apparent reason; you may have a neurological problem or another disorder of immediate concern.
- you experience chronic muscle cramps. Although most often benign, this may be a sign of serious problems such as blood clotting, restricted blood flow, or nerve damage.
- you think your swelling or puffiness is caused by a fracture, dislocation, ligament or muscle tear, or cartilage damage. If not treated by a physician in a timely manner, the affected area could suffer permanent damage.

Every family has seen its share of injuries tracing to athletic endeavors or, ironically, the pursuit of physical fitness. For the most part, athletic injuries are a result of stress put on bones or muscles. Most common are injuries to soft tissue—muscles, tendons, and ligaments.

A **dislocation** occurs when two bones are jolted apart at a joint and is often accompanied by a ligament tear in the joint. The pain is caused by the severe stretching of soft tissues.

A **fracture** is either simple (closed)—in which the broken bone remains beneath the skin surface and does minimal damage to surrounding tissues—or compound (open)—in which the bone protrudes through the skin. The ankle, hand, wrist, and collarbone are common sites of fracture.

Shoulder injuries are common in sports that require throwing motions or intense contact. Dislocations are most common in the shoulder joint. **Acromioclavicular joint (AC) separation** occurs when the ligaments that support the collarbone are torn. The rotator cuff is where four muscles meet and attach to the humerus; overuse of the shoulder may inflame or tear tendons in the area, causing **rotator cuff tendonitis.**

CHILD SPORTS INJURIES: WHAT PARENTS SHOULD KNOW

- *Each year during the high-school football season there are an estimated one million injuries; wrestling, soccer, and basketball also carry a high risk of injury.*
- *Children are at a higher risk of injury than adult athletes because those playing together may be at vastly different weights, stages of development, and strengths. Try to ensure that participants in a group are at a similar level of physical development.*

Epicondylitis affects the elbow and typically occurs in sports requiring frequent wrist manipulation and forearm rotation. The lateral (affecting the outer elbow) form is ***tennis elbow.*** Medial epicondylitis involves the inner elbow.

Lower-back injuries, such as muscle tears, are common in sports that involve a lot of bending. The high velocity and full contact nature of hockey and football frequently cause neck and spine injuries, such as a **herniated disk,** in which an intervertebral disk protrudes from the spinal column *(see **Disk Problems**).*

Intense leg movement, including twisting and spreading, may tear the adductor muscle **(groin strain),** which connects the leg with the pubic bone.

The knees are involved in some of the most common lower-body injuries. Continual jumping may result in tearing of the tendon just below the kneecap, or patella, causing **patellar tendonitis,** or jumper's knee. The knees may also suffer from other injuries, such as tears of the meniscus, a piece of cartilage in the knee joint between the femur and tibia.

The sudden tearing of muscle fibers that may occur after excessive athletic activity and the consequent accumulation of fluid in the muscle that causes pain, tenderness, and local swelling characterize a **charley horse.**

Increased interest in jogging and cross training has resulted in a parallel rise in leg injuries, including ***shin splints, tendonitis,*** and **stress fractures,** especially in the tibia or fibula bones. If continually exposed to stress from prolonged standing, running, or walking, a stress fracture may result in a larger fracture.

The foot often falls victim to injury because it must support the weight of the entire body. **Plantar fasciitis** often affects inexperienced runners, causing pain along the inner heel and along the arch of the foot, sometimes accompanied by stiffness and numbness in the heel. A similar problem, **march fracture,** develops in the bones of the foot when extreme stress (running, walking) is continually placed on the ball of the foot.

COMMON SPORTS INJURIES

The highlighted areas below show some of the sites of common injuries sustained from sports or other physical activity. The best way to prevent an athletic injury is to be in good physical condition and to stretch for several minutes before and after exercising. Never attempt to "play through" pain—doing so may cause more extensive injury and lengthen the time needed for complete healing.

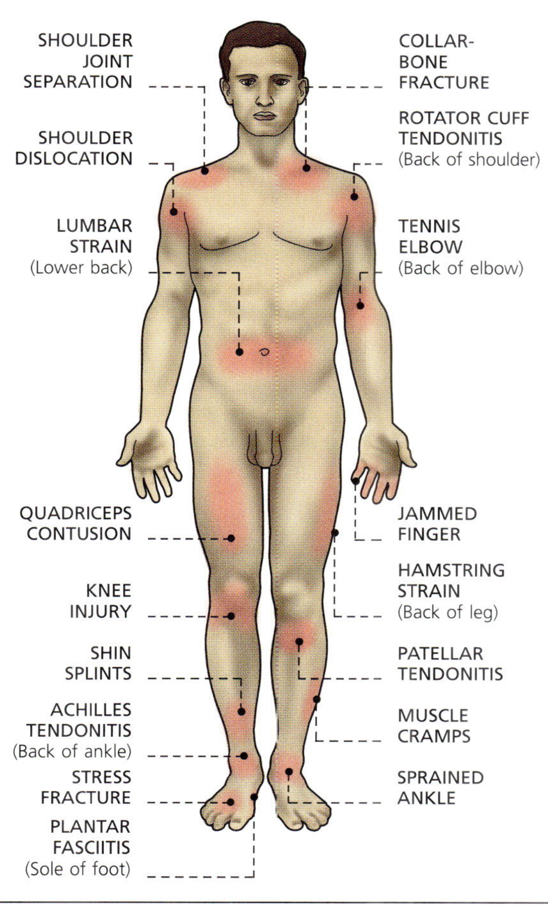

CAUSES

An **AC separation** results from sudden impact on the side of the shoulder or on an outstretched arm. Wear on the rotator cuff, causing **rotator cuff tendonitis,** may occur if you continually engage in sports that require overhead motion like that in a tennis serve. Medial **epicondylitis** is caused by traumatic, repetitive arm motion, as when pitching in baseball. Sudden, violent twisting of the elbow or continual pulling and strain on the forearm muscles can cause the condition.

A **charley horse** is usually caused by a sudden, acute strain in the leg, but mineral deficiency, hormone imbalance, calcium deposits in the muscles, or dehydration can also be causes. Muscle imbalance, a poorly aligned leg, or running on a hard road with improper footwear may cause a **stress fracture.** Tight hamstrings may contribute to lower-back problems, and tight Achilles tendons may precede cases of ***tendonitis*** of the foot and ankle.

DIAGNOSTIC AND TEST PROCEDURES

Basic assessment of an injury begins with your medical history and a physical exam. X-rays may be ordered to examine your bones for possible **fractures, dislocations,** and other injuries. A bone scan is a highly sensitive test that may detect **stress fractures** that might not show up in x-rays.

Arthroscopy, ultrasound, and magnetic resonance imaging (MRI) are generally used on joints. Arthroscopy employs a tiny camera inside a very small tube, called an arthroscope, to examine the interior of your joints; it is useful in both diagnosing and repairing some joint injuries (for example, cartilage fragments can be removed through the tube). Ultrasound scanning uses sound waves to generate an image that your doctor can view on a screen. An MRI produces excellent images of soft tissue, enabling diagnosis of damage to muscles, ligaments, and tendons.

TREATMENT

Treatment for sports injuries aims to relieve pain, repair or realign bones, and restore your body to its full athletic ability.

CONVENTIONAL MEDICINE

Most minor soft-tissue injuries are best treated with RICE: rest, ice, compression, and elevation. *(See **Sprains and Strains.**)*

Injuries such as ***tendonitis*** and **plantar fasciitis** usually require rest and a rehabilitation program to maintain flexibility and strength. ***Aspirin*** or ***ibuprofen*** may help reduce the pain and inflammation that accompany these conditions.

Depending on the severity of the pain, your physician may treat your **epicondylitis** with an injection of a ***corticosteroid,*** with ***nonsteroidal anti-inflammatory drugs (NSAIDs)*** such as ***ibuprofen,*** or with ***aspirin.*** An elbow cuff and physical therapy may also be indicated *(see **Tennis Elbow**).*

For acute pain as a result of an **AC separation,** ***codeine*** may be prescribed for the first couple of days. Thereafter, aspirin and a nonsteroidal anti-inflammatory drug may be taken for chronic pain. Your physician may immobilize the injured area with a sling.

If possible, the displaced bones of a dislocation are manipulated back into place. If this is not feasible, you may need surgery, after which the joint is immobilized until it is stable.

If necessary, a fracture is treated by reduction, a procedure in which the broken bone ends are manipulated so that they abut each other in their original position. The procedure may be

GROWING PAINS

Osgood-Schlatter disease is a condition associated with sudden growth spurts in adolescence (usually in boys ages 10 to 14). It is characterized by pain and swelling below the kneecap, where the patellar tendon attaches to the shinbone. The quadriceps muscle, located at the front of the thigh, continually pulls on the affected tendon, causing the disorder. The condition persists for six months to a year and usually clears up completely without treatment, but as long as your child suffers from symptoms, running, jumping, and squatting should be kept to a minimum, if not eliminated.

done surgically or without cutting the skin. More serious fractures are repositioned and held in place with metal pins or by screws, plates, and rods placed permanently in or on the bone.

A **march fracture** is customarily treated by placing the foot in a plaster cast or a rigid boot; you must rest it for three to six weeks.

ALTERNATIVE CHOICES

ACUPUNCTURE

Administered by a professional, acupuncture may be helpful in treating athletic injuries and soothing the body after strenuous training. It has been shown to reduce pain and swelling and should be applied as soon as possible after injury occurs.

BODY WORK

Massage relieves aches and pains, is especially helpful for ***tendonitis*** and **epicondylitis,** and can lessen the onset of muscle soreness. Administered by a professional, the **Alexander technique, Rolfing,** and the **Feldenkrais method** may be useful.

Knead the area of a **charley horse,** rubbing in the direction of the muscle fibers.

HOMEOPATHY

Arnica (30c) may be taken every 10 minutes for 1 to 2 hours, until the shock of fracture passes, and then every 8 hours for the next two to three days. Taken every 8 to 12 hours for up to three days, ***Ruta*** (30c) may aid healing after a dislocation. The symptoms of a sprained ankle may be eased with ***Rhus toxicodendron*** (30c), taken four times a day for as long as a week.

HYDROTHERAPY

Water is the perfect place for athletes recovering from injuries to work out. Aquatic movement provides muscle resistance without straining joints.

LIFESTYLE

Heat before exercise can loosen joints and soft tissue. Various types of braces and supports worn during exercise can protect joints and soft tissue and stabilize an uncomfortable joint or tendon. Consult your doctor or a physical therapist. To avoid ankle injuries, always wear appropriate shoes with ample protection and support.

NUTRITION AND DIET

Many experts advise athletes to maintain a high-carbohydrate, low-fat diet to increase energy levels and promote muscle strength.

Taken orally or topically, ***vitamin E*** may guard against muscle damage during exercise. ***Magnesium*** helps maintain muscle flexibility, which lessens susceptibility to injury.

For bone fractures, ***vitamin B complex*** and ***zinc*** may help.

AT-HOME REMEDIES

- Replacing fluids lost through perspiration with a carbohydrate-electrolyte sports drink helps prevent cramping.
- Ice packs reduce swelling; a bag of frozen vegetables can be a makeshift ice pack. Do not use chemical cold packs; they are much colder than water packs. Place a damp towel around your pack so that it is not directly on your skin.
- A warm compress may relieve muscle pain, especially before massage and stretching.
- To relieve cramping, elevate the affected area to direct blood flow toward the heart.
- If muscles are sore the day after a tough workout, soak in a hot tub and rest the affected area.

PREVENTION

Before you begin a sport or exercise routine, have a physical exam, especially if you are over 40.

Sports injuries usually result when the muscles are poorly conditioned. You should have a 10-minute warmup session—running in place or doing jumping jacks—before an athletic activity to increase your body temperature and diminish chances of muscle injury. Stretching after your workout will prevent soreness the next day.

Engage in your sport or exercise at least three times a week to maintain proper conditioning. ■

ATTENTION DEFICIT DISORDER

SYMPTOMS

Keep in mind that attention deficit disorder (ADD) is often misdiagnosed. Because so many of the symptoms are related to child development, they can be normal at one age and not at another; moreover, they may be appropriate to one child and not to another of the same age. However, ADD does exist, and it can be treated. In many cases, a child will show signs of the disorder in early childhood—even in infancy—but go undiagnosed until first or second grade, when the demands of schoolwork make them more apparent.

Symptoms include:

- habitual failure to pay attention.
- difficulties with schoolwork.
- excessive distractibility.
- an inability to organize, even with activities that are enjoyed.
- impulsiveness.
- hyperactivity—fidgeting and running about.
- excessive talking and frequent interrupting.

CALL YOUR DOCTOR IF:

- your child shows symptoms of ADD. Because the disorder is difficult to assess, you may want to consult more than one professional; a second opinion is particularly important because of evidence that ADD is sometimes diagnosed in children who do not have the genuine disorder. It is essential that those consulted have experience with ADD.

Difficulty in paying attention—the defining sign of attention deficit disorder (ADD)—is among the most common developmental problems of childhood, affecting about 20 percent of all schoolchildren, according to some estimates. (Other estimates, however, suggest a lower figure of 5 to 7 percent.) Five times as many boys suffer from ADD as girls, and the disorder can persist through adolescence, with some symptoms continuing into adulthood. Great progress has been made in treatment in recent decades. At the same time, though, much about this condition remains uncertain or ill-defined, leading to popular overuse of the term: Professionals report that it has become fashionable, especially among teenagers or their parents, to blame ADD for what may simply be negligent performance.

Most ADD children are of normal or high intelligence. Their activity levels may be normal, lower than normal (hypoactivity), or higher than normal (a version that has its own diagnostic label: attention deficit hyperactivity disorder, or ADHD). An ADD child may also have a specific learning disability that prevents him from taking in and sorting out information in the same way other children do. His brain is unable to process the messages his ears, eyes, or muscles give him.

CAUSES

Although the causes of ADD are poorly understood, biological inheritance appears to be important in many cases: The disorder seems to run in families. A number of nongenetic factors can also play a causative role. Among them: drug or alcohol abuse or other problems in a mother's pregnancy, birth trauma, early child abuse, brain injuries from accidents, ***meningitis,*** encephalitis, low-level lead poisoning *(see* ***Environmental Poisoning****),* and psychological disorders.

In the late 1970s and early 1980s, some researchers thought ADD was caused—or intensified—by sugar and artificial food additives. This theory is now controversial, but some studies still show that specific foods such as chocolate, wheat, cow's milk, and oranges may exacerbate the condition in some hyperactive children.

DIAGNOSTIC AND TEST PROCEDURES

A battery of tests—sometimes including positron emission tomography (PET) scans—may be given to assess a child's neurological and psychological status. They should be administered by a pediatrician with a special interest in school problems or a child psychiatrist. Tests include:

- a medical and social history of both the child and his family.
- a physical exam and neurological assessment including screenings of vision, hearing, and verbal and motor skills, as well as tests for blood levels of lead, a mineral that has been implicated in hyperactivity.
- a quantitative evaluation of intelligence, aptitude, personality traits, and processing skills.

You may also be advised to check with an allergist if any sensitivities are suspected.

TREATMENT

The best treatment is thought to be a combination of medication and psychological therapies. Close cooperation among therapists, physicians, teachers, and parents is very important, and team meetings are useful.

CONVENTIONAL MEDICINE

Although there is considerable controversy about their possible overuse, stimulants such as amphetamines or, more usually, ***methylphenidate*** (better known by the brand name Ritalin) are the medications often prescribed for ADD. (Strange as it seems, stimulants often calm hyperactivity.) A physician needs to monitor the dosage closely (about twice a month), both to check for the right level and to watch for side effects. Since the benefits of a Ritalin dose last only about four hours, two or three tablets may be needed each day.

Of the psychological therapies, behavior modification may be best, particularly if the therapist helps parents learn some of the techniques for behavior control. It is often given in conjunction with specific educational interventions, such as help with learning skills. Psychotherapy is a valuable option, particularly if the child suffers from low self-esteem.

ALTERNATIVE CHOICES

Several different alternative therapies may prove helpful, among them **homeopathy;** consult a homeopath for guidance. EEG **biofeedback** also shows promise as a means of behavior modification.

NUTRITION AND DIET

Although the effectiveness of dietary restrictions is controversial, some doctors recommend a high-protein, low-carbohydrate, sugar-free diet. Some children may also benefit from the B-vitamin supplements ***niacin*** (B_3), pyridoxine ***(B_6),*** and possibly thiamine ***(B_1).*** The stimulant ***caffeine***—ingested at the rate of 150 to 300 mg per day—can be helpful. Depending on the results of your child's tests for mineral blood levels, he may need supplements.

AT-HOME MANAGEMENT

- Join a support group. Connect with the national organization Children and Adults with Hyperactivity and Attention Disorders *(see **Appendix**).*
- Because an ADD child may process directions and other information in faulty ways, he is apt to be bombarded with corrections, leaving him with a low opinion of himself. Do whatever you can to promote your child's self-esteem.
- Praise and reward good behavior promptly.
- Be consistent with discipline, and make sure baby-sitters follow your methods.
- Make instructions simple and specific ("Brush your teeth; now, get dressed"), instead of general ("Get ready for school").
- Encourage your child's special strengths, particularly in sports and out-of-school activities.
- Have set routines for meals, sleep, play, and TV.
- Don't let homework monopolize all of his time after school; play and exercise are important.
- Simplify your child's room. Store toys out of sight. ■

BACKACHE

Read down this column to find your symptoms. Then read across.

SYMPTOMS	AILMENT/PROBLEM
◆ soreness after overexertion or injury; soreness that develops during the night; soreness that radiates to buttocks or thighs.	◆ Back muscle strain
◆ pain, stiffness, and tenderness in the back, buttocks, or thighs; difficulty moving or bending the back.	◆ Osteoarthritis of the spine, also called spondylosis
◆ sudden onset of pain; pain may shoot down one leg after lifting heavy objects, strenuous exercise, twisting, sneezing, or coughing; bending forward at the waist increases pain; lying down eases pain.	◆ Herniated disk (also called prolapsed disk); ruptured disk; or slipped disk
◆ chronic low-back pain that comes and goes for months or years.	◆ Misalignment of the spine
◆ sharp pain in a specific place along the spine.	◆ ***Osteoporosis***
◆ pain in the lower back in a woman who is more than four months pregnant.	◆ ***Pregnancy problem***
◆ pain in the lower back; fever of 100°F or above; painful urination; nausea or vomiting.	◆ ***Kidney infection***
◆ chronic pain and stiffness that seem worse in the morning; person with the pain is between the ages of 20 and 40.	◆ Ankylosing spondylitis
◆ pain in back, buttocks, thighs, and/or calves when walking or climbing stairs; pain is relieved by standing still or sitting.	◆ Spinal stenosis
◆ back pain, especially at night, that is unrelieved by lying down.	◆ Possibly, a tumor

WHAT TO DO	OTHER INFO
◆ See ***Back Problems*** and ***Sprains and Strains.*** Rest for a few days; use pain relievers if necessary.	◆ Physical therapy may include the application of heat and cold, gentle massage, and exercises to prevent future problems.
◆ See ***Arthritis.*** Take an anti-inflammatory drug for pain relief. Rest, heat, exercise, and physical therapy may be helpful.	◆ This condition may be caused by strain, injury, or aging.
◆ See ***Back Problems*** and ***Disk Problems.*** Treatment may include pain relievers, bed rest, physical therapy, and wearing a supportive collar.	◆ Disk problems may lead to other problems, such as ***sciatica*** or bowel or bladder ***incontinence.*** Chiropractic and acupuncture may help. If part of the disk is pressing on a nerve, surgery may be needed.
◆ See ***Back Problems.***	◆ The underlying cause may be poor muscle tone in the abdomen or back, ***obesity,*** or osteoarthritis.
◆ Hormone replacement therapy may be recommended for postmenopausal women, to prevent further bone loss.	◆ This condition is most common in women over 60 and people confined to bed or a wheelchair. Patients are encouraged not to smoke or drink alcohol, to eat less animal protein and fat, to obtain sufficient ***calcium,*** and to do weight-bearing exercise.
◆ Learning how to lift properly, wearing supportive shoes, improving posture, and sleeping on a firm mattress may help.	◆ Acupressure, massage, or chiropractic may be helpful.
◆ **Call your doctor now.** A kidney infection requires immediate treatment with ***antibiotics.***	◆ Be sure to take the antibiotics for the full length of the prescription.
◆ Usual treatment is anti-inflammatory drugs, physical therapy, massage, and prescribed exercises.	◆ Treatment is essential to prevent progression to fusion of the joints and a rigid spine.
◆ Call your doctor. Losing weight and doing abdominal exercises may help. Surgery is required in some cases.	◆ The pain is caused by a narrowing of the spinal canal at a point where a nerve passes. Modifying the posture may help.
◆ **Call your doctor without delay.** A medical evaluation is necessary for diagnosis and treatment.	◆ A tumor may be benign or malignant. By the time it causes pain, it is probably sizable. ***Cancer*** of the back is more likely in someone who already has cancer elsewhere.

Cross references are indicated by ***bold italics.***

BACK PROBLEMS

B

SYMPTOMS

- persistent aching or stiffness anywhere along your spine, from the base of the neck to the hips.
- sharp, localized pain in the neck, upper back, or lower back, especially after lifting heavy objects or engaging in other strenuous activity.
- chronic ache in the middle or lower back, especially after sitting or standing for extended periods.

CALL YOUR DOCTOR IF:

- you feel numbness, tingling, or loss of control in your arms or legs; you may have damaged your spinal cord.
- the pain in your back extends downward along the back of the leg; you may be suffering from ***sciatica.***
- the pain increases when you cough or bend forward at the waist; this may be the sign of a herniated disk *(see **Disk Problems**).*
- the pain is accompanied by fever; you may have a bacterial infection.
- you have dull pain in one area of your spine when lying in or getting out of bed, especially if you are over 50; you may be suffering from osteoarthritis *(see **Arthritis**).*

Back problems are the most common physical complaints among American adults. Nonspecific back pain is a leading cause of lost job time, to say nothing of the time and money spent in search of relief. And it's all because of one characteristic that makes us different from other animals—our upright posture.

The spinal column is an extraordinary mechanism, providing the stability we use to stand upright and the flexibility we need for active movement. The spine, or backbone, is actually a stack of 24 individual bones called vertebrae. A healthy spine is S-shaped when viewed from the side, curving back at the shoulders and inward at the neck and small of the back. As well as being the body's main structural member, it houses the spinal cord—the intricate sensory network that runs through the vertebrae to transmit feeling and control movement throughout the entire body.

The main reason late-20th-century Americans suffer from back problems is that we are increasingly defying our evolutionary heritage and becoming sedentary creatures. The upright posture is designed for walking, and for most of human history that's what people did. Only in this century, with the advent of motor vehicles, have most people gone from place to place while sitting down. In much the same way, our work habits are changing. Most of our ancestors worked standing up—hunting, gathering, working on farms or at workbenches. Today, a high proportion of people spend the better part of their working day sitting at desks, at work stations, or in cars and trucks. These recent but momentous changes in human behavior have had a profound—and largely negative—impact on human physiology.

People who walk a lot or do physical labor develop good muscle tone in their backs and legs. People who sit most of the day lose that muscle tone, and their backs are the first place to show it. To compensate, many of us turn to exercise programs: In some instinctual way, we are hearing our bodies cry out for the old ways that demanded more activity. If you are a healthy, active adult and your normal activities keep you on the go, you may not need a special exercise routine; if you work in a sedentary job or if you aren't building several hours of walking or other physi-

WHERE IT HURTS

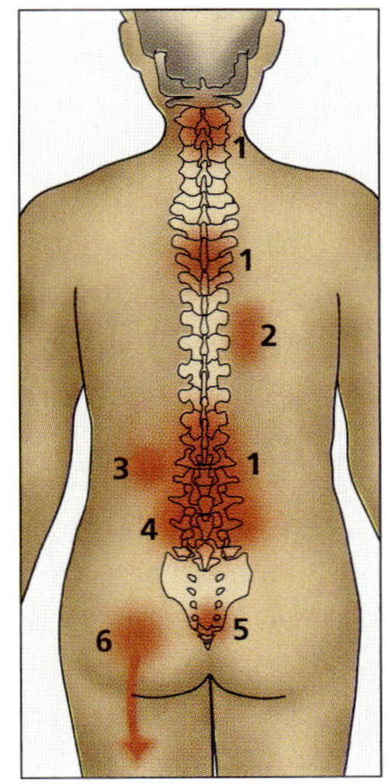

Back pain can have many causes. Pain caused by **osteoarthritis (1)** can occur anywhere along the spine. The larger back muscles can be affected by **fibrositis (2).** Pain in the loin area on either side of the spine may indicate a **kidney infection (3).** Damage to spinal disks, joints, ligaments, or muscles can be responsible for **lower back pain (4).** A fall or other injury can cause pain in the **coccyx (5).** Pain radiating from the buttock down the back or outside of the leg may be **sciatica (6).**

cal activity into your weekly routine, you should exercise regularly, with emphasis on toning up those muscles that keep your back strong.

CAUSES

Back problems rank high on the list of ailments that are self-inflicted. Most of our back troubles happen because of bad habits, generally developed over a long period of time: poor posture; overexertion in work and play; sitting incorrectly at the desk or the steering wheel; pushing, pulling, and lifting things carelessly. Sometimes the effects are immediate, but in many cases back problems develop over time. The most common type of back pain comes from straining the bands of muscles surrounding the spine. Although such strains can occur anywhere along the spine, they happen most often in the curve of the lower back; the next most common place is at the base of the neck.

Sometimes, however, ***backache*** occurs for no apparent reason. Nonspecific backache may develop from weakened muscles that cannot handle everyday walking, bending, and stretching. In other cases, the discomfort seems to come from—or is aggravated by—general tension, lack of sleep, or stress, much like a tension headache. A condition called fibrositis causes chronic backache from localized muscle tension, which may in turn be psychosomatic in origin. Whether the muscle strain is from lifting heavy objects or something as innocuous as a sneeze makes little difference to the sufferer—the pain can be agonizing.

Pregnancy commonly brings on back pain, as the developing fetus, hormonal changes, and attendant weight gain put new kinds of stresses on a pregnant woman's spine and legs. Injuries from contact sports, accidents, and falls can cause all manner of problems, from minor muscle strains to severe damage to the spinal column or to the spinal cord itself.

DIAGNOSTIC AND TEST PROCEDURES

Unless you are totally immobilized from a back injury, your doctor will probably test your range of motion and nerve function, and may use palpation to locate the area of discomfort. Blood and urine tests will make sure the pain is not due to an infection or other systemic problem. X-rays are useful in pinpointing broken bones or other skeletal defects, and can sometimes help locate problems in connective tissue. To analyze soft-tissue damage, computed tomography (CT) or magnetic resonance imaging (MRI) scans may be necessary. To determine potential abnormalities affecting nerve and muscle stimuli, an electromyogram (EMG) can be useful.

TREATMENT

Because back problems stem from a variety of causes, some of which may not be readily apparent, conventional medical treatment and alternative therapies share a common pattern of pain relief, rest, and suitable restoration of movement.

CONVENTIONAL MEDICINE

The basic treatment for relieving back pain from strain or minor injury is immediate bed rest with

B

an ice pack and ***aspirin*** or another ***nonsteroidal anti-inflammatory drug (NSAID)*** to reduce pain and inflammation. After the inflammation subsides, applying heat can soothe and restore muscles and connective tissue.

When back pain becomes truly immobilizing, the doctor will probably prescribe an appropriate over-the-counter or prescription painkiller and possibly a ***muscle relaxant.*** Some muscle relaxants such as methocarbamol or ***cyclobenzaprine*** may cause nausea, disorientation, and drowsiness as side effects, but such medications are usually recommended only for a few days. To relieve inflammation and inhibit the patient's pain perception in severe cases, therapy may include an injection of a local anesthetic such as lidocaine in combination with a ***corticosteroid*** into the tissue around the affected area or into trigger points elsewhere in the body. For relief of chronic back pain, low doses of ***antidepressant*** medications are sometimes prescribed.

Long-term bed rest is no longer considered necessary for most cases of back pain. Indeed, the lack of activity may actually contribute to recurring back problems. In most cases, you will be expected to start normal, nonstrenuous activity within 24 to 72 hours, after which controlled exercise or physical therapy should begin. Physical therapy treatments may employ massage, ultrasound, whirlpool baths, controlled application of heat, and specifically tailored exercise programs to help patients regain full use of the back.

In addition, some physicians—especially those in sports medicine—advocate using a transcutaneous electrical nerve stimulator (TENS). Electrodes taped to the body carry a mild electric current that helps relieve pain. After appropriate training, patients can use a TENS on their own to help speed recovery of strained or moderately injured backs.

Surgery for nonspecific back pain is a last resort. In cases of persistent pain from extreme nerve damage, rhizotomy—surgically severing a nerve—may be necessary to stop transmission of pain to the brain. Rhizotomy can correct the symptoms caused by friction between the surfaces in a spinal joint, but it doesn't address other problems such as herniated disks.

ALTERNATIVE CHOICES

Alternative therapies can be directed toward relieving the immediate discomfort of a back problem as well as conditioning and strengthening the body to prevent recurrence.

ACUPRESSURE

To relieve lower-back pain, apply 60 seconds of thumb pressure on either side of the spine just above the top of the pelvic bone, then massage at this point, as well as at the hip and knee joints.

ACUPUNCTURE

Some people troubled by back problems praise acupuncture for pain relief. In the hands of a trained acupuncturist, needle therapy is believed to redirect energy flow and balance throughout the body, not simply to relieve immediate or chronic back pain. Therapy involves inserting needles into points in specific muscles and on the ear to relieve blockages in the energy channels associated with back pain. Acute problems can be relieved in 1 to 4 sessions, while chronic pain problems typically require 12 or more treatments.

BODY WORK

Massage of the muscles along both sides of the spine helps relieve tension and restore mobility, especially in areas that feel tight or hard. To avoid potential damage to the spinal cord, a trained physical therapist or massage therapist is careful not to exert direct pressure on the vertebrae themselves.

The **Alexander technique** and the **Feldenkrais method** are useful for corrective whole-body positioning, not simply to correct posture but to relieve chronic tension and stress.

CHIROPRACTIC

Relief of back problems is the chiropractor's stock in trade: It is estimated that more people see chiropractors for back problems than for all other ailments combined. Chiropractic spinal manipulation has been recognized by the U.S. Agency for Health Care Policy and Research as an effective therapy for acute low-back pain.

Traditional chiropractic therapy relies on spinal manipulation to correct subluxations, or misaligned vertebrae, which may be responsible for problems anywhere along the spine. By helping restore motion to poorly functioning vertebrae, chiropractic therapy diminishes the accompanying pain and muscle spasm.

Chiropractors who use mixed therapies may rely on x-rays and other conventional diagnostic methods to treat back pain, combining spinal manipulation with muscle massage, ultrasound stimulation of deep tissue, nutritional recommendations, and exercise. For people wary of becoming dependent on painkillers and muscle relaxants for chronic back problems, modern chiropractic treatment offers a drug-free option to pain relief.

HERBAL THERAPIES

For general pain relief, drink infusions of ***white willow*** *(Salix alba)* or vervain *(Verbena officinalis).* For inflammation, try teas brewed from ***lobelia*** *(Lobelia inflata),* ***yarrow*** *(Achillea millefolium),* cramp *(Viburnum opulus),* or ***white willow. Valerian*** *(Valeriana officinalis),* available as a tincture and in capsules, is particularly recommended as a muscle relaxant and sedative.

HOMEOPATHY

Over-the-counter remedies reported to help nonspecific back problems include ***Arnica*** for bruised or sore muscles, ***Bryonia*** and ***Rhus toxicodendron*** for sharp pain that gets worse when you move, and ***Nux vomica*** for persistent backache.

MIND/BODY MEDICINE

Biofeedback therapy, using carefully monitored low-level electrical impulses, is reported to help back-pain sufferers. The special equipment translates muscle tension into audible signals. Patients learn to slow the signals and relax the muscle. **Guided imagery** treatments may have similar results without the use of electronic equipment. **Yoga** relaxes back muscles to reduce pain and inflamation.

OSTEOPATHY

Osteopathic treatment is likely to combine drug therapy with spinal manipulation or traction, followed by physical therapy and exercise. More and more doctors and physical therapists are using spinal manipulation techniques as part of back-pain therapy. The U.S. government has recognized spinal manipulation by osteopaths and chiropractors as being highly effective in treating many back problems.

PREVENTION

The most important preventive measure for lower-back pain is practicing good posture when standing and sitting.

First, analyze your posture by standing with your heels against a wall. Your calves, buttocks, shoulders, and the back of your head should touch the wall, and you should be able to slip your hand behind the small of your back. Then step forward and stand normally: If your posture changes, correct it right away. If you stand for long periods at work, wear flat shoes with good arch support and get a box or step about six inches high to rest one foot on from time to time.

Your sitting posture may be even more important. A good chair bottom supports your hips comfortably but doesn't touch the backs of your knees. Your chair back should be set at an angle of about 10 degrees and should cradle the small of your back comfortably; if necessary, use a wedge-shaped cushion or lumbar pad. Your feet should rest flat on the floor. Your forearms should rest on your desk or work surface with your elbows almost at a right angle.

When you have to lift heavy objects, don't bend at the waist. Squat with your legs, keep your back upright as you grasp the object, and stand upright again. Let your legs do the lifting, not your back. A nonprescription back brace may also give support and prevent back strain; its main benefit is that it won't let you bend over at the waist. Use a back brace sparingly: Long-term use can make you dependent on it and may eventually lead to weaker—not stronger—back muscles. ■

BAD BREATH

B

SYMPTOMS

- a stale, unpleasant odor coming from the mouth.
- a foul, putrid odor coming through the mouth from the stomach or other internal organs.

CALL YOUR DOCTOR OR DENTIST IF:

- the odor is accompanied by inflamed or bleeding gums. These may be signs of tooth decay or ***gum problems.***
- foul breath persists without any obvious cause after brushing and flossing the teeth and cleaning the gums and tongue. You may have an internal condition that requires medical diagnosis and treatment.

Most adults and many children have occasional bad breath, and some people are convinced they have it when they don't. Fear of bad breath has spawned a vast industry that promotes toothpastes, mouthwashes, and other products that promise to vanquish odors. For most of us, good oral hygiene and a balanced diet are all that's necessary for fresh-smelling breath, although in some cases bad breath—or halitosis—can signal serious health problems.

CAUSES

Plaque—a sticky coating of food particles, saliva, and bacteria on the teeth—is a major cause of bad breath. Residual traces of coffee, alcoholic drinks, tobacco smoke, and highly spiced or strong-smelling foods can also contribute to mouth odor. A regular flow of saliva helps clean the mouth, so a dry mouth after a night's sleep may smell stale. Not eating at all can cause stale breath because eating stimulates saliva flow. But when saliva collects in the mouth—particularly in depressions at the back of the tongue—and is digested by oral bacteria, powerful odors can result.

Bad breath can be caused by ***indigestion*** and such disorders as tooth decay, ***gum problems,*** and ***postnasal drip.*** Some diseases cause foul breath, including lung and gastrointestinal ailments, ***cancer, diabetes, kidney disease, tuberculosis, sinusitis,*** and ***strep throat.*** Taking certain drugs, especially some ***antidepressants,*** may cause dry mouth and bad breath. In rare cases, particularly in toddlers, prolonged bad breath may indicate a foreign body lodged in the nose. Anyone who has persistent bad breath that doesn't seem related to oral hygiene or temporary indigestion should ask a doctor about the potential cause.

TREATMENT

Good oral hygiene will take care of most bad breath. Brush and floss your teeth at least twice a day, especially after meals when food particles may be trapped in your mouth. Baking soda can substitute for toothpaste; it's a good cleanser and also deodorizes the breath. Eliminating strong-smelling food can help reduce the problem, as can stimulating the flow of saliva *(see **Nutrition and Diet,** right)* and drinking plenty of water. Mouthwashes, mints, and chewing gum are only temporary cover-ups for bad breath.

CONVENTIONAL MEDICINE

Plaque buildup is a major cause of bad breath, so have your teeth cleaned by a dental professional regularly. Chronic bad breath should be diagnosed and treated by a doctor or dentist.

ALTERNATIVE CHOICES

HOMEOPATHY

If your breath is particularly bad on awakening, after meals, or after drinking alcohol, try ***Nux vomica*** or *Kali phosphoricum.* Both are available over the counter; follow dosages on the labels.

HERBAL THERAPIES

An infusion of ***myrrh*** *(Commiphora molmol),* ***bloodroot*** *(Sanguinaria canadensis),* and ***peppermint*** *(Mentha piperita)* can be used as everyday mouthwash. To help sweeten the breath, try tea brewed from ***fenugreek*** *(Trigonella foenum-graecum)* or ***peppermint*** *(Mentha piperita).* Preparations containing cloves, aniseed, and ***fennel*** *(Foeniculum vulgare)* also are popular.

IS IT REALLY THAT BAD?

Unfortunately, the person with bad breath is often the last to know. If you aren't sure whether or not you have bad breath, ask your best friend—or your dentist. Or try this self-test: Cup your hands over your mouth, exhale deeply, then inhale through your nose to smell your breath.

NUTRITION AND DIET

A high-fiber diet with plenty of whole grains, fresh fruit, and raw, leafy vegetables helps good digestion and reduces the chance of bad breath. Eating apples, oranges, and celery can help by cleaning the teeth, dispersing bacteria in the mouth, and stimulating saliva flow. Try chewing fresh parsley or peppermint leaves, a method used by ancient Romans to sweeten their breath.

AT-HOME REMEDIES

There's no substitute for good oral hygiene. Brush your teeth with circular—not back-and-forth—movements, then floss thoroughly between your teeth all the way around your mouth.

Cleaning the tongue, which many people neglect, is very important: Use your toothbrush to brush the top of the tongue as far back as possible. A tongue blade, a device used in the Middle East and India to scrape the tongue, may be helpful. Several American companies make them, or you can try a store that sells Asian or Middle Eastern products. A soupspoon will work just as well; gently draw the inverted bowl of the spoon over your tongue to scrape off any residue. But be careful: Don't push the brush, spoon, or scraper so far back that you start to gag.

After cleaning, rinse your mouth with water. In fact, taking a few sips of water, swishing it around your mouth, and spitting it out is a good idea when brushing isn't possible. As on-the-spot breath fresheners, try mints, mouthwash, or chewing gum that contains chlorophyll, but don't rely on them to replace good oral hygiene.

PREVENTION

If you're worried about bad breath, avoid highly spiced or strong-smelling foods such as onions, hot peppers, garlic, pastrami, salami, pepperoni, and anchovies. They not only smell strong themselves but may be hard to digest, bringing on stomach gas, which can contribute to bad breath. ■

BEDSORES

B

SYMPTOMS

- an inflamed, sometimes painful, reddish patch of skin, especially on the shoulder blades, spine, lower back, hip joints, knees, ankles, or heels of a bedridden or wheelchair-bound person.
- a raw, open sore in any of the areas noted above, caused by the top layer of skin having cracked and peeled away; open bedsores can quickly become ulcerated.

CALL YOUR DOCTOR IF:

- a person is going to remain bedridden or immobile for an extended period, cannot move or is very weak, and is beginning to develop bedsores. The person may need regular attendance by a nurse or other trained healthcare provider.
- the sore produces a discharge, which may contain pus or become foul smelling; or if the sore turns black. This indicates an infection or tissue death; **get immediate medical attention.**

Anyone who cares for an immobile person at home understands the curse of bedsores. Even hospital and nursing home staffers may not be able to keep their patients from developing these irritating and sometimes debilitating skin injuries. More than a million Americans get bedsores each year, two-thirds of them being bedridden people over the age of 70.

CAUSES

A bedsore begins as a tender, inflamed area caused by unrelieved pressure on a bony, weight-bearing area of the body; it can quickly turn into a painful skin ulcer that usually heals slowly. The likely pressure points are the ankles, knees, heels, shoulder blades, and—particularly in wheelchair patients—the spine, hips, and lower back. The pressure need not be present for extended periods to cause inflammation; in some cases, bedsores form in a matter of hours. Patients with ***diabetes*** or other conditions that promote skin breakdown and infection are at risk, as are those who are underweight, paralyzed, or suffering from poor circulation, heart problems, spinal cord injury, or ***atherosclerosis.***

TREATMENT

CONVENTIONAL MEDICINE

At most hospitals and nursing homes, the standard treatment for bedsores is to clean the wound with a saline solution or hydrogen peroxide, remove any dead skin, and cover the area with a dressing that does not stick to the damaged skin. Dead tissue may need to be removed with a fine scalpel. In severe cases, when an ulcerated bedsore is deep and difficult to stabilize, plastic surgery or skin grafts may be required to restore damaged areas.

Unfortunately, some injuries and conditions prevent bedridden patients from being moved at all. Even those who can be shifted regularly risk tearing delicate skin if they are pulled over the sheets. One option for such patients is to improve

B

MOVING A BEDRIDDEN PERSON

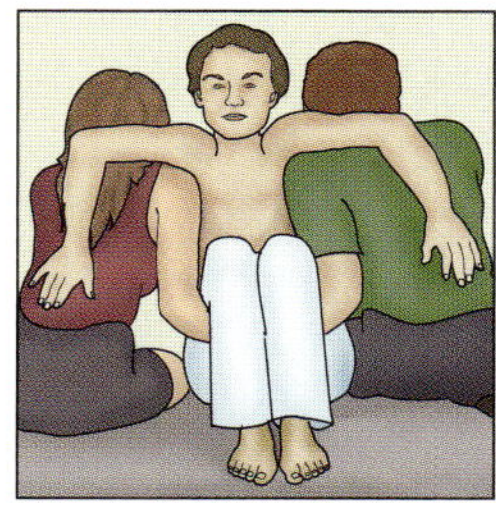

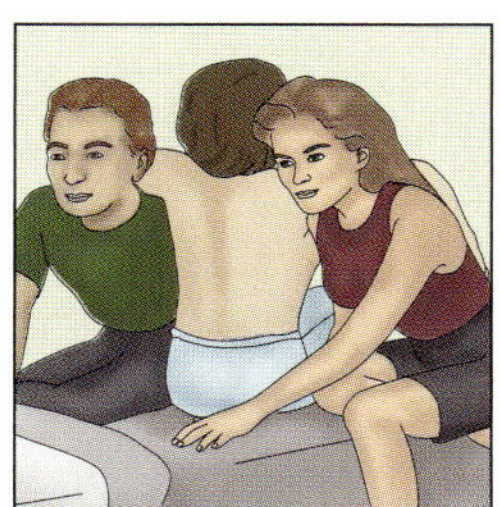

To prevent bedsores from becoming ulcerated, two people should move a bedridden patient every two waking hours. First, sit the patient up with legs bent. The movers face the head of the bed and sit on either side of the patient with one leg on the bed. Each reaches under the patient's legs and grasps the other's forearm *(top).*

With their inside shoulders under the patient's armpits, the movers put their free hands on the bed for support *(bottom).* Together they lift the patient and gently move him to a new position, adjusting the bedding as necessary.

their circulation, either by massage or by controlled, low-level electrical stimulation.

ALTERNATIVE CHOICES

Various alternative treatments can soothe inflammation and relieve pain, but they cannot replace the essential steps of moving a bedridden person often and improving the individual's diet.

HERBAL THERAPIES

Herbal treatments may relieve the discomfort of bedsores and may help fight infection. To ease minor inflammation, apply a ***marsh mallow*** *(Althaea officinalis)* root ointment; or try a poultice made from equal parts of powdered ***slippery elm*** *(Ulmus fulva)* bark, marsh mallow root, and oregon grape *(Mahonia aquifolium) root* blended with a small amount of hot water. Two drops of essential ***tea tree oil*** (*Melaleuca* spp.) in a cup of water makes an infection-fighting rinse.

NUTRITION AND DIET

Patients with bedsores need to drink plenty of water to prevent their skin from becoming dry and vulnerable to pressure. Certain vitamins and minerals, especially ***vitamins A, C, E,*** and ***B complex,*** and ***zinc,*** promote skin growth and repair. ***Vitamin C*** in particular has been shown to be effective in healing bedsores. But because some vitamins can be toxic in large doses—especially to people whose bodies are weakened by disease or injury—taking any vitamin or mineral supplements must be supervised by the attending physician.

AT-HOME CARE

Caring for invalids at home—especially aging loved ones—can be a daunting task. Some helpful tips for making each day tolerable:

- Make sure the person confined to bed or a wheelchair moves his body as often as possible when awake, but at least every two hours. If he can't move around on his own, others should move his body for him.
- Cushion the person's feet, knees, spine, and shoulders with soft pillows or cloth-covered foam pads, and adjust them frequently for comfort.
- Never pull or slide the person over bedclothes, because the friction may cause further skin damage. Always use the two-person lifting technique *(above, left).*

PREVENTION

When it comes to bedsores, prevention is clearly worth more than any cure. Wheelchair-bound or bedridden people should shift their positions regularly. They should be bathed frequently and dried thoroughly, and their skin should be lubricated with a mild, nonirritating lotion. They should have clean, dry, tight-fitting, unstarched cotton sheets; loose-fitting clothes; plenty of air circulation; a healthy diet; and some sort of regular exercise—even if a caregiver has to move their limbs.

To cushion sensitive areas, try an "eggcrate" foam mattress overlay, a water-filled mattress, or a sheepskin pad over the bedsheets. Consider a variable-pressure mattress with separate sections that can be inflated and deflated independently to adjust pressure on the patient's body. ■

BEDWETTING

B

SYMPTOMS

It is not unusual for children under the age of six to have trouble controlling their bladders at night. You should be concerned about bedwetting only if:

- your child is older than six and has never been dry at night or continues to wet the bed twice a month or more.
- your child suddenly starts wetting at night after a period of having been dry through the night.

CALL YOUR DOCTOR IF:

- your efforts to help your child learn to stay dry through the night are not working, or your child wants additional help in managing the situation.
- your child is wetting the bed and has frequent or painful urination, dark brown urine (a sign of bleeding), abdominal pain, or fever; these symptoms may indicate a urinary tract or ***bladder infection.***
- your child experiences side effects that affect his behavior or interfere with his sleep after starting a course of prescribed medication to treat bedwetting. Many drugs used in treatment cause these types of side effects.

The most important thing to remember about bedwetting is that it is a benign disorder and not a willful act. Punishment is never an answer. Between five million and seven million children suffer from bedwetting; the majority are boys.

Don't be unduly concerned about bedwetting unless your child is older than six. Before then, your child's body may not have developed enough to control bladder actions at night. Time usually cures the problem: Most children resolve any difficulties on their own by the age of seven.

CAUSES

Why bedwetting occurs is not fully understood, although most cases seem to result from some kind of developmental delay. Some experts think bedwetting is purely a behavioral issue, others believe its origins are physiological, and still others think both physiological and behavioral factors play a role. Only 2 percent of cases can be traced to neurological problems (often caused by structural spinal abnormalities) or specific diseases such as ***diabetes*** or ***bladder infections.***

Alternative therapists believe that a misalignment of muscles and joints around the pelvis can affect the activity of the sphincter muscle that controls urine release.

Any new, stressful situation may cause a child to revert to bedwetting. Once your child adjusts to the situation, the problem should resolve itself. If your child does not improve, the treatments listed here should help. In addition, you will want your child to talk through his fears.

TREATMENT

CONVENTIONAL MEDICINE

To rule out a disease-related problem, your pediatrician will perform a blood or urine test. If the test reveals diabetes or an infection, your pediatrician will treat that condition first. The doctor will also test your child to rule out nervous system problems.

There are three primary ways to treat bedwetting in an otherwise healthy child: waiting for spontaneous resolution, employing behavioral conditioning, and undertaking drug therapy.

Waiting, though often the preferred course, may make your child anxious. However, if he is old enough to benefit from motivational counseling—to learn about the condition and participate in its management—he and the rest of your family will be better able to cope. One form of motivation is to have your child place a star on a chart or calendar to mark dry nights.

Behavioral conditioning—utilizing a device with a sensor that detects wetness and sets off an alarm—has proved very effective. The child begins associating bladder distention with being awakened and in time "learns" to awaken before losing control.

Drug therapy is considered less effective because most children relapse after stopping medication. It has its place, however. For short-term help—when your child sleeps at a friend's, for example—desmopressin, an antidiuretic, works well. Doctors are moving away from the antidepressant imipramine because of side effects.

ALTERNATIVE CHOICES

ACUPRESSURE

According to proponents of acupressure, daily application of deep thumb pressure in an upward motion to the following points may help: Conception Vessel 4, Kidney 3, Spleen 6. See the ***Appendix*** for point locations. Also, try holding Heart 7, the point in the hollow of your child's wrist just below the little finger, for up to one minute and then switch sides.

BODY WORK

Shiatsu and **reflexology** may be helpful in bedwetting caused by a neurological problem. Consult a trained therapist for help.

EXERCISE

Bladder-stretching exercises may help your child increase bladder capacity. Once a day your child should hold his urine as long as possible past the first indication that his bladder is full. You and your child should measure the voided urine daily to see if capacity is increasing. Have your child practice this for up to three months to give this technique an opportunity to work.

HOMEOPATHY

Because bedwetting is a chronic problem, you need to seek help from an experienced homeopath. Common remedies include *Equisetum, Causticum,* ***Lycopodium,*** and ***Pulsatilla.***

MIND/BODY MEDICINE

Hypnotherapy can be effective with children who are highly motivated. With the help of a trained professional, your child will master a series of action statements that he will say before going to bed, such as: "When I need to urinate, I will wake up all by myself and go to the bathroom."

NUTRITION AND DIET

Sometimes bedwetting is associated with food allergies. Try eliminating milk products, citrus fruits, and chocolate—foods most frequently linked to allergies—from your child's diet.

OSTEOPATHY

If exercises or behavior-based treatments don't work, consult an osteopath for manipulation of your child's lower back and pelvic area to modify possible structural problems.

WAYS TO COPE

- Teach an older child how to change his own bed. Set out clean pajamas and sheets in his room each night. You will help him avoid embarrassment and give him a sense of being in control if he no longer has to rely on you.
- If you are using an alarm device for behavioral conditioning, avoid nylon sheets and pajamas; nylon induces sweat, which can set off the alarm.
- Prevent the mattress from getting wet by using a plastic-lined mattress cover (which may cause the child to sweat) or, better yet, provide him with a smaller, rubberized, felt-covered pad that he can place over the wet area on the bed after an accident. ■

BEE AND WASP STINGS

B

SYMPTOMS

In most cases, a bee or wasp sting causes only minor symptoms at the site of the sting, including:

- pain.
- swelling.
- redness.
- itching or burning.

Allergic reactions may produce extensive swelling. Allergies are also responsible for an even more serious, and potentially fatal, condition called **anaphylactic shock.** *(See **Emergencies/First Aid: Shock.**)* Multiple stings can produce a toxic reaction, with the same symptoms:

- rapid swelling around the eyes, lips, tongue, or throat.
- difficulty breathing.
- wheezing or hoarseness.
- itching, cramping, or numbness that is severe.
- dizziness.
- a reddish rash, or ***hives.***
- stomach cramps.
- loss of consciousness.

CALL YOUR DOCTOR IF:

- you are stung and develop any of the symptoms of anaphylactic shock listed above. **Get medical help now.**
- you are allergic to bee or wasp stings and you are stung. You are at risk of anaphylactic shock, even if your reaction to previous stings was mild; you may need emergency treatment. (See your doctor to determine if you are allergic.)

The venom from a bee or wasp sting causes local swelling, pain, and redness, which usually go away within several hours. Some people who are allergic to the venom experience larger local reactions, with more extensive swelling.

For about 3 percent of people, however, a sting can trigger a life-threatening allergic reaction called anaphylaxis (from the Greek for "nonhealing"). Painful ***hives*** and swelling may progress rapidly to block off airways, causing circulatory collapse and, sometimes, death. In the United States, about 50 people die each year from sting-induced **anaphylactic shock,** primarily people over 40 with preexisting ***heart disease.*** If you are stung by a swarm of 50 to 100 bees, the effect can be similar to that of anaphylactic shock.

The only insects with true stingers belong to the order Hymenoptera, including the Apidae (honeybees and bumblebees) and Vespidae (wasps, yellow jackets, white-faced hornets, and yellow hornets). The stinging mechanism, located in the female's abdomen, consists of a stinger attached to a venom-filled sac. The honeybee's stinger has multiple barbs so that it usually remains in the wound, causing the bee's death. Wasps, whose stingers do not have barbs, can sting more than once.

CAUSES

The venom of Hymenoptera contains toxins and inflammatory agents that cause the local pain and swelling that go away after a few hours. Some people, however, are allergic to elements in the venom and have more severe reactions, which can range from extended swelling to potentially fatal anaphylactic shock. The process of sting-induced ***allergies*** is poorly understood. Like other allergies, sting allergy appears to run in families. But scientists still don't understand why only 60 percent of allergic adults and only 8 percent of allergic children suffer shock when stung.

A person may be stung many times and have only normal reactions, then suddenly one sting will produce a strong allergic reaction. Doctors are not sure why a person suddenly develops such sensitivity or why the sensitivity may last fewer than 3 months or more than 25 years.

DIAGNOSTIC AND TEST PROCEDURES

Your doctor can determine if you are allergic to bee and wasp stings with a simple skin test, using purified, freeze-dried venom. However, only about 20 percent of people with a positive skin test suffer severe reactions to a real sting.

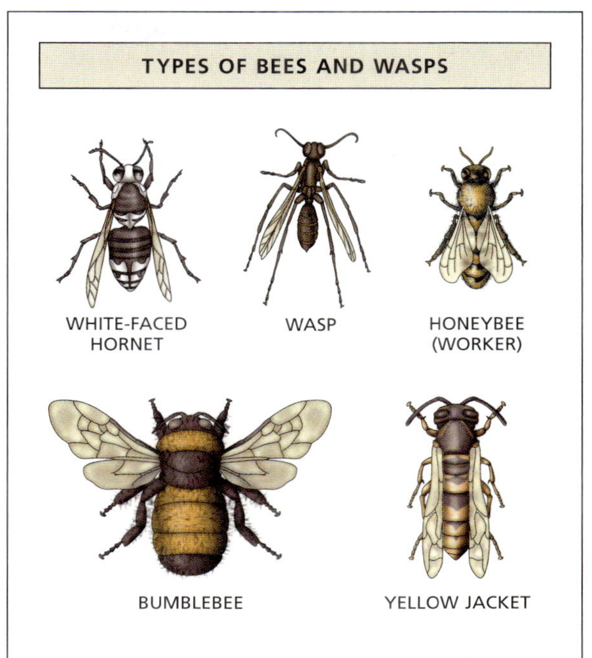

TREATMENT

For most stings, minimal treatment, such as a cold compress or ice pack, is sufficient. If you have multiple stings or a severe allergic reaction, you need medical help at once.

CONVENTIONAL MEDICINE

For pain, take ***aspirin*** or ***acetaminophen.*** For strong reactions, try ***diphenhydramine*** or another nonprescription ***antihistamine.*** For children, use cough medicine containing antihistamine (avoid aspirin because of the risk of Reye's syndrome).

For **anaphylactic shock,** the usual treatment is the bronchodilator ***epinephrine.*** You may give yourself an injection from a bee-sting kit; but after the injection, see a doctor promptly for further treatment. (Note: Bee-sting kits are now available for children; read the directions carefully.)

ALTERNATIVE CHOICES

HERBAL THERAPIES

Apply ***aloe*** *(Aloe barbadensis)* or the fresh bruised leaf or juice of ***plantain.*** Or apply ***calendula*** *(Calendula officinalis)* ointment four times a day.

HOMEOPATHY

A homeopath may recommend applying a few drops of *Pyrethrum* tincture, available over the counter, to a sting. For swelling, take ***Apis*** (30c) every 30 minutes to 2 hours.

AT-HOME REMEDIES

If the stinging apparatus remains in the skin, scrape it away with a knife or fingernail; if you use tweezers, you may squeeze more venom into the skin. For bee stings, a paste of baking soda will ease the itching. Wasp stings are alkaline and can be neutralized by vinegar or lemon juice. If you're far from home, apply mud; as it dries, it will draw out some of the toxin.

PREVENTION

To avoid sting-induced shock if you are allergic, carry a bee-sting kit (be sure you know how to administer a self-injection). You should also wear a Medic Alert bracelet or necklace describing your allergy.

If you have had a severe reaction to a sting and a positive venom skin test, venom immunotherapy—a series of weekly injections of venom—is highly effective at preventing anaphylaxis.

Reduce your chances of being stung by avoiding brightly colored, white, or pastel clothing. Don't use cosmetics or perfume with floral scents. Food odors attract insects, especially yellow jackets, so be alert when you are cooking or eating outdoors. ■

BLACK EYE

B

SYMPTOMS

- bruising and swelling of the eyelid and soft tissue around the eye, sometimes accompanied by broken blood vessels in the white of the eye. The discoloration starts out purple or blue; as the bruise heals, it may turn green or yellow before disappearing, usually in about a week.

CALL YOUR DOCTOR IF:

- a pair of black eyes occurs simultaneously; you should be examined by a doctor for possible skull fracture.

Any of the symptoms below may indicate damage to the eyeball, which should be evaluated and treated by a doctor or an ophthalmologist:

- your eyeball hurts.
- you have an open cut around the eye.
- you have blurred vision, multiple images, or floating spots.
- you see blood or other fluid in front of the iris of the eye.
- you experience unusual sensitivity to light or other vision changes.

Like many bruises, a "shiner" may be nothing to worry about and will heal of its own accord in a few days. In some cases, however, a black eye is a sign of more serious injury to the eye or the skull. Any damage to the eyeball that causes it to become red and swollen must be evaluated by an ophthalmologist or other physician; an eye injury could involve a detached retina or lead to ***glaucoma.*** A fracture in the ring of bones around the eye may trap muscle or soft tissue and can impair vision; surgery may be required to correct the condition. *(See also* ***Eye Problems, Vision Problems.****)*

CAUSES

Most black eyes are the result of a blow that causes bleeding beneath the skin, producing the characteristic blue-black discoloration. A skull fracture can cause black eyes, in which case both eyes are usually affected. People with ***sinusitis*** from allergies sometimes get "allergic shiners"—darkening under the eyes caused by inflamed and engorged blood vessels.

TREATMENT

Applying something cold to a black eye works in two ways: It helps to reduce swelling and to constrict blood vessels, which in turn stops the internal bleeding. Putting a cold steak on a black eye is a needlessly expensive variation; you can save money by using an ice pack or a package of frozen vegetables, which works just as well.

Besides cold treatment, there's not much that can be done for a black eye except to avoid doing anything that could cause further injury, such as putting pressure on the swollen eye or trying to force it open. If you need a pain reliever, take an analgesic such as ***aspirin*** or ***ibuprofen,*** either of which will also help reduce inflammation.

CONVENTIONAL MEDICINE

A doctor will recommend applying an ice pack or a cloth soaked in ice-cold water and wrung out.

Hold the ice pack or cold compress to the eye for up to 10 minutes, being careful not to apply pressure. You might try putting crushed ice in a plastic bag and taping it to the forehead. Repeat the cold treatment for 5 to 10 minutes every hour for 24 hours or as long as swelling is present.

If the eyeball itself is damaged or if vision is affected, your doctor or ophthalmologist will determine the nature and extent of the injury and give appropriate treatment. If the eye is protruding from the eye socket, surgery may be necessary.

ALTERNATIVE CHOICES

Until the beginning of this century, leeches were used to suck blood from around a black eye. That treatment actually did relieve the pressure, but it's thankfully a thing of the past. Today other nonmedical remedies may be helpful.

HERBAL THERAPY

You may want to gently apply a compress made with ***chamomile*** *(Matricaria recutita)*. Chamomile is said to reduce the fragility of tiny capillaries and to serve as an anti-inflammatory agent.

HOMEOPATHY

A homeopath may recommend various over-the-counter remedies for black eye; be sure to follow label instructions carefully. ***Arnica*** (12x) may help speed the reabsorption of escaped blood. If skin is unbroken, *Arnica* cream around the eye may help reduce bruising. If bruising is slow to clear and pain is relieved only by cold, try ***Ledum*** (12x), three doses a day for four days. If bones around the eye are very sore or the eyeball itself is injured, *Symphytum* (12x), three doses a day, up to four days, may help relieve the pain. For severe shooting or radiating pains around the eye, ***Hypericum*** (12x) once an hour for up to four hours may help relieve pain and speed healing.

NUTRITION AND DIET

A good balanced diet with plenty of protein, vitamins, and minerals is important in the healing of any injury. In particular, bromelain, the enzyme in raw pineapple, may help reduce bruising. Eat fresh pineapple or take bromelain capsules, available in health food stores.

AT-HOME REMEDIES

For a black eye that is not severely damaged, applying ice and taking a painkiller are probably all that's necessary. Boxing trainers minimize facial swelling by using a gadget that looks like a small metal iron but is cold. You can get the same effect with a cold can of soda or a bag of frozen vegetables. Be sure the can or the bag is clean, and hold it lightly against the cheek or forehead, not the eye itself.

Be careful not to go overboard with cold treatment. Even though the swelling may be painful, it is one of the body's healing responses. You want to control excessive swelling without inhibiting the repair process. Your own good sense will tell you how much cold is too much. Most swelling reactions to mild injuries last only a few hours, so you shouldn't need an ice pack after the first day. If the pain and swelling persist after an hour or two of intermittent cold application, the injury is significant and should be seen by a doctor. ■

CAUTION!

DON'T BLOW YOUR NOSE

If you have a black eye, blowing your nose may rupture more blood vessels around the damaged facial tissue. If the injury that caused your black eye also fractured the bone of the eye socket, the pressure of blowing your nose could cause additional damage to an already unstable eyeball. Also, never try to force open an eyelid that is swollen shut; doing so could further injure the skin or the eye.

BLADDER CANCER

SYMPTOMS

In its early stages, bladder cancer may not have obvious symptoms; in later stages symptoms may include:

- bloody urine, ranging in color from faintly rusty to deep red, sometimes containing blood clots. Blood traces, invisible to the naked eye, may show up in tests of urine samples.
- frequent urinary tract infections, painful urination, and a need to urinate often.
- weight or appetite loss.
- abdominal or back pain, persistent low-grade fever, ***anemia.***

CALL YOUR DOCTOR IF:

- you have any of the symptoms listed above; although they may not be cancer related, you should be screened for bladder cancer.

The bladder is a pouch in the urinary tract that stores urine after it is produced by the kidneys. The bladder is lined with specialized transitional cells, and when it is irritated, extra layers of transitional cells develop. This process increases the likelihood of a transitional cell turning cancerous, then multiplying to create a malignant tumor. Malignant tumors begin as small, superficial lumps on the inner wall of the bladder. The cancer spreads by penetrating bladder muscle, infiltrating surrounding fat and tissue, and—if untreated—eventually invading the bloodstream and lymphatic system.

The earlier the cancer is detected, the more localized it will be and the more effective the treatment. Thanks to improved procedures for early detection, five-year survival rates for this disease improved from 50 percent in the 1960s to over 70 percent in the 1990s. While bladder tumors often recur, prompt detection means they can be stopped while they are still superficial. The average age for getting bladder cancer is 68. Men are more susceptible to the disease than women, and Caucasians more susceptible than African Americans. Bladder cancer accounts for about 5 percent of cancers in the United States, or about 50,000 cases a year.

CAUSES

Chronic irritation of the bladder increases the risk of cancer. People with congenital disorders of the bladder, chronic ***bladder infections,*** or persistent cystitis—inflammation of the bladder—are more susceptible, as are people with histories of benign bladder tumors.

More than most cancers, bladder cancer is associated with exposure to cancer-promoting chemicals, or carcinogens. For example, cigarette smokers have three times more risk than nonsmokers of developing bladder cancer because of specific carcinogens in tobacco smoke. Painters, truckers, leatherworkers, machinists and metalworkers, rubber and textile workers, and people exposed to industrial dyes are at increased risk. People who have been treated with radiation or alkylating chemotherapy agents are also at higher risk. Consumption of nitrates in smoked and cured meats may also be associated with bladder cancer, as may consumption of caffeine and saccharin, but the connection is so weak that some researchers question the risk at all.

DIAGNOSTIC AND TEST PROCEDURES

The bladder can be viewed through a fiberoptic tube known as a cystoscope. If the doctor detects a tumor, a tiny tissue sample is taken through the tube and examined in the laboratory. Should the tumor be malignant, the treatment will depend on how far, if at all, the cancer has spread. Blood and urine studies and x-rays of the bladder, ureters, kidneys, and other organs provide information about tumor size, location, and the degree or amount of spread.

TREATMENT

There is no acceptable primary treatment for cancer other than medical care by a certified oncologist. Alternative therapies outside mainstream medicine may help ease the pain of the disease and the side effects of conventional treatment, but none is a proven cure for cancer. See ***Cancer*** for more information about treatment.

CONVENTIONAL MEDICINE

If detected early, superficial malignancies can usually be treated successfully by transurethral resection (TUR). In this procedure the surgeon inserts a small tube into the bladder and removes the tumor surgically or burns it out with heat or a laser beam. Combined with chemotherapy or radiation therapy, TUR may also be successful against more invasive bladder cancer. Immunotherapy with the bacillus Calmette-Guérin (BCG) vaccine is beneficial in 60 percent of cases. Injecting BCG into the bladder after the tumor has been removed significantly reduces the chance of the cancer's recurring.

Invasive cancers may require radical cystectomy, or bladder removal. The surgeon then diverts the urinary tract and creates an opening, or stoma, through which urine is passed. Patients once had to wear external urine pouches, but new techniques synthesize internal pouches from intestinal tissue. Bladder removal may also mean removing the reproductive organs in women and the prostate and seminal vesicles in men. Although this procedure renders men impotent and women infertile, men can have penile implants to overcome impotence, and women can remain sexually active.

After surgery, a combination of radiation and chemotherapy may be necessary to deter recurrence. Anyone who has had bladder cancer should have regular follow-up tests, since tumors often recur. If the cancer has metastasized, or spread beyond the urinary tract, surgery is not usually considered. Chemotherapy is the primary treatment for recurrent and metastatic cancer.

COMPLEMENTARY THERAPIES

Several scientific studies suggest that certain vitamins and minerals are beneficial in both treatment and prevention of bladder cancer. Patients receiving BCG immunotherapy may have better results with megadoses of ***vitamins A, B_6, C,*** and ***E,*** as well as ***zinc.*** Research also suggests reduced incidence of bladder cancer among people with adequate vitamin B_6, beta carotene, and ***selenium*** in their diets.

PREVENTION

To prevent bladder cancer, your best bet is to steer clear of possible carcinogens. For starters, don't smoke. Eat smoked or cured meats only occasionally and prepare fresh rather than processed foods. If you work around carcinogenic chemicals, follow safety guidelines to avoid undue exposure; take the herb ***red clover*** *(Trifolium pratense)* to help excrete the chemicals in your urine. And if you feel you may be at risk for bladder cancer, arrange regular screenings with your doctor to ensure early detection. ■

BLADDER INFECTIONS

B

SYMPTOMS

- a burning sensation when urinating; this is the most common sign of a bladder infection, but any pain or difficulty in urination may also indicate the condition.
- frequent urge to urinate.
- urine with a strong, foul odor.
- in the elderly: lethargy, incontinence, mental confusion.

In severe cases, these symptoms may be accompanied by fever and chills, abdominal pain, or blood in the urine.

CALL YOUR DOCTOR IF:

- the burning sensation persists for more than 24 hours after you begin trying self-help treatments. Untreated, bladder infections can lead to more serious conditions.
- painful urination is accompanied by vomiting, fever, chills, bloody urine, or abdominal or back pain; it may indicate potentially life-threatening ***kidney disease,*** a bladder or kidney tumor, or prostate infection. **Seek medical help immediately.**
- the burning is accompanied by a discharge from the vagina or penis, a sign of ***sexually transmitted disease, pelvic inflammatory disease (PID),*** or other serious infection. See your doctor without delay.
- you experience any persistent pain or difficulty with urination; this may also be a sign of ***sexually transmitted disease,*** a vaginal infection, a ***kidney stone,*** enlargement of the prostate *(see **Prostate Problems**),* or a bladder or prostate tumor. See your doctor without delay.

Bladder infections—generally termed cystitis, which means inflammation of the bladder—are common in women and very rare in men. In fact, about half of all women get at least one bladder infection at some time in their lives. Although doctors are not sure exactly why women have many more bladder infections than men, they suspect it may be because women have a shorter urethra, the tube that carries urine out of the bladder. This relatively short passageway—only about an inch and a half long—makes it easier for bacteria to migrate into the bladder. Also, the opening to a woman's urethra lies close to both the vagina and the anus, giving bacteria from those areas access to the urinary tract.

Bladder infections are not serious if treated promptly. But recurrences are common in susceptible people and can lead to ***kidney infections,*** which are more serious and may result in permanent kidney damage. So it's very important to treat the underlying causes of a bladder infection and to take preventive steps to avoid recurrences.

In elderly people, bladder infections are often difficult to diagnose because the symptoms are less specific and are frequently blamed on aging. Older people who suddenly become ***incontinent*** or who begin acting lethargic or confused should be checked by a doctor for a bladder infection.

CAUSES

Most bladder infections are caused by various strains of *Escherichia coli (E. coli),* the bacteria commonly found in the intestines. Women sometimes get bladder infections as a direct result of intercourse, which can push bacteria up into the bladder through the urethra. Some women contract the infection—dubbed "honeymoon cystitis"—almost every time they have sex. Women who use a diaphragm as their primary method of birth control are also particularly susceptible to bladder infections, perhaps because the device presses on the bladder and keeps it from emptying completely. Bacteria then rapidly reproduce in the stagnant urine left in the bladder. Pregnant women, whose bladders become compressed as the fetus grows, are prone to infections for the same reason. Some people develop symptoms of a bladder infection when no infection actually exists. These disorders are usually benign but are difficult to treat.

While they can be quite uncomfortable and potentially serious if complications set in, the bladder infections that most women get clear up quickly and are relatively harmless. In men, however, a bladder infection is almost always a symptom of an underlying disorder and is generally regarded as cause for more concern. Often the infection has migrated from the prostate or some other part of the body, signaling problems in those locations. Or it may indicate the presence of a tumor or other obstruction that is interfering with the urinary tract. Some studies have shown that uncircumcised boys are at somewhat greater risk of contracting a bladder infection during their first year of life because bacteria may collect under the foreskin.

In recent years, an increasing number of bladder infections in both men and women have been linked to two sexually transmitted bacteria, ***chlamydia*** and mycoplasma. And both home and hospital use of catheters—tubes inserted into the bladder to empty it—can also lead to infection.

DIAGNOSTIC AND TEST PROCEDURES

Bladder infections usually can be diagnosed readily with a urine test. If you are experiencing persistent or frequent infections, or if an anatomical defect is suspected as the cause of the problem, your physician may also want you to undergo cystoscopy, a diagnostic procedure in which a lighted tube inserted through the urethra is used to examine the inside of the bladder. And to make sure your kidneys have not been affected, your physician may order an intravenous pyelogram (IVP), a special x-ray technique for viewing kidneys, or an ultrasound scan to produce an image of the entire urinary tract system.

TREATMENT

Mild bladder infections often clear up quickly in response to simple home remedies. But if you experience no relief within 24 hours, you should consult a physician for more aggressive treatment. Delay in clearing your body of the infection can lead to more serious problems.

CONVENTIONAL MEDICINE

Bladder infections are treated with a wide variety of ***antibiotics*** to clear up the infection; with phenazopyridine, which is often given to relieve the pain and burning; and by increased intake of fluids to flush out the urinary tract. The antibiotic your physician prescribes and the number of days you will need to take it will depend on the type of bacteria that are causing the infection. Although some studies indicate that uncomplicated infections require only one to three days of treatment, your physician may prefer to treat you for a longer period of time in order to ensure that all of the bacteria are eradicated. Elderly people and those with a chronic underlying health condition, such as ***diabetes*** or HIV infection, are often prescribed a longer course of antibiotics—sometimes up to 14 days.

After the treatment has run its course, you may be asked to come in for a follow-up urine test to make sure your bladder is free of all signs of infection. People with frequently recurring bladder infections are often prescribed low daily doses of antibiotics for an additional six months or longer. Patients whose infections are related to sexual activity may be given a small dose of antibiotics to take each time they have intercourse. Some doctors prescribe the hormone ***estrogen,*** either as a topical cream or in pill form, to prevent recurrences in postmenopausal women. For cases where the infection is the result of a blockage or obstruction, such as a kidney stone or an enlarged prostate, surgery may be required.

ALTERNATIVE CHOICES

If begun promptly at the first hint of burning during urination, alternative means of treatment can be successful in getting rid of a bladder infection. But if these methods do not bring relief within 24 hours, you should call your doctor for antibiotic treatment. Consult with your doctor if you wish to continue with alternative methods while on the antibiotics to speed up the recovery process.

ACUPUNCTURE

Acupuncture treatment may help prevent recurrences of bladder infections. Consult a professional acupuncturist.

HERBAL THERAPIES

Some herbs have been found useful in both clearing up bladder infections and easing the burning that accompanies them. Perhaps the best known is cranberry, which, recent scientific studies show, has a remarkable ability to combat bladder infections and other urinary tract infections *(box, opposite).*

Another herb useful in treating bladder infections is ***nettle*** *(Urtica dioica),* which has been shown to have anti-inflammatory properties. Mix 1 tsp dried, crushed nettle leaves or root in 1 cup boiling water. Allow the infusion to cool, then drink 1 tbsp every hour or two—up to 1 cup a day.

The evergreen shrub ***uva ursi*** *(Arctostaphylos uva-ursi),* or bearberry, which acts as a diuretic and an anti-inflammatory medication, has a long history as a folk remedy for bladder infections. Soak fresh leaves in brandy or other liquor for a few hours, then add to boiling water—about 1 tsp leaves per cup of water. If you have dried leaves, you can boil them directly in the water without a preliminary alcohol soak.

Women who are prone to bladder infections after sexual activity can help prevent recurrences by washing their perineal area with a medicinal solution of the herb ***goldenseal*** *(Hydrastis canadensis)* before and after intercourse. Mix 2 tsp of the herb per cup of water, bring to a boil, and simmer for 15 minutes. Cool to room temperature before using.

HOMEOPATHY

Depending on the symptoms, homeopaths recommend a number of different remedies to help relieve the pain of a bladder infection. Here are three of the most commonly prescribed:

- If the urge to urinate is very strong and the burning is intense, ***Cantharis.***
- If you experience painful cramping with urination or your urine is very dark or bloody, *Mercurius corrosivus.*
- For women whose infections are brought on by sexual contact, *Staphysagria.*
- If you feel a dull, constant pain, *Berberis.*

Take these remedies hourly until symptoms disappear. If you experience no relief after 24 hours, seek professional help.

HYDROTHERAPY AND AROMATHERAPY

Hot sitz baths can help relieve the symptoms of a bladder infection. Adding certain pungent herbal oils to the bathwater creates a soothing, fragrant steam that aromatherapists believe makes the treatment particularly effective. Try putting in a few drops of the essential oils of ***juniper*** berry, ***eucalyptus,*** sandalwood, pine, ***parsley,*** cedarwood, ***chamomile,*** or cajuput.

You can also try a massage oil made with 1 oz vegetable oil and 5 drops each of any combination of the herbs mentioned. Massage daily, rubbing the oil over your lower back, abdomen, stomach, and hips.

REFLEXOLOGY

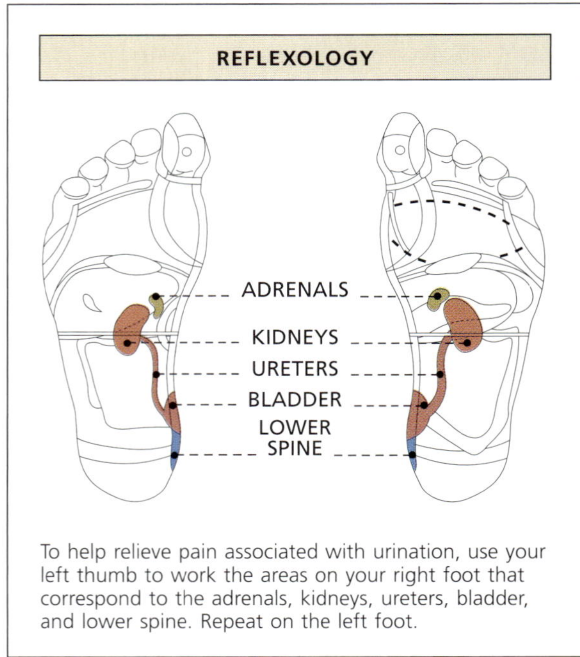

To help relieve pain associated with urination, use your left thumb to work the areas on your right foot that correspond to the adrenals, kidneys, ureters, bladder, and lower spine. Repeat on the left foot.

B

CRANBERRY JUICE: A PROVEN FOLK REMEDY

For centuries, Native Americans used crushed cranberries as a treatment for bladder and other urinary tract infections. Controlled studies now give scientific support to that ancient remedy. The research suggests that the berries' proficiency in fighting off infection is due to their high level of hippuric acid, a substance that inhibits the growth of E. coli bacteria and keeps them from adhering to the lining of the bladder.

To treat an existing bladder infection and to help prevent future ones, drink 12 to 16 oz of cranberry juice each day. Or, if you prefer, take cranberry capsules; follow the directions on the package. You can also try alternating cranberry juice with blueberry juice, which appears to have similar infection-fighting properties.

NUTRITION AND DIET

Both conventional and alternative practitioners agree that drinking plenty of fluids to keep you urinating frequently and to flush out your urinary tract thoroughly is one of the most effective means of combating a bladder infection—whatever its cause. However, you should avoid beverages that might irritate the urinary tract and aggravate the burning. Culprits include alcohol, coffee, black tea, chocolate milk, carbonated beverages, and citrus juices. Until clear of the infection, you should also avoid potentially irritating foods such as citrus fruits, tomatoes, vinegar, sugar, chocolate, artificial sweeteners, and heavily spiced dishes. Wait 10 days after the burning is gone before reintroducing these foods and drinks—one at a time—into your diet.

Supplements of ***vitamin C*** (500 mg every two hours) and ***vitamin A*** (25,000 IU each day) may also aid recovery. But check with your doctor before taking the supplements. Vitamin C increases the acidity of urine, which hampers the growth of bacteria but can also interfere with the action of some antibiotics, making them less effective.

OSTEOPATHY

Adjusting the bones and joints around the pelvis can act to strengthen the bladder muscles, helping to ward off recurrences of the infection. Consult an osteopath for treatment.

AT-HOME REMEDIES

- Drink cranberry juice daily.
- Take ***aspirin*** or ***ibuprofen*** to reduce inflammation and burning.

PREVENTION

- Practice good bathroom hygiene. Clean the anal area thoroughly after a bowel movement. Women should wipe from front to back to avoid spreading fecal bacteria to the urethra.
- Urinate as soon as possible when you feel the urge, and make sure you empty your bladder completely each time.
- Wear cotton underwear and loose, nonbinding clothing that does not trap heat and moisture in the crotch.
- Drink plenty of liquids.

Women:

- Empty your bladder as soon as possible after intercourse to wash out any bacteria that may have been pushed into the urethra.
- Avoid using perfumed soaps, bubble baths, scented douches, and vaginal deodorants. These contain substances that can irritate the urethra and make it more vulnerable to infection.
- If you use a diaphragm for birth control, make sure it fits properly, and don't leave it in too long.

BLISTERS

B

SYMPTOMS

- one or more bubbles of skin filled with clear fluid, ranging from pinpoint size to more than one-half inch in diameter. Depending on the cause, blistering may be accompanied by pain, inflammation, and itching.

CALL YOUR DOCTOR IF:

- the blistering is the result of contact with chemicals, and your skin continues to burn after flushing the area with water or saline solution. You need medical attention to counteract the irritating agent. *(See **Emergencies/First Aid: Burns**.)*
- the blistering results from a burn that has penetrated beyond the surface layer of skin. Some second-degree burns and all third- and fourth-degree burns are medical emergencies. *(See **Emergencies/First Aid: Burns,** and the **Burns** entry.)*
- your blister discharges white, yellow, or green pus, rather than clear fluid. The discharge is almost surely the result of an ***infection.***

Most blisters form as a reaction to irritation or other damage to the skin from an external source, although some can result from a disease or other ailment. A single blister is usually the result of friction or a minor burn, typically on the hands, feet, or other exposed areas. Clusters of blisters may result from extensive ***burns,*** contact ***dermatitis, insect bites,*** viral ***infections,*** drug or chemical reactions, or autoimmune disorders.

CAUSES

Friction: Blisters can be caused by excessive rubbing of exposed skin, such as a tool handle against the hand or a new pair of shoes against the ankle. Unlike ***corns and calluses,*** which develop from prolonged rubbing, friction blisters come from brief, intense contact.

Burns: Flames, steam, or contact with a hot surface can raise blisters, as can excessive ***sunburn*** or exposure to other types of radiation.

Contact dermatitis: Skin may blister when it comes in contact with chemical irritants, cosmetics, and many plant and animal toxins. *(See **Dermatitis, Poison Ivy, Insect and Spider Bites, Bee and Wasp Stings.**)*

Drug reactions: Many people develop blisters as a reaction to taking certain oral and topical drugs. The most common agents are ***penicillins*** and the ACE inhibitor ***captopril.*** Before prescribing any new drugs, a doctor should ask you about any drug reactions you may have had in the past.

Autoimmune disorders: Of the various autoimmune disorders known to cause blistering, three are most prevalent. **Pemphigus vulgaris,** a potentially fatal skin disorder, causes blisters in the mouth that sometimes spread to the head and other parts of the body; the painful blisters become raw and crusted before bursting. **Bullous pemphigoid** causes less severe eruptions that heal faster and are not life-threatening; this condition is seen chiefly in the elderly. **Dermatitis herpetiformis** causes small, itchy blisters; it is a chronic condition that usually starts in early adulthood.

Infection: Blisters are a common symptom of many infectious illnesses, including ***chickenpox, cold sores,*** herpes simplex, ***shingles,*** and ***impetigo.***

B

TREATMENT

Most blisters caused by friction or minor burns do not require a doctor's care. New skin forms underneath the affected area and the fluid is simply absorbed. Soothe ordinary friction blisters with ***vitamin E*** ointment or an ***aloe***-based cream. Do not puncture a blister unless it is large, painful, or likely to be further irritated. If you have to pop it, use a sterilized needle or razor blade; put the point or edge in a flame until it is red hot, or rinse it in alcohol. Wash the area thoroughly, then make a small hole and gently squeeze out the clear fluid. A dab of hydrogen peroxide can help protect against infection. If the fluid is white or yellow, the blister is infected and needs medical attention. Do not remove the skin over a broken blister; the new skin underneath needs this protective cover. For blisters caused by chemical contact, disease, or an autoimmune disorder, see a doctor.

CONVENTIONAL MEDICINE

While many blisters heal on their own, a few types require special care. Blistering caused by toxic agents or disease must be treated not only to relieve immediate discomfort but also to address the underlying cause. Some cases of **pemphigus,** for example, can be treated with oral ***corticosteroids*** on an outpatient basis; others require both corticosteroids and ***antibiotics*** under hospital supervision.

ALTERNATIVE CHOICES

If your blister is purely pressure- or burn-related, various ointments and rinses can be effective in relieving minor discomfort. To make good use of other therapies, you must first determine the underlying cause of the blistering.

HERBAL THERAPIES

Calendula (*Calendula officinalis*) tincture makes an excellent antiseptic to be used under a protective dressing. Blisters caused by herpes simplex respond to ***licorice*** *(Glycyrrhiza uralensis)* ointment.

HOMEOPATHY

Calendula ointment is a soothing, antiseptic dressing for closed blisters. ***Cantharis*** (12x) taken three or four times a day may help relieve the pain of a burn. ***Rhus toxicodendron*** (12x) taken three or four times a day may relieve blistering from contact ***dermatitis*** and ***cold sores.***

AT-HOME REMEDIES

- If you have a blister from friction or a minor burn, apply *Calendula* ointment to keep the skin soft and speed healing. An ordinary adhesive bandage will keep a small blister protected; cover a large blister with a gauze pad and adhesive tape.
- When a blister breaks, wash the area with soap and water, then apply a mild antiseptic such as hydrogen peroxide. Cover with *Calendula* ointment and a bandage during the day to protect the new skin from friction and dirt. Remove the bandage at night and expose the new skin to air so it hardens faster.
- If your skin is blistered by chemical contact, flush it immediately with plenty of water or a saline solution. If pain or itching persists, or if large blisters develop, call a doctor.
- Forget the old folk remedy about putting butter on burns and vinegar on blisters; both can aggravate the skin and may actually cause infection.

PREVENTION

- Jobs you do only occasionally, such as shoveling snow or raking leaves, are great for raising a blister or two; be sure to wear work gloves.
- Break in new shoes gradually, and put petroleum jelly or an adhesive bandage on areas that take the rub—before the blister happens.
- Wear socks with heels, not tube socks, which bunch up and cause blisters. Acrylic and other synthetic-fiber socks are good low-friction choices, but because they don't breathe as well as natural fibers, you should wash and dry your feet after wearing them to prevent ***athlete's foot.*** ■

BLOOD CLOTS

B

SYMPTOMS

Blood clots normally produce no obvious symptoms. Complications from abnormal clots may cause various conditions and disorders.

- Sudden and isolated pain in an arm or leg—sometimes followed by skin discoloration, tingling, numbness, or a cold feeling just below the site of pain—suggests a large clot blocking blood circulation. If left untreated, gangrene (tissue death) could result.
- A hard, bluish lump in a vein may be caused by a large blood clot.
- Sudden partial or complete blindness in one eye may be due to a blood clot blocking a retinal artery.
- Violent ***dizziness,*** or vertigo, that impairs your ability to stand or walk may be caused by a small blood clot blocking a cerebral artery.

CALL YOUR DOCTOR IF:

- you suffer from ***angina*** or have any symptoms associated with ***stroke.*** The cause may be abnormal blood clotting.
- you experience sudden or persistent sensory impairment. Among the potential causes that should be investigated is blockage of a blood vessel.

Your blood flows freely through arteries as thick as your thumb and capillaries thinner than a hair. At the first sign of injury or trauma, blood thickens, or clots, and stanches its own flow at the site of the wound. Clotting is desirable, even vital, when a blood vessel is injured, but clot formation inside healthy blood vessels is abnormal and potentially life-threatening. Such clots are frequent complications of ***heart disease*** or venous diseases such as ***phlebitis.***

A clot that forms in the heart or a blood vessel and stays there is called a **thrombus.** Tiny thrombi develop on blood vessel walls to heal minute injuries, then normally dissolve. If they don't dissolve, they not only can slow circulation but also can break loose or break apart and flow with the blood. A clot that travels and then becomes lodged at some point in a blood vessel is called an **embolus.** Emboli are less common than thrombi but potentially more dangerous.

The threat posed by an abnormal blood clot depends on both its size and its location. An obstructive clot in a cerebral artery, for example, can cause ***stroke.*** Blood clots in the arteries supplying the heart—the coronary arteries—are the major cause of ***heart attack.*** Tiny blood clots in arteries of the eye can lead to loss of vision. An embolus in the lungs that blocks a pulmonary artery can cause severe shortness of breath and even death.

CAUSES

Blood will coagulate inside blood vessels if vessel walls are damaged or if circulation becomes unusually sluggish, as in ***atherosclerosis.*** *(See also **Circulatory Problems.**)* Diseases such as ***phlebitis*** inflame the walls of blood vessels and promote abnormal clots. Clotting from sluggish blood flow is a common complication of bed rest and may even be brought on by lots of long-distance flying or driving. Pelvic vein thrombosis is an occasional complication of childbirth and is usually associated with uterine or pelvic ***infections.***

Abnormal clotting is sometimes linked to a congestive heart muscle disease that prevents the heart from pumping blood effectively. In addition, blood may clot if it is diseased or altered by certain conditions. A blood disorder called thrombocythemia, for example, causes increased production of platelets, the tiny blood cells that help clotting, resulting in overclotting. Factors that may contribute to clot formation include smoking, use of oral contraceptives, poor nutrition, ***obesity, varicose veins,*** and many other diseases.

TREATMENT

CONVENTIONAL MEDICINE

In some circumstances, drug therapy is prescribed to reduce the risk of abnormal clotting. A doctor may prescribe ***aspirin*** for patients at risk for embolisms or thrombosis. During critical care, streptokinase may be used to dissolve existing clots in areas such as the heart or lungs. After surgery, intravenous ***heparin*** may be used to prevent clotting or inhibit deep vein thrombosis. Blood clots may be removed during cardiovascular surgery, but surgery merely to remove clots is justified only in acute cases, such as impending tissue death.

ALTERNATIVE CHOICES

If you take ***anticoagulant drugs,*** ask your doctor about potential contraindications before starting any herbal or vitamin therapies.

BODY WORK

If the source of clotting is in your legs and is caused by poor circulation, **massage** therapy can be beneficial. If you have ***phlebitis,*** massage should always be done by a trained therapist to avoid dislodging a clot in a blood vessel.

HERBAL THERAPIES

Cayenne *(Capsicum frutescens)* and ***ginkgo*** *(Ginkgo biloba)* are thought to dissolve fibrin, a protein active in clot formation. ***Turmeric*** *(Curcuma longa)*, ***bilberry*** *(Vaccinium myrtillus)*, ***ginger*** *(Zingiber officinale)*, grape-skin extract, and gugulipid, an extract of ***myrrh*** *(Commiphora molmol)*, are believed to reduce platelet stickiness. ***Garlic*** *(Allium sativum)* and onion *(Allium cepa)* are said to do both, as is bromelain, a pineapple enzyme.

> **BITES THAT CURE**
>
> *Vampire bat saliva, leech saliva, and copperhead venom sound like ingredients in a witch's brew, but they may wind up saving human lives. Scientists have found enzymes in all three fluids that keep blood from clotting. The enzymes give the leech and vampire bat ample time to feed on their victims' blood; for the snake, they help venom spread quickly through the victim's bloodstream. For the rest of us, synthesized versions of the same enzymes could mean new antidotes for potentially harmful blood clots.*

NUTRITION AND DIET

If you want to condition your blood naturally, some authorities recommend eating more fish, believing that some fish oils make blood platelets less sticky. Certain vitamins and minerals may also act as natural anticoagulants. Ask your doctor or licensed nutrition therapist about supplemental ***vitamin E*** and ***magnesium*** to prevent abnormal clots from forming.

PREVENTION

- Eat a balanced diet low in saturated fats and high in fruits, vegetables, and natural fiber.
- Exercise regularly to stimulate circulation and keep extra pounds at bay.
- Some doctors recommend daily doses of ***aspirin*** for patients at risk of abnormal clotting. But because aspirin is a powerful drug, never take it on a regular basis without a doctor's prescription.
- If scheduled for surgery, ask your doctor about administering ***heparin*** during and after the operation. If possible, gentle exercise during recuperation will promote good circulation. ■

BLOOD POISONING

B

SYMPTOMS

While recovering from surgery, an infection, or a wound, a person may suffer blood poisoning or septic shock. Symptoms are described below.

- High fever and chills, rapid breathing, headache, and nausea may indicate an attack of blood poisoning, or **septicemia.**
- Severe chills, low blood pressure, loss of appetite, and possibly loss of consciousness are potential signs of **septic shock**.
- Red lines extending from a ***boil*** can be a sign of blood poisoning.

CALL YOUR DOCTOR IF:

- your symptoms suggest blood poisoning; you should have immediate medical attention to stop the spread of infection and to prevent **septic shock**.
- you experience severe chills, have a noticeable drop in blood pressure, and your skin becomes pale, cold, and clammy. You may be going into **septic shock** and need emergency medical attention.

Blood poisoning, or **septicemia,** is a serious secondary infection that occurs when bacteria from an infected site somewhere on your body invade your bloodstream. *(See **Infections.**)* If bacteria continue to multiply without being stopped by your immune system, you run the risk of **septic shock,** a potentially life-threatening condition.

Blood poisoning occurs most frequently in people who have just had surgery or other invasive treatment and in people whose immune systems are weakened by an acute or chronic ailment. Both blood poisoning and septic shock require immediate treatment to stop the spread of infection and to ensure full recovery.

CAUSES

Blood poisoning is almost always a complication of an infection and occurs when bacteria escape from the primary site and enter the bloodstream. Both the bacteria that cause the infection and endotoxins released by your body's immune system to battle those bacteria impede the blood flow to your body tissues. This triggers fever and chills—the characteristic symptoms of acute **septicemia.** If the poisoning is not brought under control by the body's immune system or by medical intervention, **septic shock** begins.

Although blood poisoning can result from infected surgical incisions, wounds, or burns, other types of infection can release enough bacteria into your blood to create septicemia. Such conditions may range from urinary tract infections or ***pneumonia*** to ***boils*** and abscessed teeth or ***gum problems.*** Unfortunately septicemia is on the rise in hospitals: As the number of patients undergoing invasive procedures for testing and surgery increases, the bacteria responsible for septicemia are continually evolving new strains that are immune to conventional antibiotics.

In rare cases, blood poisoning develops from eating unpasteurized dairy foods, including certain soft cheeses, that contain the bacterium *Listeria monocytogenes.* Eating raw oysters or other seafood that is infected with the bacterium *Vibrio vulnificus* can result in lethal septicemia for members of certain high-risk groups, such as people with liver disease, iron imbalances, and weakened immune systems.

DIAGNOSTIC AND TEST PROCEDURES

If your doctor thinks you have blood poisoning, your symptoms will be evaluated and your blood tested to identify the bacteria responsible. If symptoms indicate septic shock, you will be hospitalized; your blood will be tested for bacteria, blood gas levels, and other indicators; and you may need an electrocardiogram (ECG) to check for irregular heartbeat patterns.

TREATMENT

If you have blood poisoning or septic shock, full recovery demands professional medical treatment. Alternative treatments may help to speed your recovery and increase your resistance to bacterial infection in the future.

CONVENTIONAL MEDICINE

Once the bacteria that have caused the blood poisoning are identified, your physician will give you oral or intravenous ***antibiotics*** to fight the infection and may choose to drain and disinfect the infected area. If you develop septic shock, you will need emergency treatment and intravenous antibiotics, which may include ***penicillins, cephalosporins,*** or aminoglycosides. Until you recover completely, you will probably need to stay in a hospital so that you can be monitored for potential complications.

ALTERNATIVE CHOICES

Although you must have immediate medical treatment for blood poisoning and septic shock, alternative therapies may assist recovery and strengthen the immune system to help prevent recurrence.

HERBAL THERAPIES

To stimulate the bacteria-destroying function of your white blood cells, simmer 2 tsp ***echinacea*** (*Echinacea* spp.) in a cup of water for 15 minutes; drink a cupful three times a day. Eat ***garlic*** *(Allium sativum)* for its antibacterial and antiviral action, or take three garlic capsules three times daily.

PREVENTION

- If you develop a mouth infection, see your dentist for treatment or referral to a specialist. To speed recovery from an abscessed tooth, apply a warm-water compress, eat soft foods, floss, and rinse regularly with warm salt water.
- If you develop a boil, place a warm-water compress on it for 20 to 30 minutes three or four times daily until it bursts; this may take up to a week. Apply compresses for three days or until the boil is completely drained of pus.
- If the boil becomes infected or if red lines extend from it, see your doctor. An infected boil can cause septicemia, and squeezing an infected boil can spread the infection. ■

ACUPRESSURE

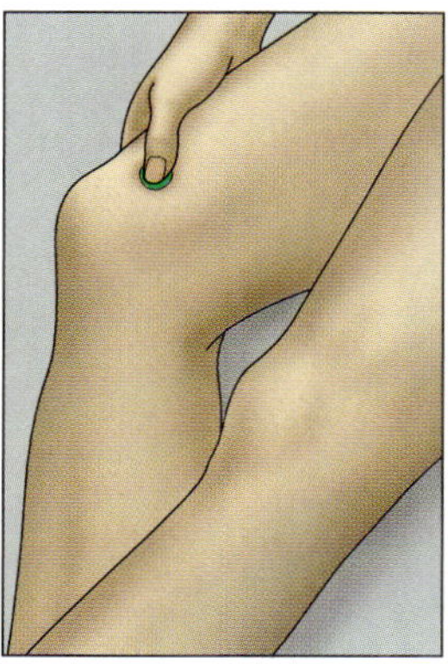

Pressure on Spleen 10 may stimulate your immune system. Bend your knee and locate the point two thumb widths from the top and in line with the inner edge of the kneecap, on the bulge of the muscle. Press with your thumb one minute. Repeat on the other leg.

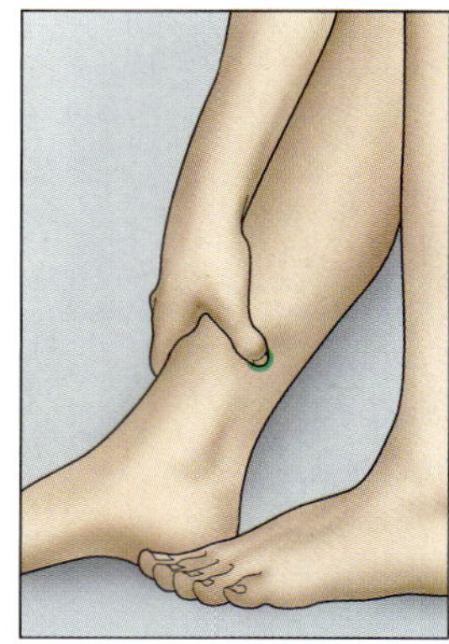

To help fight blood infection, put your thumb on Spleen 6, four finger widths above your right inner anklebone, near the edge of your shinbone. Press gently with your thumb for one minute, then switch legs. Do not use this point if you are pregnant.

BODY ODOR

B

SYMPTOMS

- a distinctive, sweaty odor, especially from the armpits, groin, and feet; usually considered unpleasant.
- any unusual odor emitted from body tissues, different from a sweaty smell, but not necessarily unpleasant.

CALL YOUR DOCTOR IF:

- the odor persists after washing, using deodorants, or trying other treatments. Body odors that are unlike the easily recognizable odor of perspiration can be signs of systemic disorders. For example, a smell like nail polish remover may indicate ***diabetes;*** an ammonia-like smell may be a sign of liver disease.

Americans have an aversion to body odor. It is the source of much self-consciousness and locker-room humor. It also supports a huge industry selling soaps, fragrances, deodorants, and antiperspirants to a willing public. Many cultures, however, don't understand the problem. They consider body odors normal, acceptable, even erotic.

Body odor is a general term for what happens to sweat and other skin secretions when they are acted upon by naturally occurring bacteria. Two types of glands produce sweat, the eccrine glands and the apocrine glands. The eccrine glands are dispersed throughout the body but are concentrated in the armpits, palms of the hands, soles of the feet, and the forehead. When the body is overheated—from hot weather, physical exertion, or fever—the eccrine glands help regulate body temperature by expelling a solution of water and salts that evaporates and cools the skin.

The apocrine glands are concentrated in the armpits and around the groin. These glands develop during puberty and have nothing to do with temperature regulation; instead, they respond to such conditions as sexual arousal, nervousness, and anger, as well as to heat and exertion. The sweat they produce is rich in organic substances that attract bacteria and produce a strong odor. Scientists believe that such odors may have been recognized as sexual signals by our ancient ancestors, just as they are in most animals.

CAUSES

By itself, sweat doesn't have an odor. Only after sweat is acted upon by naturally occurring bacteria on the skin does a person develop what we all recognize as a sweaty smell. The smell is especially noticeable in the feet, armpits, and groin, because those areas have a high concentration of sweat glands. Also, shoes and clothing trap perspiration, encouraging bacterial activity.

Eating certain foods and taking certain drugs can also cause distinctive smells; the cancer-fighting medication ***tamoxifen,*** for instance, may induce a distinctive odor. Proteins and oils from foods such as onions and certain spices may

B

cause you to give off their characteristic smells. Deficiencies in certain nutrients, such as ***zinc,*** may also contribute to body odor. Women are sometimes troubled by odors associated with menstruation, but most of these can be prevented with good hygiene.

Body odor that smells fruity—or like nail polish remover, ammonia, or maple syrup—may indicate the presence of a disease or metabolic problem. Disorders that may produce unusual body odor include fungal ***infections,*** liver disease, ***kidney disease, diabetes,*** and various gastrointestinal problems. A person who has a persistent, nonsweaty smell should be checked by a doctor to diagnose and treat the underlying cause. *(See **Sweating, Excessive.**)*

TREATMENT

The most effective way to rid your body of odors is to wash with soap and water, sometimes more than once a day. To help control the bacterial activity responsible for a sweaty smell, wash with an antibacterial soap. Deodorants containing mild antibacterial agents and scents help to slow bacterial action and cover up underarm odor, but they don't stop perspiration. To do that, you have to use an antiperspirant that blocks eccrine glands and suppresses their function. If you choose an antiperspirant, be patient; it must be used daily for about a week to provide maximum effectiveness.

You should be aware that antiperspirants contain metallic salts that can be absorbed by the skin and may cause irritation. If that happens, discontinue use and try another product, preferably one with different active ingredients. Many authorities discourage the use of antiperspirants altogether. They contend that people should not try to prevent or reduce sweating at all, since it is one of the body's natural processes.

CONVENTIONAL MEDICINE

To control unusually persistent, profuse sweating, a condition called **hyperhidrosis,** a doctor may recommend a prescription antiperspirant containing a high concentration of an ingredient such as aluminum chloride. These products must be used with care because they can cause skin irritation.

ALTERNATIVE CHOICES

Tablets containing chlorophyll, a natural plant product, are sold as a deodorant that can be taken orally. Dusting the underarms and toes with baking soda, a good natural deodorant, also helps absorb odor. Crystallized mineral salts to control body odor are sold in health and cosmetic stores.

HERBAL THERAPIES

Preparations containing essential oils of ***rosemary*** *(Rosmarinus officinalis)* and thyme *(Thymus vulgaris)* are recommended as herbal deodorants and can be used as antibacterial washes.

NUTRITION AND DIET

Excessive sweating may be linked to a ***zinc*** deficiency. Taking a 30- to 60-mg zinc supplement daily may help resolve the problem. See **Essential Vitamins and Minerals,** page 1041, for more information on zinc dosages.

AT-HOME REMEDIES

- Bathe, shower, or wash yourself thoroughly every day. Use a mild underarm deodorant or antiperspirant if you wish, or sprinkle baking soda under your arms and between your toes after drying off.
- Change, wash, and dry-clean your clothes often, especially underwear, socks or stockings, and anything worn next to the skin. In hot weather, avoid tight clothing and wear sandals, with or without socks.
- Cotton clothes and leather shoes let perspiration evaporate faster than synthetic materials.
- Excessive body hair helps to retain sweat and bacteria, so one way to minimize body odor is to shave under the arms. ■

BOILS

B

SYMPTOMS

- The first stage of a boil is an inflamed, painful, sometimes throbbing nodule under the skin, most often appearing on the face, neck, buttocks, armpits, or—rarely—a woman's nipple.
- After several days, the boil develops into a raised, reddish sore with a white or yellow center; it may be extremely painful because of pus buildup under the skin.
- A clump of boils is called a **carbuncle;** a boil on the eyelid is a ***sty.***

CALL YOUR DOCTOR IF:

- the boil causes excessive pain; you may want a doctor to lance and drain it.
- the inflammation is accompanied by a fever, or the boil appears on your lip, nose, cheeks, forehead, or spine; any infection in those locations places you at risk of a secondary infection, by spreading bacteria internally through the bloodstream to the spine or the brain.
- you think you have a **carbuncle.** This is a serious condition that should be treated with ***antibiotics.***
- You have a boil that is very tender, particularly if it has red lines radiating from it, or if you have fever and chills; the infection may have spread.

A boil, or **furuncle,** may look like a nasty pimple but in fact is the result of a ***staph infection*** that has invaded a blocked hair follicle or, occasionally, an oil gland. *(See **Acne.**)* In the beginning a boil is red and tender; after a week to 10 days pus collects under the skin, causing the center of the boil to take on a whitish color. Pus is actually a mass of white blood corpuscles—which the body's immune system has sent to fight the infection—mixed with bacteria and dead skin cells. The boil can become quite swollen and painful before the skin breaks, the pus drains, and the sore clears. A **carbuncle** is a collection of boils. Before the advent of ***antibiotics*** earlier in this century, a carbuncle was considered a potentially life-threatening condition.

CAUSES

The staph bacteria that cause boils typically enter the body through cuts, scratches, and other breaks in the skin. Various factors can cause people to be predisposed to boils, including ***immune problems; diabetes;*** exposure to certain industrial chemicals; overuse of ***corticosteroids;*** treatment of skin lesions with petroleum-based products; and general poor health, hygiene, or nutrition.

TREATMENT

Most boils can be treated at home simply by washing the infected area with antibacterial soap and applying hot compresses, which help bring the boil to a head. Over-the-counter topical ***antibiotics*** are also effective in limiting the spread of bacterial infection. Do not squeeze or lance the boil yourself; most boils burst of their own accord after about two weeks. When they do, wash the area gently until no more pus appears, then cover with an adhesive bandage to avoid reinfection and to prevent drained pus from reaching other skin areas and spreading the infection. Be sure to wash your hands thoroughly, and disinfect towels.

CONVENTIONAL MEDICINE

If the pain is severe, or if a boil refuses to break, a doctor can lance and drain it under sterile conditions. To treat a severe outbreak, a doctor may prescribe an oral ***antibiotic*** such as ***erythromycin*** or dicloxacillin.

ALTERNATIVE CHOICES

Boils have plagued humans for centuries, and humans have countered with all sorts of remedies. Use caution when trying alternative remedies on your skin, because the wrong treatment may actually aggravate an infection.

AYURVEDIC MEDICINE

Boiled onions—wrapped in a cloth to protect your skin—are said to help bring a boil to a head.

CHINESE HERBS

Chinese herbal medicine focuses on reducing heat in the body, which is thought to cause boils. Try drinking tea made from ***dandelion*** *(Taraxacum mongolicum),* ***chrysanthemum flower*** *(Chrysanthemum indicum),* or violet *(Viola yedoensis).*

HERBAL THERAPIES

Herbal remedies for boils abound. To fight inflammation, you can choose among an over-the-counter ointment made with ***calendula*** *(Calendula officinalis),* a poultice of ***slippery elm*** *(Ulmus fulva),* and a tincture of blue flag *(Iris versicolor)* or ***myrrh*** *(Commiphora molmol).*

To fight infection, apply ***tea tree oil*** (*Melaleuca* spp.) to the boil four to six times a day. Essential oils of bergamot *(Citrus bergamia),* ***lavender*** *(Lavandula officinalis),* ***chamomile*** *(Matricaria recutita),* and ***sage*** *(Salvia officinalis)* are also recommended for their antibacterial properties. ***Goldenseal*** *(Hydrastis canadensis)* contains an alkaloid known as berberine, for which bacteria-fighting properties are claimed; mix with distilled witch hazel *(Hamamelis virginiana)* to use as a wash.

HOMEOPATHY

If a boil comes up suddenly and is very red and hot, ***Belladonna*** (12x) three to four times daily may slow or halt the infection. For very painful boils try ***Hepar sulphuris,*** and for those that heal slowly use ***Silica,*** in the same potency and frequency.

NUTRITION AND DIET

Poor diet and certain nutritional deficiencies can suppress the body's immune system. Besides recommending a diet high in fresh fruits and vegetables, a nutritionist may suggest eating more ***garlic*** *(Allium sativum)* for its antiseptic properties, and foods high in ***zinc*** to enhance the immune system. You can accomplish this through your diet, or you can take up to three garlic capsules and a 45-mg zinc supplement daily.

AT-HOME REMEDIES

- Warm compresses or a warm Epsom salt bath will help draw the pus out of a boil.
- Men who get boils on the face should wash with antibacterial soap before shaving, and apply antibacterial cream when they finish.
- Resist the urge to lance or break a boil yourself; the result could be a severe secondary infection. Most boils break of their own accord; in some cases the boil heals without breaking and disperses under the skin.

PREVENTION

Breaks in the skin make a person susceptible to the infections that cause boils. Shaving nicks can cause them; so can contact sports, manual labor, insect bites, and a host of other everyday activities. Some tips:

- Wash regularly and take care of minor skin injuries promptly.
- Never share towels, bed linens, clothes, or athletic equipment with someone who has a boil or other infection. That person's clothes, bed linens, and towels should be washed daily in very hot water with detergent or bleach.
- Never squeeze a boil. The pus can spread the infection and cause complications, such as secondary infection or a **carbuncle**. ■

BONE CANCER

B

SYMPTOMS

- a hard lump felt on the surface of a bone that may or may not be painful.
- pain or swelling in bones and joints, often more intense at night, and not necessarily associated with movement; the pain may be dull and constant, or may be felt only when pressure is applied.
- spontaneous bone fractures.
- fever, weight loss, fatigue, and impaired mobility, which sometimes occur in late stages of bone cancer.

Benign bone tumors are usually painless.

CALL YOUR DOCTOR IF:

- you have any of the symptoms described above, particularly an unexplained lump on a bone or chronic pain in bones or joints. You should be tested for bone cancer.
- you have persistent, unexplained back pain. You may simply have a ***back problem*** or ***backache;*** but if the symptoms do not respond to treatment, you may want to ask your doctor about being examined for a tumor in the spine.
- you suffer one or more bone fractures for no apparent reason. After treatment for the fracture, you may want to ask your doctor about being tested for **osteosarcoma** or ***osteoporosis.***

Most primary bone tumors—those that originate in bone, cartilage, or other bone tissue—are benign, not cancerous. Primary bone cancer is rare, accounting for less than 1 percent of all cancers diagnosed in the U.S. each year. Far more common are secondary cancers that spread to bones from cancers in other parts of the body.

Primary bone cancer generally attacks young people, especially those who are unusually tall for their age. Of the main types, **osteosarcoma** accounts for nearly 60 percent of all primary bone cancers; it tends to affect teenagers, whose bones are in a stage of rapid growth. **Ewing's sarcoma** originates in bone marrow and occurs most often in children between the ages of 5 and 9 and in young adults between the ages of 20 and 30. **Chondrosarcoma** originates in cartilage and tends to attack middle-aged adults; other, less common types of bone cancer that occur in adults include fibrosarcoma, malignant giant cell tumor, and chordoma.

Primary bone cancer can be a lethal disease, but improved methods of detection and treatment have raised the five-year survival rate to more than 70 percent. The likelihood of cure depends largely on how early a tumor is detected and how rapidly the particular cancer tends to spread. The survival rate for secondary bone cancer varies. Benign tumors normally pose no long-term health risk.

CAUSES

In most cases of primary bone cancer, specific causes cannot be identified, but some cases may have genetic links. Certain chromosome abnormalities and a handful of rare, genetically linked diseases have been associated with bone cancer. Cancer is more likely to occur in bones that have been fractured or infected in the past. Exposure to specific carcinogens, such as chemicals in some kinds of dyes and paints, may increase the risk of bone cancer slightly. High-dose radiation and certain chemotherapeutic agents—particularly the so-called alkylating agents—may also be associated with some types of bone cancer.

TUMOR IN THE BONE

A bone tumor is an abnormal growth that can begin in any part of a bone—the marrow, spongy bone, or hard bone; it uses blood that would otherwise nourish healthy bone tissue. In primary bone cancer *(below)*, malignant cells have replaced normal cells in hard bone tissue. The process weakens the bone and causes pain and swelling—often the first signs of bone cancer.

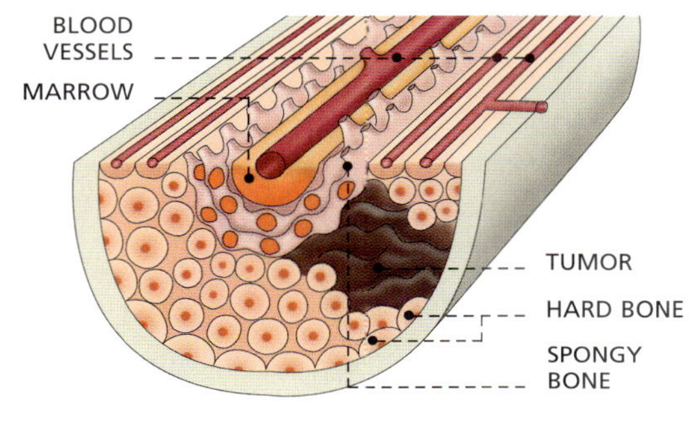

DIAGNOSTIC AND TEST PROCEDURES

When symptoms suggest bone cancer, a doctor will run blood tests to eliminate other possible causes. X-rays and other imaging tests are used to identify bone tumors, and a biopsy is taken for a positive diagnosis. If a tumor is cancerous, tests are run to check for metastasis—the spread of cancer cells from one part of the body to another.

TREATMENT

When cancer is diagnosed, there is no acceptable substitute for conventional medical treatment. Alternative therapies may complement, but cannot replace, conventional care.

CONVENTIONAL MEDICINE

When possible, bone tumors are removed surgically. If the cancer is in an arm or a leg, the tumor can be removed without amputation in about 90 percent of cases; the surgeon then reconstructs the bone using a metal prosthesis. If amputation is unavoidable, the patient is usually fitted with an artificial limb.

Patients who have had bone cancer surgery are encouraged to begin physical therapy as soon as possible in order to overcome stiffness, improve mobility, and—if necessary—learn how to use their new artificial limb.

Radiation therapy and chemotherapy may be given before surgery to reduce the size of the tumor, and radiation may be used after surgery to kill stray cancer cells. Both radiation and chemotherapy are also used to treat inoperable bone cancers. Together they may keep the cancer from spreading but rarely bring about a full cure. Some doctors are experimenting with supplemental immunotherapy so that lower doses of radiation and chemotherapy can be given without compromising the overall effectiveness of treatment. For further information on these experimental treatments, see ***Cancer.***

COMPLEMENTARY THERAPIES

Many alternative therapies have been shown to alleviate stresses associated with cancer and its treatment. Some body-work therapies, such as the **Feldenkrais** and **Aston-Patterning** methods, may be particularly beneficial to people adjusting mentally and physically to using an artificial limb. For further information on all complementary cancer therapies, see ***Cancer.***

PREVENTION

Always heed safety warnings when using paint, solvents, pesticides, household cleaners, and other products that may contain carcinogenic chemicals. If you have ever been treated with radiation in the past, be alert for bone cancer symptoms and see a doctor at once if they occur. ■

BONE SPURS

B

SYMPTOMS

- stiffness or pain in the neck or back.
- "pins-and-needles" tingling in the neck, arms, or hands.
- dizziness, headache, difficulty in maintaining balance.
- sharp pain when putting weight on one or both feet.

CALL YOUR DOCTOR IF:

- back pain persists more than two or three days after taking an over-the-counter pain reliever and resting your back; you may have a degenerated disk.
- you experience intense shooting pain in the neck or back with even slight movement; you may have a bone spur pinching a nerve.

Almost everyone has waked up with a stiff neck or a backache at one time or another, especially after an injury or strenuous physical activity. Occasionally, however, you may experience sudden shooting pains that are not linked to a particular event. Problems like these often go away on their own, but sometimes they are signs of a more serious condition, such as ***arthritis.***

A potential cause of such pains can be spurs, arising from abnormal growth in the ends of bones, especially in the spine or extremities. Bone spurs may cause excruciating pain when they interfere with nerves or muscles during normal activity.

CAUSES

Bone spurs are the result of changes over time to the ends of the bones that meet in joints, particularly the vertebrae that make up the spinal column. The fibrous cushions, or disks, between vertebrae tend to toughen and shrink with age *(see **Disk Problems**).* Meanwhile, the tough, elastic cartilage at the ends of the bones progressively hardens.

As the space between the vertebrae becomes narrower, the bone tends to compensate for the loss by growing knobby enlargements, commonly called bone spurs. These growths are often seen in older people who have disk problems, but they also can occur in young adults—especially athletes, dancers, or laborers—who put unusual stress on muscles, ligaments, and tendons.

Unlike the rounded ends of bones in normal joints, spurs do not develop a layer of protective cartilage. In some cases, the new bony surfaces eventually smooth themselves through normal movement. But when they don't, bone spurs can rub against other bony surfaces, nerves, or blood vessels, causing pain and inflammation. When such bony growths appear in the upper vertebrae of the neck, the condition is called cervical osteoarthritis. Bony spurs can also be a cause of ***sciatica***. A particularly bothersome condition occurs when a spur develops in the foot *(right),* causing pain when standing or walking.

DIAGNOSTIC AND TEST PROCEDURES

Since back pain can have various causes, the usual test for complications due to spinal bone spurs is an x-ray or a CT scan of the affected area of the spine. Magnetic resonance imaging (MRI) or electromyography (EMG) is often used to check for impairment of nerves or muscles.

TREATMENT

The discomfort caused by bone spurs can be alleviated through rest, good back support, and drug therapy.

CONVENTIONAL MEDICINE

Your doctor will probably prescribe ***aspirin, ibuprofen,*** or another anti-inflammatory painkiller. To restrict movement and take pressure off a ***pinched nerve,*** you may have to wear an orthopedic collar or back brace. Only in severe cases is surgical removal of bone spurs necessary, but even relief through surgery may be temporary, since spurs can grow back.

HEEL PAIN

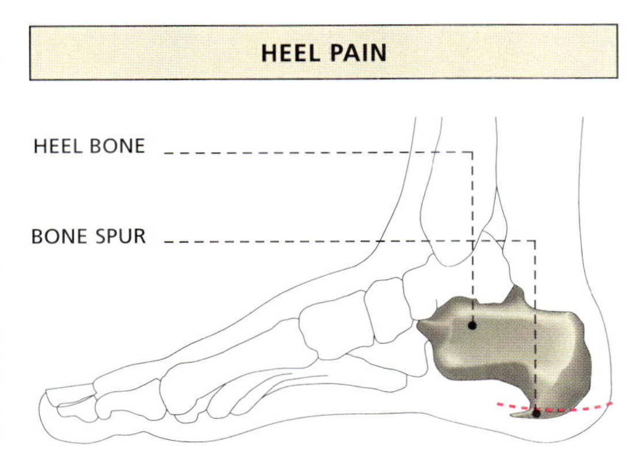

Bone spurs frequently develop at the base of the heel, where they can irritate nerves or tissue and cause pain with every step. Spurs in the foot are usually the result of unusual stress that prompts the normally smooth heel bone to sprout a knobby protrusion.

If a spur develops on a weight-bearing bone in the foot, the doctor may recommend a foam rubber pad for your shoe, with a hole cut directly under the spur to relieve pressure.

ALTERNATIVE CHOICES

Alternative therapies focus on pain relief and body work to improve range of movement.

CHIROPRACTIC

Chiropractic manipulation may help relieve the pain caused by a degenerative problem in the vertebrae. A chiropractor may also use physical therapy to relieve the discomfort of a heel spur.

HOMEOPATHY

For localized neck and back discomfort, a homeopath will typically prescribe a remedy based on whether the pain results from weather conditions, emotional stress, or mechanical strain. Before treating long-term conditions, the practitioner may conduct an analysis of the patient's genetic and psychological makeup.

YOGA

A trained instructor can prescribe effective **yoga** positions to relieve stress on affected areas and promote general relaxation and strengthening.

AT-HOME REMEDIES

When minor back pain strikes, take an over-the-counter painkiller. After inflammation has subsided, apply a heating pad or a hot-water bottle wrapped in a towel. Sleep on a firm mattress with a board under it, or on the floor with pillows beneath your head and calves.

PREVENTION

- Use your joints properly.
- Engage in moderate total-body exercises such as walking, bicycling, swimming, and tennis.
- Lose excess weight.
- Wear shoes with good ankle supports. ■

BOWEL MOVEMENT ABNORMALITIES

Read down this column to find your symptoms. Then read across.

B

SYMPTOMS	AILMENT/PROBLEM
◆ passing hard and/or infrequent stools or straining to have a bowel movement.	◆ ***Constipation***
◆ watery and/or frequent bowel movements.	◆ ***Diarrhea***
◆ ***worms*** in the stool, perhaps appearing as light-colored threads; possible itching in the anal area.	◆ Pinworm, roundworm, or tapeworm infection
◆ alternating hard/infrequent and watery/frequent stools.	◆ ***Irritable bowel syndrome;*** colon tumor; ***diabetes;*** alternating use of ***laxatives*** and ***antidiarrheal*** drugs
◆ extremely foul-smelling, large stools; weight loss despite good appetite; abdominal pain.	◆ ***Pancreatic problems,*** possibly associated with ***celiac disease***
◆ any visible blood in the stools.	◆ Many possibilities, including ***hemorrhoids, anal fissure,*** and ***colorectal cancer***
◆ persistent thin, ribbonlike stools; possible anal bleeding.	◆ Possibly, ***colorectal cancer***
◆ maroon-colored or black, tarry, metallic-smelling stools; possible abdominal pain.	◆ Bleeding from the upper or middle gastrointestinal tract, caused by any of a number of ailments or use of certain medications
◆ stools that are either too hard or too watery; abdominal pain; flatulence; nausea; vomiting; fever.	◆ ***Appendicitis***
◆ black or dark-red stools; vomiting with blood; easy bruising; spiderlike blood vessels on the skin; fatigue; yellowish skin and eyes; weight loss or gain; distended abdomen.	◆ ***Cirrhosis***
◆ pale or chalky stools; dark-orange to tea-colored urine; yellowish skin and eyes; dull abdominal pain, fever, shaking, chills.	◆ Bile duct blocked by a gallstone; gallbladder disorder; liver disorder

B

WHAT TO DO	OTHER INFO
◆ Change to a high-fiber diet and drink 6 to 8 glasses of water each day.	◆ Over 30 possible causes: ***irritable bowel, anal fissure, depression,*** and inactivity.
◆ Drink fluids copiously to replace those being lost. If diarrhea persists beyond 48 hours, call your doctor.	◆ More than a dozen causes, including ***flu*** and ***food poisoning.***
◆ See your doctor; prescription medication can cure the infection.	◆ Wormwood *(Artemisia absinthium)* taken three times daily in a pill or a tea (pour 1 cup boiling water over ½ tsp wormwood; steep for 10 minutes) is reported to cure many worm infestations.
◆ If you frequently use laxatives and antidiarrheal drugs, gradually reduce your use until you can stop; otherwise, call your doctor without delay for proper diagnosis.	◆ Laxatives can mimic the abdominal pain of irritable bowel syndrome or a colon tumor. See ***Colorectal Cancer.***
◆ See your doctor soon. You may need to eliminate all gluten-containing foods from your diet.	◆ If celiac disease prevents absorption of ***iron, vitamin*** B_{12}, or ***folic acid,*** take supplements.
◆ Call your doctor today—immediately if patient is a child or if bleeding is profuse.	◆ Never ignore ***anal bleeding;*** it can indicate colorectal cancer.
◆ Call your doctor today; an early and accurate diagnosis is essential.	◆ Treated early, colorectal cancer is curable; untreated, it can be fatal.
◆ Call your doctor today for a proper diagnosis; report any prescription or over-the-counter medications you are taking.	◆ A home test kit can determine if blood is in stools; maroon color may be from eating red foods such as beets.
◆ **Call your doctor or seek emergency care now.**	
◆ **Call your doctor or seek emergency medical help now;** cirrhosis may be life-threatening.	◆ Avoid alcohol, high-fat foods, and all drugs (except those your doctor prescribes) to enhance liver function.
◆ Adopt a low-fat diet. If abdominal pain is severe or any fever is present, see your doctor immediately. See ***Gallstones, Hepatitis.***	◆ ***Vitamin K*** supplements, or eating dark green leafy vegetables which are rich in vitamin K, may help alleviate symptoms.

Cross references are indicated by ***bold italics.***

BRAIN CANCER

B

SYMPTOMS

Most brain tumors do not show symptoms until they attain a certain size.

Symptoms associated with increased pressure on the brain from a tumor include:

- persistent headaches that get worse over a period of weeks and are often more intense when lying down.
- vomiting, sometimes but not always accompanied by nausea.
- sudden onset of seizures.
- inexplicable changes in personality or mental ability.

Symptoms that vary according to the type and location of the tumor include:

- sudden vision loss, speech problems, or other changes in the senses.
- localized weakness or paralysis, especially in the limbs.
- impaired memory.
- loss of coordination or balance.

CALL YOUR DOCTOR IF:

- you experience any of the symptoms described above. Although other ailments can cause similar symptoms, persistent headaches that occur with vomiting, convulsions, or progressive loss of speech, sight, hearing, feeling, or limb function may indicate a brain tumor.

Primary brain cancer—cancer that originates in the brain itself—is rare, accounting for only 1 percent of all cancers and about 2.5 percent of all cancer deaths. However, one in four patients with cancer elsewhere in the body eventually develops metastatic, or secondary, brain cancer. Brain cancer can occur at any age, but most often it strikes young children and middle-aged adults.

Brain tumors whose cells do not spread are considered benign, in contrast to malignant tumors, or cancers, whose cells multiply uncontrollably and can spread throughout the body. But no brain tumor is harmless: Anything that takes up space in the skull, even a noncancerous growth, can exert pressure on delicate brain tissue, produce severe pain, cause irreversible neurological damage, and threaten life. The symptoms and prognosis for recovery vary according to the location of the tumor and the type of brain cells involved.

CAUSES

The causes of primary brain cancer are unknown. Sometimes it runs in families, implying a genetic link. Other research suggests ties to chemicals such as vinyl chloride, certain herbicides and pesticides, or overexposure to electromagnetic fields. A few rare diseases, such as tuberous sclerosis and multiple intestinal polyposis, are also associated with brain cancer *(see **Colorectal Cancer**)*.

DIAGNOSTIC AND TEST PROCEDURES

Diagnosis of a brain tumor begins with a complete physical examination and neurological testing. Computed tomography (CT) and magnetic resonance imaging (MRI) scans will locate and identify a tumor. If taking a tissue biopsy is feasible, it can confirm or rule out the presence of cancer cells. X-rays and other tests determine whether cancer exists elsewhere in the body.

TREATMENT

While research for a cure continues, there is no acceptable substitute for conventional medical

TUMORS IN THE BRAIN

MENINGIOMA

GLIOBLASTOMA MULTIFORME

Several kinds of tumors can develop in the brain. Meningiomas occur in the protective membrane covering the brain, not in brain tissue itself. They are usually benign and can often be removed surgically. Glioblastoma multiformes are malignant tumors that form directly in cerebral tissue. They are usually inoperable.

treatment for cancer. Although many alternative therapies—those outside mainstream medicine—can enhance the benefits of standard care, none is a proven cancer cure. Alternative cancer therapies should be considered potential complements to, but not replacements for, conventional care.

CONVENTIONAL MEDICINE

Curing brain cancer depends on where the tumor is located and how far the malignancy has spread. Advances in computer-assisted surgery now let surgeons treat cancers that were once considered inoperable. Whenever possible, a brain tumor is treated surgically. If it can be removed, the patient may recover fully. After surgery, radiation therapy and sometimes chemotherapy are prescribed to make sure stray cancer cells are killed. But some brain tumors are located too deep in the brain to be removed even partially without causing severe brain damage. In such cases, treatment is limited to chemotherapy and a refined radiation therapy that trains laser beams on the tumor. Neither is likely to provide a cure, but they may slow the growth of cancer cells, control symptoms, and prolong the patient's life.

When cure is impossible, the main goals of treatment are to provide comfort and preserve neurological function. Various drugs, including ***analgesics, anticonvulsants,*** and ***corticosteroids,*** may be given to relieve pain, control seizures, and reduce brain swelling. Because tumors often cause residual brain damage, a patient may require physical or mental rehabilitative therapy.

For further information on radiation, chemotherapy, and other treatments, see ***Cancer.***

COMPLEMENTARY THERAPIES

While many brain cancer sufferers can handle everyday activities, the strain of the disease and the side effects of radiation and chemotherapy may eventually be debilitating. A number of alternative therapies can provide relief from such stresses, among them **hydrotherapy, Therapeutic Touch, yoga, guided imagery, meditation,** and **biofeedback.** Various forms of body work, including **massage** and **reflexology,** may also help.

GENE THERAPY

Foreign genes—not scalpels or laser beams—may prove to be the ultimate weapon against brain cancer, if promising test results are confirmed. Scientists at the National Institutes of Health have been refining a type of gene therapy that kills brain cancer cells by altering them genetically. This ingenious therapy is designed to make cancer cells vulnerable to a cell-destroying drug, while leaving healthy brain cells alone and intact. When the therapy was tested on rats, tumors virtually disappeared in 11 of 14 animals. In the first human trial, tumors shrank significantly in 5 of 8 patients, all of whom had previously failed to respond to conventional treatment. While further testing and refinement are needed, this new gene therapy may hold great promise for the future. ■

BREAST CANCER

B

SYMPTOMS

In early stages, breast cancer usually has no symptoms. As a tumor progresses, you may note the following signs:

- swelling in the armpit.
- pain or tenderness in the breast.
- a lump in the breast; often the first apparent symptom of breast cancer, breast lumps are usually painless, although some may cause a prickly sensation. Lumps are usually visible on a mammogram long before they can be seen or felt.
- a noticeable flattening or indentation on the breast, which may indicate a tumor that cannot be seen or felt.
- any change in the contour, texture, or temperature of the breast; a reddish, pitted surface like the skin of an orange is symptomatic of advanced breast cancer.
- a change in the nipple, such as an indrawn or dimpled look, itching or burning sensation, or ulceration; scaling of the nipple is symptomatic of **Paget's disease,** a localized cancer.
- unusual discharge from the nipple that may be clear, bloody, or another color—usually caused by benign conditions but possibly due to cancer.

CALL YOUR DOCTOR IF:

- one or both breasts develop an abnormal lump or persistent pain, or look or feel abnormal. The cause could be something other than cancer but should be identified.
- you have swollen lymph glands in your armpits. Any such swelling could be associated with cancer.

Each month, a woman's breasts go through temporary changes associated with menstruation, and a lump may form. While 90 percent of these are not cancerous, any lump should be examined immediately. Lumps are most common in the lobules—small sacs that produce milk—or the ducts that carry milk to the nipple, but they occasionally start in nonglandular tissue. The two main categories of breast cancer are **lobular** and **ductal carcinomas.** Each has many subtypes.

Breast cancer usually begins with formation of a small, localized tumor. Some tumors are benign, meaning they do not invade other tissue; others are malignant, or cancerous. The potential for a malignant tumor to metastasize, or spread, is common to all cancer. Once such a tumor grows to a certain size, it is more likely to shed cells that spread to other parts of the body through the bloodstream and lymphatic system. Different types of breast cancer grow and spread at different rates; some take years to spread beyond the breast, while others move quickly.

Men can get breast cancer, but they account for less than half a percent of all cases. It is the most common cancer among women, who share a lifetime risk of one in nine. It constitutes one-sixth of all U.S. cancer cases and one-third of all cancers in women. It trails only ***colorectal*** and ***lung cancers*** as a cause of cancer death. Two of every three female breast cancer patients are over 50, and most of the rest are between 39 and 49.

Fortunately, breast cancer is very treatable if detected early. Localized tumors can usually be treated successfully before the cancer spreads; 9 cases out of 10 have a 5-year survival rate. Once the cancer begins to spread, getting rid of it completely is more difficult, although treatment can often control the disease for years. Improved screening procedures and treatment options mean that at least 7 out of 10 women with breast cancer will survive more than 5 years after initial diagnosis, and fully half will survive more than 10 years.

CAUSES

Although the precise causes of breast cancer are unclear, we know what the main risk factors are.

Still, most women considered at high risk for breast cancer do not get it, while many who do have no known risk factors. Among the most significant factors are advancing age and a family history of breast cancer. Risk increases slightly for a woman who has had a benign breast lump and increases significantly for a woman who has previously had cancer of the breast or the ovaries.

A woman whose mother, sister, or daughter has had breast cancer is more likely to develop the disease, particularly if more than one so-called first-order relative has been affected. Researchers have now identified several genes that they think are responsible for familial breast cancer: About 1 woman in 200 carries them. Having these genes predisposes a woman to breast cancer, but does not ensure that she will get it.

Generally, postmenopausal women—which usually means those past age 50—are more likely to get breast cancer than premenopausal women, and statistics suggest that African American women are more likely than Caucasians to get breast cancer before menopause.

A link between breast cancer and hormones is gradually becoming clearer. Researchers think that the greater a woman's exposure to the female hormone estrogen, the more susceptible she is to breast cancer. Basically, estrogen tells cells to divide; the more the cells divide, the more likely they are to be abnormal in some way—possibly becoming cancerous. A woman's exposure to estrogen and progesterone rises and falls during her lifetime, influenced by the age she starts and stops menstruating, the average length of her menstrual cycle, and her age at first childbirth. A woman's risk for breast cancer is increased if she starts menstruating before age 12, has her first child after 30, stops menstruating after 55, or has a menstrual cycle shorter or longer than the average 26 to 29 days. Taking hormones in the form of birth-control pills or hormone replacement therapy may also increase risk, although the evidence is inconclusive. Heavy doses of radiation therapy may also be a factor, but low-dose mammograms pose almost no risk.

The diet–breast cancer link is still debated. ***Obesity*** is a noteworthy risk factor, and drinking alcohol regularly may promote the disease. Many studies have shown that women whose diets are high in fat are more likely to get the disease. Researchers suspect that if less than 20 percent of a woman's daily calories come from fat, her diet may protect her from developing breast cancer.

YOGA EXERCISE AFTER BREAST SURGERY

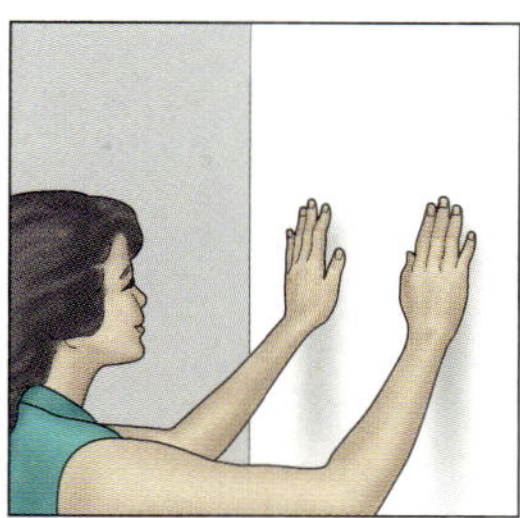

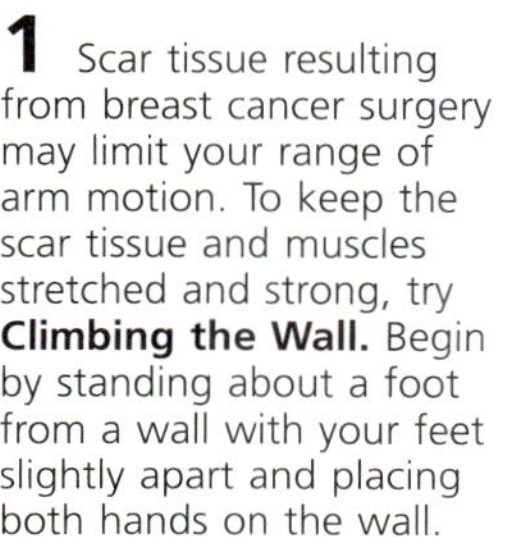

1 Scar tissue resulting from breast cancer surgery may limit your range of arm motion. To keep the scar tissue and muscles stretched and strong, try **Climbing the Wall.** Begin by standing about a foot from a wall with your feet slightly apart and placing both hands on the wall.

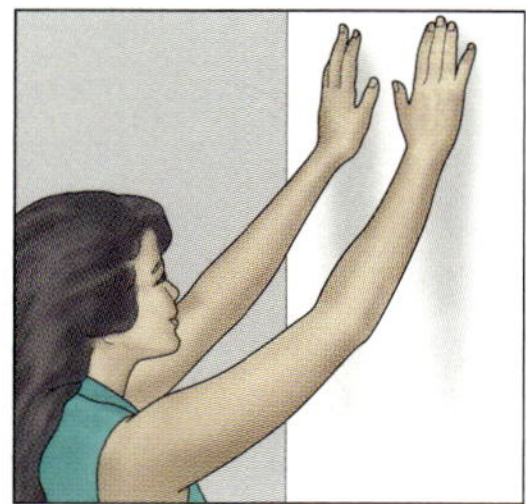

2 Slowly slide both hands up the wall as far as you can, but stop immediately if you feel any pain. Repeat five times a day, with the goal of raising both arms above your head. As with any post-surgical exercise, always have your physician's approval and guidance.

DIAGNOSTIC AND TEST PROCEDURES

Breast cancer responds to treatment best when it is detected early. In addition to having an annual medical checkup, all women should conduct monthly breast self-examinations *(see **Breast Problems**)*. A baseline mammogram—a low-dose x-ray of the breast—is recommended for women between the ages of 35 and 40. Most women should also get a mammogram every other year beginning around age 40 and every year beginning at age 50. Women at risk for breast cancer should consult their doctor for the best schedule. Any risk of developing cancer from mammography is clearly offset by the benefits: Breast lumps can be identified on a mammogram up to two years before they can be felt.

Several tests can help distinguish a benign lump from a malignant tumor. Feeling the lump may provide clues: A benign cyst may feel like a round, slippery bean, whereas a tumor may feel thicker and may cause dimpling of the skin above it. Because malignant and benign lumps tend to have different physical features, imaging tests such as mammography and ultrasonography can often rule out cancer. The only way to confirm cancer is to perform needle aspiration or a biopsy and to test the tissue sample for cancer cells.

In the event of malignancy, you and your doctor need to know how far along the cancer is. Various tests are used to check for the presence and likely sites of metastasis. Cancer cells can be analyzed for the presence or absence of hormone receptors, to find out if the cancer is likely to respond well to hormone therapy. Other tests can help predict the likelihood of metastasis and the potential for recurrence after treatment.

TREATMENT

If you have breast cancer, do what you can as soon as you can to get rid of it. But before making treatment decisions, research your options. Ask questions of your doctor, other specialists, and people who have had the disease, and seek a second opinion at a major cancer treatment center. Find a doctor you trust, and don't rush your decision. A brief delay between diagnosis and treatment will not compromise the effectiveness of treatment.

CONVENTIONAL MEDICINE

The options for treating breast cancer depend on how advanced the cancer is, how old the patient is, and how healthy she is otherwise. If possible, breast cancer is treated surgically, followed usually by some combination of radiation therapy, chemotherapy, or hormone therapy.

The standard surgical procedure for breast cancer was once **radical mastectomy**—the total removal of the breast and the surrounding fat, muscle, and lymph nodes. For breast cancer that is detected early and is still localized, **lumpectomy**—removal of the cancerous lump and the lymph nodes under the arm—or sentinel node testing—which offers better identification of malignant lymph nodes and is less invasive than surgery—are the preferred treatments.

RECONSTRUCTIVE BREAST SURGERY

Lumpectomy is not disfiguring the way breast surgery once was, but even mastectomy need not be permanently disfiguring. While some women choose to wear a prosthesis after a mastectomy, others opt for reconstructive surgery. For three decades, the most common reconstructive surgery involved implanting a silicone-filled prosthesis behind skin or muscles in the chest wall. Some women claim to have developed debilitating immune disorders from leaking silicone implants, and in 1992 such implants were removed from the market. Since then, several scientific studies have found no link between immune disorders and silicone breast implants, although they have confirmed lesser, yet undesirable, side effects. Saline-filled implants are now widely used. Surgeons can also transfer tissue from the abdomen, back, or elsewhere to construct artificial breast replacements. The cosmetic results are impressive, but the surgery is costly and complex, produces additional scarring, and may cause weakness in the area from which tissue is removed.

Faced with surgery, some women choose **modified radical mastectomy** over lumpectomy and radiation therapy. In this procedure the tumor and surrounding breast tissue are removed, but most of the muscle on the chest wall is left intact—which is less disfiguring than radical mastectomy.

For breast cancer that has metastasized and for recurrent breast cancer, radiation therapy and chemotherapy are the primary modes of treatment. Hormone therapy may also be beneficial for cancers that are hormone responsive; of the estrogen-suppressing drugs in use, ***tamoxifen*** is most widely used. Meanwhile, researchers are exploring treatment of breast cancer with various forms of immunotherapy; by manipulating the body's immune system, they hope to improve its natural resistance to cancer.

For further information on radiation, chemotherapy, and other treatments, see ***Cancer.***

COMPLEMENTARY THERAPIES

As with any cancer, there is no acceptable alternative to conventional medical treatment. The therapies listed should be considered preventive measures or complementary options to be pursued in conjunction with standard medical care.

LIFESTYLE

Regular aerobic exercise may offer some protection against a woman's developing breast cancer. Studies have found that women who exercised vigorously and often were at least half as likely as nonexercisers to get breast cancer. Exercise can also help breast cancer patients better tolerate the side effects of radiation or chemotherapy.

MIND/BODY MEDICINE

Relaxing the mind can certainly help alleviate the mental and physical stresses of cancer. Besides pursuing such individual mind/body approaches as **meditation** or **yoga,** many people benefit from structured support-group therapy. One retrospective study over 10 years of 86 women with metastatic breast cancer showed that those who participated in support-group therapy and self-hypnosis while receiving conventional treatment felt better and lived 18 months longer on average than those who got conventional care alone.

NUTRITION AND DIET

Your diet can play an important role in breast cancer prevention. In principle, dietary fats may increase your risk of developing breast cancer, and fruits, vegetables, and grains may help to reduce the risk. It's a good idea to make whole-milk dairy products, meat, and foods fried at high temperatures occasional treats rather than staples. You can enliven your menus by sampling different kinds of fresh fruits and vegetables and basing new dishes on whole grains and legumes. This way, you're bound to get plenty of body-cleansing fiber, along with vitamins and minerals thought to protect against breast cancer, specifically ***vitamins A, C, D,*** and ***E,*** and ***calcium, selenium,*** and ***iodine.*** Some doctors recommend that breast cancer patients and survivors take antioxidant supplements.

Certain plant foods contain phytoestrogens, weak plant estrogens that may be particularly useful against hormone-sensitive breast cancers. In theory, phytoestrogens block the uptake of normal estrogen in breast tissue. Withholding estrogen may reduce the likelihood of cancer and, if malignancy exists, may reduce the rate at which cancer cells multiply. Wheat, soybeans, olives, plums, carrots, apples, yams, and coconuts are among the foods that contain phytoestrogens.

AT-HOME CARE

After breast surgery, a regular routine of simple exercises *(page 205)* will help to restore your mobility and reduce muscle stiffness. To minimize potential discomfort from radiation therapy, avoid wearing a bra or clothes that may irritate the area, keep your skin clean and well aired, and use only those skin lotions, creams, and deodorants recommended by your doctor.

PREVENTION

- Check your breasts once a month, have a thorough medical checkup once a year, and have mammograms annually if you are age 50 or older. Start mammograms earlier if you have a family history of breast cancer.
- Make fruits, vegetables, grains, and fish the mainstays of your diet.
- If you practice contraception, ask your doctor about the pros and cons of estrogen-based birth-control pills.
- If you are at high risk for breast cancer, talk to your doctor or gynecologist about managing ***menopause*** symptoms without estrogen pills and about taking ***tamoxifen*** as a preventative. ■

BREAST PROBLEMS

SYMPTOMS

- pain or a feeling of fullness in one or both breasts, most likely caused by premenstrual swelling.
- pain accompanied by redness and warmth or a discharge from the nipple; this may indicate an infection. Discharge can also signal a benign growth or ***breast cancer.***
- a lump that is movable and feels unattached to the chest wall; you may have a **cyst** or a **fibroadenoma.**
- a lump that is hard, is not movable, or feels attached to the chest wall, with or without pain, perhaps with dimpling or puckering of the breast; this may be a sign of ***breast cancer.***

CALL YOUR DOCTOR IF:

- you notice any kind of new or unusual lump in your breasts, especially one that remains throughout your menstrual cycle. Although most lumps are harmless, in rare instances they may signal infection or cancer. Have your doctor check any lump.

The female breast is an organ that changes with puberty, with the monthly menstrual cycle, and with pregnancy; it also continues to change with age. Most changes in your breast are perfectly normal and no cause for concern. However, you may experience any of several conditions that require medical attention. Chief among these are **breast pain** and masses or **lumps** *(see below and page 210).*

Starting at puberty, you should examine your breasts every month, so that you are familiar with their structure and can detect any new masses or lumps. Premenstrual changes can cause temporary thickening that disappears after the period, so it is best to check your breasts about a week after your period. If you are no longer menstruating, examine your breasts monthly on a day you will remember, such as the day corresponding to your birthday.

Mammograms—detailed x-ray pictures of the breasts—can reveal tumors too tiny to be felt by hand. There is disagreement and no small controversy as to when a woman should begin getting routine mammograms: Some doctors say between ages 35 and 40; others say not until age 50. A typical pattern is every other year beginning around age 40, then increasing the frequency to once a year at age 50. If you have a family history of breast cancer, especially in your mother or sister, your physician may advise a different schedule.

BREAST PAIN

Breast pain can have many causes, including the normal swelling of breast tissue during the menstrual cycle. Other causes include infection or injury; growths, including cancer; and perhaps diet.

The general swelling of breast tissue with the menstrual period can be painful, but it is not dangerous, and no treatment is necessary if you can tolerate the discomfort. Each monthly cycle brings about hormonal changes, including increases in estrogen and progesterone, that bring more fluid into the breasts, expanding tissue, stretching nerve fibers, and producing pain. Some women experience this painful swelling just before their periods, with symptoms subsiding near the end of the menstrual flow. Others experience it as a side effect of birth-control pills.

Another possible reason for breast pain is decreased progesterone levels during the menstrual cycle. Several studies have shown a correlation between cyclic breast pain and low progesterone levels.

Trauma and infection in the breast produce the same symptoms you would see elsewhere in your body, except that in your breast, infections tend to become walled off from surrounding tissue, producing small abscesses. This may give them the appearance of cysts. Infections occur almost exclusively in breast-feeding mothers. If you suspect you have an infection, see your doctor.

Cysts may produce pain *(see **Lumps,** page 210),* but breast cancer rarely does—although pain does not rule out the possibility of cancer.

TREATMENT

Practitioners of both conventional and alternative medicine use diet and nutrition to prevent and treat monthly swelling of the breasts. Both would encourage you to maintain a healthy weight and eat a balanced diet as good preventive medicine. Because salt can contribute to fluid retention and thus worsen symptoms, you should restrict your salt intake near your period. For some women, eliminating caffeine and related substances, such as methylxanthines (found in chocolate and tea), can alleviate breast pain. Both conventional and alternative practitioners may suggest wearing a bra, even 24 hours a day, to reduce breast movement and lessen the discomfort until the tenderness passes.

CONVENTIONAL MEDICINE

In recent years, some conventional doctors have suggested ***vitamin E*** supplements, in daily doses of up to 800 IU, to treat breast pain not caused by cancer. In addition, a conventional physician may suggest relieving pain with an analgesic such as ***aspirin*** or ***ibuprofen.***

If these treatments don't help, your doctor may prescribe treatment with a hormone such as danazol, which has been shown to help relieve breast pain. You might also be given progesterone, since some studies suggest a lack of progesterone may contribute to breast pain. The anticancer drug ***tamoxifen*** is also prescribed. If one of these drugs doesn't work or gives you troublesome side effects, your doctor may switch you to another. However, do not use these drugs if you are trying to become pregnant.

All of the hormone treatments above have side effects; those of danazol, a male hormone, include headache, nausea, menstrual irregularity, and weight gain, as well as masculinization (increased hair growth and, rarely, deepening of the voice) that may not be reversible. Your doctor may be reluctant to use tamoxifen because of uncertainty about its long-term effects on cancer risk, bone density, gynecological growths, and blood clots. In fact, most patients can get relief without strong drugs; the greatest benefit comes from eliminating caffeine.

Breast infections are treated with ***antibiotics.*** If an abscess exists, your doctor may also make a small incision to drain it. If this doesn't work, minor surgery is the next step.

ALTERNATIVE CHOICES

In addition to the dietary changes and supplements cited above, alternative-medicine practitioners frequently treat breast pain with higher doses of nutritional supplements and with herbs.

In addition to the therapies listed below, **acupuncture** and **Chinese herbs** can treat breast pain effectively.

HERBAL THERAPIES

Evening primrose oil (*Oenothera biennis*), although not approved in the United States for treating breast pain, is used in Europe and has proved effective. You can take a 500 mg capsule three times a day, every day if necessary. This treatment has fewer side effects than the hormone therapies often prescribed in conventional medicine.

HOW TO CHECK YOUR BREASTS

Check your breasts monthly, 7 to 10 days after your menstrual period ends. (It's easiest in the shower, using soap to smooth your skin.) Look for dimpling, then try either the spiral or grid method below, using light pressure to check for lumps near the surface and firm pressure to explore deeper tissues. Squeeze each nipple gently; if there is any discharge—especially if it is bloody—consult your doctor.

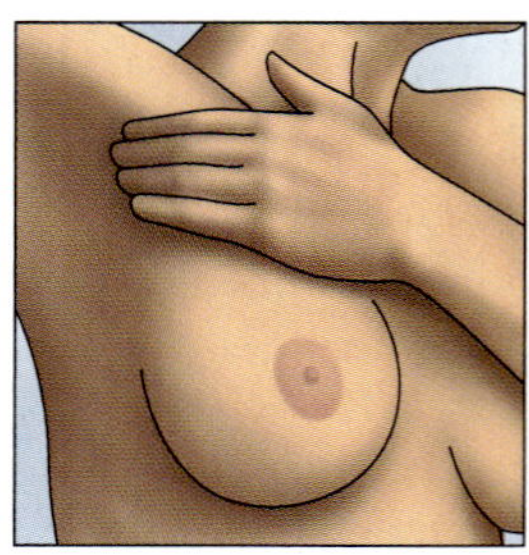

1 With either the spiral or the grid method, begin by raising your arm, and always use the flat surface of your fingers. Apply light pressure by barely depressing the surface of your skin *(left);* this will enable you to feel for any tiny lumps near the surface.

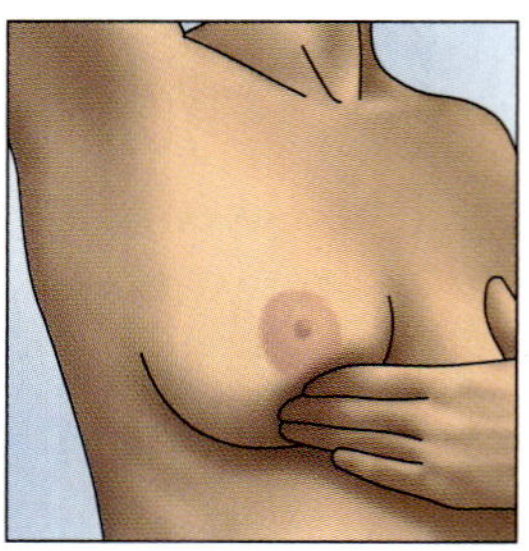

2 To apply firm pressure, press deeply into the tissue, again using the flat surface of your fingers. Be aware of any sensitive areas, unusual lumps, or thickened tissue.

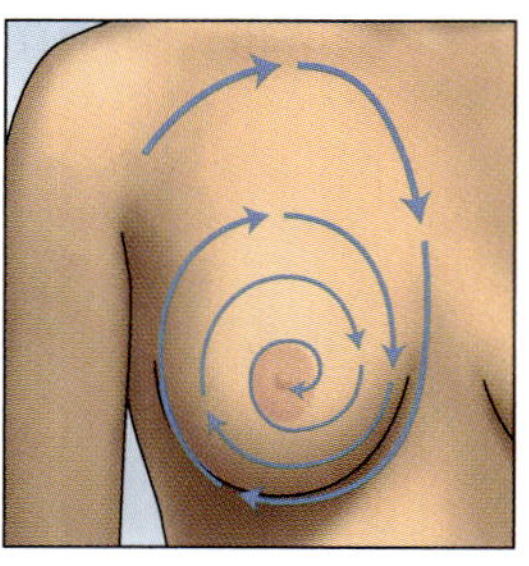

3 To use the spiral method, begin at the top of your breast near your armpit and follow the pattern illustrated at left. Apply light pressure first as you work in toward the nipple. Repeat the same pattern using firm pressure.

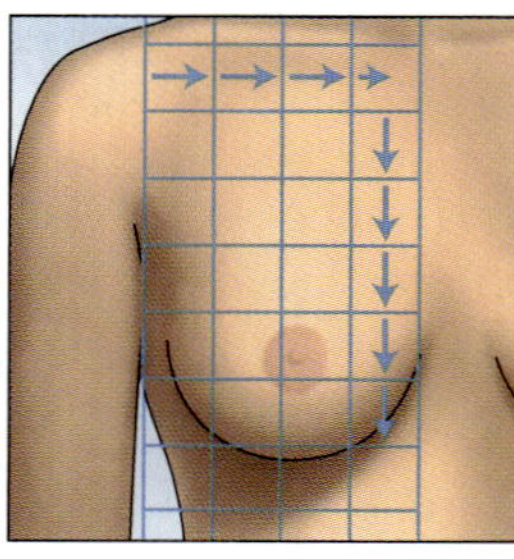

4 To use the grid method, imagine the pattern of squares illustrated at left, and follow the direction indicated by the arrows. Make a tiny spiral in each square, using first light pressure, then firm pressure.

NUTRITION AND DIET

Vitamin E effectively relieves breast pain and reduces size of breast cysts. This vitamin affects blood clotting; if you are taking a blood thinner, consult your doctor before taking any vitamin E. Although alternative practitioners sometimes recommend dosages up to 1,200 IU, many women find relief with only 400 IU daily; consult your doctor before taking more than 400 IU a day. If you have high blood pressure, consult your doctor before taking more than 100 IU a day.

Because fat in the diet is associated with estrogen production, you can reduce estrogen levels in your body by eating a low-fat diet.

AT-HOME REMEDIES

For pain relief, try applying a warm castor-oil pack to your breast. Saturate a flannel cloth with high-grade castor oil, put it on the breast, and cover it with plastic wrap and a towel; apply heat to the pack with a heating pad or hot-water bottle for 20 to 30 minutes.

LUMPS

Breast lumps come in many forms, including **cysts, adenomas,** and **papillomas.** They differ in size, shape, and location, as well as in causes and treatment. About half of all women have lumpy breasts, or fibroadenosis, which is sometimes associated with hormonal changes related to the menstrual cycle. Most lumps are benign and do not signal cancer; however, any time you find a new or unusual lump, have your doctor check it to make sure it is not cancerous or precancerous. For more information, see ***Breast Cancer.***

Researchers are studying the incidence of breast lumps in women taking birth-control pills or using hormone replacement therapy (HRT). In HRT, women take varying amounts of the hormones ***estrogen and progestin*** to alleviate the symptoms of menopause and to reduce the risk of cardiovascular disease. While the evidence is inconclusive, your doctor may have concerns about HRT and breast lumps. An additional concern is that using HRT changes breast structure, increasing the breast density and making mammograms harder to read and evaluate. This could make detecting cancer more difficult.

Cysts, which can be large or small, are benign fluid-filled sacs. They sometimes occur cyclically, and they may be painful. The best tool for distinguishing a cyst from a solid tumor is ultrasound; a needle biopsy may also be done.

With the cessation of menstruation at menopause, many cystic lumps diminish or disappear; therefore, you should immediately have your doctor check any lumps that form after menopause.

Fibroadenomas are the most common benign breast tumors seen in women under age 40 and are occasionally seen in adolescents. Fibroadenomas are usually round, several centimeters across, and mobile. They can be positively identified only by biopsy, which is recommended for anyone over age 20.

Nipple adenomas are tumors of the nipple area. They vary in appearance, sometimes recur after surgical removal, and are sometimes but not usually associated with cancer.

An intraductal **papilloma** is a relatively uncommon small growth in the lining of the milk ducts near the nipple. Usually seen in women over 40, papillomas produce a discharge, which may be bloody.

TREATMENT

CONVENTIONAL MEDICINE

For breast lumps, treatment and diagnosis are frequently related. For example, your doctor may insert a needle into a **cyst** and draw out fluid, both to examine the fluid and to eliminate the cyst. If the fluid is clear and the cyst disappears, your doctor will probably diagnose it as a benign cyst and undertake no further treatment. Many physicians take the added precaution of having the fluid checked by cytology—a pathologist's examination of the cells. If a lump does not disappear and is still present after your next menstrual period, your doctor will want to reexamine you.

If the fluid extracted from a suspected cyst is bloody or if little or no fluid can be extracted, this is a cause for concern, and a biopsy may be indicated to check for cancer.

Fibroadenomas can be diagnosed only by biopsy. Surgical removal, usually in a same-day surgical procedure, is considered the only treatment.

Nipple adenomas are surgically removed because they are sometimes associated with breast cancer. Intraductal **papillomas** are surgically removed before they grow enough to block the milk ducts.

Some conventional doctors recommend eliminating caffeine to shrink breast cysts, but the only study completed on caffeine's effect showed no connection. Some studies have suggested (although none has proved) a link between dietary fat—especially saturated fat—and benign lumps, as well as breast cancer. Limiting fat may help shrink or eliminate lumps.

ALTERNATIVE CHOICES

Alternative medicine emphasizes prevention as an effective way to manage breast problems. Diet and nutritional supplements are the first line of defense.

CHINESE HERBS

The Chinese herbs ***dong quai*** *(Angelica sinensis),* ***bupleurum*** *(bupleurum chinense),* and ***dandelion*** *(Taraxacum mongolicum)* may reduce breast lumps; consult a Chinese herbalist.

HERBAL THERAPIES

Evening primrose oil *(Oenothera biennis)*—500 mg two or three times a day—may be helpful in reducing breast lumps.

NUTRITION AND DIET

Although no studies have proved that diet causes breast tumors, some do suggest a relationship. Many practitioners of alternative medicine urge eliminating caffeine and recommend taking 400 to 1,200 IU of ***vitamin E,*** plus no more than 50 mcg (micrograms) a day of ***selenium.*** Caution: Selenium can be toxic in higher doses; you should use it only under the supervision of your health-care practitioner. ■

BREATHING PROBLEMS

Read down this column to find your symptoms. Then read across.

B

SYMPTOMS	AILMENT/PROBLEM
Breathing problems can be indicative of a wide variety of ailments. The symptoms listed below are intended as a general guide to several broad categories. For more information on specific sets of symptoms, see the entries listed in the next column.	
◆ shortness of breath, hyperventilation, or wheezing after mild or no exercise.	◆ ***Stress; allergies; asthma; emphysema; pneumonia; heart attack; lung cancer***
◆ coughing accompanied by yellowish or greenish phlegm.	◆ Acute or chronic ***bronchitis***
◆ coughing accompanied by frothy white, pink, rust-colored, or bloody phlegm.	◆ ***Heart disease; pneumonia; tuberculosis; lung cancer;*** lung abscess; pulmonary edema
◆ dry cough with pain in chest.	◆ ***Heart disease; lung cancer; pleurisy; pneumonia;*** reaction to heart medication

B

WHAT TO DO	OTHER INFO
◆ **Call 911 or your emergency number now** if you suspect a heart attack. See also ***Emergencies/First Aid: Heart Attack.***	◆ If you suspect that your shortness of breath is caused by stress due to poor physical shape or to anxiety, you can remedy the problem by exercising regularly and practicing mind/body techniques such as yoga or meditation.
◆ See ***Bronchitis.*** Your doctor will prescribe ***antibiotics*** if the cause is a bacterial infection.	◆ If the cough is accompanied by a fever and has lasted only a few days, you probably have acute bronchitis. If the cough has persisted for several weeks, and you smoke, you may have chronic bronchitis.
◆ **Call your doctor now.** Treat coughs accompanied by this type of sputum as medical emergencies.	◆ Frothy white or pinkish sputum is nearly always a sign of heart disease, while rust-colored phlegm points to pneumonia. Strenuous coughing can rupture small blood vessels in the back of your throat and cause bleeding, but you should still see a doctor immediately if you are coughing up bloody sputum.
◆ Call your doctor for a proper diagnosis.	◆ If a dry cough comes on very suddenly in a child, it may mean that a small object is lodged in the throat. See ***Emergencies/First Aid: Choking.*** Also, the class of heart medications known as ***angiotensin-converting enzyme (ACE) inhibitors*** can produce the side effect of a dry cough in some people.

BRONCHITIS

B

SYMPTOMS

Acute Bronchitis:

- hacking cough.
- yellow, white, or green phlegm, usually appearing 24 to 48 hours after a cough.
- fever, chills.
- soreness and tightness in chest.
- some pain below breastbone during deep breathing.

Chronic Bronchitis:

- persistent cough producing yellow, white, or green phlegm (for at least three months of the year, and for more than two consecutive years).
- wheezing, some breathlessness.

CALL YOUR DOCTOR IF:

- your cough is so persistent or severe that it interferes with sleep or daily activities; you could be damaging sensitive air sacs in your lungs.
- your symptoms last more than a week, and your mucus becomes darker, thicker, or increases in volume; most likely, you have an infection requiring ***antibiotics.***
- you display symptoms of acute bronchitis and have chronic lung or heart problems or are infected with the virus that causes ***AIDS;*** respiratory infections can leave you vulnerable to more serious lung diseases, such as ***pneumonia.***
- you have great difficulty breathing. This symptom, sometimes mistakenly associated with bronchitis, could signal ***asthma, emphysema, tuberculosis, heart disease,*** a serious ***allergic*** reaction, or ***cancer.***

Bronchitis is an upper respiratory disease in which the mucous membrane in the lungs' upper bronchial passages becomes inflamed. As the irritated membrane swells and grows thicker, it narrows or shuts off the tiny airways in the lungs, resulting in coughing spells accompanied by thick phlegm and breathlessness. The disease comes in two forms: acute and chronic.

Acute bronchitis is responsible for the hacking cough and phlegm production that sometimes accompany an upper respiratory infection; in most cases the infection is viral in origin, but sometimes it is caused by bacteria. If you are otherwise in good health, the mucous membrane will return to normal after you've recovered from the initial lung infection, which usually lasts for several days.

Chronic bronchitis, like the lung disease ***emphysema,*** is a serious long-term disorder that requires regular medical treatment. People who have chronic bronchitis tend to be obese and lead sedentary lives, and most are heavy smokers; they typically have emphysema as well, which accounts for some of the overlapping symptoms.

If you are a smoker and come down with acute bronchitis, it will be much harder for you to recover. Even one puff on a cigarette is enough to cause temporary paralysis of the tiny hairs, known as cilia, on the lining of your lungs that are responsible for brushing out debris, irritants, and excess mucus. If you continue smoking, you may do sufficient damage to the cilia to prevent them from functioning properly, increasing your chances of developing chronic bronchitis. In some heavy smokers, the membrane stays inflamed and the cilia eventually stop functioning altogether. Clogged with mucus, the lungs are then vulnerable to viral and bacterial infections, which over time distort and permanently damage the lungs' airways.

Acute bronchitis is very common among both children and adults. Although the disorder often can be treated effectively without professional medical assistance, you will need to see a doctor for a prescription of ***antibiotics*** if the underlying lung infection is bacterial. If you suffer from **chronic bronchitis,** you are at risk for developing cardiovascular problems as well as more serious lung diseases and infections, so you should be monitored by a doctor.

CAUSES

Acute bronchitis is generally caused by lung infections; approximately 90 percent of these infections are viral in origin, 10 percent bacterial. **Chronic bronchitis** may be caused by one or several factors. Repeated attacks of acute bronchitis, which weaken and irritate bronchial airways over time, can result in chronic bronchitis. Industrial pollution is another culprit. Chronic bronchitis is found in higher-than-normal rates among coal miners, grain handlers, metal molders, and other people who are continually exposed to dust. But the chief cause is heavy, long-term cigarette smoking, which irritates the bronchial tubes and causes them to produce excess mucus. The symptoms of chronic bronchitis are also worsened by high concentrations of sulfur dioxide and other pollutants in the atmosphere.

DIAGNOSTIC AND TEST PROCEDURES

Tests are usually unnecessary in the case of **acute bronchitis,** as the disease is easy to detect on examination. Your doctor will simply use a stethoscope to listen for the rattling sound in your lungs' upper airways that typically accompanies the problem. If your symptoms persist for a week or more, your doctor may also take a culture of the phlegm you produce when you cough, to determine if you have a bacterial or viral infection. In cases of **chronic bronchitis,** the doctor will almost certainly augment these procedures with an x-ray of your chest to check the extent of the lung damage, as well as with pulmonary function tests to measure your lung capacity.

THE BRONCHIAL TUBES

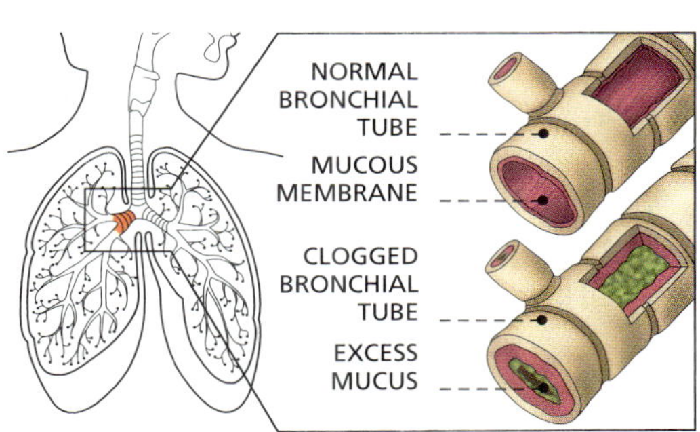

Air flows down the windpipe and into the lungs through branching conduits called the bronchial tubes, or bronchioles, which normally are lined with only a thin mucous membrane. In bronchitis, however, this membrane becomes inflamed, resulting in stepped-up mucus production. Over time, excess mucus can clog the bronchioles, cutting off air flow to the lungs. Coughing is the body's way of ridding the lungs of this mucus buildup.

TREATMENT

Conventional treatment for both acute and chronic bronchitis may consist of antibiotics and a prescription cough syrup. In severe cases of chronic bronchitis, supplemental oxygen may be necessary. Alternative choices, by and large, help relieve the accompanying discomfort but do not treat infections.

CONVENTIONAL MEDICINE

If your **acute bronchitis** is caused by a bacterial infection, your doctor probably will prescribe ***antibiotics,*** which should help clear up the symptoms in several days. Even if the cause is viral, your doctor may prescribe antibiotics as a preventive measure, because your lungs are susceptible to bacterial infections in their weakened state. The productive (phlegm-producing) coughing that comes with acute bronchitis is to be expected and, in most cases, encouraged; coughing is your body's way of getting rid of excess mucus. However, if your cough is truly disruptive—that is, it keeps you from sleeping or is so violent it becomes painful—or nonproductive (dry and raspy sounding), your doctor may prescribe a ***cough suppressant.*** In most cases, you should simply do all the things you normally would do for a cold: Take ***aspirin*** for fever and drink lots of liquids.

If you have **chronic bronchitis,** your lungs are

vulnerable to infections. Unless your doctor counsels against it, get a yearly flu shot as well as a vaccination against ***pneumonia.*** The pneumonia vaccine is typically a one-shot procedure: One vaccination should protect you for life against all the common strains of the disease. Only in very rare cases is a second shot required.

Do not take an over-the-counter ***cough suppressant*** to treat chronic bronchitis unless your doctor directs you to do so. As with acute bronchitis, the productive coughing associated with chronic bronchitis is helpful in ridding the lungs of excess mucus. In fact, your doctor may even prescribe an ***expectorant*** if your cough is relatively dry. However, if you notice any changes in the color, volume, or thickness of the phlegm, you may be coming down with an infection. In that case, your physician may prescribe a weeklong or 10-day course of broad-spectrum antibiotics, which fight a range of bacteria.

If you are overweight, your doctor may insist that you diet to avoid putting excessive strain on your heart. Many doctors also prescribe ***bronchodilators,*** drugs that help dilate the lungs' constricted airways, or anti-inflammatory drugs to reduce spasm and inflammation in the airways. For people with chronic bronchitis, inhaled bronchodilators, available in aerosol or metered-dose inhalers, are generally preferred over oral medications. In most cases, one or two puffs will relieve the breathlessness that accompanies chronic bronchitis. Special circumstances may require a greater dosage, but you should never increase your intake unless instructed to do so by your doctor. Bronchodilators are potent drugs; overuse can cause dangerous side effects, such as ***high blood pressure.***

If your body's ability to transfer oxygen from your lungs into the bloodstream is significantly handicapped, your doctor may prescribe **oxygen therapy,** either on a continuous or on an as-needed basis. Oxygen-delivering devices are widely available. If you use an oxygen tank at home, be sure to take special care not to expose the apparatus to flammable materials (alcohol and aerosol sprays, for example) or to sources of direct heat, such as hair dryers or radiators.

If you smoke, your doctor will urge you to quit. Studies show that people who kick the habit even in the advanced stages of chronic bronchitis not only can reduce the severity of their symptoms but also can increase their life expectancy.

ALTERNATIVE CHOICES

A number of alternative therapies can be used to complement—but never to replace—a conventional doctor's care. These remedies may help ease some of the symptoms of acute and chronic bronchitis, but they do not treat infections.

ACUPUNCTURE

Studies suggest that acupuncture may relieve the symptoms associated with bronchitis. The technique should be performed only by a licensed acupuncturist.

AROMATHERAPY

Essential oils such as ***eucalyptus*** *(Eucalyptus globulus),* ***hyssop*** *(Hyssopus officinalis),* aniseed *(Pimpinella anisum),* ***lavender*** *(Lavandula officinalis),* pine *(Pinus sylvestris),* and ***rosemary*** *(Rosmarinus officinalis)* may help ease breathing and relieve nasal congestion. Inhaling deeply through your nose, breathe the aroma from a few drops of one or more of these oils dabbed on a handkerchief, or sniff directly from the bottle. Try mixing a few drops of essential oil in a sink full of hot water; cover your head with a towel and breathe in the fragrant steam.

CHINESE HERBS

The Chinese herb ***ephedra*** *(Ephedra sinica)* is a potent bronchodilator. CAUTION: Large quantities of this herb have the same effect as large quantities of the hormone ***epinephrine;*** do not use ephedra if you have ***high blood pressure*** or ***heart disease.*** Prepare an infusion by combining 5 grams ephedra, 4 grams ***cinnamon*** sticks *(Cinnamomum cassia),* 1.5 grams ***licorice*** *(Glycyrrhiza uralensis),* and 5 grams ***apricot seed*** *(Prunus armeniaca).* Steep the mixture in cold water, then bring it to a boil. Drink it hot. Do not use this mixture if you have yellow or greenish mucus. Consult a Chinese herbalist for other remedies.

B

HERBAL THERAPIES

A wide variety of herbs act as soothing expectorants, making them appropriate in the treatment of bronchitis. A sampling of therapies follows; for more, seek the advice of a professional herbalist or homeopath.

In the case of **acute** or **chronic bronchitis,** the herb ***coltsfoot*** *(Tussilago farfara)* may relax constricted or spasming bronchial tubes and gently help to loosen phlegm. To prepare an infusion, add a cup of boiling water to 1 or 2 tsp of coltsfoot; let the infusion steep for 10 minutes. Drink it as hot as possible, three times daily. ***Mullein*** *(Verbascum thapsus),* believed to have an anti-inflammatory effect on mucous membranes, can also be prepared as an infusion by following the directions above.

To treat **acute bronchitis,** use the same directions to prepare an infusion from the herb ***hyssop*** *(Hyssopus officinalis),* which may encourage sweating (thus lowering fever) and lessen inflammation. Osha *(Ligusticum porteri)* tincture has anti-viral properties; take 15 to 20 drops, 3 times a day, for 10 to 14 days. Herbal expectorants appropriate for **chronic bronchitis** include aniseed *(Pimpinella anisum),* elecampane *(Inula helenium),* and ***garlic*** *(Allium sativum).*

STEAMING TOWARD RECOVERY

Humidity is helpful in treating both acute and chronic bronchitis, as moisture in the air can loosen phlegm inside the lungs and make it easier for you to expectorate. To be effective, however, humidifying devices must be used properly.

The warm steam distributed by vaporizers works well when used in a relatively small space, such as a bathroom; in an average-size room, most vaporizers aren't powerful enough to generate the density of steam necessary to be truly helpful. Be sure to clean the vaporizer regularly for the duration of your infection, to prevent the distribution of germs.

Some devices can actually be hazardous to your health. Cold humidifiers, used frequently in homes with dry air, must be cleaned daily with bleach; otherwise, they can spread germs and encourage mold or mildew growth, increasing your chances of developing lung infections.

HOMEOPATHY

For **acute** and **chronic bronchitis,** take the following three times a day, for up to four days: To treat fever, cough, and tightness in the chest, use ***Aconite*** (6c). For loose white phlegm, cough, and irritability, use ***Kali bichromicum*** (6c). For loss of voice, cough, thirst, and sore throat, use ***Phosphorus*** (6c).

NUTRITION AND DIET

To strengthen the immune system and protect against infection, nutritionists often recommend ***vitamins A, B complex, C,*** and ***E,*** along with the minerals ***selenium*** and ***zinc.*** Some experts suggest that you also avoid mucus-producing foods, found mainly in the dairy group (although goat's milk generally causes less mucus production than cow's milk), as well as in refined starches (white-flour–based products) and processed foods.

AT-HOME REMEDIES

For acute bronchitis:

Throughout the duration of your infection, stay at home and keep warm. You don't necessarily need to stay in bed, but don't overextend yourself. Consider using a vaporizer, or try inhaling steam over a sink full of hot water.

For chronic bronchitis:

Avoid exposure to paint or exhaust fumes, dust, and people with colds. Consider using a vaporizer or inhaling steam over a sink full of hot water. Dress warmly in cold, dry weather. ■

BULIMIA

B

SYMPTOMS

- recurrent episodes of binge eating and purging.
- unrealistic fear of becoming fat.
- weight fluctuation (although relatively normal weight may be maintained).
- food cravings.
- overuse of laxatives.
- ***depression.***
- tooth enamel erosion, gum infections, cavities, and tooth discoloration (caused by stomach acids from frequent vomiting).
- gastrointestinal upset.

CALL YOUR DOCTOR IF:

- you find yourself secretly binging, then vomiting or using laxatives.
- you avoid eating in front of other people.
- your child has an unreasonable fear of being fat and thinks she's fat when she's not.
- your child avoids eating with others or frequents the bathroom immediately after meals.

Bulimia is an eating disorder that, like ***anorexia nervosa,*** is psychological in origin and can have dire physical consequences. While anorexics simply starve themselves, bulimics binge on food and then purge by self-induced vomiting. Bulimics also frequently use diet pills, laxatives, and diuretics to reduce their weight. The purging may serve two purposes: preventing weight gain and also temporarily relieving ***depression*** and other negative feelings.

Like anorexia, bulimia mostly afflicts young women. Because binging and purging are practiced in secret, the incidence of the disorder is uncertain, but researchers estimate that as many as one-fifth of all U.S. women in high school and college display at least temporary bulimic symptoms. The average age of onset is 18.

Bulimia can occur on its own or intermittently with anorexia. In the intermittent pattern—which occurs in about 1 case out of 5—a young woman will not eat for some time, setting herself up for a binge; she may use appetite suppressants in the noneating phase. Despite their overlap, the two disorders are associated with some different personality traits: Anorexics are apt to suppress all urges, including sexual ones; bulimics, on the other hand, tend to indulge their cravings, impulsively getting into trouble with drugs, sexual promiscuity, shoplifting, or binge buying.

A bulimic's overall health depends on how often she binges and purges. She may vomit occasionally (once a month) or very frequently (many times a day). Physical repercussions include swelling of the stomach or pancreas, inflammation of the esophagus, enlarged salivary glands, and tooth decay and gum disease from vomiting stomach acids. Frequent vomiting also depletes the water and potassium in bodily tissues, causing abnormal heart rhythms, muscle spasms, and even paralysis. In severe cases, some of these physical problems can lead to death. Another danger is suicidal depression.

Bulimia is a real illness and usually cannot be controlled voluntarily by its sufferers without professional help. Admonitions from family and friends to stop are at best useless, at worst counterproductive.

B

CAUSES

Pressures and conflicts within the family are thought to be the primary cause of bulimia. A bulimic is apt to be an overachiever and perfectionist who feels she can't live up to her parents' expectations. She has low self-esteem and often suffers from depression. She may have been physically or sexually abused as a child: About half of all bulimics report a history of abuse.

TREATMENT

Psychotherapy—often combined with ***antidepressants***—is the primary treatment, together with nutritional counseling. Be sure to find a psychologist or psychiatrist experienced in dealing with eating disorders. The same is true for nutritional counseling, whether the patient sees the family doctor or another health professional. Clinics that specialize in eating disorders can often provide psychiatrists, psychotherapists, and nutritionists. All therapists involved should work in close cooperation with one another.

CONVENTIONAL MEDICINE

Psychological treatments for bulimia may involve individual, family, or group psychotherapy. Behavior or cognitive therapies are also often prescribed. Behavior therapy focuses on altering habits (binging and purging, in this case); sessions are usually devoted to analyzing the behavior and devising ways to change it, and the patient follows specific instructions between sessions. Cognitive therapy also concentrates on habitual behavior; it aims at exploring and countering the negative thoughts that underlie destructive habits. Individual or group psychotherapy focuses on the underlying emotional experiences and relationships that have caused the bulimia.

Antidepressants, used in conjunction with psychological therapies, are now a mainstay in bulimia therapy. ***Selective serotonin reuptake inhibitors,*** such as ***sertraline*** and ***fluoxetine,*** appear to be more helpful than ***tricyclic antidepressants,*** such as ***amitriptyline*** and imipramine.

ALTERNATIVE CHOICES

Most alternative therapies for bulimia do not address the root causes of the disorder, but they can be helpful in relieving some of the physical distress resulting from it. It is important to consult practitioners who are experienced in dealing with eating disorders.

HERBAL THERAPIES

Use any herbal therapies that reduce ***anxiety*** or ***depression.*** To soothe stomach pains or mouth inflammation, try ***marsh mallow*** *(Althaea officinalis)* root or ***slippery elm*** *(Ulmus fulva)* powder. *(See also **Canker Sores** and **Gastritis.**)*

HOMEOPATHY

Homeopathic medicine offers potentially beneficial prescriptions for eating disorders. In difficult cases, where conventional medicine has not been successful, consider seeking out a homeopath who has experience in treating bulimia.

MIND/BODY MEDICINE

Body exercises such as **yoga, t'ai chi, qigong,** and dance can help bulimics with their problems of body image. Reprogramming mental processes to gain control over the binge-and-purge cycles is another approach. Either **hypnotherapy** or EEG **biofeedback** may help. Be sure to interview hypnotherapists or biofeedback practitioners about their experience in treating eating disorders.

NUTRITION AND DIET

A nutrient-dense, sugar-free diet may help reduce binge eating. Also eliminate alcohol, caffeine, flavor enhancers, most salt, and cigarettes. Eat a balanced diet, supplemented daily with ***vitamin C*** (1,000 mg), ***vitamin B complex*** (50 mg), and a multivitamin/multimineral supplement. ■

BUNION

B

SYMPTOMS

- an angular protrusion at the side of the foot behind the big toe, sometimes accompanied by hardened skin or a callus.
- swelling, redness, unusual tenderness, or pain at the base of the big toe and in the ball of the foot, especially if the area becomes shiny and cool to the touch.

CALL YOUR DOCTOR IF:

- you have persistent pain when walking normally in otherwise comfortable, flat-soled shoes; you may be developing ***bursitis*** or a ***bone spur*** in your foot.

A bunion is an unnatural bump or bend in the bone that forms the ball of the foot at the base of the big toe. The result is an unsightly swelling at the inside of the foot, sometimes pushing the big toe inward so it overlaps one or more other toes. A similar condition on the little toe is called a bunionette.

Because a bunion occurs at the joint where the toe bends in normal walking, your entire body weight rests on it at each step. While most bunions don't affect normal walking, they can be extremely painful.

CAUSES

Foot problems typically develop in early adulthood, becoming more pronounced as the foot spreads with aging. In many people, bunions are hereditary and occur along with other problems associated with weak or poor foot structure, as well as with ***corns and calluses***, ***bone spurs***, and ***bursitis***. Bunions sometimes develop with ***arthritis*** and can be associated with other progressive deformation of bones in the foot.

Bunions can also be brought on by years of wearing tight, poorly fitting shoes—especially high-heeled, pointed shoes styled more for fashion than for comfort and good support. As the bones gradually assume an unnatural shape, pressure on the other bones of the foot can lead to bursitis.

DIAGNOSTIC AND TEST PROCEDURES

Most of the time, bunions are so obvious from the pain and the unusual shape of the toe that further diagnosis is unnecessary. Even so, a doctor will usually take x-rays to determine the extent of the deformity and to see if orthopedic shoes or surgery is needed.

TREATMENT

Relieving a bunion's discomfort generally consists of steps to reduce pain and inflammation, followed by measures to prevent recurrence.

B

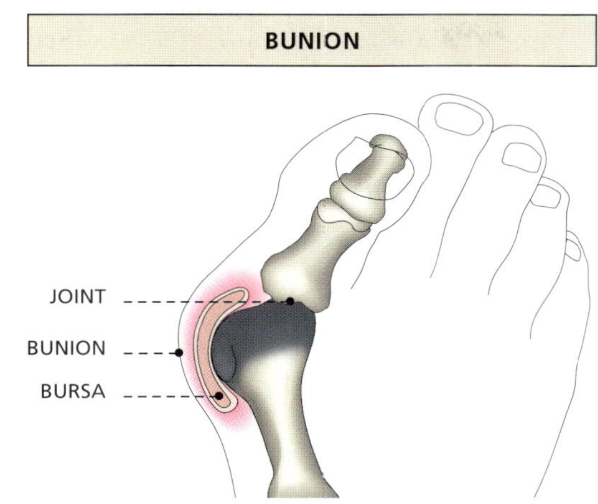

Weakness in the structure of the foot, exacerbated by poorly fitting shoes or some sports, can force the large joint of the big toe outward, resulting in a knobby protrusion called a bunion. Pain occurs when the bursa, a fluid-filled sac overlying the joint, becomes inflamed and swollen.

CONVENTIONAL MEDICINE

Your doctor may recommend ***aspirin*** or another over-the-counter pain remedy, or may prescribe a specific medication to relieve the swelling and inflammation. A heating pad or warm footbath may also help relieve the immediate pain and discomfort, as may an analgesic cream containing capsaicin, a chili-pepper extract.

If your bunion isn't persistently painful and you catch it early, wearing well-made, well-fitting shoes may be all the therapy you need. Most doctors don't advise bunion pads, splints, or other shoe inserts, which can exert pressure elsewhere on the foot and aggravate foot problems.

In some cases, an orthotic specialist can prescribe shoes with specially designed insoles and uppers that take the pressure off affected joints and help the foot regain its proper shape.

Most physicians are reluctant to recommend surgery for bunions, since many patients remain dissatisfied with the results. Done in a hospital under local anesthesia, a bunionectomy realigns the metatarsal bone behind the big toe by cutting the ligament at the joint. Wires may be temporarily inserted to keep the bones in line, and excess bone may be removed.

ALTERNATIVE CHOICES

Various therapies for reducing pain and inflammation can be used effectively on bunions.

BODY WORK

In certain cases, especially if bone degeneration is not advanced, **Rolfing** and Reiki techniques have been reported to alleviate the discomfort.

CHIROPRACTIC

Professional manipulation can help change the positioning of deformed bones. Practitioners can also help lessen the pain of bunions by having patients alter the way they walk.

HOMEOPATHY

Following an analysis of your overall situation, a homeopath can prescribe remedies that may relieve the pain of a bunion and may stabilize bone degeneration. For acute pain, try ***Apis, Cantharis,*** or ***Bryonia.***

AT-HOME REMEDIES

- When a bunion causes sore feet, a hot compress or a good soak in warm water will ease the pain.
- Sacrifice a pair of old but comfortable shoes: Cut away the leather or fabric upper—not the sole—to take pressure off a bunion.

PREVENTION

Because bunions develop slowly, taking precautions as your feet grow in childhood and early adulthood can pay off later in life. Closely monitor the shape of your feet as they develop, especially if foot problems run in your family. Exercising your feet can strengthen them, particularly if you learn to pick up small objects with your toes. Wear shoes that fit properly and that do not cramp or pinch your toes. Women should avoid shoes with high heels or pointed toes. ■

BURNS

B

SYMPTOMS

If the burn is:

- red, tender, and possibly swollen and blistering, it is probably a **first-degree burn** (which can include ***sunburn***).
- red, painful, and blistering, it is probably a **second-degree burn** (which can include severe sunburn).
- severely painful, the burned skin looks white or charred and blood vessels are exposed, or nerve damage is so substantial that there is no pain, it is probably a **third-degree burn.**
- characteristic of a third-degree burn, and muscle or bone is exposed, it is a **fourth-degree burn.**

CALL YOUR DOCTOR IF:

- you have a large first-degree burn.
- you have a second-degree burn on your hands, face, feet, groin, buttocks, or a major joint, or the burn is larger than three inches in diameter; or you have a third- or fourth-degree burn. You may suffer from shock, low blood pressure, and rapid pulse, and the area could become infected. **Get medical help immediately.**
- you have a chemical burn. This type of burn can cause serious secondary symptoms such as seizures and loss of consciousness. **Get medical help immediately.**
- you have an electrical burn. This type of burn can also cause injuries that might not be apparent. All electrical burns should be checked by a doctor.

See also ***Emergencies/First Aid: Burns.***

The skin is sensitive, living tissue composed of three primary layers: the epidermis, the dermis, and subcutaneous tissue. Any exposure to heat above 120°F will damage its cells and cause some degree of burning. Every year in the United States two million people are burned: 300,000 seriously, 70,000 requiring admission to a hospital, and 6,000 fatally. Children and the elderly are more susceptible to more serious forms of burning because their skin is thinner.

Minor burns include **first-degree burns,** limited **second-degree burns,** and ***sunburns*** (which may be classified as first- or second-degree burns depending on severity). **First-degree burns** affect the top layer of skin, the epidermis. Such burns are generally not serious and heal quickly. Within two days the damaged skin from a first-degree burn will peel away. **Second-degree burns** affect the epidermis and some of the underlying dermis layer of skin. Unless a second-degree burn covers a large area or has developed a secondary ***infection*** (which may be avoided with proper treatment), it is not serious and will heal in a short time.

Major burns include widespread **second-degree** and all **third-** and **fourth-degree burns**. Third- and fourth-degree burns are always serious and involve all three layers of skin. The area may appear white, or blackened and charred. Such severe burns affect fat tissue and nerves. **Fourth-degree burns** penetrate to muscle and bone.

Electrical burns can be deceiving. Although burning of the skin may be minimal, interior damage can be extensive and may include damage to

DON'T BUTTER THAT BURN

Don't try to soothe any kind of burn by putting butter or margarine on it. Such greasy substances can actually hold heat in the wound and slow down healing; they can also lead to ***infection.***

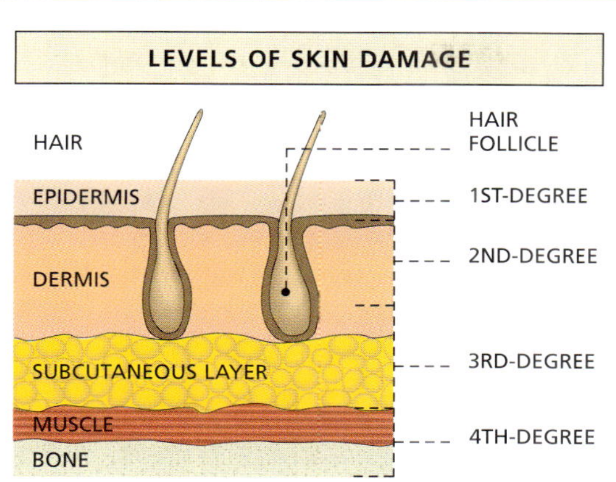

First-degree burns damage the thin epidermal layer and usually heal quickly. Second-degree burns damage some of the dermis, but not enough to destroy hair follicles and cells that generate new skin. Third-degree burns penetrate the subcutaneous layer, usually requiring skin grafts for new growth. Fourth-degree burns, by far the most severe, destroy the skin and damage muscle and bone.

the heart. High-voltage electric shock can cause cardiac arrest. *(See **Emergencies/First Aid: Cardiac and Respiratory Arrest** and **Electric Shock.**)*

TREATMENT

For any type of burn, immediate, aggressive care is essential to speed healing and recovery.

CONVENTIONAL MEDICINE

After at-home first-aid treatment has been applied to minor burns, any persisting pain may be alleviated with ***aspirin*** or ***acetaminophen.*** If your burn requires medical treatment, your doctor will cover the area with an antibacterial dressing or leave it exposed to promote healing (in which case the burn must diligently be kept clean). Avoid breaking blisters; exposure of the tissue underneath increases your likelihood of infection. ***Analgesics*** may be prescribed, or ***antibiotics*** if there are signs of infection. Any shock resulting from major burns will be treated with the administration of intravenous fluids. Severe major burns may require skin grafting or plastic surgery for repair and to avoid extensive scarring.

ALTERNATIVE CHOICES

All major burns should be treated by a medical professional. In addition to the therapies mentioned below, Chinese herbs, homeopathy, aromatherapy, and Ayurvedic medicine may also be helpful in treating minor burns.

HERBAL THERAPIES

Apply ***calendula*** *(Calendula officinalis)* ointment or ***aloe*** *(Aloe barbadensis)* to reduce pain, promote healing, and prevent infection in minor burns. Herbalists believe that honey is an effective healing agent. Spread a thin layer on your minor burn, cover with a loose dressing, and repeat daily until healed.

MIND/BODY MEDICINE

In some cases of major burns, concentrated healing thoughts and a positive attitude toward recovery have minimized symptoms such as pain, inflammation, and scarring. The most dramatic results have occurred when this technique has been applied within a few hours of injury.

AT-HOME REMEDIES

Flush minor burns with running water, then apply a cool compress. When your burn begins to heal, pierce a ***vitamin E*** capsule and rub the liquid onto the affected area to help prevent scarring. If your burn is major, drink lots of fluids during recovery; such burns cause loss of body fluids.

PREVENTION

Burns are frequently caused by preventable accidents in the home. Each floor should have a working smoke detector, and a fire extinguisher should be kept in the kitchen. All detectors and extinguishers should be tested at least annually. When cooking, turn pot handles to the inside of the stove, and if you have small children in the home, place covers over all unused electrical outlets. ■

BURSITIS

B

SYMPTOMS

- pain, inflammation, and swelling in the shoulders, elbows, hips, knees, or joints of the hands or feet, particularly during stretching or extension when exercising, lifting, or otherwise pushing the joint beyond its normal limits.
- restricted range of motion in a joint, with or without immediate pain.

CALL YOUR DOCTOR IF:

- pain in a joint persists more than a few days; you may be experiencing ***tendonitis,*** a strained ligament or tendon, or the onset of ***arthritis.***
- swelling persists after taking a painkiller or anti-inflammatory agent as prescribed; you may need to have a physician drain fluid from the affected joint or to undergo ***corticosteroid*** treatment.

Wherever your bones, tendons, and ligaments move against each other, particularly near joints, the points of contact are cushioned by small fluid-filled sacs called bursae. By reducing friction, each of the more than 150 bursae in your body helps joints operate smoothly through the full range of natural movement.

When a joint is overused, or when it stays under pressure or tension for extended periods of time, a nearby bursa can become inflamed. The sac fills with excess fluid, causing pressure on surrounding tissue. The immediate signal is pain, often accompanied by inflammation, swelling, and tenderness in the area.

One of the most common sites for bursitis to strike is the shoulder, which has the greatest range of motion of all the body's major joints. The pain is generally felt along the outside top of the shoulder. The discomfort of bursitis tends to be most severe after a night's sleep and will typically subside somewhat with normal activity. Other places that are prone to bursitis are the elbows, hips, and knees.

Bursitis is associated with strenuous activity, particularly among manual workers and athletes, as well as in otherwise sedentary people who push their bodies past reasonable limits. While you may be tempted to "tough out" the pain, it's not a good idea. Chronic bursitis left untreated can lead to the formation of calcium deposits in normally soft tissues, sometimes causing permanent reduction of motion in the affected joint.

CAUSES

The immediate cause of bursitis is typically an injury to or sustained pressure on a joint, resulting in inflammation of the bursal sac. Professional and amateur athletes alike recognize bursitis in the form of the sore shoulder that comes from running, throwing, and jumping, or the exaggerated arm swings used in tennis, baseball, and bowling. Heavy lifting, repetitive motion, or working for extended periods in unusual positions can also bring on a bursitis attack.

TREATMENT

Although bursitis generally disappears in a few days or weeks, you must take measures to avoid further strain or injury.

CONVENTIONAL MEDICINE

Initial treatment typically consists of ***aspirin*** or over-the-counter ***nonsteroidal anti-inflammatory drugs (NSAIDs).*** These pain relievers also tend to reduce inflammation. Heat and ultrasound can help relax the joint and promote tissue repair.

Diathermy (deep-heat therapy), under the direction of a sports physician, licensed physical therapist, or trainer, not only can relieve the discomfort and inflammation of bursitis but also can soothe tense muscles, nerves, and tendons.

Bursitis may recur, particularly if you engage regularly in strenuous exercise or physical labor. In such cases your doctor may prescribe ***corticosteroid*** treatment, in the form of either oral medication, topical creams, or injections to the affected joints. In severe cases, it may be necessary to draw fluid from inflamed and swollen bursae with a hypodermic syringe to relieve the pressure. In persistent conditions, bursae can be surgically removed.

ALTERNATIVE CHOICES

Bursitis tends to heal itself with rest, but in the meantime the pain and inflammation can be relieved through a variety of remedies.

ACUPUNCTURE

Treatment by a trained acupuncturist can bring quick relief of bursitis pain.

BODY WORK

An injured or strained joint needs rest and immobilization for natural healing to occur. In the short term, **massage** of the affected area stimulates circulation and relaxes surrounding muscles. After the initial therapy, exercise—such as **yoga**—is a practical long-term method of loosening and strengthening affected joints.

CHIROPRACTIC

Following conventional methods of pain relief, a chiropractor can use mobilization techniques to restore a joint's active range of motion.

HERBAL THERAPIES

To increase blood circulation, reduce inflammation, and alleviate muscle tension, an herbalist might recommend 2 to 8 ml daily of a tincture of the following herbs, taken orally three times a day: 2 parts each of willow (*Salix* spp.) bark, cramp bark *(Viburnum opulus),* and celery *(Apium graveolens)* seed, along with 1 part prickly ash *(Zanthoxylum americanum).*

Mix equal parts ***lobelia*** *(Lobelia inflata)* and cramp bark to make a tincture that you can rub into your muscles as needed to ease the tension associated with bursitis pain.

HOMEOPATHY

After evaluating the nature of the bursitis pain, a homeopath may prescribe regimens of ***Belladonna, Bryonia,*** or ***Rhus toxicodendron.***

NUTRITION AND DIET

Vitamin C (ascorbic acid), ***vitamin A,*** and ***zinc*** are recommended for making tissue-building collagen and for repairing injured tendons and bursa tissue. Good dietary sources of vitamin C are citrus fruits and potatoes; cod-liver oil is a good source of vitamin A. In addition, ***vitamin E*** is considered effective in promoting the healing of damaged tissue. Follow the recommendations of a trained dietitian for amounts and duration when taking vitamin supplements. Another approach reported to be helpful in recurring cases of bursitis involves ***vitamin*** B_{12} injections, administered by a licensed healthcare practitioner.

PREVENTION

Warming up before strenuous exercise and cooling down afterward is the most effective way to avoid bursitis and other strains affecting the bones, muscles, and ligaments. ■

CANCER

SYMPTOMS

In its early stages cancer usually has no symptoms, but eventually a malignant tumor will grow large enough to be detected. As it continues to grow, it may press on nerves and produce pain, penetrate blood vessels and cause bleeding, or interfere with the function of a body organ or system. The following symptoms may signal the presence of some form of cancer:

- change in the size, color, shape, or thickness of a ***wart,*** mole, or mouth sore.
- a sore that resists healing.
- persistent ***cough,*** hoarseness, or ***sore throat.***
- thickening or lumps in the breasts, testicles, or elsewhere.
- a change in bowel or bladder habits.
- any unusual bleeding or discharge.
- chronic ***indigestion*** or difficulty swallowing.
- persistent ***headaches.***
- unexplained loss of weight or appetite.
- chronic pain in bones.
- persistent ***fatigue, nausea,*** or ***vomiting.***
- persistent low-grade ***fever,*** either constant or intermittent.
- repeated instances of ***infection.***

CALL YOUR DOCTOR IF:

- you develop symptoms that may signal cancer, are not clearly linked to another cause, and persist for more than two weeks. You should schedule a medical examination. If the cause of your symptoms is cancer, early diagnosis and treatment will offer a better chance of cure.

Throughout our lives, healthy cells in our bodies divide and replace themselves in a controlled fashion. Cancer starts when a cell is somehow altered so that it multiplies out of control. A tumor is a cluster of abnormal cells: Most cancers form tumors, but not all tumors are cancerous. Benign, or noncancerous, tumors—such as freckles and moles—stop growing, do not spread to other parts of the body, and do not create new tumors. Malignant, or cancerous, tumors crowd out healthy cells, interfere with body functions, and draw nutrients from body tissues. Cancers continue to grow and spread in a process called metastasis—eventually forming new tumors in other parts of the body.

The term "cancer" encompasses more than 100 diseases affecting nearly every part of the body, and all are potentially life-threatening. The four major types are **carcinoma, sarcoma, *lymphoma,*** and ***leukemia.*** **Carcinomas**—the most commonly diagnosed cancers—originate in the skin, lungs, breasts, pancreas, and other organs and glands. **Lymphomas** are cancers of the lymphatic system. **Leukemias** are cancers of the blood and do not form solid tumors. **Sarcomas** arise in bone, muscle, or cartilage, and are relatively rare. *(See entries for specific types of cancers.)*

Cancer has been recognized for thousands of years as a human ailment, yet only in the past century has medical science understood what cancer really is and how it progresses. Cancer specialists, called oncologists, have made remarkable advances in cancer diagnosis, prevention, and treatment. Today, more than half of all people diagnosed with cancer are cured. However, some forms of the disease remain frustratingly difficult to treat. For those people who cannot be cured, modern treatment can significantly improve quality of life and may extend survival.

CAUSES

The fundamental cause of all cancer is a change, or mutation, in the nucleus of a cell. For a healthy cell to turn malignant, its genetic code must be reprogrammed for constant, uncontrolled cell division. Substances that either start or promote

THE SEVEN WARNING SIGNS

To remember the seven early warning signs of cancer (as designated by the American Cancer Society), think of the word CAUTION:

C *hange in bowel or bladder habits*

A *sore that does not heal*

U *nusual bleeding or discharge*

T *hickening or lump in the breast or elsewhere*

I *ndigestion or difficulty swallowing*

O *bvious change in a wart or mole*

N *agging cough or hoarseness*

the process are called carcinogens, and there are many types. Scientists theorize that about 10 million of the 300 trillion cells in a human body die and are replaced every second. With such a high rate of cell activity, the potential for occasional malignant cell mutation is high. In a healthy person, special cells from the body's immune system can somehow recognize mutant cells and destroy them before they multiply. Nevertheless, some mutant cells may occasionally evade such detection and survive, causing cancer.

Because the causes of cancer are complicated, experts speak in terms of "risk factors." Any habit, trait, or use of a substance that increases the odds of getting cancer is a risk factor, and the risk for nearly all cancers increases with age. Inherited, or familial, predisposition is a risk factor, although its influence varies from case to case. Researchers continue to identify genes that, when flawed, strongly predispose a person to getting a particular type of cancer. Such genetic predisposition is considered an influential risk factor but by no means guarantees that the person will develop the cancer.

Environmental risk factors relate to where and how we live. Most common cancers are linked to one of three environmental risk factors: smoking, sunlight, and diet. Smoking is linked to cancer of the ***lung,*** head-and-neck area, ***bladder, kidney, stomach, cervix,*** and ***pancreas,*** as well as to some ***leukemias.*** Excessive exposure to sunlight is linked to ***skin cancer.*** Dietary factors are associated with some cancers of the gastrointestinal tract, and may be linked to others, such as cancer of the ***breast, prostate,*** and ***uterus.*** Eating habits suspected of promoting cancer include overconsumption of alcohol, fat, and foods that have been smoked, cured, pickled, or charred. Lack of dietary fiber or antioxidant vitamins and minerals is also believed to be a risk factor.

Many substances in the environment have been identified as carcinogens, but in most cases a very high level of exposure is needed to cause cancer. Environmental carcinogens include various chemicals, gases, and other substances found in air, water, foods, pesticides, tobacco smoke, cleaning products, paints, and many industrial settings; excessive ionizing radiation—the type in x-rays, nuclear radiation, and radioactive waste; and certain viruses, such as the HIV, hepatitis B, papilloma, and Epstein-Barr viruses. Although ***stress*** and certain personality types have been suggested as cancer risk factors, there is no hard scientific evidence to confirm such ideas.

All these factors may contribute to cancer causation, yet cancer is not caused by any single factor. Cancer results from a "multifactor hit" of age, inherited predisposition, general health, and carcinogenic exposure. For example, some people exposed to particular carcinogens will develop cancer, while others, exposed just as intensely to the same carcinogens, will not. And as far as we know, most people who get a particular form of cancer are not strongly predisposed genetically to the specific disease. Thus, everyone's cancer risk profile is complex and unique.

DIAGNOSTIC AND TEST PROCEDURES

The earlier cancer is diagnosed and treated, the better the chance of its being cured. Some types of cancer—such as those of the skin, breast, mouth, testicles, prostate, and rectum—may be detected by routine self-examination or other screening measures before the symptoms become serious. Most cases of cancer are detected and diagnosed after a tumor can be felt or when other symptoms develop. In a few cases cancer is diagnosed incidentally as a result of diagnosis or treatment for other medical conditions.

Diagnosis begins with a thorough physical examination and a complete medical history. Lab studies of blood, urine, and stool can detect abnormalities that may indicate cancer. When a tumor is suspected, imaging tests such as x-rays, computed tomography (CT), magnetic resonance imaging (MRI), ultrasound, and fiberoptic scope examinations help doctors determine its location and size. To confirm the cancer diagnosis, a biopsy is performed: A tissue sample is surgically removed from the suspected malignancy and studied under a microscope to check for cancer cells.

If the diagnosis is positive (meaning cancer is present), other tests are performed to provide specific information about the cancer; this essential follow-up phase of diagnosis is called staging. The most important thing doctors need to know is whether cancer has spread from one area of the body to another. If your initial diagnosis is made by a primary care physician, or if symptoms persist even though you are told that you do not have cancer, seek a second opinion. In any event, before the actual treatment begins, it is extremely important that you get a confirming opinion by a doctor who specializes in cancer treatment.

TREATMENT

A comprehensive cancer program combines both curative and supportive treatment. Curative treatment attempts to terminate or slow the disease with some combination of surgery, radiation therapy, chemotherapy, and possibly hormone therapy or immunotherapy. When cancer is no longer detected, a patient is said to be in remission. Generally, patients who remain cancer free for five or more years are considered cured. Some cancers cannot be cured, but all can be treated, and in most cases the patient will improve.

Supportive treatment by nurses and other professionals accompanies cancer treatment. The goal is to relieve pain and other symptoms; maintain general health; and provide emotional, psychological, and logistical support to patients and their families. Similar supportive treatment is available to rehabilitate patients after curative treatment. Supportive therapy such as hospice care for cancer patients nearing the end of their lives provides relief from pain and other irreversible symptoms. Most mainstream care is geared toward providing supportive treatment through the broad resources of a cancer treatment center. The best complementary cancer therapies, which are generally provided outside a hospital, also provide excellent supportive care.

CONVENTIONAL MEDICINE

Goals of treatment vary according to how advanced a cancer is at diagnosis and whether it is considered curable. If cure seems likely, the patient is treated aggressively in the hope of long-term remission and cure. Cancer not considered curable can still be treated in an effort to prolong life and help make the patient comfortable.

The three standard cancer treatments are **surgery, radiation,** and **chemotherapy.** Each is designed to remove or kill the malignant cells and can be used either to effect a cure or to relieve severe symptoms. Surgery and radiation destroy cancer cells locally, while chemotherapy uses drugs to kill cancer cells that spread through the body. Surgery can treat localized tumors successfully but only rarely cures metastatic cancer. Radiation and chemotherapy are used mainly to reduce tumor size before surgery, as well as to minimize the chance of recurrence after surgery and to treat metastatic cancer.

Because chemotherapy and radiation can affect healthy as well as diseased cells, they typically cause side effects. With chemotherapy, side effects may include nausea, vomiting, fatigue, temporary hair loss, mouth sores or dryness, difficulty swallowing, diarrhea, and increased vulnerability to infection. Radiation may have some of the same effects, depending on the area of the body that is irradiated. Medication and other complementary therapy can help curb side effects during treatment, and most side effects disappear when the treatment is concluded.

WARNING!

BEWARE OF CANCER QUACKERY

Sadly, the sale of bogus cancer treatments to vulnerable people is a multi-billion-dollar-a-year business. To protect yourself from cancer quackery, be an educated consumer. Research unproven therapies critically, skeptically, and thoroughly. Do not accept anecdotes and testimonials in place of scientific proof. Interview critics as well as supporters. Ask the following questions when assessing a treatment—and get satisfactory answers:

- **Has it been objectively shown in peer-reviewed scientific literature to be safe and effective?**
- **Does its potential for benefit outweigh its potential for harm?**
- **Is it logical and understandable? If it relies on a secret formula or technique, avoid it.**
- **Does the practitioner claim that the treatment is experimental, yet still ask you to pay for it? If so, it's probably a scam.**
- **Does the practitioner have legitimate degrees and licenses from accredited institutions?**
- **Does the practitioner claim to be a victim of a conspiracy by the mainstream medical community? If so, look into such charges further rather than accept them as adequate explanations for lack of proof or endorsement.**
- **Do you have any doubts? If so, resolve them before you spend any money or begin treatment.**

Hormone therapy is standard treatment for some types of cancer that grow faster in the presence of particular hormones—for example, cancer of the breast, prostate, or uterus. By blocking either the production or the action of the hormones, this therapy slows tumor growth and may extend survival for several months or even years.

Although still largely experimental, **immunotherapy** is emerging as another mode of cancer treatment, with the goal of destroying cancer cells without affecting healthy cells. It does not attack cancer cells directly but employs various techniques to manipulate the body's immune system into fighting cancer more aggressively. **Gene therapy**—a promising subcategory of immunotherapy—manipulates genetic material inside either cancerous cells or the immune cells intended to attack them, in order to make the cancer cells easier targets. Immunotherapy and other experimental treatments generally are reserved for patients with metastatic or recurrent disease who do not respond well to standard treatment.

Patients who have practiced good nutrition tend to respond better to treatment, with fewer side effects. Because weight loss and malnutrition may become problems for cancer patients, clinical nutrition programs are fundamental parts of mainstream care. Most hospitals also offer support groups or individual counseling to help patients deal with mental and emotional difficulties.

As cancer advances, pain may become a significant problem. Fortunately, moderate to severe cancer pain can be managed effectively with prescription medication, such as ***codeine*** and morphine. Addiction does not occur with drugs given for advanced care, and research shows that people with reduced pain respond better to treatment and enjoy better quality of life.

COMPLEMENTARY THERAPIES

Alternative and unconventional treatments for cancer are numerous and varied. While some legitimate therapies offer real support, many questionable therapies have no benefits, may be dangerous, and may harm patients by delaying appropriate care. Even the most promising unconventional therapies do not cure cancer and should never replace standard treatment. Instead, supportive therapies should complement conventional care.

Appropriate complementary therapies improve quality of life and may relieve physical and emotional stress. The act of seeking complementary therapy is beneficial in its own right: It gives patients a sense of control over their illness and the opportunity to play a role in their own care. Before trying any complementary cancer therapy, research it thoroughly to make sure it is potentially beneficial and absolutely safe. Then check with your doctor to be sure it will not compromise standard treatment.

ACUPUNCTURE

Acupuncture has proved to relieve pain associated with many major illnesses. Although scientific study has not fully documented its effectiveness in treating cancer pain and side effects such as nausea and vomiting, it is a safe therapy that many cancer patients find beneficial.

BODY WORK

By promoting relaxation, body-work therapies such as **massage, qigong,** and **reflexology** ease muscle tension and may alleviate other symptoms such as nausea and chronic pain. Because many body-work therapies provide comforting physical contact, they can lessen the anxiety, depression, and isolation that cancer patients often feel.

CHINESE HERBS

Some cancer sufferers report relief from pain, nausea, and vomiting using traditional Chinese medicine. Most practitioners recommend herbal remedies not to cure cancer but to relieve side effects of conventional treatment. Researchers are studying plants used in traditional Chinese medicine to identify constituents that may combat cancer cells directly or stimulate the immune system to do so, among them ***astragalus*** *(Astragalus membranaceus),* ***dong quai*** *(Angelica sinensis),* and ***Asian ginseng*** *(Panax ginseng).*

EXERCISE

Exercise can help control fatigue, muscle tension, and anxiety. Patients tend to feel better if they do exercises such as walking or swimming, which calm the mind as well as strengthen the body.

HERBAL THERAPIES

Thousands of herbs are used by folk healers worldwide to treat cancer, but no herbal remedy cures cancer, despite claims to the contrary. Some nontoxic herbs can be used to relieve symptoms and support general health, but because some herbs contain toxic ingredients, check with your doctor before taking any herb to relieve cancer symptoms.

HOMEOPATHY

Homeopathic remedies do not treat cancer directly, but some can alleviate side effects of radiation and chemotherapy. Consult a professional homeopath for safe and appropriate remedies.

MIND/BODY MEDICINE

Some mind/body therapies work to improve quality of life through behavior modification; others encourage expression of emotions. Behavior therapies such as **guided imagery,** progressive muscle **relaxation, hypnotherapy,** and **biofeedback** are used to alleviate pain, nausea, vomiting, and the anxiety that may occur in anticipation of or after cancer treatment. Individual or group counseling and art or music therapy let patients confront problems and emotions caused by cancer and receive support from fellow patients. Patients who pursue these types of therapies tend to feel less lonely, less anxious about death, and more optimistic about recovery.

NUTRITION AND DIET

Scientific evidence suggests that nutrition can play a role in cancer prevention. But no diet has been shown to slow or reverse cancer—and no diet cures cancer. Vitamins, minerals, and other nutrients may inhibit cancer by neutralizing carcinogens, ensuring proper immune function, or preventing tissue and cell damage. Researchers are particularly interested in antioxidants—***vitamins A*** (particularly beta carotene), ***C,*** and ***E,*** and ***selenium***—but are also studying ***folic acid, vitamin*** $\boldsymbol{B_6}$***, magnesium, zinc,*** and coenzyme Q10, among others.

Because too much of some vitamins can be harmful, many experts are cautious about dietary supplements. Instead, they advise a varied diet that includes lots of fresh fruits, vegetables, and whole grains; avoids processed, smoked, cured, fried, or barbecued foods; emphasizes lean cuts of meat and low-fat seafood; and minimizes sugar, fats, and alcohol.

Many customized diets for cancer emphasize vegetarianism, and patients who follow a nutritionally sound vegetarian diet tend to feel better. Unfortunately, many anticancer diets also promote fasting, purging, and taking supplemental "immune-boosting" vitamins, minerals, and other concoctions that do not treat cancer and may be both harmful and expensive. As a rule, patients should avoid any diet that claims to cure cancer, advocates abandoning standard treatment, causes severe weight loss or weakness, requires severe food restriction, or costs a lot of money.

CONTROVERSIAL CANCER TREATMENTS

The search for new cancer treatments is a vigorous and highly controversial branch of medical research. All treatments must be thoroughly tested and proved effective before they are authorized for general use. Supporters of some experimental treatments claim remarkable recoveries; critics insist that objective trials, not anecdotal claims, are the only true measure of their worth.

The following treatments have their share of advocates but have thus far been deemed ineffective or unproven in independent tests and clinical trials: hydrazine sulfate, studied by Dr. Joseph Gold as a cancer therapy since the 1970s; Dr. Stanislaw Burzynski's treatment with antineoplastons, originally synthesized from human urine; the "immuno-augmentative therapy" of the late Dr. Lawrence Burton; Dr. Emanuel Revici's "biologically guided chemotherapy"; Dr. Gaston Naessens's "714X" therapy; and shark cartilage supplements.

AT-HOME CARE

Relieving side effects of treatment:

- After radiation therapy, be gentle to your skin. Do not scrub it, expose it to sunlight, or wear tight clothing. Aloe vera ointment is gentle and soothing, and you can ask your radiation oncologist about other nonirritating lotions.
- Eat light snacks throughout the day rather than three heavy meals. Also try eating food cold or at room temperature to avoid nausea.
- If your treatment involves lowering your white blood cell count, steer clear of sick people; tell your doctor about any fever or unusual symptoms.

Relieving pain:

- In addition to taking prescribed medication, try relaxation techniques such as **yoga, meditation,** or **massage** given by a friend or spouse.

Other tips:

- Join a cancer support group.
- Get plenty of rest.
- Rather than feeling compelled to maintain a "positive attitude," express your emotions honestly. Don't worry if you sometimes feel depressed or afraid: These are normal and legitimate reactions that will not make your cancer worse.
- Fill your days with activities you enjoy. Reading a good book, listening to music, and talking with friends are simple pleasures, but surprisingly therapeutic.
- Contact the American Cancer Society and the National Cancer Institute for free information about cancer prevention, diagnosis, treatment, and tips for managing cancer symptoms. *(See the **Appendix.**)*

PREVENTION

- Do not smoke or use chewing tobacco.
- Stay out of the sun. Use sunscreen outdoors to protect your skin from ultraviolet rays.
- Follow the diet tips under **Nutrition and Diet.**
- Drink alcohol only in moderation.
- Exercise regularly to keep your body active.
- Get regular screening for cancer as part of your annual physical checkup.
- If your work exposes you to known carcinogens, be sure to follow all safety guidelines.
- To limit exposure to carcinogenic chemicals at home, avoid aerosol cleaning products; clean up spills and wash hands after using cleaning products; wear gloves when using pesticides; and open doors and windows to allow fumes to escape when using chemicals, stains, or paints indoors. ■

CANKER SORES

SYMPTOMS

- small, painful, craterlike ulcers that appear singly or in clusters on the inside of the mouth, usually lasting 5 to 10 days. The sores are grayish white or pale yellow with red borders; they may occur on the inside of the cheeks and lips, on the tongue, at the base of the gums, or on the soft palate.
- tingling or burning in the mouth; this sensation often occurs 6 to 24 hours before sores appear.

CALL YOUR DOCTOR IF:

- your canker sores are extremely painful; your doctor can give you medication to alleviate pain.
- the sores last more than 14 days; this may indicate a more serious condition that needs treatment.
- you have persistent multiple mouth sores, which may indicate an underlying problem, such as a drug reaction or, in rare cases, ***oral cancer*** or ***leukemia.***

Canker sores, also known as aphthous ulcers, are annoying infections of the mouth that afflict up to 50 percent of Americans each year. They appear most commonly in adolescents, whose immune systems are not fully developed, and in women just before the onset of menstrual periods. In fact, women are twice as likely as men to get them. If your parents suffered from canker sores, you have a 90 percent chance of developing them. Often canker sores occur when you are under stress or run down.

Traumatic ulcers, which are caused by injuries, result in similar sores. These injuries are often caused by rough dentures, a slip of the toothbrush, or hot food.

CAUSES

No one knows what causes most canker sores, or why women are more likely to get them. Their appearance, however, often seems related to ***stress.*** Some doctors think that canker sores may result from deficiencies in ***iron, folic acid, vitamin*** B_{12}, or a combination. Canker sores may also be caused by an immune system defect, such as a food ***allergy.*** Canker sores are not thought to be contagious.

TREATMENT

Canker sores generally go away by themselves, and in most cases, you can safely ignore them. Over-the-counter remedies may help the healing process. Some alternative therapies reduce stress and soothe the inflamed area. If a sore is extremely painful or doesn't clear up, see your doctor.

CONVENTIONAL MEDICINE

Many physicians suggest the use of over-the-counter ointments to relieve the discomfort of a canker sore. Look for a medicine that contains glycerin, which protects the sore, and peroxide, which fights bacteria. If your sore does not respond to over-the-counter or at-home treatments, your doctor may prescribe a medication containing ***diphenhydramine*** to dry up the sore and lidocaine to relieve pain. If you have an infection, your doctor may treat it with an ***antibiotic*** such as ***tetracycline.*** If the sore is the result of another medical condition, such as a food sensitivity, the underlying condition should be diagnosed and treated.

ALTERNATIVE CHOICES

Alternative therapies are aimed both at healing sores and at preventing them from recurring.

ACUPRESSURE

To relieve stress, press Gall Bladder 21, the highest point of the shoulder muscle, midway between the outer tip of the shoulder and the spine. If you do this as soon as you notice a tingling in the mouth, before a sore develops, it may help reduce its severity. See the ***Appendix*** for more information on point location.

AROMATHERAPY

Aromatherapists recommend applying antiseptic oils of ***myrrh*** *(Commiphora molmol),* ***tea tree*** (*Melaleuca* spp.), and geranium *(Pelargonium odoratissimum).* You may also rinse your mouth four times a day with ½ cup water mixed with 1 drop each of the oils of geranium and ***lavender*** *(Lavandula officinalis).*

CHINESE HERBS

A practitioner of Chinese medicine may create an herbal formula to strengthen your entire system, heal sores, and prevent them from recurring.

HERBAL THERAPIES

To heal sores and prevent them from recurring, drink ***marsh mallow*** *(Althaea officinalis)* and ***slippery elm*** *(Ulmus fulva)* tea 3 times a day until the sores are healed. You may also apply compresses made from teas of ***calendula*** *(Calendula officinalis),* ***goldenseal*** *(Hydrastis canadensis),* or ***myrrh*** *(Commiphora molmol).*

MIND/BODY MEDICINE

Canker sores are often brought about by stress. Learn to **meditate,** listen to **guided-imagery** cassettes, and visualize yourself as a healthy, relaxed person. The most important thing is to find a relaxation technique you enjoy and will keep doing.

NUTRITION AND DIET

If you're prone to develop canker sores, avoid coffee, spices, citrus fruits, and other foods that may irritate your mouth.

If your sores are caused by a vitamin or mineral deficiency, supplements of ***vitamins C*** and ***B complex,*** as well as ***folic acid, iron,*** and ***zinc,*** may help. If you suffer from recurrent mouth ulcers caused by a food sensitivity, avoid the foods that set off the allergic reactions.

AT-HOME REMEDIES

- Rinse your mouth four times a day with a combination of 2 oz hydrogen peroxide, 2 oz water, and 1 tsp each of salt and baking soda. Do not swallow.
- Rinse your mouth with milk of magnesia to coat sores.
- Try mouthwashes that contain the pain-relieving medication ***chlorhexidine.***
- Cover the ulcer with a wet tea bag; the tannin will help dry up the sore.
- Use over-the-counter salves containing glycerin and peroxide.
- Try stress-relieving acupressure exercises.

PREVENTION

- Brush your teeth with disinfecting baking soda.
- Eat 4 tbsp live-culture yogurt a day; it contains bacteria that can keep your system healthy.
- Avoid foods that are spicy, salty, or acidic.
- Take vitamin and mineral supplements ***C, B complex, folic acid, iron,*** and ***zinc.*** ■

CARPAL TUNNEL SYNDROME

SYMPTOMS

- a tingling or numb feeling in the hand, usually just in the thumb and first three fingers.
- shooting pains in the wrist, forearm, and sometimes extending to the shoulder, neck, and chest, or foot.
- difficulty clenching the fist or grasping small objects.
- sometimes, dry skin and fingernail deterioration.

CALL YOUR DOCTOR IF:

- you feel pain in your wrist, hand, or fingers after a fall or other accident; you may have a broken bone.
- your hands or fingers feel painful and stiff, especially if the joints become swollen; you may be suffering from a form of ***arthritis.***
- the skin on your hands and fingers becomes white and then bright red, especially in cold weather; you may be in the early stages of ***Raynaud's syndrome.***
- pain in the hands and fingers is more intense at night; this may signal late-onset ***diabetes.***

Carpal tunnel syndrome (CTS) is one of several names for painful and disabling injuries to the thumb and fingers, and sometimes to the wrists, elbows, and other joints. Your doctor may call it **cumulative trauma disorder, occupational neuritis, repetitive stress injury (RSI),** or **overuse injury.** The warning signs are tingling and numbness in the affected joints—typically the fingers—especially after the regular workday, or when you're ready to go to sleep, or on wakening.

Left untreated, the symptoms progress to persistent pain and aching in other areas such as the hands and arms. CTS can eventually lead to the inability to grip things firmly and to use your hands in a normal way. If you experience similar tingling and numbness in your feet, ankles, and lower legs, the condition is called **tarsal tunnel syndrome.**

Many people think CTS came in with the computer keyboard. In fact, injuries to the carpal tunnel and other major nerve passages have been around a long time; but with so many fingers tapping away at computer keyboards, the problem is more widespread than ever. The same symptoms can develop from any repetitive manual activity.

CTS and other forms of RSI are most common in middle age and tend to affect women more than men, especially if the women are overweight, pregnant, or menopausal. Whether the causes are systemic or the result of repetitive stress, most injuries to the carpal and tarsal tunnels are easily prevented and entirely correctable if recognized early. The critical factor in injuries involving repetitive stress is for the patient to stop or change the activity that brings on the discomfort. Failure to do so can result in permanent, irreversible damage to the nerves and muscles in the hand, wrist, or other parts of the body.

CAUSES

Repetitive stress injuries can happen to anyone whose work calls for long periods of steady hand movement, from musicians to meat cutters. They tend to come with work that demands repeated grasping, turning, and twisting; they are especially likely if the work requires repeated twisting or involves repetitive vibration, as in hammering nails or operating a power tool. Stressful hand, arm, and neck positions—whether from working at a desk, long-distance driving, or waiting on tables—only aggravate the potential for damage.

A number of sports can bring on repetitive stress injuries: Rowing, golf, tennis, downhill skiing, archery, competitive shooting, and rock climbing are just a sampling of activities that stress the hand and wrist joints. Injuries and ailments that cause swelling or compression of soft tissue on nerves, such as ***sprains, leukemia,*** and rheumatoid ***arthritis,*** can lead to stress injuries. ***Diabetes, thyroid problems,*** and other systemic disorders are also associated with discomfort from stressed nerves, as is the fluid accumulation that sometimes accompanies pregnancy. Some authorities believe that a pyridoxine ***(vitamin*** B_6***)*** deficiency can also induce the symptoms.

DIAGNOSTIC AND TEST PROCEDURES

Your doctor will first check for swelling, inflammation, weakness, poor reflexes, and limited range of movement in the hand and arm. Numbness will affect the thumb, first two fingers, and inside of the ring finger; the little finger usually is not affected. The Tinel's sign test, which involves tapping the front of the wrist, will cause numbness in the forearm of an RSI sufferer.

The classic procedure for identifying RSI is the Phalen wrist flexion test—sometimes called the reverse prayer test: Holding the hands together back to back, with fingernails touching, induces tingling in a patient suffering from RSI. The doctor may want to confirm the condition by inducing pain or numbness with compression, using a blood-pressure cuff inflated above systolic pressure on the forearm. To check for potential abnormalities in the joint itself, a physician may call for an x-ray, magnetic resonance imaging (MRI), nerve-conducting velocity (NCV) studies, or an electromyograph (EMG).

TREATMENT

An instinctive reaction to numbness or tingling in the fingers is to drop the hands to the sides and shake the wrists and fingers. This natural response often provides immediate relief and—if the symptoms occur only occasionally—may be all that's needed. But if you continue doing the activity that brings on tingling and numbness, the symptoms will continue, and you can suffer permanent damage to the affected nerves. The following treatments, ranging from conservative to radical, can help prevent, counteract, or cure that damage.

CONVENTIONAL MEDICINE

You can expect your doctor to recommend rest, cool baths, or cold compresses, and to show you how to use a splint to keep your wrist from bending, especially while sleeping. You may need to wear the wrist splint for a week or two, but normally it does not keep you from using the hand. In some cases, however, the doctor may recommend that you stop typing or doing hand/finger work until the symptoms subside. You can also change your hand position on the job, use a wrist support in front of your computer keyboard, take frequent breaks to relieve stress, and do regular

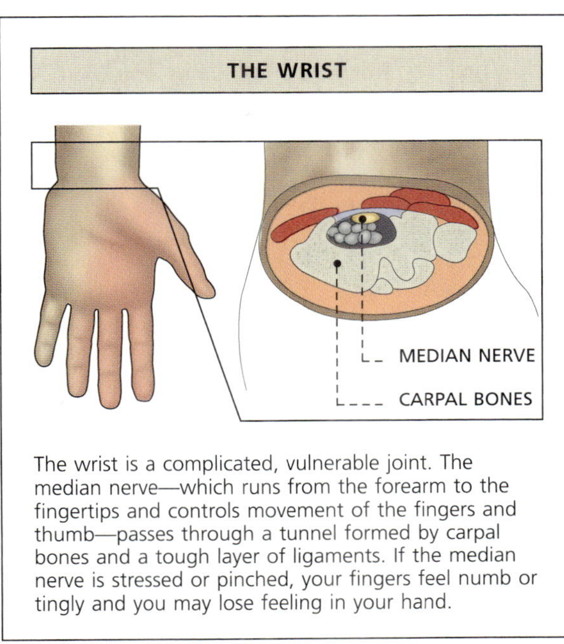

The wrist is a complicated, vulnerable joint. The median nerve—which runs from the forearm to the fingertips and controls movement of the fingers and thumb—passes through a tunnel formed by carpal bones and a tough layer of ligaments. If the median nerve is stressed or pinched, your fingers feel numb or tingly and you may lose feeling in your hand.

hand and arm exercises. The doctor may also recommend treatment for ***arthritis, obesity,*** or other associated disorders.

To relieve long-term pain, the doctor may prescribe ***aspirin*** or another ***nonsteroidal anti-inflammatory drug (NSAID)*** such as ***ibuprofen.*** Cortisone cream, or other externally applied analgesic preparations, can be helpful in relieving pain and counteracting the dry skin and cracked nails that sometimes accompany RSI. ***Corticosteroid*** injections can help reduce inflammation in severe cases. If the symptoms occur during pregnancy or are associated with obesity, you may be given a ***diuretic*** to get rid of excess fluid in the soft tissues.

To rebuild strength and normal movement, you may need physical therapy involving deep soft-tissue massage, stretching, and gentle range-of-motion exercises. To activate the body's own painkilling mechanisms, your doctor may recommend that you use a self-administered transcutaneous electric nerve stimulation (TENS) device, which sends low-intensity electrical pulses to the affected area.

If you have had persistent or intermittent symptoms of carpal tunnel syndrome for a year or more—or if you have a pinched or entrapped nerve—more aggressive medical intervention may be necessary. In some cases, your forearm and hand may have to be immobilized in a cast for several weeks. As a last resort, you may need surgery to relieve pressure on the nerve and remove any scar tissue. While the surgery is generally an outpatient procedure, recovery may take from several weeks to a month or more.

ALTERNATIVE CHOICES

Nonconventional treatments for carpal tunnel syndrome complement the need to reduce inflammation, rest the damaged wrist, and take the necessary steps to correct the habits or activities that caused the problem in the first place.

ACUPUNCTURE

Acupuncture may provide symptomatic pain relief by stimulating healthy circulation, calming nerves, and releasing the body's own painkilling agents. In addition to inserting needles around the sore wrist, an experienced acupuncturist may treat the back, shoulders, and neck. Chinese herb therapy is often recommended as a complement to acupuncture.

BODY WORK

A physical therapist may offer a combination of **massage, hydrotherapy,** low-level electrical stimulation, and ultrasound to help reduce inflammation and swelling. Massage combined with ultrasound stimulates blood circulation while relaxing muscles and reducing tension, not only in the affected area but in the entire body.

Exercises that strengthen the hand and wrist can be useful in preventing further stress injuries. If the injury was caused by repetitive stress, a few minutes of warmup exercises before beginning work and regular tension-relieving exercises throughout the workday can have a positive, preventive effect.

CHIROPRACTIC

Conventional chiropractic therapy adjusts the bones in your hand and wrist to restore normal nerve activity. A chiropractor may also advise ultrasound, massage, and nutritional therapy.

HERBAL THERAPY

Make a soothing compress by grating 1 to 2 oz of fresh ***ginger*** *(Zingiber officinale)* and making an infusion with half a cup of hot, but not boiling, water. Dip a soft, folded cloth into the infusion and apply the compress to the affected area, covering it with a dry cloth to retain the heat.

HOMEOPATHY

Over-the-counter homeopathic remedies may provide relief of carpal tunnel symptoms: ***Arnica*** (6x to 30c) for swelling and bruising caused by overuse or misuse of the joints; ***Ruta*** (12x or 30c) for tendon inflammation; and ***Rhus toxicodendron*** (12x or 30c) for pain. If these remedies do not relieve symptoms within a week, see a licensed homeopath for a more specific analysis and remedies appropriate to your condition.

NUTRITION AND DIET
Supplemental ***vitamin E*** in amounts up to 800 IU daily is reported to help improve circulation. ***Vitamin C*** supplements up to 1,000 mg may be beneficial in tissue restoration. ***Vitamin B_6***, or pyridoxine, is reported to help nerve inflammation and enhance blood circulation, and serves as a mild diuretic. Because high-protein diets inhibit the absorption of B_6, reduce your protein intake. Start with 50 mg a day, or try a ***vitamin B complex*** supplement; symptoms should ease within the month.

Cutting down on sugar and sweets in general may be helpful, since a diet high in refined sugar is thought to weaken the body's ability to combat inflammation.

OSTEOPATHY
Osteopathic physicians may recommend manipulation of the joint and surrounding soft tissue to improve circulation and nerve function, as well as appropriate drugs.

YOGA
If you are suffering from carpal tunnel syndrome or other stress-related problems, yoga positions that relax the neck and back may be advisable. The spider exercise *(see **Gallery of Yoga Positions**, page 1091)* may also be helpful. Avoid hand and neck stands, as well as positions that include arm twists, any of which could harm already sensitive nerves.

AT-HOME REMEDIES
A few simple exercises and a cold pack may be the most effective on-the-spot treatment for reducing the discomfort and numbness of a repetitive stress injury. For most of us, the quickest source of cold is a few ice cubes or a pack of frozen vegetables wrapped in a towel. Use the cold pack for about an hour at a time, 10 minutes on the affected area and 10 minutes off.

An effective exercise you can do anytime and anywhere is opening and closing your fist a dozen or more times. Other quick hand routines:

- With palms facing each other, press your fingertips together 20 times, rest, then repeat.
- Holding your hands over your head, rotate them at the wrists clockwise for 20 seconds, then do the same exercise counterclockwise.
- Strengthen hand and forearm muscles with a spring-style or foam-rubber grip exerciser.

For **tarsal tunnel syndrome,** some people find that walking barefoot whenever possible alleviates the discomfort and helps prevent recurrence.

PREVENTION
The natural position of the hand in most normal activities is straight or slightly bent at the wrist, with the thumb more or less in line with the forearm. Bending the hand forward or backward at the wrist for extended periods stresses the carpal nerves, so learn to keep your wrist and hand as straight as possible as you work.

If your job calls for repetitive hand or finger work, take breaks and exercise your hands and wrists every hour. If you work at an office keyboard, use a wrist support to help prevent unnatural bending and make sure your desk and chair height are correct for your stature.

Interior architects and designers now realize that the science of ergonomics—human engineering—is essential not just to make the home and workplace efficient, but to maintain the well-being of the inhabitants. Fortunately, ergonomically designed offices and factories are fast becoming the norm.

Finally, if carpal tunnel symptoms begin, don't work through the pain. Get a professional diagnosis and follow the recommendations. ■

CATARACTS

SYMPTOMS

Because everyone's eyesight changes later in life, and because cataract development is usually a gradual process, your first symptom may be having trouble passing the vision test when renewing your driver's license or having a regular eye exam. Physical symptoms include:

- hazy vision that might be worse in bright light.
- impaired vision at night; difficulty in discerning movements, details, or objects.
- blinding or uncomfortable glare from automobile headlights or bright sunlight.
- seeing halos around lights.
- unexpected improvement in near vision.
- double or triple vision in one eye only.
- a milky white or opaque appearance to the normally transparent lens of the eye (advanced case).
- painful inflammation and pressure within the eye (very advanced case).

CALL YOUR DOCTOR IF:

- you have any of the above symptoms or if your vision deteriorates or becomes distorted in any way. Cataracts are not visible to a casual observer until they are quite advanced, so it is essential that you see an ophthalmologist for evaluation.

The lens of the human eye focuses light so that you can see objects clearly at various distances. It must remain transparent for clear vision. The clouding of this lens is called a cataract. As the developing cataract blocks or distorts the light entering the eye, you will experience a gradual, persistent, painless blurring of vision, as though you were looking through a haze.

Cataracts are the leading cause of blindness, accounting for almost 20 million cases worldwide and at least 40,000 cases in the United States. Despite these numbers, the disease is actually one of the less serious eye disorders, because surgery can restore the lost sight in most cases. Yet in the U.S. alone, some 5,000 people go blind each year because of ignorance, fear, or refusal to undergo a relatively painless operation.

CAUSES

Cataracts are the result of changes in the chemical structure of proteins in the cells of the lens. The usually clear protein becomes cloudy, primarily as a result of the protein's aging over the course of a lifetime; about 75 percent of all cataracts arise from this natural aging. Called **senile cataracts,** they are most prevalent in people over the age of 70.

A variety of ordinary stresses can contribute to senile cataracts. One major factor is exposure to sunlight, particularly ultraviolet B (UVB) radiation, which reacts with the lens protein. Other risk factors, according to some specialists, are cigarette smoke, air pollution, vitamin deficiencies, and heavy alcohol consumption.

The most common type of senile cataract, and one with a surprising side effect, is known as **nuclear sclerosis,** in which the cataract develops in the nucleus (center) of the lens. During the early stages of cataract formation, the lens swells slightly, which increases its focusing power and improves near vision to such an extent that some people find they can suddenly read without eyeglasses. But the improvement doesn't last long; as clouding increases, vision deteriorates again.

Cataracts may also develop as a secondary effect of other eye ailments such as ***glaucoma*** or

THROUGH A LENS DARKLY

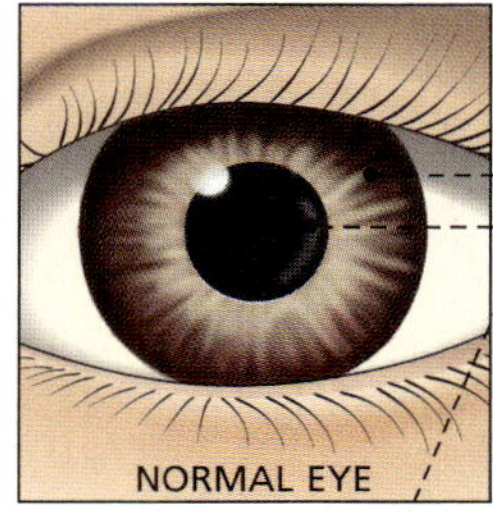

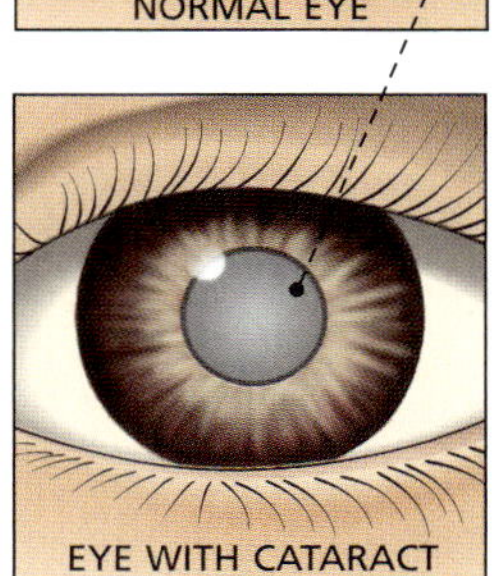

In a normal eye, the lens is clear and appears black in the center of the pupil *(top)*. As a person ages, natural changes in the lens fibers cause a clouding of the lens known as a cataract, which in severe cases appears opaque in the pupil *(bottom)*. Progressive clouding leads to blurred, dim, hazy vision. Fortunately, surgery can correct most cataracts and restore near-normal vision.

of systemic diseases such as ***diabetes*** mellitus. Other causes include physical injury to the lens, large amounts of radiation, chemical and drug toxicity, and hereditary disorders.

DIAGNOSTIC AND TEST PROCEDURES

By shining a penlight on your pupil, your doctor may detect the cataract. Using special instruments and techniques, your ophthalmologist will identify its precise character, location, and extent.

TREATMENT

At present the only corrective treatment for a developed cataract is surgery. However, both conventional and alternative therapies are seeking ways to prevent cataract formation.

CONVENTIONAL MEDICINE

Cataract surgery is one of the most successful of all operations. More than 500,000 cataract operations are performed each year in the United States, and approximately 95 percent of the patients report improved vision.

The operation, usually performed under local anesthesia on an outpatient basis, is safe, fast, and nearly painless. The clouded lens may be removed through a small incision made at the outer edge of the cornea or with an ultrasonic needle called a phacoemulsifier using a technique that reduces the size of the incision, making sutures unnecessary. The next step often is the implantation of a clear plastic replacement lens. In cases where lens removal is not followed by an artificial lens implant, strong or thick corrective eyeglasses or contact lenses are necessary.

Following surgery, you will usually wear a protective eye shield or glasses during the day and an eye shield at night. To prevent infection and reduce inflammation, your physician may recommend that you apply ***antibiotic*** and steroid ointments or drops to your eye.

Over time, 20 to 50 percent of patients experience a recurrence of visual clouding caused by a cellophane-thin membrane that sometimes develops behind the artificial lens implant. The membrane can be easily removed by laser.

PREVENTION

The single most important thing you can do to prevent cataract development is to avoid bright sunlight outdoors by wearing sunglasses that filter out UVB. Dark glasses that do not filter out UVB can actually increase your risk, because your pupils widen to adjust to the decreased light, thus exposing your eyes to more of the dangerous UVB radiation.

Some ophthalmologists think that antioxidants, which reduce free radicals (unstable chemical compounds) that can damage lens protein, offer protection against cataract development by lessening or retarding protein deterioration in the lens brought on by environmental factors. Naturopaths recommend a diet high in fruits and vegetables containing antioxidants such as beta carotene ***(vitamin A), selenium,*** and ***vitamins C*** and ***E,*** including citrus fruits, spinach, sweet potatoes, carrots, and broccoli. ■

CELIAC DISEASE

C

SYMPTOMS

- abdominal pain and swelling.
- flatulence and a bloated feeling.
- ***diarrhea.***
- pale, foul-smelling stools that may float in water, sometimes with yellow fat globules floating on the surface of water in the toilet.
- fatigue, loss of appetite, and eventual loss of weight.
- itchy, blistering skin on elbows and knees in people with dermatitis herpetiformis.
- in children, delayed growth and muscle weakness.
- in infants, signs of extreme gastrointestinal distress within a few weeks after starting to eat cereal.

CALL YOUR DOCTOR IF:

- you have celiac disease and you begin to have new abdominal pain, diarrhea, or weight loss; these could be early signs of intestinal ***cancer.***
- your infant does not appear to improve within a few days after cereal is eliminated from the diet.

Celiac disease—sometimes called celiac-sprue—is a sensitivity of the small intestine to gluten, a protein found in most cereal grains but not in corn and rice. The intolerance to gluten irritates the small intestine and leads to deterioration of the tiny fingerlike villi (essential for the absorption of food) on the mucous lining.

The term *celiac* simply refers to the abdominal cavity, but the disease can have complications beyond the stomach and intestines. Women with untreated celiac disease often fail to conceive and, if they do, tend to miscarry more frequently than the normal population. Even after treatment, conception may not occur for 18 months or more. The disease can cause ***impotence*** in men, who may take up to two years to regain full sexual potency after starting treatment.

Celiac disease often appears in infancy or early childhood but may occur at any age. It seems to have a strong genetic component and affects twice as many women as it does men, especially women of northern European ancestry. In Iceland, for example, where virtually the entire population is Scandinavian, 1 out of 300 infants has the disease, but it is relatively rare in the more varied population of the United States.

Most people with celiac disease accept a lifelong ban on baked goods, pasta, and other foods made from whole-grain or processed wheat flour. Celiac patients who fail to eliminate gluten from their diets are 10 to 15 percent more likely than the norm to develop ***cancer*** of the small intestine.

CAUSES

Sensitivity to gluten seems to be hereditary and frequently affects siblings, but its exact cause is unknown. Some research suggests it stems from a deficiency of an enzyme that digests gluten. Other research points to a defect in the immune system that causes certain cells to attack the intestinal mucous membrane when gluten is in the diet.

DIAGNOSTIC AND TEST PROCEDURES

To diagnose celiac disease, your doctor may first test your blood for antibodies that will be present if you are sensitive to gluten. The doctor may order a barium x-ray to detect abnormalities on the intestinal lining. A final diagnosis requires a biopsy so that a tiny sample of the intestinal lining can be examined under a microscope.

TREATMENT

Corrective treatment for celiac disease is almost entirely dietary, and in most cases the patient responds without the need for additional measures.

CONVENTIONAL MEDICINE

Primary treatment consists in changing your diet. Your doctor will direct you to eliminate foods that contain wheat, rye, barley, and oats. You can probably eat foods made with corn, rice, and millet, and with gluten-free wheat, which some patients tolerate well. A dietitian can identify products that contain gluten in unlikely forms such as soy sauce and modified food starch, which is added to a number of packaged foods. In families known to carry celiac disease, breast-feeding babies for at least four months and not giving them wheat products until they are a year old lower their chances of developing the disease.

Until the intestine is well on its way back to health, doctors frequently advise celiac patients to avoid fatty foods and dairy products, which are relatively difficult to digest. If you are constipated because you're not getting enough fiber on the gluten-free diet, your doctor may suggest you try a spoonful of rice bran mixed with juice or fruit. If you have lost weight and appear very ill, your doctor may prescribe steroids, such as ***prednisone,*** to help the intestine heal.

ALTERNATIVE CHOICES

The information that follows includes suggestions for relieving uncomfortable symptoms and complementing the gluten-free diet.

HERBAL THERAPIES

Slippery elm *(Ulmus fulva)* bark has long been used to soothe the bowels. Mix 2 tsp of the powder in a cup of warm water and drink promptly, four times a day. One tbsp of meadowsweet *(Filipendula ulmaria)* infused in a cup of warm water may soothe the bowels and reduce the likelihood of diarrhea.

NUTRITION AND DIET

You may need supplemental ***folic acid, vitamin A,*** and ***zinc*** to speed healing and maintain a healthy gastrointestinal tract. Papain, a protein-digesting enzyme, may help you digest any gluten that sneaks into your diet; take 500 to 1,000 mg daily with meals.

REFLEXOLOGY

For celiac-associated diarrhea, a reflexologist will massage areas on the bottoms of the feet associated with the ascending colon, transverse colon, diaphragm, liver, and adrenal glands. *(See page 25 for area locations.)*

YOGA

Many different yoga positions can help tone the intestinal tract, including abdominal massage *(see* ***Gallery of Yoga Positions,*** *page 1085),* knee down twist *(page 1088),* spinal *(page 1091),* and yoga mudra *(page 1093).*

AT-HOME REMEDIES

People rarely "grow out of" celiac disease. The key to controlling the illness is to stop eating foods made from or containing gluten, which means cutting out all wheat, rye, and barley, and usually oats. Some patients need dietary supplements to offset deficiencies in iron and folic acid caused by the disease. If the gluten-free regimen is strictly followed, people usually begin feeling better within days. Complete recovery may take several months, as the intestines regain their normal lining. Thereafter, most people can digest any food permitted in the gluten-free diet. ■

CERVICAL CANCER

SYMPTOMS

In its early stages, cervical cancer causes no pain or other symptoms. The first identifiable symptoms of the disease are likely to include:

- watery or bloody vaginal discharge, sometimes heavy and foul smelling.
- vaginal bleeding after intercourse, between menstrual periods, or after menopause; menstrual periods may be heavier and last longer than normal.

If the cancer has spread to nearby tissues, symptoms may include:

- difficult urination and possible kidney failure.
- painful urination, sometimes with blood in urine.
- dull backache or swelling in the legs.
- diarrhea, or pain or bleeding from the rectum upon defecation.
- fatigue, loss of weight and appetite, and general feeling of illness.

CALL YOUR DOCTOR IF:

- abnormal bleeding, vaginal discharge, or any other symptoms last more than two weeks without explanation. You should have a complete gynecological examination that includes a Pap smear.
- NOTE: Any vaginal bleeding after menopause should be brought to your doctor's attention right away. The cause may simply be vaginal dryness or a benign uterine polyp, but vaginal bleeding is the most common symptom of cervical and ***uterine cancer.*** *(See also **Cervical Problems**.)*

The cervix is the narrow neck of a woman's uterus, just above the vagina. More than 9 out of 10 cervical cancers originate in surface cells lining the cervix. In some women, healthy cells enter an abnormal phase called **dysplasia;** although these cells are not cancerous, they can become so. When dysplastic cells turn malignant, the first detectable stage is **carcinoma in situ.** As cancer cells multiply, some may invade the lining of the cervix itself, spread to nearby tissue, and enter the bloodstream or lymphatic system.

Just as it usually takes many years for **dysplasia** to become **carcinoma in situ,** it often takes months or even years for cervical cancer to become invasive. For this reason, and because of the Pap smear—a highly effective, widely available screening test—cervical cancer is one of the least threatening kinds. When caught early, it is curable; even in advanced cases, the chance of surviving at least five years, with likelihood of full cure, is still better than 60 percent. Only when the cancer spreads to distant organs does prognosis for five-year survival dip below 20 percent.

Dysplasia is most likely to occur in women between the ages of 25 and 35, **carcinoma in situ** between ages 30 and 40, and invasive cancer between ages 40 and 60. Cervical cancer constitutes about 2.5 percent of all cancers afflicting American women; each year some 55,000 cases of **carcinoma in situ** and about 15,000 cases of invasive cancer are diagnosed.

CAUSES

Four out of five cervical cancer cases are linked to sexually transmitted viral infections, such as ***genital herpes*** and a few of the 60 or so human papilloma viruses (HPV) that often cause ***genital warts.*** But many women who have a sexually transmitted viral infection do not develop cervical cancer, while others who get cancer have never had such infections. Women who began having sexual intercourse before age 18, have had multiple sex partners, have had several full-term pregnancies, or have a history of ***sexually transmitted disease*** are most likely to develop **dysplasia** or cervical cancer. Apparently genetic makeup and other factors are also part of the complex interactions that cause cervical cancer.

Cervical cancer is also more common among women who smoke. Many researchers doubt that smoking causes cervical cancer on its own but feel that it may heighten one's vulnerability to other illnesses, such as viral infections. Women whose immune system is severely suppressed by other diseases, by treatments, or by organ transplants are more vulnerable to cervical cancer, as are women whose mother took diethylstilbestrol (DES) while pregnant; DES is a drug once prescribed to prevent miscarriage but no longer marketed. Women who are obese or who use birth-control pills may be at slightly increased risk.

DIAGNOSTIC AND TEST PROCEDURES

Every woman should have an annual pelvic exam and Pap smear, which tests a cervical cell sample for abnormalities. Together these procedures detect cervical cancer 95 percent of the time, often long before the disease produces symptoms. If your Pap smear is abnormal, your doctor may prescribe antibiotics and test you again, since a minor infection can affect the results. If the second test is abnormal, your doctor will visually examine your cervix and take a tissue sample of any apparent abnormality for biopsy. If the biopsy confirms cancer, further tests will determine whether the disease has spread. These tests might include x-rays of the bladder, rectum, bowels, and abdominal cavity; blood and urine tests; and liver and kidney function studies. If you have ever had a sexually transmitted viral infection, your doctor will need to know what strain you were infected with to determine the most appropriate treatment for the cervical cancer.

TREATMENT

Most cases of cervical cancer are cured or controlled by a combination of surgery, chemotherapy, and radiation therapy. A variety of alternative therapies might prove useful in easing side effects and improving overall health. See ***Cancer*** for more information on therapies.

CONVENTIONAL MEDICINE

Women with ***genital warts*** and mild **dysplasia** should be carefully monitored for signs of cancer but usually require no immediate treatment. **Carcinoma in situ,** severe **dysplasia,** and mildly invasive cancers are normally treated surgically. Superficial tumors can be treated with radiation but are more often removed with a scalpel, a laser beam, controlled freezing, or cauterization.

If cancer has advanced deep into the cervix or spread to neighboring organs, hysterectomy—removal of the cervix, uterus, and possibly other organs—is imperative. If cancer spreads beyond the pelvic area, radiation therapy and perhaps chemotherapy may relieve symptoms and suppress the spread but rarely result in cure. Any woman who has had **dysplasia** or cervical cancer should see her doctor regularly for at least five years after treatment to check for recurrence.

COMPLEMENTARY THERAPIES

One promising field of cancer prevention research is **nutrition and diet.** Some evidence suggests that ***folic acid*** and beta carotene *(see **vitamin A**)* help ward off precancerous and cancerous conditions of the cervix. Patients undergoing radiation therapy may benefit from supplements of ***vitamin B_6.*** Ask your doctor about other dietary recommendations or nutritional supplements.

PREVENTION

- If you are a woman over age 18, or are under 18 and sexually active, have a pelvic exam and Pap smear yearly. If your Pap smear is normal several years in a row, your doctor may recommend the test less often.
- If you practice contraception, consider barrier or spermicidal contraceptives, which—according to one study—may lower the risk of cervical cancer compared with hormone-based contraceptives.
- If you have more than one sexual partner, be sure to use condoms to protect yourself from ***sexually transmitted diseases.*** ■

CERVICAL PROBLEMS

C

SYMPTOMS

- vaginal discharge that is green, gray, white, or yellow.
- pain during intercourse.
- vaginal bleeding, sometimes during or after intercourse.
- unusually heavy menstrual periods.
- crampy pelvic pain or a feeling of heaviness.

Many cervical problems have no symptoms.

CALL YOUR DOCTOR IF:

- you have a smelly or colored discharge; you may have an ***infection.***
- you have bleeding between your periods or after menopause; you may have an infection, hormone problem, **cervical polyps, cervical erosion, *cervical cancer,* uterine fibroids,** or ***uterine cancer*** *(see **Uterine Problems**).* You should seek a medical diagnosis as soon as possible.

The cervix is the knoblike lower portion of the uterus that connects the uterus to the vagina. At its center is a small opening, known as the cervical os, that provides an exit for uterine tissue and blood during menstruation and allows sperm to enter. On the uterine side of the os is the cervical canal, a narrow, inch-long passageway leading into the uterus. During childbirth the cervix thins and gradually opens, or dilates, to allow for the delivery of the child.

The part of the cervix that protrudes into the vagina is covered with pink tissue called squamous cell epithelium. The part that extends into the cervical canal is covered with red, mucus-producing tissue called columnar epithelium. The place where these two parts meet is known as the squamocolumnar junction.

Inflammations of the cervix, both acute and chronic, are known by the general term **cervicitis.** The main symptom of cervicitis is abundant vaginal discharge that is grayish, green, white, or yellow, depending on the type of infection. Other symptoms may include pain during intercourse. Some women with cervicitis experience backache or a feeling of pelvic heaviness caused by the drainage of the infection-fighting lymph nodes along the ligaments in the back that support the uterus.

Two other common conditions of the cervix are **cervical eversion** and **cervical erosion.** Cervical eversion occurs when the red columnar cells lining the inner cervical canal begin to form on the outer vaginal part of the cervix. This condition is common among teenagers and women who are pregnant or on birth-control pills. Cervical erosion occurs when the pink squamous cell tissue of the cervix has been worn away, leaving red exposed sores on its surface. Many women with cervical eversion or erosion have no symptoms, although occasionally the conditions may cause a whitish or slightly bloody vaginal discharge.

Other conditions involving the cervix include **cervical stenosis**—partial or total narrowing of the cervix, which can lead to obstruction—and **cervical incompetence,** the premature opening of the cervix during pregnancy, which creates a high risk of miscarriage.

Cysts and polyps can form on the cervix. **Cer-**

vical cysts** occur without symptoms and require no treatment. **Cervical polyps** are also usually harmless, although they may cause irregular bleeding and discharge. Because of these discomforts and because they sometimes affect fertility, cervical polyps are often removed surgically.

Genital warts can also infect the cervix, producing flat, benign lesions. These warts are caused by the human papilloma virus, and there are many subtypes, several of which are associated with an increased risk of ***cervical cancer.***

Another potentially serious cervical problem is **dysplasia,** the abnormal development of cervical cells. Dysplasia is considered a precancerous condition because, if untreated, it leads to cervical cancer in 30 to 50 percent of cases. Although cervical dysplasia strikes women of all ages, it most commonly afflicts women aged 25 to 35. Dysplasia produces no obvious symptoms. The only way to detect the condition is with a test known as a Pap smear *(see **Diagnostic and Test Procedures,** page 246).*

CERVICAL POLYPS

Cervical polyps are benign growths on the cervix, the lower portion of the uterus that connects to the vagina. Two common types of polyps are endocervical polyps *(above, left),* found within the cervix itself, and ectocervical polyps *(above, right),* found outside the mouth of the cervix. The polyps are usually harmless, but in some cases they may be removed in a minor surgical procedure.

CAUSES

The causes of cervical problems vary. **Cervicitis** is usually associated with other infections of the vaginal cavity caused by ***sexually transmitted diseases,*** such as ***genital herpes, chlamydia, trichomoniasis,*** and ***gonorrhea.*** In some instances lacerations or tears to the cervix during childbirth may also lead to an infection.

What causes **cervical eversion** and **erosion** is not always clear; however, about 20 percent of women are born with eversions, and the friction of intercourse appears to be a factor in erosions. Some doctors believe that the hormones in birth-control pills and the strings of intrauterine devices (IUDs) may cause cervical eversion and erosion, as well as cervicitis. It is estimated that 95 percent of women have an erosion on their cervix at some point during their lives, although often without any symptoms.

Cervical stenosis has a variety of causes. Some women are born with the blockage; others develop it as the result of infections or abnormal growths, such as **polyps** or **uterine fibroids** *(see **Uterine Problems**).* Surgical procedures involving the cervix, such as biopsies and curettage (or scraping) of the cervical canal, can also lead to blockages.

The cause of **cervical incompetence,** which can result in loss of a pregnancy, is unknown, although it has been associated with surgical procedures, such as therapeutic abortions and dilation and curettage (D and C). Abnormal development of the cervix can also lead to cervical incompetence. Women whose mothers took the synthetic estrogen hormone diethylstilbestrol (DES), which was once given in an effort to prevent miscarriage during pregnancy, are at greater risk for cervical and vaginal abnormalities.

A nabothian **cyst,** the most common type of cyst that forms on the cervix, occurs when a mucus gland on the cervix becomes obstructed. ***Endometriosis,*** the growth of endometrial tissue outside the uterine cavity, can also cause cysts, known as endometriomas, to form on the cervix.

Cervical polyps often develop after an infection as the body tries to heal itself by growing

C

new cells to cover the old, inflamed ones. Polyps also form during pregnancy and in women who take birth-control pills, as a result of hormonal changes that stimulate the overgrowth of tissue.

Cervical warts are caused by the human papilloma virus (HPV), which is transmitted by sexual contact.

Cervical dysplasia is caused by a subtype of the human papilloma virus, which also causes ***cervical cancer,*** but not everyone who is exposed to the virus develops dysplasia or cancer, indicating that other factors are also at work.

DIAGNOSTIC AND TEST PROCEDURES

The first test used to diagnose cervical problems is the Pap smear, a simple procedure in which cells are collected from the cervix with a brush or wooden spatula and examined under a microscope. If the Pap smear indicates a precancerous or cancerous condition, a cervical biopsy—removal of tissue from the cervix for examination—will also be done. The biopsy is performed with a colposcope, a special magnifying instrument. In cases where the area of abnormal tissue extends into the cervical canal, a procedure known as a conization, which removes a cone-shaped piece of tissue from the center of the cervix for analysis, may also be needed. Depending on the procedure, conizations are done in a hospital under a general anesthetic or in your gynecologist's office under a local anesthetic.

TREATMENT

Some harmless and symptomless cervical problems, such as erosion and nabothian cysts, often require no treatment. Other conditions can be treated with both alternative and conventional methods. For serious cervical problems, such as dysplasia or cancer, however, you should always seek conventional treatment.

CONVENTIONAL MEDICINE

Conventional medical treatments for cervical problems depend on the condition.

ACUPRESSURE

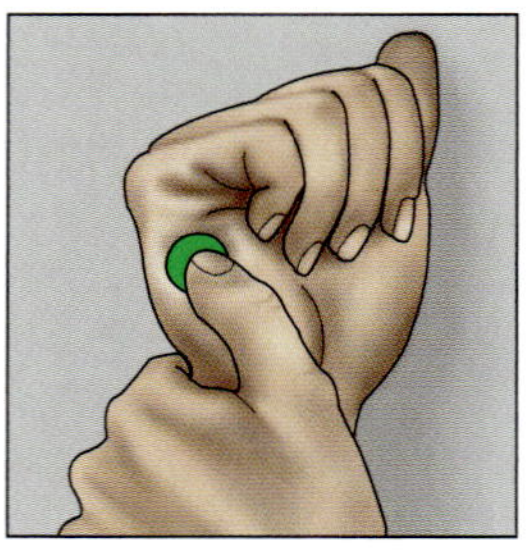

1 Pressing Small Intestine 3 may help provide relief from back stiffness that sometimes accompanies cervical problems. Place your thumb on the side of the hand, just below the knuckle of the little finger, between the bone and the muscle. Apply pressure for one minute.

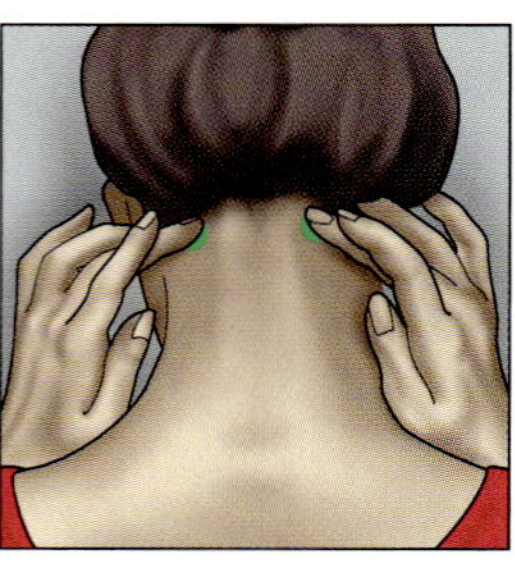

2 To reduce neck-muscle stress that may be associated with cervical problems, try pressing Gall Bladder 20. Place the tips of both middle fingers in the hollows at the base of your skull, about two inches apart, on either side of the spine. Press firmly for one minute.

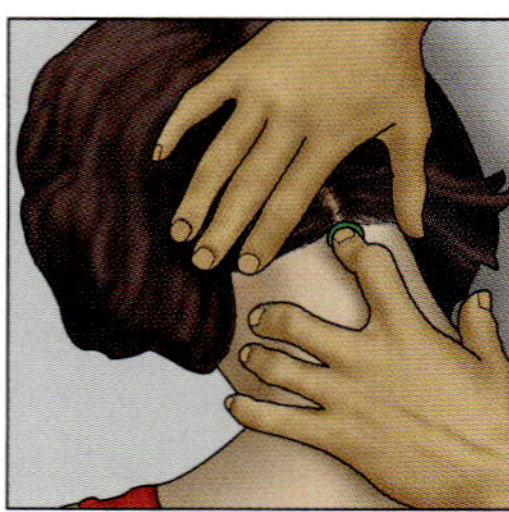

3 Applying pressure to Bladder 10 may provide relief from the stress and tension associated with cervical problems. Press on the ropy muscles a half inch below the base of the skull for one minute.

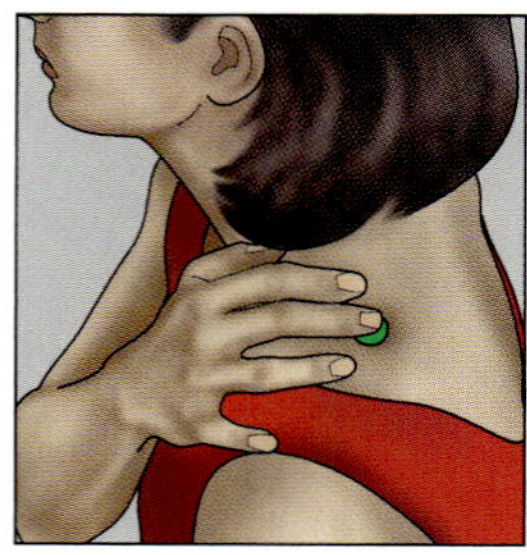

4 To relieve nervousness and irritability, try pressing Gall Bladder 21. For one minute, use your middle finger to press on the highest point of the shoulders, one or two inches out from the base of the neck. Pregnant women should press lightly on this point.

Cervicitis is usually treated with an ***antibiotic*** or sulfa drug. Your doctor will probably recommend that you refrain from intercourse until the infection has cleared up to keep it from spreading. In chronic cases of cervicitis antibiotics are not always effective. Your doctor may recommend that the infected tissue be destroyed by either electric cauterization or cryosurgery, which removes the tissue by freezing it with liquid nitrogen. These procedures, which cause only minor cramping and require no anesthetics, can usually be done in a doctor's office.

If necessary, **cervical cysts** and **polyps** can be removed surgically in your doctor's office under local anesthesia. Surgery to remove blockage caused by **cervical stenosis** is usually done in the hospital. If your cervix begins to close after the surgery, a follow-up procedure to keep it open may be necessary.

Pregnant women with **incompetent cervixes** used to be confined to their beds for their entire pregnancy. Today, the condition is more commonly treated with a procedure called cerclage, which involves stitching the cervix closed, usually during the 12th to 16th week of pregnancy. The stitches are removed in the ninth month of pregnancy. Most women who have the procedure are able to deliver their babies vaginally.

Mild cases of **cervical dysplasia** are treated with cauterization, cryosurgery, or laser surgery, which uses a high-energy beam of light to vaporize the affected tissue. In more advanced cases conization is used. Some doctors recommend a hysterectomy for women with severe cervical dysplasia; however, this is almost always unnecessary. If you have recurring dysplasia that fails to respond to treatment, you should be screened for HIV infection *(see* ***AIDS****)*.

ALTERNATIVE CHOICES

Alternative treatments may help to heal minor cervical problems.

HERBAL THERAPIES

Goldenseal *(Hydrastis canadensis)* douches are recommended for **cervicitis** and **cervical erosion.** Pour 1 cup of boiling water over 1 tbsp of the herb. Steep the liquid for 15 minutes, then strain and use warm. Pour into a douche container and use as directed on the container package. Repeat every day until symptoms are gone.

HYDROTHERAPY

To stimulate the flow of blood to the cervix and help **cervical erosions** heal, try taking alternating hot and cold sitz baths. Fill one bathtub or large bowl with hot water and another with cold water. Sit in the hot water for 3 minutes, followed by 1 minute in the cold water. Repeat three times, ending with the cold bath, then immediately dress in warm clothing. Take the sitz baths every other day until the cervical erosion heals.

AT-HOME REMEDIES

To help treat **cervical eversion,** douche with a vinegar-and-water solution. By changing the pH of the vagina, the douche may help stop the red columnar cells normally found in the uterus from forming on the vaginal side of the cervical os. To make the douche, mix 2 tbsp white vinegar in a quart of warm water. Use daily until symptoms are gone. To treat **cervical dysplasia,** take 5 mg of ***folic acid*** each day for 6 months.

PREVENTION

- Practice sexual abstinence or use condoms. Studies have shown that the more exposure to semen a woman has, the greater her risk of **dysplasia** and other cervical problems.
- Use barrier methods of birth control—condoms, diaphragms, or cervical caps—when having sex. Such methods offer some protection against ***sexually transmitted diseases,*** which can lead to cervical problems.
- To help prevent **cervicitis,** eat plenty of fresh vegetables and fruits. These foods are rich in ***vitamin C,*** beta carotene *(see* ***vitamin A****)*, ***folic acid,*** and other nutrients that strengthen the immune system and help fight off some infections.
- If you smoke, quit. Women who smoke have a greater incidence of dysplasia and cervical cancer.
- Women with **erosion** or inflammation of the cervix should be screened for conditions that may cause infertility. ■

CHEST PAIN

Read down this column to find your symptoms. Then read across.

SYMPTOMS	AILMENT/PROBLEM
◆ chest pain that may radiate to jaw, neck, left arm, or elsewhere; possibly, sweating, shortness of breath, nausea, vomiting, anxiety.	◆ ***Heart attack*** (damage to the heart muscle)
◆ sudden chest pain with shortness of breath; worsening of pain with deep breathing or cough, which may produce blood-streaked sputum; sweating; fainting.	◆ ***Blood clot*** in lung (pulmonary embolism)
◆ sudden chest pain with increasing shortness of breath; worsening of pain with breathing; possibly, recent chest injury.	◆ Collapsed lung (pneumothorax)
◆ severe chest pain beginning during exercise and subsiding after a short rest; possibly, radiation of pain to other areas.	◆ ***Angina***
◆ chest pain with shortness of breath or chest rattle; fever and coughing up of phlegm; worsening pain with deep breathing or cough.	◆ ***Pneumonia***
◆ pain and tenderness on one side of chest after recent severe cough, injury, or chest surgery.	◆ Injured muscle or rib
◆ pain and tightening in chest; possibly, frequent deep breaths; rapid heartbeat; tingling and numbness of lips, arms, or legs.	◆ ***Stress; anxiety; panic attack***
◆ burning pain, usually in lower chest, that worsens on reclining; acid or sour taste in mouth; pain relieved by belching or antacids.	◆ ***Heartburn*** (a gastrointestinal problem)

WHAT TO DO	OTHER INFO
◆ **Call 911 or your emergency number now.** *(See **Heart Attack.**)*	◆ Loosen clothing; try to stay calm. If someone with you has a heart attack and stops breathing, use CPR *(see **Emergencies/First Aid: Cardiac and Respiratory Arrest**).*
◆ **Call 911 or your emergency number now.** You will be treated to dissolve the blockage.	◆ Hospitalization is usually required for extensive diagnostic testing, including a lung scan.
◆ **Call 911 or your emergency number now.** You may require a chest tube to reinflate the lung.	◆ The cause may be injury, or the lung may collapse spontaneously for an unknown reason.
◆ **Call your doctor now** if you are not already under a doctor's care for ***angina.*** See also ***Heart Disease.***	◆ Stop smoking, decrease fat in the diet, and increase exercise, but avoid overexertion.
◆ Call your doctor, who will probably prescribe ***antibiotics*** (if the cause is bacterial), plus rest, fluids, and ***analgesics.***	◆ You must get a professional diagnosis and treatment plan for pneumonia.
◆ Rest; apply warm compresses. For pain, wrap chest with a pressure bandage and/or take ***analgesics.*** If pain persists, call your doctor to check the possibility of a broken rib.	◆ Chest wall movement tends to worsen chest pain caused by injury, but you must breathe deeply enough to keep lungs inflated.
◆ See the related entries.	◆ Persistent stress (which may also be associated with ***heart disease***) may be relieved by relaxation techniques.
◆ Try an ***antacid,*** or consult your doctor about taking other or stronger medication, or if additional symptoms occur. See ***Heartburn, Gas and Gas Pains, Hiatal Hernia, Indigestion.***	

CHICKENPOX

C

SYMPTOMS

- a very itchy rash that spreads from the torso to the neck, face, and limbs. The rash, lasting 7 to 10 days, progresses from red spots to fluid-filled blisters (vesicles) that drain and scab over. Vesicles may also appear in the mouth, around the eyes, or on the genitals, and can be very painful. See also the ***Visual Diagnostic Guide.***

CALL YOUR DOCTOR IF:

- you think your child has chickenpox; a doctor can confirm your diagnosis.
- chickenpox is accompanied by severe skin pain, and the rash produces a greenish discharge and looks inflamed—signs of a secondary bacterial skin infection.
- chickenpox is accompanied by a stiff neck, persistent sleepiness, or lethargy—symptoms of acute encephalitis, a serious illness. **Get medical help immediately.**
- your child is recovering from chickenpox and begins running a fever, vomiting, has convulsions, or is somnolent; these are signs of Reye's syndrome, a dangerous, potentially fatal disease that sometimes follows viral infections, particularly if ***aspirin*** has been used in treatment. **Get medical help immediately.**
- an adult family member gets chickenpox; in adults, the illness can lead to complications such as ***pneumonia.*** See your doctor without delay.
- you are pregnant, have never had chickenpox, and are exposed to the disease; your unborn child may be at risk for birth defects. See your doctor without delay.

Chickenpox, a viral illness characterized by a very itchy red rash, is one of the most common infectious diseases of childhood. It is usually mild in children, but adults run the risk of serious complications, such as bacterial ***pneumonia.***

People who have had chickenpox develop lifetime immunity. But the virus remains dormant in the body, and if you had chickenpox as a child, you may later develop ***shingles.*** Because chickenpox can pass from a pregnant woman to her unborn child, possibly causing birth defects, doctors often advise women considering pregnancy to confirm their immunity with a blood test.

CAUSES

Chickenpox is caused by the herpes zoster virus, also known as the varicella zoster virus. It is spread by droplets from a sneeze or cough, or by contact with the clothing, bed linens, or oozing

IDENTIFYING THE RASH

Small, red bumps appear on the chest and back and soon form a rash of itchy, fluid-filled blisters that burst and form scabs. Within days the rash spreads to the face, arms, and legs *(right).* Scabs will dry and drop off about a week after they appear, and the rash should be gone in two weeks. Avoid scratching the scabs; they may become infected and even leave scars if scratched.

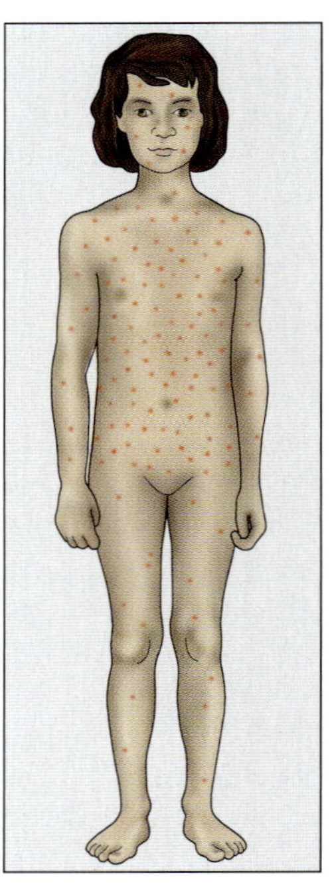

vesicles of an infected person. The incubation period is 7 to 21 days; the disease is most contagious a day before the rash appears and up to 7 days after, or until the rash forms scabs.

TREATMENT

Chickenpox is extremely contagious. Keep your child home until most of the vesicles are dry and scabs have fallen off.

CONVENTIONAL MEDICINE

Your pediatrician may prescribe an ***antihistamine,*** such as ***diphenhydramine,*** to relieve pain and swelling. ***Antibiotics*** are called for if a secondary bacterial skin infection arises or if an adult with chickenpox contracts bacterial ***pneumonia. Acyclovir,*** an ***antiviral drug,*** is sometimes prescribed in severe cases, although some doctors question its effectiveness.

ALTERNATIVE CHOICES

HERBAL THERAPIES

For itching, herbalists recommend the following wash: Add 1 oz each dried gumweed (*Grindelia* spp.) and ***calendula*** *(Calendula officinalis)* to 1 qt water. Bring to a boil, then simmer for five minutes. Strain, discard the herbs, and allow the wash to cool. Press a washcloth dampened in the solution to the child's skin after a bath. The wash can be reused for three days if refrigerated.

HOMEOPATHY

Consult a homeopath for appropriate remedies and dosages for children. To relieve itching, your practitioner may prescribe ***Rhus toxicodendron,*** especially if itching is worse at night. ***Sulphur*** may help when the vesicles are burning.

AT-HOME REMEDIES

- Trim your child's fingernails or cover her hands with socks or mittens to keep her from scratching, which could lead to infection as well as to possible scarring.
- To ease itching, add a handful of oatmeal or baking soda to bathwater; apply cool, wet towels to the skin and allow them to dry.
- Dab calamine or witch hazel on the lesions to relieve itching. Do not use lotions with ***diphenhydramine,*** which may sensitize your child to antihistamines.
- Leave your baby's diaper off as much as possible to allow the vesicles to dry out and scab.
- Dissolve ½ tsp salt in a glass of warm water and use as a gargle to ease mouth sores.

PREVENTION

A vaccine to prevent chickenpox received FDA approval in 1995, and many doctors now recommend that children be immunized, usually after the child is a year old, as a protection to vulnerable people such as pregnant women. Consult your pediatrician for advice.

PREGNANCY CONCERNS

If you have not had chickenpox and are exposed to the virus while pregnant, contact your doctor immediately. A varicella zoster immunoglobulin injection, given within 72 hours of exposure, may help lessen the severity of the disease. The virus can still pass to your unborn child through the umbilical cord, but possible complications such as fetal malformation or retarded growth may be less likely to occur. If you give birth while you have chickenpox, the baby should also receive immunoglobulin.

CAUTION!

Never give *aspirin*—even baby aspirin—or other products containing the salt called salicylate to a child who has chickenpox. Aspirin has been linked to Reye's syndrome, a rare but very dangerous illness that causes inflammation of the liver and brain. ■

CHLAMYDIA

SYMPTOMS

In men:

- a whitish yellow discharge from the penis.
- a frequent urge to urinate or a burning sensation while urinating.
- redness at the tip of the penis.

In women:

- no symptoms, or mild discomfort that you may mistake for vaginitis or menstrual cramps.

CALL YOUR DOCTOR IF:

- you develop any of the symptoms listed above; chlamydia requires immediate medical treatment to avoid serious complications that can lead to sterility in both men and women.
- you are a woman and you experience high fever and other flulike symptoms, such as chills, backache, weight loss, and diarrhea, along with severe pelvic pain, bleeding after intercourse, severe nausea, or recurring back pain; you may have developed ***pelvic inflammatory disease,*** a serious complication of chlamydia that can result in sterility.

Chlamydia, which strikes about three million to five million Americans a year, is the most common bacterial sexually transmitted disease in the United States. Epidemiologists believe it's twice as common as ***gonorrhea,*** 6 times as common as ***genital herpes,*** and 30 times as common as ***syphilis.***

The good news is that chlamydia is easily cured by ***antibiotics.*** The bad news is that 80 percent of women who contract the disease don't know they are infected until they develop serious complications such as ***pelvic inflammatory disease,*** which strikes 500,000 women a year and may result in sterility. Men with chlamydia may also develop epididymitis, an inflammation of the scrotal tubes that can cause sterility.

If you're a sexually active woman who is not in a monogamous relationship, ask your doctor to test you for chlamydia during your annual physical. This is especially important if you are pregnant or planning to have a baby. Chlamydia has been linked to ectopic pregnancy and premature birth. Each year in the United States 180,000 babies born to infected mothers suffer ***conjunctivitis***—an inflammation of membranes in the eye—or ***pneumonia.***

CAUSES

Chlamydia is caused by *Chlamydia trachomatis,* a microscopic organism that has the characteristics of both a virus and a bacterium. The disease is spread by vaginal or anal sex, and if you touch your eyes with a contaminated hand, you may also develop ***conjunctivitis.***

C A U T I O N !

If you're a woman who is pregnant or planning to have a baby, get tested for chlamydia, even if you have no symptoms. Infected infants can develop conjunctivitis, a serious eye disease that could result in blindness.

DIAGNOSTIC AND TEST PROCEDURES

If you suspect you have chlamydia, your doctor may want to test your cervical fluid or penile discharge with a special culture medium, examining the fluids microscopically with a substance that makes bacteria glow. The doctor may draw blood to check for antibodies to the disease.

TREATMENT

In uncomplicated cases of chlamydia, the cure rate is 95 percent. However, because most women don't know they have the disease until it has caused serious complications such as pelvic inflammatory disease, sexually active women should be tested for chlamydia once a year.

CONVENTIONAL MEDICINE

If you are diagnosed with chlamydia, your doctor will prescribe ***antibiotics*** such as ***tetracycline, doxycycline, erythromycin,*** or sulfa-based drugs such as ***sulfamethoxazole.*** If you have pelvic inflammatory disease, you'll need stronger doses of doxycycline, cefoxitin, or ***penicillin*** derivatives.

ALTERNATIVE CHOICES

Never attempt to treat chlamydia yourself. You must take the antibiotics your doctor prescribes. However, several alternative remedies may help to reduce symptoms and speed healing.

ACUPRESSURE

Doctors of Chinese medicine believe that sexually transmitted diseases result from the buildup of toxins. They may suggest that you manipulate the chi, or energy flow, of the liver meridian by massaging acupressure points Liver 3, on top of the foot between the big and second toes, and Liver 8, on the inside of the leg above the knee. You may also want to try kneading Kidney 3, on the inside of the leg between the anklebone and the Achilles tendon. *(See the* ***Appendix*** *for more information about point locations.)*

CHINESE HERBS

A doctor of Chinese medicine will prescribe a remedy that is uniquely suited to your symptoms and body chemistry. A typical prescription may include 10 to 20 herbs, such as ***Chinese foxglove root*** *(Rehmannia glutinosa)* and ***dong quai*** *(Angelica sinensis).*

HERBAL THERAPIES

Oregon grape *(Mahonia aguifolium)* root and ***goldenseal*** *(Hydrastis candensis),* which support the immune system, may be useful in treating genital infections. You may take capsules or tincture.

NUTRITION AND DIET

With any infectious genital disease, it's helpful to cleanse your system and boost its ability to fight off infection. In addition to taking antibiotics prescribed by your physician, you might consider fasting for one to three days. Be sure to ask your physician's advice before beginning a fast.

Juices that may help to rid your body of toxins by stimulating urine flow include pomegranate-cranberry and celery-parsley-cucumber. To increase your body's resistance to chlamydial infection, supplement your daily diet with ***vitamin E*** (200 IU) and ***zinc*** (15 mg).

To restore healthy intestinal flora after you have taken antibiotics, try eating yogurt with live *Lactobacillus acidophilus* cultures, or take ½ tsp *Lactobacillus acidophilus* powder, 1 tsp *Bifidobacterium* powder, and ½ tsp *Lactobacillus bulgaricus* in a glass of water, three times a day. The preparations are also available in capsules and tablets from health food stores.

PREVENTION

Use a condom to prevent transmission of chlamydia. Women whose partners have symptoms of chlamydia should be tested as well. ■

CHOLESTEROL PROBLEMS

SYMPTOMS

A high level of cholesterol in the blood does not have obvious symptoms but can be a risk factor for other conditions that do have recognizable symptoms, including ***angina, atherosclerosis, heart disease, high blood pressure, stroke,*** and other circulatory ailments.

- Soft, yellowish skin growths or lesions called xanthomas may indicate a genetic predisposition to the body's inability to process cholesterol and triglycerides normally.
- ***Obesity*** and ***diabetes*** may be associated with high cholesterol levels.
- In men, ***impotence*** may be due to arteries affected by excessive blood cholesterol.

CALL YOUR DOCTOR IF:

- you detect soft, yellowish skin growths on yourself or on your children. You should ask about being tested for a predisposition to high cholesterol.
- you develop symptoms of ***atherosclerosis, angina,*** or ***heart disease,*** such as pain in the lower legs, kidney failure, dizziness, unsteady gait, or thick speech. Any of these conditions may be associated with high blood cholesterol, and each requires medical intervention.

Cholesterol is a paradox: Everyone needs it, but for some people it's a potential killer. A naturally occurring fat, cholesterol contributes to such vital bodily functions as building new cells, insulating nerves, and producing hormones. The liver makes all the cholesterol the body normally needs, but because this waxy substance is found in all animal products, you ingest it whenever you eat meat and dairy foods. For people genetically predisposed to cholesterol problems, a diet high in saturated fats is the chief cause of high cholesterol levels.

In the bloodstream, cholesterol binds with protein molecules to form various types of so-called lipoproteins. High-density lipoprotein (HDL) is a dense, compact microparticle that transports excess cholesterol to the liver, where it is altered and expelled in the bile. Low-density lipoprotein (LDL) is a larger, less dense particle that tends to remain in the body. Very-low-density lipoproteins (VLDLs) are molecules that transport triglycerides—chemical compounds that store fatty acids, an essential source of energy for the body.

The amount of cholesterol in your bloodstream would not be of such significance were it not for its association with various cardiovascular diseases. The risk of developing these conditions is complex and depends on not only how much cholesterol but also what kind of cholesterol you have in your blood. Generally speaking, LDL—the so-called bad cholesterol—is associated with increased risk of dying from coronary ***heart disease;*** HDL—or "good cholesterol"—is associated with decreased risk. However, the risk of cardiovascular ailments posed by high LDL cholesterol varies widely from one person to the next.

Specifically, LDL cholesterol is the type that infiltrates arterial walls, initiating the inflammatory disease known as ***atherosclerosis;*** people with atherosclerosis are in turn vulnerable to ***heart disease, stroke,*** and other cardiovascular disorders. Even so, most people who have high cholesterol never actually get heart disease, and most heart attack victims do not suffer abnormally high cholesterol levels. Since no one can predict with certainty which people with high cholesterol will develop heart disease, play it safe and keep your cholesterol levels in check.

CAUSES

Having high cholesterol may be determined by the luck of the genetic draw. Some families are genetically blessed with low total cholesterol or high HDL-cholesterol levels regardless of diet or lifestyle. Other families suffer from various hereditary disorders that significantly increase the risk for high cholesterol; the most prevalent of these disorders are also associated with ***obesity*** and ***diabetes.*** People with such a genetic predisposition who eat a diet high in saturated fats are very likely to have high blood cholesterol.

On the positive side, vigorous exercisers, such as long-distance runners, tend to have high HDL-cholesterol levels. Before menopause, women tend to have higher HDL cholesterol than men their age. Because some researchers deduce that estrogen may raise HDL, or "good," cholesterol and VLDL while lowering LDL, doctors can weigh the potential benefits when considering hormone replacement therapy for postmenopausal women. *(See **Menopausal Problems**.)*

DIAGNOSTIC AND TEST PROCEDURES

A laboratory test to determine your blood cholesterol level is now a routine part of most physical checkups. When you have your blood tested you will typically get three readings expressed in milligrams per deciliter: one for total or serum cholesterol, one for HDL cholesterol, and one for triglycerides. Often, a reading for LDL cholesterol will also be included, as well as a figure for the ratio of total cholesterol to HDL cholesterol.

The first concern is your serum cholesterol level: Total cholesterol below 200 is considered normal and safe. Cholesterol levels between 200 and 240 are considered borderline, and a level of 240 or more is definitely high. HDL cholesterol for a man should be above 35, and for a woman it should be above 45. As for LDL cholesterol—the dangerous kind—ideally your level should be below 130; between 130 and 160 is borderline, and above 160 is high. Your triglyceride level should be below 200. Finally, for the ratio of total cholesterol to HDL cholesterol, the lower the number, the better. For men, 4.2 to 7.3 is average; for women, 3.9 to 5.7 is average. In general, then, any ratio reading below 4 (which means you have more HDL relative to your total cholesterol) is good.

TREATMENT

Advice from your doctor about cholesterol reduction is likely to echo that of nutritionists and most alternative practitioners: Adopt a diet low in fat and cholesterol, lose weight, exercise regularly, and if you smoke, quit.

CONVENTIONAL MEDICINE

For people in the high-normal to borderline serum-cholesterol range—about 40 percent of American men and an even higher percentage of American women—diet and lifestyle changes may reduce cholesterol levels or keep them in a desirable range. If your cholesterol level is close to or above 240, adjusting diet and lifestyle may not be enough. Instead, your doctor may prescribe either a natural cholesterol-reduction plan based on a high-fiber dietary supplement, such as bran or ***psyllium,*** or a synthetic ***cholesterol-reducing drug.***

Of the many cholesterol-reducing drugs available, members of the statin family—fluvastatin, ***lovastatin, simvastatin,*** and ***pravastatin***—are among the more widely prescribed. They operate by blocking an enzyme that the liver uses to manufacture cholesterol. They are tolerated well by most patients, although they are expensive and can sometimes produce unwanted side effects such as liver inflammation. For some people, ***niacin*** (vitamin B_3) is an alternative, but to be effective it must be taken in large doses. It is often a poorly tolerated drug and can cause such side effects as skin flushing and stomach irritation. Slow-release or timed-release niacin products may minimize side effects but must always be taken under a doctor's supervision.

C

A blood-cleansing procedure called LDL apheresis may help people with severe genetic cholesterol disorders. Over several hours, blood is removed from the body, chemically cleansed of LDL cholesterol, then returned to the body. Treatments every two to three weeks can reduce average LDL-cholesterol level by 50 to 80 percent but are costly in terms of both time and money.

ALTERNATIVE CHOICES

Alternative therapists offer a range of natural ways to control your cholesterol levels. All can be pursued independently, many in conjunction with drug therapy. The following list of treatments will let you customize your own program. To be safe, advise your doctor if you are using any alternative therapeutic substances or methods before mixing them with prescription drugs.

AYURVEDIC MEDICINE

Ayurvedic healers have traditionally employed Malabar tamarind, also known as Brindall berry, a yellowish fruit from India used extensively in curries, to treat ***obesity.*** Some studies suggest that the fruit may also help reduce total cholesterol and triglyceride levels.

CHINESE MEDICINE

Traditional Chinese healers treat various forms of chronic heart disease, along with factors like high cholesterol, with **acupuncture** and an herbal therapy that employs ***polygonum*** *(Polygonum multiflorum).* Because Chinese herbs almost always work in combinations rather than individually, you should consult a trained herbalist for an appropriate prescription.

HERBAL THERAPIES

A highly touted remedy for fighting high cholesterol is gugulipid *(Commiphora mukul),* an extract of the mukul myrrh tree of southern India. Gugulipid's ability to control cholesterol and triglyceride levels has been compared to that of some synthetic drugs, with claims that it lowers LDL- and raises HDL-cholesterol levels without side effects.

Other herbs reputed to have cholesterol-lowering properties include ***alfalfa*** *(Medicago sativa),* ***turmeric*** *(Curcuma longa),* ***Asian ginseng*** *(Panax ginseng),* and ***fenugreek*** *(Trigonella foenum-graecum).* You might also consult a nutritionally oriented doctor about the benefits of phytosterol tablets. Phytosterols are plant compounds structurally comparable to cholesterol that effectively block uptake of cholesterol in the liver.

YOGA

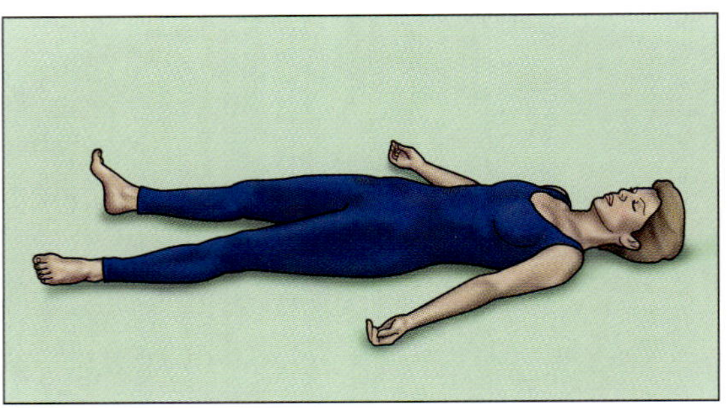

Try the **Corpse** position to promote relaxation. Lie on your back with your feet about 18 inches apart and turned out slightly. Place your hands about 6 inches from your hips, with your palms up. Close your eyes and breathe deeply for 8 to 10 minutes.

LIFESTYLE

Evidence suggests that even though exercise alone cannot lower total cholesterol, moderate exercise several times a week can help raise HDL-cholesterol levels in many people. Vigorous exercise may raise HDL levels even higher, although at some point athletes apparently reach an "HDL plateau."

MIND/BODY MEDICINE

Stress is believed to contribute to elevated cholesterol, so relaxation techniques that combat stress may help lower cholesterol levels. Progressive relaxation with **guided imagery** is something you can try anywhere, anytime. You might also try **massage** therapy, **yoga** *(above),* **meditation,** or **biofeedback.**

NUTRITION AND DIET

The basic dietary rules for lowering cholesterol

are simple: Avoid saturated fats and dietary cholesterol. Experts recommend a diet with not more than 30 percent of your daily calories from fat; some say 20 percent. Saturated fats derived from animal products and tropical oils should be kept to a minimum, so avoid eating red meat, pork, and deep-fried foods and pay attention to nutrition labels on packaged foods. Eat more vegetables, fruits, and grains, which are cholesterol free, virtually fat free, and rich in fiber.

Garlic *(Allium sativum)* and onion *(Allium cepa)* are believed to lower cholesterol, but reports vary on how much you should eat in order to benefit. It's safe to say that the more you eat, preferably raw, the better the effect. For other useful nutritional tips, see **Make Healthy Food Your Ally,** below.

PREVENTION

- Keep your weight in check.
- Eat wisely every day—no more than 300 mg of cholesterol and at the very most 30 percent of calories from fat.
- Exercise several times a week—vigorously if you can, but moderate exercise is better than none at all.
- If you smoke, quit.
- Practice relaxation techniques, **yoga,** and other stress reduction techniques on a daily basis.
- Track your progress. Have your blood cholesterol level tested periodically by your doctor or a reputable lab. At-home test kits, like many consumer health devices, are generally unreliable.

MAKE HEALTHY FOOD YOUR ALLY

People who have a genetic predisposition to cholesterol problems should follow their doctor's dietary recommendations. The rest of us should be able to keep cholesterol levels in check by a self-imposed goal of not more than 30 percent of daily calories from fat.

If you know your foods well, you can distinguish friend from foe. First, cut back on red meat, especially organ meat, because of its high saturated fat and cholesterol content. Eat poultry sparingly and avoid the skin; chicken has less saturated fat than red meat but still contains significant cholesterol. Most fish contains less fat and cholesterol than red meat. Most shellfish is also low in fat, and although it is high in cholesterol, for most people it is preferable to red meat and poultry. Whenever possible, go easy on whole dairy products, mayonnaise, chocolate, tropical oils, and hydrogenated or partially hydrogenated oils or fats such as margarine.

For cooking, replace saturated fats that are solid at room temperature, such as butter and shortening, with liquid monounsaturated fats such as olive, canola, or flax oil. There is evidence that consuming moderate amounts of monounsaturated fat—found in such foods as nuts, seeds, and avocados—may actually lower LDL cholesterol. Avoid tropical oils such as palm and coconut; they contain no cholesterol but are high in saturated fat. Eating grapes may help reduce blood cholesterol, thanks to flavonoid compounds in their skins. Look for grape-seed oil—squeezed from grape seeds after wine pressing—for cooking and for salad dressings.

Limit yourself to three eggs a week: One egg yolk contains almost an entire daily recommended allowance of cholesterol. Vitamins, minerals, and nutrients that have reputed cholesterol-reducing properties include ***vitamins E, C,*** and ***A*** (beta carotene), L-carnitine, pantethine, ***chromium, calcium, copper,*** and ***zinc.*** To keep your menus lively, try incorporating rice bran, artichokes, shiitake mushrooms, and chili peppers—all believed to help lower cholesterol.

Finally, select foods that contain water-soluble fiber, which offers an excellent defense against high blood cholesterol. Foods on the high-fiber list are grapefruit, apples, beans and other legumes, psyllium seed, barley, carrots, cabbage, and oatmeal. ■

CHRONIC FATIGUE SYNDROME

SYMPTOMS

- recent onset of debilitating fatigue.
- fatigue that is not a result of exertion and that is unrelieved by rest.
- persistent low-grade fever.
- muscle soreness and weakness.
- sleep disorders (***insomnia*** or oversleeping).
- swollen, tender lymph nodes.
- migrating joint pain without swelling or redness.
- forgetfulness, confusion, inability to concentrate.
- recurrent sore throat.
- headaches.
- long-lasting malaise following physical exertion.
- symptoms that persist for six months and result in a substantial reduction of activities.

CALL YOUR DOCTOR IF:

- you have overwhelming fatigue and no identifiable, obvious reason for it, such as ***stress.*** Your doctor will need to rule out other illnesses that share symptoms with chronic fatigue syndrome, such as ***depression, thyroid problems, mononucleosis, arthritis, lupus,*** and ***cancer.***

Chronic fatigue syndrome, or CFS—also known as chronic fatigue and immune dysfunction syndrome (CFIDS), chronic Epstein-Barr virus (CEBV), and myalgic encephalomyelitis (ME)—first came to public attention in the mid-1980s. It primarily strikes young urban professionals, with Caucasian women under the age of 45 accounting for 80 percent of cases; however, all segments of the population, including children, are susceptible.

CFS is characterized by overwhelming fatigue and other flulike symptoms, but it is not contagious. Typically, the onset is sudden and debilitating. The exhaustion felt by CFS sufferers doesn't result from overexertion and isn't alleviated by rest or medications; indeed, it tends to become worse over time.

CFS is not a progressive degenerative or fatal disease, although it may linger one or more years. The symptoms wax and wane and often become disabling before improving, but the vast majority of people do eventually recuperate.

CAUSES

The cause of CFS is not known, but researchers are investigating a variety of possibilities. For example, CFS may be an autoimmune disease that results from a combination of viruses, allergies, and hormonal imbalances. One theory holds that excessive reliance on ***antibiotics*** or long-term exposure to pesticides or chemical toxins may be at fault. *(See also* ***Environmental Poisoning.****)* Studies also suggest a dysfunction of the immune system. In addition, some scientists are studying enteroviruses such as polio; human herpes viruses; and the recently discovered retroviruses such as HIV, although there is no link between CFS and HIV or ***AIDS.*** Others see a link between CFS and chronic yeast infections *(see* ***Yeast Infections****)*.

Current theory holds that CFS may develop when an opportunistic virus or other agent invades the body at a time when the immune system is already suppressed. Factors that might contribute to this state include physical, emotional, or environmental stress, or a combination of the three.

Although many people, including some physicians, are skeptical and believe that CFS is psychological rather than physiological, research shows that CFS sufferers have disturbances in immunological functioning that make their bodies unable either to eradicate invading viruses or to prevent the reactivation of viruses previously dormant in their systems.

The Epstein-Barr virus, which causes ***mononucleosis,*** was once viewed as the cause of CFS but is now known to be an unrelated problem.

DIAGNOSTIC AND TEST PROCEDURES

Your doctor will take your medical history, perform a physical exam, and do a complete blood count to rule out other disorders that share symptoms with CFS, such as HIV, ***mononucleosis, multiple sclerosis,*** fibromyalgia (a disease causing muscle pain), ***Lyme disease,*** and ***depression.*** You may also be given an antinuclear antibody (ANA) test for ***arthritis, lupus,*** and other connective tissue diseases. Your thyroid function may be tested to check for an underactive thyroid. An erythrocyte sedimentation rate (ESR) test will show elevated readings if there is any inflammation in your body.

Once other possibilities have been ruled out, your doctor will apply specific guidelines set forth by the Centers for Disease Control and Prevention to determine whether you have CFS. Your symptoms must have been present for at least six months and must meet these guidelines for the diagnosis to be definitive.

TREATMENT

Given that the cause of CFS is unknown, treatment is restricted to relief of symptoms. A number of conventional and alternative therapies can help you weather the course of the disease.

CONVENTIONAL MEDICINE

An often recommended first step with chronic fatigue syndrome is to maintain general good health while avoiding situations that are physically or psychologically stressful, and to balance rest and nonvigorous exercise.

The flulike symptoms of CFS can be temporarily alleviated with a variety of medicines. Your doctor may prescribe a short course of ***nonsteroidal anti-inflammatory drugs (NSAIDs)*** or ***aspirin*** to counteract your low-grade fever, headaches, and joint or muscle soreness. Low doses of ***monoamine oxidase (MAO) inhibitors, fluoxetine,*** or ***tricyclic antidepressants*** have improved patients' quality of sleep and helped relieve both fatigue and muscle pain. Studies have shown varying degrees of success in treating other CFS symptoms with intravenous injections of gamma globulin, an age-old blood derivative product. And some doctors are attempting to modulate the immune system with ***histamine H_2 blockers*** (a subclass of ***antiulcer drugs***) such as ***cimetidine*** and ***ranitidine,*** although this form of treatment is still considered experimental.

Sensitivity to a chemical, pesticide, household cleaning product, or another potential environmental toxin may also be contributing to CFS. Try eliminating suspected items, then reintroducing them one by one, to pinpoint what may be causing your symptoms. If you discover that a special sensitivity is your problem, you also might want to consider asking your pharmacist to use preservative-free dilutions in preparing any medications you may be taking.

ALTERNATIVE CHOICES

A number of alternative therapies can help control the various symptoms of CFS. But be sure to check with your doctor for an accurate diagnosis before embarking on a course of treatment.

ACUPRESSURE

Applying gentle pressure to the gallbladder points may help relieve fatigue and depression while strengthening your immune system. See the ***Appendix*** for help in locating the points on your shoulders and neck known as Gall Bladder 20 and Gall Bladder 21. This sequence can be repeated one or more times a day or whenever CFS symptoms appear. Pregnant women should be careful to press Gall Bladder 21 lightly.

YOGA

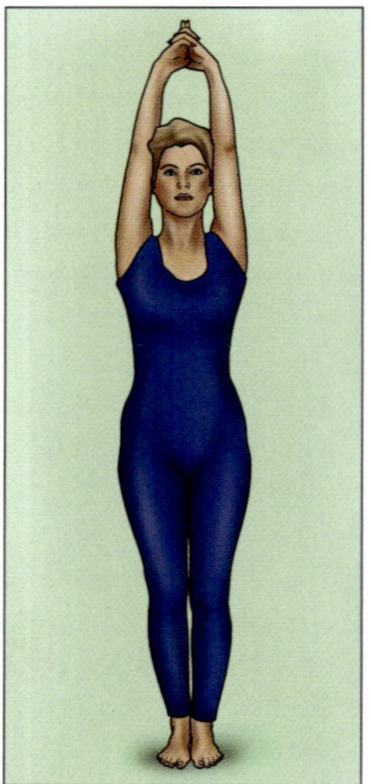

1 Stress-reducing exercises may help chronic fatigue. For the **Mountain,** stand with your feet together. Inhale and raise your arms straight out from your sides and join them over your head. Hold for 20 seconds while breathing deeply, then exhale and slowly lower your arms. Do once or twice a day.

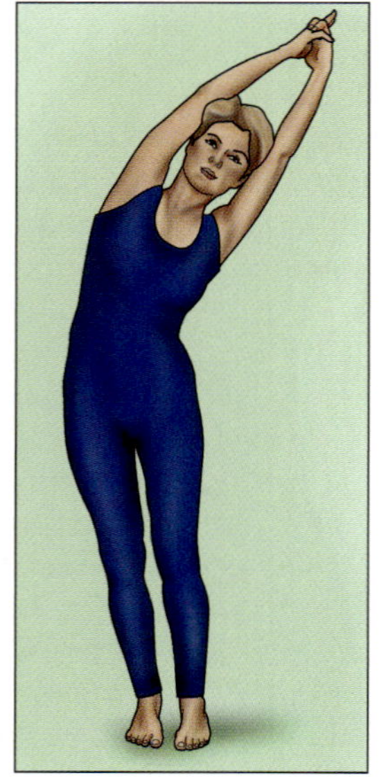

2 To do the **Half Moon,** inhale and clasp your hands over your head. Exhale and stretch to the right, pushing out your left hip. Breathe deeply, keeping your shoulders and hips on the same plane. Inhale and return to center. Repeat on the left side. Do once or twice a day.

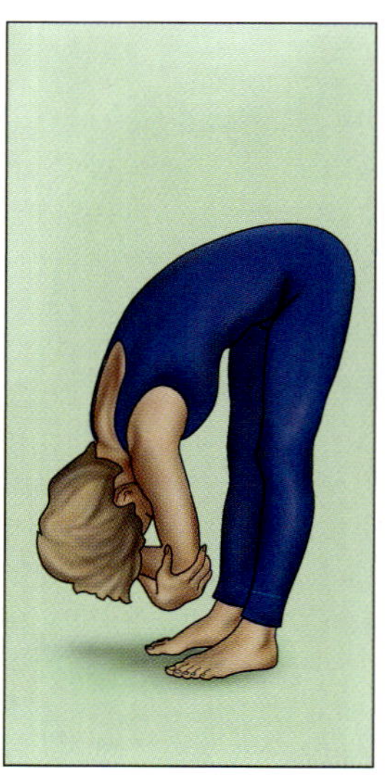

3 For the **Rag Doll,** stand with your arms at your sides, then exhale and bend forward from the waist. Let the top of your head drop toward the floor (do not force the stretch). Cup your elbows in your palms and relax, breathing deeply. Hold for 20 seconds, then inhale and slowly stand up. Do once or twice a day.

ACUPUNCTURE

An acupuncturist may undertake a series of treatments to attempt to normalize and balance the immune system. In Chinese medicine, enhancing vital energy, nourishing the blood, and strengthening the spirit can be part of therapeutic strategy.

CHINESE HERBS

A commercially prepared mixture called the Astragalus Ten Formula combines ***Asian ginseng*** *(Panax ginseng),* ***licorice*** *(Glycyrrhiza uralensis),* ***astragalus*** *(Astragalus membranaceus),* and other herbs in powder or tablet form. Anecdotal reports describe improvement among CFS patients after taking this formula regularly. Consult an herbalist specializing in Chinese medicine for the proper administration of this herbal remedy or for other suggested herbal formulas.

HERBAL THERAPIES

Shiitake *(Lentinus edodes)* mushrooms contain oligosaccharides, known to be extremely potent immune stimulators; take in moderate doses only, as advised by a qualified herbalist. ***Licorice*** *(Glycyrrhiza glabra)* is said to have antiviral properties. Silymarin, a component of ***milk thistle*** *(Silybum marianum),* may help with the liver problems that sometimes affect people with CFS. ***Astragalus*** *(Astragalus membranaceus),* ***ashwaganda*** *(Withania somnifera),* ***Siberian ginseng*** *(Eleutherococcus senticosus),* ***burdock*** *(Arctium lappa),* and ***Asian ginseng*** *(Panax ginseng)* are all said to stimulate immune activity and may be beneficial to CFS sufferers if taken regularly. ***Gotu kola*** *(Centelle asiatica)* may slowly but surely increase your energy levels. Consult a qualified herbalist for more specific guidelines.

HOMEOPATHY

Some homeopathic practitioners have reported success in treating the symptoms of CFS. As with all chronic ailments, it's best to seek the advice of a homeopathic physician or specialist who can accurately diagnose and treat the specific symptoms of your particular case.

C

MIND/BODY MEDICINE

Meditation, progressive **relaxation, guided imagery, qigong,** and **yoga** are techniques that may help alleviate CFS symptoms without being tiring. In fact, they may provide you with additional energy because they reduce stress.

NUTRITION AND DIET

One theory holds that a nutritional deficiency may be a contributing factor causing CFS, so it's important to maintain a healthful diet. Avoid caffeine, decaffeinated coffee, alcohol, refined sugar, white flour, salt, and fried, preserved, high-fat foods in favor of whole grains, beans, rice, fish, and fresh fruits and vegetables. Add edible seaweeds, ***shiitake*** *(Lentinus edodes)* mushrooms, and ***licorice*** *(Glycyrrhiza glabra)* to your diet. Eating two cloves of ***garlic*** *(Allium sativum)* a day may help boost your immune system's antiviral and antibacterial activity. When garlic is crushed or sliced, a sulfur compound called alliin is converted into allicin, which some people have a difficult time tolerating. If you can't digest fresh garlic, you might want to try one of the commercially prepared aged garlic extract tablets that are available.

Coenzyme Q10 and ***vitamin*** B_{12} are nutritional supplements that may lessen symptoms. Some evidence suggests that a combination of malic acid and ***magnesium*** may help relieve fatigue and muscle pain. Egg lecithin taken with meals may enhance immunity and promote energy. Other immune system-enhancing vitamins include ***vitamin C*** and beta carotene *(see* ***Vitamin A****)*, which is also a natural antioxidant. ***Vitamins*** B_5 and B_6, ***zinc, selenium, manganese,*** and ***chromium*** all play a role in strengthening the immune system as well.

The amino acid tryptophan, found in various foods, may be helpful for some symptoms, and since it helps the body produce serotonin, a natural sedative, it may aid in sleep. However, don't take it in supplement form if you have high blood pressure or are taking antidepressants.

It's not uncommon for people with CFS to have food sensitivities or to have had them as children. These sensitivities may manifest themselves as an allergic reaction or other intolerance to a particular food or several different foods.

When a food that you're allergic to enters your body, your immune system views it as an invader, like a virus or bacterium, and attacks it by flooding your bloodstream with antibodies. The overabundance of these antibodies, in conjunction with the release of histamines and other body chemicals, results in such symptoms as increased mucus production, tissue swelling, headache, sore throat, and sometimes mental confusion.

The simplest way to figure out which food or foods are to blame is to try an elimination diet: For a week or two, stop eating things you think may be causing an allergic reaction. Typical culprits include dairy products, nuts, eggs, shellfish, and preservatives in prepared foods, but other foods can also be the source of your problems. If your symptoms disappear, reintroduce each food, one at a time, and see how your body responds. If your symptoms come back, you will have determined at least one of the foods to which you are sensitive and can then eliminate it in all its variations from your diet.

AT-HOME REMEDIES

Make sure you don't attempt more activity during the day than you can handle. Get plenty of rest, pay close attention to your diet, and exercise lightly on a regular basis.

PREVENTION

Because no one knows what causes CFS, there is no sure way to prevent it. However, you may be able to avoid CFS and any worsening of symptoms by strengthening your immune system with vitamins, a proper diet (including avoiding allergens), reducing stress with relaxation techniques or **yoga,** mild exercise, avoiding environmental toxins, and keeping any allergies you may have under control. You might also want to consider experimenting with various alternative therapies to determine which ones work best for you. ■

CIRCULATORY PROBLEMS

SYMPTOMS

- cramplike pain, muscle fatigue, and aching in the legs; the blood vessels in your calves, thighs, feet, or hips may be blocked, possibly due to hardening of the arteries *(see* ***Atherosclerosis****).*
- bulging, bluish vessels in an aching leg; you may have ***varicose veins***.
- a painful vein; you may have ***phlebitis.***
- a finger, toe, or other body part that feels numb after exposure to cold weather, then becomes red and painful once warmed; you could be suffering from ***frostbite*** *(see page 69 in* ***Emergencies/First Aid****).*

CALL YOUR DOCTOR IF:

- you experience sudden and severe localized pain, and tissue in the affected area turns pale and cold; you may have a fully blocked blood vessel, which can lead to tissue death.
- you develop skin ulcers, localized skin discoloration, or nonhealing sores; these may be signs of obstructed blood flow.
- you are experiencing pain in leg muscles while walking or resting; your blood flow may be dangerously restricted.

Most of us experience the discomfort of tired, stiff, aching legs every now and then. Many people, however, must cope with this sensation on a daily basis. This condition, called **intermittent claudication,** results from blocked arteries in the pelvis, thighs, or calves and most often is caused by ***atherosclerosis,*** commonly known as hardening of the arteries. But circulatory problems come in many other forms as well. Most can be treated effectively at home and in consultation with a doctor. In severe cases, though, a corrective surgical procedure may be appropriate.

Blood circulates through the body via a complex system of vessels. Arteries carry oxygen-rich blood from the heart to the rest of the body; veins return oxygen-depleted blood from distant reaches of the body to the heart. Circulatory problems arise when these vessels become blocked or overly constricted. Such interruptions in normal blood flow can be brought on by a variety of conditions. Weakened arterial walls, for example, can balloon out and form pockets that trap blood. Veins can stretch, causing their internal valves to malfunction, and vascular disease can cause vessels to constrict. Most of the time, the discomfort caused by circulatory irregularities is confined to the buttocks and legs, but it can also affect other parts of the body.

CAUSES

Circulatory problems are rarely linked to a single cause. Rather, they usually come as a consequence of multiple risk factors. The incidence of poor circulation rises with age, as hardening of the arteries becomes more common. Gender also seems to play a role in determining who gets certain circulatory problems. Women, for example, are more likely than men to develop ***varicose veins***. Many circulatory disorders run in families. Lifestyle also wields significant influence. Among the risk factors linked to poor circulation are smoking, ***obesity,*** and prolonged periods of sitting or standing. Women taking birth-control pills exhibit a higher incidence of circulatory problems, as do people with ***diabetes.***

TREATMENT

The path to improved circulation usually begins at home. Beyond self-improvement measures, many treatment options are available to those who suffer from circulatory problems. Take the time to learn about your options, then decide which treatment program will work best for you.

CONVENTIONAL MEDICINE

Before suggesting a treatment, your doctor will need to diagnose the underlying cause of your circulatory disorder. You can help in this process by providing information about your lifestyle, family medical history, and personal medical history. If you have ***diabetes,*** for example, you stand a greater risk of developing circulatory trouble.

In most cases, a doctor will advise a program of regular aerobic exercise and good nutrition. You may be told to lose weight and to abandon old habits that interfere with circulation. If you are bothered by swelling or inflammation, your doctor may also advise a daily dose of ***aspirin,*** which inhibits blood clotting *(see* ***Blood Clots****)*.

For more severe cases, treatment options range from drug therapy to surgery. Many doctors prescribe ***pentoxifylline*** to improve blood flow to the extremities. In a procedure called angioplasty, doctors insert a small catheter into a blocked blood vessel and inflate a tiny balloon to widen the channel. Another technique is rotational atherectomy, in which a tiny diamond-studded drill is used to break up deposits in peripheral blood vessels. Other, more invasive surgical procedures include revascularization—bypassing blocked vessels with healthy ones taken from elsewhere in the body—and endarterectomy, in which portions of diseased vessels are opened to remove obstructing deposits.

ALTERNATIVE CHOICES

Many nonconventional treatments for poor circulation are attempts to strengthen weak blood vessels or widen their openings, thus allowing greater blood flow to distant parts of the body. Some alternative therapies also help to ease the discomfort or reduce the inflammation and swelling associated with circulatory problems.

BODY WORK

Manipulative techniques such as **massage** and **yoga** can promote blood flow and help to alleviate the discomfort caused by poor circulation.

CHELATION THERAPY

Many people seek relief through chelation therapy, which involves injecting the chemical EDTA into the bloodstream. But this form of treatment is controversial and far from universally accepted. *(For more information, see* ***Atherosclerosis.****)*

CHINESE MEDICINE

A traditional healer may advise a combined program of **acupuncture, herbal therapy,** and **massage.** Chinese herbs are also used in specific combinations to treat circulatory problems. Consult a specialist for the combination that is most appropriate for your condition.

HERBAL THERAPIES

An extract of the small, thorny ***hawthorn*** *(Crataegus oxyacantha)* tree promotes circulation by improving blood flow through the coronary arteries. And ***ginkgo*** *(Ginkgo biloba)* has a well-documented record of medicinal success. *(See "The Medicinal History of Ginkgo," overleaf.)* Studies show that concentrated extracts from the leaves of the ginkgo tree may help improve circulation by dilating the arteries. If you have a blood-clotting disorder, consult a doctor before using ginkgo, since the plant contains a substance thought to suppress the blood's clotting ability. Ginkgo has also been shown to cause mild side effects, including excitability and digestive problems.

Taken orally, an Asian herb called ***gotu kola*** *(Centella asiatica)* appears to benefit circulation by strengthening and toning blood vessel walls. ***Cayenne*** *(Capsicum frutescens)* and ***ginger*** *(Zingiber officinale)* may stimulate circulation by dilating arterioles and capillaries near the skin's surface. ***Butcher's-broom*** *(Ruscus aculeatus)* is believed to alleviate swelling and inflammation caused by many circulatory disorders. Butcher's-

C

broom can be prepared and eaten much like its cousin, asparagus, or brewed into a tea.

HYDROTHERAPY

A long soak in a warm bath, followed by a brisk rub with a towel dipped in cold water, can ease general discomfort caused by poor circulation. You might add a decoction of thyme leaves or larch needles (larch is a type of pine) to the bathwater for a stimulating effect. Soak cold feet in a warm footbath for 15 minutes. To promote circulation in the legs, alternate hot and cold footbaths (1 to 2 minutes in hot water, 30 seconds in cold water) for 15 minutes; end with cold.

MAGNETIC FIELD THERAPY

This controversial technique is based on the assumption that magnetic fields have an influence on the functioning of the body. Practitioners use magnets and electromagnetic equipment—including magnetic blankets and beds—in treatment sessions that can last from just a few minutes to overnight. Most often used to promote bone healing, magnetic field therapy may also be useful in the treatment of circulatory problems. WARNING: Do not use this technique if you are pregnant.

NEURAL THERAPY

Intended to restore electrical conductivity within the body through injections of ***anesthetics,*** neural therapy is an especially popular treatment option in Germany for a range of painful conditions, including some circulatory problems. WARNING: Neural therapy should be used only as a complement to orthodox medical treatment, not as a substitute. This technique is not recommended for patients who have cancer, diabetes, or renal failure, or for people who are allergic to local anesthetics.

NUTRITION AND DIET

As a general rule, your diet should be low in fat and high in fiber. Emphasize whole grains and fresh fruits and vegetables. Avoid caffeinated drinks, since caffeine causes blood vessels to constrict. And if you suffer from cold hands and feet,

THE MEDICINAL HISTORY OF GINKGO

The ginkgo, which first took root in northern China about 200 million years ago, is the oldest living tree species on Earth. Almost all of these plants were wiped out during the last ice age. But the few that survived became forebears of an ancient medicinal legacy. Approximately 4,000 years ago, Asian herbalists began investigating the healing properties of ginkgo. Earliest mention of the plant appears in a major Chinese herbal text dating to 1436 and the Ming Dynasty. Ever since, the ginkgo has been prized throughout China for its medicinal properties, particularly as a treatment for ***asthma.***

In 1730 the ginkgo was exported to Europe, where it became popular not for its medicinal properties but for its value as an ornamental tree. Only recently did the plant, also known as the maidenhair-tree, begin to excite scientific curiosity in the West. Over the past two decades, hundreds of scientific studies have been published extolling the benefits of ginkgo. A standardized ginkgo extract was developed in Germany to treat a number of conditions, ranging from circulatory problems to poor memory.

Today ginkgos are grown on plantations in the United States, Europe, Japan, and South Korea. After drying and milling, the leaves are converted into a concentrated extract that can be marketed in both solid and liquid form.

don't fall for the "warming" properties of hot toddies. Alcohol can make you feel warmer, but it ultimately impairs your ability to stay warm. Alcohol makes it more difficult for you to maintain your body temperature in cold weather and may even promote hypothermia.

If you suffer from hardened arteries, eat more fish. Not only is fish low in fat and high in nutritional value, but it also boosts levels of high-density lipoprotein (HDL), the "good" cholesterol that purges blood vessels of fatty deposits. For dessert, try pineapple. Studies suggest that an enzyme in pineapple called bromelain enhances circulation while reducing inflammation.

Healthful doses of certain vitamins and minerals may also improve your circulation. ***Vitamin C, vitamin E,*** and ***niacin,*** all of which are believed to have a dilating effect on blood vessels, may help to get the blood flowing and make walking less painful. However, consult a doctor or nutritionist before using niacin, as it can cause uncomfortable flushing. ***Magnesium*** supplements also may help dilate the vessels and alleviate arterial spasms. Note: Carbonated beverages usually contain large amounts of phosphate, which robs the body of magnesium.

REFLEXOLOGY

Stimulating reflexology areas on the feet for the adrenal glands, in addition to reflexology areas analogous to the localized problem area, may enhance circulation. *(See illustration below, left.)*

REFLEXOLOGY

Improve poor circulation in an area by working its corresponding reflexology area. To enhance overall circulation, also work the adrenal area: Push back your big toe and walk the thumb of your other hand along the extended tendon from the waistline to the adrenals.

AT-HOME REMEDIES

- Take regular walks or bike rides to enhance circulation in your legs. Do simple exercises, such as arm windmills, to get the blood flowing elsewhere.
- If you are taking birth-control pills, switch to another form of contraception. Stay away from over-the-counter ***decongestants;*** most of these drugs are vasoconstrictors, which can increase heart rate and blood pressure as well as constrict blood vessels.
- If you smoke, quit.
- Dress appropriately for cold weather. Layer your clothing and wear a warm hat, wool mittens (rather than gloves), and socks made of polypropylene or a polyester blend rather than all cotton.
- Take especially good care of your feet, keeping them warm, dry, and comfortable, as even minor problems can turn to major infections in cases of poor circulation.

PREVENTION

- Make sure that the food you eat is high in fiber and low in fat and includes plenty of whole grains, fresh fruits, vegetables, and fish. If necessary, supplement your diet with ***vitamin C, vitamin E, niacin,*** and ***magnesium.***
- If your job requires long hours of sitting, schedule regular breaks into your daily routine; stand up, stretch, and walk around for a few minutes every hour or so to get blood circulating in your legs and feet.
- If you smoke, now's the time to stop. And if you are overweight, try trimming down. ■

CIRRHOSIS

SYMPTOMS

Often no symptoms appear until the disease has entered the late stages. When they occur, symptoms can include:

- nausea, vomiting, and loss of appetite.
- unusual gain or loss of weight.
- yellow coloration of the skin and eyes *(see **Jaundice**).*
- dark urine.
- bloody, black stools, or unusually light-colored stools.
- vomiting of blood.
- abdominal swelling.
- prolonged generalized itching.
- swollen feet or legs.
- red palms.
- sleep disturbances and confusion.
- fatigue or loss of stamina.
- enlarged breasts in men.
- loss of sex drive.
- menstrual disturbances in women.
- spiderlike blood vessels on chest and shoulders.

CALL YOUR DOCTOR IF:

- you notice any of the above symptoms; without proper treatment, cirrhosis can be fatal.

Cirrhosis is a serious degenerative disease that occurs when healthy cells in the liver are damaged—usually as a result of ***alcohol abuse*** or ***hepatitis***—and replaced by scar tissue. As liver cells give way to tough scar tissue, the organ loses its ability to function properly. Severe damage can lead to liver failure and possibly death. Cirrhosis poses another danger as well: Dense scarring slows the normal flow of blood through the liver, causing pressure to build up in supplying blood vessels. In some cases this pressure becomes so great that the vessels in the esophagus rupture.

Every year about 26,000 people in the United States die from cirrhosis. The disease cannot be reversed or cured except, in some cases, through a liver transplant. It can often be slowed or halted, however, especially if the disease is detected in the early stages of development. Patients who think they might have cirrhosis should see a physician without delay.

Cirrhosis is serious because of the importance of the organ it affects. The liver, weighing about three pounds and roughly the size of a football, is the largest of the body's internal organs. Among its many functions, the liver serves as an essential part of the digestive system by producing bile, which is stored in the gallbladder, then released into the small intestine, where it helps break down fatty food. The liver also helps maintain the proper composition of the blood by regulating the amounts of fat, protein, and sugar that enter the bloodstream. As the body's primary blood filter, the liver works to detoxify alcohol, drugs, and other potentially harmful chemicals. Along with the spleen, the liver traps and disposes of worn-out red blood cells. And because it aids in the removal of bacteria and viruses from the blood, the liver is a vital component of the immune system. If your liver is not functioning properly, you are more susceptible to infection.

The liver is remarkably tolerant of disease and injury. Even after 70 percent of its mass has been destroyed or removed, the organ can still function, albeit with decreased effectiveness. If the conditions that caused the destruction have been removed or corrected, the liver usually can bounce back. Although function can never be restored to parts of your liver that have turned to scar tissue, you can live a healthy life with the remaining portion if the disease is caught in time. However, there is a point of no return with cirrhosis. As more cells are replaced by scar tissue, fewer healthy cells are left to handle the liver's many tasks. Eventually function problems arise and may remain. This is why it's important to identify the underlying causes as soon as possible and begin taking steps to eliminate them.

CAUSES

Cirrhosis occurs as the result of long-term injury to the liver. Possible causes include viruses, genetic deficiencies, prolonged obstruction of bile flow, and long periods of exposure to drugs and other toxic substances. In the majority of cases, however, the culprit is excessive consumption of alcohol *(see **Alcohol Abuse**)*.

The link between alcohol and cirrhosis is well documented. Studies show that while moderate drinking may actually help prevent ***strokes*** and ***heart disease,*** heavy drinking has a clearly harmful effect on the liver. For example, the French—famous for their wine consumption—have a relatively low incidence of heart disease, but the rate of cirrhosis in France is very high. Many physicians believe that more drinkers die from cirrhosis than are protected from heart disease.

Simply put, the more alcohol you drink—and the greater the frequency of drinks—the more likely you are to develop cirrhosis. Because the bodies of men and women process alcohol differently, the amount that you can safely imbibe depends largely on your sex. In general, men can have two or three alcoholic drinks a day without suffering liver damage. Women, on the other hand, can safely consume only one or two drinks daily.

These guidelines notwithstanding, it's important to note that alcohol tolerance may vary from one person to the next. For some people, one drink per day is enough to leave permanent scars in the liver. If you drink—especially if you do so heavily and often—have a physician examine you for signs of cirrhosis. This is necessary even if you feel healthy, since the symptoms of cirrhosis often do not appear until it is too late to arrest the development of the disease or slow its progress.

Excessive drinking almost inevitably causes some liver damage, but it does not always lead to cirrhosis. Some people who drink heavily develop **alcoholic hepatitis,** an inflammation of the liver that can last a week or two, producing symptoms of nausea, fever, loss of appetite, ***jaundice,*** and confusion. Over time, the condition can also lead to cirrhosis. Even light drinkers who go on a bender for several days can develop a condition known as **fatty liver,** caused when cells of the liver become swollen with accumulated fat and water. This condition can cause pain or tenderness in the liver, temporary jaundice, and abnormalities in other liver functions. (Fatty liver can also result from ***diabetes, obesity,*** and severe malnutrition.)

After alcoholism, the most frequent cause of cirrhosis is ***hepatitis,*** a general term meaning inflammation of the liver. Of the various forms of this disease, only two—hepatitis B and hepatitis C—are likely to result in cirrhosis. Scarring usually occurs after hepatitis has become chronic (lasting six months or more). The symptoms may be so mild at first that patients with chronic hepatitis do not even realize their livers are scarring. Meanwhile, the damage continues, perhaps resulting in a serious case of cirrhosis later in life. Therefore, it is important for people with hepatitis to have regular medical checkups. And because hepatitis is contagious, family members of an infected person should also be tested.

Cirrhosis sometimes, though rarely, occurs because of an inherited liver disorder. In **Wilson's disease,** for example, a genetic deficiency inhibits the body's ability to metabolize copper. As a result, excessive amounts of the metal accumulate in various body organs, particularly the liver, where it destroys tissue. Similarly, in **hemochromatosis** the body absorbs excess amounts of iron, which damages the liver and causes scarring. This disorder mostly strikes men between the ages of 40 and 60; women are usually not affected because their bodies lose iron during menstruation.

Children born with **galactosemia** lack an enzyme needed to digest milk sugar. Normally, milk sugar passes harmlessly through the digestive system and out of the body. But in people with galactosemia, the substance accumulates in the liver at levels that become toxic and potentially fatal without proper treatment. Infants with this disorder should be taken off milk and given a substitute formula.

Some babies are born with no bile ducts, or with ducts that are malformed. Because bile is unable to drain out of the body, it accumulates in the liver and eventually poisons it. Although the problem can sometimes be corrected through surgery, most children with this disorder die from cirrhosis before they reach the age of two.

Cirrhosis can result when ***gallstones*** block the flow of bile and cause it to back up into the liver for long periods of time. The disease may also come as a consequence of long-term exposure to certain drugs, including methotrexate and isoniazid, and to toxic substances in the environment, such as pesticides and arsenic-based compounds.

DIAGNOSTIC AND TEST PROCEDURES

A patient's history and symptoms, along with the results of a physical examination, are usually enough to determine a case of cirrhosis. Once the diagnosis has been made, the physician may order one or more liver function tests, which use blood samples to identify specific liver diseases and assess the organ's overall health. The doctor may also require a liver biopsy, or tissue sample, to ascertain the cause of the cirrhosis. In this procedure, a needle is inserted into the liver to draw out a fragment of tissue, which is then sent to a lab for analysis.

TREATMENT

The best way to treat cirrhosis is to correct the underlying cause. This could involve giving up alcohol, seeking treatment for ***hepatitis*** or an inherited disorder, or eliminating certain substances from your diet or environment.

CONVENTIONAL MEDICINE

Specific remedies for cirrhosis depend on the underlying cause and its stage of development. Besides halting the progress of the disease, conventional treatment also aims at correcting any complications, such as internal bleeding, which in themselves can be disabling or life-threatening.

If your cirrhosis is caused by alcoholism, you simply must stop drinking—immediately and completely. If you continue to drink after you have been diagnosed with cirrhosis, you have less than a 40 percent chance of living longer than five more years. If you stop drinking, however, those chances increase to 60 to 70 percent.

Corking the bottle is also the best way to remedy **alcoholic hepatitis** and alcohol-induced **fatty liver.** Both of these conditions usually clear up when the patient stops drinking long enough for the liver to heal. Conventional treatment of cirrhosis caused by chronic ***hepatitis*** emphasizes rest, proper nutrition, and possibly the use of the drug interferon. Some types of hepatitis, however, cannot be cured.

For **Wilson's disease,** doctors generally prescribe medications that rid the body of accumulated copper. It may be necessary to continue these medications for life. In the case of **hemochromatosis,** the best way to dispose of excess iron is to draw blood from the patient once or twice a week. This should be kept up for as long as two years, or until the iron level reaches its normal range. Treatment then continues every two to four months.

Severe cirrhosis may require a liver transplant—a serious procedure usually regarded as a last resort. Transplants are not appropriate for

CAUTION!

Because the liver plays a key role in processing drugs, alcohol, and toxins in the body, people with cirrhosis must avoid anything that will cause further damage to the organ. If you have cirrhosis, your liver may not be able to process drugs properly. Be sure to consult your doctor before taking any medication, including birth-control pills, *antibiotics*, and over-the-counter drugs such as *acetaminophen.*

everyone: Some patients are too old, too young, or too sick for the procedure. And people whose cirrhosis is due to alcohol abuse must demonstrate a prolonged period of abstinence before the operation. Doctors generally are hesitant to transplant a liver if the patient is just going to abuse it.

As with any form of major surgery, liver transplants can be risky. The new liver may not function properly, or the body may reject the transplanted organ. There's also the danger that infection will set in after surgery. Still, the procedure has a promising success rate overall. In the United States, 60 percent to 75 percent of adult patients and 90 percent of children survive the operation. Transplant patients live an average of five years after surgery.

ALTERNATIVE CHOICES

Alternative therapies for cirrhosis generally attempt to support the functioning of healthy liver cells as well as relieve some of the discomfort and disability associated with the disease.

CHINESE MEDICINE

Various Chinese herbs, used in combination, may promote healthy liver function. However, self-medication can be dangerous; remedies should be prescribed only by a licensed practitioner.

HERBAL THERAPY

Milk thistle *(Silybum marianum)* is believed to promote healthy liver function. However, consult a licensed practitioner before using this remedy.

HOMEOPATHY

Certain homeopathic remedies, including *Taraxacum officinale* and *Chelidonium majus,* may help improve the efficiency of healthy liver cells in cases of cirrhosis. Consult a licensed practitioner for their proper use.

NUTRITION AND DIET

Good nutrition often plays a vital role in the treatment of cirrhosis. Although parts of the liver that have given way to scar tissue can't be restored, a balanced diet—including plenty of fruits, vegetables, grains, milk, and protein—can help promote regeneration among cells in the intact portion. Adults with the disease need to monitor their intake of protein. Too little protein can slow cell regeneration, and too much can raise the amount of ammonia in your bloodstream, possibly leading to mental impairment. Check with a doctor or nutritionist for the amount of protein that's right for you.

Because the liver must filter and refine substances that are introduced into the body, patients with cirrhosis are often told to seek medical advice before taking large doses of vitamins or other dietary supplements. Cirrhosis patients should also avoid eating uncooked shellfish, which are sometimes harvested in polluted estuaries and may carry organisms that cause hepatitis or other diseases.

PREVENTION

- If you drink, know your limits and do not exceed them. Generally speaking, men can have two or three drinks a day without suffering liver damage. The safe limit for women is one or two drinks daily. Keep in mind, though, that alcohol tolerance can vary greatly from one person to the next. Doctors often advise people to set a daily limit of one or two drinks and to avoid drinking every day.
- Avoid uncooked shellfish.
- Never mix alcohol and drugs. Some medications, including ***acetaminophen,*** react with alcohol and can damage the liver.
- Avoid exposure to industrial chemicals, which can enter the bloodstream and cause liver damage.
- Maintain a healthy, balanced diet.
- Take precautions to avoid contracting ***hepatitis.*** Practice safe sex and—if you use intravenous drugs—be especially careful to avoid dirty needles. Before traveling to countries where the disease is prevalent, ask your doctor about hepatitis vaccinations and immune serum globulin shots. (Immune serum globulin shots provide ready-made defender proteins called antibodies, whereas vaccinations prompt the body to produce its own.) ■

COLD SORES

C

SYMPTOMS

- fluid-filled blisters or red, painful sores on or near the mouth, or on fingers.
- swollen, sensitive gums of a deep red color.
- a fever, flulike symptoms, and swollen lymph nodes in the neck often accompanying the first attack; recurrent sores usually don't produce these symptoms.

CALL YOUR DOCTOR IF:

- you develop a high fever and/or chills; high fevers can be dangerous.
- your sores are very painful; you may be able to get prescription relief.

Cold sores, also called fever blisters, are a painful infection caused by the herpes simplex virus. They may show up anywhere on your body but are most likely to appear on your gums, the outside of your mouth and lips, your nose, cheeks, or fingers. Blisters form, then break and ooze; a yellow crust develops and eventually sloughs off, revealing new skin underneath. The sores usually last 7 to 10 days.

Ninety percent of all people get at least one cold sore in their lives. This first occurrence is often the worst. Some children who are affected may become seriously ill. After the first infection, many people develop antibodies and never have another cold sore. About 40 percent of American adults, however, have repeated cold sores.

Although cold sores generally are not serious, the infection may be life-threatening for anyone who has ***AIDS*** or whose immune system is depressed by other disorders or medications. In infants, who usually contract the virus during birth, the infection may spread to other organs, causing serious complications or even death.

The infection from a cold sore may cause blindness if it spreads to the eye; herpes is a frequent cause of infectious blindness.

CAUSES

Cold sores are caused by the herpes simplex virus, which is transmitted by such forms of contact as kissing an infected person or sharing eating utensils, towels, or razors. A person with a cold sore who performs oral sex on another person can give that person ***genital herpes.***

Sores may develop as late as 20 days after exposure to the virus. Once the virus enters your body, it may emerge years later at or near the original site of entry. Before an attack you may experience itching or sensitivity at the site. The virus may be triggered by certain foods, stress, fever, colds, allergies, sunburn, and menstruation.

DIAGNOSTIC AND TEST PROCEDURES

Your doctor may take a culture from your sore or simply examine it to see if you have the virus.

TREATMENT

You can't cure a cold sore, but you can alleviate the pain it causes by avoiding spicy or acidic foods, applying ice, and using over-the-counter remedies. Look for medicines that contain numbing agents such as ***phenol,*** and emollients to reduce cracking and soften scabs. To speed healing, apply a water-based ***zinc*** ointment as soon as you feel the tingling that precedes a sore.

CONVENTIONAL MEDICINE

If your cold sore is especially painful or irritating, your doctor may prescribe an anesthetic gel to alleviate pain.

ALTERNATIVE CHOICES

Several alternative therapies may help to speed healing and prevent sores from coming back.

AROMATHERAPY

Applying geranium *(Pelargonium odoratissimum)* or ***eucalyptus*** *(Eucalyptus globulus)* oils to cold sores every hour may help reduce pain and speed healing of the sores. Aromatherapists believe that ***tea tree oil*** (*Melaleuca* spp.) has antiseptic properties.

HERBAL THERAPIES

To dry up a cold sore, herbalists recommend applying lemon balm *(Melissa officinalis).* Herbalists also recommend applying ***calendula*** *(Calendula officinalis)* ointment, 3 to 4 times a day, to relieve pain, and speed healing.

MIND/BODY MEDICINE

Cold sores often are triggered by ***stress.*** Try deep muscle **relaxation, biofeedback, guided imagery,** and **meditation.** Don't forget to exercise; activity bolsters your immune system so you can defend yourself against the virus.

NUTRITION AND DIET

The herpesvirus thrives on the amino acid arginine. Stay away from nuts, chocolate, and seeds. Instead, eat foods high in lysine, such as kidney beans, split peas, and corn.

If you have more than three cold sores a year, take 500-mg lysine supplements every day. Triple the dosage when you feel yourself developing another sore.

AT-HOME REMEDIES

- Apply ice for 15 minutes to relieve pain.
- Apply ***vitamin E*** oil to help sores heal.
- Use lip balm sunscreen with an SPF of 15 or higher.
- Cover your cold sore with petroleum jelly.

PREVENTION

- Don't kiss someone who has a cold sore or use the same utensils, towels, or razors.
- Wash your hands after touching a cold sore.
- Don't rub your eyes after touching your cold sore; you could develop corneal herpes, which may lead to blindness if left untreated.
- Don't touch your genitals after touching your cold sore; you could develop ***genital herpes.***
- Replace your toothbrush.
- Avoid foods that contain arginine.
- Eat foods high in lysine, or take supplements.■

C A U T I O N !

Cold sore infections can spread to other organs in infants and cause serious illnesses. If your infant develops a sore with a fever, call the doctor. If you have *AIDS* or a depressed immune system, or are on medication following an organ transplant, guard against developing cold sores. If you touch a cold sore and then touch your eye, you could develop a serious corneal ulcer, a manifestation of herpes.

COLIC

C

SYMPTOMS

Colic is not a disease but a pattern of persistent, prolonged crying. Doctors consider it colic if an otherwise healthy infant up to three months old exhibits the following behavior:

- loud crying lasting three hours or more for three or more days a week, over a period of more than three weeks.
- prolonged crying between 6:00 p.m. and midnight in a baby that has been fed.
- while crying, the baby draws his legs to his abdomen and clenches his hands and curls his toes; his face alternately flushes and pales with the effort of crying.
- episodes of crying that sometimes begin or end with a bowel movement or the passing of gas.

CALL YOUR DOCTOR IF:

- your baby has not had colic before and you suspect he is colicky; your physician will want to rule out other causes.
- bouts of colic are accompanied by fever, diarrhea, vomiting, or constipation—all possible signs of illness.
- your baby's crying sounds painful, not fussy—indicating injury or illness is causing the distress.
- your baby is older than three months and still acting colicky; behavioral problems or illness may be the cause.
- your colicky child fails to gain weight and is not hungry, which suggests illness.
- you're exhausted or fear stress might lead you to hurt your baby.

About 20 percent of all infants suffer from colic—spates of crying that go on for hours for no apparent reason. Although distressing for the child and exhausting and emotionally draining for parents, the condition itself is benign and usually ends by the time a child is four months old.

CAUSES

The cause of colic is not known. Experts attribute it to any number of things, including an infant's immature digestive system, ***allergies,*** hormones in breast milk, cow's milk, and overfeeding.

TREATMENT

There is no cure for colic, although many at-home remedies have proved helpful in soothing colicky babies. Any of those listed on page 273 may work for your child. It is important to remain calm; communication of your own anxiety or frustration to a colicky child will probably result in more crying. Above all, never punish a colicky baby. If you feel yourself near the breaking point, ask someone else to stay with your child while you rest or get away to compose yourself.

CONVENTIONAL MEDICINE

If you suspect your child has colic, call your pediatrician. After ruling out possible medical causes

COMFORT FOR QUICK RELIEF

Fearing that catering to a colicky baby would spoil the child, doctors used to counsel parents to ignore their baby's cries or to delay in responding to them. Physicians now encourage early, sympathetic response to colic.

of prolonged crying, such as ***otitis media*** or ***respiratory problems,*** most doctors recommend simple home-management techniques. Some encourage parents to talk with other parents for support. If you have gone through colic with an older child, you may decide to call the doctor only if you think your colicky infant is sick.

ALTERNATIVE CHOICES

ACUPRESSURE

Manipulating certain acupressure points may soothe a crying child. See the ***Appendix*** for help in locating these points. Apply pressure to the webbed area between your child's thumb and index finger (Large Intestine 4) on either hand. Gently massage Conception Vessel 12, above your child's navel, and the corresponding points near the spine (Bladder 20, 21). Applying pressure to Stomach 36 may also quiet your child.

HERBAL THERAPIES

Teas made with herbs containing carminative oils, which reduce inflammation in the bowels and lessen gas production, may help a colicky child. Try teas made of ***chamomile*** *(Matricaria recutita),* lemon balm *(Melissa officinalis),* ***peppermint*** *(Mentha piperita),* or anise *(Pimpinella anisum).*

HOMEOPATHY

Homeopathic medicine offers several over-the-counter colic remedies that are considered safe to use without prior consultation with a homeopath. Seek help from a professional if your child does not respond to a remedy within 24 hours.

AT-HOME REMEDIES

Maintain a consistent pattern of comfort. Consistency will help you avoid getting locked into a behavioral problem with your child later. If one of these methods brings the child relief, stick with it.

- Give your baby a pacifier.
- Motion can relieve colic. Walk with the baby; rock him in your arms or in a swing; go for a car ride; or put him in an infant seat near a clothes dryer, where the vibration can be felt.

COMFORTING A COLICKY BABY

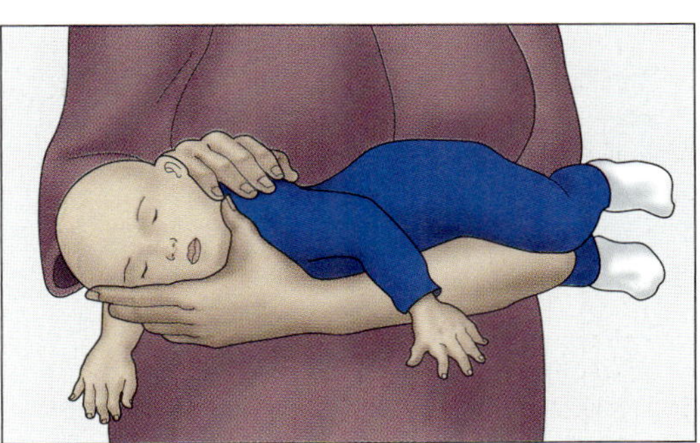

Holding a colicky baby in a secure, restful position can have a calming effect. Hold the baby, stomach down, along your forearm, with head facing outward on your palm and legs on either side of your elbow. You can gently pat the baby on the back with your free hand. This technique may be more effective if you rock in a rocking chair or walk quietly until the baby falls asleep.

- White noise may soothe your child. Try running a vacuum cleaner or hair dryer where your infant can hear it.
- Wrap the child snugly in a blanket to provide a sense of security and comfort.
- Place the baby, stomach down, on a warm water bottle in your lap. Test the temperature of the bottle against your inner wrist.
- Ask a relative or friend to take over when you feel yourself getting frustrated or exhausted.

PREVENTION

You can't prevent colic, but if the distress is related to feeding, you may lessen the frequency of episodes by trying the following: Hold your baby upright when feeding; burp often. Feed smaller amounts more frequently. To prevent him from swallowing air, feed your baby slowly. If you are breast-feeding, try eliminating from your own diet cow's milk, caffeinated drinks, and broccoli and other cabbage family vegetables, all of which can promote gas pains in your child. If you are bottle-feeding, try a formula free of cow's milk.■

COLITIS

C

SYMPTOMS

- persistent or recurrent ***diarrhea*** with blood or pus in the stool.
- ***abdominal pain.***
- bowel movements or diarrhea during the night.
- fever, fatigue, weakness, weight loss, pains or soreness in joints.

CALL YOUR DOCTOR IF:

- you are having heavy, persistent diarrhea; you may be at risk of dehydration.
- you have rectal bleeding, with clots of blood in your stool; your colitis has reached a severe stage.
- you have constant pain and a high fever; you might have **toxic megacolon,** a severely dilated and inflamed colon. **Get medical help immediately.**

Colitis is a general term for inflammatory ailments of the lower intestine, which include ***Crohn's disease*** and chronic ulcerative proctitis. **Ischemic colitis** is an intestinal disorder that affects mainly the elderly. One of the most serious forms of colitis is **ulcerative colitis,** a chronic disease that requires close medical attention.

In **ulcerative colitis,** the colon develops tiny ulcers and other inflammations that flare up periodically and cause attacks of bloody stools or diarrhea that may be painful. It is usually diagnosed in young adults but can occur at any age, and may be associated with various other disorders ranging from ***eye problems*** to ***arthritis*** in the arm and leg joints. Attacks of ulcerative colitis tend to recur, and the risk of ***colorectal cancer*** increases rapidly 8 to 10 years after onset. With regular medical treatment, however, the disease is rarely fatal, and most sufferers can lead fairly normal lives. Doctors recognize several levels of severity:

- With a mild case you will have up to four loose, possibly bloody, bowel movements a day, which may temporarily relieve abdominal pain.
- With a moderate case you will have abdominal pain and four to eight bloody stools daily, as well as a low fever and weight loss.
- With a severe case you will have six or more bloody stools or diarrhea daily and during the night, with fever of 100°F or higher, as well as symptoms of ***anemia.***

CAUSES

Although several theories have been put forward about the causes of colitis, none has been proved conclusively. Colitis-like symptoms can also occur in conjunction with bacterial and parasitic infections, such as salmonella poisoning. Temporary colitis-like symptoms strike some people after they take certain ***antibiotics,*** such as ***amoxicillin,*** ampicillin, ***cephalosporins,*** chloramphenicol, ***clindamycin,*** lincomycin, ***penicillin, tetracycline,*** or ***trimethoprim.*** When the drugs are discontinued, the symptoms tend to disappear.

DIAGNOSTIC AND TEST PROCEDURES

Doctors look for signs of **ulcerative colitis** by examining the inside of the colon with a sigmoidoscope, a flexible tube inserted through the rectum. A diagnosis is often made by taking a biopsy, removing a tiny sample of the colon lining for testing under the microscope.

TREATMENT

Ulcerative colitis is among the most serious systemic illnesses. If left untreated, it can lead to complications in other body systems and is potentially fatal. Prompt diagnosis and appropriate medical treatment are essential. ***Diarrhea*** in infants and young children is always a serious matter and must be diagnosed and treated as quickly as possible.

CONVENTIONAL MEDICINE

Doctors focus first on controlling inflammation and stopping diarrhea, and eventually on improving nutrition. If you have intense diarrhea and bleeding, your doctor will probably recommend immediate hospitalization, intravenous feeding, and treatment with appropriate drugs—probably intravenous methylprednisolone or ***hydrocortisone.*** Azathioprine, an immunosuppressant, is an option for those who do not tolerate steroids well. When the disease is stable but diarrhea is still a problem, you may need an ***antidiarrheal*** remedy such as a ***loperamide*** and ***codeine*** compound. Because diarrhea tends to dehydrate the body, you need to replace the water you are losing. In severe cases, surgery to remove the colon may be necessary. After the immediate symptoms of colitis are under control, your doctor will probably recommend a high-fiber, lactose-free diet and will encourage you to get regular exercise and to stop smoking.

ALTERNATIVE CHOICES

Because **ulcerative colitis** is a serious, potentially life-threatening illness, you should see a doctor at the first sign of diarrhea with bloody stools. If the medical diagnosis rules out ulcerative or other infectious forms of colitis, however, you may find that alternative therapies are helpful in relieving your symptoms.

ACUPUNCTURE

To provide relief from diarrhea and colitis-like symptoms, your acupuncturist will ask you specific questions about your condition to determine which points to stimulate. The likely points are along the foot-stomach and conception meridians, near the navel and left knee. *(See the **Appendix** for point locations.)*

HERBAL THERAPIES

For soothing an irritated intestine and reducing inflammation, many herbalists recommend a combination of ***marsh mallow*** *(Athaea officinalis)*, ***slippery elm*** *(Ulmas fulva)*, and geranium *(Geranium maculatum)*. *(See also **Celiac Disease**.)*

HOMEOPATHY

Homeopathy is considered appropriate for relief of colitis and colitis-like symptoms, not only in adults but in infants and children as well. Consult a homeopath for specific treatments; among the commonly prescribed homeopathic remedies for colitis are ***Arsenicum album*** and ***Nux vomica.***

NUTRITION AND DIET

Omega-3 fatty acids, found naturally in fish oil and flaxseed oil and available in capsule form at health food stores, may help reduce intestinal inflammation. Consult a knowledgeable health-care practitioner for the dosage appropriate to your condition. Avoid foods that may irritate the bowel, including dairy products, hot spices, caffeine, nuts, and seeds.

REFLEXOLOGY

In order to relieve the discomfort of intestinal problems, massage the colon, liver, adrenal, lower spine, diaphragm, and gallbladder areas on the bottom of your foot. *(See page 25 for area locations.)* ■

COLORECTAL CANCER

SYMPTOMS

In its early stage, colorectal cancer usually produces no symptoms. The most likely warning signs include:

- changes in bowel movements, including persistent ***constipation*** or ***diarrhea,*** a feeling of not being able to empty the bowel completely, or rectal bleeding.
- dark patches of blood in or on stool; or long, thin, "pencil stools."
- stomach discomfort, intermittent cramps, frequent gas pains, heartburn, nausea, vomiting, bloating, or difficulty swallowing.
- unexplained fatigue, or loss of appetite or weight.

CALL YOUR DOCTOR IF:

- you notice a change in your bowel movements, experience bleeding from the rectum, or notice blood in or on your stool. Don't assume you have ***hemorrhoids;*** schedule a rectal examination and possibly a sigmoidoscopy.
- you experience persistent ***abdominal pain,*** unusual weight loss, or fatigue. These symptoms may be due to other causes, but they could also be linked to cancer.
- you are diagnosed with ***anemia.*** In determining its cause, your doctor should check for bleeding from the digestive tract because of colorectal cancer.

Coiled inside your abdominal cavity is a long, tubular digestive tract. The muscular second half of this tube—the large intestine, or bowel—is composed of the colon, which stretches several feet, and the rectum, which is only a few inches long. Together, the colon and rectum act as a waste processor: Digested food moves into the colon, the body absorbs any remaining water, and the solid waste is pushed through the rectum and out of the anus in the form of stool.

The inner lining of the colorectal tube can be a fertile breeding ground for small tumors called **polyps.** About half of all adults over the age of 40 grow at least one colorectal polyp. Most polyps are benign, but at least one type is known to be precancerous. Nine out of ten malignant colorectal tumors develop from polyps in glandular tissue of the intestinal lining, although a few rare types of colorectal cancer arise from nonglandular tissue.

If colorectal cancer is diagnosed and treated while the tumor is still localized, the disease is highly curable, with five-year survival rates of about 90 percent. If the tumor continues to grow, cancer can spread directly through the bowel wall to surrounding tissues and organs, as well as into the bloodstream or lymphatic system. Once the cancer spreads to lymph nodes or other organs, successful treatment becomes more difficult. Depending on how advanced the disease is, five-year survival rates range anywhere from 70 percent to 5 percent.

Cancers of the colon and rectum are jointly responsible for about 12 percent of cancers in the United States, with approximately 150,000 cases diagnosed each year. Like many cancers, colorectal cancer is a particular concern for the elderly. Although detection is often possible at an early stage, many people delay seeking medical care because they are embarrassed or fearful of symptoms related to their bowels. Risk increases significantly after 50 and continues to increase with age. Colorectal cancer is characteristically an urban disease, affecting city dwellers more often than rural dwellers, and Caucasians more than African Americans.

INTESTINAL TUMORS

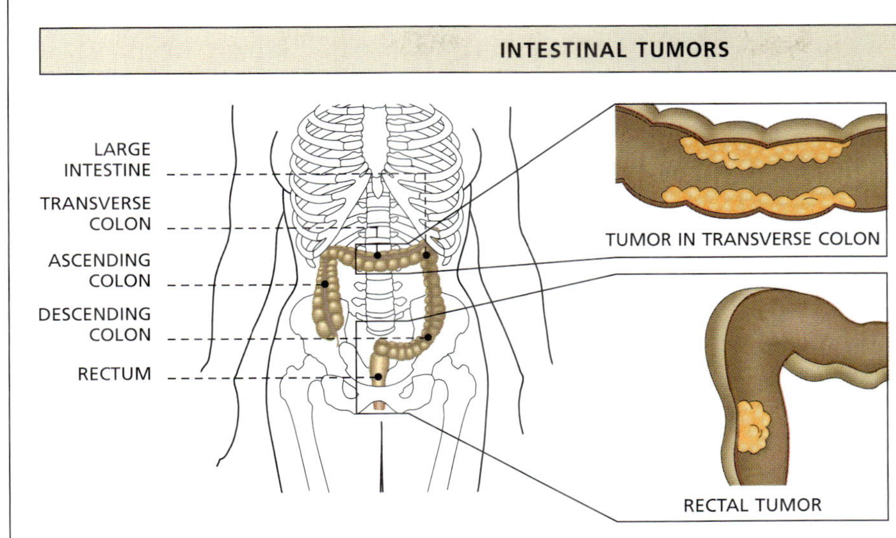

The lower digestive tract, or large intestine *(far left),* includes the colon and the rectum. The large intestine has three main parts: the ascending, transverse, and descending colons. A tumor in the transverse colon *(inset, top left)* can result in abdominal pain, irregular bowel movements, and occult blood in the stool. With a rectal tumor *(inset, bottom left)* blood may be visible in bowel movements.

CAUSES

Colorectal cancer is strongly associated with certain other diseases. Those people considered at high risk include anyone with a personal or family history of colon polyps, inflammatory disease of the colon such as ulcerative ***colitis*** or ***Crohn's disease,*** and ***cancers*** of the ***pancreas, breast, ovaries,*** colon, or rectum—especially in a parent or sibling. If you develop ulcerative colitis, the risk of getting colorectal cancer is 20 times greater than average. As with any cancer, potential susceptibility to colorectal cancer is at least partly determined by genetic makeup. A few people inherit a condition called familial polyposis, in which colon polyps develop at an early age; unless treated, these people are almost certain to develop colorectal cancer. *(See box, overleaf.)*

Diet also seems to contribute to the risk, although the cause-and-effect relationship is still unclear. People whose diets are low in fiber because they do not eat enough fruits, vegetables, and grains are known to be at increased risk. Many studies implicate animal fat and protein as promoters of colorectal cancer, although researchers are cautious about drawing any definite conclusions. Some studies show that regularly eating red meat, which is rich in saturated fat and protein, increases risk, while others find no connection. Some scientists think that fat is the main culprit, while others suspect protein. Others contend that it's not the fat and protein themselves, but the way they are cooked. They note that fats and protein cooked at high temperatures—especially when broiled and barbecued—can produce a host of potentially carcinogenic substances linked to colorectal cancer.

Heavy exposure to certain chemicals, including chlorine—which in small amounts is commonly used to purify drinking water—may increase the risk of colorectal cancer. Exposure to asbestos is thought to be potentially harmful, because it has been implicated in causing formation of polyps in the colon.

DIAGNOSTIC AND TEST PROCEDURES

Beginning about the age of 50, everyone should be screened regularly for colorectal cancer. Once a year, your doctor should perform a digital rectal examination and check your abdomen and lymph nodes for signs of swelling or a mass. As part of your annual checkup, a stool sample should be analyzed for occult blood—microscopic traces that could signal bleeding in the digestive tract. Every three to five years, you should

C

THE GENETIC LINK

*Researchers have found that many colorectal cancer patients share certain genetic defects. Having one of these defects means that you are predisposed—but not necessarily bound—to get the disease. For example, scientists have identified a specific gene for hereditary nonpolyposis colorectal cancer (HNPCC), or Lynch syndrome. Presence of the gene—which is extremely rare—predisposes a person to colorectal, **stomach, uterine,** and certain other **cancers** of the abdominal organs. Scientists can now test people with a family history of these cancers to find out if an individual carries the flawed gene. Those individuals can then be screened regularly to ensure early cancer detection.*

have a sigmoidoscopy, an examination of your rectum and lower, or sigmoid, colon using a flexible, lighted tube called a sigmoidoscope. While this screening technique may not be altogether pleasant, it is extremely valuable for detecting early cancer and other gastrointestinal disorders. *(See also **Colitis** and **Crohn's Disease.**)* A noninvasive screening procedure called virtual colonoscopy does away with the tube, instead using spiral computed tomography, which produces a three-dimensional image of the colon after it has been emptied and partially inflated with air.

Any suspicious symptoms or abnormalities will alert your doctor to perform a colonoscopy, a procedure much like sigmoidoscopy that allows a closer view of the inner lining of the bowel. If your doctor finds a polyp or tumor, a biopsy will determine whether or not it is malignant. You may also have x-rays taken of the colon and rectum to view potential masses, along with blood and urine studies to check for characteristic chemical abnormalities. Should a biopsy confirm cancer, other tests are run to find out whether it has spread to likely sites such as the liver, using x-ray, ultrasound, or CT scans. Further blood tests might be ordered to find out how well the liver is functioning and to measure the blood level of a substance called carcinoembryonic antigen (CEA), often found in higher-than-normal concentration in the presence of colorectal cancer, especially if it has spread.

TREATMENT

Cancer treatment involves not only specific therapies for curing or controlling the disease, but also strategies for meeting a patient's emotional and physical needs. Restoring and maintaining quality of life is a central issue for physicians, as it should be for family members and friends as well. Many complementary cancer therapies can be valuable adjuncts when pursued along with standard medical treatment to help make the stresses of cancer and its treatment more tolerable. However, complementary therapies should never replace standard care.

CONVENTIONAL MEDICINE

Surgery is the most effective treatment for local colorectal tumors. Very small tumors can be removed through a colonoscope, but even with small tumors the surgeon usually prefers to do a laparotomy—removing a significant portion of the bowel and nearby lymph nodes. Often, the surgeon can reconnect the healthy sections of the colon and rectum; when this is not possible, the surgeon forms an opening—known as a stoma—in the abdomen and reroutes the severed colon to it. Waste is collected in a bag worn over the stoma. This procedure, known as a colostomy, often is only temporary; once the bowel has had time to heal, a second operation reconnects the colon and rectum. The need for permanent colostomy is more common with rectal cancer, since retaining the rectum may be difficult. *(See **Crohn's Disease.**)*

In the treatment of rectal cancer, preoperative radiation or chemotherapy may be advised to shrink the tumor. Radiation and chemotherapy may also be recommended to prevent local tumor recurrence and to lengthen survival time. Radiation is rarely recommended after colon cancer. Instead, doctors have found that chemotherapy combined with immunotherapy can improve the period of survival in patients whose cancer has spread from the colon to surrounding lymph nodes. Chemotherapy may be helpful for patients with rectal or colon cancer that has metastasized to organs in other parts of the body, even though it is not likely to offer a cure. *(See **Cancer** for more information on therapies.)*

In the immediate postoperative period, the patient can expect to receive painkillers and other medication to ease temporary diarrhea or constipation. Postop patients will be encouraged to eat nutritious foods, rich in calories and proteins, in order to foster strength and healing.

Once cancer of either the colon or rectum achieves remission, follow-up exams to check for recurrence are essential indefinitely. But hundreds of thousands of people are living comfortable, normal lives even after colorectal surgery and a colostomy. Although adjusting to life after a colostomy requires time, support, and understanding, people with stomata have discovered for the most part they can eat, play, and work as well as they did before.

COMPLEMENTARY THERAPIES

Studies published since the 1970s have essentially confirmed that a high-fiber diet substantially reduces the risk for colorectal cancer. Dietary fiber seems to protect the bowel from prolonged exposure to carcinogens by moving waste quickly and by inhibiting formation of some carcinogens. Major studies also show that a diet high in whole grains, fruits, and vegetables reduces risk for colorectal cancer, largely because of the fiber and other nutrients they provide.

While some studies indicate that ***folic acid, calcium, vitamin D,*** and the antioxidant ***vitamins C, E,*** and ***A*** (beta carotene) offer protection against developing colorectal cancer, other studies have failed to confirm these findings and in some cases have flatly contradicted them. For now, the best advice regarding colorectal cancer and nutrition is to include in your daily diet whole grains—especially brown rice—and at least five fresh fruits and vegetables—especially cruciferous vegetables like cauliflower and broccoli—to ensure that you get ample fiber and many nutrients that may be protective.

PREVENTION

Eat plenty of fresh fruits, vegetables, and whole grains; cut back on red meat and other high-fat foods such as eggs and most dairy products. You can get the protein you need from low-fat dairy products, nuts, beans, lentils, and soybean products. Avoid overcooking or barbecuing meats and fish. To get more fiber, you can add wheat bran to your breakfast cereal.

Speak with your doctor about the latest evidence on ***aspirin*** and colorectal cancer. Some studies show that people who regularly take aspirin significantly reduce their risk for colorectal cancer, although other studies find no correlation. In any event, don't start taking aspirin on your own; it is a drug and can cause health problems if taken without a doctor's advice.

If you are over 50, make sure that you are being properly screened for colorectal cancer, especially if you are at high risk for the disease. Home test kits that check for blood in the stool are available at many drugstores. If such a test is positive, see your doctor. If your doctor finds a polyp, have it removed. ■

COMMON COLD

C

SYMPTOMS

- head and chest congestion, perhaps with a runny nose and difficulty breathing.
- sore throat.
- sneezing.
- dry cough that may occur only at night.
- chills.
- burning, watery eyes.
- allover, vague achiness.
- headache.
- constant fatigue.

CALL YOUR DOCTOR IF:

- your newborn (two months or younger) has cold symptoms. For infants, the common cold can be a serious illness.
- congestion makes it hard to breathe, or your chest makes a whistling sound (a wheeze) when you breathe. You may have ***asthma.***
- your throat hurts and your temperature is 101°F or higher; or your cold symptoms worsen after the third day. You may have a bacterial ***infection*** (such as ***strep throat***), ***sinusitis,*** or ***bronchitis.***
- your temperature is 103°F or higher. You may have ***pneumonia.* Seek medical care immediately.**
- your cold symptoms occur suddenly with exposure to certain triggers—such as pollen, cats, or perfume—and/or the symptoms continue for weeks. You probably have an ***allergy.***

The aptly named common cold is the most frequent ***infection*** in all age groups in the United States. Cold symptoms are triggered when a virus attaches itself to the lining of your nasal passages or throat. Your immune system responds by attacking the germ with white blood cells called neutrophils. If your immune system cannot recognize the virus, the response is "nonspecific," meaning your body produces as many neutrophils as possible (usually more than are needed) and circulates them to the infected sites. This all-out attack kills many viruses, but it doesn't affect the 200 or so viruses that cause colds. Extra neutrophils clumping together at infection sites is what causes the achiness and ***inflammation*** of a cold, complete with vast amounts of mucus in the nose and throat.

Cold symptoms settle in between one and four days after you are infected by a cold virus and typically last for about three days. At that point the worst is over, but you may feel congested for a week or more. During the first three days that you have symptoms, you are contagious (meaning you can pass the cold to others), so take preventive measures. *(See **Prevention,** page 283.)*

Although everyone catches colds, children have them more often than adults. Cold infections are most common during "cold season," which in the United States begins in late fall and runs through spring. During this time of the year people are more likely to congregate indoors, usually with some form of centralized heating on. Closer contact with others, which increases your chances of being exposed to contagious viruses, and hot, dry air, which dries the nose and throat tissues, help create a perfect environment for a viral infection.

Except in newborns, colds themselves are not dangerous. They usually go away in a week or so without any special medicine. Unfortunately, colds do wear down your body's resistance, making you more susceptible to bacterial infections.

CAUSES

More than 200 viruses can infect your nose and throat and cause the common cold. Unfortunately, there is no absolute cure for any of them, so determining which one is causing your cold won't help you recover any quicker. You "catch" a cold virus by breathing minute, airborne droplets from a cold sufferer's cough or sneeze, or by touching a virus-infected surface—such as a doorknob or telephone—and then transferring the germs to your nose or mouth.

DIAGNOSTIC AND TEST PROCEDURES

If your cold is nasty enough to send you to the doctor, your physician will likely examine your throat and ears and may take a throat culture (brushing your throat with a long cotton-tipped swab) to determine if you have a bacterial infection, which requires treatment with ***antibiotics.***

TREATMENT

Conventional and alternative medicine seek the same ends: to make it as easy as possible for your body to fight the cold virus while alleviating the aches and congestion as much as possible. Adequate rest is key to cold recovery; you may find you need 12 hours or more of sleep per night while you're fighting the cold. Drinking water is also important. Mucus flows freely in a well-hydrated body, helping you avoid or recover from infection; and healthy, moist tissues are harder for a virus to infect than dry tissues. If you have a fever, your body is using heat to help kill the cold virus. Giving medication to lower a fever can actually undermine your body's defense efforts. A temperature of 103°F or higher warrants a call to your physician, however.

Pregnant or nursing mothers should check with their doctor before using any type of cold therapy whatsoever, including over-the-counter drugs and herbal remedies.

CONVENTIONAL MEDICINE

No specific treatment exists for the virus that is causing your cold, but in treating your symptoms you can find relief. ***Ibuprofen*** can relieve achiness, but ***acetaminophen*** and ***aspirin*** may make congestion worse. Never give aspirin to a child with a fever; give acetaminophen instead *(see **Caution** below).* If your throat is sore, gargle as often as you like with salt water (½ tsp salt in 1 cup water).

It's tempting to acquiesce to an advertiser's claims and try one of the many over-the-counter "cold and flu" preparations, but think twice. These multisymptom drugs likely contain medications for symptoms you don't have, and therefore may result in needless overtreatment. Avoid them entirely for children under 13; even those cold preparations marketed especially for children don't seem to work for this age group, and the drugs commonly induce drowsiness, making everything worse. Over-the-counter ***decongestants*** (such as those containing ***pseudoephedrine***) can help break up nasal congestion, but only temporarily: If these drugs are taken regularly for more than five days, your body may "rebound" from them and produce even more mucus—and worse congestion. Pseudoephedrine increases blood pressure and heart rate; do not take it without first checking with your doctor if you have ***heart disease, high blood pressure, prostate problems, diabetes,*** or ***thyroid problems.***

Over-the-counter ***cough suppressants,*** such as those containing ***dextromethorphan,*** can be helpful if your cough is so severe that it interferes

CAUTION!

Never give *aspirin* to a child with a fever; give *acetaminophen* instead. Reye's syndrome, a neurological disease that can cause coma, brain damage, and death, has been linked to aspirin use in children aged 4 to 15. Reye's syndrome is rare, but typically follows a viral infection: One to three days after the virus has set in, the child becomes extremely tired, vomits heavily, and may be agitated, delirious, and/or confused. Reye's syndrome is an emergency that requires urgent intravenous fluid replacement.

C

with sleeping or talking. Otherwise, allow yourself to cough as you need to (always covering your mouth as you do), because coughing removes mucus and germs from your throat and lungs. Over-the-counter ***antihistamines*** can temporarily make breathing easier, but at a cost: They clear the nose by drying it up, making nasal mucus thicker and harder to drain.

ALTERNATIVE CHOICES

Time is of the essence: Begin to treat your cold as soon as you feel the first symptom. Especially with herbal remedies, an early response often results in a faster and more comfortable recovery.

AROMATHERAPY

Herbal steam can reduce congestion, and if the vapor temperature is 110°F or higher, it will also kill cold germs on contact. Choose ***eucalyptus*** *(Eucalyptus globulus),* wintergreen *(Gaultheria procumbens),* or ***peppermint*** *(Mentha piperita).* Place either fresh leaves or a few drops of the herb's oil in a bowl and pour in boiling water. Place a towel over your head, lean over the bowl to create a steam tent, and breathe the vapors.

HERBAL THERAPIES

Taken at the first sign of symptoms, osha *(Ligusticum porteri)* and ***echinacea*** (*Echinacea* spp.) can reduce a cold's intensity and duration, often even preventing it from becoming a full-fledged infection. Osha's anti-viral properties fight the cold virus directly. Take 15 to 20 drops of osha tincture three times a day for 7 to 10 days. Echinacea apparently stimulates the immune response, enhancing resistance to all infection. Take two capsules, or 15 drops of glycerated tincture, twice a day for 7 to 10 days. ***Goldenseal*** *(Hydrastis canadensis)* helps clear mucus from the throat. It also contains the natural antibiotic berberine, which can help prevent bacterial infections that often follow colds. Take two capsules, or 15 drops of glycerated tincture, twice a day for 7 to 10 days.

For a good "cold tea," combine equal parts of elder *(Sambucus nigra),* ***peppermint*** *(Mentha piperita),* and ***yarrow*** *(Achillea millefolium)* and steep 1 to 2 tsp of the mixture in 1 cup hot water. This blend can help the body handle fever and reduce achiness, congestion, and inflammation.

Garlic *(Allium sativum)* appears to shorten a cold's duration and severity. Any form seems to work: capsules or tablets, oil rubbed on the skin, or whole garlic roasted or cooked in other foods. If you elect capsules, take 3, three times daily, until the cold is over.

HOMEOPATHY

Cold symptoms often respond well to homeopathic remedies. The dosage is 12c or 30c, taken every two hours for a maximum of four doses. ***Gelsemium*** may help if you have chills, aching arms and legs, and fatigue, or if your throat hurts. When your runny nose feels as though it burns, your eyes water constantly, and you sneeze often, try ***Allium cepa.*** If you feel irritable and have a runny nose that becomes congested at night, take ***Nux vomica.*** For a barking cough, a burning sore throat, and a bitter taste that lingers in your mouth, try ***Aconite.***

LIFESTYLE

Refrain from smoking, especially when you have a cold. Smoking assaults the mucous membranes and lungs, increasing your susceptibility to all sorts of respiratory infections, including colds. Once you have a cold, smoke irritates the already-inflamed tissues, making healing and recovery more difficult.

NUTRITION AND DIET

Good nutrition is essential for resisting and recovering from a cold. Eat a balanced diet. Drink plenty of fluids. Take supplements as needed to ensure you are receiving the recommended dietary allowances for ***vitamin A,*** the ***vitamin B complex (vitamins B_1, B_2, B_5, B_6, folic acid),*** and ***vitamin C,*** as well as the minerals ***zinc*** and ***copper.*** If your diet is deficient in zinc, your body is low in neutrophils, and you're an easy mark for all types of infections, including colds. Zinc is available as a tablet or throat lozenge.

While you have a cold, avoid dairy products and white sugar, which tend to make mucus thicker.

COLD MYTHS

There may be as many myths about colds as there are viruses that cause them. To set the record straight, it's not prudent to starve—or feed—a cold. Let common sense and your appetite be your guide: If you are hungry, eat; if you aren't, don't. Low temperatures and dampness or moisture do not cause colds. For example, you will not catch cold from getting soaking wet and chilled in a rainstorm, going out in winter with wet hair, or sleeping near an open window. Antibiotics cannot cure colds, because they are only effective against bacteria, and colds are caused by viruses.

The last 20 years have witnessed much research into whether or not taking megadoses (1 gram or more each day) of ***vitamin C*** will prevent colds. The jury is still out. Results have varied, but it doesn't appear that megadoses of vitamin C can prevent colds. However, this dosage may lessen the duration and the severity of cold symptoms, possibly because vitamin C is essential for healthy neutrophils.

"Jewish penicillin," also known as chicken soup, has been heralded as a cold therapy since the 12th century. Recent scientific evidence supports the notion that chicken soup reduces cold symptoms, especially congestion. Something (yet to be determined) in the chicken soup keeps neutrophils from clumping together and causing inflammation.

Any food spicy enough to make your eyes water will have the same effect on your nose, promoting drainage. If you feel like eating, a hot, spicy choice will help your body fight your cold.

AT-HOME REMEDIES

- Eat honey-based hard candies or cough drops to soothe your sore throat, but stay away from minty ones; they can be drying. Sugar-based candies can increase mucus.
- Dab ***calendula*** *(Calendula officinalis)* ointment or petroleum jelly in and around your nostrils to protect against chafing and burning.
- Keep your body hydrated by drinking at least 10 glasses of water each day; this will replace the fluids lost through perspiration and your runny nose and minimize nasal and chest congestion. Keep a glass of water on your bedside table to sip during the night.
- Humidify your room (especially during the colder months when central heating dries the air) to keep your nose and throat tissues moist.

PREVENTION

A strong immune system is the best defense against all infections, colds included. Boost your body's natural resistance by eating well, not smoking, and drinking plenty of water every day. Minimize contact with people who have colds, or at the very least don't share towels, silverware, or beverages with them. Cold viruses often survive for hours in the open, on doorknobs, money, and other surfaces, so wash your hands frequently.

When you have a cold, do your best to keep it to yourself. A hearty sneeze can carry your cold virus up to 12 feet away, so always cover your mouth when you sneeze (or cough).

Regular, moderate exercise (such as walking for 45 minutes, five times a week) appears to strengthen the immune system and make you less likely to get colds and other infections. Saunas may also help: Swedish researchers have evidence that taking at least two saunas each week can keep you from succumbing to a cold. The reason is unclear, although the sauna's heat may prevent cold germs from reproducing. ■

CONGESTION

Read down this column to find your symptoms. Then read across.

SYMPTOMS	AILMENT/PROBLEM
◆ runny or stuffed nose; scratchy or sore throat; sneezing; head, muscle, and bone aches; thin, clear nasal discharge that turns thick and greenish yellow.	◆ ***Common Cold***
◆ stuffed nose; headache; increasing pressure and pain in the face behind or over the eyebrows, between or over the eyes, on the bridge of the nose, or in the cheeks, upper jaw, or teeth; possible puslike nasal discharge.	◆ Sinus infection
◆ high fever; sometimes, sudden chills, headache, muscle and joint aches, and exhaustion; may be followed by a runny or stuffed nose, nosebleeds, hoarseness, dry cough, and watery eyes.	◆ ***Flu***
◆ stuffed nose with watery discharge; frequent sneezing; itchy eyes and roof of mouth; headache, irritability, exhaustion, possible insomnia.	◆ ***Hay Fever***
◆ a deep, hacking cough that, a day or two later, produces phlegm; tightness or soreness in the chest; possible pain beneath the breastbone when breathing deeply; slight fever, chills, and fatigue.	◆ Acute ***Bronchitis***
◆ difficulty in breathing caused by excess mucus in the lungs; persistent, long-lasting cough with white, yellow, or green phlegm; some wheezing.	◆ Chronic ***Bronchitis***
◆ labored breathing caused by inflamed lung tissue; fever, chills, chest pain, muscle aches, sore throat, cough, and enlarged lymph glands in the neck.	◆ ***Pneumonia***
◆ cough with up to ½ cup of thick, puslike, greenish or blood-streaked, foul-smelling sputum; fever of 101°F or above; sweating, chills, bad breath, and loss of appetite.	◆ Lung abscess

WHAT TO DO	OTHER INFO
◆ See ***Common Cold.*** In some people, ***vitamin C*** may alleviate symptoms. Colds usually last a week or so; call your doctor if symptoms persist.	◆ Sometimes the first signs of a cold are irritability and restlessness.
◆ See ***Sinusitis.***	◆ Sinus pain may be even worse if you bend forward. Tapping, jolting, or jarring the tender area will hurt. Other symptoms include bad breath, high fever, and a feeling of the "blahs." A sinus infection may occasionally be caused by an abscessed or badly decayed tooth.
◆ See ***Flu.*** Call your doctor if symptoms worsen or new symptoms develop.	◆ Different strains of the flu produce different symptoms, including diarrhea, vomiting, and upset stomach. Children may develop swollen neck glands and respiratory problems such as choking and harsh breathing.
◆ See ***Hay Fever.*** Try to avoid, eliminate, and protect yourself from airborne substances, such as pollen, dust, mold, and pet dander, that might induce an allergic reaction.	◆ Many medications can relieve the symptoms of hay fever. Be aware of possible side effects, such as drowsiness.
◆ See ***Bronchitis,*** especially those sections dealing with the acute form. Call your doctor if your phlegm is blood streaked, your symptoms last more than a week, or your cough interferes with your normal activities and sleep.	◆ Repeated attacks of acute bronchitis may be caused by your environment. The combination of polluted air and cold and damp may increase your susceptibility. Recurrent attacks of acute bronchitis may lead to chronic bronchitis.
◆ See ***Bronchitis.*** Call your doctor now if you have symptoms of chronic bronchitis. Stop smoking and avoid irritants.	◆ Chronic bronchitis is a serious form of chronic obstructive pulmonary disease (COPD).
◆ See ***Pneumonia.*** There are several types of pneumonia (all serious). Call your doctor now for proper diagnosis and treatment.	◆ Although most people recover completely, pneumonia can be deadly for infants and the very old.
◆ Lung abscesses result from dental disease, ***pneumonia,*** or other infection and can be treated with ***antibiotics.*** Call your doctor for appropriate diagnosis and treatment.	◆ When treated appropriately, an acute lung abscess can be completely cured without surgery. If it is not treated correctly, an acute lung abscess can become chronic.

CONJUNCTIVITIS

SYMPTOMS

- Burning itchy eyes that discharge a heavy, sticky mucus may indicate **bacterial conjunctivitis.**
- Copious tears, a swollen lymph node, and a light discharge of mucus from one eye are signs of **viral conjunctivitis.**
- Redness, intense itching, and tears in the eyes may indicate **allergic conjunctivitis.**

See also ***Eye Problems*** and the ***Visual Diagnostic Guide.***

CALL YOUR DOCTOR IF:

- you physically injure your eye. Eye injuries can become infected and lead to corneal ulcers, which can endanger your eyesight.
- your eyes become red when you wear contact lenses. Remove the lenses immediately and see your ophthalmologist; you may have a corneal infection.
- the redness in your eye is affecting your vision and is accompanied by severe pain or excessive yellow or green discharge. You may have a ***staph infection*** or a streptococcal infection *(see **Strep Throat**).*
- your conjunctivitis frequently recurs or appears to be getting worse after a week of home treatment; you may have a bacterial or viral infection.
- your newborn baby's eyes are inflamed and are not producing tears; this may indicate **ophthalmia neonatorum,** which must be treated immediately to prevent permanent eye damage.

The conjunctiva—the transparent membrane that lines your eyeball and your eyelid—can become inflamed for various reasons. Most cases of conjunctivitis run a predictable course, and the inflammation usually clears up in a few days. Although conjunctivitis can be highly contagious, it is rarely serious and will not damage your vision if detected and treated promptly.

Bacterial conjunctivitis, commonly known as **pinkeye,** usually infects both eyes and produces a heavy discharge of mucus.

Viral conjunctivitis is usually limited to one eye, causing copious tears and a light discharge.

Allergic conjunctivitis produces tears, itching, and redness in the eyes, and sometimes an itchy, runny nose.

Ophthalmia neonatorum is an acute form of **inclusion conjunctivitis** in newborn babies. It must be treated immediately by a physician to prevent permanent eye damage or blindness.

CAUSES

Conjunctivitis is caused by a bacterial or viral infection or by an allergic reaction to pollen, smoke, or other material that irritates your eyes. Children sometimes contract conjunctivitis after a cold or sore throat. Redness and inflammation of the conjunctiva can also be brought on by eyestrain, ***stress,*** and poor nutrient levels.

Ophthalmia neonatorum may occur if the baby's tear ducts are not completely opened or if the infant is exposed to bacteria when passing through the birth canal of a mother infected with ***chlamydia*** or ***gonorrhea.*** The herpesvirus may also be associated with conjunctivitis and corneal infection.

TREATMENT

Traditionally, at-home remedies have been sufficient for soothing conjunctivitis associated with uncomplicated colds, minor infections, or allergies. Treatment consists primarily of cleansing the eyes and preventing the condition from spreading.

A PROTECTIVE LAYER

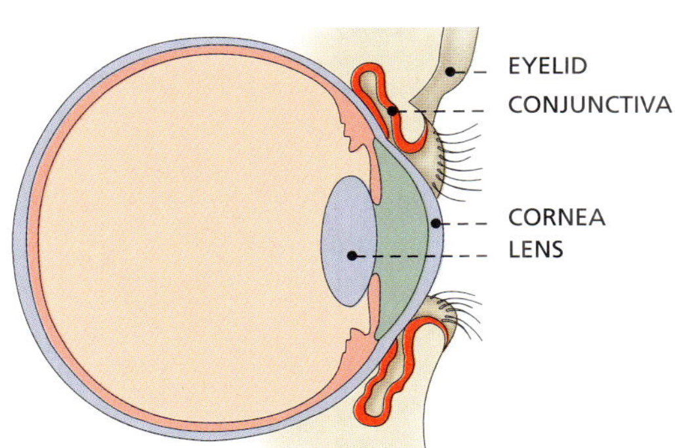

The conjunctiva is a thin, protective membrane that covers the exposed white of the eye and the inside of the eyelid. Bacterial conjunctivitis—sometimes called pinkeye—is the result of an infection that makes the conjunctiva red, teary, and itchy, with a thick, greenish yellow discharge. When conjunctivitis is caused by an allergy, the discharge is clear and watery.

CONVENTIONAL MEDICINE

If your conjunctivitis symptoms do not appear to be associated with a cold or allergy, you may want to see your doctor or an ophthalmologist for a medical diagnosis. For **bacterial conjunctivitis,** the treatment will probably call for ***antibiotic*** eye drops or ointment. **Allergic conjunctivitis** may respond to ***antihistamine*** or steroid eye drops, but you should not use steroid drops for either **bacterial** or **viral conjunctivitis.**

ALTERNATIVE CHOICES

Alternative therapies rely on natural remedies to soothe your irritated eyes and ease the itching and inflammation.

HERBAL THERAPIES

Using an eyecup, wash the eye several times a day with one of the following solutions. In each case, cool and strain the eyewash through coffee filter paper before using.

◆ 1 tsp dried ***eyebright*** *(Euphrasia officinalis)* steeped in 1 pt boiling water.

◆ 2 to 3 tsp ***chamomile*** *(Matricaria recutita)* in 1 pt boiling water.

HOMEOPATHY

Depending on your symptoms, take the following remedies four times daily for one or two days:

◆ for stinging eyes and red, puffy eyelids, ***Apis*** 12x or 30c.

◆ for bloodshot eyes and a gritty feeling, *Argentum nitricum* 12x or 30c.

◆ for itchy eyes with a sticky, yellow discharge, ***Pulsatilla*** 12x or 30c.

AT-HOME REMEDIES

You can cleanse and soothe irritated eyes with a prepared boric acid eyewash, or try the herbal eyewashes above. To relieve discomfort of **bacterial** or **viral conjunctivitis,** apply a warm compress for 5 to 10 minutes, three to four times a day. For **allergic conjunctivitis,** place a cool compress or a cool, moist tea bag on your closed eye. If the condition does not improve in five days, consult an ophthalmologist.

PREVENTION

Bacterial and **viral conjunctivitis** are highly contagious. Unless you take preventive measures, the condition may spread to your other eye or to other people.

◆ Wash your hands often and well.

◆ Keep your hands away from the infected eye.

◆ Do not share washcloths, towels, pillowcases, or handkerchiefs with other family members.

◆ Change your washcloth, towel, and pillowcase after each use, and wash them thoroughly.

◆ Do not use other people's eye cosmetics, particularly eye pencils and mascara.

If your child gets **pinkeye,** keep him or her out of school for a few days. Once one student comes down with conjunctivitis, it is not uncommon for it to spread to an entire class. ■

CONSTIPATION

C

SYMPTOMS

- hard, compacted stools that are difficult or painful to pass.
- no bowel movements in three days for adults, four days for children.

CALL YOUR DOCTOR IF:

- your constipation is associated with fever and lower abdominal pain, and your stools are thin or loose; these symptoms may be an indication of ***diverticulitis.***
- you have blood in your stools; this may be from a fissure or ***hemorrhoid*** but could also be a sign of ***colorectal cancer;*** changes in your bowel movement pattern, such as passing pencil-thin stools, may also signal colorectal cancer.
- your constipation develops after you start a new prescription drug or take vitamin or mineral supplements; you may need to discontinue or change dosage.
- you or your child has been constipated for two weeks, with recurrent abdominal pain; this could be a sign of lead poisoning or other serious ailment *(see **Environmental Poisoning**).*
- you are elderly or disabled and have been constipated for a week or more; you may have an impacted stool.

Your digestive system is remarkably efficient: In the space of a few hours it extracts nutrients from the foods you eat and drink, processes them into the bloodstream, and prepares leftover material for disposal. That material passes through 20 or more feet of intestine before being stored temporarily in the colon, where water is removed. The residue is excreted through the bowels, normally within a day or two.

Some people—including many alternative therapists—say we should move our bowels one to three times a day to remain healthy, but this opinion is not backed by scientific studies. Depending on your diet, your age, and your daily activity, regularity can mean anything from three bowel movements a day to one every three days. Nonetheless, the longer fecal material sits in the colon, the harder the stool becomes and the more difficult it is to pass. A normal stool should not be either unusually hard or soft, and you shouldn't have to strain unreasonably to pass it.

CAUSES

Our busy, modern lifestyles may be responsible for most cases of constipation: not eating enough fiber or drinking enough water, not getting enough exercise, and not taking the time to respond to an unmistakable urge to defecate. Emotional and psychological problems can contribute to the problem. Persistent, chronic constipation may also be a symptom of more serious disorders, including ***irritable bowel syndrome,*** diverticulosis *(see **Diverticulitis**),* ***colorectal cancer, diabetes, Parkinson's disease, multiple sclerosis,*** and ***depression.***

Bowel habits tend to vary with age and circumstances. Bottle-fed babies, for example, tend to have firmer stools and more bouts of constipation than breast-fed babies. Some children become constipated when they start school or other activities because they are embarrassed to ask permission to use the toilet. Being sensitive to pain, children may avoid the toilet if they have minor splits or tears in the anus from straining or other irritations.

For various reasons, constipation tends to be more common among women, especially during pregnancy. Constipation in the elderly usually occurs for lack of dietary fiber and lack of exercise. Some drugs and vitamin supplements can cause constipation: opiates such as morphine and ***codeine;*** aluminum salts in ***antacids;*** some dietary ***iron*** and ***calcium*** supplements; and certain ***antihistamines, diuretics, antidepressants,*** antipsychotics, and blood-pressure medications. If you are susceptible to constipation, pay particular attention to the potential side effects of recommended or prescribed medications, and ask your doctor or pharmacist about alternatives if constipation strikes.

DIAGNOSTIC AND TEST PROCEDURES

Occasional constipation does not justify visiting a doctor, but you should seek professional advice for a persistent problem. The doctor will first examine your abdomen for any sign of a hardened mass and may conduct a rectal exam. To check for systemic problems, your doctor may take blood samples. The doctor may examine your colon with a sigmoidoscope, a flexible tube with a magnifying viewer, which is inserted into the rectum. You might also need a barium enema, which coats the intestinal lining so it can be seen on an x-ray.

TREATMENT

Most cases of constipation respond to conservative treatment, such as dietary changes or mild laxatives. Severe or chronic cases will prompt your physician to test for systemic causes and other diseases.

CONVENTIONAL MEDICINE

Your doctor will probably start treatment by getting more fiber or bulk into your diet. For stubborn constipation in older children or adults, the doctor may recommend a nondigestible sugar called lactulose or specially formulated electrolyte solutions. Except for fiber or bulking agents, over-the-counter laxatives should be avoided. Your doctor will also encourage you to take adequate time for moving your bowels and not to suppress the urge to have a bowel movement.

Fecal impaction is a more serious form of constipation that sometimes affects the elderly and disabled. To release hardened material in the rectum, a doctor inserts a gloved finger and manually breaks up the solidified stool. A gentle enema using warm water or mineral oil may also be helpful.

ALTERNATIVE CHOICES

Like many conventional doctors, most practitioners of alternative medicine approach constipation as a lifestyle problem. Corrective measures include increasing fiber consumption, exercising regularly, and setting a routine time to move your bowels. In addition to the following treatments, acupuncture may relieve chronic constipation.

EXERCISE

Walking for 20 to 30 minutes at a pace fast enough to "get the heart pumping," or a good session at some other exercise, helps stimulate the bowels. Doctors say regular exercise, besides offering cardiac benefits, is an excellent way to correct chronic constipation. People should become accustomed to regular exercise when they are young, so it becomes a healthy, lifelong habit.

HERBAL THERAPIES

Your health food store will have a selection of potentially useful herbal remedies. Try small amounts to test the effect they have on you or take them as recommended by a naturopath. Avoid herbal laxatives containing ***senna*** *(Cassia senna)* or ***buckthorn*** *(Rhamnus purshiana);* they can damage the lining and injure the nerves of the colon, and you can become dependent on them.

HOMEOPATHY

For relief of mild constipation, you can find prepared remedies at a health food store. If your stools are soft but you have to strain to pass them, try remedies containing ***Bryonia.***

C

LIFESTYLE

Simply recognizing the need to move the bowels solves many cases of constipation. Children respond to praise for sitting on the toilet and having regular bowel movements, and they can be trained at an early age.

For people who are convinced that regular bowel habits are important, the treatment is easy: Sit on the toilet every day at the same time for about 10 minutes, even if you don't have an urge to move your bowels. The best time is after a meal, because food in the stomach stimulates the colon to move. Be patient: It may take a couple of months before this new habit begins to work for you. Remember, however, to heed your body's own signals and never resist the urge to move your bowels at other times.

NUTRITION AND DIET

Almost all Americans should eat more fiber. The American Dietetic Association recommends 30 grams of fiber a day, yet many people consume less than half that amount. Increasing your fiber intake is easy: Eat more raw fruits and vegetables—especially peas, beans, and broccoli—bran cereals, whole grains, whole-wheat bread, and dried fruits such as raisins, figs, and prunes. A bonus is that most of these foods are rich in vitamins and minerals, yet lower in calories than most processed foods.

It is never too early to start a healthy diet. Children as young as six months can be fed whole-grain cereals, which have more fiber and more nutrients than processed cereals. Even fast-food addicts can be tempted into snacking on fruit and raw vegetables. Otherwise, try a soluble or insoluble fiber supplement like ***psyllium*** *(Plantago psyllium),* which becomes gelatinous when combined with water and adds bulk to the stool. Drink 1 to 2 rounded tsp of powdered psyllium a day, stirred into a glass of cold water or juice, or include an equal amount of powdered flaxseed *(Linum usitatissimum),* available in many health food stores. Follow with 8 oz of plain water. Psyllium generally works within two days, but you can take it every day and not become dependent on it.

The insoluble fiber wheat bran works as well

ACUPRESSURE

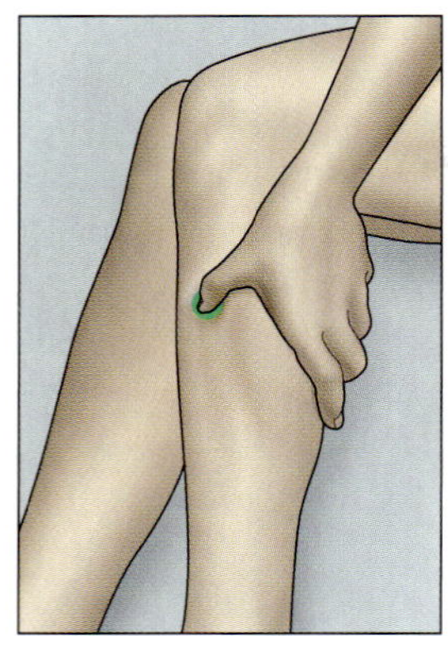

1 Digestion may be improved by steady finger pressure on Stomach 36, four finger widths below the kneecap just outside the shinbone. Maintain pressure for one minute, then switch legs. To verify the location, flex your foot; you should feel a muscle bulge at the point site.

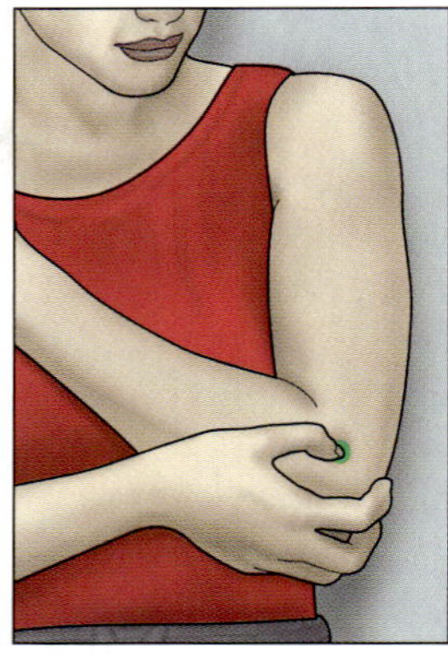

2 As an aid to relieving constipation, try applying pressure to Large Intestine 11, on the outer edge of the inside elbow crease. With the arm bent, press deeply into the point with your thumb for one minute, then repeat on the other arm.

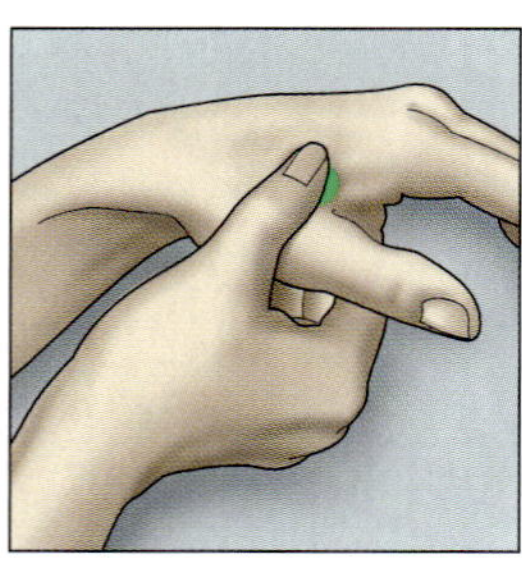

3 Pressing Large Intestine 4 in the web between your thumb and index finger may help relieve constipation. Use the thumb and index finger of your right hand to squeeze the web of your left hand for one minute. Repeat on the right hand. Do not use this point if you are pregnant.

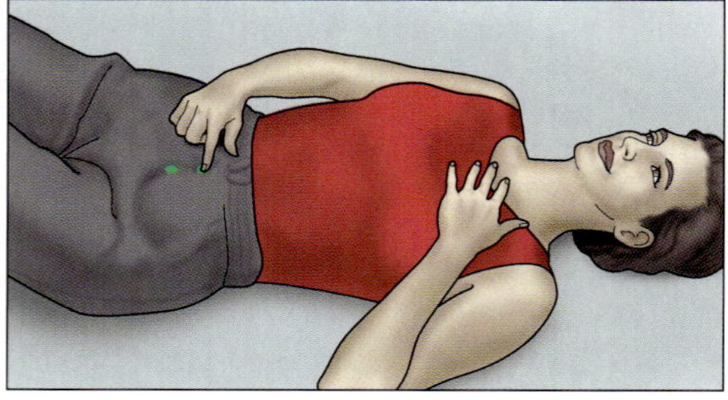

4 Pressure on Conception Vessel 6 may help ease abdominal pains from constipation. The point is about three finger widths below the navel. Using the index finger of one hand, press inward as far as you can, then inhale slowly and deeply. Relax and exhale.

as psyllium but may give you gas for a few weeks until your system adjusts to the change. You can mix wheat bran with fruit juice, canned fruit or cereal, or sprinkle it into sandwiches. Start by taking 1 tbsp a day, and gradually increase it to 3 or 4 spoonfuls.

Take one *Lactobacillus acidophilus* capsule, twice a day for 30 days. The cultures in the capsules aid digestion by helping break down food. Finally, an old folk remedy for stimulating the bowels is drinking a glass of warm water with the juice of a whole lemon in it after waking up in the morning.

YOGA

The Cobra position is considered one of the best for toning the abdominal organs. Lie on your stomach, with the your forehead resting on the ground and your legs together. Place your hands, palms down, just beneath your shoulders, keeping your elbows close to your body. Inhale and lift your head and chest off the floor with your head aligned with your spine. Only your torso should be raised; your pelvis should touch the floor. Look forward and hold this position for 15 to 20 seconds. Exhale and slowly bring your torso and head back down. Do this up to three times a day.

The knee-to-chest pose is intended to activate the abdominal organs and relieve gas. Lie on your back with your arms at your sides. Lift your right knee up toward the chest. Grasp your right knee with your hands, and pull your leg in, squeezing your abdomen; hold for 15 to 20 seconds. Repeat with the other leg. Do this up to three times a day.

AT-HOME REMEDIES

- ◆ Eat 30 grams of dietary fiber a day. Some good sources are bran, whole grains such as brown rice, and other whole-grain cereals, raw or cooked dried fruits like raisins and prunes, cooked dried beans, popcorn, and nuts.
- ◆ Drink six to eight glasses of water daily, in addition to your regular beverages with meals.

BREAK THE LAXATIVE HABIT

Constipation—real or imagined—is one of the most common medical complaints. In the United States alone, people spend hundreds of millions of dollars a year on laxatives. In many cases, it's not money well spent.

If you take laxative products regularly, your body may become dependent on them, and your constipation is likely to get worse. If you must take laxatives, however, the best ones are fiber-based. They may take a bit longer to work than patent purgatives, but they don't abuse your digestive system.

In any case, don't take over-the-counter laxatives for more than a few days at any one time, and never take a laxative if you have abdominal pain or nausea, if you are vomiting, or if you are pregnant.

- ◆ Go to the toilet at the same time every day—preferably after a meal—and take enough time to let your bowels move fully. If you need to move your bowels at other times, don't resist the urge.

PREVENTION

The key to preventing constipation is simple enough: Drink adequate amounts of water—six to eight glasses a day is a good rule—and get sufficient fiber by eating fruits, vegetables, and grains. Fiber is critical because most of our stool is actually made up of bacteria, and fiber gives bacteria a good foundation to grow on. Ample bacterial action results in a larger volume of stool and better bowel function. ■

CORNS AND CALLUSES

SYMPTOMS

- A **hard corn** is a compact patch of hard skin with a dense core, located on the top of a toe, the outside of the little toe, or the sole of the foot.
- A **soft corn** is a reddened area of skin up to one-half inch in diameter, with a thin, smooth center, on the side of a toe.
- A **seed corn** is a pluglike circle of dead skin on the heel or ball of the foot.
- A **callus** is a patch of compact, dead skin up to an inch wide on the soles of the feet, the palms of the hands, or any area subject to friction.
- A **plantar callus** is compact dead skin up to an inch wide on the sole of the foot, with a distinctive white center.
- A **hereditary callus** is an area of dead skin up to an inch wide occurring where there is no apparent friction or pressure, such as on the sole of the foot or palm of the hand. This condition runs in families and is usually seen in children.

See also the ***Visual Diagnostic Guide.***

CALL YOUR DOCTOR IF:

- you cut a corn or callus; the break in the skin invites ***infection.***
- a corn discharges pus or clear fluid; it is infected or ulcerated. Either condition requires medical attention.
- you develop a corn and you suffer from ***diabetes, atherosclerosis,*** or other ***circulatory problems.*** You run the risk of developing a secondary infection.

As annoying as corns and calluses can be, the reason your body forms them is to protect sensitive skin that presses or rubs against underlying bone. Corns generally occur on the toes and balls of the feet, while calluses can develop on hands, feet, or anywhere there is repeated friction—even on a violinist's chin.

A **hard corn** is a small patch of thickened, dead skin with a packed nucleus; a **soft corn** has a much thinner surface and usually occurs between the toes. A **seed corn,** the least common type, is a patch of stiff skin around a tiny plug of cholesterol; a seed corn occurs only on the sole of the foot and often accompanies anhidrosis, or lack of perspiration.

Like corns, calluses have several variants. Besides the **common callus,** usually caused by friction on the hands or feet, there's the **plantar callus** on the sole of the foot and the **hereditary callus,** found on the soles or palms. All are larger than corns—up to an inch in diameter—and lack the corn's telltale center.

CAUSES

Although some corns and calluses on the feet develop from improper walking motion, most are caused by ill-fitting shoes. High-heeled shoes are the worst offenders, putting pressure on the toes and making women four times as likely as men to experience foot problems. **Soft corns** and **plantar calluses** may be caused by either friction or pressure. If your child develops a callus that has no clear source of pressure, it is probably a genetically determined **hereditary callus.** Feet spend most of their time in a closed, moist environment ideal for breeding bacteria; ***staph infections*** can start when bacteria enter corns through breaks in the skin and cause the infected corn to give off fluid or pus.

To find out whether a hard patch of skin is a callus or a ***wart,*** your doctor will scrape some skin off the affected area. Warts bleed, but calluses just reveal more dead skin. The distinction is useful, because warts are viral and resist treatment, while most calluses (except the hereditary kind) are easily correctable.

TREATMENT

Most corns and calluses gradually disappear when the friction or pressure is removed. To keep corns and calluses on the feet away, wear correctly fitted shoes.

CONVENTIONAL MEDICINE

Most podiatrists discourage the use of over-the-counter salicylic-acid corn remedies; applied improperly, corn plasters can kill healthy tissue around the corn. Properly positioned moleskin pads can help relieve pressure on a corn. Oral ***antibiotics*** generally clear up infected corns, but sometimes pus has to be drained through an incision; over-the-counter antibacterial ointments are not effective against infected corns, because most staph bacteria are resistant to them.

Hydrocortisone creams may help remove cracked calluses. Apply the cream and cover the area overnight with a plastic bag or a sock. In the morning, rub off as much of the callus as you can with a coarse towel or brush. Using a pumice to rub the dead skin from a callus after showering, then applying urea-based cream, can also be effective. Do not try this with corns; rubbing will just make them more tender and painful.

You can consider surgery to remove a **plantar callus,** but it is likely to come back anyway. A better approach is to keep your feet dry and friction free. Wear properly fitted shoes and cotton socks, not wool or synthetic fibers that might irritate the skin. If a podiatrist or orthopedist thinks your corn or callus is caused by abnormal foot placement or hip rotation, orthopedic shoe inserts may help correct the problem.

ALTERNATIVE CHOICES

BODY WORK

Some practitioners of alternative medicine work to correct your body imbalance when standing and walking. Types of body work that might help people who suffer from chronic corns and calluses include **Rolfing, Aston-Patterning,** and the **Feldenkrais method**.

HERBAL THERAPIES

Apply a ***calendula*** *(Calendula officinalis)* salve two or three times a day to corns or calluses to soften tissue and prevent inflammation.

HYDROTHERAPY

To soothe irritated feet, try a good soak in warm water with Epsom salt. To soften tender corns, rub them with lemon juice.

AT-HOME REMEDIES

The best therapy for corns and calluses is to find the cause of the friction and remove it. In the meantime, be kind to your feet:

- Soak your feet in an Epsom salt footbath every day to soothe and soften the skin.
- Apply ***hydrocortisone cream*** or a ***calendula-*** based ointment to a cracked callus. ***Aloe*** *(Aloe barbadensis)* cream is also good for soothing and healing the skin.
- Elevate your feet and expose them to fresh air whenever possible.
- Use pumice or a callus file to gently rub dead skin off a callus, but never rub a corn.
- Don't cut or pare away dead skin yourself. Cutting a corn or callus may lead to ***infection.***

PREVENTION

When it comes to corns and calluses, prevention is better than cure. Have both feet professionally measured and buy only properly fitting shoes. Be sure the width is correct and allow up to half an inch between your longest toe and the front of the shoe. Avoid pointed shoes and high heels. Women who wear stylish shoes at work can take some of the pressure off their feet by walking to and from the office in correctly fitted athletic shoes.

Have your shoes repaired regularly. Worn soles give little protection from the shock of walking on hard surfaces, and worn linings can chafe the skin and harbor bacteria. Worn heels increase uneven pressure on the heel bone, which supports 25 percent of your weight. If the soles or heels of your shoes tend to wear unevenly, see an orthopedist about corrective shoes or insoles. ■

COUGH

SYMPTOMS

More important than the cough itself are aspects of it that provide clues to its cause:

- frequency and duration of the cough.
- length of the coughing spell.
- type of material being coughed up (mucus or phlegm, blood).
- color of the sputum (white, clear, green, yellow, pink, blood-specked).
- consistency of the material coughed up (thick, thin, frothy).
- presence or absence of accompanying pain.

CALL YOUR DOCTOR IF:

- your cough lasts for more than 7 to 10 days; it may be a sign of a serious disease.
- your cough produces yellow, green, pink, or rust-colored sputum.
- your cough is exhausting, persistent, and accompanied by any of the following signs: hoarseness, sore throat, shortness of breath, wheezing, chest pains or tightness, fever of 101°F or higher, headache, back and leg aches, fatigue, rashes, or weight loss. A cough combined with one or more of these symptoms indicates an underlying ailment.

Although it is usually unwelcome and involuntary, a cough is not itself an illness, but rather a protective reflex. Generally, the reflex kicks in when the membranes lining the respiratory tract secrete excessive mucus or phlegm. These secretions help to protect your airways from infections and irritants by trapping and flushing out viruses, bacteria, and foreign particles. Coughing is your body's way of getting rid of this accumulation. The sudden burst of air in a cough not only helps to keep the breathing passages open, but also may prevent infectious mucus from falling into your lungs and bronchial tubes, where it could lead to such serious infections as ***pneumonia*** or ***bronchitis.*** *(See also* ***Respiratory Problems****.)*

Although coughs have many different patterns, they may be categorized according to two characteristics—duration and productivity. Duration refers to how long the person needs to cough. A cough can come and go quickly, as when you cough up something stuck in your throat; it can last for several days if you have a cold; or it can be persistent and chronic, as when you have chronic ***bronchitis.***

A productive cough is one that produces some of the sputum (mucus or phlegm) that protects the lungs and other parts of the lower respiratory tract. A nonproductive, or dry, cough is often the result of irritation caused by mucus running from the nasal passages to the throat.

Although coughing is usually an involuntary act, it can also be voluntary—the result of a conscious decision. In addition, some people cough more often than others because individuals vary in the amount of irritation they can tolerate.

CAUSES

A cough can be caused by anything that irritates the respiratory airways enough to elicit the protective cough reflex. The most common cause is an acute respiratory tract infection, such as the ***common cold, flu,*** and ***sinusitis.*** In these cases the excessive mucus produced in response to the infection triggers the cough.

Coughs can also be triggered when you accidentally inhale small objects, such as pieces of food, or breathe in irritants such as dust, cigarette smoke, and noxious fumes.

A harsh or forceful cough can itself be an irritant. Coughing causes the airways to contract; repeated contractions lead to irritation of the upper airways, and this prolongs the cough in a sort of vicious cycle.

A dry, nonproductive cough can be a side effect of drugs prescribed for other ailments. There are, for example, five types of ***angiotensin-converting enzyme (ACE) inhibitors,*** used in the treatment of ***high blood pressure*** and ***heart disease,*** that sometimes cause a dry cough. If you are taking one of these drugs and find you are coughing, ask your doctor to prescribe another. A persistent nonproductive cough that interferes with your sleep may indicate a condition called esophageal reflux, in which you involuntarily bring the acidic contents of your stomach back up into the esophagus and then inhale this material.

A chronic, persistent cough should always be considered abnormal. The cough may be caused by smoking, ***allergies, asthma,*** or chronic ***bronchitis,*** but it may also be an indication of ***emphysema, tuberculosis,*** or ***lung cancer.***

DIAGNOSTIC AND TEST PROCEDURES

Any persistent cough may be a symptom of an underlying illness. Your doctor will make the diagnosis based on the frequency, duration, and severity of the cough; breathing difficulties; the type of material being coughed up (the color and consistency of the mucus, phlegm, or blood); and the presence and location of any accompanying pain, swelling, or rash. The doctor may wish to obtain a chest x-ray and a sputum specimen to test for infection.

Although some of the chronic obstructive lung diseases in which coughing may be a symptom are incurable (***emphysema,*** some types of ***lung cancer,*** and occupation-related lung diseases, for example), most are treatable. If you have a dry cough along with leg and back aches, fever above 101°F, headache, and a sore throat, you may be diagnosed with ***flu.*** A productive cough in which the color of the sputum changes from white (which is normal) to yellow or green may signal infection, possibly ***bronchitis*** or ***sinusitis.*** If your cough is accompanied by difficulty in breathing, wheezing, and tightness in the chest, you may be diagnosed with bronchial ***asthma.*** A cough that produces blood, or pink, yellow, or rust-colored mucus, accompanied by chest pains, headache, fever, and difficulty in breathing, may be diagnosed as ***pneumonia.*** And if you have a hacking cough along with a pink rash, muscle aches, fever, and red eyes, you may be diagnosed with ***measles*** or ***German measles.***

TREATMENT

Most coughs are not dangerous. Therefore, if you have a nonproductive (dry) cough, along with a runny or stuffed-up nose, sore throat, and sneezing, you have all the classic symptoms of a com-

ATTENTION!

COUGHING UP BLOOD

Any cough that produces blood should be evaluated immediately. The underlying cause may or may not be serious, but you should have it checked. Be sure, however, that you are not confusing coughing up blood with blood in your mouth from bleeding gums or a nosebleed.

Hemoptysis (the medical term for coughing up blood) is caused by the rupturing of a blood vessel in the nose, throat, breathing passages, or lungs. The most common cause of a rupture is an infection such as bronchitis, tuberculosis, or pneumonia. Other causes include ailments that produce persistent coughing; blood clots in the lungs; lung cancer; and bleeding disorders such as hemophilia, a hereditary ailment characterized by spontaneous, excessive bleeding.

C

mon cold, and you should let it run its course.

Since coughing is a protective response by the body, suppressing it with cough medicine, particularly if it is a productive cough, not only reduces the protective clearing action but may serve to mask a more serious underlying problem. Use conventional or alternative cough remedies for no longer than 7 to 10 days and preferably only for temporary relief from nighttime coughing.

CONVENTIONAL MEDICINE

An ***antibiotic*** might be prescribed for an underlying bacterial infection. Antibiotics would not be prescribed for a viral infection such as the common cold, however. In that case, your doctor would just prescribe bed rest, ***aspirin*** or ***acetaminophen,*** plenty of fluids, and moist air (from a humidifier, vaporizer, or teakettle). If your cold or flu produces thick, sticky sputum, an ***expectorant*** may help to clear your lungs.

A nonproductive cough can be treated by one or more common therapies: throat soothers and ***cough suppressants,*** or ***antihistamines*** if your cough is caused by allergies. To relieve a cough's irritation, try cough drops, lozenges, and syrups. Your doctor might recommend a cough suppressant containing the narcotic drug ***codeine*** and requiring a physician's prescription, or nonprescription cough drops containing ***dextromethorphan.*** Many over-the-counter products contain topical anesthetics that will slightly numb your irritated throat and may provide temporary relief.

Ultimately, for any cough that persists for more than 7 to 10 days, seek medical advice. Based on the diagnosis, your doctor will prescribe the appropriate treatment for the underlying illness or problem.

COUGH MEDICATIONS

*Because coughing is a normal, protective attempt to clear your breathing passages of secretions, irritants, foreign objects, and blockages, it seldom should be stopped. Indeed, unless a physician so orders, children under the age of two should never be given any type of cough medicine. Coughing protects their sensitive lungs (see **Croup** and **Whooping Cough**).*

If your cough is productive, use a cough suppressant only for temporary relief. An expectorant cough medication may help to loosen the mucus or phlegm and clear your throat, but consuming large quantities of water will have the same effect. Dry, irritating coughs can be controlled by prescribed antitussives and some over-the-counter products. If your throat is dry and sore from coughing, you can try the various throat soothers, such as honey, lozenges, and cough drops.

ALTERNATIVE CHOICES

The following alternative therapies may ease the discomfort of acute or chronic respiratory infections. They do not treat the infection itself, but they may complement conventional care.

ACUPRESSURE

Sometimes a coughing fit can make the muscles in the upper back contract or go into spasm. To relieve the pain this causes, apply pressure to Lung 5 *(above, right).*

CHINESE HERBS

Sang ju yin, a decoction of mulberry leaf *(Folium mori albae)* and chrysanthemum *(Flos chrysanthemi morifolii),* is a classic cough treatment. It contains a number of other ingredients as well and is available in prepared form. Drink as directed for two to three days. If your cough does not improve, see a practitioner.

HERBAL THERAPIES

A wide variety of herbs act as stimulating or relaxing expectorants that help the body remove

ACUPRESSURE

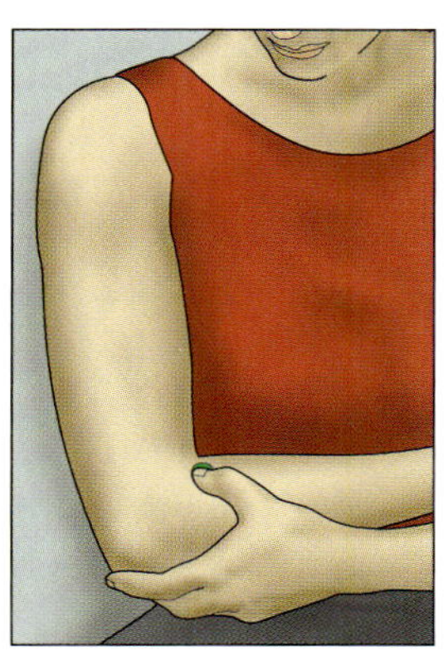

Pressing Lung 5 may help ease coughing spasms. Bend your left elbow and make a fist; place your right thumb on the outside crease of the elbow alongside the taut tendon. Press firmly for one minute, and repeat on the other arm. Do three times.

excess mucus from the airways. Stimulating expectorants increase the quantity and then liquefy viscous sputum so it can be cleared out by coughing. Relaxing expectorants loosen the sputum and are soothing if you have a dry, irritating cough.

Since most herbal traditions have remedies for specific types of coughs, you might want to check the many possibilities with an herbalist. However, a basic herbal cough tea that can be taken several times a day for three days consists of 2 parts ***coltsfoot*** *(Tussilago farfara)*, 2 parts ***marsh mallow*** *(Althaea officinalis)*, 2 parts ***hyssop*** *(Hyssopus officinalis)*, 1 part aniseed *(Pimpinella anisum)*, and 1 part ***licorice*** *(Glycyrrhiza glabra)*. Add 1 tbsp herb mix to 1 cup boiling water, steep for 20 minutes, and drink while hot.

HOMEOPATHY

Homeopaths recommend different remedies and dosage schedules for the beginning and later stages of various types of coughs. For relief of early symptoms, take one dose four times a day; for relief of persistent symptoms, take two doses a day for four days. If you are often thirsty and have painful bouts of dry coughs that intensify with the slightest movement, try ***Bryonia*** (12c). If your cough is accompanied by hoarseness, difficulty in breathing, and considerable rattling in the chest, take *Antimonium tartaricum* (12c). If your throat tickles and you get violent coughing fits whenever you lie down, try *Drosera* (12c). If the slightest draft of cool air initiates a tickling cough, take *Rumex crispus* (12c). If you happen to get chilled and develop a fever and a barking cough, try ***Aconite*** (12c).

NUTRITION AND DIET

The best thing to do for a cough is to drink plenty of liquids, four to six large glasses a day. A large intake of fluids will loosen the mucus and make coughing it up easier. Warm liquids, or just plain water, are best for this purpose. Try to avoid caffeinated or alcoholic beverages, which are diuretics that cause you to lose more liquid than you take in.

Conventional and alternative practitioners agree that you might speed recovery by drinking fresh fruit and vegetable juices. Some physicians recommend ***vitamin C*** supplements; others consider a well-balanced diet just as effective.

AT-HOME REMEDIES

Most of the treatments referred to above can be used at home. In addition to drinking plenty of liquids, including herbal teas, you may find relief by rubbing your throat and chest with essential oil of ***eucalyptus*** *(Eucalyptus globulus)* or ***myrrh*** *(Commiphora molmol)*. A simple rub might help you breathe more easily, cough less, and get a good night's sleep.

During the winter when the heat is on, use a vaporizer to keep the air from getting too dry, which can aggravate a cough.

Another way to reduce persistent night coughing is to sleep with the head of your bed raised six to eight inches. This prevents the pooling of secretions and the return of the irritating acidic contents from your stomach to your esophagus, which you may be breathing in *(see **Sore Throat**)*. Try to avoid caffeine and peppermint.

You can make an effective expectorant with a large onion and organic honey. Slice the onion into rings, place in a deep bowl, cover with honey, and let stand 10 to 12 hours. Strain and take a tablespoon of this mixture four or five times a day. ■

CROHN'S DISEASE

SYMPTOMS

- severe ***abdominal pain*** and ***diarrhea.***
- cramps or pain after eating, especially in the lower right side of the abdomen.
- chronic low-grade fever, loss of appetite, fatigue, or weight loss, especially if accompanied by persistent nausea and vomiting.
- ***arthritis,*** with the symptoms above.
- in young children, any of the symptoms above, plus failure to thrive; in older children, failure to grow at a normal rate.

CALL YOUR DOCTOR IF:

- you have a sudden attack of abdominal pain, fever, and the urge to pass gas or have a bowel movement; you may be in the initial stage of ***appendicitis*** or ***colitis.***
- you experience prolonged diarrhea, especially if you have had an ileostomy; you may become dangerously dehydrated.
- you have any of the symptoms above accompanied by vomiting; these may signal partial or complete intestinal blockage.

In Crohn's disease, a chronic disorder of the intestines, the gastrointestinal tract becomes inflamed and weak, making digestion difficult and leading to general physical debility. The symptoms are similar to ulcerative ***colitis;*** to distinguish between them, your doctor may need to examine a sample of intestinal tissue. The inflammation of Crohn's disease can occur anywhere in the intestinal tract, although it usually strikes the end of the small intestine or the colon.

Crohn's disease is typically diagnosed among people in their twenties and thirties, but the disease can also occur in infants and children. It is more common in women than in men, and it is rare in people of Asian or African descent. The disease is a lifelong ailment that can be controlled but not cured: Crohn's patients usually experience a roller-coaster ride of attacks of abdominal pain and diarrhea followed by weeks or months of remission.

A common complication of Crohn's disease is the development of fistulas that channel through the intestine or the skin itself, often near the anus. Surgery may be required to close the fistulas. Some Crohn's patients show a tendency toward nonintestinal disorders, such as inflammation of the eye, skin eruptions, ***kidney stones,*** or ***arthritis*** in the knees, ankles, and wrists. People who have had Crohn's for 20 years or more are at risk of developing ***colorectal cancer,*** so if you have Crohn's disease and are over 30, you should get regular checkups.

CAUSES

The actual cause of Crohn's disease is unknown, but it may be an autoimmune disorder. The inflammation apparently occurs when the body's own immune system—for reasons not yet understood—attacks a part of the intestine. *(See* ***Immune Problems.****)* Some scientists are studying whether a virus causes Crohn's, but no specific viral agent has been identified. Less likely suspects include food additives such as silica, a chalky substance added to toothpaste and some dietary supplements, and carrageenan, a seaweed derivative widely used as a thickening agent in ice cream and many other dairy products. It is clear, however, that smokers have a greater risk of developing Crohn's than nonsmokers and a poorer prognosis if they continue smoking after developing the disease.

Some ***antibiotics*** can cause fever, abdominal pain, and diarrhea—symptoms similar to those of Crohn's disease. Parasitic illnesses such as giardiasis, which can be contracted by drinking water from springs and streams, also cause Crohn's-like symptoms.

DIAGNOSTIC AND TEST PROCEDURES

Crohn's disease can usually be diagnosed from x-rays of the large and small intestines. Your physician may also do a sigmoidoscopy to view the intestines and may take a tiny sample of tissue from the intestinal lining for examination under the microscope.

TREATMENT

At present, Crohn's disease is not curable. Medical treatment typically involves a three-stage approach to controlling the disease—depending on the severity of the symptoms—beginning with drug therapy and a restricted diet, then hospital treatment, and if necessary, surgery.

CONVENTIONAL MEDICINE

You and your doctor will work together to minimize attacks by finding the combination of medications and dosages that works best for you. Some doctors believe Crohn's patients remain free from attacks longer if they take maintenance doses of drugs even when the symptoms are not present; others wait until the patient has recognizable symptoms before prescribing anything. Children with Crohn's disease may need high-protein, high-calorie liquid supplements to keep their growth on track.

Sulfasalazine, an intestinal anti-inflammatory agent, is the cornerstone of conventional medical treatment. It may be prescribed for years at a stretch and is given in varying dosages depending on the severity of the symptoms. Steroids such as ***prednisone*** are often prescribed with sulfasalazine to reduce the inflammation of the intestines. Most doctors are wary of prescribing steroids for longer than a few months, however, because of the potentially severe side effects. To reduce the need for steroids, an immunosuppressant such as azathioprine may be substituted. Your doctor may also prescribe an ***antidiarrheal*** agent containing ***codeine*** for mild bouts of diarrhea. You will probably be put on a bland, well-balanced diet.

If you become severely ill with diarrhea and are losing weight, your doctor may want you to be hospitalized while you receive steroids intravenously. Your doctor may also recommend intravenous (IV) feedings, which allow the intestines to rest. After stabilization, some patients may need IV feedings at home with the help of a visiting nurse.

If the disease does not respond to drugs and diet, your doctor may recommend surgery. A partial colectomy removes the damaged section of the colon but preserves the bowel if possible. In

THE ILEUM AND COLON

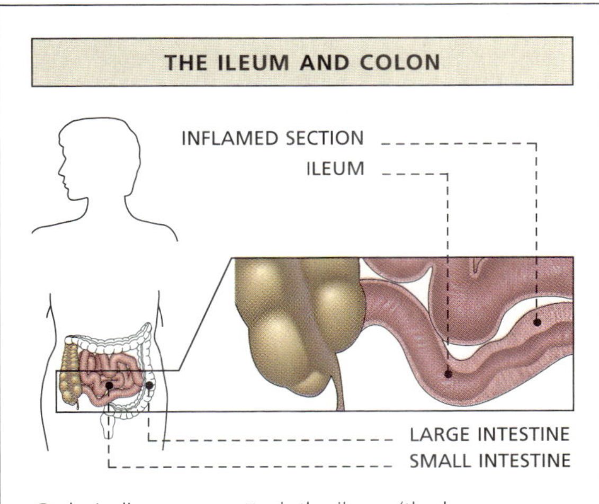

Crohn's disease can attack the ileum (the lower portion of the small intestine) or the colon (large intestine). Ulcers form on the inner intestinal lining and eventually spread through the intestinal wall. As the affected part of the intestine becomes scarred and thick, the passage narrows, disrupting nutrient absorption and normal bowel function.

a total colectomy, the entire colon is removed and the end of the small intestine is brought to the surface with an ostomy bag for evacuation. (This part of the procedure is known as an ileostomy.) Although the disease may recur after surgery, the symptoms are likely to be less severe and less debilitating than before.

To help you cope with the stresses of having Crohn's disease, your doctor may suggest group therapy, sponsored by the Crohn's and Colitis Foundation or by a local hospital. If you have undergone an ileostomy, you can receive support and tips from your local chapter of the United Ostomy Association.

ALTERNATIVE CHOICES

While Crohn's disease is not curable, many people with mild forms of the disease or Crohn's-like symptoms have found ways to relieve intestinal distress short of drugs or surgery.

ACUPUNCTURE

A trained acupuncturist will ask detailed questions about you and your symptoms of pain and diarrhea. Points near the navel along the foot-stomach meridian are used to treat acute diarrhea. To treat chronic intestinal discomfort, the practitioner may choose points along the liver, spleen, or kidney meridians. *(See pages 22-23 and the **Appendix** for more information.)*

CHINESE HERBS

Consult a practitioner of Chinese medicine for an appropriate herbal combination.

HERBAL THERAPIES

Powdered ***slippery elm*** *(Ulmus fulva)* bark is soothing to the intestines. Dissolve ¼ tsp in a glass of warm water and drink four times a day. Tea made with ***chamomile*** *(Matricaria recutita)*, ***marsh mallow*** *(Althaea officinalis)* root, or meadowsweet *(Filipendula ulmavia)* is also soothing. Steep 1 tbsp of the herb in a cup of boiling water and drink three times a day. A half cup of aloe vera juice, taken 2 or 3 times a day, is soothing too. The juice is available at many health food stores.

HOMEOPATHY

A homeopath will try to determine the origin of the disease and may want to assess your constitutional makeup before prescribing remedies. For symptomatic relief of diarrhea, try the following remedies every 60 minutes, up to four doses a day:

- *Mercurius corrosivus* 12x or 30c if your stool contains blood and mucus and you have a feeling that the bowel has not emptied.
- ***Arsenicum album*** 12x or 30c if you have profuse diarrhea with a burning or colicky stomach, anxiety, and chills.
- *Podophyllum* 12x or 30c if you have greenish, painless diarrhea with gurgling and stomach cramps that are worst in the morning.

MIND/BODY MEDICINE

Practices that relax the body such as **meditation,** gentle **yoga** positions, **t'ai chi,** and relaxation techniques can help calm the bowel and lessen diarrhea and pain. Positive affirmation and **guided imagery** can also help relax the bowel.

NUTRITION AND DIET

When the disease is active, you may speed the healing process by drinking juice squeezed from green, leafy vegetables such as cabbage, which are loaded with chlorophyll, or by taking tablets of chlorella, a freshwater alga. Drinking broth made from seaweeds such as ***kelp*** (*Fucus* spp.) may also be helpful.

Some doctors recommend a high-protein, high-fiber, low-fat diet to speed healing, with extra ***B vitamins, vitamin A, magnesium, calcium, zinc,*** and ***copper.*** Be sure to check with your doctor or a licensed nutritionist before taking vitamin and mineral supplements, however, because some have laxative or constipating effects.

Omega-3 fatty acids from fish and flaxseed oils are said to help reduce inflammation. Flavonoids such as quercetin may also reduce inflammation. You can find omega-3 oil and flavonoid supplements in health food stores. Follow the directions on the label or ask your doctor about dosage. Your doctor may also recommend powdered ***psyllium*** *(Plantago psyllium)* seed, a soluble fiber, to give your stools more bulk. Mix powdered psyllium in cold water, drink it quickly, and drink another glass of water to increase its effectiveness.

REFLEXOLOGY

To soothe a troubled digestive tract, massage the colon, liver, adrenal, lower spine, diaphragm, and gall bladder areas on the foot *(see pages 24-25 for information and area locations)*.

AT-HOME REMEDIES

Use a juicer to squeeze your own cabbage and other green, leafy vegetable juices, and drink at least one glass every day. A snack of celery sticks is another quick way to get an extra measure of fiber. When the occasional bout of diarrhea strikes, take time to sit down with a cup of chamomile or marsh mallow root tea.

LIVING WITH AN ILEOSTOMY

After surgery to remove the diseased part of the colon, or large intestine, the cut end of the small intestine—the ileum—is led through an opening in the lower abdomen and surgically reconstructed to form a new opening—a stoma—for waste matter. A small plastic bag fastens against the opening to catch waste from the remaining intestine. Because the waste is only partially digested, it is liquid and has a mild acidic odor. A nurse will teach you how to wear and care for the ileostomy bag. Some people change the bag every day; others can go for about a week.

Your body will quickly adapt to having a shorter intestine, and the waste matter will eventually resemble more normal feces. To counteract any unpleasant odors, you can add an aspirin tablet or a little baking soda to each new bag. The stoma eventually shrinks to about the size of a nickel, but the skin around it may remain sensitive and require attention to prevent it from becoming irritated.

People with ileostomies are surprised that the bag hardly interferes with their normal lives. After recovery from an ileostomy, you will probably be able to do everything you could before, even swimming and having normal sexual relations. You can also enjoy a normal diet, although you may have to cut out certain foods, such as popcorn and very fibrous vegetables, that may tend to clog the stoma.

PREVENTION

There is no evidence that food allergies cause Crohn's, but food sensitivities may add to the irritation of the colon. To check for sensitivities, avoid a suspected food for 10 to 30 days, then try it. If a reaction occurs, eliminate the food from your diet. Common allergens are dairy products, eggs, and wheat.

C A U T I O N !

THE DANGER OF DEHYDRATION

If you ever have repeated bouts of diarrhea, be very careful not to let yourself get dehydrated. Taking fluids may not seem sensible after a liquid bowel movement, but it's precisely what you need. A quick antidehydration remedy is drinking several glasses of water mixed with either ½ tsp salt or with baking soda.

Infants and small children with diarrhea should be checked by a doctor as soon as possible after more than two runny bowel movements. Young children tend to become dehydrated quickly and can suffer serious damage to the digestive tract, and in extreme cases, death. In elderly people, severe dehydration has been known to bring on temporary dementia. ■

CROUP

C

SYMPTOMS

- a sharp, barking cough, usually accompanied by trouble inhaling and sometimes by a hoarse voice caused by inflamed vocal cords.
- labored breathing that seems to put strain on the neck muscles, ribs, or breastbone, making these areas retract noticeably with each breath.

CALL YOUR DOCTOR IF:

- your child has croup accompanied by a high fever (103°F or more).
- home remedies are not working and the croup symptoms seem to be worsening; hospitalization may be required.
- your child has croup and his respiratory rate exceeds 50, he is having extreme difficulty breathing, he cannot talk, or he is turning pale or blue. These are all symptoms of severe respiratory distress. **Call 911 or your emergency number for immediate emergency help.**
- your child is younger than the age of five and has noisy, rapid breathing; a foreign object may be stuck in his throat.
- your child suddenly begins drooling or can't swallow, has a high fever but no cough, and is leaning forward but can't bend his neck and can't talk. Your child may have a dangerous bacterial infection called epiglottitis, which causes a blocked airway. Do not open the mouth to look inside; doing so can completely close the throat and shut down the child's breathing. **Call 911 or your emergency number for immediate emergency help.**

Croup, a viral infection of the voice box (larynx) associated with signs of a respiratory infection, such as a runny nose or cough, is a relatively common ailment of childhood. Usually the first indication is a cough that sounds like the bark of a seal. Your child may have trouble breathing because the tissue around the larynx is inflamed, constricting the windpipe, and because the bronchial passages are blocked with mucus. The sound of air being forced through the narrowed airways may produce hollow raspy noises, or stridor, with each inhaled breath.

Croup lasts for five or six days and is highly contagious. It usually affects children between three months and six years old (the average age is two), whose small windpipes and bronchial passages are vulnerable to blockage. Most cases are mild and can be managed at home. In severe cases or in the case of epiglottitis—an unrelated bacterial infection of the epiglottis (the flap covering the trachea), whose symptoms mimic croup—your child may need to be hospitalized.

CAUSES

Most croup cases are caused by a parainfluenza virus. The disease is transmitted by airborne droplets from an infected child's cough.

TREATMENT

You and your child may be panicked by the apparent sudden onset of a croup attack. Try to

WARNING!

If your child can't breathe, cough, or speak and he is leaning forward with his neck thrust out, do not open his mouth or tilt his head back to look inside. His throat could close completely, causing respiratory arrest. Call 911 or your emergency number. If your child stops breathing, begin CPR immediately ***(see pages 50-53).***

ACUPRESSURE

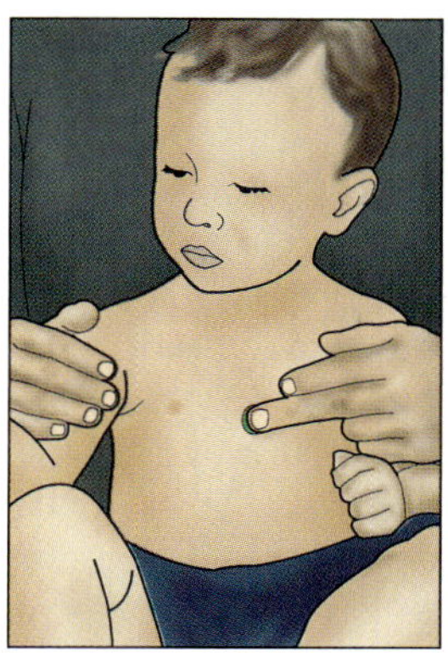

1 Gentle pressure on Conception Vessel 17 may help to calm a baby suffering from croup. Place your finger in the center of the child's chest, midway between the nipples, and press lightly. Hold for one minute and release.

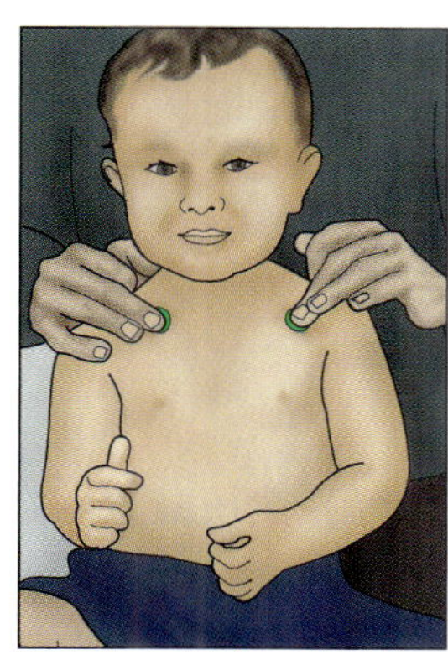

2 Coughing spasms may be eased by pressure on Lung 1. Place one finger of each hand about ½ inch below the large hollow under the collarbone, on the outer part of the chest near the shoulder. Apply pressure gently for one minute.

keep your child calm; crying will only make breathing more difficult. Croup usually can be managed with mist or steam therapy, which dissolves sticky or dried mucus in the child's breathing passages. Because the condition commonly worsens at night, many doctors recommend that you sleep in the same room with your child or use a baby-monitoring device to listen for any change in the child's condition. Be ready to get medical help if your child doesn't improve.

CONVENTIONAL MEDICINE

Doctors recommend home care for all but the most serious cases of croup. If the symptoms are severe enough, your pediatrician may take x-rays to check for epiglottitis—which would be treated with ***antibiotics*** during a short hospital stay. Severe cases of croup may also require hospitalization; the child will be given inhaled medications such as racemic ***epinephrine*** or oral ***corticosteroids*** to counter swelling.

ALTERNATIVE CHOICES

ACUPRESSURE

Practitioners suggest pressing at least four of the following points in succession: Large Intestine 4; Triple Warmer 5; Bladder 12, 13; Lung 1, 2; Conception Vessel 17; and Governing Vessel 24. *(See the **Appendix** for information on point locations.)*

HERBAL THERAPIES

To alleviate a persistent cough, herbalists use aniseed *(Pimpinella anisum),* sundew *(Drosera rotundifolia),* thyme *(Thymus vulgaris),* or wild cherry *(Prunus serotina)* bark, which are said to act as mild cough suppressants.

HOMEOPATHY

Aconite, favored by homeopaths for croup, can be given in the 12x or 30c dosage at the beginning of an attack and then every 30 minutes until the child can sleep. If Aconite doesn't work or if the child's breathing sounds like wood being sawed, try *Spongia* in the same dosage and intervals. For a more mucus-filled bronchial cough, ***Hepar sulphuris*** is the third choice for acute croup.

AT-HOME REMEDIES

- A cool-mist humidifier may help your child breathe. Direct the mist away from the face and don't put medications in the water; they can irritate your child's throat.
- Steam may help loosen phlegm and relax the throat. Turn on the shower and let steam accumulate in your bathroom. Carry your child around in the room (but not under the shower) until the child's breathing becomes easier.
- Cold air sometimes offsets croup. If the night is cool, take your child for a ride in the car with the windows down.
- ***Acetaminophen*** will bring down a fever and lower your child's respiratory rate.
- Offer plenty of noncitric liquids to restore fluids and to loosen phlegm.
- Keep your child away from cigarette smoke.■

CUTS, SCRATCHES, AND WOUNDS

SYMPTOMS

With most cuts and scratches, the primary danger is infection, particularly if the wound is caused by an animal or a human bite, or if it is deep or ragged, or if it cannot be cleaned completely. Signs of infection include:

- increased pain, redness, or swelling, or discharge from the wound.
- fever, swollen lymph nodes.
- red streaks spreading from the wound site toward the heart.

CALL YOUR DOCTOR IF:

- the bleeding cannot be stopped with pressure. The wound should be stitched or taped within a few hours.
- you suspect **internal bleeding.** Signs include weakness, perspiration, and pain out of proportion to the injury. See ***Emergencies/First Aid,*** page 70.
- you believe the victim has suffered a broken bone or a penetrating blow to the body, particularly to the abdomen.
- the victim has a head injury.
- the injury affects a joint or the functioning of the fingers.
- the site of the wound is the face or some other area where scarring would be a concern.
- the victim has not been immunized against tetanus during the last five years.
- signs of ***infection*** (swelling, increased pain, increased or smelly discharge) appear.

Cuts, scratches, and minor wounds are an inescapable part of life. Fortunately, the damage usually heals quickly, but two steps should be taken immediately: You must clean the wound and stop the bleeding. *(For severe, persistent bleeding,* *see* ***Emergencies/First Aid,*** *page 48.)*
Injuries can occur in several forms:

A **cut,** or **incision,** typically caused by a knife, has clean edges. If deep, it can bleed profusely and damage muscles, tendons, and nerves beneath the skin. If contaminated, it may become infected. If spread open, there is a risk of scarring.

A **laceration,** perhaps caused by broken glass or sharp metal, has jagged edges and is likely to involve more damage to deeper tissue than a cut. The risks of infection and scarring are greater.

A **scrape,** or **abrasion,** occurs when skin is rubbed against a hard surface; small blood vessels in the skin are torn and ooze blood. Because of their large surface area, scrapes are easily contaminated by dirt and bacteria.

A **puncture** wound is a narrow, deep hole produced by a nail, tooth, or other penetrating object. Punctures seldom bleed heavily, but they may cause internal injury and carry a risk of tetanus or other infections.

TREATMENT

Before treating yourself or someone else, wash your hands with soap and warm water; even clean-looking skin carries bacteria that can infect.

Commercial healing agents are seldom needed. Antibiotic ointments may help for wounds such as abrasions, but many over-the-counter remedies—including iodine—actually delay healing.

CONVENTIONAL MEDICINE

Cuts and **lacerations:** Let the wound bleed a little; the flowing blood will carry dirt out of the wound. Wash the wound with mild soap and a washcloth under running water. Then use antiseptic wipes, stroking from the wound outward, using a clean section of the wipe for each stroke.

After the wound is clean, blot it dry with sterile gauze or a clean cloth. Put a sterile, absorbent

REMOVING A FISHHOOK

A fishhook embedded just under the surface of the skin *(1)* can usually be removed without the aid of a doctor. Loop a string around the curve of the hook and grasp the string with one hand. With the other hand, gently press down on the hook's shaft *(2)* to free the barb from surrounding tissue. Once the barb is disengaged, yank quickly on the string to pull the hook from the wound *(3)*.

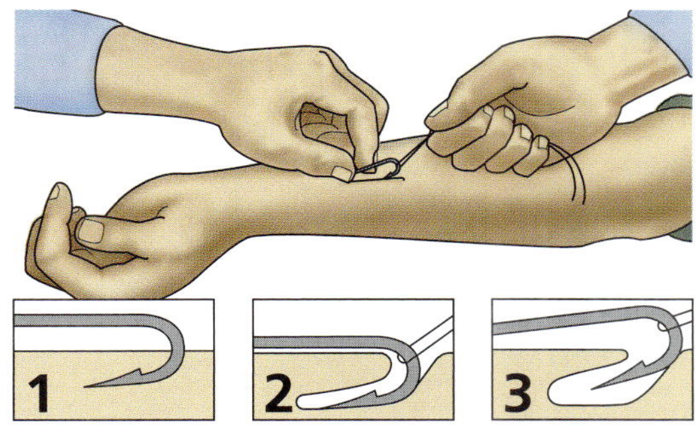

dressing or cloth directly on the cut and apply gentle pressure. Once bleeding has stopped, apply a bandage or tape to hold the dressing in place. In addition to protecting the wound from contaminants, the dressing will minimize drying; cells regenerate more rapidly and produce less scarring when kept moist.

Abrasions: Follow the same steps, but because infection is so common, pay extra attention to cleaning the wound; scrub gently but thoroughly. ***Antibiotic*** ointment may be helpful.

Punctures: Wash the wound thoroughly with soap and a strong stream of water, apply an ***antiseptic*** solution, and bandage the hole with a sterile gauze pad. Do not tape the hole closed and do not apply antibiotic ointment; sealing the wound can increase the likelihood of infection.

For more serious wounds, your most important job is to stop the flow of blood. Pressure is the surest method. Follow these steps:

- Wash your hands if possible, and use sterile gloves; or put a few layers of dressing or a layer of plastic wrap between your hands and the wound.
- Try to calm and reassure the victim. Lay the person flat, head slightly lower than the torso, or with legs elevated, to reduce the chance of fainting.
- Elevate the site of bleeding above heart level if possible; this will slow the flow of blood.
- Apply sterile gauze or a cloth dressing (or a piece of clean clothing) and maintain pressure until the bleeding stops. Your goal is to compress the bleeding vessels enough to allow clots to form. When the bleeding has stopped, bind the dressing firmly with adhesive or other tape.

ALTERNATIVE CHOICES

Honey or granulated sugar applied to minor cuts may assist healing. They both inhibit the growth of bacteria and thus retard infection.

AROMATHERAPY

Tea tree oil (*Melaleuca* spp.) provides topical therapy as an antiseptic, similar to hydrogen peroxide. Add a few drops to water when washing a wound.

HERBAL THERAPIES

Topical ***aloe*** *(Aloe barbadensis)* soothes the skin and may assist healing of superficial **abrasions** and tissue that is healing or scarred. ***Calendula*** *(Calendula officinalis)* is antiseptic and can be applied as a lotion or ointment.

HOMEOPATHY

Ledum is effective at reducing pain in **puncture** wounds and may help ward off infection. *Staphysagria* has been reported of value for lacerations, and ***Hypericum*** for cuts in painful areas, such as the lips. ***Aconite*** (30c) every 30 minutes for three to five doses may help calm a frightened individual.

NUTRITION

For small wounds, or after healing has begun, ***vitamin E*** taken orally (or the oil applied topically) may speed healing. ***Vitamins A, C,*** and ***B complex*** and the amino acids arginine and glycine (between meals) may also help; bromelain (from pineapple) may reduce inflammation. ■

DANDRUFF

D

SYMPTOMS

- flakes of skin that range from small and white to large, greasy, and yellow.
- itchy flaking that appears on the scalp or eyebrows, or around the hairline, ears, or nose.

CALL YOUR DOCTOR IF:

- scaling is greasy and yellow, and does not respond to over-the-counter dandruff shampoos and lotions; you may have seborrheic ***dermatitis*** and need more aggressive treatment to relieve the itching and flaking.
- your dandruff is localized in a few patches and is very itchy; you may have a fungal infection, which requires treatment with prescription medication.

Dandruff—those dry, white flakes of skin you constantly find yourself brushing off your collar or shoulders—typically poses no health risk whatsoever. But it can be a source of embarrassment, and the itchiness that may come with it is a genuine nuisance. Many people incorrectly assume that the problem has something to do with hygiene and how often you wash your hair. Although it's true that shampooing infrequently can aggravate an existing case of dandruff, it will not bring one on. What actually lies behind dandruff is a simple difference between people in a natural process we all undergo every day: shedding skin cells. The difference is that some of us shed more than others.

CAUSES

Skin cells that grow and die off too fast are the cause of dandruff, but doctors do not know why this happens. Some people with severe flaking have overactive sebaceous glands (whose task is to lubricate the skin with oils); others have an elevated level of the fungus *Pityrosporum ovale,* which is present in most people but to excess in dandruff sufferers. Other causative factors include family history, food allergies, excessive sweating, use of alkaline soaps, yeast infections, and stress. Even the season of the year can contribute to the problem: Cold, dry winters are notorious for bringing on dandruff or making it worse.

If dandruff flakes are greasy and yellow, the probable cause is the skin condition known as seborrheic ***dermatitis;*** dry, thick lesions consisting of large, silvery scales may be traced to the less common ***psoriasis*** of the scalp. These forms of dandruff—as well as the run-of-the-mill variety—become a hazard only if you scratch to the point of causing breaks in the skin, which can place you at greater risk for infections, particularly from staph and strep bacteria.

TREATMENT

Many over-the-counter shampoos can keep moderate dandruff in check, but consult your doctor about more stubborn forms such as seborrheic ***dermatitis.*** Some herbal remedies may relieve the itching and dryness, but it usually takes a tar-based product to subdue the greasy scales.

The U.S. Food and Drug Administration (FDA) has approved only five active ingredients as safe and effective for treating dandruff: coal-tar preparations, pyrithione zinc, salicylic acid, ***selenium*** sulfide, and ***sulfur*** (the FDA also recognizes a combination of salicylic acid and sulfur as an effective preparation). All other substances have been banned as active ingredients in dandruff shampoos, so read the label.

CONVENTIONAL MEDICINE

If you find that you are still scratching and shedding after trying over-the-counter preparations, see your doctor. You may be using the wrong shampoo for your condition. For really stubborn dandruff cases you may need to use a prescription steroid lotion.

Most doctors recommend that dandruff sufferers use a medicated shampoo daily, leaving the lather on for at least 10 minutes. Be sure to rinse thoroughly; shampoo and soap residue can actually aggravate skin problems. After your dandruff has cleared up, use the medicated shampoo no more than once or twice a week, because it is too harsh for daily use. When possible, let your hair dry naturally instead of blowing it dry.

Brushing your hair with a natural-bristle brush can also prove beneficial. Brush your hair from your scalp outward with steady, firm strokes. This will carry oil from your scalp, where it can cause dandruff, along the hair strands, which need the oil to stay shiny and healthy.

ALTERNATIVE CHOICES

In addition to herbal preparations, other alternative options—including a careful diet, stress-reducing **mind/body** exercises, and **massage**—may prove to be of some benefit in treating dandruff.

HERBAL THERAPIES

To prevent flaking and protect against infection, try massaging ***tea tree oil*** (*Melaleuca* spp.) into your scalp. Some practitioners believe it is as effective as prescription steroid creams.

Dried thyme *(Thymus vulgaris),* ***rosemary*** *(Rosmarinus officinalis),* or ***sage*** *(Salvia officinalis)* may make an effective rinse. Boil 2 heaping tbsp of one of these herbs in 1 cup of water for 10 minutes. Strain and cool. Pour the liquid on damp, clean hair and massage it into your scalp. Do not rinse.

MIND/BODY MEDICINE

Stress may aggravate dandruff. Regular exercise is not only good for your overall health but is also one of the most effective ways to relieve stress. You might also consider adding a relaxation technique such as **yoga** to your weekly routine.

NUTRITION AND DIET

Dandruff is a common symptom of food allergies, often resulting from a cumulative effect that can make it somewhat difficult to identify the source of the allergic reaction. For example, you drink milk every day and never think to associate the milk with the thickening scales on your head, though it could be the cause.

If standard dandruff treatments don't seem to be working for you, try cutting fatty foods (such as nuts and chocolate), dairy products, excessive sugar, and seafood out of your diet. Supplements of vitamins, such as ***biotin,*** thiamine ***(vitamin*** B_1***),*** ***niacin*** (vitamin B_3), and cobalamin ***(vitamin*** B_{12}***),*** may help eliminate dandruff by improving your body's ability to break down fatty acids.

AT-HOME REMEDIES

- Briskly massaging your scalp—either when you shampoo or when you use an herbal preparation such as tea tree oil—will improve the circulation in your scalp; the improved blood flow will help prevent the skin from drying and cracking.
- Watch your diet. Dairy products, fatty foods, seafood, and excessive sugar have all been shown to make dandruff worse.
- Wash your hair and scalp at least once a week with a medicated dandruff shampoo to prevent recurrences. ■

DEPRESSION

D

SYMPTOMS

For **major depression,** you may experience four or more of the following:

- persistent sadness, pessimism.
- feelings of guilt, worthlessness, helplessness, or hopelessness.
- loss of interest or pleasure in usual activities, including sex.
- difficulty concentrating.
- insomnia or oversleeping.
- weight gain or loss.
- fatigue, lack of energy.
- anxiety, agitation, irritability.
- thoughts of suicide or death.
- slow speech; slow movements.

In children and adolescents:

- insomnia, fatigue, headache, stomachache, dizziness.
- apathy, social withdrawal, weight loss.
- drug or alcohol abuse, a drop in school performance, difficulty concentrating.
- isolation from family and friends.

For **dysthymia** (minor but chronic depression), your symptoms will be less intense, fewer in number, but longer-lasting.

CALL YOUR DOCTOR IF:

- you or your child has suicidal thoughts, or has other signs of either **major depression** or **dysthymia;** help is available.

Note: There is a distinct difference between feeling "depressed" and having a depressive illness. If you have low spirits for a while, don't be concerned. However, if you feel you can't lift yourself out of your misery, seek help.

Almost all of us feel low sometimes, usually because of a disturbing event in our lives. But ongoing depression—suffering a period of what is known as **major depression**—is another matter. Depression in some form affects 25 percent of all women, 10 percent of all men, and 5 percent of all adolescents worldwide. It is the most common psychological problem in the United States, afflicting some 17.6 million people each year.

Depressive reaction (minor and often temporary depression) encompasses the normal depressed feelings that arise because of a specific life situation. The symptoms can be severe, but they usually do not need treatment and abate over time—anywhere from two weeks to six months.

Dysthymia (minor, chronic depression), similar to depressive reaction in its symptoms and degree of suffering, lasts longer—at least two years.

Major depression, or depressive illness, is a serious condition that can lead to an inability to function or even to suicide. Sufferers experience not only a depressed mood but also more harmful symptoms, including disinterest in their usual activities, extreme fatigue, sleep problems, or feelings of guilt and helplessness. They are more likely to lose touch with reality, sometimes having delusions or hallucinations. Depressive illness can be treated but often goes undiagnosed because it is confused with depressive reaction. It is a cyclical illness, so though most patients recover from their first depressive episode, the recurrence rate is high—perhaps as high as 60 percent within 2 years and 75 percent within 10 years. Major depression often appears spontaneously, is seemingly unprovoked, and often disappears spontaneously as well, usually in 6 to 12 months. Because of its disabling effects or the possibility of suicide, major depression needs treatment.

Depression can strike at any age, including in childhood. Studies in the United States show that 1.8 percent of prepubertal children and 4.7 percent of 14- to 17-year-olds have some form of depression. However, the common time of onset is early middle age, and depression is particularly rife among the elderly, as a reaction to the facts of growing older—the death of a spouse or friends, the physical limitations of age, and the impending confrontation with death. Elderly widowers are particularly susceptible to suicide.

CAUSES

Depression is an illness that seems to have different causes. **Depressive reaction,** or "normal depression," occurs as a result of a particular event. Depressed moods can also be a side effect of medication, hormonal changes (such as before menstrual periods or after childbirth), or a physical illness, such as the ***flu*** or a viral ***infection.***

Although the exact causes of **major depression** and **dysthymia** are unknown, researchers currently believe that both forms are caused by a malfunction of the brain's neurotransmitters, chemicals (particularly serotonin) that modulate moods. This malfunction seems to have a large genetic component: In one study, 27 percent of depressed children had close relatives who suffered from mood disorders.

DIAGNOSTIC AND TEST PROCEDURES

Although very common, depression is often ignored or misdiagnosed and left untreated. Such inattention can be life-threatening; **major depression** in particular has a high suicide rate.

Studies show that 74 percent of people seeking help for depression go to their primary care physician, and that 50 percent of these cases are misdiagnosed. Of the cases that are correctly diagnosed by a general practitioner, 80 percent are given too little medication for too short a time. Some of this mishandling may occur because patients seek a doctor's help with—and physicians prescribe for—physical symptoms, such as sleep problems, fatigue, or weight loss, without considering depression as a possible root cause. Tests should also be made to rule out any organic factors—such as nutrient deficiencies, hypothyroidism *(see **Thyroid Problems**),* reactions to drugs (either prescription or recreational)—that can produce similar symptoms.

The elderly are at greatest risk of being overlooked or misdiagnosed. Frequently, primary care physicians, and the elderly themselves, dismiss symptoms of depression as a part of growing old or categorize it as senile dementia—an irreversible condition that causes loss of memory and concentration. This is unfortunate because depression, unlike dementia, is reversible and can be treated successfully.

For all of these reasons, you should consult a psychiatrist or psychopharmacologist (a psychiatrist who specializes in drug therapies for mental illness) for diagnosis and treatment.

TREATMENT

Many therapies—both conventional and alternative—are available for depression. Treatments may vary according to the cause of the depression and its severity. Conventional methods include psychotherapy, antidepressant drugs, and electroconvulsive therapy (ECT).

CONVENTIONAL MEDICINE

Major depression and **dysthymia** are usually treated with a combination of psychotherapy and ***antidepressants.*** Psychotherapy aims to teach patients how to overcome negative attitudes and feelings and to encourage them to return to normal activities. Drug therapy is intended to moderate or correct neurochemical imbalances that affect moods.

The group of antidepressants most frequently prescribed today are drugs that regulate the neurochemical serotonin. Known as ***selective serotonin reuptake inhibitors (SSRIs),*** the group

IMPORTANT!

Depression is not a sign of emotional weakness. It is an illness with physiological as well as psychological causes. Most depression goes undiagnosed and untreated, often because people report only some of their symptoms and primary care doctors fail to consider it as a possibility. If you are suffering from persistent symptoms, do not hesitate to seek help from a psychiatrist or psychopharmacologist who can diagnose and treat your problem correctly.

includes ***fluoxetine,*** nefazodone, ***paroxetine, sertraline,*** and trazodone. ***Bupropion***, a drug from another class, is also used to regulate neurotransmitters. For children and adolescents, paroxetine may be suggested.

The ***tricyclics,*** which have been used to treat depression since the 1950s, are another option, although they are apt to have more unpleasant side effects than the SSRIs. Because adolescents do not tolerate side effects well and tend to stop taking their medication, tricyclics are not recommended for them. Tricyclics include imipramine and ***amitriptyline,*** as well as ***nortriptyline, doxepin,*** and desipramine.

The third group of antidepressants, the ***monoamine oxidase (MAO) inhibitors,*** have also proved effective. MAO inhibitors work more quickly than the tricyclics, but they have more severe side effects and require a change in diet; severe hypertension can occur if patients on MAO inhibitors eat foods containing tyramine—such as cheese, many beans, and various alcoholic beverages. MAO inhibitors are usually prescribed only if the SSRIs and the tricyclics fail to bring improvement.

Lithium carbonate, which is the drug commonly used for ***manic-depression,*** is used to treat depression as well.

Electroconvulsive therapy (ECT) involves the application of an electric shock of about 80 volts through electrodes on the head. The shock is not felt by the patient, who is anesthetized. Although doctors are still uncertain exactly how ECT works, its controversial techniques have been refined in the past 20 years and it is thought to be as safe as drugs—and in some cases more effective. Still, ECT should be used only after all other options have been considered—because it requires hospitalization and general anesthesia—or when rapid results are vital, as with suicidal patients or those who refuse to eat or drink. Usually given three times a week for two weeks, treatments generally don't extend beyond 6 to 10 sessions.

ALTERNATIVE CHOICES

Many alternative therapies are effective, particularly for minor depression. For more serious depressions, though, they should be considered as complementary treatments, not replacements for conventional methods; major or chronic depression should be treated by a psychiatrist.

In addition to the remedies mentioned below, you may want to consider **acupressure, acupuncture,** or **homeopathy,** which may be helpful in relieving some symptoms; see a qualified, experienced practitioner. **Massage,** which is both soothing and energizing and enlivens the body, may also help. Try it once a week, if possible.

ACUPRESSURE

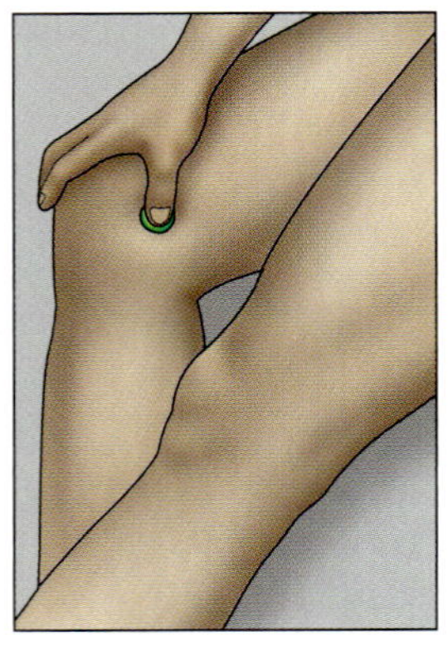

Pressing Liver 8 may help relieve the effects of depression. Bending your right knee, place your thumb above the inside knee crease, just below the joint of the knee (swing your leg a few times to find it). Press for one minute, two or three times, then repeat on your left leg.

AROMATHERAPY

Aromatherapy may ease mental fatigue and help with sleep. The essential oils that may benefit depression are basil, clary, jasmine, rose, and ***chamomile*** *(Matricaria recutita).* The oil may be placed in a bowl of steaming water (2 or 3 drops), in a bath (5 or 6 drops), or on the edge of your pillow (1 or 2 drops).

BIOFEEDBACK

Anecdotal evidence suggests that EEG (brain-wave) biofeedback (also known as neurotherapy) is effective in reducing the intensity of all types of depression. Neurotherapy attempts to change brain-wave patterns through training—thus doing what drugs do chemically. The number of training sessions depends on the severity of the depression. **Depressive reaction** may need only 6 sessions, **dysthymia** may average 20, and **major depression** may need 30 to 60. Because it is, in effect, self-training, biofeedback has the advantage of putting the depressed person in charge of his own therapy; he can use it at will whenever it is needed.

CHINESE HERBS

"Aspiration" is a combination of several Chinese and Western herbs believed to help lift depression. The formula addresses physical symptoms as well as psychological ones, including loss of appetite, chest constriction, and constipation. It is most effective when taken in conjunction with regular aerobic exercise, daily practice of a **relaxation** technique, and a good diet *(see **Nutrition and Diet,** right).* Another Chinese herbal formula, "Gather Vitality," may help with insomnia or oversleeping, aching limbs, and fatigue.

EXERCISE

Exercise should be a part of any therapy for depression; it improves blood flow to the brain, elevates mood, and relieves stress. Even if used alone, it can often bring startling results. Studies show that jogging for 30 minutes three times a week can be as effective as psychotherapy in treating depression. Pick an exercise you like and do it daily, if possible. Any exercise is fine; the more energetic and aerobic, the better.

HERBAL THERAPIES

An experienced herbalist will recommend a particular combination of herbs tailored to your specific symptoms. For a general prescription for depression, one suggestion is: 2 parts ***St.-John's-wort*** *(Hypericum perforatum),* 1 part oat *(Avena sativa)* straw, and 1 part ***lavender*** *(Lavandula officinalis).* Take 4 ml of the tincture each day for at least one month. St.-John's-wort, taken in any of its forms, is a traditional depression remedy in Europe. However, some herbalists report that its effects are unpredictable: Sometimes the herb gets remarkable results, other times it has no effect at all.

MIND/BODY MEDICINE

Many mind/body practices are helpful with depression. Music and dance can lift the spirits and energize the body. **Meditation** and relaxation techniques, such as progressive muscle relaxation, both stimulate and relax. Other choices include transcendental **meditation** and the Asian exercise techniques of **yoga, t'ai chi,** and **qigong.** Choose one or two that suit you and practice daily.

NUTRITION AND DIET

Because depressive symptoms are exacerbated by nutritional deficiencies, good nutrition is important. Increase your intake of healthful foods such as whole-grain cereals, lean meats, fruits and vegetables, fish, and low-fat dairy products. It's very important to avoid alcohol, but also stay away from junk food, sugar, aspartame, and caffeine, which give you a sudden spurt of energy or a high feeling but then let you down.

Recent clinical studies strongly suggest that ***vitamin B complex, folic acid*** (400 mcg daily), and S-adenosylmethionine (two doses of 800 mg daily) are useful in treating depression. The antioxidant ***selenium*** (100 mcg daily) was shown to have a mood-elevating effect in regions where food is deficient in selenium.

Many European studies show that the amino acid supplement L-tryptophan, known to increase the synthesis of serotonin, is of value in relieving depression. A natural form of this amino acid is available by prescription; consult your naturopathic physician. You can also find tryptophan in certain foods, such as turkey, chicken, fish, cooked dried beans and peas, brewer's yeast, peanut butter, nuts, and soybeans. Eat plenty of these foods together with a carbohydrate (potatoes, pasta, rice), which will ease the brain's uptake of tryptophan.

PREVENTION

Some forms of depression may not be preventable since current theory suggests that they may be triggered by neurochemical malfunctioning in the brain. However, there is good evidence that depression may often be alleviated or prevented with good health habits. Proper diet, exercise, vacations, no overwork, and saving time to do things you enjoy all help keep the blues at bay. ■

DERMATITIS

SYMPTOMS

Dry, reddish, itchy skin indicates some type of dermatitis, or skin inflammation, of which there are many types.

- A red rash that is limited to the area of skin exposed to an irritant is probably **contact dermatitis,** an allergic reaction.
- Red, itchy, circular patches of weeping, scaly, or encrusted skin signal **nummular dermatitis,** common in older people who have dry skin or live in dry environments.
- Greasy, yellowish scales on the scalp and eyebrows, behind the ears, and around the nose indicate **seborrheic dermatitis;** in infants it is called **cradle cap.**
- Scaling, greasy-looking, sometimes ulcerated skin appearing inside the lower legs and around the ankles may indicate **stasis dermatitis.**
- Extreme, persistent itchiness may signal **atopic dermatitis,** or ***eczema.***

See also the ***Visual Diagnostic Guide.***

CALL YOUR DOCTOR IF:

- your skin has oozing sores or other signs of ***infection.*** You may need treatment with ***antibiotics*** or other drugs.
- the affected skin does not respond to treatment with over-the-counter creams or medicated shampoos. You should have a medical diagnosis and treatment.
- during a flareup of ***eczema*** you are exposed to anyone with a viral skin disease such as ***cold sores*** or ***warts.*** You are at increased risk of contracting the viral disorder.

Dermatitis simply means skin inflammation, but it embraces a range of ailments. In most cases the early stages are characterized by dry, red, itchy skin, although acute attacks may result in crusty scales or ***blisters*** that ooze fluid. Since many agents can irritate the skin, a doctor will try to narrow the diagnosis to a specific category of dermatitis, even though treatment is similar for most types of skin irritation and inflammation.

CAUSES

The following are the most common general types of dermatitis and their typical causes:

Contact dermatitis typically causes the skin to develop a pink or red rash, which may or may not itch. Pinpointing the exact cause of contact dermatitis can be difficult. Among plants, the leading culprits are ***poison ivy,*** poison oak, and poison sumac, although contact with certain flowers, herbs, fruits, and vegetables irritates some people. Common chemical irritants include detergents, soaps, chlorine, some synthetic fibers, nail polish remover, antiperspirants, and formaldehyde (found in permanent-press fabrics, polishes, artificial-fingernail adhesive, particle board, and foam insulation). Wearing rubber gloves, unwashed new clothes, or plated jewelry can also cause contact dermatitis. The inflammation is frequently caused by cosmetics and skin-care products.

Nummular dermatitis consists of distinctive coin-shaped red patches that are most commonly seen on the legs, buttocks, hands, and arms of people 55 or older. Living in a dry environment or taking very hot showers can cause this condition, as can ***stress*** and other skin disorders.

Seborrheic dermatitis consists of greasy, yellowish scaling on the scalp and other hairy areas, as well as on the face or genitals, and in skin creases along the nose, under the breasts, and elsewhere. This ailment can be associated with a biotin deficiency in infants—where it is known as **cradle cap**—or with overproduction and blockage of oil glands in adults. It may be aggravated by ***stress*** and is common in ***AIDS*** patients.

Stasis dermatitis is caused by poor circulation. Veins in the lower legs fail to return blood efficiently, causing pooling of blood and fluid buildup. This leads to unhealthy skin growth and irritation, especially around the ankles.

Atopic dermatitis, or ***eczema,*** causes the skin to itch, scale, swell, and sometimes blister. Eczema usually runs in families and is often associated with food ***allergies, asthma,*** and ***stress.***

For information about other types of skin disorders, see also ***Diaper Rash, Hives, Impetigo, Psoriasis, Rashes, Scabies,*** and ***Shingles.***

DIAGNOSTIC AND TEST PROCEDURES

Most types of dermatitis can be diagnosed by a doctor's observation of the irritation and its location on the body. Sometimes a skin scraping will be taken for microscopic analysis. To identify causes of **contact dermatitis,** a doctor may try patch tests, applying suspected irritants to areas of skin on the back. If no inflammation develops after two to four days, the doctor applies other potential irritants until the cause is clear.

TREATMENT

The first step in treating dermatitis is identifying and eliminating the cause. Most mild skin inflammations respond well to warm baths followed by application of petroleum jelly or over-the-counter ***hydrocortisone*** cream. **Seborrheic dermatitis** may respond to coal-tar-based shampoo; avoid sunlight for the first few hours after using it, since it increases the risk of ***sunburn*** on the scalp. Once irritants causing **contact dermatitis** are identified, treatment will be based on avoidance, ***allergy*** relief, or other coping mechanisms. To help dry the sores of **nummular dermatitis,** soak the area in salt water, then apply a ***corticosteroid*** cream. If you suffer from **stasis dermatitis,** wear support stockings and rest frequently with your legs elevated to help improve circulation.

CONVENTIONAL MEDICINE

To reduce inflammation and heal the irritation of most types of dermatitis, a doctor usually recommends over-the-counter or prescription ***corticosteroid*** cream, and might prescribe an oral ***antihistamine*** to relieve severe itching and an ***antibiotic*** if a secondary infection develops. Severe cases of **seborrheic dermatitis** may call for corticosteroid injections. **Stasis dermatitis** may involve treatment with tar or zinc paste, which must stay on the sores for up to two weeks; this technique requires bandaging by a trained professional.

ALTERNATIVE CHOICES

Because many forms of dermatitis are chronic, most alternative therapies seek only to relieve the symptoms—itchiness, burning, and swelling.

HERBAL THERAPIES

Over the centuries, countless herbs have been used to treat skin ailments. Picking out what's right for your condition can be difficult, so seek help from a trained practitioner. Here are some

CAUTION!

THE COSMETIC CONNECTION

If a rash develops on your face, neck, lips, scalp, or hairline, the prime suspects could be among your cosmetics or other skin-care aids, including perfume, deodorants, antiperspirants, shampoos, toothpaste, mouthwash, and aftershave lotion. The irritating ingredient in makeup and skin products is usually a scent or a preservative, but be wary of "unscented" products, too; they may contain chemicals that neutralize natural odors but that can also irritate your skin.

The claim that a cosmetic or skin-care product is "hypoallergenic," "organic," or "nonallergic" can be similarly misleading, since no product can be risk free for everyone. If you have sensitive skin, keep your cosmetics and skin-care aids simple and rely on unscented products.

substances herbalists consistently recommend:

Burdock *(Arctium lappa)* boosts the immune system and helps reduce inflammation. Brew tea using 1 to 3 tsp of dried root per cup of boiling water, or take up to 1½ tsp of tincture daily.

Some practitioners believe ***evening primrose oil*** *(Oenothera biennis)* works as well as ***corticosteroids*** for itchy skin and has fewer potential side effects, but the recommended dose of 500 mg three times a day can be costly. People with liver disease or high cholesterol should use it only under medical supervision; pregnant women should not use this treatment because it can affect their estrogen and progesterone levels.

Topical ointments made with ***calendula*** *(Calendula officinalis)* or ***chamomile*** *(Matricaria recutita)* are effective for treating many types of dermatitis. You can make another herbal remedy by mixing tinctures of ***nettle*** *(Urtica dioica)*, cleavers (*Galium* spp.), and either ***goldenseal*** *(Hydrastis canadensis)* or ***myrrh*** *(Commiphora molmol)* in equal parts; take up to 1½ tsp a day. You can also make a tea from fresh nettles or fresh cleavers—1 tbsp of the herb steeped in a cup of boiling water—and drink three or four cups a day. WARNING: In some cases an allergy to nettle will worsen **atopic dermatitis *(eczema).***

MEN JUST DON'T GET SOME TYPES OF RASHES

Paradoxically, unisex fashion trends have uncovered an unsuspected difference between the sexes. Men who wear pierced earrings or other forms of jewelry are far less likely than women to develop contact dermatitis from the nickel in plated jewelry. A team of scientists found that 12 percent of the 15-year-old girls in their study were sensitive to nickel, while less than 2 percent of the young men in a later study had a similar problem. Differences in the types of jewelry the two groups wear may account for some of the disparity, but the researchers also suspect that male and female hormones may play a real but undetermined role.

HOMEOPATHY

For benign, short-term skin problems, an over-the-counter *Calendula* cream may soothe the inflammation. Taking ***Rhus toxicodendron*** (12x or 30x)) three or four times a day may relieve the itching of **contact dermatitis** caused by poison ivy or other plants. If you have a chronic form of dermatitis, a homeopath will investigate everything from your sleep patterns to your family history before recommending a remedy.

LIGHT THERAPY

When certain chronic types of dermatitis do not respond to conventional ***corticosteroid*** or coal-tar treatment, many doctors recommend using ultraviolet (UV) rays from an artificial light source. In light-therapy treatments, patients expose the affected areas under a sunlamp, which emits UV radiation, for a prescribed period of time over several sessions. In nearly all cases, the skin clears considerably in a matter of weeks.

Despite its apparent effectiveness, light therapy has its drawbacks. At four to eight sittings a month, treatment can be time-consuming for the patient and relatively expensive. Light therapy may cause premature aging of the skin and increase a person's risk of developing ***skin cancer.*** In some instances, the dermatitis can recur within a year.

In severe or persistent cases, the treatment can be supported with drug therapy. Light therapy supported with an oral medication called psoralen has good long-term results but carries additional risks. Treatment with psoralen can cause liver problems in some patients; close monitoring by a physician is necessary. Pregnant women should avoid drug-supported light therapy altogether, since psoralen can cause fetal deformities. Women undergoing such therapy should wait several months after stopping treatment before trying to become pregnant.

Some people try to avoid the doctor's office or hospital by using a tanning salon as their source of UV radiation. They won't find the healing rays they seek, however. Because of concerns about the risks of skin cancer, tanning salons must filter out the type of UV rays used in light therapy. Even patients who own a sunlamp or who can find UV radiation commercially should rely on a doctor's care. Only a qualified physician can tell you how much UV radiation you can tolerate without risking long-term damage to your skin.

MIND/BODY MEDICINE

Since some cases of dermatitis may be stress related, relaxation techniques such as **yoga** may be effective, particularly for **atopic** and **seborrheic dermatitis**. **Guided imagery** can also help: You create and control an image opposite to the physical manifestation of the ailment. For example, if you have a red, dry rash, imagine applying a soothing blue ointment to the affected area. This technique works best if you close your eyes and ears to outside stimuli and concentrate all your senses on the image in your mind; you need to smell the ointment, see the healing, and feel the relief.

NUTRITION AND DIET

Because some patients with **seborrheic dermatitis** are believed to have difficulty metabolizing fatty acids necessary for promoting the body's anti-inflammatory response, a doctor may suggest 50 mg of ***vitamin B complex*** twice daily. ***Vitamin A*** (25,000 IU a day) and ***zinc*** (50 to 100 mg a day) may aid in skin healing, while ***vitamin E*** ointment or capsules (200 to 400 IU a day) can help relieve itching and dryness. To avoid the risk of overdose, particularly of fat-soluble vitamins, have your doctor check dosages carefully and monitor your progress; a pediatrician must assess any vitamin supplements given to a child.

AT-HOME REMEDIES

- Over-the-counter oatmeal or cornstarch preparations mixed into a warm bath may soothe the skin and relieve itching. Take care not to stay in the bath too long; lengthy immersion can strip sensitive skin of essential oils.
- For dryness, rub petroleum jelly or vegetable shortening on affected areas after a bath, or use a topical ointment containing ***aloe*** *(Aloe barbadensis)* or zinc.
- Avoid eating potential allergens, such as milk, eggs, and wheat. You may get help from supplemental ***vitamins A, B complex,*** and ***E,*** as well as ***zinc.***
- If you suspect an ***allergy*** to a chemical or cosmetic, try an at-home patch test. Apply a small amount of the suspected irritant to a spot on your arm or back for seven days. If you have a reaction, you know it is a potential irritant.

PREVENTION

The best way to prevent a rash caused by contact with toxic plants like ***poison ivy*** is to wash the exposed skin with soap and water as soon as possible after contact. Most other cases of dermatitis develop in people with sensitive skin and can be prevented only by avoiding the irritant. If you have **atopic** or **seborrheic dermatitis,** for example, you have a higher-than-average chance of being allergic to nickel in jewelry or to getting dry skin during the winter. Fair-skinned people seem especially prone to skin problems. If you feel you are at risk, consider these preventive steps:

- Use a humidifier at home and at work to keep the air from getting too dry.
- Wear loose-fitting, natural-fiber clothing; untreated cotton is ideal.
- Avoid plated jewelry, especially in your ears, to prevent nickel-related rashes. Surgical steel or 14-karat gold earring posts are safer choices.
- Don't wear a watchband that presses against your skin for long periods; the friction and sweat buildup can cause rashes.
- Supplement your diet with ***vitamins A, B complex,*** and ***E,*** and ***zinc.***
- Lubricate your skin after a bath using an unscented, preservative-free lotion or ointment.■

DIABETES

D

SYMPTOMS

- excessive thirst and appetite.
- increased urination (sometimes as often as every hour).
- weight loss.
- fatigue.
- nausea, perhaps vomiting.
- blurred vision.
- in women, frequent vaginal infections and perhaps the cessation of menstruation.
- in men, ***impotence.***
- in men and women, ***yeast infections.***

CALL YOUR DOCTOR IF:

- you feel nauseated, weak, and excessively thirsty; are urinating very frequently; have abdominal pain; and are breathing more deeply and rapidly than normal—perhaps with sweet breath that smells like nail polish remover. You may need immediate medical attention for ketoacidosis.
- you feel weak or faint; are experiencing a rapid heartbeat, trembling, and excessive sweating; and feel irritable, hungry, or suddenly drowsy. You could be developing ***hypoglycemia,*** and may need to eat or drink something quickly to avoid more serious complications.

Diabetes mellitus, the most common disorder of the endocrine system, affects between 10 million and 20 million people in the United States alone. The disease is brought on by disorders in blood levels of insulin, a pancreatic hormone that helps your system convert blood glucose, or blood sugar, into energy. **Type 1 diabetes**—sometimes called insulin-dependent diabetes mellitus (IDDM) or juvenile or juvenile-onset diabetes—results from a shortage of insulin. **Type 2 diabetes**—also known as non-insulin-dependent diabetes mellitus (NIDDM) or adult-onset or stable diabetes—results from the body's inability to process the hormone effectively. About 90 percent of all diabetics have this form.

Regardless of what type of diabetes you have, you need to work closely with your doctor to manage your diet, medication, and activity on a day-to-day basis. Your ability to oversee your own care will make a huge difference in whether you can control the condition and avoid its potentially serious effects.

The many short- and long-term complications of diabetes can demand as much attention as the disease itself. Most important, you need to watch your blood sugar levels every day to prevent an attack of ***hypoglycemia,*** in which available levels of blood sugar are too low to fulfill your body's energy needs. Hypoglycemia can easily be remedied, however, once you recognize its symptoms.

Hyperglycemia, or high blood sugar, can bring on a serious diabetic condition known as ketoacidosis, in which the blood becomes increasingly acidic from the accumulation of toxic by-products called ketones that are produced as the body breaks down fat for energy. Ketoacidosis occurs in Type 1 diabetics if they do not receive adequate supplementary insulin and their bodies are starved for energy sources. Ketoacidosis can also occur in diabetics if glucose and insulin levels are not properly balanced, or if the body comes under sudden physical stress, perhaps from an accident or illness. (Any sort of illness increases the body's need for insulin to process blood glucose into the energy required to fight illness or infection.)

If you are diabetic, be especially alert for the warning signs of ketoacidosis: nausea, excessive thirst, frequent urination, extreme weakness, abdominal pain, and rapid deep breathing. Failure to respond immediately with injections of insulin and intravenous salt solutions (to replenish lost body fluids) can result in coma or death.

Long-term complications of diabetes can damage the eyes, nervous system, kidneys, and cardiovascular and circulatory systems, as well as hinder the body's overall resistance to infections. Cuts and sores heal more slowly for people with diabetes, and diabetics are also prone to ***gum problems,*** urinary tract infections, and mouth infections such as thrush, caused by an overgrowth of yeast organisms. *(See also* ***Urinary Problems*** *and* ***Yeast Infections.****)*

Complications from diabetes are the primary cause of adult blindness in the United States. Within 10 years after their condition is diagnosed, about half of all diabetics develop an eye disorder called diabetic retinopathy, which can weaken the capillaries that supply blood to the retina, and eventually affect vision. Almost all of those who have had the disease for at least 30 years experience some degree of diabetic retinopathy. Diabetics are also more likely to develop ***cataracts*** and ***glaucoma.***

People with diabetes stand a higher than normal chance of developing ***heart disease*** and circulatory problems such as ***high blood pressure,*** hardening of the arteries *(see* ***Atherosclerosis****),* ***heart attacks,*** and ***strokes.*** Poor circulation also makes diabetics more susceptible to skin ulcers, cramps, and gangrenous (tissue-destroying) infections. Damage to the blood vessels in the kidneys from diabetes may lead to kidney failure.

A number of people with diabetes suffer from a condition known as diabetic neuropathy, which causes a gradual deterioration of the nervous system. The condition appears to begin early in both types of diabetes mellitus and affects motor nerves as well as sensory nerves. As a result, diabetics commonly experience a variety of aches and pains. Some develop slowed reflexes, loss of sensation, numbness and tingling in the legs, ***impotence,*** and ***circulatory problems.***

ATTENTION!

LURKING DANGERS

Some over-the-counter remedies that are safe for nondiabetics contain ingredients that can cause problems for diabetics. For example, *aspirin* taken in large amounts can alter blood glucose levels. Diabetics seeking relief from respiratory ailments must be careful when using phenylephrine, *epinephrine,* or *ephedrine,* all of which can raise blood sugar levels. Type 2 diabetics tempted to use appetite suppressants to control their weight need to know that these drugs usually contain caffeine, which boosts blood sugar. Fish oil, commonly taken as a way to improve cholesterol levels, also raises blood sugar. To learn about potential hazards lurking in nonprescription medications, talk to your doctor and your pharmacist, and read labels carefully.

CAUSES

In **Type 1 diabetes,** the pancreas secretes little or no insulin. Unable to use glucose in the blood, the body tries to produce energy by burning fat and muscle. Type 1 diabetes develops fairly quickly, usually striking people under age 30. Recent research suggests that many Type 1 diabetics may have had a genetic predisposition to the disease that was triggered by a viral infection.

Type 2 diabetes usually develops in people over age 40, and there appears to be a strong link between obesity and the development of Type 2 diabetes. Although this particular group of diabetics may have sufficient or even excessive amounts of insulin in their systems, their bodies are unable to use the hormone effectively. Excessive food intake boosts blood glucose levels, and the pancreas cannot produce enough insulin to convert the extra sugar into energy. Sometimes a similar form of this disease, called gestational diabetes, occurs as a temporary condition in women who are pregnant.

D

FIRST AID FOR DIABETICS

You can take steps to help someone who is experiencing a diabetic emergency. First, check to see if the victim is wearing or carrying a Medic Alert tag. If the person has diabetes, the tag should indicate this, and possibly the type of diabetes as well. Hyperglycemia (high blood sugar) can occur in either Type 1 or Type 2 diabetics. Hypoglycemia (low blood sugar) can also strike all diabetics and, in some cases, people who don't have the disease.

Hyperglycemia symptoms include rapid, heavy breathing; abdominal pain; sweet-smelling breath; frequent urination; vomiting; drowsiness; and possibly unconsciousness. What you should do: If the person is conscious and can swallow, give him something to drink that contains no sugar (to prevent dehydration), then take him to the hospital. ***If the victim is unconscious, call 911 immediately.***

Hypoglycemia symptoms include pale, clammy skin; excessive hunger; disorientation; aggressive behavior; and possibly unconsciousness. What you should do: If the victim is conscious and can swallow, give him something to eat or drink that contains sugar—such as fruit juice, candy, a soft drink, or plain sugar—then take him to the hospital. ***If the victim is unconscious, call 911 immediately.***

If the victim is conscious and you are unsure whether he is hyper- or hypoglycemic, give him something to eat or drink that contains sugar, such as fruit juice, candy, a soft drink, or even plain sugar, then take him to the hospital. (Even if the person has hyperglycemia, the additional sugar will do no harm.) ***If the victim is unconscious, call 911.***

DIAGNOSTIC AND TEST PROCEDURES

Your doctor may suspect that you have diabetes if a routine physical examination indicates that excess sugar in your body is being flushed out in your urine. Actual diagnosis begins with an examination of your glucose levels, which the doctor does by taking a blood sample in the morning before you have had anything to eat; if your pancreas is producing little or no insulin (Type 1), or if the body is not producing enough insulin to process blood sugar (Type 2), your glucose levels will be elevated. Additional tests for diabetes include a glucose tolerance test, which measures the body's ability to convert glucose into energy. After fasting for a period, you drink a very sweet beverage containing glucose, then have your blood glucose levels checked.

TREATMENT

Treatment for both forms of diabetes mellitus requires adjustment of insulin levels in the body and strict management of diet and exercise. By paying close attention to the content and timing of your meals, you can minimize or avoid the "seesaw effect" of rapidly changing blood sugar levels, which can require quick changes in insulin dosages.

CONVENTIONAL MEDICINE

If you have **Type 1 diabetes,** it is essential that you receive supplementary insulin every day, at least twice a day, to promote your body's use of blood glucose. Since insulin is a protein and is destroyed by digestive enzymes, it cannot be taken orally. Rather, it must be injected directly into the body at set intervals. While some diabetics use a computerized pump that administers insulin on a set basis, most doctors advise direct injections. Learning to give injections to yourself or to your infant or child may at first seem daunting, but the process quickly becomes routine.

Most insulin in use today is processed synthetically, although some is still derived from animal hormone. The medication comes in three varieties: short-acting (taking effect within 30 or 40 minutes and lasting for 6 hours); intermediate-acting (taking effect in 2 to 4 hours and lasting up to 24 hours); and long-acting (taking effect in 6 to 8 hours and lasting up to 32 hours). Each injection plan is tailored for the individual diabetic and adjusted to accommodate events such as periods of stress, adolescent growth, and the premenstrual period of a woman's monthly cycle.

By monitoring your own blood glucose levels, you can track your body's fluctuating insulin demand and help your doctor calculate the most appropriate insulin dosage. One self-monitoring technique involves a special meter that reads glucose levels in a sample of your blood dabbed on a strip of treated paper. Another method uses paper strips that change color when exposed to a drop of blood to indicate glucose levels.

For some **Type 2 diabetics,** diet and exercise are sufficient to keep the disease under control; others require drug therapy, which may include insulin, an oral hypoglycemia medication such as tolbutamide, acetohexamide, glimepiride, ***glipizide, glyburide,*** or chlorpropamide, or an antihyperglycemic such as acarbose or metformin. If you take any of these drugs for Type 2 diabetes, ask your doctor about possible interactions with other prescription drugs.

Maintaining a balanced diet is vital in both Type 1 and Type 2 diabetes, so work with your doctor to set up a menu plan. If you have Type 1 diabetes, and the timing of your insulin dosage is determined by activity and diet, when you eat and how much you eat are just as important as what you eat. Usually, doctors recommend three small meals and three to four snacks every day to maintain the proper balance between glucose and insulin in the blood. Carbohydrates—especially some starches and other complex carbohydrates, which release glucose relatively slowly into the bloodstream—should make up 50 to 60 percent of your total caloric intake; proteins should compose from 20 to 25 percent; and fats, from 20 to 30 percent.

Recommended proportions of carbohydrates, proteins, and fats for Type 2 diabetics are essentially the same, although patients who are overweight are encouraged to lower their intake of fat and eat more complex carbohydrates and fiber. Since Type 2 diabetics are usually not concerned with scheduled doses of insulin, they do not need to time their meals so carefully.

Another crucial element in a diabetic's daily program is exercise, which can help Type 2 diabetics in particular lose excess weight. For people with either type, exercise can also help mitigate cardiovascular complications of the disease, and it may offer stress relief as well. Type 1 diabetics need to remember, however, that exercise lowers blood glucose levels. To prevent an attack of hypoglycemia, plan to eat a carbohydrate snack approximately half an hour before you begin exercising, and make sure you have something to eat or drink if you start to feel hypoglycemic symptoms. With either type, check with your doctor before starting an exercise program.

It is also a good idea to wear a Medic Alert bracelet or tag indicating that you have diabetes; this will make others aware of your condition in case you have a severe hypoglycemic attack and are not able to make yourself understood, or if you are in an accident or another situation and need emergency medical care. Identifying yourself as a diabetic is important because hypoglycemic attacks can be mistaken for drunkenness, and victims often aren't able to care for themselves. Without prompt treatment, hypoglycemia can result in a coma or seizures. And since your body is under increased stress when you are ill or injured, your glucose levels will need to be monitored by any medical personnel who give you emergency care.

ALTERNATIVE CHOICES

Since diabetes that is incorrectly treated can be life-threatening, you should never try to treat the disease without the help of a doctor, and you should always discuss any possible treatments thoroughly. Some alternative remedies offer variations of diabetic diets. Others emphasize supplemental vitamins and minerals, prescribe herbs to restore blood sugar levels, or treat secondary effects. Stress-reduction practices may also help lower blood glucose levels.

ACUPUNCTURE
Stimulation of certain points may relieve pain associated with diabetic neuropathy, boost the immune system, and minimize circulatory system complications. Consult a licensed practitioner.

CHINESE HERBS
Chinese herbal medicines, including ***ginseng root*** *(Panax ginseng),* are frequently used to alleviate some symptoms of diabetes; consult a practitioner for a comprehensive treatment plan.

HERBAL THERAPIES
Check with a practitioner to make sure herbs are appropriate for your condition. Remember: If you need insulin to manage your diabetes, there is no herbal substitute for the hormone.

Blueberry *(Vaccinium myrtillus)* leaves in a decoction may lower blood glucose levels and help maintain the vascular system. This remedy may also help to keep the blood vessels of the eye from hemorrhaging if you develop diabetic retinopathy. Diabetics in one study who ate crackers made from the powdered form of ***burdock*** *(Arctium lappa)* after a starchy meal had a lowered incidence of hyperglycemia. A cream made with ***cayenne*** *(Capsicum frutescens)* may relieve pain associated with peripheral neuropathy, a type of diabetic neuropathy.

Supplementing the diet with ***fenugreek*** *(Trigonella foenum-graecum)* seeds has been shown in clinical and experimental studies to reduce blood glucose and insulin levels while lowering blood cholesterol. ***Garlic*** *(Allium sativum)* may lower blood pressure as well as levels of blood sugar and cholesterol.

Ginkgo *(Ginkgo biloba)* extracts have been used to stem deteriorating vision in patients by maintaining adequate blood flow to the retina. Other reported benefits of ginkgo include reducing the risk of heart disease, hypertension, and elevated cholesterol levels.

Onion *(Allium cepa)* may free up insulin to help metabolize glucose in the blood, thus lowering blood glucose levels. Both raw and boiled onion extracts have been found to have this effect. Onion is also considered beneficial in maintaining a healthy cardiovascular system.

LIFESTYLE
In laboratory tests, exercise has been shown to increase the tissue levels of ***chromium,*** which the body uses to regulate blood glucose and cholesterol levels. For **Type 1 diabetics,** exercise has also been found to increase the body's ability to use available insulin so that fewer insulin injections are needed. WARNING: If you have Type 1 diabetes, keep in mind that exercise lowers your blood glucose; eat a carbohydrate snack before exercising, and eat or drink again if you feel the warning symptoms of a hypoglycemic attack.

Type 2 diabetics who need to lose weight can benefit from moderate exercise. However, if you are a Type 2 diabetic, you should avoid weightlifting or other forms of exertion that involve pushing or pulling heavy objects; these activities raise blood pressure and may aggravate any eye problems that stem from diabetes.

If you are diabetic, be sure to take good care of your teeth and floss regularly; diabetes can exacerbate gum disease.

MIND/BODY MEDICINE
Any sort of practice that will lower your stress level, such as **biofeedback, meditation, hypnotherapy, yoga,** or other relaxation techniques, may help lessen your insulin requirements.

NUTRITION AND DIET
Some practitioners claim that diabetes is a disorder of Western lifestyles, pointing out that when people in other cultures abandon native foods for a diet of refined and processed foods, diabetes rates begin to rise. The high-carbohydrate high-plant-fiber diet (HCF diet) is an alternative to the conventional diet plan for diabetics.

The HCF diet calls for diabetics to follow these daily guidelines in planning their meals: Eat 70 to 75 percent complex carbohydrates, 15 to 20 percent proteins, and only 5 to 10 percent fats. The HCF diet is said to boost insulin's ability to promote blood glucose as an energy source, improve cholesterol levels, reduce the incidence of hyperglycemia and hypoglycemia, and help with weight loss for Type 2 diabetics.

A modified version of the HCF diet further restricts what foods may be eaten but increases the

Essential Foot Care

If you are diabetic, your foot is your Achilles heel, so to speak. This is because nerve damage from diabetic neuropathy can deaden your perception of pain and allow small injuries such as blisters to develop into major infections before you notice anything is wrong. Diabetics need to examine their feet closely every day, looking for red spots, bruises, cuts, blisters, swelling, or any sign of infection. Watch out for dry skin, which can crack and allow bacteria and fungi to invade. Cut toenails straight across to avoid ingrown toenails. Wear comfortable shoes, and don't risk injuring your feet by walking barefoot or wearing sandals.

allowable amount of complex carbohydrates. One university study indicated that a high-carbohydrate, high-fiber diet could reduce the insulin demands of Type 1 diabetics by 30 to 40 percent, and of Type 2 diabetics by 75 to 100 percent.

Diabetics should avoid sugar, as it can lower the body's glucose tolerance and worsen circulatory problems. Nutritionists also emphasize the importance of certain foods, vitamins, and minerals, including the following:

Chromium supplements can be very helpful for people with diabetes. Chromium not only lowers blood glucose levels and improves glucose tolerance but it also lowers insulin levels and helps hold down blood cholesterol levels.

Inositol, a B-complex vitamin, has been shown to help protect diabetics from peripheral neuropathy by relieving numbness and tingling in the hands and feet. However, since inositol might alter blood sugar levels, make sure to check with your practitioner before starting supplements. ***Biotin,*** also called vitamin H, may improve glucose metabolism in diabetics.

Vitamin B_6 may help decrease the severity of diabetic neuropathy and reduce insulin demands in Type 2 diabetics. ***Vitamin*** B_{12} may help treat diabetic neuropathy; injections may prove more beneficial than oral doses.

Diabetics may need supplements of ***vitamin C*** to make up for low blood levels of insulin, which normally works to help cells absorb the vitamin. Proper amounts of vitamin C help the body maintain good cholesterol levels, fight off infection by bolstering the immune system, and prevent cataracts. Although some practitioners recommend supplementing your diet with up to 1 gram of vitamin C per day, you should consult your practitioner to make sure this is a safe dosage for you to take. ***Vitamin E*** may help limit damage to the vascular system and improve blood cholesterol levels.

Manganese helps the body metabolize glucose; diabetics often have a serious manganese deficiency. ***Magnesium*** supplements may help control diabetic retinopathy and reduce the possibility of cardiovascular damage.

Zinc may help increase glucose tolerance, and ***potassium*** may improve a diabetic's ability to utilize insulin. ***Copper*** supplements may help improve cardiovascular fitness.

Okra and peas can help stabilize blood sugar levels and provide fiber in a high-complex-carbohydrate diet. Some research suggests that cinnamon can lower insulin requirements in Type 2 diabetics; seasoning your food with as much as ¼ tsp at every meal may help regulate blood sugar levels.

PREVENTION

Because of the apparent link between obesity and Type 2 diabetes, you can do a great deal to help reduce your chances of developing the disease by slimming down if you are overweight. This is especially true if diabetes runs in your family.

A good exercise program and a nutritionally balanced diet can greatly limit the effects of both Type 1 and Type 2 diabetes. If you smoke, quit; smoking can significantly increase the risk of heart disease, particularly for diabetics. ■

DIAPER RASH

SYMPTOMS

- redness over the diaper area—around the genitals, buttocks, and thighs, but not on the abdomen.
- tight, papery skin, or skin that is shiny and bright red.
- a strong smell of ammonia.
- in boys, an inflamed penis.

See also the ***Visual Diagnostic Guide.***

CALL YOUR DOCTOR IF:

- you see no improvement after four days of home treatment, or you also see white patches inside the mouth that appear red after being wiped with a clean cloth; your child may have a ***yeast infection*** called candidiasis, or sometimes thrush.
- the rash is scaly and has a yellowish hue and appears not only in the diaper area, but elsewhere on the body, such as behind the ears or under the arms; your child may have seborrheic ***dermatitis.***
- the diaper rash does not go away within a few days or worsens; your child may have developed a strep or ***staph infection*** or a local reaction to a particular lotion, soap, or laundry detergent.
- the diaper area is covered with blisters that leave shallow red sores; your child may have ***impetigo,*** which requires treatment with ***antibiotics.***
- your son's penis is swollen and red and you can't retract the foreskin, or you notice a greenish discharge from the penis; your child may have a painful condition called balanitis, which requires antibiotics.

Almost all babies develop a diaper rash—an inflammation of the skin on the buttocks, genitals, and thighs—at some time in their young lives. Although a diaper rash may cause a baby discomfort and even some pain, it is rarely serious. Most cases are of short duration, lasting only three or four days. But sometimes a rash will persist, an indication that a secondary skin condition or infection has developed.

Your baby can get diaper rash whether you use disposable or cloth diapers; moisture, not the diaper itself, is the culprit. Keeping your child clean and changing a diaper soon after it is soiled is the key to battling diaper rash.

CAUSES

Diaper rash can be caused by anything that irritates your baby's sensitive skin. The most common source of the problem is urine and stool left in contact with the skin for too long, but a rash can also be caused by inadequate drying of the baby's skin after a bath or by an allergic reaction to lotions or soaps used directly on the baby's skin or to chemicals in the laundry detergent used to clean fabric diapers. Seborrhea, an inflammatory skin condition that affects the oil glands, can trigger a diaper rash as can thrush, a type of ***yeast infection***. Babies receiving ***antibiotics*** for other illnesses are particularly susceptible to thrush-related diaper rash because the drugs allow fun-

C A U T I O N !

When baby powder or talc comes in contact with broken skin, it may cause an inflammatory reaction called granulation. If inhaled, the fine powder may cause lung damage. To help keep diapered areas dry, most pediatricians now recommend barrier creams or cornstarch, which is coarser and heavier than powder. Do not use cornstarch if your baby has a yeast infection, however: Yeast thrives on cornstarch.

gal growth. ***Eczema,*** an allergic skin condition, can also occur as a diaper rash in reaction to foods or other allergens.

TREATMENT

Most diaper rashes respond well to home treatments and require no medical care. If your baby's rash fails to improve after three or four days, see a pediatrician. The rash should be diagnosed to rule out the presence of a more serious infection.

CONVENTIONAL MEDICINE

For an ordinary rash, the doctor may recommend an over-the-counter ointment containing zinc oxide to protect the skin. If your child has developed a bacterial infection, a topical or oral ***antibiotic*** may be prescribed. For thrush, your pediatrician will prescribe an ***antifungal*** cream for the rash and possibly an oral antifungal liquid to clear up patches of thrush in your baby's mouth. For diaper rashes involving seborrheic ***dermatitis*** or ***eczema,*** doctors sometimes prescribe hydrocortisone cream. Over-the-counter antifungal and ***hydrocortisone*** creams are also available; however, you should check with your child's pediatrician before using them instead of prescription creams.

ALTERNATIVE CHOICES

Alternative remedies can be very effective in treating and preventing common diaper rashes. Seek professional medical care, however, if your child's rash does not improve within several days.

AROMATHERAPY

Mix 2 drops each of essential oils of sandalwood, ***peppermint*** *(Mentha piperita)*, and ***lavender*** *(Lavandula officinalis)* in 4 tbsp of a carrier lotion or oil such as sweet almond oil; gently apply the lotion to the reddened area of skin.

HERBAL THERAPIES

Calendula *(Calendula officinalis)* cream may relieve diaper rash. Herbalists also recommend the following ointment, which you can make at home:

- 1 tbsp each: dried ***chickweed*** *(Stellaria media)* leaves, powdered ***marsh mallow*** *(Althaea officinalis)* root, and powdered ***comfrey*** *(Symphytum officinale)* root.
- 1/8 tsp ***goldenseal*** *(Hydrastis canadensis)* root powder.
- 1 cup sweet almond oil.
- 1/4 cup beeswax.

In a cast-iron pan, heat the herbs in the oil for 5 to 10 minutes. Don't let them burn. Add beeswax and let it melt. Strain the mixture through cheesecloth into a jar with a tight-fitting lid. Refrigerate until solid. Apply when you diaper your baby. The rash should improve after three or four applications. Discard after two months.

AT-HOME REMEDIES

- ◆ At the first sign of redness, wash your baby's bottom with warm water, and dry it thoroughly. Then apply an antiseptic cream and a barrier ointment, such as zinc oxide, to protect the skin.
- ◆ Change your baby's diaper as soon as it becomes soiled. Let your baby go without diapers as often as possible.
- ◆ Use disposable diaper liners, which allow urine to pass through to the diaper while keeping the baby's skin dry.
- ◆ Until the rash clears up, avoid plastic pants or diaper covers, which trap moisture.

PREVENTION

You can't prevent diaper rash, but you can limit its duration or severity by keeping your baby dry and clean and by changing the baby's diaper as soon as it becomes soiled. Wash cloth diapers in hot water, use bleach or vinegar in the rinse water, and add extra rinse cycles to help kill bacteria and remove traces of soap. If the entire diaper area is red and irritated, the child may be allergic to your detergent. Try another brand to see if the rash clears. The best preventive measure is to let your baby go without diapers as much as possible. ■

DIARRHEA

Read down this column to find your symptoms. Then read across.

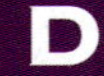

SYMPTOMS	AILMENT/PROBLEM
◆ frequent or watery stools; possible abdominal cramping after eating or drinking coffee.	◆ Overeating fiber-rich foods such as whole grains, vegetables, and/or fruit, or drinking too much coffee
◆ frequent or watery bowel movements after beginning a new medication.	◆ Side effect of drugs such as ***antibiotics, antacids, cimetidine,*** quinine, and others
◆ frequent or watery stools during times of stress or depression.	◆ Emotion-induced diarrhea
◆ recurrent stools with mucus; lower abdominal pain that worsens with eating or stress.	◆ ***Irritable bowel syndrome***
◆ recurrent, foul-smelling, watery stools that are pale or yellowish; flatulence; stomach cramps; weakness.	◆ Malabsorption, a digestive disorder in which fats and nutrients are not properly absorbed by the intestines
◆ relentless watery bowel movements; nervousness; insomnia; excessive sweating.	◆ An overactive thyroid gland, ***diabetes,*** or an underactive adrenal gland
◆ loose stools, possibly with visible blood.	◆ Many possibilities, including ***colorectal cancer***
◆ sudden attack of watery, frequent stools that may be bloody; nausea; fever; abdominal cramping.	◆ ***Gastroenteritis,*** such as intestinal ***flu,*** traveler's diarrhea, ***food poisoning;*** or ***gastritis***
◆ frequent, watery stools (perhaps with blood or pus); abdominal pain; weakness; lack of appetite; possible vomiting, mild fever, joint pain.	◆ ***Colitis*** or ***Crohn's disease***
◆ episodes of frequent, watery stools; coughing; wheezing; flushed face.	◆ A carcinoid tumor (a growth in the intestine that may be benign or malignant)
◆ watery stools that may be black; center or left abdominal pain; possible bright red anal bleeding.	◆ ***Diverticulitis***

WHAT TO DO	OTHER INFO
◆ Drink plenty of water, continue to eat a normal diet, avoid coffee.	◆ Diarrhea should resolve itself in less than 48 hours. The over-the-counter drug ***loperamide*** may help alleviate symptoms.
◆ Ask your doctor about changing or stopping your medication.	
◆ Experiment with ***stress***-reducing techniques until you find one that works and fits into your daily life. Seek treatment for ***depression.***	
◆ Anything that reduces ***stress,*** such as regular meditation, yoga, or moderate exercise, often relieves this diarrhea.	◆ Taken 3 times daily, ***peppermint*** *(Mentha piperita)* or ***chamomile*** *(Matricaria recutita)* tea may ease intestinal spasms and cramps.
◆ Call your doctor today; see ***Anemia, Celiac Disease, Lactose Intolerance, Pancreatic Problems.***	◆ Malabsorption is common after bowel surgery. Dietary changes alone can often relieve symptoms.
◆ See your doctor for treatment. See ***Diabetes, Thyroid Problems.***	
◆ Call your doctor today. The many causes of ***anal bleeding*** range from harmless to dangerous.	◆ Any anal bleeding should be examined by a doctor. If you are over age 50, get a routine check every three years for hidden anal bleeding (and ***colorectal cancer***).
◆ Keep your body well hydrated by drinking plenty of water, fruit juice, and/or prepared electrolyte solutions (available at the drugstore).	◆ Most gastroenteritis resolves itself in a day or two. If it persists, consult your doctor.
◆ Avoid stressful situations and foods that disagree with you.	◆ Avoid spicy and high-fat foods, as they worsen colitis-induced diarrhea.
◆ See your doctor for diagnosis and treatment, which may include ***anticancer drugs*** and/or surgery.	◆ Carcinoid tumors spread very rapidly and should not be ignored.
◆ Call your doctor today to get a proper diagnosis.	

DISK PROBLEMS

D

SYMPTOMS

Many cases of damaged spinal disks have no physical symptoms. However, if your disk problem directly affects spinal nerves, you may have one or more of the following symptoms:

- sharp pain in the back, sometimes going down the back of one or both legs, immediately upon or shortly after exertion or injury.
- inability to bend or straighten your back, accompanied by severe pain.
- gradual development of neck or lower-back pain, possibly intense on arising or when sneezing or coughing.
- numbness or tingling in an arm or leg, and possibly a progressive loss of strength in one or both legs.

CALL YOUR DOCTOR IF:

- you experience persistent pain in the upper or lower back; you may be suffering from ankylosing spondylitis or a form of ***arthritis.***
- back pain is accompanied by fever; you may have a viral or bacterial ***infection.***
- you have sudden loss of feeling or weakness in your extremities; you may have an injury to your spinal cord.

Only a person who has experienced it understands the agony and helplessness that come with a damaged spinal disk. The pain is excruciating, and every movement makes it worse. Like most kinds of pain, however, it is actually a valuable warning signal. If you heed the warning and take proper action—or, more appropriately, inaction—the discomfort usually stops and the problem can be corrected. If you ignore the warning, you could suffer permanent physical and neurological damage.

As children, some of us may have heard parents or relatives grumble about the pain of a slipped disk. We may have pictured a wobbly stack of pennies with one sticking out enough to tip the rest over. As with other myths and mysteries of childhood, there was a little truth in the image, but not much. Intervertebral disks are actually flexible pads tightly fixed between the vertebrae—the specialized bones that make up the spinal column *(see **Back Problems**)*. Each is a flat, circular capsule roughly an inch in diameter and perhaps one-quarter-inch thick, made of a tough, fibrous outer membrane called the annulus fibrosus, surrounding an elastic core called the nucleus pulposus.

The disks are firmly embedded between the vertebrae and are held in place by the ligaments connecting the spinal bones and by the surrounding sheaths of muscle. There is really little if any room for them to slip or move. The points on which the vertebrae actually turn are called facet joints, which stick out like arched wings on either side of the vertebrae and keep the vertebrae from bending and twisting far enough to damage the spinal cord, the vital network of nerves that runs through the center of each bone.

The disk is sometimes described as a shock absorber for the spine, which makes it sound more flexible or pliable than it really is. While the disks separate the vertebrae and keep them from rubbing together, they are far from pneumatic or springlike. In children they are actually gel- or fluid-filled sacs, but they begin to solidify as part of the normal aging process. By early adulthood, the blood supply to the disk has stopped, the soft inner material has begun to harden, and the disk is less elastic. In middle-aged adults the disks are tough and quite unyielding, with a consistency similar to that of a piece of hard rubber.

Under stress, it is possible for the inner material to swell and herniate, pushing through the tough outer membrane of the disk. The entire disk becomes distorted, and all or part of the core material actually protrudes through the outer casing at a weak spot, causing pressure against surrounding nerves. If further activity or injury causes the membrane to rupture or tear, the disk material can injure the spinal cord or the nerves that radiate from it, producing extreme, debilitating pain—an unmistakable signal to stop all movement immediately. Such damage to a disk can be irreversible.

By far the majority of disk injuries occur in the lumbar region of the lower back, with less than 10 percent affecting the neck and shoulders. Not all herniated disks press on nerves, however, and it is entirely possible for a person to have deformed disks without any pain or discomfort. For that reason, an x-ray or MRI scan showing a distorted disk can sometimes misdiagnose pain that has an entirely different cause.

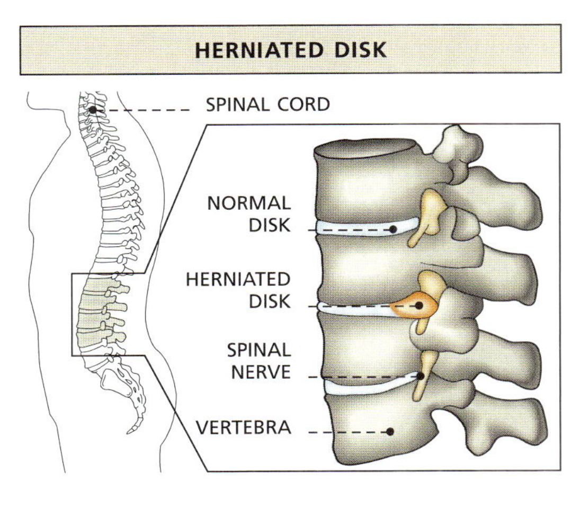

A normal intervertebral disk acts as a cushion between the bones in the spinal column. A disk is said to be herniated or prolapsed when the soft inner core pushes through the weakened or ruptured outer layer. If it touches a nerve, the result is immediate, excruciating pain.

Herniated disks are most common in men under 50, although they can occur in active children and young adults. Older people, whose disks no longer have fluid cores, are much less likely to encounter the problem. People who do regular, moderate exercise are much less likely to suffer from disk problems than their sedentary counterparts. They also tend to stay flexible considerably longer, without the annoying stiffness that many people take for granted as they grow older.

CAUSES

Although a violent injury can damage a disk, problems with disks are often brought on by everyday activities—lifting heavy objects the wrong way, stretching too hard during a tennis volley, or slipping on an icy sidewalk. Any such event can cause the fibrous outer covering of the disk to break or distort to the point that it impinges on a spinal nerve. Sometimes, however, a disk swells, tears, or degenerates without any apparent cause.

Disk problems are sometimes lumped together under the term **degenerative disk disease.** Change in the condition of the disk is a natural result of aging, and it contributes to a gradual loss of flexibility as we grow older. But disk degeneration is far more serious in some people than in others. Severe cases may be the result of a deficiency in collagen, the material that makes up cartilage. Poor muscle tone and obesity also put excessive strain on the spine and the ligaments that hold the disks in place.

DIAGNOSTIC AND TEST PROCEDURES

The classic procedure for identifying a herniated disk is the straight-leg-raising test. The patient lies on his or her back while the doctor holds the ankle and slowly raises the leg; pain in the back of the leg often—though not always—indicates a herniated disk in the lower back. The doctor will also look for weakness and loss of reflexes in legs and feet. Locating the site of the pain may be enough to identify the herniated disk.

A spinal x-ray may eliminate other potential

causes, but because x-rays do not show soft tissue clearly, magnetic resonance imaging (MRI), computed tomography (CT) scans, or myelography—a radiological technique for viewing the spinal cord—may be used to identify and determine the extent of a herniated disk.

TREATMENT

Both conventional and alternative therapies call for pain relief, rest, steps to reduce inflammation, and measures to restore strength and normal activity. Except in severe cases of disk degeneration's affecting nerves that control muscle movement, herniated disks generally heal themselves, and surgery is rarely necessary.

CONVENTIONAL MEDICINE

Doctors usually prescribe bed rest and painkilling medication such as ***aspirin, ibuprofen*** or another ***nonsteroidal anti-inflammatory drug (NSAID),*** and in some cases ***corticosteroids*** and ***muscle relaxants.*** With a herniated disk, any movement of the back can heighten the pain and potentially aggravate the injury, so full bed rest is a must, at least for the first few days after the onset. Once the patient is well enough to move, the doctor may call for a back brace or neck collar to limit movement and ease the pressure on sensitive nerves while the disk heals. In severe cases, full or partial traction may be needed.

If the disk is just temporarily distorted, the potential for complete recovery is excellent. If the outer membrane actually breaks or ruptures and loses some of its gelatinous center, however, the damage may be permanent unless more aggressive steps are taken.

When the herniated disk causes weakness or paralysis of the nerves that control muscles of the back and limbs, the doctor may recommend epidural injections or surgery. Epidural injection consists of a combination of an anesthetic and corticosteroids injected through a long needle into the space between the affected disk and the covering of the nerve and spinal cord. Surgery may be performed to remove some of the soft core of a swollen disk with a hollow needle so that the disk no longer impinges on a nerve. Other microsurgical procedures can remove fragments of core material that have broken through the fibrous outer wall. Discectomy is the surgical removal of part of a herniated disk, and is done to relieve pressure on the nerve. In this procedure, the core of the disk is removed, leaving the tough outer casing in place between the vertebrae. Like epidural injection, it sometimes brings long-term relief, but there is no guarantee of permanent recovery. Because any invasive therapy near the spinal cord is potentially dangerous, surgery should be undertaken only in extreme cases, when the herniated disk is causing weakness or paralysis of nerves going to muscles.

Injections of the drug colchicine may be helpful in relieving acute pain and inflammation of a ruptured disk. A somewhat controversial treatment, now largely out of favor, is chemonucleolysis, which is said to dissolve material in a herniated disk by an injection of the enzyme chymopapain.

Just as artificial replacements for damaged or worn parts are being surgically implanted in other parts of the body, intervertebral disk replacement has passed the experimental stage and is being performed in other countries. The safety and long-term success of disk replacement remain to be seen, but like stainless-steel hip joints and plastic heart valves, synthetic versions of intervertebral disks may offer yet another medical option in the not-so-distant future.

ALTERNATIVE CHOICES

Besides pain relief and rest immediately following an episode of a herniated disk, alternative therapies tend to focus on relaxation and gentle exercise to restore full movement.

ACUPRESSURE

While acupressure can be highly effective for treating lower-back pain, acupressure therapists exercise caution when dealing with pain from spinal disks. Rather than applying pressure to the spine or to points on meridians next to the spinal column, an acupressure therapist may recom-

YOGA EXERCISES

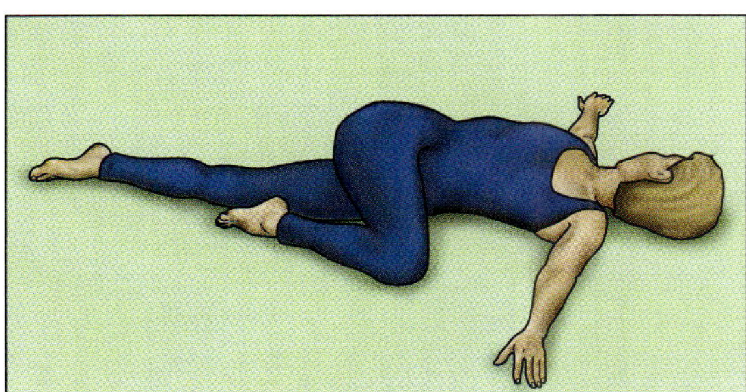

1 The **Knee Down Twist** stretches lower-back muscles. Lie on your back with arms out, inhale, and put your right foot on your left knee. Exhale, turn your head to the right, and bring your right knee toward the floor to your left. Hold 15 to 20 seconds, while breathing deeply. Repeat on the other side.

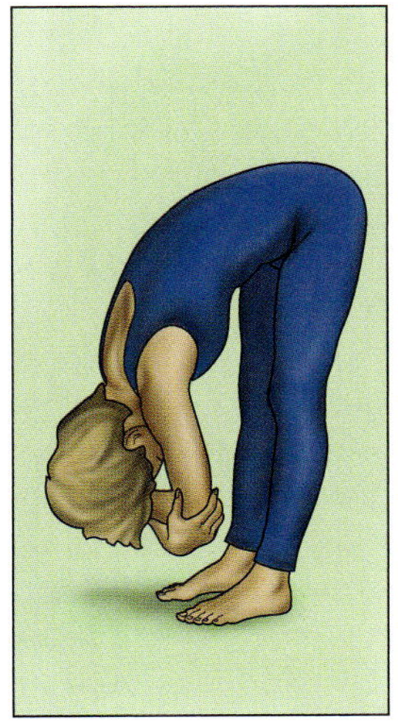

2 The **Rag Doll** restores flexibility. From a standing position, slowly bend forward from your hips, head down, as far as you can go without straining your back or bending your legs. If your back is painful, slightly bend your knees. Hold 15 to 20 seconds as you breathe slowly. Inhale and come back to an upright position.

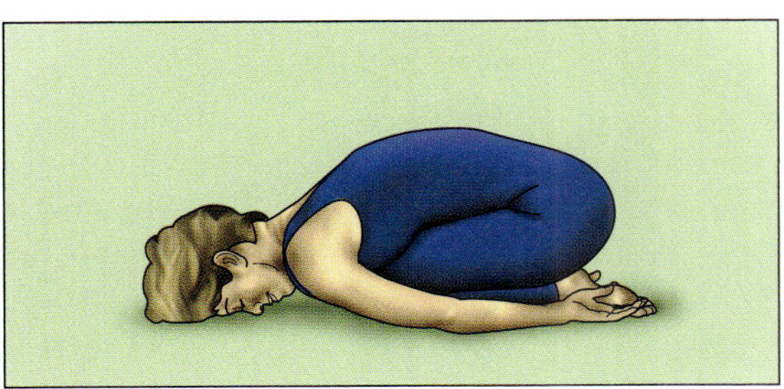

3 The **Child** stretches low-back muscles. Sit on your heels, knees together. Exhale and bend from the hips. Extend your upper body over your knees with arms at your sides, palms up. Move your forehead toward the floor. Breathe slowly, hold 15 to 20 seconds, then sit up again.

mend preventive treatment to relax the back muscles before a problem occurs. One such recommendation is sleeping in the shrimp position, lying on your side with the back curled, and using warm compresses or moist heat to improve circulation.

D

ACUPUNCTURE

An acupuncturist will determine the precise location of the nerve or nerves affected by a herniated disk and will most likely treat points along the governing vessel meridian. *(See pages 22 and 23 and the **Appendix** for more information.)*

BODY WORK

Alternative therapists focus on the body mechanics that have led to stress on the disk. **Reflexology** manipulates certain areas in the hands and feet. For pain and tension relief in the lower back, advocates of reflexology cite positive results from applying firm pressure behind the anklebone and at the outer edge of the instep.

After initial symptoms are under control, a practitioner trained in the **Alexander technique** or the **Feldenkrais method** may help people with chronic problems reestablish good posture and body control, which in turn can help prevent the recurrence of disk problems.

CHIROPRACTIC

Today's chiropractic treatment for chronic disk problems is likely to include manual examination or x-ray diagnosis to determine the location of the affected vertebra. Hands-on procedures to correct muscle and joint malfunction—with due caution not to exacerbate the disk strain—are likely to be followed by a regimen of massage and exercise that will soothe and strengthen the surrounding muscles.

PREVENTION

Yoga is a well-established, long-term approach to relaxing and conditioning both the body and the mind. The exercises at left are recommended for strengthening the back and neck, relaxing the back muscles, and relieving overall bodily stress. ■

DIVERTICULITIS

D

SYMPTOMS

- severe, cramping abdominal pain that is usually more severe on the left side.
- nausea.
- fever.
- constipation, thin stools, diarrhea.
- pain in the lower left quadrant of the abdomen that increases when the sore spot is touched.

CALL YOUR DOCTOR IF:

- you have fever, chills, and abdominal swelling, or are vomiting; you could have peritonitis, an infection of the membrane that lines the abdominal cavity. **Get medical help immediately.**
- blood appears in stools; this indicates **internal bleeding.** *(See also page 70 in **Emergencies/First Aid.**)*
- you have a fever; you may have an infection that requires medication.
- severe pain continues despite treatment; you may have another abdominal disorder.

Diverticulitis is the inflammation or infection of small pouches, called diverticula, that develop along the walls of your intestines. The formation of the pouches themselves is a relatively benign condition known as diverticulosis. The pouches can develop anywhere on the digestive tract, but they most commonly form at the end of the descending and sigmoid colons, and they also frequently occur on the first section of the small intestine (although they rarely cause problems there). If you have diverticulosis, you may not even be aware of it, because the diverticula are usually painless and cause few, if any, symptoms. You may experience some cramping on your left side that disappears when you pass gas or move your bowels. And because diverticula sometimes bleed, bright red blood may appear in your stool.

The more serious disease, diverticulitis, may involve anything from a small abscess in one or more of the pouches to a massive infection or perforation of the bowel. The symptoms are similar to those of ***appendicitis,*** except that the pain is located in the lower left side rather than the lower right side.

Diverticulitis may be acute or chronic. The acute form can manifest itself with one or more severe attacks of infection and inflammation. In chronic diverticulitis, inflammation and infection may subside, but they may never clear up completely. The inflammation of diverticulitis can eventually result in a bowel obstruction, which is indicated by constipation, thin stools, diarrhea, abdominal distention, and abdominal pain. If the obstruction persists, abdominal pain and tenderness will increase, and you may experience nausea and vomiting.

If it is left untreated, diverticulitis can lead to serious complications requiring extensive surgery. Abscesses may form around the infected diverticula, and if these go through the intestinal wall, you may develop peritonitis, a potentially fatal infection that requires immediate treatment. An infected diverticulum can also reach an adjoining organ and form a connection, or fistula, between them. This most frequently occurs between the large intestine and the bladder, and it can lead to an infection of the neighboring kidneys. Another potential complication is severe internal and colonic bleeding.

CAUSES

Aging and heredity are primary factors in the development of diverticulosis and diverticulitis, but diet also plays a role; eating a lot of low-fiber, refined foods can greatly increase the risk. Indeed, in Western societies, an estimated 20 to 50 percent of people over 50 eventually develop diverticular disorders; the figure may be higher than 50 percent in the United States.

If you are often constipated and usually strain at bowel movements, you may create enough pressure in the intestinal walls to begin the development of diverticular pouches. If the diverticula then become filled with fecal material or with undigested food, they are vulnerable to bacterial infection, leading to the inflammation of diverticulitis.

THE DIVERTICULA

If the lining of the colon is weakened for some reason, internal pressure can force small pockets of the lining to bulge through the muscle wall. Undigested food or fecal matter lodged in the bulges—or diverticula—can become infected. If the condition is not treated, the resulting inflammation—called diverticulitis—may cause abscesses that can break through the intestinal wall into the abdominal cavity.

DIAGNOSTIC AND TEST PROCEDURES

If you think you have either diverticulosis or diverticulitis, your doctor will probably have tests done on both your blood and stool to help diagnose possible infection. Because ***cancer, irritable bowel syndrome,*** and diverticulitis can share the same symptoms, your doctor will need to thoroughly examine your intestines. A barium enema, which fills the colon with barium and allows an x-ray to show an outline of the inside of the intestines, can help confirm a diagnosis of diverticulitis. You may also have the insides of your intestines examined with a flexible lighted tube in a procedure called a sigmoidoscopy. Sometimes a bit of tissue may also be removed for a biopsy, to test for cancerous growth. If you have an acute case of diverticulitis, both barium enemas and biopsies can injure your intestine, so your doctor may choose instead a CT scan, which shows the bowel wall and the outside of the colon and can also confirm the diagnosis.

TREATMENT

Diverticulosis can be treated at home, but if you have diverticulitis, you need to see a physician to make sure you fully recover and to avoid possibly life-threatening complications. Conventional medicine treats diverticulitis using diet modifications, antibiotics, and possibly surgery. Alternative treatments for diverticulitis may be used in conjunction with conventional treatment to help ease the symptoms and bolster the digestive tract.

CONVENTIONAL MEDICINE

If you have a mild case of diverticulosis, your doctor may have you eat a high-fiber diet to make sure your bowels move regularly and to reduce your odds of getting diverticulitis. If you do go on to develop diverticulitis but have only a mild infection, you may need just bed rest, stool softeners, a liquid diet, ***antibiotics*** to fight the inflammation, and possibly ***antispasmodic drugs.***

However, if you have had a perforation or develop a more severe infection, you will probably be put in the hospital for intravenous antibiotic therapy. You may also be fed intravenously to give your colon time to recuperate. In some cases, your doctor may want to drain infected abscesses and give your intestinal tract a rest by performing a temporary colostomy. A colostomy creates an opening so your intestine will empty into a bag that is attached to the front of your abdomen. Depending on the success of your recovery, this procedure may be reversed during a second operation. *(See also* ***Colorectal Cancer.****)*

If you have several attacks of acute diverticulitis, your doctor may want to remove the infected section of the intestine when you are free of symptoms. You may also need surgery if intravenous therapy does not effectively treat your acute attack of diverticulitis. Whatever your treatment, your chances for a full recovery are very good if you receive prompt medical attention.

ALTERNATIVE CHOICES

Alternative practitioners may treat some mild cases of diverticulitis, but more serious cases require conventional treatment in order to prevent dangerous health complications.

ACUPUNCTURE

To treat diverticulitis, an acupuncturist will target points intended to relieve pain and distention, reduce inflammation, regulate intestinal peristalsis, and improve the tone of the intestinal wall. Treatments are performed once or twice a week depending on the severity of the condition, with a full course of treatment requiring about 10 visits. It's very important to observe good dietary habits while undergoing acupuncture therapy.

AROMATHERAPY

Inhaling two drops of ***hyssop*** *(Hyssopus officinalis)* three times daily may serve as an abdominal relaxant.

CHINESE HERBS

Some Chinese herbs that are used to treat systemic disorders may prove helpful for diverticulitis. See a practitioner of Chinese medicine for recommendations and treatment.

HERBAL THERAPIES

Slippery elm *(Ulmus fulva)* may be soothing to infected diverticula: Put 1 tsp powder into ½ cup water, bring to a boil, and simmer 15 minutes. Drink three times daily.

Always check with a practitioner first to see if using this herb is appropriate for your particular illness.

HOMEOPATHY

Many homeopathic remedies, such as ***Belladonna, Bryonia,*** and *Colocynthis,* may be used to treat diverticulitis. Check with a homeopathic physician to see which medicines and dosages might be appropriate for you.

MASSAGE

Use a light vegetable oil to massage your lower abdomen with circular clockwise strokes for five minutes while you are lying down each morning. Follow the massage by drinking an herbal tea such as ***chamomile*** *(Matricaria recutita),* which may help promote relaxation.

MIND/BODY MEDICINE

Relaxation techniques may help you deal with the stress and pain of diverticulitis.

NUTRITION AND DIET

Drink at least six glasses of water daily to prevent constipation. If you do become constipated, prunes, prune juice, or herbal teas specifically formulated for constipation may serve as natural laxatives. Keep to a low-fat, high fiber diet; fat slows down passage of food through the intestine, while fiber will speed it up. Get yourself tested for food allergies to identify foods that irritate your system and that you should avoid.

During acute attacks of diverticulitis, try a one- to three-day water or vegetable-juice fast. Eat low-bulk foods (broths and low-fiber breads) while diverticula are still inflamed and sensitive. During an attack of acute diverticulitis, make the following foods a significant part of your diet: cooked vegetables, cooked fruits, and apples—all of which will be soothing to the inflamed intestine. Avoid milk and milk products (yogurts and cheeses), which could worsen your illness, especially if you have diarrhea. Iron supplements may irritate the colon; consult your health-care practitioner.

REFLEXOLOGY

To stimulate secretion of norepinephrine and hydrocortisone (which help your body deal with stress and reduce infection) and maintain intestinal muscle tone, a practitioner will massage adrenal gland areas on the foot. Stimulating intestine areas helps intestines contract regularly and remove wastes as will stimulating areas corresponding to the location of the inflamed diverticula in the intestine (the descending colon area). Stimulating the diaphragm/solar plexus area may help with stress and tension.

AT-HOME REMEDIES

- ◆ Use a heating pad to treat mild pain and spasms in your abdomen. However, do not use high settings for prolonged periods, and never sleep on a heating pad; you could burn yourself.
- ◆ To promote regularity, try to move your bowels at the same time every day (after meals is usually easier).
- ◆ Stay in bed if you are feverish or having a great deal of pain, and get medical help soon.

PREVENTION

The best preventive action you can take against diverticulitis, of course, is to keep from developing the small intestinal sacs called diverticula. You have a good chance of doing that simply by modifying your diet and lifestyle. Eat whole-grain brown rice and buckwheat, whole-grain breads, oatmeal, bran cereals, fibrous fresh fruits, and vegetables, or try an over-the-counter preparation containing ***psyllium*** *(Plantago psyllium)* to increase the bulk in your diet. You can also try ground psyllium seed: Add 1 tsp over any cold liquid, and drink once a day—within a few minutes of preparing, before the mixture gels. Make sure you drink plenty of fluids if you increase your intake of fiber, and take care to add fiber gradually; a sudden switch to a high-fiber diet can cause your abdomen to become distended and create an uncomfortable amount of intestinal gas. Adjust your diet to remove foods that are difficult for you to digest.

Avoid refined foods such as white flour, white sugar, white rice, and other processed foods. Contrary to popular wisdom, however, it is not necessary to avoid nuts and seeds; they are no more likely than other foods to become caught in diverticula.

Try over-the-counter stool softeners to fight constipation. If you have the urge to move your bowels, don't delay or ignore it. Regular exercise and **yoga** can help the muscles in your intestine retain their tone, which encourages regular bowel movements. Don't use suppositories for constipation, because your system may become addicted to them. Prunes, prune juice, and psyllium seed are all good natural laxatives. Specially formulated teas to fight constipation are available in health food stores, but some may be very strong, so use them only as directed; avoid products containing ***senna*** *(Cassia senna),* which is an especially strong herbal laxative. ■

D

DIZZINESS

Read down this column to find your symptoms. Then read across.

SYMPTOMS	AILMENT/PROBLEM
◆ dizziness (your head or everything around you seems to spin) with no obvious associated symptoms.	◆ Dizziness (general)
◆ dizziness with weakness, paralysis, or numbness in arms or legs; possibly, blurred or temporary loss of vision or difficulty speaking.	◆ ***Stroke*** or transient ischemic attack
◆ dizziness with persistent or recurrent headache; less commonly, nausea, vomiting, seizures, personality change, vision loss, speech problems, weakness or paralysis, memory impairment, or coordination or balance problems.	◆ Brain tumor or bleeding
◆ dizziness when turning the head, with pain and stiffness in joints, in a person older than 50.	◆ Cervical osteoarthritis
◆ continuous severe dizziness that worsens with movement; loss of hearing, ringing in ears; possibly, nausea, vomiting; previous viral infection.	◆ Inflamed inner ear and/or nerve (labyrinthitis)
◆ attacks of intermittent dizziness; loss of hearing, ringing in ears; possibly, headache, nausea and vomiting, pallor, or exhaustion.	◆ ***Ménière's disease***
◆ dizziness when changing the position of your head.	◆ Postural dizziness (benign positional vertigo)

WHAT TO DO	OTHER INFO
◆ Sit, close your eyes, bow your head, and breathe deeply. If attacks are severe, call your doctor to check on possible causes that could be treated; you may need to change a medication you're taking.	◆ Many drugs can cause dizziness, such as ***nonsteroidal anti-inflammatory drugs (NSAIDs), antibiotics,*** and ***antihypertensives.***
◆ **Call 911 or your emergency number now.** The usual procedure is hospitalization for tests, medication to prevent further strokes, and possibly surgery. See ***Stroke.***	◆ A stroke is a sudden loss of brain function caused by blockage of or damage to a blood vessel to the brain. In transient ischemic attack, the disruption of blood supply is temporary and the symptoms subside.
◆ **Call your doctor, 911, or your emergency number now.** A brain tumor may require surgical removal, radiation therapy, and/or chemotherapy. Bleeding within the skull is an emergency and may require surgery. See ***Brain Cancer.***	◆ A tumor develops slowly over a period of time, whereas bleeding may begin suddenly as the result of trauma or abnormalities of the blood vessels.
◆ Call your doctor, who may prescribe a neck collar or anti-inflammatory drugs to relieve pain. See ***Arthritis.***	◆ Dizziness may be caused by bony outgrowths and inflammation of neck joints, which put pressure on nerves and blood vessels.
◆ The usual treatment is bed rest, the ***antihistamine*** meclizine, and possibly, ***antianxiety drugs.***	◆ With or without treatment, recovery usually takes several days to three weeks. The cause of this inflammation is believed to be viral.
◆ Call your doctor. The usual treatment is bed rest and the ***antihistamine*** meclizine for relief of vertigo.	◆ Sometimes a tube is inserted to equalize air pressure on both sides of the eardrum. ***Vitamin*** B_6 (50 mg, three times a day) may be helpful.
◆ Call your doctor if the symptoms are troublesome. Head-tilting exercises may help to bring on and then blunt the vertigo.	◆ Postural dizziness usually subsides in a few seconds without treatment.

D

SYMPTOMS

- changes in appearance and behavior that affect relationships and work performance.
- in children, abrupt changes in mood or attitude, poor school performance, temper flareups, or increased secrecy.

Specific symptoms depend on the drug:
- Extreme energy, weight loss, dilated pupils, insomnia, and trembling may indicate abuse of **stimulants,** or "uppers."
- Lethargy, slurred or confused speech, lack of balance, constricted pupils, or excessive sleep may point to abuse of **sedatives,** or "downers."
- Mood swings, red eyes, dilated pupils, slowed time sense and reflexes, dizziness, and lethargy may indicate **marijuana** use.
- Ulcerated nostrils are typical of **cocaine** sniffing; a runny nose or sniffles are typical of smoking crack cocaine; needle marks on the arms may indicate intravenous cocaine abuse.
- Weight loss, lethargy, mood swings, excessive sweating, slurred speech, constricted pupils, and poor appetite suggest **opiate** abuse.
- Hallucinations, dilated pupils, trembling, and sweating indicate abuse of **psychedelic** drugs.

CALL YOUR DOCTOR IF:

- you detect any of the above symptoms in a family member—especially a child or teenager—and suspect drug abuse. The abuser will often deny the problem; you will need professional guidance to deal with the situation.

Drug abuse is the use of a psychoactive drug—legal or illegal—enough to cause the abuser physical, mental, emotional, or social harm. Addiction or dependence is the compulsive, continued use of a drug. *(See also **Alcohol Abuse** and **Nicotine Withdrawal.**)* While the term "drug abuse" conjures up violent images of the illegal drug trade, abuse of legal drugs is an even larger health problem. Between two and three million Americans are addicted to prescription drugs, and hospitals report as many emergencies from abuse of legal drugs as from illegal drugs. Like alcohol abusers, drug abusers commonly deny their problem by playing down the extent of drug use or blaming external factors, such as job or family stress. Families may join in denial in a misguided effort to defend the abuser, creating a powerful barrier to treatment and recovery.

Commonly abused drugs fall into several broad categories:

Central nervous system (CNS) depressants. Sleeping pills and ***antianxiety drugs*** are among the most prescribed medications in the United States; about seven million people take some form of CNS depressant at least once a week. Barbiturates bring on effects like those of alcohol: Small doses are relaxing, but large amounts can damage both mind and body. Taken with alcohol, barbiturates can be fatal. The risks of addiction and overdose are so well known that doctors prescribe barbiturates with extreme caution.

Benzodiazepines are safer than barbiturates but can cause dependence as patients develop tolerance to them after a few weeks of use. This class includes the popular antianxiety agents ***diazepam, alprazolam,*** and ***triazolam.*** Their abuse brings on drowsiness, slurred speech, and lack of coordination, which may progress to memory impairment, tremors, and paranoia. A drug abuser being treated with benzodiazepines for anxiety during withdrawal is quite likely to start abusing a benzodiazepine.

Stimulants. Addictive stimulants cause rapid speech, agitation, and a debilitating pattern of highs followed by crashes. People addicted to amphetamines, or uppers, often try to calm themselves down with CNS depressants, or downers, and become caught in an up-and-down cycle. A more powerful and more habit-forming stimulant is cocaine; the smoked version called crack is highly addictive. There are an estimated two million cocaine addicts in the U.S.

Opiates. About half a million people in the U.S. are addicted to opium, morphine, or heroin. The addiction typically causes ***depression, anxiety,*** low self-esteem, and reduced coping ability. Intravenous injection of these drugs carries the additional risk of ***hepatitis, AIDS,*** and other transmissible diseases.

Cannabis. Smoking marijuana can depress short-term memory, motivation, and energy levels. Chronic use brings increased heart rate, ***vision problems,*** poor lung function, changes in sex hormones, and increased risk of ***lung cancer.*** Marijuana and other forms of cannabis such as "hash" are not highly addictive but are considered entry drugs: Marijuana users are significantly more likely to use cocaine than are nonusers.

Other commonly abused substances range from **tobacco** and **alcohol** to **psychedelic drugs** like LSD. Athletes who use **anabolic steroids** to add muscle face the possibility of violent behavior, ***heart disease,*** and severe liver and hormone damage. Babies of pregnant women who abuse either legal or illegal drugs face special dangers, ranging from premature birth and malnutrition to life-threatening birth defects. Many adolescents are tempted to experiment with drugs and are highly vulnerable to peer pressure—especially those in poverty or with nonsupportive families.

MISUSE OF LEGAL DRUGS

Millions of Americans abuse legal prescription and nonprescription drugs. Even mild, "everyday" drugs such as cough medicines and diet pills can be abused to the point of dependence and physical harm. ***Aspirin*** *and* ***ibuprofen*** *can cause bleeding* ***stomach ulcers,*** *long-term use of* ***laxatives*** *can damage the bowels, and nasal sprays can produce a dependence that actually increases congestion. All medications should be taken only as directed; if a drug is not achieving the desired effect, consult your doctor before taking more.*

CAUSES

There is little agreement on the underlying cause of substance abuse, but experts are more likely to regard it as a disease than a lack of will power. Chronic alcohol and drug abusers may have a genetic predisposition to addiction, but environmental and social factors such as poverty, family dysfunction, and peer pressure are also significant. Certainly the social context can be crucial: One cannot become addicted to drugs without starting to use them in the first place.

Many people consider that drug dependence comes from a natural desire to alter a person's consciousness or an effort to achieve wholeness. One reason addictive drugs are so dangerous is that most people who use them believe they are immune to addiction. Once drug dependence is established, the pattern is hard to break—whether or not the abuser is aware of the problem. Tolerance to opiates and stimulants increases with use, so chronic abusers have to take more to get the same effect. For the most addictive drugs, such as heroin and cocaine, continued use is often reinforced by the desire to avoid the pain of withdrawal.

TREATMENT

Treatment is a two-step process. **Withdrawal** from drug use may require only days or weeks, but can be unpleasant and even dangerous without professional supervision. **Recovery** is the extended stage of remaining drug free.

CONVENTIONAL MEDICINE

The first step in treating drug abuse is awareness. Some addicts may not know they are drug dependent; others deny it. At this stage, family, friends, or a trusted professional must make the case for abstinence and treatment.

No single treatment fits all abusers; appropriate treatment depends on the type and severity of the addiction. Approaches range from outpatient maintenance programs, psychotherapy, and self-help groups like Narcotics Anonymous to residential programs lasting weeks or months. An addicted person may need not just drug treatment but also medical care, welfare support, and psychiatric or social counseling. Successful recovery programs strive to establish social support, raise self-esteem and a sense of spirituality, and help the addict avoid situations that can trigger relapse. For many abusers, the key to success may involve finding regular employment, drug-free housing, and friendships with people who do not use drugs.

Withdrawal from **CNS depressants,** or downers, can be painful and even life-threatening. Stopping the chronic use of barbiturates and some ***benzodiazepines*** can produce delirium tremens, rapid pulse, weakness, convulsions, and hallucinations. Because of the danger of seizures, withdrawal should be done under a doctor's care if the drugs have been used for more than four to six weeks.

Breaking away from **stimulants,** or uppers, can produce lethargy, anxiety, fatigue, hallucinations, and depression. Because most stimulants do not produce physical addiction as strong as that of barbiturates or heroin, withdrawal symptoms may not be as severe. The exception is cocaine, which is very difficult to relinquish. Post-withdrawal treatment of chronic cocaine abuse often requires extensive counseling, along with group and family support. Therapy and group support are equally essential for abusers of amphetamines; patients may become depressed and even suicidal after withdrawal.

Withdrawal from an addiction to **opiates**—with shakes, sweats, tremors, and acute craving for the drug—has been widely dramatized. As disagreeable as the symptoms are, they are not as dangerous to the addict as those of alcohol or barbiturate withdrawal. While opiate addiction was once thought almost impossible to break, the experience of many Vietnam War veterans who voluntarily quit their drug habits on returning home has shown that self-initiated cure is possible. After withdrawal from heroin or morphine, some users are "maintained" on prescribed dos-

DRUGS AND THE ELDERLY

Older people often suffer adverse drug effects or become unwitting abusers for several reasons. We metabolize and excrete drugs more slowly as we age, so it is easier to take an overdose. Many people do not even realize that cough medicines, sleeping aids, diet pills, and laxatives are drugs. Older people often increase the risk of dangerous interactions and side effects by simultaneously taking several prescription drugs for different ailments or combining prescription and nonprescription drugs without their physicians' knowledge.

In older people, symptoms of drug intoxication are easily mistaken for mental illness or other ailments. Complications of drug abuse are more common in the elderly, and detoxification is more complex. Certain drugs are of special concern. ***Diuretics,*** *commonly used to lower blood pressure, can deplete the body's store of* ***potassium*** *and other minerals, causing weakness and appetite loss. Some* ***antihypertensive drugs*** *may bring depression, fatigue, or fainting.* ***Antianxiety drugs*** *may cause drowsiness, shakiness, confusion, and amnesia if taken to excess. While anyone taking medication should follow dosages meticulously, it is especially important for older people to do so and to tell their physicians about all the medications they take. Supervising or helping an older person with medications is not just a kindness—it may be a lifesaver.*

es of methadone, a less addictive narcotic, under a doctor's care. While controversial, methadone maintenance is still customary because stress or depression can easily trigger a return to more harmful drugs even after years of nonuse.

Recovery is the stage after withdrawal when the individual must strive to remain drug free. This stage is often very difficult because it requires the addicted person to change habits and lifestyle, and to control the use of potentially addicting substances throughout life. The backing of family, friends, employers, and drug-support groups can be a powerful—often vital—part of an addict's recovery. For adolescents, group treatment is often more successful than individual therapy. Since a child's addiction is often part of a family problem, treatment should involve all family members. Because of the power of peer pressure, an adolescent may need more reinforcement than an adult to stay with a recovery regimen.

ALTERNATIVE CHOICES

Many alternative therapies can help reduce the stress that accompanies or underlies drug abuse, strengthen the body, and reduce cravings.

ACUPUNCTURE

Acupuncturists report success in treating addicts of heroin, cocaine, and other drugs. In particular, acupuncture on several points of the ear is reported to reduce withdrawal symptoms and cravings, prevent relapse, and raise recovery rates.

HERBAL THERAPIES

Cleansing the body of toxins is an important step in healing. Silymarin, found in ***milk thistle*** *(Silybum marianum),* is taken to strengthen the liver. Wild oat extract, ***burdock*** *(Arctium lappa)* root, ***licorice*** *(Glycyrrhiza glabra), and* ***red clover*** *(Trifolium pratense)* are said to cleanse the blood, while ***skullcap*** *(Scutellaria lateriflora),* ***valerian*** *(Valeriana officinalis),* and vervain reduce anxiety. See a professional herbalist for dosages.

HYDROTHERAPY

Some therapists believe that cleansing the body of drugs takes months. A daily 10- to 20-minute bath containing half a cup of baking soda or sea salt can be a powerful aid to detoxification.

MIND/BODY MEDICINE

Biofeedback, meditation, relaxation response, and **guided imagery** techniques can help reduce stress and bring about behavioral changes as aids to recovery. For specific techniques, see ***Stress.***

NUTRITION AND DIET

Drug abusers tend to eat poorly and may overuse sugar. For lasting recovery, eat at least three regular meals a day with a good balance of protein, vegetables, and complex carbohydrates. If you have an irresistible craving for sweets, use barley malt or rice syrup instead of sugar, and take a 250 mcg capsule of ***chromium*** picolinate daily to help stabilize erratic blood sugar levels. Ask your doctor about the potential benefits of supplemental ***vitamins C*** and ***E***, pantothenic acid ***(vitamin*** B_5***),*** adrenal extract, ***magnesium, calcium, potassium,*** choline, ***zinc, folic acid,*** and L-tyrosine.

PREVENTION

While efforts to eradicate illegal drugs have shown little success, both treatment and public education make a difference. One study found that a dollar spent on treatment of cocaine users was seven times as effective in cutting cocaine consumption as a dollar spent on law enforcement.

Parent groups, community efforts, public education and prevention programs, drug-free workplaces, and strong national leadership have all played a role in discouraging illegal drug use. Parents may not be able to stop their children from experimenting with drugs, but they can give them accurate information about drug abuse—especially the genetic risk to their own unborn children. Lectures and scare tactics are rarely successful, but adolescents should understand the internal and external pressures that make people start using drugs, hear rebuttals to pro-drug arguments, and learn techniques for resisting peer pressure. But if you don't want your children to abuse drugs—including alcohol and tobacco—the best first step is to set the right example. ■

EARACHE

Read down this column to find your symptoms. Then read across.

SYMPTOMS	AILMENT/PROBLEM
See ***Otitis Media*** or the ***Atlas of the Body*** for an illustration of the anatomy of the ear.	
◆ earache that gets worse over weeks or months; blocked feeling and ringing in the ears; partial hearing loss.	◆ Excess earwax that has hardened in the outer ear canal, blocking the eardrum
◆ following air travel or scuba diving, ear pain that may radiate into the cheeks and forehead; dizziness; ringing in the ears; ears feel blocked.	◆ Barotrauma (strained or damaged eardrum, due to large changes in atmospheric pressure)
◆ feeling that something is in your ear; hearing loss; ear pain.	◆ Presence of a foreign object, such as a bug, a seed, or an earplug, in the ear
◆ itching in the ear, later becoming sharp or dull ear pain; pain worsens if you pull on your earlobe; yellowish discharge; possibly, fever and temporary hearing loss.	◆ ***Swimmer's ear***
◆ ear pain that is either sharp and sudden or dull and throbbing; fever; nasal congestion; muffled hearing.	◆ ***Otitis media***
◆ pressure in the ear; a lump outside or inside the ear canal; excessive earwax; possibly, hearing loss and infection (fever, ear pain, and swelling).	◆ A benign (noncancerous) cyst or tumor in or just outside the ear canal
◆ earache; persistent tooth or jaw pain.	◆ Tooth or gum trouble, such as tooth decay or abscess; ***temporomandibular joint syndrome***
◆ dull pain, redness, and swelling both within and behind the ear; mild fever; thick pus discharge from ear; possibly, partial hearing loss.	◆ Mastoiditis (***infection*** of the mastoid process, the honeycomb-like bone behind the ear)
◆ sudden ear pain, usually after an injury or an infection; bleeding or pus discharge from the ear; dizziness; ringing in the ear; partial hearing loss.	◆ Ruptured eardrum

WHAT TO DO	OTHER INFO
◆ For three days, place a few drops of warm baby oil or olive oil in the ear twice daily to soften wax. Then use a bulb syringe to flush out the wax with warm water.	◆ Flushing the ear may cause dizziness. Never try to remove wax by inserting an object—even a cotton-tipped swab—in your ear; you could damage your eardrum.
◆ Symptoms should dissipate within a few hours without treatment. If they don't, consult your doctor.	◆ During flight, hold your nose and gently blow air into it, or constantly suck hard candy or chew gum; this may help equalize the pressure on either side of your eardrum.
◆ See ***Emergencies/First Aid: Ear Emergencies.***	◆ Never try to remove an object that is lodged in your ear; you risk perforating your eardrum. See your doctor.
◆ Take ***acetaminophen*** for pain. Your doctor may also prescribe ear drops containing an ***antibiotic,*** an ***antifungal drug,*** or cortisone (to reduce inflammation).	◆ Keep water out of your ears (when swimming and showering) for at least three weeks after symptoms have subsided. Don't use earplugs; they can be harmful.
◆ Place a warm compress over the ear and take ***acetaminophen.*** Call your doctor; you may need prescription ***antibiotics.***	◆ A few drops of warm ***garlic*** *(Allium sativum)* or ***mullein*** *(Verbascum thapsus)* oil in your ear may lessen pain.
◆ Often no treatment is needed. If the cyst or tumor becomes extremely large or infected, your doctor will remove it.	◆ The homeopathic remedy ***Silica*** (6x) may help shrink the cyst or tumor.
◆ Call your dentist today. An abscessed tooth is an emergency. See also ***Gum Problems; Toothache.***	◆ Relaxation techniques may ease mild cases of temporomandibular joint syndrome.
◆ Call your doctor today. You need aggressive ***antibiotic*** therapy, perhaps for several weeks. Persistent infection may call for surgical removal of the mastoid process.	◆ Without treatment, mastoiditis can cause serious problems, such as ***meningitis*** and facial paralysis.
◆ Take ***acetaminophen*** for pain until you can see a doctor. You may need a patch for the eardrum (to speed healing) and ***antibiotics.*** Large tears can be surgically repaired.	◆ Don't blow your nose or allow water in your ear until the rupture has healed (which should take two months or so).

ECZEMA

SYMPTOMS

- patches of chronically itchy, dry, thickened skin, usually on wrists, face, and inner creases of the knees and elbows.
- skin lesions, patches of redness, scaling, and—in dark-skinned people—changes in skin color; sometimes small bumps or ***blisters*** that may ooze fluid.

See also the ***Visual Diagnostic Guide.***

CALL YOUR DOCTOR IF:

- you develop an otherwise unexplained ***rash*** and have a family history of eczema or ***asthma.*** You should have a medical diagnosis of the condition.
- the inflammation does not respond within a week to treatment with over-the-counter coal-tar preparations or steroid-based creams. A physician may suggest more aggressive forms of treatment.
- you develop yellowish to light brown crust or pus-filled blisters over existing patches of eczema. This may indicate a ***staph*** or other bacterial infection that should be treated with an ***antibiotic.***
- during a flareup of eczema you are exposed to anyone with a viral skin disease such as ***cold sores, genital warts,*** or ***genital herpes.*** Having eczema puts you at increased risk of contracting the viral disorder.
- you develop numerous small, pus-filled blisters. You may have **eczema herpeticum,** a rare but potentially serious complication caused by the herpes simplex II virus.

Strictly speaking, eczema is a form of ***dermatitis*** characterized by chronically itchy, inflamed skin. The affected area typically becomes dry, the skin flakes off, and occasionally ***blisters*** develop. When eczema appears on fair-skinned people, the affected areas typically turn a brownish gray color; on people with dark skin, it generally alters their natural pigmentation, making the affected area either lighter or darker. Eczema appears most frequently on the face, wrists, elbows, and knees but is not limited to those areas.

Eczema—also known as **atopic dermatitis**—afflicts between 3 and 7 percent of the population to some degree, and in more than 70 percent of patients, it runs in the family. It is most common among infants, many of whom grow out of it before their second birthday. If it persists, the child is likely to be a chronic sufferer and may develop distinctive thickened, brownish gray skin in the areas that break out most frequently. Eczema is often associated with ***asthma,*** so children with that disorder may be at greater risk of skin problems. Since eczema may be in part an internal response to some sort of external ***stress,*** initial treatment focuses on identifying and reducing the possible cause.

CAUSES

Many cases of eczema are ***allergy*** related. In susceptible people, outbreaks can be caused by ingesting certain foods, such as cow's milk, eggs, wheat, and nuts—as well as by inhaling airborne irritants like dust mites and pollen. Eczema is also caused by contact with irritants in common substances, such as woolen and synthetic fabrics, latex rubber, certain detergents, chlorine-based products, the mineral nickel used in plated earrings and other jewelry, and chemicals like formaldehyde, found in permanent-press fabrics, polishes, rugs, foam insulation, and particle board.

In people predisposed to eczema, doctors think outbreaks may be caused by a change in the way a person's immune system reacts to certain kinds of physically, chemically, or emotionally induced ***stress.*** Besides contact with potential allergens, any emotionally charged event—from a move to a new job—may trigger a flareup of the disorder. *(See **Immune Problems** and **Stress.**)*

DIAGNOSTIC AND TEST PROCEDURES

To determine whether an allergy is the underlying cause of the inflammation, ask your doctor about taking a radioallergosorbent test (RAST).

TREATMENT

Because eczema is generally a benign disorder, and because the underlying causes differ from person to person, primary treatment is directed at alleviating symptoms. At-home remedies and over-the-counter medications are usually sufficient. For chronic eczema, a doctor will focus on identifying allergens, building up the immune system, or relaxing the patient. For information on light therapy for eczema, see ***Dermatitis.***

CONVENTIONAL MEDICINE

To relieve itchiness, most doctors will start patients on such basic therapies as a warm bath to remove crusted skin followed by immediate application of petroleum jelly or vegetable shortening, which helps conserve the skin's natural moisture. Topical coal-tar preparations also work, but they can be messy and smelly; they should not be used by pregnant women, and their prolonged use may increase the risk of ***skin cancer.***

If symptoms persist, the doctor may recommend application of an over-the-counter steroid-based ***hydrocortisone*** cream. ***Doxepin*** cream, available with a prescription, may also be effective at relieving itchiness associated with eczema. Apply the ointment as a thin film four times a day for up to eight days. Most patients report no side effects, but the cream may cause a burning sensation in some cases.

If the eczema is allergy related, taking oral ***antihistamines*** may help. In severe cases, the doctor may prescribe oral ***corticosteroid*** medication; steroids should always be taken with caution and never without medical supervision.

For extreme cases of eczema, particularly in children, a wet body wrap can be effective in getting moisture back into the skin. The patient sleeps in wet pajamas covered with dry clothes or a nylon sweat suit; some doctors suggest covering the face with wet gauze wrapped with an elastic bandage, and covering the hands and feet with a pair of wet, then a pair of dry, tube socks. The patient's room must be kept warm.

ALTERNATIVE CHOICES

Alternative therapies are available to address both the symptoms of eczema and some of the underlying causes. Patients should be aware, however, that some herbal therapies can cause allergic reactions and that certain Chinese herbs can be toxic to the liver and immune system. Long-term treatment with herbs should be undertaken only with thorough knowledge of the potential effects and under the guidance of trained therapists. Use extreme caution when giving herbs to children, pregnant women, and the elderly.

ACUPRESSURE

Acupressure is not intended to cure eczema, but applying deep pressure several times a week to

C A U T I O N !

Although steroid creams or oral steroids may be appropriate for acute outbreaks or severe episodes of eczema, long-term use is not advisable because of the considerable risk of side effects. Topical steroid creams can cause thinning and spotting of the skin, *acne,* and permanent stretch marks. If used around the eyes, topical steroid medications can, in rare cases, lead to *glaucoma.* Eczema patients who take oral steroids for longer than the usual two-week cycle and then stop using the drug face the additional risk of severe relapse. For these reasons, steroid therapy is advised only under a doctor's supervision.

E

Liver 3, on top of the foot, and Stomach 36, below the knee, may relieve the tension that can bring on episodes of inflammation. *(See the **Appendix** for more information on point locations.)*

AROMATHERAPY

Essential oils of ***lavender*** *(Lavandula officinalis),* thyme *(Thymus vulgaris),* jasmine *(Jasminum officinale),* and ***chamomile*** *(Matricaria recutita)* may be effective in soothing allergy-related eczema. Add a few drops of one of these oils to a bowl of hot water to scent a room.

BODY WORK

Among the many forms of alternative therapy that relieve tension, **shiatsu** and **reflexology** are the most widely used body work techniques. Consult licensed practitioners about appropriate treatment for your condition.

CHINESE HERBS

Studies suggest that a particular traditional Chinese herbal tea mixture can be beneficial to certain eczema patients. The herbs include siler *(Ledebouriella divaricata)* root, ***Chinese foxglove*** *(Rehmannia glutinosa),* and ***licorice*** *(Glycyrrhiza uralensis),* which are said to be anti-inflammatories, and peony *(Paeonia lactiflora),* which is said to affect the immune system. The researchers caution against long-term use of such mixtures, however, because of potential liver toxicity and because the skin condition may return after patients stop drinking the tea. Because of the wide range of Chinese herbal products, a licensed professional should monitor your use of any long-term treatment.

HERBAL THERAPIES

Evidence suggests that ***evening primrose oil*** *(Oenothera biennis)* may effectively treat itching associated with eczema. Some practitioners consider it as effective as ***corticosteroids*** without their potential side effects. However, people with liver disease or high cholesterol should use this treatment only under medical supervision, and pregnant women should not use it at all because of its effect on estrogen and progesterone levels.

Burdock *(Arctium lappa)* root and ***dandelion*** *(Taraxacum officinale)* root may also be effective in treating some forms of eczema. Take up to 1½ tsp of the fluid extract a day. You can also brew teas from either of these roots: Simmer 1 tbsp of the dried root in a cup of boiling water for 10 minutes, strain, and drink up to three cups a day. ***Chamomile*** *(Matricaria recutita)* ointment soothes dry, flaky skin and helps to combat inflammation and itching. Do not take any of these herbs for longer than one month without supervision by a medical herbalist or other trained practitioner.

HOMEOPATHY

A homeopathic remedy to soothe inflamed skin that patients can apply safely at home is topical *Calendula* cream. Do not attempt to treat eczema with other homeopathic remedies, however, without consulting a licensed homeopath. Because eczema is a chronic, systemic problem, a homeopath will make a complete examination of all your symptoms—including sleep patterns, food cravings, body temperature, moods, and family history—before deciding on a plan of action. During homeopathic treatment, eczema may actually get worse before it gets better, so professional supervision is important.

NUTRITION AND DIET

Since many eczema patients have ***allergy*** problems, they should pay particular attention to their diets. In addition to avoiding the traditional suspects—cow's milk, eggs, wheat flour, sugar, and nuts—patients should be wary of eating too much red meat, because animal fats contain fatty acids that promote the body's inflammatory response.

The oils of mackerel, herring, and salmon are high in eicosapentaenoic acid (EPA), shown to reduce skin inflammation and itchiness. Since you would have to eat up to two pounds of fresh fish a day to get the necessary amount of EPA, it's more convenient to take 1 tbsp cod-liver oil or four 1,000-mg fish-oil capsules, with food, a day.

Patients may benefit from a daily 50-mg ***zinc*** supplement; many eczema sufferers have a zinc deficiency, and zinc helps the body metabolize fatty acids. Your doctor may recommend taking ***vitamin A,*** also found in cod-liver oil, which is essential for the repair and renewal of skin. Adults can take doses of up to 25,000 IU a day. To avoid the risk of overdose, particularly with fat-soluble vitamins, ask your doctor to monitor your progress.

MIND/BODY MEDICINE

With all the possible causes of eczema, many patients overlook the key element of emotional or physical ***stress.*** A Swedish study of adult eczema patients found that those who used relaxation techniques along with their regular regimen of topical preparations improved much faster than those who received topical medication alone.

AT-HOME REMEDIES

- To soothe itchiness and help the skin retain moisture in mild forms of eczema, try a warm bath followed by an application of topical ointment. Use simple creams or ointments made with zinc oxide, ***vitamin E, burdock, chamomile,*** or ***calendula***—and no additives, preservatives, oils, or perfumes.
- Relax. To relieve stress and improve circulation, take a brisk walk or exercise on a regular basis. Come home to a warm bath sprinkled with a few drops of essential oil of ***lavender.***
- Drink plenty of fluids to keep your skin hydrated.
- Eat little or no red meat. Be wary of highly allergenic foods such as cow's milk, wheat, and eggs. Take daily supplements of fish oil, ***vitamin A,*** and ***zinc.***
- If your baby has eczema, keep her from scratching by putting mittens on her hands when she goes to bed. To avoid the possibility of loose threads wrapping around the baby's wrists or fingers and cutting off circulation, always put the mittens on inside out.

PREVENTION

Since eczema often runs in families, parents may have a good idea whether their own children may be at risk. But even if your baby inherits the predisposition, you may be able to lower her chances of being a chronic sufferer. One study suggests that children weaned from breast milk before the age of four months were nearly three times as likely to develop recurrent eczema as children who were weaned later. If possible, babies should live on their mothers' milk exclusively for the first three months, and doctors advise continuing breast milk for at least up to six months as you introduce your baby to solid food. To avoid triggering food allergies that might bring on eczema, do not offer any eggs or fish until the child is at least a year old. Babies should also be protected from such potential allergens as tobacco smoke and pet hairs, and from airborne irritants such as mites and molds. ■

A T T E N T I O N !

BEWARE OF SECONDARY INFECTIONS

Eczema sores can create tiny openings in the skin through which moisture is lost and bacteria and viruses can enter the body. Scratching the skin affected by eczema creates more openings. This is a particular problem with babies, who tend to develop eczema on the cheeks and forehead. If your baby has eczema, keep her nails cut short and—if she tends to scratch the sores—put mittens on her hands inside out, especially at bedtime.

Open eczema sores make a person more susceptible than normal to highly contagious viral skin diseases. Anyone with eczema must be careful to avoid exposure to people with *cold sores, warts,* and other diseases caused by viruses. In particular, the herpes simplex II virus causes eczema herpeticum, a rare but potentially serious complication of adult or infant eczema. It is recognizable by numerous small, pus-filled blisters, which require immediate medical attention.

E

EMPHYSEMA

SYMPTOMS

Emphysema progresses slowly over time and is often mistaken for other ailments, ranging from ***asthma*** to ***heart disease.*** Typical symptoms of emphysema include:

- shortness of breath, worsening over the years.
- a chronic, mild cough, sometimes accompanied by a small amount of phlegm.
- a distended, "barrel-shaped" chest.

CALL YOUR DOCTOR IF:

- your cough produces unusual amounts of phlegm, especially if the phlegm is dark in color and thick. This is a symptom of ***bronchitis*** and an accompanying upper respiratory infection that may require ***antibiotics.***
- you have a lingering, mild cough (sometimes dismissed as "smoker's cough") that does not go away after several months. This symptom points to emphysema, but it could also signal the early stages of ***lung cancer.***
- you begin to lose weight inexplicably. This symptom is associated with emphysema, but it is also characteristic of ***cancer.***
- you regularly become breathless after simple activities, such as climbing a flight of stairs. Again, breathlessness is associated with emphysema, but it could also be a sign of ***cancer*** or ***heart disease.***

Emphysema, a potentially fatal lung disease characterized by increasing loss of elasticity in the lungs, typically causes chronic, mild ***coughing*** and shortness of breath. Although a number of factors—including heredity, pollution, and a preexisting chronic lung disease such as ***asthma***—can play a role in its development, emphysema is most often caused by long-term, heavy smoking. In many cases, emphysema patients also suffer from chronic ***bronchitis,*** which accounts for some of the overlapping symptoms.

More people in the United States die from emphysema than from any other respiratory disease. To date, no cure has been found and no treatment can reverse its effects. However, by seeking professional medical help in the beginning stages of the disease, you can substantially slow its advance.

Emphysema results when the alveoli—tiny, thin-walled air sacs clustered at the ends of the airways deep within the lungs—become damaged or enlarged. Healthy lungs contain about 300 million of these spongy sacs, which are responsible for delivering oxygen into the bloodstream and drawing out carbon dioxide waste. But when the lungs' airways become constricted or damaged, usually from smoking, breathing becomes more forced and difficult. Long periods of labored breathing put pressure on the lungs that eventually stretches the alveoli beyond their normal limits. Over time they lose their natural elasticity and sometimes they burst. Such damage not only prevents the alveoli from working efficiently; it also significantly reduces the surface area and overall elasticity of the lungs. As emphysema develops, sufferers are often unable to carry out even the simplest forms of exercise, such as walking up a flight of stairs, without becoming breathless.

Emphysema is most common in men between the ages of 50 and 70 who have smoked heavily for years, but the disease is becoming more common in women as they join the ranks of heavy smokers. People with emphysema are particularly vulnerable to ***pneumonia, bronchitis,*** and other lung infections, as well as to cardiovascular problems such as heart failure. Although emphysema patients need to be monitored by a medical professional, they can make changes in their lifestyle, learn breathing techniques, and supplement their doctor's care with a number of other therapies to make their lives more comfortable.

CAUSES

By far the most common cause of emphysema is heavy, long-term smoking. Cigarette smoke is thought to break down the elastic fibers in the walls of the alveoli, making the air sacs more susceptible to rupture. Smoking also has the effect of weakening the walls of the lungs' branching airways, causing them to collapse on exhalation, trapping stale air. Besides its role in the development of emphysema, smoking also makes people with the disease more vulnerable to lung infections and other serious disorders, such as chronic ***bronchitis.***

Even one puff on a cigarette is enough to cause temporary paralysis in the tiny, hairlike cells known as cilia that are responsible for brushing debris and excess mucus from the lungs. Cilia damaged by continued smoking function only poorly and eventually may stop working altogether. Clogged with mucus, the lungs are then vulnerable to viral and bacterial infections, which over time distort and permanently damage the lungs' airways.

Any lung disease that causes the narrowing of the respiratory airways—such as chronic bronchitis or ***asthma***—may contribute to the development of emphysema, since the resulting pressure on the lungs may exhaust and ultimately damage the alveoli. In rare cases, emphysema can also be caused by the lack of a cellular enzyme that helps to maintain the elasticity of fibers in the walls of the alveoli. People who have inherited this enzyme deficiency have an increased chance of coming down with emphysema sometime in their thirties or forties, even if they don't smoke.

ALVEOLI

HEALTHY ALVEOLI

STRETCHED AND DAMAGED ALVEOLI

LUNG

Deep in the lungs, the job of delivering oxygen to the bloodstream and removing carbon dioxide is carried out by tiny, thin-walled air sacs called alveoli. When airways become constricted, usually because of smoking, the lungs are forced to work harder, and this puts tremendous pressure on the fragile alveoli. Over time, the sacs may swell or even burst, hampering the vital exchange of gases.

DIAGNOSTIC AND TEST PROCEDURES

A doctor can diagnose emphysema by simply tapping on your chest and listening with a stethoscope. If the tapping produces a hollow sound, more than likely the lungs' air sacs are enlarged or ruptured—the telltale signs of emphysema. After diagnosis, the doctor will probably take an x-ray of your chest to help gauge the extent of the lung damage.

TREATMENT

No treatment will restore your lungs to a healthy state, but there are things you can do to keep your emphysema from getting worse. The first important step is to see a doctor if you develop any of the symptoms listed on page 346. Never dismiss a "smoker's cough" as harmless or merely bothersome; if you smoke, and if you have coughed steadily for more than a month or have suffered chronic breathlessness, chances are your lungs are already damaged. You must stop smoking immediately. If you don't, your condition will almost certainly deteriorate. Breathing techniques, aromatherapy, and oxygen therapy (usually necessary in advanced emphysema) may help you cope with the disease.

CONVENTIONAL MEDICINE

It is important to see a physician regularly if you have emphysema. Your doctor can teach you how to do breathing exercises correctly and how to practice controlled coughing as a way to remove excess mucus from your lungs. Mild physical exercise is also recommended for people with emphysema. A doctor may also prescribe ***bronchodilators*** to help ease breathing.

In severe cases of emphysema, at-home oxygen therapy may be necessary; oxygen-delivering devices are widely available for at-home use in both stationary and mobile tanks. In some cases, surgery may be an option. One procedure—in which damaged portions of the lungs are removed—has been shown to alleviate some of the symptoms of emphysema.

ALTERNATIVE CHOICES

If you have emphysema, you should think of alternative choices only as supplements to supervised medical care. The following remedies may provide some relief from the discomfort associated with the disease.

AROMATHERAPY

Essential oils such as ***eucalyptus*** *(Eucalyptus globulus),* ***hyssop*** *(Hyssopus officinalis),* aniseed *(Pimpinella anisum),* ***lavender*** *(Lavandula officinalis),* pine *(Pinus sylvestris),* and ***rosemary*** *(Rosmarinus officinalis)* may help ease breathing and relieve nasal congestion. Inhale through your nose directly from the bottle, or from a tissue dabbed with a few drops of one or more essential oils. You might also try massaging your chest with 2 tsp of light vegetable oil mixed with 2 drops of essential oil.

CHINESE HERBS

The Chinese herb ***ephedra*** *(Ephedra sinica),* also called *ma huang,* is a potent bronchodilator. Note, however, that large quantities of ephedra have the same effect as large quantities of ***epinephrine;*** do not use this herb if you have ***high blood pressure*** or ***heart disease.*** Prepare an infusion by combining 5 grams ephedra, 4 grams ***cinnamon*** *(Cinnamomum cassia)* sticks, 1.5 grams ***licorice*** *(Glycyrrhiza uralensis),* and 5 grams ***apricot seeds*** *(Prunus armeniaca).* Let the mixture steep in cold water, then bring it to a boil. Drink it hot. Do not use this remedy for a long period of time.

HERBAL THERAPIES

A number of herbs act as soothing expectorants and may be appropriate in the treatment of emphysema. Elecampane *(Inula helenium),* for example, is believed to help clear excess mucus from the lungs. To prepare an infusion, shred the root to yield 1 tsp and add a full cup of cold water. Let the infusion stand for 10 hours, then strain and drink it hot three times daily.

Mullein *(Verbascum thapsus)* tea is recommended for soothing the mucous membranes, especially during episodes of nighttime breathlessness. Other herbs that may help relieve shortness of breath include grindelia (*Grindelia* spp.), *Euphorbia pilulifera,* ***lobelia*** *(Lobelia inflata),* wild black cherry *(Prunus serotina)* bark, ***licorice*** *(Glycyrrhiza glabra),* motherwort *(Leonurus cardiaca),* and aniseed *(Pimpinella anisum).*

HOMEOPATHY

To treat emphysema, a homeopath might recommend the following substances, taken twice a day for a week or as needed. For wheezing and congestion, *Antimonium tartaricum* (12c). For symptoms that worsen on damp days, in stuffy rooms, or early in the morning, *Ammonium carbonicum* (12c). For symptoms that grow worse at night or in cold air and drafts, ***Hepar sulphuris*** (12c).

NUTRITION AND DIET

Some nutritionists recommend avoiding foods that cause excess mucus production, such as dairy products, processed foods, white flour products and white sugar.

REFLEXOLOGY

Toes outstretched, massage the upper surface of both feet, just below the second and fourth toes; this area corresponds to the lungs and chest.

YOGA

The following **yoga** exercises can help you learn

to breathe more efficiently and relieve symptoms.

- With your fingertips on your shoulders, breathe out and join your elbows together in front of you. Inhale as you bring your elbows back as far as you can go, opening your chest and throat fully. Repeat 4 or 5 times, 3 times a day.
- While sitting on a stool or standing, make a breaststroke motion with your arms; slowly stretch them behind you. Clasp your hands, lowering your arms below your buttocks, and pull your shoulders back. Then, still clasping your hands behind you, breathe in and lift your arms up as far as you can. Breathe out, lower your arms, and unclasp your hands. Repeat 4 or 5 times, 3 times a day.

AT-HOME REMEDIES

Inhaling steam can help loosen phlegm in your lungs. First, fill a sink with boiling water. Keeping your eyes closed, drape a towel over your head and inhale the steam for four to five minutes. To further ease breathing and help relieve nasal congestion, try adding a few drops of one or more essential oils to the hot water. *(For a list of suggested oils, see **Aromatherapy**.)*

The moist air distributed by vaporizers can also help clear the lungs. However, in an average-sized room, most vaporizers aren't powerful enough to generate the density of moisture necessary to be truly helpful. If you want to use a vaporizer, place it in a smaller space, such as a bathroom. Don't use warm air vaporizors or humidifiers: They must be scrubbed daily with bleach; otherwise, they can spread germs and encourage mold or mildew growth, increasing your chances of developing lung infections. Rinse cool air vaporizers and humidifiers daily.

PREVENTION

If you smoke, the best way to prevent emphysema is to stop right away. Organizations such as Smokenders and the American Lung Association offer programs that will help you kick the habit. There are also a number of alternative smoking-cessation techniques available *(see **Nicotine Withdrawal**)*.

LEARNING TO BREATHE EASIER

Although there is no cure for emphysema, you can practice some simple exercises and breathing techniques that will help you cope with the disease. *(See **Yoga** for more breathing exercises.)*

Take a walk. Physical fitness is very important for people with emphysema, and daily walking is one of the best means to that end. Begin with a short walk and increase your distance every day. Try to avoid highly polluted areas, or do your walking indoors, perhaps at a local shopping mall.

Arm lift. From a standing position, lift both arms high over your head while breathing deeply. When your lungs are completely filled, slowly lower your arms and exhale. Repeat the exercise three times at first, then increase the number of repetitions each day.

Leg lift. Lie comfortably on your back with knees bent and feet on the floor. Inhale deeply. Slowly raise one knee toward your chest as you exhale; lower your leg as you breathe in. Repeat three times with the same leg, then switch.

Sitting stretch. While seated in a chair, lean back, inhale deeply, and raise your arms high over your head. With your chin tucked into your chest, breathe out as you slowly slump forward; bring your head to your knees and let your arms hang loosely by your sides. Repeat three times.

Diaphragmatic breathing. (This exercise can help increase the efficiency of your lungs and strengthen the muscles that control breathing.) While lying on your back, put the fingertips of one hand over your diaphragm, which lies immediately below your rib cage in the top center of your abdomen. Inhale deeply through your nose and concentrate on pushing your diaphragm against your fingers while expanding your chest. Count slowly to three, then exhale through your nose to the count of six. When you can take about a dozen breaths this way without tiring, try diaphragmatic breathing while sitting, then while walking, and eventually while climbing stairs. ■

ENDOMETRIOSIS

SYMPTOMS

- sharp abdominal pains before, during, or just after menstrual periods.
- sharp abdominal pain during intercourse.
- menstrual periods that are abnormally heavy, especially if they produce large clots and last more than seven days.
- ***infertility.***

CALL YOUR DOCTOR IF:

- you suspect you are suffering from endometriosis; a proper diagnosis is essential to treatment.

Normally, the tissue that lines a woman's uterus, known as the endometrium, is found only in the uterus. However, in a woman suffering from endometriosis, microscopic bits of this tissue migrate outside the uterus, become implanted on other organs and tissues, and grow there. These lesions, or areas of abnormal tissue, usually develop within the abdominal cavity—often involving other portions of the reproductive system, such as the ovaries or the muscular wall of the uterus—but in rare cases they can affect other organs, such as the lungs.

Like the endometrium itself, the transplanted tissue responds to the hormones estrogen and progesterone by thickening and then bleeding every month. But because the transplanted tissue is embedded in other tissue, the blood it produces cannot escape and ends up irritating the surrounding tissue, causing cysts, scars, and adhesions to form. These can eventually bind the reproductive organs together so that they move as one mass when manipulated by a physician.

Cases of endometriosis are classified as minimal, mild, moderate, or severe, depending on

ENDOMETRIAL TISSUE

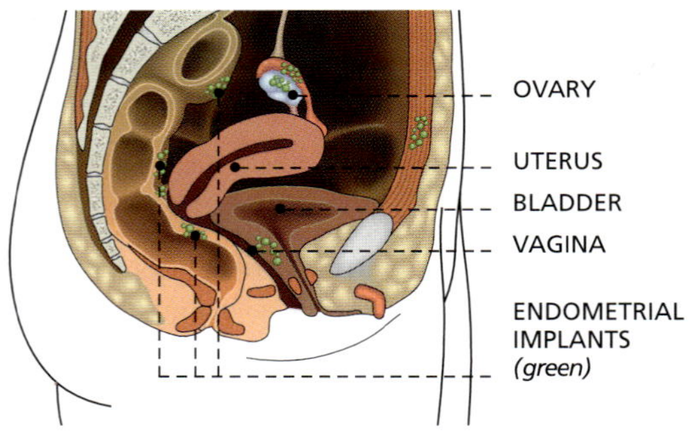

Special tissue called endometrium is flushed out of the uterus as part of the natural menstrual process. If fragments of endometrial tissue become implanted in other organs in the pelvic cavity, they can grow, become irritated, and cause pain and abnormal bleeding. Left untreated, the tissue growths can eventually form cysts that disrupt the function of the reproductive organs.

the size of the lesions and how deeply they reach into host organs. Symptoms vary, and about 10 percent of patients have no noticeable symptoms at all. Others experience abnormally heavy and painful periods and sharp, deep abdominal pain during intercourse. Endometriosis accounts for 30 to 40 percent of female infertility. In women who are able to conceive, symptoms may diminish or disappear during pregnancy, but they may return a year or two later.

Endometriosis is most likely to strike women in their thirties and forties; it usually stops at menopause with the marked decline in the production of estrogen.

CAUSES

Researchers do not know definitively how endometrial tissue reaches other parts of the body. One likely possibility involves a condition known as retrograde, or backward, menstruation. Normally during menstruation, portions of the sloughed-off uterine lining exit the uterus through the cervix and the vagina. But in retrograde menstruation, fragments of the endometrium flow back into the fallopian tubes and may then be carried into the abdominal cavity, giving rise to endometriosis. Indeed, doctors have found that endometriosis occurs more often in women with physical conditions that increase retrograde menstruation, such as obstructions in the vagina and cervix.

There is some controversy as to whether tampon use can cause retrograde flow. Evidence seems to suggest that it does not, but some women who have endometriosis avoid tampons, just to be on the safe side. *(See also **Toxic Shock Syndrome** for guidelines on tampon use.)*

In the rare cases of endometriosis affecting the lungs or other tissue far from the uterus, researchers speculate that the stray endometrial fragments travel through the bloodstream or the lymphatic system, although no one knows just how this happens.

Another theory suggests that endometrial tissue migrates outside the uterus on a fairly routine basis but develops into endometriosis only in women who have an immune system problem that prevents the body from destroying the displaced fragments.

Despite uncertainty about the specific mechanisms behind endometriosis, researchers can point to correlations. The fact that the condition tends to run in families suggests that genetic influences may play a role. Studies have also shown that endometriosis occurs more often in women who have a shorter-than-normal menstrual cycle or a longer-than-normal flow: Women who have fewer than 25 days between periods or who menstruate for more than 7 days are twice as likely to develop endometriosis. Recent evidence also points to exposure to dioxin, an industrial chemical, as a possible cause.

There seems to be no direct relationship between the size of lesions and the severity of pelvic pain. Some women with small lesions report debilitating pain, while others with extensive lesions have no symptoms. Pain probably comes from the scarring and irritation caused by bleeding, or from endometrial tissue invading or growing on a nerve.

How the disease causes infertility is also unclear, but it doesn't appear to be related to the severity of the case; many women with tiny lesions are infertile. Some investigators think the endometrial implants upset the process of ovulation. The implants may also hinder passage of the egg through the fallopian tubes by interfering with the cilia responsible for moving the egg. Other research suggests that endometrial implants secrete chemicals that create an environment hostile to fertilization.

TREATMENT

Endometriosis may respond to both conventional and alternative treatments, ranging from hormonal drugs and surgery to herbal remedies. However, the condition is managed, not cured; symptoms often return when treatment is stopped. Menopause usually ends the symptoms, but in women who take estrogen during and after menopause, symptoms may continue.

Since endometriosis often recurs and often

causes infertility, you may wish to join an endometriosis support group to get help in coping with the uncertainties of the condition. Many hospitals can refer you to a support group.

CONVENTIONAL MEDICINE

Your doctor will usually perform a pelvic examination in order to rule out other potential causes of your symptoms. However, diagnosis can be made only by laparoscopy—visual examination with a slim, lighted instrument that the doctor inserts into the abdominal cavity through a small incision. This procedure is usually done under general anesthesia; many doctors also do a biopsy to confirm the diagnosis.

For women who can conceive and want a child, pregnancy is thought by many doctors to be a good treatment. Pregnancy alleviates symptoms, probably because it temporarily stops menstrual cycles. In some women endometriosis does not return after they have given birth. Alternatively, your doctor may have you take birth-control pills continuously for nine months or more, producing a pseudopregnancy that halts the menstrual cycle and stops the bleeding of the endometrial lesions. This treatment can be effective, but it does not work as well as actual pregnancy; symptoms frequently return.

If a continuous course of birth-control pills fails to bring relief, your doctor may advise treatment with androgens—male hormones. Drugs with hormonal effects such as danazol and nafarelin work by stopping the menstrual cycle, thus keeping uterine tissue from bleeding. Danazol, however, has masculinizing side effects that may not be reversible, such as increased body hair growth and—rarely—deepening of the voice, and it cannot be taken for long periods of time. Indeed, with all such drug therapies, complete cure is uncommon, since the implants remain attached to organs and may resume monthly bleeding when therapy ends.

Analgesics such as ***ibuprofen*** and ***naproxen*** may relieve the discomfort of cramps but will not affect the implants' cyclic changes, so again they address the symptoms without addressing the underlying cause.

YOGA

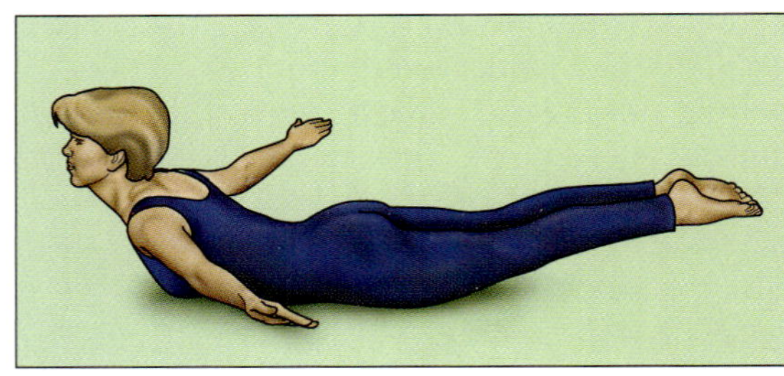

1 The **Boat** strengthens the spine and conditions the pelvic area. Lying on your stomach, inhale and lift your head, chest, arms, and legs off the floor. Stretch your arms behind you and hold the position for 15 to 20 seconds, then exhale and relax back onto the floor. Do once or twice a day.

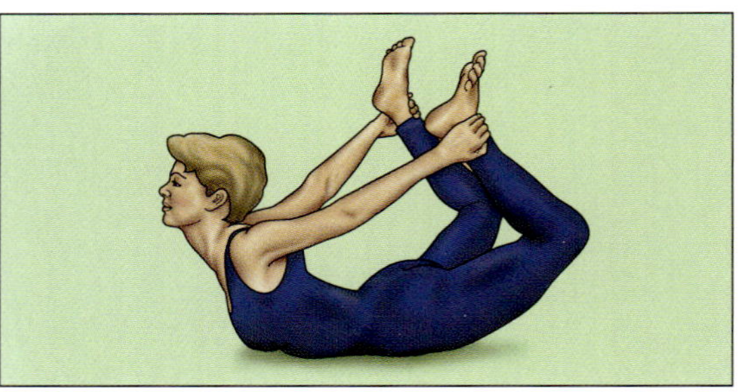

2 The **Bow** increases the elasticity of the spine. Lie on your stomach and grasp both ankles. While inhaling, press your pelvis down and slowly raise your head, chest, and thighs off the floor. Hold for 15 seconds, breathing slowly. Exhale, then release. Do once or twice a day.

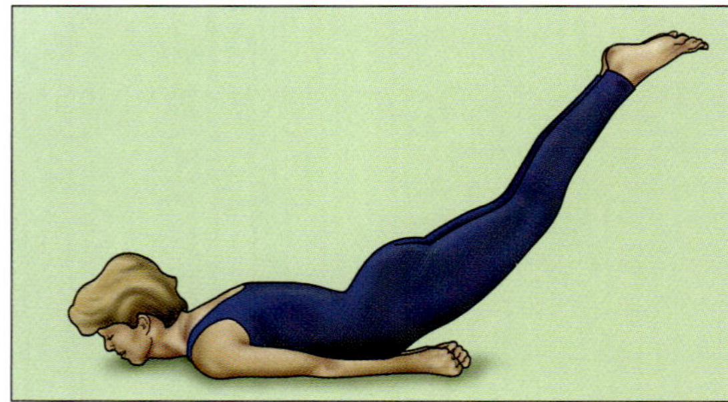

3 The **Locust** tones the muscles in the pelvic area. Lie on your stomach with your arms at your sides. Squeeze your buttocks as you press down with your arms. While inhaling, raise your legs, keeping them straight as you press outward through the toes and heels. Hold for 15 seconds, then exhale and release. Do once or twice a day.

If tissue growth is rampant and drug treatment is ineffective, your doctor may advise surgery. If all the implanted tissue is removed, your symptoms should disappear. However, some tissue fragments may remain and regrow, and your symptoms may recur, even after a hysterectomy. Your doctor may thus combine surgery with continued drug therapy.

ALTERNATIVE CHOICES

Most alternative remedies aim at relieving symptoms; but since they tend not to affect lesions directly, they may be less effective than comparable conventional treatment.

ACUPRESSURE

You may be able to alleviate cramping by applying pressure to Spleen 6, located on the inside of the leg two inches above the ankle. Do not use this point if you are pregnant. (See the ***Appendix*** for more information on point locations.)

HERBAL THERAPIES

Some herbal formulas may relieve pain. ***Skullcap*** *(Scutellaria lateriflora),* ***black cohosh*** *(Cimicifuga racemosa),* and ***wild yam*** *(Dioscorea villosa)* may address underlying hormonal problems. ***Valerian*** *(Valeriana officinalis)* may help you relax, but do not take it for longer than a month unless directed by your healthcare practitioner. Life root *(Senecio aureus)* and black cohosh enhance the health of pelvic organs. Consult a medical herbalist for specific formulas.

NUTRITION AND DIET

The body contains hormonelike substances called prostaglandins that, among other things, play a role in muscle contractions and thus contribute to menstrual cramping. Eating foods rich in natural antiprostaglandins—including mackerel, sardines, salmon, and tuna—may therefore help reduce symptoms. You may choose to take these nutrients in the form of fish-oil supplements and cod-liver oil.

A daily multivitamin-multimineral supplement containing ***vitamin B complex*** (50 to 100 mg), ***vitamin E*** (400 to 600 IU), ***calcium*** (1,000 mg), and ***magnesium*** (400 to 600 mg) may help balance estrogen and prostaglandin levels and reduce menstrual cramps.

AT-HOME REMEDIES

- In addition to taking an ***analgesic*** for pain relief, apply a heating pad or moist heat, and drink warm beverages to help relax cramping muscles. Exercise moderately to increase endorphins, your body's natural painkillers.
- To reduce tension, drink soothing herbal teas made with herbs such as ***hops*** *(Humulus lupulus)* and ***valerian*** *(Valeriana officinalis).*

PREVENTION

- Avoid exposure to dioxin, which recent evidence has shown may play a role in causing some instances of endometriosis.
- If you use tampons, change them frequently, especially when your flow is heavy, and consider alternating tampons with sanitary napkins; these measures may help prevent menstrual flow from backing up—which is one theory for the cause of endometriosis.

RISK FACTORS!

Several factors correlate with increased risk of endometriosis. Be aware of the greater likelihood that you will get this disease if:

- you have a close relative with endometriosis, especially a mother or a sister.
- your menstrual cycle is consistently short—fewer than 25 days.
- your menstrual flow during each period is long—more than a week.
- you experience heavy flow during periods.
- you use tampons and change them less often than every eight hours.
- you use an IUD.
- you have a medical condition that blocks or constricts your cervix or vagina.
- you have a congenital anomaly of the uterus, such as a double uterus or a double cervix.
- you have been exposed to dioxin. ■

ENVIRONMENTAL POISONING

SYMPTOMS

For **acute environmental poisoning,** see ***Emergencies/First Aid: Poisoning.***

The symptoms of **chronic environmental poisoning** are wide ranging and often vague. Among the most common:

- cough, headache, nose and eye irritation, diarrhea, dizziness, blurred vision, anxiety, lightheadedness, memory loss, drowsiness, tingling in extremities, aching in muscles and joints, difficulty concentrating, fatigue.
- in severe cases, depression, an overwhelming feeling of weakness, and difficulty breathing.
- disappearance of symptoms when you are not around the possible toxic agent (for example, during the weekend when you are not at your workplace).

CALL YOUR DOCTOR IF:

- your symptoms are persistent, and you can think of no obvious explanation for them but have reason to believe you've been exposed to a toxic substance; you need to be checked and tested to see whether you are indeed suffering from environmental poisoning.

NOTE: **Acute environmental poisoning,** which usually occurs as a result of a catastrophic accident or a one-time event such as a child ingesting a toxic chemical, requires immediate help. **Call 911 or a poison control center now.**

The human body is remarkable for its ability to handle the onslaughts of what can at times be a hostile environment. It is capable of neutralizing or expelling many potentially harmful agents, whether they are organic microbes or industrial chemicals or minerals. However, if your body absorbs low levels of some chemicals or minerals over a period of months or even years, you may develop **chronic environmental poisoning.** (Another form of environmental poisoning is **acute environmental poisoning,** which results from exposure to or ingestion of dangerous amounts of a toxic substance; for information on how to deal with acute poisoning, see ***Emergencies/First Aid: Poisoning.***) Symptoms of chronic environmental poisoning are often vague and can vary in severity; the condition is thus sometimes mistaken for another ailment or remains undetected altogether.

Some people cannot tolerate even minimal exposure to certain chemicals because a genetic malfunction interferes with the production of enzymes that would normally metabolize the toxins and neutralize their damaging effects. Other people are just more sensitive to toxins in the environment: This increased sensitivity can be due to age (both the very young and the elderly being more susceptible to environmental poisoning) and health factors (including smoking, drinking, diet, exercise, and existing chronic disease).

Many conditions fall into the category of environmental poisoning. In some people, for example, environmental poisoning may take the form of an ***allergy,*** a physical reaction to a substance that most people are able to tolerate. People who work in poorly ventilated buildings with unhealthy levels of airborne toxins may develop what is known popularly as **sick building syndrome,** while agricultural workers who use pesticides day after day are at risk for **pesticide poisoning.** Although not universally accepted in the medical community as a physical illness, **multiple chemical sensitivity**—in which the body reacts adversely to a wide range of substances, from plastics to perfumes, that do not normally trouble most people—is yet another condition attributed to chronic exposure to potential environmental toxins.

Studies suggest that, once lodged in the body, toxic substances are a factor in the development of many other diseases and conditions that may not at first glance seem directly related to environmental poisoning. Among these are birth defects, ***endometriosis, infertility,*** other reproductive and developmental problems, coronary ***heart disease,*** respiratory illness, and many types of ***cancer,*** especially of the lung, skin, and breast.

Because we encounter low levels of so many environmental toxins in daily life, identifying the toxin or toxins that may be responsible for environmental poisoning can be difficult. Some of the most common and hazardous toxins are lead, asbestos, gasoline and other petroleum distillates, radon, carbon monoxide, organophosphates, formaldehyde, and drinking-water contaminants.

Benzene is one hazardous substance that is found in many forms. It is used in the production of deodorant, oven cleaner, soap, and perfume, and it is a component of paints, pesticides, asphalt, and gasoline and jet fuel. It can contaminate ground-water and surface-water supplies and pollute the air via auto exhaust, manufacturing processes, and cigarette smoke. Yet despite its widespread presence in the environment and its classification as a cancer-causing agent (carcinogen) in the United States, benzene is generally considered a hazard only for the two million or so industrial workers who are exposed to elevated benzene levels at their jobs.

Another common industrial chemical is formaldehyde, which is found in a wide variety of products, including plastics, paper, cosmetics, and carpets. Construction materials, such as particle board, building insulation, and plywood, can emit formaldehyde gas for several years after their manufacture and installation. Several studies since the 1980s have indicated that long-term exposure to formaldehyde is a health risk. The Environmental Protection Agency (EPA) classifies the chemical as a probable carcinogen, although only industrial workers are considered at risk. Some researchers claim that much lower levels of exposure can irritate the eyes and respiratory tract, but many people routinely exposed to formaldehyde at such levels do not develop even these milder symptoms of toxicity.

Cleansing Your System

To cleanse your body, eat a high-fiber diet, which helps the gastrointestinal tract move out toxins that have not been absorbed into the bloodstream or stored in other parts of the body. Also, to help the kidneys flush toxins from your system, drink at least two quarts of purified water each day.

Two substances that have received public notice as known carcinogens are asbestos and radon. Asbestos is a fine, fiberlike mineral that until recently was used in construction. Radon and its breakdown products, which are present in the Earth's crust, are released naturally into the air via radioactive decay. Both radon and asbestos are indoor air pollutants that have been significantly linked to the development of ***lung cancer.*** Not all buildings contain asbestos, however; and only certain areas of the United States emit radon at levels considered health-threatening.

Carbon monoxide is a common, yet poisonous, gas that is released into the air whenever fuel, wood, or tobacco products are burned. Heavy rush-hour traffic can generate high levels of carbon monoxide, and dangerous, sometimes lethal levels can build up in poorly ventilated garages or houses where faulty heating devices emit exhaust fumes that stay trapped indoors. When carbon monoxide enters the bloodstream, it disrupts the body's usual mechanisms for transporting and absorbing oxygen. Mild cases of carbon monoxide poisoning may cause headaches, nausea, or dizziness; severe cases can lead to respiratory failure and death.

The mineral lead is another contaminant of the air, water, soil, and food. Poisonous at even low levels, lead is known to have a damaging effect on the reproductive system, the kidneys, the nervous system, and the production of blood cells. Since the use of lead-free gasoline has become widespread, lead levels in the air have been significantly reduced. The EPA sets permissible limits for lead in drinking water. However, young children are still at risk of developing lead poisoning from ingesting particles of lead-based paint, which was used in most homes and buildings until it was banned in 1978.

Organophosphates are a potential toxic hazard for farm workers, gardeners, veterinarians, and other people who work with pesticides or insecticides. These chemicals, which are usually absorbed by the skin, retain their potency for several days after they have been applied to field crops. Their toxic effects can range from extreme fatigue, skin irritations, and nausea to depression, breathing problems, seizures, or coma. Agricultural workers who are routinely exposed to high levels of pesticides are considered at greatest risk of developing serious side effects, but some researchers believe that homeowners who use these products regularly in their houses or gardens may also be at risk.

Taking preventive actions, from checking your home for radon emissions to wearing protective gear when exposed on the job to hazardous chemicals, is the key to combating any level of environmental poisoning. The more you know about the particular risks involved, the better you can avoid toxic substances before they become a problem.

CAUSES

Toxic chemicals can get into the body through inhalation (for instance, carbon monoxide), penetration of the skin (pesticides), or ingestion (lead). Some substances can affect the human fetus by crossing the placenta; some also contaminate breast milk and thus may be ingested by a nursing infant.

Once inside the body, toxins can act in a number of ways. Despite how or where a toxin enters the body, it may have its greatest effect on certain target organs. The liver and kidneys, which filter impurities from the body, are often the most susceptible to toxins, especially inhaled industrial solvents. Some chemicals and minerals are stored in the body's fat or bones and may be released later. Lead, for example, is stored in the bones and may be released when a woman becomes pregnant and her body draws on its stores of bone calcium. Some hazardous agents may be effectively broken down by metabolic processes once they are in the body, but others may become even more harmful as a result.

DIAGNOSTIC AND TEST PROCEDURES

A doctor will probably give you a complete physical examination and take a detailed medical history. You may be asked to keep a diary of your diet and other behavior. Your blood, urine, hair, and fatty tissue may be analyzed for chemical content, and you may also have a liver function test to see how it responds to certain chemicals.

Some doctors are currently studying the usefulness of "environmental control units," special chemically sterile chambers in which patients suspected of having **multiple chemical sensitivity** are exposed to various substances until those specifically linked to their illness are identified.

TREATMENT

CONVENTIONAL MEDICINE

The treatment you receive will depend on which toxic substances are identified as causing your illness. For instance, lead poisoning is often treated with chelation therapy, which involves injections of chemicals that bind with lead in the blood; the lead is later eliminated in urine. However, most treatments for environmental poisoning focus on monitoring symptoms and identifying and eliminating offending substances from the patient's immediate environment.

ALTERNATIVE CHOICES

Regular exercise, a balanced diet, and stress-reduction techniques, such as **yoga** and **meditation,** can help strengthen your immune system, enabling your body to be more resilient to environmental toxins.

HERBAL THERAPIES

Milk thistle *(Silybum marianum),* ***burdock*** *(Arctium lappa),* and ***dandelion*** *(Taraxacum officinale)* may help detoxify the liver; ***red clover*** *(Trifolium pratense)* may help detoxify the blood. For general immune support try ***Siberian ginseng*** *(Eleutherococcus senticosus),* ***astragalus*** *(Astragalus membranaceus),* and cleavers (*Galium* spp.). For advice on how best to treat your specific condition, consult an herbal practitioner.

PREVENTION

Be aware of your environment. Ask questions. Pay close attention to what you are eating and breathing. A recent study—the largest ever on the health effects of airborne particles from smokestacks and traffic—found that people in the most polluted U.S. cities are about 15 percent more likely to die prematurely than those living in cities with the cleanest air.

Here are some specific preventive steps that you can take:

- Talk to your state environmental office to see if your house is located in an area known for radon contamination; if so, have it tested.
- If you are removing paint from your house, have it tested for lead content. Painting over the old paint may be preferable to removing it, because sanding can release lead particles into the air. Some communities have regulations for removing lead paint; check with your local environmental or health department before beginning the job.
- When using hazardous products, always follow the instructions, and wear protective clothing and eye gear.
- Keep your children and pets off lawns that have recently been treated with pesticides. (Some communities require that homeowners post a notice when chemicals have been applied.) Stay indoors with the windows closed if trees in your neighborhood are being sprayed with chemicals.
- Use nontoxic cleaning products and insecticides around your house. Many of these products are now available in stores or through catalogs.
- In buildings, be alert to obvious—or overpowering—chemical odors that may be emitted by paints, pesticides, new carpets, office machines, or other offenders. Make sure the ventilation in your office meets or exceeds standards.
- Some studies indicate that certain houseplants can help remove impurities such as benzene, carpet chemicals, and formaldehyde from the air. Consult your local horticultural society or garden center.
- To help avoid pesticides, thoroughly wash fruits and vegetables, peel produce, and consider buying organic.
- Avoid walking or running near streets with heavy automobile traffic; your increased respiration will increase the amount of carbon monoxide and other toxins that you inhale.
- Install a carbon monoxide detector in your home. Without a detector, you may remain unaware of a buildup of the gas, which is colorless, tasteless, and odorless and may not cause any physical irritation.
- A balanced diet will help your body maintain its ability to fight toxins. Vitamin deficiencies have been linked to increasing the toxic effects of several substances. Your susceptibility to lead poisoning, for example, increases if your body is deficient in ***calcium, zinc, phosphorus, copper, magnesium, iron, vitamin C,*** or ***vitamin E.*** However, because some vitamins and minerals can be toxic in large doses, never exceed the amounts recommended on the label for your daily requirements, without first consulting a nutritionist.
- Weight-loss diets, which make your body metabolize existing fat for energy, will also result in the release of any chemicals that have been stored in those fat cells. If you want to lose weight, do so slowly so that your system does not become flooded with a sudden release of these substances. ■

EPILEPSY

SYMPTOMS

Seizures—episodes of abnormal mental or muscular activity—are the basic indicator of epilepsy. They vary widely:

- Staring straight ahead and lapsing into complete immobility for a few seconds characterize a **petit mal seizure.**
- Loss of consciousness, rhythmic jerking motions, and incontinence are among the signs of a **grand mal seizure**, which may last up to 30 minutes.
- Repetitive lip smacking, aimless fiddling movements, and a sense of detachment from surroundings may indicate a **temporal lobe seizure.**
- Rhythmic twitching of a hand, a foot, or the face, often followed by a period of weakness or paralysis, indicates a **Jacksonian seizure.**
- Convulsions in an already ill child three months to three years old, resulting from a sudden climb in fever, indicate a **febrile seizure**. See page 74 for guidelines on how to help someone having a seizure.

CALL YOUR DOCTOR IF:

- you or someone without a prior history of epilepsy experiences a seizure for the first time. You need a doctor's diagnosis; the cause could also be poisoning, ***stroke,*** or drug overdose. In feverish infants, convulsions could be a sign of ***meningitis;*** **get medical help immediately.**
- one seizure follows another without a return to consciousness; the brain could be deprived of oxygen—**call 911 or your emergency number now.**

Epilepsy is an elusive neurological disorder with a broad range of symptoms, widely differing degrees of severity, and much mystery about why it strikes. In all cases, however, it results from electrical storms in the brain—erratic discharging by neurons. The electrical misfiring of brain cells produces epilepsy's characteristic seizures, which may occur infrequently or in rapid succession.

While every case of epilepsy is distinct, a standardized classification scheme has been developed to describe seizures. The attacks are divided into two main types: generalized (involving the entire brain) and partial (misfirings originating in one area of the brain). Within these categories, seizures are further identified according to the pattern of the attack. The two most common forms of seizure are both of the general type: a **petit mal seizure,** which may include such symptoms as swallowing motions or staring, and can recur many times in a day; and a **grand mal seizure,** which may begin with a cry, a loss of consciousness, and a fall, followed by rigidity, then jerking motions, a period of confusion, and sometimes deep sleep. Among the partial types are **temporal lobe seizures,** which may be preceded by a vague feeling of abdominal discomfort, sensory hallucination, and distorted perceptions such as déjà vu; and **Jacksonian seizures,** with localized twitching of muscles that sometimes spreads to the whole body.

The first signs of epilepsy are usually seen in childhood or adolescence. Very young children with high fevers may have convulsions, but this is not true epilepsy, and such seizures generally disappear after the age of three.

CAUSES

Most cases of epilepsy are of unknown origin. Sometimes, however, a genetic basis is indicated, and other cases may be traceable to birth trauma, lead poisoning, congenital brain infection, head injury, alcohol or drug addiction, or the effects of organ disease. Triggers for the attacks also vary widely. Among the factors that can bring on attacks are certain chemicals or foods, sleep deprivation, ***stress,*** flashing lights, menstruation, some prescription and over-the-counter medications, illegal drugs, and possibly oral contraceptives.

DIAGNOSTIC AND TEST PROCEDURES

An electroencephalogram (EEG) performed on a sleep-deprived individual can reveal abnormal brain waves characteristic of epilepsy, and imaging tests such as an MRI or CT scan can identify physical trauma that may be causing seizures.

TREATMENT

Epilepsy can often be well controlled by medication. A recommended precaution for epileptics is to wear a Medic Alert bracelet so that other people can quickly recognize what is happening during a seizure and lend effective assistance.

CONVENTIONAL MEDICINE

In the great majority of cases, seizures can be reduced in frequency and severity or eliminated altogether with regular medication; side effects vary, but most are mild. ***Anticonvulsants*** commonly prescribed include ***phenytoin,*** phenobarbital, ***valproic acid, carbamazepine,*** and gabapentin.

ALTERNATIVE CHOICES

Self-medication should never be practiced in place of a doctor's care, and your doctor should be aware of all separate treatments to avoid any drug incompatibility. There is no substitute for the benefits of prescribed drug therapy.

HOMEOPATHY

You may want to consider consulting a homeopath if conventional prescription drugs are not completely controlling seizures. Homeopathic remedies can serve as an effective adjunct to conventional drugs, but don't expect results overnight; the homeopath will advise you on how long it will be before treatments begin to work.

MIND/BODY MEDICINE

Electroencephalogram **biofeedback** may be effective in helping epileptics alter their brain waves to prevent seizures. With guidance, they learn to control their own brain waves by watching them on a computer screen. Stress reduction techniques and relaxation may help reduce seizure frequency.

NUTRITION AND DIET

The amino acid taurine may help reduce the frequency of seizures; consult a naturopathic physician.

OSTEOPATHY

When epilepsy appears to have resulted from a physical injury, cranial osteopathy or craniosacral therapy may help; consult an osteopath.

AT-HOME REMEDIES

- Regularly practice biofeedback techniques, learned from a trainer, to ward off epileptic attacks.
- Make sure you get ample sleep; too little can increase the likelihood of seizures.

PREVENTION

Identify and watch for particular foods, environments, or physical and emotional signs that precede attacks. It's not uncommon, for example, to feel annoyed or elated several hours prior to a **grand mal seizure**, and immediately before the attack, to become aware of a warning "aura"—perhaps a taste or smell; this warning may allow you to lie down in time to avoid falling. In cases where the aura is a smell, some people are able to fight off seizures by sniffing a strong odor, such as garlic or roses. When the preliminary signs include depression, irritability, or headache, an extra dose of medication (with a doctor's approval) may help prevent an attack. In the case of a **Jacksonian seizure**, firmly squeezing the muscles around those that are twitching can sometimes halt the attack. ■

EYE PROBLEMS

Read down this column to find your symptoms. Then read across.

SYMPTOMS	AILMENT/PROBLEM
For more information about eye problems specifically related to your vision, see ***Vision Problems.***	
◆ eye is red and painful; upper and lower eyelids may be swollen.	◆ Corneal abrasion or other corneal injury
◆ eyes feel tired, may burn and water; usually occurs in older people and contact lens wearers; is more common in women.	◆ Dry eyes
◆ both eyes are turned inward (crossed eyes); one eye is turned outward (walleye); one eye holds the line of sight while the other wanders.	◆ Strabismus (inability of both eyes to be directed at the same object at the same time; usually caused by weakness or defect in one of six muscles controlling eye movement)
◆ inflammation at one point along the edge of the eyelid, usually at the base of an eyelash; the area reddens and may be painful, a pimple may form, and the pimple may discharge pus.	◆ ***Sty***

WHAT TO DO	OTHER INFO
◆ Call your doctor, who may prescribe an ***antibiotic*** and a painkiller, remove any foreign matter, and place a patch over the eye. **Call your doctor immediately** if your vision is impaired; these symptoms could indicate a variety of eye problems, some of which can be very serious.	◆ To avoid scratching the cornea, do not rub your eye if you think you have something in it. See ***Emergencies/First Aid: Eye Emergencies*** for instructions on how to remove a foreign object from your eye. Always see your doctor if you have suffered an eye injury.
◆ Try using artificial tears, found in over-the-counter eye drops. Avoid those with vasoconstrictors, which constrict blood vessels in tissues overlying the eye. For an herbal therapy, try bathing your eyes in a solution made with ***eyebright*** *(Euphrasia officinalis).* A homeopath can recommend eyedrops to soothe and heal your eyes.	◆ Use a humidifier in winter to avoid too much dry heat. Protect your eyes from sun and wind with wraparound sunglasses.
◆ Call your doctor or ophthalmologist. Treatment aims to correct unbalanced eye muscles, and may include eye drops or ointment, corrective lenses, or surgery. Eye exercises may help balance the muscles.	◆ Eye muscle problems are usually congenital but may also result from a loss of vision in one eye from any cause. Treatment is most effective in young children.
◆ In most cases a sty will clear up on its own. See your doctor if the inflammation recurs; you may need an ***antibiotic.*** A homeopath can suggest an appropriate remedy.	◆ Apply a hot compress to the area periodically to help bring the sty to a head. *(See also the **Visual Diagnostic Guide.**)*

FACIAL PAIN

Read down this column to find your symptoms. Then read across.

SYMPTOMS	AILMENT/PROBLEM
◆ stabs of intense pain in lip, gum, cheek, or chin, usually triggered by touch, in people over 50.	◆ Trigeminal ***neuralgia***
◆ dull pain around eyes and cheeks that worsens on bending forward; possibly, thick discharge from nose, temporary loss of smell, nasal speech, headache, malaise, sore throat, fever, toothache.	◆ ***Sinusitis***
◆ throbbing forehead pain; the artery crossing your temple may be swollen and painful to the touch; possibly, mild fever, loss of vision.	◆ Inflamed artery (temporal arteritis, giant cell arteritis)
◆ continuous throbbing pain on one side of face when tooth is touched; tooth feels loose; possibly, swollen glands in neck, fever.	◆ Tooth abscess
◆ pain or bruised feeling on one side of face; red, blistery rash on face, ear, or throat; inability to move facial muscles; tingling, itching, prickly sensation of skin; low fever.	◆ ***Shingles*** (herpes zoster nerve infection)
◆ throbbing pain around one eye, subsiding and recurring; usually accompanied by nasal congestion; sweating; tearing and reddening of eye.	◆ Cluster ***headache***
◆ clicking or popping around jaw joint and pain on opening mouth; jaw pain; possibly, recurrent headaches and pain radiating through face and around the neck and shoulders.	◆ ***Temporomandibular joint (TMJ) syndrome***

WHAT TO DO	OTHER INFO
◆ Call your doctor, who may prescribe ***analgesics*** to kill the pain, possibly with low doses of an ***anticonvulsant*** or ***antidepressant*** drug to maximize pain relief.	◆ This nerve inflammation could be caused by a blood vessel pressing on a nerve. Deep-tissue massage and acupuncture may help relieve pain. Surgery is sometimes required.
◆ The usual treatment is an ***analgesic, decongestant,*** or ***antibiotic*** (if cause is bacterial); or ***antihistamines,*** immunotherapy, or inhaled ***corticosteroids*** (if cause is allergy).	◆ Allergies and dental abscesses may predispose you to sinusitis. Acupuncture, Chinese herbs, and homeopathy may be helpful for acute pain or to prevent recurrence. Homeopathic sinus sprays can decrease swelling.
◆ Call your doctor, who may prescribe ***corticosteroids*** to reduce inflammation and prevent loss of vision.	◆ Treatment brings a 75 percent chance of complete recovery.
◆ **Call your dentist now;** treatment is essential. Take an ***analgesic;*** rinse mouth hourly with warm salted water. See ***Toothache.***	◆ Emergency dental treatment is essential to prevent damage to the jawbone through spread of ***infection.***
◆ Call your doctor for treatment that may include prescribed pain relievers, an ***antiviral*** medication, or rarely, an ***antibiotic.***	◆ High doses of ***vitamin E*** (500 IU, three times a day, taken under a doctor's supervision) may be helpful. Shingles is caused by a recurrence of the same virus that causes ***chickenpox.***
◆ Call your doctor if you have not yet been diagnosed. See ***Headache.***	◆ The trigger may be alcohol or medications that dilate blood vessels, such as ***nitroglycerin.*** Inner nasal applications of ***cayenne*** *(Capsicum frutescens)* ointment may relieve pain.
◆ Call your dentist for treatment that may include correction of jaw misalignment or of other dental problems.	◆ Treatment may include anti-inflammatory drugs, moist heat, physical therapy, and soft foods. Acupuncture, shiatsu, and relaxation techniques such as biofeedback are especially effective.

FAINTING

Read down this column to find your symptoms. Then read across.

SYMPTOMS	AILMENT/PROBLEM
◆ brief loss of consciousness, possibly preceded by pallor and lightheadedness, usually lasting several minutes.	◆ Fainting (general)
◆ faintness or fainting after exertion or several hours spent in hot (usually humid) air; fatigue; possibly, nausea, vomiting, headache, weakness, rapid heartbeat.	◆ **Heat exhaustion** or **heatstroke**
◆ faintness or fainting in someone who is vomiting blood or passing bloody or black, tarry stool.	◆ Digestive tract bleeding (ulcer, polyps, inflammatory or infectious diseases, ***cancer***)
◆ faintness or fainting when standing abruptly after sitting, lying, or bending, especially in persons taking ***antihypertensive drugs.***	◆ Low blood pressure (hypotension)
◆ faintness or fainting in a person who has ***diabetes*** or who has not eaten recently; possibly, weakness, tingling in hands, feet, and lips, trembling, nausea, headache, rapid heartbeat.	◆ Low blood sugar ***(diabetes, hypoglycemia)***
◆ faintness or fainting after an emotional shock or other stressful event or in a person with a panic disorder.	◆ ***Stress; anxiety***
◆ sudden faintness or fainting with numbness and weakness; possibly, blurred vision, confusion, difficulty speaking, or paralysis.	◆ ***Stroke;*** transient ischemic attack
◆ sudden fainting in someone with irregular pulse or ***heart disease.***	◆ ***Heart disease; heart attack***

WHAT TO DO	OTHER INFO
◆ **Call 911 or your emergency number** if someone is unconscious for more than five minutes or has no pulse; start CPR (*see* ***Emergencies/First Aid: Loss of Consciousness***). Otherwise, make the person comfortable after consciousness returns.	◆ Brief, infrequent fainting with no other symptoms usually is not a cause for concern.
◆ **Call 911 or your emergency number now.** Move to a cool place; drink water; apply cool compresses. See ***Emergencies/First Aid: Heatstroke and Heat Exhaustion.***	◆ A victim of heatstroke does not sweat, despite a body temperature of 100°F or higher; pulse may be rapid and strong.
◆ Call your doctor without delay; proper diagnosis is essential.	◆ Your doctor will order tests to detect the cause of bleeding.
◆ Rise more slowly. If you frequently faint when standing, call your doctor to check for underlying ailments.	◆ If you take ***antihypertensive drugs,*** your doctor may reduce dosage. If fainting recurs, seek evaluation for another condition.
◆ Call your doctor if fainting recurs. Anyone with low blood sugar should carry a sweet or protein snack to eat when feeling faint.	◆ Treatment for ***diabetes*** is designed to normalize blood levels of glucose and ***insulin*** through diet and sometimes medication.
◆ You may benefit from counseling or psychotherapy. See also ***Phobias, Panic Attack, Posttraumatic Stress Disorder.***	◆ You may benefit from relaxation exercises such as biofeedback, meditation, or yoga. Acupuncture or massage may also reduce anxiety.
◆ **Call 911 or your emergency number now;** immediate medication may prevent further damage.	◆ Stroke rehabilitation may include speech and physical therapy, including gentle aerobic exercise. Acupuncture and Chinese herbs may also be helpful.
◆ **Call your doctor or 911 or your emergency number now** unless you have a chronic, stable, benign ***heart arrhythmia.*** See also ***Heart Disease*** and ***Heart Attack.***	◆ Fainting can follow pump failure, arrhythmia, valve problems, and other factors that lower blood flow. Smoking cessation, changes in diet, exercise, and stress reduction may help prevent heart disease.

F

FATIGUE

Read down this column to find your symptoms. Then read across.

SYMPTOMS	AILMENT/PROBLEM
◆ following recent travel, persistent fatigue; sleeplessness; hunger at seemingly odd times.	◆ Jet lag (disruption of your body's normal rhythms for sleeping and eating)
◆ general lethargy that somewhat limits daily activities; possibly, obesity; tendency to feel stressed.	◆ Your lifestyle is working against you and needs change
◆ fatigue that develops after starting a new medication.	◆ Side effect of prescription or over-the-counter medication such as sleeping pills, cough and cold preparations, and blood pressure drugs
◆ fatigue during the day; trouble falling asleep, and/or difficulty sleeping through the night.	◆ ***Insomnia***
◆ persistent sadness, fatigue, and pessimism; sudden change in appetite; difficulty sleeping, or tendency to oversleep; sometimes, thoughts of death or suicide.	◆ ***Depression***
◆ nighttime sleep that is interrupted by sudden awakenings from a choking sensation, followed by drowsiness and more sleep; fatigue during the day.	◆ Sleep apnea (episodes of interrupted breathing—for up to one or two minutes at a time—during sleep)
◆ debilitating fatigue that lasts for six months or more; fatigue is not from exertion and is not relieved by rest; persistent low-grade fever; aching, weak muscles; swollen lymph nodes; joint pain; headache; confusion; sore throat.	◆ ***Chronic fatigue syndrome***
◆ weakness and fatigue; dizziness; faintness; pale skin; heart palpitations; loss of appetite.	◆ ***Anemia***

WHAT TO DO	OTHER INFO
◆ Keep your body well hydrated: Drink water and avoid alcoholic beverages. When you arrive at your destination, force your body to adjust to the local time zone quickly.	◆ The hormone melatonin is believed to help regulate the body's rhythms; melatonin supplements may help fight jet lag. Discuss with your doctor.
◆ Determine what lifestyle patterns (overworking, not exercising enough) are contributing to your fatigue, and make changes; begin a diet to lose weight, and/or adopt a stress-reduction technique—such as yoga—that you're comfortable with and will do regularly.	◆ Aromatherapy may help reduce stress: Place 2 drops of essential oil of ***peppermint*** *(Mentha piperita)* on a handkerchief, and inhale.
◆ Talk to your doctor or pharmacist about the side effects of any medications you are taking. Also check in the ***Index of Conventional and Natural Medicines*** beginning on page 882.	
◆ If your insomnia lasts longer than a month, visit your doctor; you may have an underlying problem such as hypothyroidism. Mild insomnia is normal during pregnancy.	◆ Use different strategies to help yourself sleep; before bed, try taking a warm bath, reading a book for pleasure, practicing deep breathing, or having a cup of ***chamomile*** *(Matricaria recutita)* tea.
◆ Depression often responds to both conventional and alternative treatments. Consult your doctor, a psychotherapist, or a counselor such as a member of the clergy.	◆ Regular exercise is a significant aid to recovering from depression.
◆ See your doctor for an accurate diagnosis. Treatments are available for mild cases *(see **Snoring**)*, but surgery to keep airways open is sometimes necessary.	◆ Other disorders that can mimic sleep apnea include ***asthma*** and slight heart failure.
◆ See your doctor; this condition is easily confused with ***AIDS, mononucleosis,*** and other ailments.	◆ The cause for this syndrome is not clear; chronic ***stress,*** viruses, allergies, and hormonal imbalances have all been implicated.
◆ See your doctor without delay. Anemia can have serious complications.	◆ Treatment will depend on the cause and extent of your anemia, and may include dietary changes, nutritional supplements, and/or surgery.

Read down this column to find your symptoms. Then read across.

SYMPTOMS	AILMENT/PROBLEM
◆ extreme fatigue; fever; sore throat; chills; headache; body aches; nasal congestion; cough.	◆ ***Flu***
◆ severe fatigue, headache, sore throat that may be severe, chills, muscle aches, fever, cough; possibly followed by swollen lymph nodes, yellowish skin, rash that resembles ***measles,*** soreness in upper-left abdomen.	◆ ***Mononucleosis***
◆ lack of appetite; fatigue; mild fever; muscle or joint aches; nausea and vomiting; abdominal pain; possibly, dark-colored urine, light-colored stools, yellowish, itching skin.	◆ The liver is either inflamed ***(hepatitis)*** or degenerating ***(cirrhosis)***
◆ fatigue, weight loss, cough (occasionally with bloody sputum), slight fever, nighttime perspiration; sometimes, pain in the chest, back, and/or kidneys.	◆ ***Tuberculosis;*** possibly, ***lung cancer***
◆ fatigue; weight gain; numbness and tingling in hands; constipation; dry skin and hair; increased sensitivity to cold; persistently low body temperature.	◆ Hypothyroidism (failure of the body to produce enough thyroid hormones)
◆ fatigue; excessive thirst and frequent urination; increased appetite; weight loss; recurring ***yeast infections.***	◆ ***Diabetes***
◆ weakness; fatigue; weight loss; salt cravings; darkening skin; hair loss.	◆ Addison's disease (a potentially fatal illness that occurs when the adrenal glands cannot produce adequate amounts of the hormone cortisone)
◆ frequent waking during the night to urinate; persistent fatigue; weight loss; dry, itching skin; pallor; shortness of breath; swelling of hands and feet; unpleasant taste in mouth.	◆ ***Kidney disease***
◆ shortness of breath; fatigue and weakness; coughing; swelling in abdomen or legs; rapid heartbeat.	◆ Congestive heart failure (heart not pumping at full capacity, causing fluid to accumulate in other areas of the body)

WHAT TO DO	OTHER INFO
◆ Rest as much as possible and drink plenty of water. Take an anti-inflammatory painkiller such as ***ibuprofen*** if necessary.	◆ Vaccines for some forms of flu are offered each year and are recommended for anyone over 65, as well as for other groups at high risk for developing serious complications.
◆ See your doctor. Complete bed rest is essential, with a gradual return to normal activity; no other treatment is usually given.	◆ Most people feel better within two or three weeks, but the fatigue may last for months.
◆ See your doctor without delay. Treatment will depend on the type and severity of your illness. See ***Hepatitis*** and ***Cirrhosis.***	◆ Cirrhosis may be caused by one of several viruses, by overuse of alcohol or drugs, or by ingesting one of many toxins.
◆ See your doctor today. For ***tuberculosis,*** you will need one or several ***antibiotics. Lung cancer*** therapy is wholly dependent on the extent of the disease.	◆ Taken as an infusion or in capsule form, ***echinacea*** (*Echinacea* spp.) is reputed to stimulate immune system activity, thereby helping to fight ***infection.***
◆ You will likely need hormone replacement therapy; consult your doctor. See ***Thyroid Problems.***	◆ Avoid foods that interfere with thyroid hormone production, including cabbage, peaches, spinach, and peanuts.
◆ See your doctor for a diet and medication regimen to avoid serious (and possibly lethal) complications.	◆ Type 1 diabetes requires ***insulin*** injections; Type 2 does not and can be controlled through diet and exercise alone.
◆ **Call your doctor now.** You will need regular cortisone supplements to avoid going into adrenal shock.	◆ Once Addison's disease develops, it is a lifelong condition that requires regular cortisone-like supplements.
◆ **Get medical care immediately.** Kidney disease is a life-threatening condition that often requires emergency care.	◆ Ask your doctor or nutritionist for dietary guidelines for minimizing stress on your kidneys.
◆ **Get emergency medical care.** You may be hospitalized to stabilize your condition; treatment may include surgery, medication, changes in diet, and specific exercises.	

F

Cross references are indicated by ***bold italics.***

FEET, ACHES AND PAINS

Read down this column to find your symptoms. Then read across.

SYMPTOMS	AILMENT/PROBLEM
◆ pain when putting weight on your foot; hard, flat lump of roughened skin on sole; mild pain when the lump is squeezed; possibly, tiny black dots on the lump's surface.	◆ ***Plantar wart***
◆ pain at the base of your big toe and the ball of your foot; bony protrusion at the side of your foot near your big toe; swelling, redness, tenderness, and limited joint motion.	◆ ***Bunion***
◆ pain under the heel and arch of your foot, especially if you walk or run a lot; possibly, stiffness and numbness in your heel.	◆ Plantar fasciitis (inflammation of connective tissue in the foot)
◆ persistent, shooting pains between your third and fourth toes.	◆ Morton's neuroma (a benign mass of nerve tissue)
◆ sharp pain when you put weight on your foot or heel.	◆ ***Bone spur***
◆ pain, swelling, redness, warmth, and stiffness in joints of your foot and elsewhere.	◆ Rheumatoid ***arthritis***
◆ intense pain in your big toe; swelling, warmth; possibly, alternating chills and fever.	◆ ***Gout***
◆ pain in your foot following an injury or sudden movement; possibly, swelling and the inability to put weight on the foot.	◆ Broken bone or other injury

F

WHAT TO DO	OTHER INFO
◆ Most warts go away on their own, so you may choose to do nothing. But if the wart is especially troublesome, see your doctor about removal methods.	◆ To prevent the spread of this highly contagious virus on your own feet or to others, do not pick at the warts; wear rubber shoes in the shower.
◆ Wear soft, wide shoes; consider made-to-order shoes. If the pain is severe, your doctor or podiatrist may recommend surgery.	◆ Although you may inherit a tendency to get bunions, the condition is worsened by wearing tight shoes. ***Bursitis*** or osteoarthritis may also be present, causing pain and stiffness.
◆ Try an over-the-counter arch support; call your doctor for diagnosis and rehabilitation recommendations.	◆ This so-called overuse injury causes tissues in the sole of your foot to become inflamed.
◆ For quick relief, remove your shoes and massage the area. If the pain persists, your doctor may suggest ***corticosteroid*** injections or surgery.	◆ A neuroma is typically caused by an inflamed, pinched nerve. Avoid tight shoes and high heels. Over-the-counter metatarsal arch supports may help.
◆ Avoid tight shoes; try putting a foam rubber pad, with a hole cut out under the spur, in your shoe. Take an anti-inflammatory painkiller such as ***ibuprofen.***	◆ Acupuncture or physical therapy may help to relieve the discomfort.
◆ Try taking an anti-inflammatory painkiller such as ***ibuprofen.*** Arthritic joints require a balance of rest and exercise. See ***Arthritis.***	◆ The pain of arthritis may be helped by acupuncture, homeopathy, and various relaxation techniques.
◆ The usual treatment is a ***nonsteroidal anti-inflammatory drug (NSAID)*** and/or the drug colchicine.	◆ The homeopathic remedy *Colchicum,* from the plant from which colchicine is extracted, may relieve the pain.
◆ **Call your doctor or get emergency care now** if you cannot walk or move your foot or if you are unsure of the severity of injury. If there is no fracture, rest with the foot raised and apply an ice bag. See ***Sprains and Strains*** and ***Emergencies/ First Aid: Fractures and Dislocations.***	◆ A fracture may require a firm bandage or plaster cast or, possibly, surgery to reposition bones. Soft-tissue injuries may be massaged with an over-the-counter anti-inflammatory cream or ***Arnica*** cream, provided there is no break in the skin.

F

Cross references are indicated by ***bold italics.***

FEVER AND CHILLS

Read down this column to find your symptoms. Then read across.

F

SYMPTOMS	AILMENT/PROBLEM
◆ fever (a higher-than-normal body temperature, usually above 98.6°F), with or without other symptoms; possibly, chills, especially while fever is climbing.	◆ Fever (general)
◆ fever with severe headache and stiff neck; possibly, nausea, vomiting, light sensitivity, drowsiness, confusion.	◆ ***Meningitis***
◆ fever with convulsions, shaking, and/or blue color to face, usually in a baby or child.	◆ Fever with convulsions
◆ fever in a child under 12, accompanied by earache, rash, swollen jaw , noisy breathing, runny nose, red eyes, or dry cough.	◆ Various illnesses of infancy and childhood, such as ear infection, ***croup, measles, German measles, chickenpox, mumps***
◆ abrupt onset of fever (102°F to 106°F); possibly, chills, headache, malaise, diarrhea, runny nose, dry cough, sore throat, or aches in muscles or joints.	◆ ***Flu*** or other viral ***infection***
◆ fever after several hours in heat or strong sun; fever in a baby dressed too warmly.	◆ Overheating or **heat exhaustion**
◆ fever with sore throat; pain in back and painful urination; pelvic pain; nausea, vomiting, and diarrhea; chest pain when taking a breath, cough, and shortness of breath.	◆ Various ***infections,*** such as ***tonsillitis,*** pharyngitis, or ***laryngitis; bladder*** or ***kidney infection; pelvic inflammatory disease; gastroenteritis; bronchitis*** or ***pneumonia; malaria; AIDS***
◆ fever after taking medication.	◆ Drug reaction
◆ fever with throbbing face pain, especially when tooth is touched; possibly, swollen glands in neck.	◆ Tooth abscess

WHAT TO DO	OTHER INFO
◆ Call doctor if fever lasts longer than 48 hours or if fever in an infant between three and six months exceeds 100.5°F (rectal). Take fluids and ***aspirin, acetaminophen,*** or ***ibuprofen*** (do not give aspirin to a child).	◆ Most fevers are caused by bacterial or viral ***infections.*** A baby who won't drink liquids may need intravenous rehydration.
◆ **Call your doctor now.** Unless treated, meningitis can cause permanent neurological damage.	◆ The usual treatment is ***antibiotics*** for bacterial infection, or intravenous fluids and ***analgesics*** for viral infection.
◆ **Call 911 or your emergency number** if child's skin turns blue or if patient is adult. Sponge with tepid water to lower fever.	◆ Fever convulsions do not represent a seizure disorder, but infants should be examined for an underlying problem.
◆ Call your doctor; treatment depends on the illness. See related entries.	◆ Adults should not be exposed to measles, chickenpox, or mumps if they have not had them. Childhood diseases are more serious in adults.
◆ Rest; increase fluid intake. Call your doctor if you have shortness of breath or if fever lasts more than 48 hours. See ***Flu.***	◆ Flu may lead to secondary infections, such as ***pneumonia,*** especially in patients who are elderly, very young, chronically ill, or smokers.
◆ Rest in a cool place. Call your doctor if temperature continues to rise. See ***Emergencies/First Aid: Heatstroke and Heat Exhaustion.***	◆ Vigorous exercise can temporarily raise your temperature well above normal.
◆ Call your doctor for a proper diagnosis. The usual treatment is ***antibiotics*** if the infection is bacterial. Otherwise, treatment depends on the disease. See related entries.	◆ Seek treatment for fever with back or pelvic pain (possibly ***kidney infection*** or ***pelvic inflammatory disease***) or ***chest pain*** with shortness of breath (possibly ***pneumonia***).
◆ Check on changing your prescription.	◆ ***Penicillin*** and some ***antihypertensives*** may cause fever.
◆ **Call your dentist now** for emergency treatment. See ***Toothache.***	◆ Treatment is needed to prevent spread of infection, possible damage to jaw, and ***blood poisoning.***

FLU

SYMPTOMS

- fever—usually between 101°F and 102°F, but occasionally as high as 106°F—sometimes alternating with chills.
- ***sore throat.***
- dry, hacking ***cough.***
- aching muscles.
- general fatigue and weakness.
- nasal congestion, ***sneezing.***
- ***headache.***

CALL YOUR DOCTOR IF:

- you experience any of these symptoms and your immune system is already weakened by ***cancer, diabetes, AIDS,*** or other conditions; or if you have a serious illness like chronic ***heart*** or ***kidney disease,*** impaired breathing, cystic fibrosis, or chronic ***anemia.*** You may be at risk of developing serious secondary complications and need to be carefully monitored as long as symptoms last.
- your fever lasts more than three or four days, you become short of breath while resting, or you have chest pain. You may have developed ***pneumonia.***

Influenza—commonly shortened to "flu"—is an extremely contagious viral disease that appears most frequently in winter and early spring. The infection spreads through your upper respiratory tract and sometimes goes into your lungs. The virus typically sweeps through large groups of people who share indoor space, such as schools, offices, and nursing homes. The global influenza epidemic of 1918—which started in a military training camp in Kansas—eventually killed some 500,000 people throughout the United States.

Although both colds and influenza stem from viruses that infect the upper respiratory tract, the symptoms of influenza are more pronounced and its complications more severe. Influenza occurs most commonly in school-age children, but its most severe effects are felt by infants, the elderly, and people with chronic ailments. Despite advances in prevention and treatment, influenza and its complications are still fatal to about 20,000 people in the U.S. annually. Specific strains of the disease can be prevented by injections of antibodies in a flu vaccine, but after influenza—or any other viral infection, for that matter—has started, there is no cure except to let it run its course.

CAUSES

The flu virus is transmitted by inhaling droplets in the air that contain the virus, or by handling items contaminated by an infected person. The symptoms start to develop from one to four days after infection with the virus.

Researchers divide influenza viruses into three general categories: types A, B, and C. While all three types can mutate, or change into new strains, type A influenza mutates constantly, yielding new strains of the virus every few years. This means that you can never develop a permanent immunity to influenza. Even if you develop antibodies against a flu virus one year, those antibodies are unlikely to protect you against a new strain of the virus the next year. Type A mutations are responsible for major epidemics every several years. Types B and C are less common and result in local outbreaks and milder cases. Type B has also been linked to the development of Reye's syndrome, a potentially fatal complication of influenza and other viral infections—such as ***chickenpox***—that usually affect children.

Most influenza viruses that infect humans seem to originate in parts of Asia where close contact between livestock and people creates a hospitable environment for the mutation and transmission of viruses. Swine, or pigs, can catch both avian (meaning from birds or poultry) and human forms of a virus, and act as hosts for these different viral strains to meet and mutate into new forms. The swine then infect people with the new form of the virus in the same way in which people infect each other—by transmitting viruses through exchange of droplets in the air.

DIAGNOSTIC AND TEST PROCEDURES

All three types of influenza mimic the basic symptoms of the ***common cold,*** such as ***cough*** and ***headache.*** Your doctor may take a throat culture or blood test to rule out the possibility of other ailments such as ***strep throat*** or, if public-health officials are gathering statistics on an influenza outbreak, to identify the specific viral strain.

TREATMENT

Influenza will run its course regardless of how you treat it. Because it is a viral disease, it does not respond to antibiotics. If you are in good health, influenza will probably pass with no complications after a week or so of bed rest and self-care at home. If you are over 65, are a diabetic, or have another chronic disease, talk to your physician about being immunized before winter sets in *(see **Prevention,** page 377).* If you then come down with flu anyway, make sure your doctor monitors your progress so that any complications can be caught and treated appropriately.

CONVENTIONAL MEDICINE

Doctors have no single treatment that applies to all cases of influenza. You will probably be told to rest in bed, eat nourishing food, and drink lots of liquids. Fluids are especially important to help avoid dehydration from fever and for loosening up respiratory tract secretions.

You can try over-the-counter medicines to ease the discomfort of your ***cough,*** nasal congestion, and ***sore throat.*** A steam vaporizer in your room puts moisture into the air and may make breathing easier. If you are feverish and have muscle aches, ***analgesics*** like ***aspirin, ibuprofen,*** or ***acetaminophen*** may help you feel better. Because it has been linked to Reye's syndrome, you should not give aspirin to children.

If these remedies don't help a severe bout of flu, your physician may give you an oral ***antiviral***

A COLD OR THE FLU: WHICH IS IT?

The common cold and influenza are both contagious viral infections of the respiratory tract. Although the symptoms can be similar, influenza is worse: A cold may drag you down a bit, but influenza can make you shudder at the very thought of getting out of bed.

Congestion, sore throat, and sneezing are common with colds, and both ailments bring coughing, headache, and chest discomfort. With influenza you are likely to run a high fever for several days, and your head and body will ache. Usually, complications from colds are relatively minor, but a severe case of influenza can lead to a life-threatening illness like **pneumonia.**

Over 100 types of cold viruses are known, and new strains of influenza evolve every few years. Since both diseases are viral, neither can be conquered by antibiotics; those drugs are useful only against a secondary bacterial infection that may cause **sinusitis** *or* **pneumonia.**

drug that is active against type A influenza. You need to give yourself time to fully recuperate from influenza and prevent the development of secondary infections that can cause ***bronchitis, sinusitis,*** or ***pneumonia.***

ALTERNATIVE CHOICES

Alternative therapies may help strengthen your body's ability to fight the virus and recover from the illness as well as ease temporary flu symptoms.

ACUPRESSURE

Pressure on a number of points can be recommended for various flu symptoms; refer to the ***Appendix*** for the location of acupressure points. Bladder 36 is recommended for stimulating natural resistance to colds and flu. Bladder 2, Stomach 3, Large Intestine 20, Gall Bladder 20, and Governing Vessels 16 and 24 may be helpful for relieving nasal congestion, headaches, and eyestrain. Large Intestine 11 may help fight fever and strengthen your immune system. Large Intestine 4 may offer general relief from flu symptoms, but do not press it if you are pregnant. Conception Vessel 22 and Kidney 27 may help relieve chest congestion and coughing. Finally, try Bladder 38 to relieve coughing, breathing difficulties, and other respiratory complications.

AROMATHERAPY

In flu season, when those around you are coming down with the virus, protect yourself by gargling daily with one drop each of the essential oils of ***tea tree*** (*Melaleuca* spp.) and lemon in a glass of warm water; stir well before each mouthful. If you come down with the flu despite your best preventive measures, 2 drops of tea tree oil in a hot bath may help your immune system fight the viral infection and ease your symptoms. Tea tree oil can be irritating to the skin, however, so don't use more than 2 drops in a full bath.

If you have a congested nose or chest, add a few drops of essential oils of ***eucalyptus*** *(Eucalyptus globulus)* or ***peppermint*** *(Mentha piperita)* to a steam vaporizer. If you are asthmatic, do not use steam; instead, sprinkle a few drops of these essential oils on a handkerchief and inhale.

HERBAL THERAPIES

For an herbal approach to stimulating your immune system, try taking 20 drops each of tincture of osha *(Ligusticum porteri)* and ***echinacea*** (*Echinacea* spp.) twice a day. If flu symptoms appear, chew a clove of raw ***garlic*** *(Allium sativum)* for its antiviral properties, but do not eat raw garlic on an empty stomach.

An infusion of ***boneset*** *(Eupatorium perfoliatum)* may relieve aches and fever and clear congestion: Simmer 1 cup boiling water with 2 tsp of the herb for 10 to 15 minutes; drink a cupful every hour, as hot as you can stand it. To combat chills, try taking 30 drops of ***yarrow*** *(Achillea millefolium)* or elder *(Sambucus nigra)* flower tincture every four hours until your chills are gone.

HOMEOPATHY

For homeopathic self-care, try one of the following remedies in 12c or 30c dosages every 3 to 4 hours for a day or two. If you don't notice an improvement in your condition after 24 hours, try another homeopathic remedy.

- If you feel tired, weak, "heavy," and chilled, with headache and stuffy nose, try ***Gelsemium.***
- If you feel general achiness in your muscles, with headache and irritability that are worse when you move around, and if you are thirsty for cold fluids and have a dry hacking cough, try ***Bryonia.***
- If you are restless, chilled, and thirsty with a dry mouth, hoarse voice, and aching joints, try ***Rhus toxicodendron.***
- If you have a dry cough with achiness, or if your body feels bruised and chilled, and you are thirsty for cold drinks although they upset your stomach, try *Eupatorium perfoliatum.*

NUTRITION AND DIET

Eat ***vitamin C***-rich fresh fruits and vegetables like citrus fruits, Brussels sprouts, and strawberries; or take 1,000 mg of vitamin C two to three times a day. Increase ***zinc*** intake with lean meats, fish, and whole-grain breads and cereals.

REFLEXOLOGY

To support your respiratory system, press your thumb into the solar plexus/diaphragm point for a few seconds, or massage the point with your thumb. *(See page 25 for information about locating this point.)*

AT-HOME REMEDIES

- Take two tablets of ***aspirin, acetaminophen,*** or ***ibuprofen*** every four hours to reduce fever, headache, and body aches: These symptoms are usually worst in the afternoon and evening. Do not give ***aspirin*** to anyone under 21, because some people in this age group may be at risk of developing Reye's syndrome.
- If you have a sore or scratchy throat, try a saltwater gargle. Dissolve 1 tsp salt in 1 pt warm water. Gargle whenever your throat is uncomfortable, but don't swallow the mixture.
- Use a heating pad on body aches.
- When you feel like eating, try bland, starchy food like dry toast, bananas, applesauce, boiled rice, rice pudding, cooked cereal, and baked potatoes. These foods provide a gentle transition for your digestive system when you have not been eating regularly.
- Don't drink alcoholic beverages; they leave you dehydrated and can lower your body's ability to fight illness and secondary infection. Avoid over-the-counter flu remedies that contain alcohol.
- If you take over-the-counter pain relievers, make sure your symptoms are actually diminishing, not just temporarily suppressed, before you get out of bed. If you don't give yourself enough time to recover fully, you may end up prolonging your illness or developing complications.

PREVENTION

An effective preventive measure against influenza is to be inoculated every fall against strains that have developed since the previous outbreak. If you are vaccinated against one or more type A and B strains, you may still come down with flu, but your symptoms are likely to be milder than they would have been had you not had a vaccination.

Influenza vaccine is available through physicians and public-health facilities. Because influenza is a serious threat, the U.S. Centers for Disease Control and Prevention recommend vaccination for everyone over 65; nursing home residents and employees; anyone whose immune system is compromised by AIDS, cancer, or other chronic ailments; and people who work in medical facilities. The vaccine is usually given as a single injection, although children may receive two; a nasal form will soon be available. If you are pregnant, wait until your second trimester and make sure your doctor approves of the vaccination. Some people develop low fever and muscle aches as side effects of the vaccine. Because the vaccine is grown in chicken embryos, it is not recommended for people allergic to eggs.

Oral antiviral medications may lessen your risk of contracting type A flu, but they are most effective if you begin to take them a few weeks before flu season begins or within two days after symptoms appear. Usually these drugs are prescribed for people at high risk for developing complications from flu, such as people with chronic lung disease or the elderly. If the virus has already begun to circulate in your community, a doctor may also prescribe amantadine while you are waiting for a vaccination. If so, continue taking it for two weeks after you are vaccinated to ensure that you are adequately protected while your body builds up its immune response to the vaccine. Other preventive measures you can take during flu season are to:

- Give up smoking—which damages your respiratory tract—and alcohol, since both substances lower your resistance to infection in general.
- Avoid sleeping in a room with someone who has flu; the virus is easily spread in the air.
- Wash your hands often to kill viruses you may have picked up by touching contaminated objects like doorknobs or phone receivers.
- Try to avoid crowds, and give people who are coughing or sneezing a wide berth. Airplanes are especially effective at exposing people to flu viruses because cabin air is recirculated.
- Stay warm and dry so that your body can fight off infection by flu and other viruses. ■

FLUID RETENTION

Read down this column to find your symptoms. Then read across.

SYMPTOMS	AILMENT/PROBLEM
◆ painless swelling of the ankles and/or feet; no other symptoms.	◆ Edema (fluid accumulating in ankles and/or feet)
◆ prominent dark blue blood vessels in the legs and feet; aching or tender legs that often swell after standing for any length of time; possibly, discolored, peeling skin or skin ulcers.	◆ ***Varicose veins***
◆ in women, bloating; headache; painful breasts, muscle aches, irritability; anxiety; depression; anger; fatigue; insomnia; food cravings.	◆ ***Premenstrual syndrome*** (PMS), a group of symptoms related to the hormonal changes of the menstrual cycle
◆ fatigue and nausea followed by swelling in the abdomen and legs; abdominal pain; dark-colored urine; light-colored stools; yellowish, itching skin.	◆ Severe ***cirrhosis;*** substantial degeneration of the liver
◆ swelling in the hands and feet; frequent waking during the night to urinate; persistent fatigue; weight loss; elevated blood pressure; pallor; unpleasant taste in mouth.	◆ ***Kidney disease***
◆ swelling in the feet and legs; rapid weight gain; headache; shortness of breath; little or no urination.	◆ Acute renal failure
◆ shortness of breath; fatigue; cough; swollen abdomen, legs, and ankles; rapid or irregular heartbeat; low blood pressure.	◆ Congestive heart failure (heart not pumping at full capacity, causing fluid to accumulate in other parts of the body)
◆ in pregnant women, swelling in hands and face; sudden weight gain; possibly, headache, blurred vision, confusion, irritability, and/or stomach pain.	◆ Preeclampsia, also called toxemia; a form of ***high blood pressure*** that occurs in 5 to 10 percent of all pregnancies

WHAT TO DO	OTHER INFO
◆ Elevate your feet to encourage fluids to circulate, and avoid sitting for long periods of time. If swelling is persistent, call your doctor.	◆ Causes may include weak veins in the legs, staying seated for long periods of time, and/or pregnancy.
◆ See your doctor for advice. Your treatment will depend on the severity of your problem, and will likely include over-the-counter ***aspirin*** or ***ibuprofen*** for pain.	◆ Special elastic support stockings can help minimize discomfort.
◆ See your doctor for an accurate diagnosis. Treat your symptoms as needed. (Try over-the-counter ***analgesics*** for achiness; avoid salt, and drink plenty of fluids to minimize bloating.) If PMS is debilitating, your doctor may suggest medication.	◆ If you are deficient in ***magnesium, zinc,*** or ***vitamin*** B_6, supplements may alleviate your symptoms. ◆ Acupuncture, Chinese herbs, and homeopathy may relieve symptoms.
◆ **Get emergency medical care.** You may need to stay in the hospital until your condition stabilizes.	◆ A diet of small, frequent meals with low salt, no alcohol, and as few medications as possible will minimize stress on the liver.
◆ **Get medical care immediately.** Kidney disease can be a life-threatening condition that requires emergency care.	◆ Consult your doctor before taking any drugs, including over-the-counter medications such as ***ibuprofen*** and ***acetaminophen,*** which may contribute to kidney disease.
◆ **Get emergency care immediately.** With proper treatment, the kidneys often become functional again.	◆ Causes may include the worsening of a long-term ***kidney disease;*** shock; an ***infection;*** or a reaction to drugs.
◆ **Get emergency medical care.** You may be hospitalized to stabilize your condition; treatment may include surgery, medication, changes in diet, and specific exercises. See ***Heart Disease.***	◆ Risk of developing congestive heart failure is highest if you have existing heart disease, you smoke, or you abuse alcohol.
◆ **Get emergency medical care.** Mild cases respond well to treatment, and a full-term delivery is likely; severe situations may require an early delivery to save the baby's and the mother's lives.	◆ The elevated blood pressure of preeclampsia usually drops to normal within 24 hours of the baby's birth. If you did not have chronic ***high blood pressure*** before becoming pregnant, you'll most likely not have it after your pregnancy, either.

F

FLUSHED FACE

Read down this column to find your symptoms. Then read across.

SYMPTOMS	AILMENT/PROBLEM
◆ flushed face accompanied by fatigue, nausea, and/or headache.	◆ Most likely a result of excessive alcohol consumption
◆ flushed face; warm, dry skin; excessive thirst and hunger; possibly also frequent urination, rapid breathing, vomiting, confusion.	◆ ***Diabetes***
◆ face flushes easily during emotional stress or during exercise; in the case of exercise, may be accompanied by a headache, possibly a migraine.	◆ A natural propensity to blush; a physiological response to exertion
◆ fatigue, dizziness, nausea, extreme sweating, and headaches followed by flushed face, hot and dry skin, and rapid but weak pulse.	◆ Heatstroke (sunstroke)
◆ flushed face accompanied by gas, belching, possibly nausea, gurgling stomach, and acidic and bitter-tasting regurgitation rising to the throat and mouth.	◆ ***Indigestion***
◆ abnormally flushed cheeks and nose that may progress to pus-filled pimples; aggravated by spicy foods, hot drinks, or alcohol; most common in women over 30.	◆ Rosacea
◆ Flushing of the face often accompanies a high fever (104°F or above); see ***Fever and Chills*** for more information. A rosy glow in the cheeks and face is common in pregnant women.	

F

WHAT TO DO	OTHER INFO
◆ Avoid drinking more than one or two alcohol-based drinks per day. See ***Alcohol Abuse.***	◆ Dilated blood vessels associated with a flushed face cause the body to lose heat more rapidly than normal and during cold weather can put you at risk for hypothermia; drinking alcohol is thus not a good way to try to warm someone up.
◆ See ***Diabetes.*** Consult your physician as soon as possible.	◆ Avoid sugar and caffeinated beverages. Exercise regularly.
◆ Blushing is not a health problem, and it is also normal to flush in the face when exercising. If you are troubled by how easily you flush, consider seeing a specialist in Chinese medicine, who will focus on correcting a presumed energy imbalance between the upper and lower halves of your body. See also ***Headache.***	◆ Some alternative practitioners associate quick flushing of the face with a disturbed physiology that could be a signal of potential health problems; you may want to consider seeing an acupuncturist or homeopath for an evaluation.
◆ Cool down with a cold shower or wet washcloths; ***get medical help immediately.*** See also ***Heatstroke*** in ***Emergencies/ First Aid.***	◆ Homeopaths often suggest ***Belladonna*** or Glonoine as a complement to emergency care for heatstroke.
◆ Try an over-the-counter ***antacid*** or upset-stomach remedy. See ***Heartburn*** and ***Indigestion.***	◆ Ayurvedic, herbal, and homeopathic therapies offer several viable alternatives.
◆ See ***Acne.***	◆ If left untreated, rosacea can develop into sebaceous hyperplasia, in which enlarged oil glands create a bulbous nose. Rosacea responds particularly well to ***antibiotics,*** dietary changes, or large doses of ***B vitamins,*** especially riboflavin ***(vitamin B_2).***

FOOD POISONING

SYMPTOMS

Generally, food poisoning causes some combination of ***nausea, vomiting,*** and ***diarrhea*** that may or may not be bloody, sometimes with other symptoms.

- Abdominal cramps, diarrhea, and vomiting, starting from one hour to four days after eating tainted food and lasting up to four days, usually indicate **bacterial food poisoning.**
- Vomiting, diarrhea, abdominal cramps, headaches, and fever and chills, beginning from 12 to 48 hours after eating contaminated food—particularly seafood—usually indicate **viral food poisoning.**
- Vomiting, diarrhea, sweating, dizziness, tearing in the eyes, excessive salivation, mental confusion, and stomach pain, beginning about 30 minutes after eating contaminated food, are typical indications of **chemical food poisoning.**
- Partial loss of speech or vision, muscle paralysis from the head down through the body, and vomiting may indicate **botulism,** a severe but very rare type of bacterial food poisoning.

CALL YOUR DOCTOR IF:

- you recognize symptoms of **botulism.** You need immediate medical treatment for a life-threatening illness.
- you recognize symptoms of **chemical food poisoning.** You need immediate medical treatment to avoid potential damage to one or more of your vital organs. *(See also* ***Emergencies/First Aid,*** *page 73.)*
- the vomiting or diarrhea is severe and lasts for more than two days. You are at risk of becoming dehydrated.

You can get food poisoning after eating food contaminated by viral, bacterial, or chemical agents. Food poisoning causes mild to acute discomfort and may leave you temporarily dehydrated. Mild cases last only a few hours and at worst a day or two, but some types—such as **botulism** or certain forms of **chemical poisoning**—are severe and possibly life-threatening unless you get medical treatment.

CAUSES

Many bacteria can cause food poisoning. People who are ill or infected can transmit ***staph*** bacteria to food they are preparing. People who eat or drink contaminated food or water can get **travelers' diarrhea,** usually caused by the bacterium *E. coli*. Bacteria can contaminate poultry, eggs, and meat, causing **salmonella** poisoning; though potentially fatal, most cases cause only mild discomfort. Harmful bacteria grow in cooked and raw meat and fish, dairy products, and prepared foods left at room temperature too long; dishes made with mayonnaise are notorious culprits.

Canned goods—especially home-canned produce—can harbor a bacterium that needs no oxygen to multiply and is not destroyed by cooking. This bacterium causes **botulism,** a rare but potentially fatal food poisoning. Infants may develop botulism from eating honey because their immature digestive systems, unlike those of adults, cannot neutralize its naturally occurring bacteria.

Raw seafood—especially contaminated shellfish—may bring on **viral food poisoning.** Certain mushrooms, berries, and other plants are naturally poisonous to humans and should never be eaten; potato sprouts and eyes also contain natural toxins. Toxic mold can form on improperly stored fruit, vegetables, grains, and nuts. **Chemical food poisoning** can be caused by pesticides or by keeping food in unsanitary containers.

DIAGNOSTIC AND TEST PROCEDURES

If your symptoms are mild, you probably don't need a doctor. If symptoms last beyond two days, you may need your stool, blood, or vomited material tested to identify the cause of your illness.

Botulism is diagnosed from a description of symptoms and by tests for the bacteria in samples of blood, stool, or the suspect food. **Chemical food poisoning** can usually be diagnosed by a description of symptoms and by testing food potentially responsible for the poisoning.

TREATMENT

Vomiting and diarrhea are the body's way of flushing poison out of your system, so don't take any antiemetic or antidiarrheal medicine for 24 hours after your symptoms develop. Once you can keep fluid in your stomach, drink clear liquids for about 12 hours. Then eat bland foods like rice, cooked cereals, and clear soups for a full day.

Because repeated vomiting or diarrhea can remove large amounts of water from your system, dehydration is a potentially dangerous complication, especially in children and older adults. You must see that lost fluids are replaced promptly and completely. If you cannot keep liquids down, intravenous fluid replacement may be necessary.

CONVENTIONAL MEDICINE

If symptoms are severe or persistent, your doctor may prescribe ***antidiarrheal*** or antiemetic drugs until the condition is under control. Infants, children, elderly people, and anyone with ***diabetes*** or other chronic conditions will be monitored for dehydration and other potential complications.

If you have **botulism,** you will be hospitalized immediately. Although botulism can lead to respiratory failure and even death, prompt treatment greatly increases your chance for full recovery. If symptoms indicate **chemical poisoning,** you should have your stomach pumped out as soon as possible, or the poison could affect other organs by the time you receive treatment for the specific toxin. *(See **Emergencies/First Aid,** page 73.)*

ALTERNATIVE CHOICES

Try one or more of these alternative remedies while the body rids itself of the poison.

ACUPRESSURE

To relieve general nausea, try pressing Pericardium 6 on your inner forearm, two finger widths from the wrist crease, for one minute.

HERBAL THERAPIES

Ginger *(Zingiber officinale)* can be an effective remedy for nausea: Take two capsules or a cup of ginger tea every two hours as needed. An infusion of meadowsweet *(Filipendula ulmaria),* ***catnip*** *(Nepeta cataria),* or ***slippery elm*** *(Ulmus fulva)* may help soothe stomach and intestinal membranes: Steep 2 tsp of the herb in a cup of boiling water for 15 minutes; drink three times daily.

HOMEOPATHY

Try any of the following over-the-counter remedies in 12c or 30c potency every three to four hours until symptoms improve: ***Arsenicum album,*** *Veratrum album,* ***Nux vomica,*** or *Podophyllum.*

NUTRITION AND DIET

After symptoms subside, restore strength by eating foods like white rice, bland vegetables, and ripe bananas. To restore essential bacteria to your digestive tract, eat plain yogurt with active *Lactobacillus acidophilus* cultures, or take *Lactobacillus acidophilus* capsules. Avoid unfermented milk products, which may be difficult to digest.

PREVENTION

- Always wash your hands before preparing any food; wash utensils with hot soapy water after using them to prepare any meat or fish.
- Don't thaw frozen meat at room temperature. Let meat thaw gradually in a refrigerator, or thaw it quickly in a microwave oven and cook immediately.
- Avoid uncooked marinated food and raw meat, fish, or eggs; cook all such food thoroughly.
- Don't eat any food that looks or smells spoiled, or any food from bulging cans or cracked jars.
- Set your refrigerator at 37°F; never eat cooked meat or dairy products that have been out of a refrigerator more than two hours. ■

GALLSTONES

SYMPTOMS

Gallstones most frequently make their presence known when they become lodged in one of the ducts that carry bile, a digestive juice, from the gallbladder to the small intestine. When such an obstruction occurs, you might experience the following:

- severe and sudden pain in the upper right abdomen and possibly extending to the upper back.
- intermittent or recurring indigestion.
- fever and shivering.
- severe nausea and vomiting.
- ***jaundice.***

CALL YOUR DOCTOR IF:

- your abdominal pain begins quite suddenly, lasts more than three hours, and is followed by a mild aching sensation in the right upper abdomen; you may have gallstones or a bile-duct infection.
- you notice ***jaundice;*** gallstones may be obstructing the bile duct, causing bile to back up into the liver and seep into your bloodstream.

Gallstones are crystal-like deposits that develop in the gallbladder—a small, pear-shaped organ that stores bile, a digestive juice produced by the liver. These deposits may be as small as a grain of sand or as large as a golf ball; they may be hard or soft, smooth or jagged. You may have several gallstones or just one.

One out of every 10 people in the United States has gallstones or will develop them at some time in life, yet most of those who have the condition do not realize it. In this case, what you don't know probably won't hurt you; gallstones that are simply floating around inside the gallbladder generally cause no symptoms and no harm. These "silent" stones usually go unnoticed unless they show up in an ultrasound examination conducted for some other reason. However, the longer a stone exists in the gallbladder, the more likely it is to become problematic. It may take as long as 25 years for a gallstone to start causing trouble.

When symptoms do occur, it's usually because the gallstone has moved and become lodged within the cystic duct, a small conduit that connects the gallbladder to another tube called the common bile duct. The typical symptom is abdominal pain, perhaps accompanied by nausea, indigestion, or fever. The pain, caused by the gallbladder's contraction against the lodged stone, generally occurs within an hour of eating a large meal or in the middle of the night. Stones can also clog the common bile duct, which carries bile into the small intestine.

Obstructions in the bile pathway can cause a duct to become inflamed and possibly infected. If the problem continues for a number of years, liver damage and possibly liver failure may result. Blockage of the common bile duct, which merges with the pancreatic duct at the small intestine, can also lead to inflammation of the pancreas *(see **Pancreatic Problems**).*

In a rare but dangerous condition that occurs most often in older women, gallstones migrate into the small intestine and block the passageway into the large intestine; symptoms include severe and frequent vomiting. Gallstone problems can also lead to cancer of the gallbladder or bile duct.

DISRUPTION OF BILE FLOW

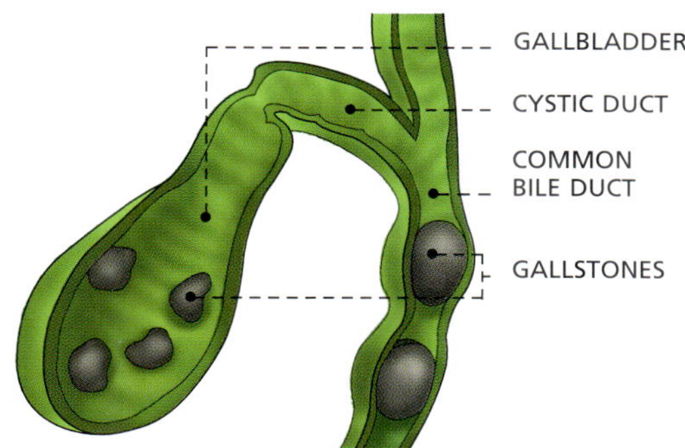

Crystal-like deposits called gallstones often go unnoticed if they remain in the gallbladder, which stores bile produced by the liver. But a stone that exits the gallbladder and becomes lodged in the cystic duct or the common bile duct *(above)* can cause intense pain and inflammation. Prolonged blockage can lead to infection, liver damage, or severe pancreatic problems.

Approximately a million new cases of gallstones are diagnosed in the United States each year. For reasons that are still unclear, women are four times as likely as men to be afflicted. Gallstones are also more common in people over the age of 40, in those who are obese or have lost a lot of weight in a short amount of time, and in women who have had multiple pregnancies.

CAUSES

The primary function of the gallbladder is to store bile, a brown or greenish fluid that helps the body break down fatty food. When you eat a meal, the gallbladder releases its stored bile into the cystic duct. From there the fluid passes through the common bile duct and into the small intestine.

Chief among the ingredients of bile are cholesterol and bile acids. Normally, the concentration of bile acids is high enough to break down the cholesterol in the mixture and keep it in liquid form. However, a diet high in fat can tip this delicate balance, causing the liver to produce more cholesterol than the bile acids are able to handle. As a result, some of this excess cholesterol begins to solidify into crystals, which we call gallstones. About 80 percent of all gallstones are created this way. The remaining 20 percent consist of calcium mixed with the bile pigment bilirubin.

If the liver fails to produce adequate amounts of bile acids, gallstones can form even in people who eat properly. And as researchers have found, a diet extremely low in fat can also contribute to gallstone formation: With little fatty food to digest, the gallbladder is called into play less frequently than usual, so the cholesterol has more time to solidify. Other factors that can reduce activity in the gallbladder, possibly leading to gallstone formation, include ***cirrhosis,*** the use of oral contraceptives, and pregnancy.

DIAGNOSTIC AND TEST PROCEDURES

If your symptoms suggest a gallstone-obstructed duct, your doctor might first examine your skin for ***jaundice,*** then feel your abdomen to check for tenderness. A blood test may reveal evidence of an obstruction.

Because other digestive problems, such as an infection of the duct, can produce symptoms similar to those of a gallstone attack, the doctor may also run other tests to determine if gallstones are in fact the culprit. The most common technique is an ultrasound examination. This quick, painless procedure uses high-frequency sound waves to create pictures of the gallbladder, bile duct, and their contents.

A more complicated test may be used if the doctor suspects that a gallstone is lodged in the bile duct. Commonly known by the acronym ERCP, this test allows the physician to look at the bile duct through a small flexible tube called an endoscope. The doctor sprays the back of the patient's throat with an anesthetic drug to prevent gagging, then passes the endoscope into the mouth, through the stomach, and into the area of the small intestine where the bile duct enters. Dye is injected through the tube and into the bile duct, then x-rays are taken. The procedure takes about an hour and can be done in the doctor's office.

TREATMENT

In most cases, treatment of gallstones is considered necessary only if they are symptomatic. Of the various conventional treatments that are available, surgical removal of the gallbladder is the most widely used. Some alternative treatments have also been found to be effective in alleviating the symptoms of troublesome gallstones.

CONVENTIONAL MEDICINE

When deciding what course of action to take for symptomatic gallstones, doctors usually choose from among three main treatment options: watchful waiting, nonsurgical therapy, and surgical removal of the gallbladder.

Watchful Waiting. While a gallstone episode can be extremely painful or frightening, almost a third of all people who experience an attack never have a recurrence. In some cases, the stone dissolves or becomes dislodged and thereby resumes its "silence." Because the problem may solve itself without intervention, many doctors take a wait-and-see approach following the initial episode.

Even when the patient has had repeated gallstone episodes, the physician may postpone treatment or surgery because of other health concerns. If your surgery has been delayed, you should remain under a doctor's care and report any recurrences of gallstone symptoms immediately.

Nonsurgical Therapy. If you are unable or unwilling to go through surgery for a gallstone problem that requires treatment, your physician may recommend one of several noninvasive techniques. Note: While these methods may destroy symptom-causing gallstones, they can do nothing to prevent others from forming.

Some gallstones can be dissolved through the use of a bile salt, although the procedure can be used only with stones formed from cholesterol and not from bile pigments. Taken as a tablet, the salt dissolves the stone by increasing the level of bile acids in the gallbladder. Depending on its size, the gallstone may take months or even years to go away. Another nonsurgical technique, shock wave therapy, uses high-frequency sound waves to fragment the stones. Bile salt is administered afterward to dissolve the small pieces.

A method called contact dissolution can also be used to dissolve gallstones. Not strictly speaking a nonsurgical therapy because it involves an incision, this procedure is less invasive than direct surgical removal of the gallbladder. The doctor inserts a catheter through the abdomen, then injects a special drug directly into the gallbladder. In many cases, the stone disappears within a few hours.

Surgical Removal of the Gallbladder. While the gallbladder serves an important function, it is not essential for a normal, healthy life. When gallstones are persistently troublesome, doctors often recommend removing the organ entirely. This operation is considered among the safest of all surgical procedures. It is also the only treatment method that eliminates the possibility that other gallstones will develop in the future.

When the gallbladder has been removed, bile flows directly from the liver into the small intestine, and this sometimes leads to digestion problems. Because bile no longer accumulates in the gallbladder, quantities of the digestive fluid cannot be stored up and used to break down an especially fatty meal. This condition is not considered serious, however, and can be corrected by simply limiting fat in the diet.

Until recently, removal of the gallbladder was done through traditional "open" surgery, which requires surgeons to make a large incision in the abdomen. Patients faced a two- or three-day hospital stay plus several weeks of recovery at home.

Today, however, the most commonly used surgical technique is a much simpler approach known as laparoscopic cholecystectomy. The doctor makes a half-inch incision in the abdomen, then uses special pencil-thin instruments to remove the gallbladder. A tiny microscope and video camera, snaked through the incision to the site, allow the physician to view the operation.

Laparoscopic surgery is highly effective and very safe. It has reduced the hospital stay to a day or two. Patients report less pain and are generally able to resume a normal lifestyle in a short period of time. However, people who are obese or who have a severe infection or inflammation in the gallbladder may still be considered candidates for traditional open surgery.

ALTERNATIVE CHOICES

Some alternative therapies, administered by a skilled practitioner, may help alleviate gallstone symptoms. Like most nonsurgical conventional treatments, however, alternative therapies do not necessarily prevent future gallstone problems.

ACUPUNCTURE

Some patients have found that acupuncture, if administered by a licensed practitioner, can relieve the pain associated with gallstones.

CHINESE HERBS

Very small gallstones may be dissolved through the ingestion of Chinese herbs such as pyrrosia leaf *(Pyrrosia lingua)* and rhubarb *(Rheum palmatum).* These herbs must be blended carefully by a skilled practitioner.

HOMEOPATHY

A number of homeopathic remedies can be used to treat gallstone-related symptoms. For acute pain, a homeopath might prescribe *Dioscorea, Colocynthis,* or ***Belladonna.*** Inflammation of gallbladder tissue may call for *Berberis vulgaris, Hydrastis,* or *Chelidonium majus.* You should consult a professional homeopath for exact medicine and dosages.

NUTRITION AND DIET

Depending on the severity of your condition, an improved diet may help relieve gallstone symptoms. Gallstones occur more frequently in people who are obese than in those at or near their proper weight. Though a reduction in the intake of fat may help prevent gallstones, general weight reduction seems to be the best way to avoid their development and to relieve the painful symptoms once gallstones have formed. If you are overweight, a balanced diet and exercise will help you trim down and reduce your chances of developing gallstones.

PREVENTION

A sensible diet is the best way to prevent gallstones. Seek out good sources of fiber—raw fruits and vegetables, whole grains, cooked dried beans and peas, whole-grain cereals, and bran, for example—and avoid eating too much fat. A high-fiber, low-fat diet helps keep bile cholesterol in liquid form. However, don't cut out fats abruptly or eliminate them altogether, as too little fat can also result in gallstone formation.

Recent studies have found that moderate consumption of olive oil (about 2 tbsp a day) may actually lower your chances of developing gallstones. An ingredient in olive oil evidently helps reduce cholesterol levels in the blood and gallbladder. Researchers have found that the incidence of gallstones is relatively low among people who live in areas where olive oil consumption is high.

Studies suggest that lecithin—a natural substance used as a thickener in ice cream, mayonnaise, and other foods—may help prevent gallstones by keeping cholesterol from solidifying in the gallbladder. Lecithin is found in a number of foods, including soybeans, oatmeal, eggs, milk, peanuts, cabbage, and chocolate. Even though most people get plenty of lecithin in their normal diet, supplements are available in tablet or liquid form at health food shops and drugstores. Take one tablet or 1 tbsp before each meal, or follow the instructions on the label. WARNING: Over time, large amounts of choline, a chemical in lecithin, could lead to liver problems or other complications. Check with your doctor or nutritionist before taking lecithin supplements. ■

GAS AND GAS PAINS

SYMPTOMS

- abdominal bloating and pain.
- belching.
- flatulence (passing rectal gas).

CALL YOUR DOCTOR IF:

- you have persistent, unexplained bloating for more than three days; you may have a more severe abdominal disorder.
- you have severe abdominal pain; you may have ***appendicitis***.
- you have pain in your upper right abdomen; you might have ***gallstones*** or a ***stomach ulcer.***
- you are flatulent and have lower abdominal pain that decreases when you pass gas or have a bowel movement; you may have ***irritable bowel syndrome***.
- you are flatulent, are losing weight, and have pale, foul bowel movements; you might have a malabsorption disorder, in which your intestines are not able to digest fat.

G

Gas and gas pains are a normal part of your digestive process. People may typically pass gas more than 10 times a day, but you can greatly exceed that average and still be perfectly healthy. You can usually prevent and treat gas and gas pains without professional care, but if you have other symptoms, you should consult with a doctor to find out if you have a more serious health problem.

CAUSES

When air enters your stomach, you may expel it through belching. You can take in air when you eat or drink, especially if you eat quickly. Drinking through a straw, drinking carbonated beverages, chewing gum, wearing false teeth, or swallowing air from nervous habit may also increase the amount of air that gets into your stomach.

If you eat too much high-fiber foods such as beans, vegetables, fruit, or grains, the partially digested cell walls of these foods will pass into your intestines, where bacteria begin a fermentation process that produces gas. If you have ***lactose intolerance,*** you do not produce enough lactase, a digestive enzyme that breaks down milk sugars, and you are more likely to produce gas after eating dairy foods. A gastrointestinal infection may also produce intestinal gas.

TREATMENT

You can usually treat gas and gas pains without the active involvement of a healthcare professional. Conventional medicine suggests decreasing excessive gas through changes in diet and use of over-the-counter preparations. Alternative medicines offer a wide variety of treatments.

CONVENTIONAL MEDICINE

A doctor will probably suggest you treat gas problems by changing what you eat. Avoid high-fiber foods like beans, milk products, alcohol, and carbonated beverages. Moderate exercise after meals can help move gas through your system more quickly. You may also decide to try over-the-counter preparations for gas pains. ***Simethicone,*** the active ingredient in most of these over-the-counter preparations, appears to help break up gas bubbles in the large intestine. Activated charcoal tablets absorb intestinal gas, but check with your doctor before using them, because they also absorb medications. If you are lactose intolerant, lactase supplements can help you to digest milk products more effectively. An over-the-counter product containing alpha-galactosidase may reduce the gas that is produced in digesting beans.

ALTERNATIVE CHOICES

There are many alternative therapies for gas problems. Most of them can be practiced at home, but you should check with a practitioner to make sure a particular therapy is suitable for your needs.

ACUPRESSURE

Pressing the following points may help to alleviate gas pains: Conception Vessel 6, Large Intestine 4, Spleen 6, and Stomach 36. *(See the **Appendix** for information on point locations.)*

ACUPUNCTURE

A practitioner can provide treatment for gas using the same points used in acupressure except for Conception Vessel 8, where heat might be applied instead.

HERBAL THERAPIES

Anise water, made by steeping 1 tsp of aniseeds in 1 cup of water for 10 minutes, may be helpful. Teas made with ***peppermint*** *(Mentha piperita) or* ***chamomile*** *(Matricaria recutita),* or ***fennel*** *(Foeniculum vulgare)* seeds, may also relieve gas pains.

HOMEOPATHY

Carbo vegetabilis is the most commonly used homeopathic remedy, but ***Lycopodium*** is used as well. ***Nux vomica*** is used for gas associated with constipation, and ***Chamomilla*** is preferred for gas in infants. Talk to a homeopath about which is most suitable for you.

LIFESTYLE

Regular exercise stimulates digestion and promotes the reabsorption and expulsion of gas.

MIND/BODY MEDICINE

Biofeedback and **qigong** can relieve stress and reduce gas production.

NUTRITION AND DIET

Increase your fiber intake slowly and try avoiding beans, peas, and fermented foods such as cheese, soy sauce, and alcohol. Asafetida powder dispels intestinal gas and may be used as a spice with beans. Drink fewer carbonated drinks. Avoid mixing two or more proteins at the same meal. Do not overeat, and eat fewer different food items at one sitting. For people who are lactose intolerant, replacing cow's milk with soy milk may help.

REFLEXOLOGY

Stimulate stomach areas to encourage stomach digestion, liver area to trigger bile secretion, gallbladder area to trigger release of stored bile, intestine areas to stimulate regular contractions in both intestines, and pancreas area to encourage secretion of digestive enzymes. *(See page 25 for area locations.)*

AT-HOME REMEDIES

Dissolve a teaspoon or two of superfine white, green, or yellow French clay (available at health food stores) in water and drink at least once daily (but not with meals). The clay absorbs impurities and intestinal gas; check with your doctor to make sure it won't absorb medications you may be taking as well.

PREVENTION

One of the main methods of preventing gas and gas pains is also the primary treatment: Avoid overeating and foods that generate gas in your system. Try to become more aware of the air that you swallow; you can avoid some gas, for instance, by not gulping your food. ■

G

GASTRITIS

SYMPTOMS

Any of a variety of mild-to-severe stomach symptoms may indicate gastritis. The most common are:

- upper abdominal discomfort or pain.
- nausea.
- vomiting.
- diarrhea.
- loss of appetite.

G

CALL YOUR DOCTOR IF:

- you are vomiting blood or have bloody, black, or tarry stools; you have **internal bleeding** and need immediate medical attention. *(See page 70.)*
- stomach pain becomes severe; you may have a gastric or duodenal ulcer *(see **stomach ulcers**).*
- you have excessive thirst, a dry mouth, or decreased urination; you may be dehydrated and need fluid replacement.

Gastritis is a general medical term for inflammation of the stomach lining. Attacks of **acute gastritis,** marked by discomfort, nausea, vomiting, or diarrhea, usually last only one or two days. The term "acute" means that the attacks are short, not necessarily that the symptoms are severe. People with **chronic gastritis** may have no pain but may experience appetite loss or nausea. Chronic gastritis can lead to pernicious ***anemia,*** a deficiency in blood cells caused by a lack of ***vitamin B_{12}.***

Gastritis occurs most often among the elderly, but it can affect anyone at any age. Self-care is often the best treatment for mild gastritis. For more-severe cases the treatment offered by your practitioner will depend on the underlying cause of the inflammation.

CAUSES

Many conditions can irritate your stomach and cause acute or chronic gastritis. ***Aspirin*** and other over-the-counter and prescription drugs may cause erosion of the stomach lining. Viral or bacterial infections, as well as ingested substances and alcohol abuse, may cause stomach inflammation.

DIAGNOSTIC AND TEST PROCEDURES

Your doctor may suspect acute gastritis from your symptoms and order tests to confirm the diagnosis. A barium x-ray, for instance, may show stomach lesions. Another possible procedure is gastroscopy, a visual examination of the stomach's interior. A confirmed diagnosis of chronic gastritis requires a biopsy.

TREATMENT

In both conventional and alternative medical practices, treatment for gastritis depends upon the type of gastritis you have. Conventional medicine uses over-the-counter antacids, prescription drugs, antibiotics, and in rare cases, surgery to treat gastritis. Both conventional and alternative practitioners frequently suggest changes in lifestyle—such as stopping smoking—that reduce your risk of developing gastritis.

CONVENTIONAL MEDICINE

For a mild case of gastritis, over-the-counter antacids are recommended. If you find these are not effective, your doctor may prescribe ***cimetidine, ranitidine,*** or ***famotidine,*** which reduce production of stomach acid. Gastritis caused by bacteria can be treated with ***antibiotics*** and with over-the-counter preparations that contain ***bismuth subsalicylate.*** Chronic gastritis can also usually be treated with over-the-counter antacids. If your stomach lining has been seriously eroded by excess stomach acid and you have internal bleeding, you may need blood transfusions and other intravenous fluids. Surgery may be needed to control the bleeding if other treatments don't work or if you have ulcers or perforations through the stomach wall.

ALTERNATIVE CHOICES

Alternative treatments focus on treating gastritis with both physical and mental techniques. Some require a practitioner's care, but you can try some at home as well.

DRUGS AND GASTRITIS

Anti-inflammatory drugs, often used for arthritis and other disorders, can irritate your stomach lining to the point that gastritis and other stomach problems develop. ***Aspirin*** *and many* ***nonsteroidal anti-inflammatory drugs (NSAIDs)*** *like* ***ibuprofen, naproxen,*** *indomethacin, and tolmetin are among the drugs that can be harsh on your stomach. Avoid them if you have been diagnosed with gastritis.*

ACUPRESSURE AND ACUPUNCTURE

A practitioner can treat gastritis by using many points, depending on your symptoms, or you can press the points associated with digestive system problems, such as Conception Vessel 6 and 12, Pericardium 6, Spleen 34, and Stomach 36. *(See the* ***Appendix*** *for point locations.)*

HERBAL THERAPIES

To soothe your stomach, drink a tea made of 1 tbsp ***chamomile*** *(Matricaria recutita)* steeped in 1 cup boiling water for 10 minutes. ***Licorice*** *(Glycyrrhiza glabra)* extract in capsule or liquid form may also help.

HOMEOPATHY

For acute gastritis, try one of the following remedies every hour for up to four doses; if that one doesn't work, try one of the others, and if the gastritis persists, consult a homeopath for other possibilities.

- Burning pains and vomiting that are relieved by cold food and drinks: ***Phosphorus*** (12x).
- Nausea, tender stomach, and a sensation like a stone in your stomach: ***Bryonia*** (12x).
- A sensation like a knot in your stomach, acid reflux, hiccups, and increased discomfort after eating and drinking: ***Nux vomica*** (12x).
- Stomach pain that is better after eating but returns two hours later: *Anacardium* (12x).

NUTRITION AND DIET

Limit or eliminate alcohol, caffeine, and carbonated drinks from your diet; contrary to popular belief, though, you do not need to avoid spicy foods in particular. Eat more noncitrus fruits, cooked vegetables, and bland foods, and eat fewer refined carbohydrates such as white bread and white rice. Supplements of ***zinc*** and ***vitamin A*** may help heal the stomach lining.

AT-HOME REMEDIES

Over-the-counter antacids and ***acetaminophen*** may offer relief. Don't eat solid food on the first day gastritis develops; drink lots of water and other liquids—but not milk, which increases acid secretion—to prevent dehydration. ■

GASTROENTERITIS

SYMPTOMS

Gastroenteritis is also often called stomach flu or intestinal flu. Its symptoms generally last less than 48 hours. They include:

- nausea and vomiting.
- diarrhea.
- abdominal cramps and pain.
- fever.
- weakness.

G

CALL YOUR DOCTOR IF:

- symptoms last longer than two days, your fever is 102°F or higher, or your symptoms recur after treatment; you may have a more serious gastrointestinal disorder.
- you have mucus or blood in your stool, or are vomiting blood; this indicates internal bleeding *(see also **Emergencies/First Aid,** page 70)*.
- you have excessive thirst, are urinating less frequently, have a dry mouth, and feel confused; you may be dehydrated and need fluid replacement.
- you have severe pain or swelling in the abdomen; you may have ***appendicitis*** or another abdominal disorder.

Gastroenteritis is a general term that applies to many types of irritation and infection of the digestive tract. Unless you have a severe case or complications set in, you probably don't need a professional diagnosis or treatment. However, children, the elderly, and people with chronic health conditions need to be watched for complications such as dehydration.

CAUSES

Gastroenteritis may be caused by many things. The most common cause is a virus that can spread quickly through an office, school, or day-care center. ***Food poisoning,*** bacteria, and parasites also can cause gastroenteritis. Bacterial infection in the digestive tract is often responsible for travelers' diarrhea. Sometimes taking certain medications or drinking excessive amounts of alcohol can irritate your digestive tract enough to cause gastroenteritis.

DIAGNOSTIC AND TEST PROCEDURES

A doctor can usually diagnose gastroenteritis by your symptoms alone. Lab tests of your stool can show if you have a parasitic or bacterial infection.

TREATMENT

Unless you have a bacterial form of gastroenteritis, or develop complications, you probably don't need professional care. Alternative methods treat nausea, vomiting, diarrhea, and other symptoms.

CONVENTIONAL MEDICINE

If you have a simple case of gastroenteritis, your doctor will probably recommend rest, drinking lots of liquids, and eating bland foods if you can tolerate them. Over-the-counter remedies that contain ***bismuth subsalicylate*** or absorbent clays may help control diarrhea. Other drugs may be prescribed to treat severe diarrhea. If your vomiting is severe, your doctor may prescribe ***prochlorperazine*** or trimethobenzamide. If your gastroenteritis is caused by a bacterial agent, ***antibiotics*** may also be prescribed; they may make your diarrhea worse but are necessary to kill the harmful bacteria. If you become dehydrated from vomiting and diarrhea, you may be put in the hospital to have the lost fluids replaced intravenously. This happens most frequently to infants, elderly people, and people with chronic diseases such as ***diabetes.***

ALTERNATIVE CHOICES

Like most conventional medical treatment, alternative choices mainly offer self-help treatments for the symptoms of gastroenteritis.

ACUPRESSURE AND ACUPUNCTURE

In addition to using the acupressure techniques illustrated at right, press Pericardium 5 for vomiting and nausea *(see the **Appendix** for point locations).* See a practitioner for acupuncture treatment to harmonize the digestive organs.

ACUPRESSURE

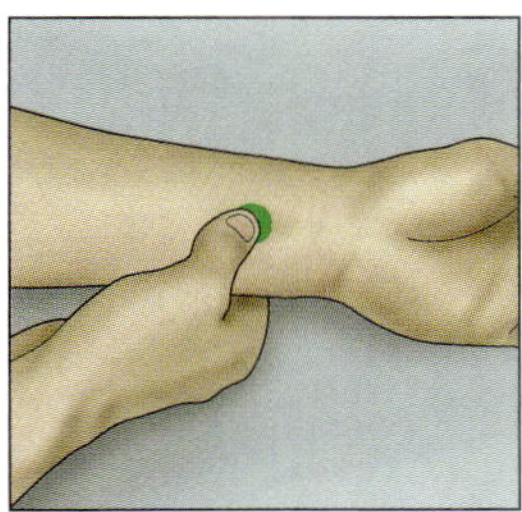

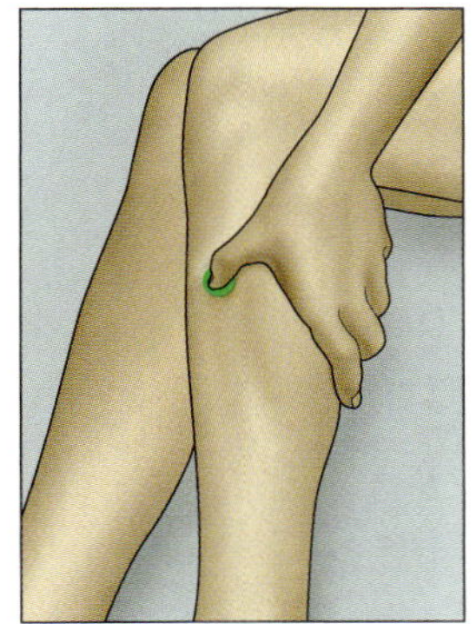

Acupressure on points PE 6 and ST 36 may help relieve nausea, stomach disorders, and indigestion. PE 6 is located between the two bones of the forearm, two finger widths from the center of the inner wrist crease *(top).* ST 36 is located four finger widths below the bottom of the kneecap on the outside of the large leg bone *(bottom).* Press your thumb firmly into each point and hold for one minute. Repeat on the other arm and leg; press on each point three to five times.

HERBAL THERAPIES

Meadowsweet *(Filipendula ulmaria)* can reduce nausea and stomach acidity: Pour 1 cup boiling water on 2 tsp dried meadowsweet and steep for 15 minutes; drink three times daily. ***Slippery elm*** *(Ulmus fulva)* may also help calm your digestive tract when the worst symptoms have passed: Mix 1 part powdered slippery elm with 8 parts water and bring to a boil; simmer for 15 minutes, and drink half a cup three times a day.

HOMEOPATHY

If symptoms are severe, take 12x dosages of one of the following homeopathic preparations every two hours until symptoms improve. If you do not feel any better after two or three doses, try another preparation.

- ***Arsenicum album*** for restlessness, exhaustion, chills, thirst, vomiting, diarrhea, and burning pains.
- ***Ipecac*** for extreme nausea and vomiting.
- ***Nux vomica*** for symptoms caused by exhaustion, overeating, or drinking too much alcohol or coffee.

NUTRITION AND DIET

Drink lots of fluids. After symptoms are gone, 2 capsules, twice a day, of *Lactobacillus acidophilus,* and eating ripe bananas, whole-grain foods, and vegetables help soothe the stomach and restore protective bacteria in your digestive system. Avoid milk products for two weeks after diarrhea ends; they can cause a recurrence of diarrhea while your system readjusts to absorbing milk.

REFLEXOLOGY

Stimulate the adrenal areas to fight infection and the stomach areas to restore normal function. See page 25 for area locations.

PREVENTION

- Wash your hands frequently to avoid picking up or passing along germs that cause gastroenteritis.
- See ***Food Poisoning*** for important safeguards about preparing and storing food. ■

GENITAL HERPES

SYMPTOMS

- numbness, tingling, or burning in the genitals.
- burning sensation while urinating or having intercourse.
- painful urination or frequent need to urinate.
- watery blisters in the genital area.
- flulike symptoms.

G

CALL YOUR DOCTOR IF:

- you have any of the symptoms listed above; your condition needs to be properly evaluated and diagnosed.

Herpes is the most common viral sexually transmitted disease in the United States, affecting more than 20 million people. The disease is both highly contagious and incurable, but it is not fatal, and you can learn to live with it.

Usually, herpes spreads only if the infected person is experiencing an outbreak of blisters. However, people can sometimes spread it even if they have no symptoms; it can also be spread through oral sex if one partner has a herpes sore on the mouth or genitals.

The first outbreak is usually the most extensive and painful, and can last from five days to three weeks. As much as 30 percent of those who have one outbreak never have another. Many people experience precursor signals several hours prior to an outbreak of blisters: pain running down the buttocks or in the knees, and/or itching in the genital area.

CAUSES

Genital herpes is caused by a virus that invades the body through tiny breaks in the skin. After symptoms disappear, the virus travels to deep nerve centers at the base of the spinal cord near the buttocks. When reactivated, the virus moves out along the nerves, resulting in a new outbreak.

People who are chronically ill or under severe stress seem to have the most attacks, and many kinds of stimuli or stress may reactivate the virus, including sunburn, sexual intercourse, and menstruation. Outbreaks may also occur in response to certain foods or medications.

TREATMENT

There is no cure for herpes, but there are ways to lessen the discomfort and speed healing.

CONVENTIONAL MEDICINE

A doctor may prescribe ***acyclovir,*** either as a pill taken orally or applied as a cream. The drug can prevent recurrences or lessen them in up to 90 percent of people who have herpes. If you are pregnant, however, the doctor will recommend another medication, because acyclovir may cause fetal damage. ***Analgesics*** such as ***aspirin*** or ***acetaminophen*** may lessen the pain, and drying agents such as calamine lotion may help heal the sores.

ALTERNATIVE CHOICES

There are several things you can do yourself to alleviate herpes symptoms and prevent recurrences. For example, because herpes outbreaks are often brought on by ***stress,*** the disease responds well to **relaxation** techniques. Changes in diet and vitamin supplements may also help.

ACUPRESSURE

Acupressure massage is said to relieve fatigue and tension, which may trigger outbreaks. Press the highest point of the shoulder muscle midway between the outer tip of the shoulder and the spine. Do this several times a day.

CHINESE HERBS

A doctor of Chinese medicine will prescribe a formula tailored to your needs. It may include herbs such as **gentiana** *(Gentiana scabra)* and ***dong quai*** *(Angelica sinensis).*

HERBAL THERAPIES

Research suggests that glycyrrhizic acid, a constituent of ***licorice*** *(Glycyrrhiza glabra),* inactivates the herpesvirus. Drink herbal teas or take capsules as directed by your physician or an herbalist. Lemon balm *(Melissa officinalis)* may also be effective against the herpesvirus; apply lemon balm tea directly to the sores. ***Calendula*** *(Calendula officinalis)* ointment, applied to the sores 3 times a day, will soothe the pain and help kill the virus.

HOMEOPATHY

A homeopath will prescribe a specific combination of remedies that may include ***Rhus toxicodendron, Sepia, Natrum muriaticum, Hepar sulphuris,*** and *Thuja occidentalis.*

MIND/BODY MEDICINE

By reducing stress, you can prevent outbreaks or lessen their severity. See page 27 for descriptions of various techniques, such as **meditation,** that help relieve stress.

NUTRITION AND DIET

The herpesvirus needs the amino acid arginine to thrive; conversely, the amino acid lysine prevents it from flourishing. Avoid arginine-rich foods such as peanuts, cashews, and chocolate. Lysine-rich foods include beef, lamb, fish, milk, and cheese. You can also take 500 mg of lysine in capsule form daily to help prevent outbreaks; as soon as you notice symptoms, take 1,000 mg every four hours. In addition, ***vitamin E*** may decrease pain and speed the healing of lesions.

AT-HOME REMEDIES

- Apply diluted lemon juice, ***vitamin E,*** or ***tea tree oil*** (*Melaleuca* spp.) to dry up sores.
- Apply ice 10 minutes on, 5 minutes off to relieve pain.
- Use zinc sulfate ointment to heal sores.
- Soothe lesions with baking soda compresses.
- Add 3 tbsp salt to a warm bath; follow with a cold bath. Soak about 15 minutes in each.

PREVENTION

If an infected partner is having a herpes outbreak, don't have intercourse, even if you use a condom. If the infected person is symptom free, use a condom anyway; he or she may still be contagious. Don't practice oral sex if one of you has a cold sore.

CAUTION!

If you are pregnant and have herpes, follow your doctor's advice carefully. If you deliver your child while you're having an outbreak, you could pass the disease to the baby. In such cases, your doctor may recommend that you undergo a Cesarean section. ■

GENITAL WARTS

SYMPTOMS

- painless flesh-colored or grayish white growths on the vulva, anus, or penis that may develop a cauliflower-like appearance.
- growths that are itchy or mildly sore.

CALL YOUR DOCTOR IF:

- you develop any of the symptoms listed above; although genital warts are harmless, they are contagious and require medical treatment.

G

Genital warts *(Condylomata acuminata)* affect an estimated 10 million to 20 million Americans. As many as a million people contract genital warts each year; pregnant women and people with impaired immune systems are more susceptible than is the general population to this infection.

Sometimes what appear to be genital warts are merely accumulations of normal skin that have no medical significance; about 1 in 100 men has these. But because genital warts are contagious, you should see a doctor if you discover any such growths.

Although the warts are harmless in themselves, there appears to be some link between genital warts and ***cervical cancer.*** Several studies have shown that 90 percent of women who have cervical cancer also had genital warts. This doesn't mean cancer is inevitable, but if you have genital warts you should probably play it safe and get a Pap smear every six months.

CAUSES

Genital warts are caused by the human papilloma virus, or HPV, the same virus that causes warts on the hands, feet, and face. The virus lives inside your body's cells, where it replicates; eventually the virus breaks out of its original host cell to infect other cells.

DIAGNOSTIC AND TEST PROCEDURES

Your doctor may want to take a culture to determine whether your warts are contagious. If you are a woman and are diagnosed with warts, make sure to be tested for cervical irregularities during your regular gynecological exams. Your doctor may take a Pap smear or insert a colposcope, a device to microscopically inspect the vaginal walls and cervix for abnormal cells.

TREATMENT

Although there is no cure and no vaccine for genital warts, they are easily controlled and should in no way disrupt your life. About one-fifth of all warts disappear spontaneously within six months, and two-thirds go away after two years. Nevertheless, unlike warts on other areas of the body, genital warts should not be left untreated because they are much more contagious. And even though conventional treatments will remove the warts themselves, the virus remains in the body and may cause later outbreaks.

CONVENTIONAL MEDICINE

Don't attempt to get rid of genital warts with over-the-counter remedies. The genital area is too sensitive for these products and you could damage your skin. Instead, let your doctor remove warts with a chemical "paint" called podophyllin. Podophyllin treatment usually is effective within a few weeks. If you're pregnant, your doctor will want to use another treatment, since podophyllin may be absorbed into the bloodstream and cause fetal abnormalities. Warts may also be frozen with liquid nitrogen or solid carbon dioxide (dry ice), burned off with lasers, or surgically removed. Another treatment involves injections of interferon alpha, or Intron A. In some studies, the drug eliminated warts in half the subjects.

ALTERNATIVE CHOICES

Because genital warts are contagious, you should see a physician before exploring alternative methods to help alleviate symptoms and prevent warts from coming back.

CHINESE HERBS

A doctor of Chinese medicine will give you a unique herbal prescription to cleanse your liver and build up your immune system. Ingredients may include ***Chinese foxglove root*** *(Rehmannia glutinosa)* and ***gentiana*** *(Gentiana scabra).*

HERBAL THERAPIES

To help heal warts, apply ***garlic*** *(Allium sativum),* or the juice of a sour apple, a dandelion stalk, a fresh pineapple, or fresh green figs. Preparations made from the herbs lomatium *(Lomatium dissectum)* and thuja *(Thuja occidentalis)* are useful against genital warts.

HOMEOPATHY

A homeopathic physician will prescribe a treatment to strengthen your immune system. *Sabina* is a common remedy.

MIND/BODY MEDICINE

Several studies have shown that **hypnotherapy** may be effective in reducing or eliminating warts. Ask your physician if hypnotherapy might help you. ***Stress*** may also contribute to outbreaks, so find a relaxation technique that works for you. Many forms of **meditation** and self-hypnosis can be practiced at home.

NUTRITION AND DIET

To prevent HPV infections from recurring, eat plenty of foods that contain ***vitamins A*** and ***C,*** which help the body fight off infections, and ***folic acid,*** which strengthens the immune system. Both broccoli and spinach are good sources of these nutrients.

AT-HOME REMEDIES

- Apply thuja *(Thuja occidentalis)* ointment to warts to help them heal.
- Eat a balanced diet with plenty of fruits and vegetables.
- Meditate regularly. Try listening to guided meditation cassettes.

PREVENTION

The best way to prevent genital warts is to use condoms. If your partner discovers a wart, insist that he or she see a doctor, and if the warts prove to be venereal, get tested yourself—even if you have no symptoms. ■

G

GERMAN MEASLES

SYMPTOMS

A child with German measles may not look or act sick, but symptoms may include:

- a low-grade fever and swollen glands behind the ears and at the back and sides of the neck.
- loss of appetite, irritability, loss of interest in personal care.
- in an older child or teenager, joint pain.

A rash appears in only about half the cases of German measles. When it does appear, it starts on the face and torso and spreads to the arms and legs. Over the course of about four days, the rash fades. See also the ***Visual Diagnostic Guide.***

CALL YOUR DOCTOR IF:

- you are pregnant and you think you have been exposed to German measles; the virus can pass from you through the umbilical cord to your unborn child, possibly causing birth defects.
- your child has German measles and is having trouble staying fully awake or is extremely lethargic. This may indicate encephalitis, a rare complication.
- your child has German measles and has abdominal pain accompanied by vomiting; these are possible symptoms of pancreatic or liver inflammation.

German measles, or rubella, is a mild illness, in many cases no more uncomfortable for your child than a cold. People who have had German measles once develop a lifetime immunity.

The danger of German measles is to the unborn child, especially during the first trimester. A pregnant woman who contracts German measles runs a 20 percent to 50 percent risk of bearing a child with birth defects, including blindness, deafness, and congenital heart defects. Before becoming pregnant, a woman should confirm that she is protected *(see **Prevention,** opposite).*

Many states require children to be immunized before entering public school *(see page 33).*

CAUSES

German measles is caused by a virus and transmitted by droplets from a sneeze or cough. The incubation period—when the virus multiplies and the child is not contagious—is 14 to 21 days from exposure. Infected children are contagious from 2 days before to 7 days after any rash is visible.

TREATMENT

Your child should stay at home while sick or up to a week after any rash disappears.

CONVENTIONAL MEDICINE

No medical treatment of a child with German measles is required. If you are pregnant and are exposed to rubella, you should contact your doctor immediately. The risk of birth defects is higher the earlier in your pregnancy the exposure occurs, and in some cases your doctor may advise you to consider a therapeutic termination of your pregnancy. However, after the 20th week of your pregnancy the risk of a defect being caused by exposure to German measles drops to zero.

ALTERNATIVE CHOICES

Many alternative practitioners believe it is better for an otherwise healthy child to contract Ger-

IDENTIFYING THE RASH

The first signs of German measles are fever and swollen glands in the neck. In about half of all cases, tiny, pinkish spots develop on the face and trunk two or three days later *(right)*. Unlike measles, the spots do not merge into a solid, uniform rash.

After several days the rash on the face subsides, and the spots spread to the arms and legs. They last up to five days and do not itch.

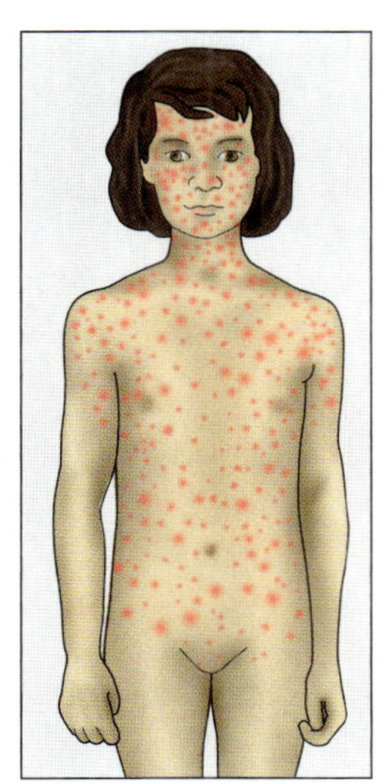

man measles than to be vaccinated, because immunity is then permanent. However, since an infected child can pass the disease to others at risk, especially pregnant women, you should seriously consider immunization.

HOMEOPATHY

Always consult a homeopathic physician for appropriate dosages and remedies for children. ***Belladonna, Pulsatilla,*** and *Phytolacca* are three remedies often prescribed; the choice depends on your child's symptoms and temperament.

OSTEOPATHY

Gentle, rhythmic pressure applied over the spleen, a procedure known as spleen pumping, may enhance the release of white blood cells into the blood. Seek help from an osteopath.

AT-HOME CARE

- Keep your child quiet, especially if she has a fever; confinement to bed is not necessary. Children should be kept home while any rash is visible and for a week thereafter.
- Cool sponging will help relieve fever and discomfort from a rash. An ***acetaminophen-*** based pain reliever may also help.

PREVENTION

Immunization of children as a protection to others is strongly recommended by most healthcare practitioners, but be aware that vaccination does not always provide lifetime immunity. The homeopathic version is not an accepted equivalent and will not provide adequate protection.

The MMR (measles, mumps, and rubella vaccine) is now given at 12 or 15 months, with a booster at the age of 4 to 6 or 10 to 12. If a household member is pregnant and there is any question of her not being immune, your doctor will recommend delaying immunization of your children to prevent exposing the mother-to-be to the live, though weakened, virus in the vaccine.

At least three months before trying to become pregnant, a woman should have a blood test to see if the rubella antibodies are present; if not, she should be immunized or reimmunized.

PREGNANCY CONCERNS

If you are pregnant, are not sure of your immunity to rubella, and suspect you have been exposed, contact your doctor immediately, because the virus can pass to your unborn child. If your child has German measles, notify any at-risk individuals who have had contact with your child during the illness and up to 10 days before symptoms appeared, so they can seek appropriate care.

C A U T I O N !

Never give a child *aspirin*—even baby aspirin—or other products containing the salt called salicylate to reduce a fever or to relieve pain. Aspirin has been linked to Reye's syndrome, a rare but very dangerous illness that causes inflammation of the liver and brain. ■

G

GLAUCOMA

SYMPTOMS

- Teary, aching eyes, blurred vision, occasional headaches, and progressive loss of peripheral vision are signs of **chronic glaucoma.**
- A sudden onset of severe throbbing pain, headaches, blurred vision, rainbow halos around lights, redness in the eye, dilated pupils, and sometimes nausea and vomiting are signs of **acute glaucoma.**
- Blurred vision, headaches, and halos around lights following an eye injury are signs of **secondary glaucoma.**
- In infants, teary or cloudy eyes, unusual sensitivity to light, and enlarged corneas are signs of **congenital glaucoma.**

CALL YOUR DOCTOR IF:

- you have symptoms of **acute glaucoma.** You need immediate medical attention to prevent potentially permanent eye damage or blindness.
- you become drowsy, fatigued, or short of breath after using eye drops containing ***beta-adrenergic blockers*** such as ***timolol,*** betaxolol, or bunolol. The medication may be aggravating a heart or lung problem.
- you are prescribed drugs for other ailments. Many medications, especially those used to treat stomach and intestinal disorders, may aggravate glaucoma.

G

More than two million adult Americans suffer from glaucoma, making it one of the leading causes of blindness. **Chronic glaucoma,** which accounts for 90 percent of cases in the United States, usually appears in middle age and seems to have a genetic component: 1 out of 5 sufferers has a close relative with the condition. Doctors often refer to **chronic glaucoma** as the "sneak thief in the night" because it comes on gradually to steal your vision. It may be well established before you notice the warning signs: You have headaches, you need new glasses, you start losing side vision, and eventually you develop blank spots where you can't see anything.

Other forms of glaucoma are less common but no less serious. If you have sudden, severe pain in the eyes, blurred vision, and dilated pupils—sometimes with nausea or vomiting—it may be an attack of **acute,** or **narrow-angle, glaucoma.** This type accounts for less than 10 percent of reported cases, but it comes on quickly and requires urgent medical attention. If left untreated, it can irreversibly damage the optic nerve, which carries visual images from the eye to the brain, causing blindness—sometimes in a matter of days.

Secondary glaucoma is usually associated with another eye disease or disorder, such as an enlarged ***cataract,*** uveitis (an inner-eye inflammation), an eye tumor, or an eye injury. People suffering from ***diabetes*** are also susceptible to **neovascular glaucoma,** a particularly severe form of the disease. **Congenital glaucoma** is an extremely rare, inborn condition affecting babies; 80 percent of cases occur by the age of one.

CAUSES

The eye's lens, iris, and cornea are continuously bathed and nourished by a water-based fluid called aqueous humor. As new fluid is produced by cells inside the eye, excess fluid normally drains out through a complex network of tissue called the drainage angle, where the cornea and iris meet *(illustration above, right).* An imbalance between the rate of production of aqueous humor and the rate of drainage will bring on **chronic,** or **open-angle, glaucoma.** This is the most

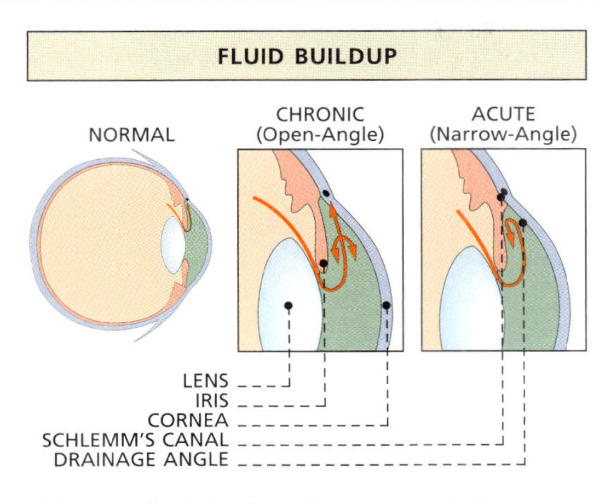

Fluid normally drains from the eye through the drainage angle—located between the cornea and the iris—and out through the tiny Schlemm's canal. **Chronic,** or **open-angle, glaucoma** *(inset, left)* occurs when fluid is produced faster than it can drain out. **Acute,** or **narrow-angle, glaucoma** *(inset, right)* occurs when the iris blocks the drainage angle.

prevalent form of the ailment and generally develops slowly with age.

Some people apparently inherit a condition of the inner eye in which the iris can block normal drainage channels. When this happens, the fluid does not drain out of the eye fast enough, and the sudden pressure from fluid buildup causes **acute glaucoma.** In newborns, defects in the drainage angle are the cause of **congenital glaucoma.** Both conditions need prompt medical attention to prevent potential loss of sight.

Depending on the individual, the onset of glaucoma may be related to gradual changes in drainage-angle tissue, increased fluid production, or a congenital abnormality. Whatever the specific cause, the effect is the same: The increase in pressure from excess fluid damages the optic nerve, which relays visual messages to the brain. As the optic nerve deteriorates, your field of vision narrows and you have difficulty discerning things at either side. If nerve damage continues, it can affect your central vision and lead ultimately to total blindness.

Researchers are not certain what triggers these abnormalities, but they do know some things that may induce or aggravate them. Using certain ***antidepressants, antihypertensives,*** and steroids for a long period may increase pressure within the eye. A change in the body's collagen metabolism may also contribute to glaucoma. Collagen, one of the most abundant proteins in the body, plays an integral role in maintaining the strength and utility of your eye tissue. ***Corticosteroid*** eye drops, sometimes prescribed for other eye disorders, are thought to destroy collagen balance in certain situations *(see **Eye Problems** and **Vision Problems**)*. Stress and allergies may aggravate symptoms of chronic glaucoma.

DIAGNOSTIC AND TEST PROCEDURES

Procedures for glaucoma screening are brief and painless. Your optometrist will routinely measure your inner-eye pressure with an air-puff tonometer; an ophthalmologist may use a more sensitive instrument called an applanation tonometer. But the mere presence of higher-than-normal pressure within the eye does not mean that you have glaucoma: Slight pressure in your eye without evidence of damage to your optic nerve is called **ocular hypertension.** In most cases, this condition calls only for repeat testing at regular intervals to check for early signs of nerve damage.

If glaucoma is suspected, your ophthalmologist may dilate your eyes and examine the optic nerve with a hand-held ophthalmoscope. You should have a visual field test, which measures your peripheral, or side, vision.

Congenital glaucoma is difficult to diagnose because a child under a year old cannot describe the symptoms. If the cornea in your child's eye appears cloudy, a congenital condition may be present. Babies are routinely checked for the disorder at birth, but if you suspect congenital glaucoma, see a pediatric ophthalmologist at once.

TREATMENT

Treatment of glaucoma requires measures to control the flow and drainage of aqueous humor in the eye, restoring the normal balance of inner-eye pressure. **Chronic glaucoma** may not be noticed until it has progressed to a relatively advanced stage, but it can usually be controlled. Both medical and surgical approaches have high rates of success in treating **chronic glaucoma,** but you can help yourself by relieving stress and maintaining collagen production. **Acute glaucoma** is different: If the pressure of excess fluid in the eye is not relieved quickly, the result can be blindness.

CONVENTIONAL MEDICINE

Appropriate therapy depends on the nature and stage of the ailment. Your ophthalmologist may not prescribe any therapy for **ocular hypertension** when the pressure in your eye is minimal; periodic evaluation with close monitoring of your peripheral vision and of the appearance of the optic nerve may be sufficient.

Chronic glaucoma is typically managed with eye drops. Those that contain ***epinephrine*** or pilocarpine help increase fluid outflow but may have undesirable side effects: Pilocarpine may cause headaches and blurred vision; epinephrine may cause excessively red, teary eyes and in rare cases may aggravate heart problems. Eye drops containing ***beta-adrenergic blockers*** such as ***timolol,*** betaxolol, and bunolol may have heart or lung side effects. Latanoprost relieves eye pressure but may cause blurred vision. Oral carbonic anhydrase inhibitors help decrease fluid production but may cause stomach upset or tingling hands and feet. Because of potential drug interactions, your ophthalmologist should know before prescribing eye drops about any other medications you take.

If your chronic glaucoma does not respond to medication, or if you cannot tolerate the side effects, your doctor may recommend one of several surgical techniques:

- Trabeculoplasty creates 50 to 100 small laser burns at the drainage angle, where the iris and cornea meet, increasing the outflow rate of aqueous fluid. This relatively brief procedure can be done in an ophthalmologist's office.
- Trabeculectomy creates an artificial channel for fluid outflow in advanced cases in which the inner-eye pressure is high and the optic nerve continues to be damaged. Results vary, but generally the success rate is high.

When glaucoma is unresponsive to surgery or when the risks of a surgical procedure are too high, other options are available to destroy the cells that produce too much aqueous fluid: Ultrasound treatment uses high-frequency sound waves, diathermy uses heat, and cryosurgery uses a freezing process.

Many medications, especially those used to treat stomach and intestinal disorders, may aggravate your glaucoma by actually increasing inner-eye pressure. Always make sure your physician and ophthalmologist are each aware of what the other prescribes for you.

ALTERNATIVE CHOICES

Alternative approaches to treating glaucoma emphasize prevention and good eye maintenance. Natural remedies may help keep glaucoma at bay or—if you are already under a doctor's care—may complement conventional treatment. Some therapies seek to relieve stress in order to control inner-eye pressure. Herbal and dietary applications attempt to maintain collagen balance and replenish any nutrient deficiencies.

ACUPUNCTURE

Performed in conjunction with herbal therapy and a nutritious diet, acupuncture may help relieve tension and reduce pressure in the eye. The acupuncturist will concentrate on points along the bladder, gallbladder, liver, and kidney meridians. *(See **Appendix** for point locations.)*

BODY WORK

According to **reflexology** therapists, the nerve endings where your toes meet the rest of your foot influence the nerves in your visual system. Therapeutic **massage** and manipulation of your foot in this area relieve stress and tension, which may help reduce eye pressure.

HERBAL THERAPIES

A variety of herbs have properties that address the factors contributing to glaucoma.

- ***Bilberry*** *(Vaccinium myrtillus)*—or its American equivalent, huckleberry—helps maintain collagen balance and prevents the breakdown of ***vitamin C.*** Eat 2 to 4 oz three times a day whenever the fresh berries are available.

- *Cannabis sativa,* also known as marijuana, contains the chemical compound tetrahydrocannabinol (THC). Clinical studies have demonstrated that it reduces the inner-eye pressure that causes glaucoma. Though a controlled substance, cannabis can be prescribed by a licensed professional to treat glaucoma.

MIND/BODY MEDICINE

Eye exercises may relieve stress and eyestrain caused by overworked eyes and many eye problems, including glaucoma. *(See **Vision Problems**.)*

Hydrotherapy may be used to stimulate circulation in the eye. Soak a cloth in hot water, wring it out, and place it on your eyes for up to three minutes. Then do the same with a cold compress, and alternate each compress three times.

NUTRITION AND DIET

Studies suggest that ***vitamin C*** lowers inner-eye pressure and restores collagen balance, making it especially useful if you are unresponsive to oral medications or eye drops. Foods high in vitamin C include cauliflower, broccoli, turnip greens, strawberries, grapefruits, and oranges. Alternatively, take up to 3,000 mg of a vitamin C supplement daily. ***Chromium*** and ***zinc*** may also deter glaucoma, as most people with the disease exhibit deficiencies of these minerals, as well as of thiamine ***(vitamin B_1).***

When used in conjunction with traditional drug therapies, rutin is said to reduce inner-eye pressure and restore collagen balance. It can be found in supplement form in varying strengths at health food stores. See the product label or ask your doctor for appropriate dosages.

It is important to identify and avoid any foods and other substances you may be allergic to, since an allergic reaction may induce excess pressure within the eye.

AT-HOME REMEDIES

Early detection is crucial. Only an ophthalmologist can diagnose the condition, but you must be aware of the warning signs. So if you sense that your vision is deteriorating—especially if you are over 40—a complete eye examination is a must.

If you are already near- or farsighted, a balanced diet and eye exercises may be effective preventive measures against glaucoma. If you have ***diabetes*** or ***high blood pressure,*** you should diligently stick to your prescribed treatment to reduce the inherent risk of developing glaucoma. Once you have been diagnosed with glaucoma, however, you may remain under the regular care of your physician or ophthalmologist. You may also have to use eye drops for the rest of your life. The alternative treatments listed above can complement your professional medical care. ■

RISK FACTORS

The following factors increase the risk of developing glaucoma. If one or more apply to you, have your eyes examined annually.

- ***Chronic glaucoma*** *usually develops after the age of 40.*
- *Diabetics are three times as likely to develop glaucoma as are nondiabetics.* ***Neovascular glaucoma,*** *a severe form of the disease, is linked to diabetes.*
- ***High blood pressure,*** *migraine* ***headaches,*** *and nearsightedness are associated with the onset of glaucoma.*
- *Glaucoma is sometimes inherited, although a person may have a genetic predisposition to the disorder without developing it.*
- *African Americans develop glaucoma-induced blindness at a rate several times higher than that of Caucasians. Researchers have yet to find the reason for a greater incidence of glaucoma in certain racial groups.*

GOITER

SYMPTOMS

- swelling at the base of the neck, ranging from a small lump to a general enlargement *(see illustration opposite).*
- If you have **hyperthyroidism** (an overactive thyroid gland), you may also experience weight loss despite an increased appetite, an increased heart rate, elevated blood pressure, nervousness, diarrhea, muscle weakness, and hand tremors.
- If you have **hypothyroidism** (an underactive thyroid gland), you may also experience lethargy, slowed physical and mental functions, depression, a lower heart rate, an intolerance to cold, constipation, easy weight gain, and tingling or numbness in your hands.

CALL YOUR DOCTOR IF:

- you have a large goiter and experience dizziness, hoarseness, or difficulty in swallowing; the goiter may be pressing on your jugular vein, windpipe, esophagus, or the nerve that runs to your larynx. The growth requires treatment and may need to be surgically removed.

G

Goiters can be any one of several types of growths in the thyroid gland, located at the base of the neck. In the case of ***Graves' disease,*** the entire thyroid gland becomes enlarged. Another type, called **nodular goiter,** results when one or more nodules, or adenomas, develop in the thyroid and trigger excess production of thyroid hormone. A goiter may be a temporary problem that will remedy itself over time without medical intervention, or a symptom of another, possibly severe, thyroid condition that requires medical attention *(see **Thyroid Problems**).*

CAUSES

Goiters can occur when the thyroid gland produces either too much thyroid hormone **(hyperthyroidism)** or not enough **(hypothyroidism).** The problem may arise when the pituitary gland stimulates thyroid growth to boost production of the hormone. But most goiters are caused by insufficient iodide, a key ingredient in the manufacture of thyroid hormone. To make up for the resulting shortfall of the hormone, the gland begins to grow. Sometimes a slight swelling is enough to correct the problem, but if the goiter interferes with breathing, it must be treated or removed.

Another type of thyroid growth, called a **sporadic goiter,** can form if your diet includes too many goitrogenic (goiter-promoting) foods, such as soybeans, rutabagas, cabbage, peaches, peanuts, and spinach. These foods can suppress the manufacture of thyroid hormone by interfering with your thyroid's ability to process iodide. Drugs such as iodides, propylthiouracil, and phenylbutazone may have the same effect.

DIAGNOSTIC AND TEST PROCEDURES

A goiter may be large enough for you to see or to feel with your hand, or it may remain unnoticed until a physician discovers it, perhaps during a routine exam. In any case, the first step is to determine whether the goiter is a symptom of another thyroid condition. Radioactive iodide uptake tests track how much iodide the thyroid takes in within a certain time period. Higher-than-normal

THE THYROID GLAND

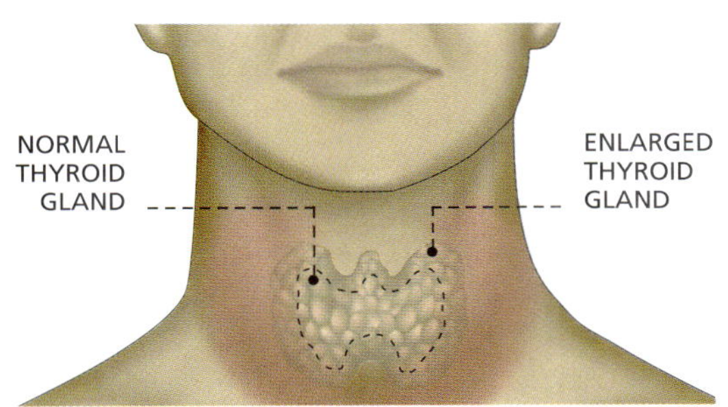

The thyroid gland, located at the base of the neck in front of the windpipe, needs iodide to produce necessary quantities of a vital bodily hormone. If the diet does not contain enough iodide, the gland simply begins to grow in an effort to meet its production quota. In some cases the enlarged thyroid, known as a goiter, becomes uncomfortable or overproductive and must be surgically removed.

amounts indicate possible **hyperthyroidism;** low levels indicate **hypothyroidism.** Blood tests also can measure levels of thyroid hormone.

TREATMENT

A goiter may require no treatment, especially if it is small and has succeeded in boosting production of thyroid hormone. However, if the goiter develops because of excessive thyroid hormone production, fails to produce enough hormone, or causes discomfort, you should seek medical help.

CONVENTIONAL MEDICINE

If your goiter requires treatment, supplementary iodide or a synthetic hormone such as ***levothyroxine*** may stop the pituitary gland from secreting the excess hormone that is causing the goiter to grow. When the medication takes effect, the thyroid will begin to return to its normal size. However, a large **nodular goiter** with a lot of internal scar tissue will not shrink with hormone treatment. If the goiter is uncomfortable, causes overproduction of thyroid hormone, or becomes cancerous, the entire thyroid gland may have to be surgically removed.

ALTERNATIVE CHOICES

Alternative therapies treat goiters by attempting to boost production of thyroid hormone and correct the body's chemical imbalance.

CHINESE HERBS

Notoginseng root *(Panax notoginseng)* and tang-kuei formula may help reduce the size of a goiter. Consult a practitioner for appropriate dosages.

HERBAL THERAPIES

To improve an underactive-thyroid condition, try bladder wrack *(Fucus vesiculosus)* three times a day. Take it in tablet form or as an infusion, which is prepared by steeping 2 to 3 tsp dried bladder wrack in 1 cup boiling water for 10 minutes.

A PINCH OF PREVENTION

Dietary supplements of iodide, which the body uses to make thyroid hormone, have proved to be an effective weapon in the war against goiters. People who live in coastal areas usually get plenty of iodide from their food and drinking water—even from ocean mists. But in mountainous or inland regions, the amount of available iodide is normally very low. In the United States the incidence of goiters dropped dramatically after manufacturers began adding iodide to table salt in 1924. In fact, no cases of iodide deficiency have been reported in the U.S. since 1970. By contrast, in developing countries—such as India—that have not implemented iodide supplements, goiters remain a common medical complaint. ■

GONORRHEA

SYMPTOMS

- a puslike urethral discharge that may be yellowish, cloudy, green, white, or bloodstained.
- frequent need to urinate.
- burning sensation while urinating.
- severe pelvic and lower abdominal pain.
- constant urge to move bowels **(anal gonorrhea).**
- nausea, vomiting, fever, chills.
- pain during intercourse.
- reddened, irritated tip of penis.
- severe sore throat, pain on swallowing **(pharyngeal gonorrhea).**

CALL YOUR DOCTOR IF:

- you have any of the above symptoms. Gonorrhea is a serious contagious disease that can lead to severe complications.

Incidents of gonorrhea—a bacterial infection of the genitourinary tract and, occasionally, the rectum, pharynx, and eyes—are on the rise in the United States, especially among teenagers and young adults. Approximately 2.5 million cases of gonorrhea are reported annually.

If you're a woman and you have gonorrhea, there's a good chance you won't know it; women often experience no symptoms until the infection has done serious damage. On the other hand, 95 percent of men develop symptoms within days or weeks. If your partner has symptoms, both of you should see a doctor and seek treatment. Because the disease is so contagious, doctors must report cases of gonorrhea to local public-health officials; you should be prepared to answer questions concerning your recent sexual contacts.

Left untreated, gonorrhea may spread and damage the heart or cause gonococcal ***arthritis.*** In men, it can lead to prostatitis, urethritis *(see* ***Prostate Problems*** *and* ***Urinary Problems****),* or epididymitis, an inflammation of the scrotal tubes. In women, the infection may spread to the uterus and fallopian tubes, causing ***pelvic inflammatory disease,*** which may result in scarring of the tubes and sterility.

Even if you have no symptoms, you should ask your doctor to perform a gonorrhea test once a year. This is especially important for women who are pregnant or plan to be; newborns may be permanently blinded as a result of exposure to the organism during birth.

CAUSES

Gonorrhea is caused by a bacterium called *Neisseria gonorrhoeae,* which is transmitted sexually.

DIAGNOSTIC AND TEST PROCEDURES

Your gynecologist may discover gonorrhea during a routine pelvic exam if your cervix is red or there is a discharge coming from the center of it. The doctor will culture any discharge from the infected area—cervix, urethra, pharynx, or rectum—and may examine the sample under a microscope after it is stained with a special dye.

TREATMENT

Because gonorrhea is a contagious disease with serious consequences, you must seek conventional medical treatment first.

CONVENTIONAL MEDICINE

Your doctor will prescribe ***analgesics*** to relieve pain, as well as ***antibiotics*** such as ceftriaxone, ***doxycycline,*** ampicillin, or ***erythromycin*** to kill the bacteria. Because of the advent of newer, drug-resistant strains, the doctor may also treat you with probenecid, a drug that enables antibiotics to remain active longer in your system. If the infection has spread to other organs, you may be treated with ***amoxicillin.***

ALTERNATIVE CHOICES

In addition to conventional treatment, a number of alternative therapies may speed healing.

ACUPRESSURE

In Chinese medicine, a white discharge is said to be due to lack of chi, or energy. To cleanse your system and build up energy, try massaging acupressure points Liver 3, on top of the foot between the big and second toes, and Liver 8, on the inside of the leg above the knee. Also try kneading Kidney 3, on the inside of the leg between the anklebone and the Achilles tendon. *(See the **Appendix** for more information about point locations.)*

CHINESE HERBS

To cleanse your system, a doctor of Chinese medicine may prescribe an herbal formula tailored to your body's needs. This might include ***gentiana*** *(Gentiana scabra),* ***Chinese foxglove root*** *(Rehmannia glutinosa),* ***dong quai*** *(Angelica sinensis),* ***bupleurum*** *(Bupleurum chinense),* and ***licorice*** *(Glycyrrhiza uralensis).* Herbs such as ***coptis*** *(Coptis chinensis)* are considered helpful in strengthening the urinary and reproductive systems, especially when pelvic inflammatory disease is a complication.

HERBAL THERAPIES

Calendula *(Calendula officinalis),* ***myrrh*** *(Commiphora molmol),* and thuja *(Thuja occidentalis)* may reduce the inflammation and discharge that accompany gonorrhea; use these herbs as a tea or douche. Pipsissewa *(Chimaphila umbellata),* a woodland wildflower once used to flavor soft drinks, may also help, as could ***uva ursi*** *(Arctostaphylos uva-ursi),* ***goldenseal*** *(Hydrastis canadensis),* and ***burdock*** *(Arctium lappa).*

HOMEOPATHY

A homeopathic physician may want to attack the gonorrhea bacteria with antibiotic herbs and then prescribe a remedy to strengthen your immune system and prevent recurrences.

NUTRITION AND DIET

If your doctor approves, try fasting for one to three days to clean out your system. Drink the juices of pomegranate and cranberry or a mixture of celery, parsley, and cucumber to flush out toxins from the urinary tract. Because antibiotics destroy beneficial intestinal bacteria as well as pathogenic kinds, eat yogurt containing live cultures or take acidophilus supplements.

AT-HOME REMEDIES

- Take hot baths to help reduce pain and inflammation.
- Eat a balanced diet, including live-culture yogurt.
- Supplement antibiotic therapy with the herbs listed above.
- Use ice packs to reduce abdominal pain.
- Apply moist heat to infected joints to ease the pain of gonococcal arthritis.

PREVENTION

Always use a condom. If your partner develops symptoms, both of you should be tested and treated by a doctor. ■

GOUT

SYMPTOMS

- sudden, intense pain in a joint, typically the big toe or ankle, sometimes the knee.
- swelling, inflammation, and a feeling that the joint is very hot.
- in extreme cases, alternating chills and fever.
- usually strikes unexpectedly and may recur, but the symptoms typically do not last more than a week.

CALL YOUR DOCTOR IF:

- severe pain in a joint recurs or lasts more than a few days, especially if the pain is accompanied by chills or fever; you may be experiencing the early signs of rheumatoid ***arthritis*** or, in rare cases, lead poisoning.
- symptoms of gout increase or other side effects occur while you are taking allopurinol to reduce uric acid production or colchicine to relieve pain; these drugs may be interacting adversely with other medication.

Without warning and, for some reason, in the middle of the night, it strikes—an intense pain in a joint, most often the big toe, but sometimes other joints, including knees, elbows, thumbs or fingers. Attacks of gout can be unexpected and excruciatingly painful. With prompt treatment, the pain and inflammation disappear after a few days, but they may recur at any time.

Nine out of ten gout sufferers are middle-aged men, and about half of them have a hereditary predisposition to the ailment. Gout is uncommon in women and very rare in children. Men who are overweight or suffering from ***high blood pressure*** are particularly prone to gout—especially if they are taking thiazide ***diuretics*** to lower the body's water retention.

Gout is actually a form of arthritis; specifically, it is the body's reaction to irritating crystalline deposits in the space between the bones in a joint. In spite of the extreme pain at onset, gout responds well to prompt treatment; mild cases may be controlled by diet alone. Chronic attacks of gout, however, may require long-term medication to prevent damage to bone and cartilage, as well as deterioration of the kidneys because of excess uric acid production.

Chronic gout sufferers may feel tiny, hard lumps accumulating over time in the soft flesh of the hands, feet, or earlobes. These harmless deposits, called tophi, are concentrations of uric acid crystals that can eventually cause aching, stiffness, and protrusions. If similar deposits form in the kidneys, they can lead to painful and potentially dangerous ***kidney stones***.

CAUSES

Gout is brought on by an excessively high level of uric acid in the blood. Uric acid is essential to the digestive process, and the excess is filtered through the kidneys and eliminated in urine. If the body produces too much uric acid or fails to excrete it, crystals of sodium urate become concentrated in the joints and tendons, causing inflammation, pressure, and severe pain.

Although the precise mechanism that causes

gout to develop is unknown, the disorder is often associated with an injury or surgical procedure, periods of stress, diet, or reactions to alcohol and certain drugs, including antibiotics. Gout may also occur in the presence of some tumors or cancers. Research shows a relation between gout and kidney disorders, enzyme deficiencies, and lead poisoning. Gout may also accompany ***psoriasis*** or ***anemia.*** Susceptibility to gout can be inherited, and repeat attacks are common if the body's uric acid level is not kept under control.

Pseudogout, or false gout, is a similar but generally less painful condition caused by calcium crystals in the joints. More common after age 60 in both sexes, pseudogout is treated with anti-inflammatory agents or, in severe cases, surgery followed by cortisone injections.

DIAGNOSTIC AND TEST PROCEDURES

Because other diseases may masquerade as gout, it is important to see a physician for an accurate diagnosis of any kind of joint pain.

Blood and urine tests may or may not be useful diagnostic tools, since you can have a high level of uric acid without having gout, or the level may appear normal after an attack. To confirm the presence of uric acid crystals in persistent cases, a specialist may take x-rays or draw fluid from the synovial sac that cushions the joint.

JOINT PROBLEMS

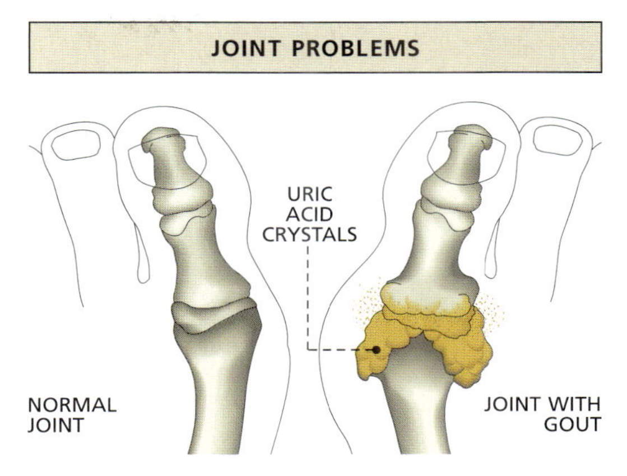

Gout occurs when the body is unable to rid the blood of excess uric acid. Crystals of the chemical accumulate between the bones of certain joints, most commonly in the big toe. The result can be sudden and severe pain, inflammation, and in severe cases, joint deformity.

TREATMENT

Anyone who experiences a gout attack quickly realizes that the first order of business is to ease the pain. Clothing or other covering only aggravates the discomfort of the swollen, sensitive joint, so most doctors advise keeping the foot or affected extremity bare, even when sleeping. The next stage of treatment will be an oral pain-killer, typically a ***nonsteroidal anti-inflammatory drug (NSAID).***

After the initial discomfort is relieved, the answer to controlling gout is keeping the body's level of uric acid in balance.

Even without conventional or alternative treatment to relieve pain and inflammation, the immediate symptoms of gout will disappear in a few days or a week. Nonetheless, all incidents of suspected gout should be diagnosed and treated by a physician. Left untreated, uric acid deposits can eventually cause irreversible damage to the kidneys and other tissues.

CONVENTIONAL MEDICINE

Many doctors recommend oral doses of ***ibuprofen,*** available in both prescription and nonprescription versions, or other anti-inflammatory agents. Low doses of ***aspirin,*** which may have been recommended for other conditions, should be discontinued, as it can slow the elimination of uric acid.

Corticosteroid injections in the affected joint may be helpful in reducing pain and inflammation in severe attacks or chronic cases. However, steroids such as ***hydrocortisone*** can have undesirable side effects in some patients and must always be administered by a licensed specialist. *(See also **Bursitis.**)*

The standard treatment favored by many physicians to treat acute or chronic gout attacks is colchicine, a medication that prevents uric

GOUT ATTACKS

Although gout is most likely to strike the big toe, the disorder can also affect other joints, including the elbows, hands, and knees. Recurrent attacks of gout may affect several areas at once.

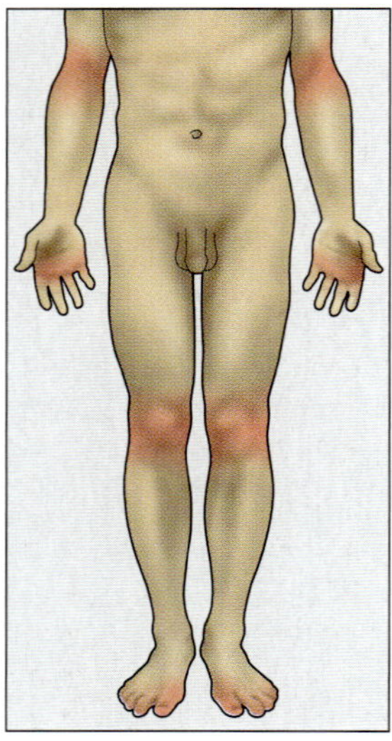

acid crystal deposits and has been in use for centuries. CAUTION: Colchicine may cause adverse side effects or interact with a number of ***antidepressants,*** tranquilizers, or ***antihistamines;*** it should not be taken by pregnant women because of the risk of birth defects.

Your physician will probably recommend that you cut out certain protein-rich foods, especially those high in purines, chemicals essential for the body's production of uric acid. These foods include organ meats, shellfish, fatty fish, asparagus, spinach, and most dried beans. Although you should drink plenty of liquids, you should avoid alcohol, which retards the elimination of uric acid. Obese patients may be put on an even stricter regimen.

Keeping the body's level of uric acid in balance can be done through the diet and, if necessary, by one of several drugs, such as allopurinol, that reduce the body's production of uric acid. Allopurinol may cause rashes, drowsiness, and disorientation, and it can have adverse reactions with other medications, particularly ***anticoagulants*** and ***diuretics.***

To encourage excretion of excess uric acid in the long term, the drugs of choice are probenecid and sulfinpyrazone. But like other medications used to combat gout, they may cause adverse interactions with other drugs or complications with existing ailments such as blood disorders, ulcers, and kidney problems.

In many cases, prompt treatment with appropriate drugs solves the problem permanently. Since recurring attacks are possible, however, chronic sufferers may have to remain on low-level drug therapy for extended periods, sometimes for life.

ALTERNATIVE CHOICES

Nonconventional approaches to treating gout begin with reducing the immediate pain and inflammation, then continue with therapies to control excessive uric acid production.

ACUPRESSURE

Among recommended acupressure points for relieving the pain of a gouty toe are several locations on the affected foot itself: Spleen 3, at the side of the metatarsal joint just behind the big toe; Stomach 42, at the center of the top of the instep; and Liver 2, just behind the space between the big and second toes. Press each of these points firmly for 60 seconds. If the pain permits, you can also use two other points at the back corners of the big toenail. *(See the **Appendix** for more information about point locations.)*

ACUPUNCTURE

Because acupuncture can be administered to areas other than the swollen joint, this procedure may be more tolerable than direct treatments, such as **massage,** to patients in the initial stages of gout. See a professional for treatment.

HERBAL THERAPY

Drink an infusion of 1 tbsp ***burdock*** *(Arctium lappa)* or gravelroot *(Eupatorium purpureum)* in a cup of water, three times a day, to stimulate elimination of uric acid. Do not take herbal teas if colchicine has been prescribed.

HOMEOPATHY

A homeopath may consider predisposition to gout in an overall constitutional treatment. *Colchicum,* or autumn crocus, the plant from which colchicine is extracted, can be effective in relieving the pain of an attack. Other mixed homeopathic remedies may include dilute doses of ***Arnica, Ledum,*** *Urtica urens, Benzoicum acidum,* ***Lycopodium,*** and ***Pulsatilla.***

NUTRITION AND DIET

In general, gout seems more common with diets that include meat and animal fats but is unusual in people following vegetarian diets. Dietary regimens for preventing attacks of gout in people showing a hereditary predisposition to the disease usually eliminate red meat and meat extracts such as bouillon and gravies; yeast and other enzyme-producing products; organ meats such as liver, sweetbreads, and kidneys; shellfish and certain kinds of preserved fish, including sardines, herring, and anchovies; caffeine and alcohol.

Foods that appear to suppress the immediate symptoms of gout include complex carbohydrates, particularly from cereals, fruits, and leafy green vegetables. Simple carbohydrates, such as those in refined sugar, are likely to increase uric acid production and should be avoided.

Several authorities report favorable results in treating the pain of chronic gout by having patients eat fresh cherries—up to 8 oz a day—or drink cherry juice without added sugar. Similar effects are claimed for blueberries and other red-blue berries.

Some practitioners recommend a teaspoon of activated charcoal three times a day to stimulate uric acid elimination.

Drinking plenty of clear, nonalcoholic fluids—fruit juices, herbal teas, or water—helps to dilute the urine and promote excretion of uric acid through continued flushing of the kidneys.

REFLEXOLOGY

To help restore balance to the kidneys and spleen, the organs responsible for uric acid production, a reflexology practitioner will massage the appropriate area at the center of the sole of the foot. Some advocates of reflexology assert that this direct massage technique serves to break up deposits of uric acid crystals that have become concentrated in the feet.

AT-HOME REMEDIES

The first concern in an attack of gout is to reduce pain and inflammation. If you can stand it, apply a plastic bag containing a few ice cubes or a bag of frozen vegetables to the joint; this will help relieve painful swelling. Wrap the cold bag in a soft cloth or towel and hold it against the painful area for up to five minutes at a time, then repeat as needed.

Because even the pressure of a sheet or blanket can be painful to a gout-afflicted joint, at bedtime rest the gouty foot inside a cardboard box or a plastic laundry basket that has been placed on its side.

PREVENTION

If gouty arthritis runs in the family, men in particular should moderate their intake of alcohol, fats, and high-purine foods, and should keep their weight within recommended ranges. Blood and urine tests during routine checkups will signal potential susceptibility to gout attack. ■

THE PRICE OF HIGH LIVING

The old image of the gout sufferer as a rotund, aging aristocrat, surrounded by roast beef and flagons of ale, swollen foot propped on a cushion, wasn't entirely mythical. While gout isn't simply a sign of "high living" and can occur anytime in adulthood, we now know that rich foods and alcohol can contribute to the real cause of gout and will certainly aggravate the disease after the initial attack.

G

GRAVES' DISEASE

SYMPTOMS

- weight loss despite increased appetite.
- faster heart rate, higher blood pressure, and increased nervousness.
- excessive perspiration.
- increased sensitivity to heat.
- more frequent bowel movements, sometimes with diarrhea.
- muscle weakness, trembling hands.
- development of a ***goiter*** (enlargement of the thyroid gland, causing a swelling at the base of the neck).
- bulging eyes.
- in women, change in frequency or total cessation of menstrual periods.

CALL YOUR DOCTOR IF:

- you are feverish, agitated, or delirious, and have a rapid pulse. You could be having a **thyrotoxic crisis,** in which the effects of too much thyroid hormone suddenly become life-threatening.

G

First described by Sir Robert Graves in the early 19th century, Graves' disease is one of the most common of all ***thyroid problems.*** It is also the leading cause of **hyperthyroidism,** a condition marked by excessive production of thyroid hormones. Once the disorder has been correctly diagnosed, it is quite easy to treat. In some cases, Graves' disease goes into remission or disappears completely after several months or years. Left untreated, however, it can lead to serious complications—even death. Although the symptoms can cause discomfort, Graves' disease generally has no long-term adverse health consequences if the patient receives prompt and proper medical care.

CAUSES

Hormones secreted by the thyroid gland control metabolism, or the speed at which the body converts food into energy. The metabolic rate is directly linked to the amount of hormone "fuel" that circulates in the bloodstream. If, for some reason, the thyroid gland secretes an overabundance of this fuel, the body's metabolism goes into high gear, producing the pounding heart, sweating, trembling, and weight loss typically experienced by hyperthyroid people. Normally, the thyroid gets its production orders through another chemical, called thyroid-stimulating hormone (TSH), released by the pituitary gland in the brain. But in Graves' disease, a malfunction in the body's immune system results in the manufacture of abnormal antibodies, or defender proteins, that mimic the pituitary's messenger chemicals. *(See **Immune Problems.**)* Spurred by these false signals to produce, the thyroid's hormone factories work overtime and exceed their normal quota.

Exactly why the immune system begins to produce these aberrant antibodies is unclear. Heredity and other characteristics seem to play a role in determining susceptibility. Studies show, for example, that if one identical twin contracts Graves' disease, there is a 50 percent likelihood that the other twin will get it too. Also, women are more likely than men to develop the disease. And smokers who develop Graves' are more prone to eye problems than nonsmokers with the disease.

Eye trouble—usually in the form of inflamed and swollen eye muscles and tissues that can cause the eyeballs to protrude from their sockets—is a distinguishing complication of Graves' disease. However, only a small percentage of all Graves' patients will experience this condition, known as exophthalmos. Even among those who do, the severity of their bout with Graves' has no bearing on the seriousness of the eye problem or how far the eyeballs protrude. In fact, it isn't clear whether such eye complications stem from Graves' disease itself or from a totally separate, yet closely linked, disorder. If you have developed exophthalmos, your eyes may ache and feel dry and irritated. Protruding eyeballs are prone to excessive tearing and redness, partly because the eyelids no longer can shelter them effectively from injury.

In severe cases of exophthalmos, which are rare, swollen eye muscles can put tremendous pressure on the optic nerve, possibly leading to partial color blindness or a decrease in visual acuity. Eye muscles weakened by long periods of inflammation can lose their ability to control movement, resulting in double vision.

DIAGNOSTIC AND TEST PROCEDURES

Although Graves' disease can be diagnosed from the results of one or two tests, your doctor may use several methods to double-check the findings and rule out other disorders. An analysis of your blood will show if the levels of two hormones—thyroxine and triiodothyronine, which are produced or regulated by the thyroid—are higher than normal. If they are, and if levels of thyroid-stimulating hormone in your blood are abnormally low, you are hyperthyroid, and Graves' disease is the likely culprit. Blood analysis can also detect the presence of the abnormal antibody associated with Graves' disease, but this test is somewhat expensive and generally not necessary.

To confirm a diagnosis of Graves' disease, your doctor may conduct a radioactive iodide uptake test, which shows whether large quantities of iodide are collecting in the thyroid. The gland needs iodide to make thyroid hormones, so if it is absorbing unusually large amounts of iodide, it obviously is producing too much hormone.

IMPACT ON THE EYES

Protruding eyeballs are an occasional symptom of Graves' disease. When tissues lining the eye socket become inflamed, they can swell and force the eyeball forward, a condition known as exophthalmos. If the lid cannot close over it, the eye may become dry and irritated. Prolonged inflammation can weaken eye muscles, impairing eyeball movement and causing vision problems.

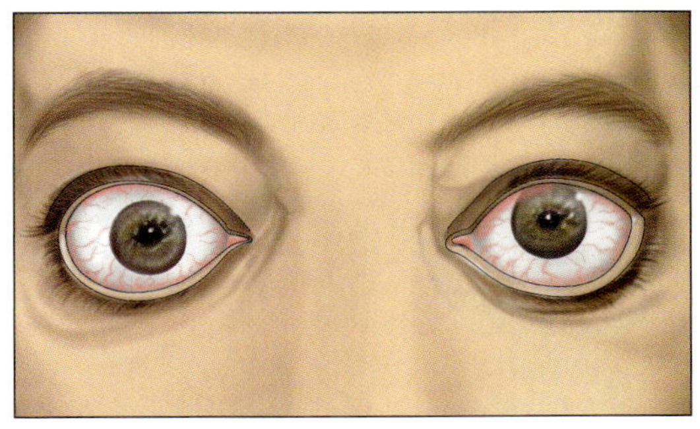

If exophthalmos is your only symptom, your physician will probably run blood tests to check for hyperthyroidism, since this eye disorder can occur apart from Graves' disease. The doctor may also evaluate your eye muscles using ultrasound, a CT scan, or magnetic resonance imaging (MRI). Signs of swelling in any one of these tests will confirm a diagnosis of Graves' disease.

TREATMENT

If you have Graves' disease, or even suspect that you have it, you should have a professional diagnosis and, if necessary, a treatment plan that suits your particular condition. Although the disorder is rooted in a malfunctioning immune system, the goal of both conventional and alternative approaches is to restore thyroid hormone levels to their correct balance and to relieve discomfort.

CONVENTIONAL MEDICINE

If you have a mild case of Graves' disease, you and your practitioner may simply decide to see how the disease develops before initiating any treatment. Should medical intervention be necessary, the two most frequently used conventional treatments involve disabling the thyroid's ability to produce hormones.

One common approach uses a strong dose of radioactive iodide to destroy certain cells in the thyroid gland. This procedure attempts to halt excess hormone production by thinning the ranks of cells responsible for manufacturing the chemicals. The amount of radioactive iodide you receive depends on the estimated size of your thyroid—determined either through a physical exam or by ultrasound—and on the gland's level of activity, as indicated by the results of an iodide uptake test. Despite its destructive effect on thyroid cells, the iodide used in this procedure will not harm surrounding tissues and organs.

At the beginning of the treatment, you will be given a capsule or liquid containing the radioactive iodide. Either way you take it, you should not feel any effects as the substance enters your system. Most of the iodide will gather and remain in your thyroid; excess amounts will be excreted in your urine. It is a good idea to drink several extra glasses of water per day for about a week after the treatment to help flush the material out of your body as quickly as possible. To be on the safe side, you should also limit contact with infants, children, and pregnant women for at least seven days after you ingest the iodide.

You probably won't notice any changes in your body for several days after taking the radioactive iodide, but if your thyroid gland feels inflamed and sore, ***acetaminophen, ibuprofen,*** or ***aspirin*** can offer some relief. Over the next several months, the thyroid's hormone secretion should gradually begin to drop. During this time you need to see your doctor for periodic checkups to determine how well the treatment is progressing. Chances are good that a single dose of radioactive iodide will be sufficient to correct your hyperthyroidism. However, if your condition hasn't improved three months or so after your initial treatment, your practitioner may give you a second dose of iodide. Once the doctor has decided that your Graves' disease is effectively under control, you will still need to have routine checkups to make sure that your thyroid levels remain within the normal range.

Although radioactive iodide treatments are generally safe, they cannot be given to pregnant women because the chemical may destroy the thyroid gland in the fetus. Therefore, you must make sure that you are not pregnant before you take radioactive iodide for Graves' disease. It is best to let several months pass after your last dose of radioactive iodide before you become pregnant; confirm the length of time you should wait with your practitioner. Except during these periods following the treatment, radioactive iodide poses no health risks for women who want to become pregnant, and it will not affect the fertility of either women or men.

Antithyroid drugs such as propylthiouracil and methimazole, which interfere with thyroid hormone production, can be used to treat Graves' disease. After you begin treatment, it may take several months for your hyperthyroid symptoms to subside. This is because the thyroid has already generated and stored enough hormone to keep it circulating at elevated levels. Once the stores are drained, hormone production should drop to its normal level. Although your disease may seem to go away entirely, you might still need drug therapy to keep your thyroid operating properly. Even if your case of Graves' disease does go into remission and your doctor says it's safe to stop taking your medication, you will need to be evaluated every year or so to make sure your hyperthyroidism has not returned.

Beta-adrenergic blockers such as ***atenolol*** and ***propranolol,*** frequently prescribed to treat heart disease and hypertension, are also used by some patients to alleviate the heart palpitations and muscle tremors that characterize Graves' disease. Before prescribing beta blockers for this condition, however, your doctor needs to know if you are asthmatic or have any kind of heart trouble.

Radioactive iodide treatments and antithyroid drugs are usually effective in slowing down thyroid hormone output, but in some cases surgery is the best approach for Graves' disease. If you develop the disorder before or during pregnancy, for example, or if you are reluctant or unable to undergo radioactive treatment or are allergic to antithyroid medication, your doctor may recommend subtotal thyroidectomy, a relatively safe and simple procedure in which most of the thyroid gland is removed.

Because many conventional remedies severely limit the thyroid's ability to manufacture thyroid hormone, they increase the chances that you will develop **hypothyroidism,** a potentially serious condition marked by insufficient thyroid hormone production *(see **Thyroid Problems**).* Therefore, if you have undergone any of the aforementioned treatments for Graves' disease, you must continue to see your doctor for periodic checkups to make sure the problem has not been overcorrected, causing your thyroid hormone levels to drop too low.

Only about 5 percent of people with Graves' disease will develop eye problems severe enough to warrant professional treatment. And almost half of those who develop exophthalmos, the condition that causes the eyeballs to protrude, will have mild cases that can be helped with simple treatments *(see **At-Home Remedies,** right).*

Graves' disease patients with eye problems can find temporary relief from the redness, swelling, and pain through a number of drugs, including ***prednisone,*** methylprednisolone, and dexamethasone. However, these medications should not be used for long periods of time, as they can lead to bone loss, muscle weakness, and weight gain. Vision problems and severe cases of eye protrusion can often be corrected through radiation therapy and surgery. Make sure to ask your doctor about any possible complications before undergoing surgery.

ALTERNATIVE CHOICES

Alternative treatments generally serve to complement conventional medicine's more direct goal of thyroid hormone suppression. Some of these therapies help alleviate the unpleasant symptoms of Graves' disease, while others seek to improve general thyroid function.

In addition to the treatments listed below, **acupuncture, homeopathy, meditation,** relaxation techniques, and **yoga** can address Graves' disease. Consult a qualified practitioner.

HERBAL THERAPIES

For relief from the symptoms of Graves' disease, try a combination of 4 parts bugleweed (*Lycopus* spp.), 2 parts motherwort *(Leonurus cardiaca),* 2 parts ***skullcap*** *(Scutellaria lateriflora),* and 1 part ***hawthorn*** *(Crataegus laevigata)* in a tincture, three times a day.

LIFESTYLE

After the heart rate has stabilized, aerobic exercise for 15 to 20 minutes a day is thought to be very good for maintaining good thyroid function.

NUTRITION AND DIET

If you are hyperthyroid, eating foods that inhibit the manufacture of thyroid hormones might help lower hormone secretion. These include cabbage, peaches, radishes, peanuts, rutabagas, soybeans, and spinach. ***Vitamin B complex*** injections may also prove useful.

AT-HOME REMEDIES

- If your lids cannot close completely over your eyes, use eye patches at night. This will help keep your corneas from drying out.
- Use over-the-counter or prescription artificial tears to moisten your eyes whenever they feel dry.
- If your eyes are red and swollen in the morning, sleep with your head elevated.
- Wear tinted glasses to protect your eyes from bright light, sunlight, and wind. ■

GROIN STRAIN

SYMPTOMS

- pain and stiffness in one or both sides of the groin when you try to walk or sit; may be accompanied by swelling or black-and-blue discoloration.

CALL YOUR DOCTOR IF:

- you detect a swelling or bulge along the crease between your leg and stomach, especially if you are overweight or have been engaging in strenuous activity; you could have a ***hernia.***
- you run a high temperature or have chills associated with pain in the groin; these may be symptoms of a bone or ***kidney infection.***
- the pain extends to the small of the back, whether or not your temperature is high; you may be suffering from a ***kidney stone*** or a ***prostate problem.***
- the pain extends to the lower abdomen; you may have a digestive or (if you are a woman) gynecological disorder, or a viral ***infection.*** If the pain happens during a menstrual period, discuss the symptoms with your gynecologist.

By definition, the groin is where your torso joins your legs. It's the place where your trunk and your legs can bend forward, backward, and to the sides. Because the groin is the center of a lot of body movement, it is subject to potential strain, particularly in athletes, dancers, and people who do physical labor. Less active people can also suffer groin injury: Ordinary lifting, stretching, running, and weekend sports can put great strain on the bones and muscles of the groin.

The effect of a strain to these key muscles and tendons—sometimes called a groin pull—is immediate and often immobilizing. The pain is intense, and you cannot walk, sit, or put weight on your leg without extreme discomfort. As a protective reflex, you tend to stiffen up and limp, favoring the injured side of the groin. In some cases you may have to be carried to a place where you can lie down, relax, and ease the pain.

CAUSES

The immediate cause of a groin pull is bruising or tearing the muscles that run from the pelvis down the thighs. It may also involve a torn tendon connecting the ends of the muscle to a bone. Groin pulls are usually caused by overexertion, lifting heavy objects improperly, or failing to warm up before a strenuous activity. Sometimes a strained groin muscle comes from external causes, such as falling against a solid object or being struck with great force, as in an accident.

TREATMENT

A minor groin pull will generally heal itself with rest in a matter of hours or a few days. If the muscle tissue is actually torn, the healing process may take a week or more. In severe or recurring cases, surgery may be necessary to repair the damage to muscles and tendons.

CONVENTIONAL MEDICINE

To reduce the swelling and inflammation of your groin strain, apply an ice pack as quickly as pos-

REFLEXOLOGY

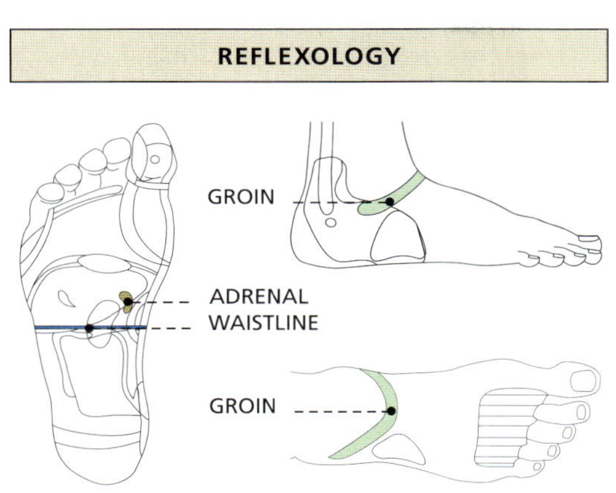

To reduce muscle tension in the groin, work the groin and adrenal areas. Holding your foot straight back, walk your left index finger from one side of the groin area to the other; walk back with your right finger. Repeat several times. Then push the big toe back and walk your thumb along the inside of the main tendon on the bottom of your foot from the waistline area to the adrenal area.

sible after the injury. You might also take ***aspirin*** or a ***nonsteroidal anti-inflammatory drug (NSAID)*** to relieve pain. Rest the affected muscle until the swelling and inflammation subside. Later you can apply a warm compress to relax the damaged muscle tissue and encourage the body's natural healing processes.

If your groin pull is due to an ***athletic injury,*** you may want to see a specialist in sports medicine, not just to relieve the pain but also to advise you on how to prevent a pull from happening again. Among young people who play team or individual sports, groin pulls are fairly common and tend to heal quickly—as long as the victim resists the urge to "play through the pain." Older people with groin strain—especially those who are not athletically inclined—should allow plenty of time to let the natural healing process work.

ALTERNATIVE CHOICES

Like conventional approaches, alternative treatments center on pain relief and rest until the muscles and tendons restore themselves to their normal condition and capability.

ACUPRESSURE

To relieve immediate pain in the thigh and groin, try pressure at the Gall Bladder 34 point, between the outside edge of the anklebone and the Achilles tendon. *(See the **Appendix** for more information on point locations.)*

BODY WORK

After relieving the immediate pain of a minor groin pull with a cold compress and rest, massaging the area using a warm body oil is an excellent way to relax muscles.

A **reflexology** therapist will manipulate the area along the front of the ankle where it joins the foot—a technique intended to stimulate circulation and lymphatic activity and to help relieve muscle tension in the groin.

HOMEOPATHY

Arnica is the homeopath's first-aid remedy for muscle injuries. It can be taken orally and applied as a salve to the painful area. ***Rhus toxicodendron*** and ***Ruta*** may also be useful for muscle strains.

AT-HOME REMEDIES

If you suffer a groin pull, lie down in a comfortable place and let your body relax. Apply a cold pack—a plastic bag of ice cubes or a packet of frozen vegetables wrapped in a towel—for 10 minutes on and 10 off until the pain recedes. Avoid exertion for several days, until you can use the affected muscles without pain.

PREVENTION

The single most important factor in avoiding muscle strain—in the groin or anywhere else in your body—is to warm up your muscles with moderate exercises or **yoga** before starting any strenuous activity. When a warmup period is not possible, work into the activity gradually, letting your muscles and tendons stretch and become more elastic. Make sure you stretch afterward to prevent post-activity spasms. ■

GUM PROBLEMS

SYMPTOMS

- swollen, red gums that may bleed easily.
- localized pain, loose teeth, and bad breath, which suggest **periodontitis;** x-rays may reveal some bone loss in the jaw area.
- extremely painful, inflamed gums coated with a gray-white mucus; sometimes accompanied by a mild fever, malaise, bad breath, excess saliva, and painful swallowing. These are signs of **Vincent's angina.**
- sudden and unexplained severe bone loss around molars and incisors, especially in young African American girls; this is indicative of **juvenile periodontitis.**
- extremely sore, swollen gums that bleed easily; perhaps accompanied by earaches, sinuslike infection, nosebleeds, fever, weight loss, and malaise. You may have **Wegener's granulomatosis,** a rare but potentially fatal disease.

CALL YOUR DENTIST IF:

- you have any of the groups of symptoms listed above; timely treatment can help prevent the spread of infection and potentially save teeth.

Periodontal disease (gum disease) is one of the most prevalent chronic diseases, with an estimated 98 percent of Americans over 60 affected by some form. A diet rich in refined sugars is largely to blame, but modern dentistry and good toothbrushes and toothpastes have helped offset some of the pernicious effects of our eating habits; as a result, just 8 percent of adults ever develop severe gum problems. That rate would be even lower if people made an effort to cut back on highly processed foods—notorious for the quantities of refined sugars they contain—and took dental hygiene more seriously. As it is, though, fewer than half of Americans see a dentist every year.

CAUSES

Periodontal disease is an infection of the gums and other tissues that support the teeth. The stage is set for problems when food particles, saliva, and bacteria are allowed to accumulate around the gum line, which encourages the formation of a soft bacterial mass known as plaque. Pockets can form as increasing amounts of plaque push between teeth and the surrounding membranes; these pockets and the decayed material in them create a good breeding ground for the bacteria already present. Excess sugar in the diet decreases saliva production (the body's best defense against bacteria in the mouth) and impairs disease-fighting white blood cells. The earliest stage of the resulting infection, known as **gingivitis,** is marked by painless inflammation, swelling, redness, and possibly bleeding. Certain vitamin deficiencies, medication, glandular disorders, and blood diseases may make you more susceptible to gingivitis; but in general, poor dental hygiene is the primary cause.

If the pockets around your teeth deepen and your gums turn an intense red, the problem may have become **periodontitis,** an inflammation of the periodontal ligament, which helps hold your teeth in their sockets of bone. If the infection worsens, it can cause bone and tooth loss. Periodontitis progresses slowly and often imperceptibly. Dentists used to think that bleeding gums

PERIODONTAL DISEASE

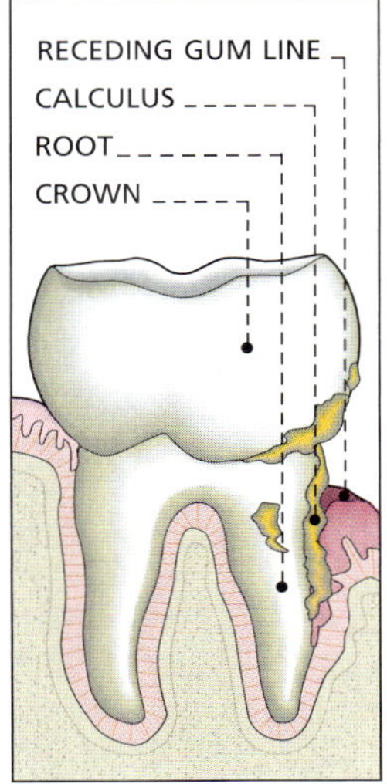

A bacterial film called plaque can accumulate along the gum line at the base of the teeth if not brushed away. Plaque hardens into calculus, which irritates the gums and causes them to recede. Pockets that form between the gums and teeth collect more plaque and calculus, causing destruction of the bone and ligament supporting the tooth, eventually resulting in tooth loss.

were a reliable indicator of periodontitis, but current research suggests this is not the case. You are at no greater risk for periodontitis if routine brushing causes your gums to bleed than if your gums almost never bleed.

In those rare instances when periodontitis comes on suddenly, it may be another form of the disease—either **juvenile periodontitis** or **Vincent's angina.** Juvenile periodontitis, which can lead to severe bone loss around the permanent molars and sometimes the incisors, occurs most often in African American girls, for reasons that are not entirely clear to researchers but that suggest some sort of genetic link. As in other gum problems, poor dental hygiene seems to be a contributing factor.

Vincent's angina (also known as trench mouth, because a large number of World War I soldiers fighting in the trenches contracted it) is caused by a combination of poor diet, ***stress,*** and of course, bacteria. Particularly common in teenagers with poor dental hygiene and a high-sugar diet, Vincent's angina is characterized by extreme pain, some bleeding, and a distinctive gray-white mucus that covers the gums. It is sometimes accompanied by a mild fever, malaise, bad breath, excess saliva, and painful swallowing.

A condition known as **strawberry gingivitis**—in which the gums become inflamed to the point of looking like overripe strawberries—can be the earliest sign of an uncommon though potentially fatal disease called **Wegener's granulomatosis.** The gums will be extremely sore and swollen, and they will bleed easily. Other symptoms include earaches, a sinuslike infection, nosebleeds, fever, weight loss, a cough, and malaise. Although the exact cause of the disease remains unknown, it progresses like a bacterial infection. It affects all ages and both sexes, although it is more prevalent in men; if left untreated, it can eventually damage the heart, lungs, and kidneys and cause renal failure.

In general, smokers are more than twice as likely to develop some kind of gum disease as nonsmokers. Other at-risk groups include people with ***diabetes, leukemia,*** and ***Crohn's disease,*** and pregnant women. Studies have shown that certain bacteria thrive on elevated hormone levels, which spells trouble not only for pregnant women but also for women taking oral contraceptives.

Chemotherapy and radiation treatments can also increase your risk for gum problems, as can exposure to toxic heavy metals such as mercury.

TREATMENT

The best treatment for periodontal disease is prevention. If you do develop gum problems, seek professional treatment and advice.

CONVENTIONAL MEDICINE

A proper daily dental regimen of thorough brushing and flossing—supplemented by regular trips to the dentist, who will clean areas you miss or perhaps can't reach—is the best way to prevent and to address most gum problems. Occasionally **gingivitis** is aggravated by an external factor that a dentist or orthodontist may be able to correct, such as poorly aligned teeth, excessive grinding, or ill-fitted crowns or bridges.

For aggressive forms of gingivitis, the dentist would first remove all plaque and calcified plaque (calculus) and then, perhaps, prescribe ***doxycycline*** or a ***chlorhexidine***-based mouthwash. More effective than common commercial brands, such a mouthwash may have some unwelcome side effects, including staining the teeth or bringing on an allergic reaction.

Dentists typically follow a similar routine to treat **periodontitis,** though in some cases surgery is required to clean out the pockets of infection and to remove damaged bone. It's up to the patient to follow through with solid brushing, flossing, and rinsing.

For **Vincent's angina,** the dentist or periodontist will clear out damaged or dead tissue and usually also prescribe a painkiller. Occasionally an ***antibiotic*** is also necessary; but in most cases, a good diet, high fluid intake, plenty of rest, and good oral hygiene (including no smoking) should suffice.

In those rare instances when **Wegener's granulomatosis** develops, immediate treatment is crucial. Cytotoxic agents such as cyclophosphamide, when combined with ***corticosteroids,*** have dramatically cut the fatality rate (as high as 90 percent if left untreated) for this disease.

Some of the latest advances in technology have made dental visits a lot less painful and noisy, and more effective. Ultrasound lasers have not yet completely replaced scrapers and picks and other such implements, but they are more and more often the preferred cleaning tool for removing plaque and other material. And in the past, dentists often had difficulty identifying the exact bacteria responsible for any given case of periodontitis, but improved testing methods have made precise diagnosis and more effective treatment possible.

ALTERNATIVE CHOICES

Many alternative therapies exist for gum problems, including rinses and pastes that will reduce plaque, fight infection and inflammation, and slow bleeding. But these therapies are no better than conventional commercial products at reaching below the gum line to areas where periodontitis blossoms. You still need to see a dentist regularly to ward off the risk of severe gum disease and tooth loss.

ATTENTION!

HEART DISEASE AND PERIODONTITIS

Young men who don't take care of their teeth and gums may be slipping into a lifestyle that places them at greater risk for heart disease. A 1993 study of nearly 10,000 subjects (men and women) found a 25 percent increase in heart disease among those with periodontitis. The connection was most remarkable in men under 50 with periodontitis, who had nearly double the risk of coronary heart disease as men who had little or no periodontal disease. Researchers could not determine if the gum problems were just a general indicator of poor hygiene and diet that led to other health problems or whether some direct correlation exists between heart problems and periodontitis. Either way, gum disease is a red flag.

ACUPUNCTURE

A professional acupuncturist would work with the stomach and large intestine meridians to stimulate energy in the gum area.

AYURVEDIC MEDICINE

Massage bleeding gums with a mixture of lemon juice (half a lemon) and a cup of water; the acid can help reduce bacteria.

HERBAL THERAPIES

Massage gums with ***goldenseal*** *(Hydrastis canadensis)* or powdered ***myrrh*** *(Commiphora molmol)* to fight infection. Gargle with ***bayberry*** (*Myrica* spp.) or prickly ash *(Zanthoxylum americanum)* to stimulate circulation, especially for bleeding gums. A combination of ***sage*** *(Salvia officinalis)* and ***chamomile*** *(Matricaria recutita)* makes an excellent mouthwash. Take ***echinacea*** (*Echinacea* spp.) to fight infection: Make a tea by boiling 1 to 2 tsp of the root in 1 cup of water; simmer for 10 minutes, then drink three times a day. Or you can use 1 to 4 ml in tincture form. Drink Roman chamomile *(Anthemis nobilis)* to fight inflammation in the gums. CAUTION: Do not use myrrh if you are pregnant.

HOMEOPATHY

For tender, bleeding gums and excessive salivation try ***Mercurius vivus;*** take orally twice a day for three days. If you continue to have problems, see a professional homeopath.

MASSAGE

Massaging the gums and jaws can improve circulation and speed healing. Use the rounded part of your fingertips and move along your gum line or the outside of your jaw in small circular motions. A stimulator brush, which has only two rows of bristles and is used without toothpaste, can also be therapeutic.

MIND/BOBY MEDICINE

The stress reduction effects of **yoga, meditation,** and other relaxation techniques help the jaw relax, increasing circulation to the gums and aiding in the healing and prevention of disease.

NUTRITION AND DIET

Crucial for healthy gums is a diet low in refined sugars and high in fiber. (Fiber works much like a dog's bone or biscuit to help cleanse the teeth.) Other important nutritional elements include ***vitamins A*** (especially beta carotene), ***C,*** and ***E,*** as well as ***zinc,*** flavonoids (present in onions), and ***folic acid*** (particularly for pregnant women and women on oral contraceptives). Gingivitis is common in scurvy patients, a reflection of vitamin C's vital role in maintaining a healthy mouth.

AT-HOME REMEDIES

You can make a wide assortment of mouthwashes and toothpastes at home. Some of the most effective ingredients include:

- a combination of baking soda and hydrogen peroxide, for brushing your teeth or as a mouth rinse.
- a mixture of ***bayberry*** and prickly ash as a gargle.
- cashew oil, ***vitamin E*** oil, or poultices of ***goldenseal*** or ***myrrh*** massaged into the gums, to speed healing and protect against infection.

PREVENTION

Prevention of periodontal disease begins at home, with good routine dental hygiene. Too many of us give our teeth a quick brush twice a day and only occasionally a good flossing. For really proper care you need to floss daily, brush longer, rinse with a mouthwash, and massage your gum line. Always floss first, to loosen food particles and plaque, then brush your teeth gently but thoroughly with a soft brush using a circular motion. Rigorous horizontal brushing with hard bristles can cause your gums to recede. Mouthwashes combat bacteria, but they should not be substituted for brushing, which you should do two or three times a day. A ***myrrh***-based toothpaste will help strengthen gums and fight infection each time you brush.

The American Dental Association (ADA) recommends that you visit your dentist once or twice a year to get rid of intractable plaque and calculus, but some dentists believe that excellent at-home dental hygiene keeps the plaque and calculus from ever forming. To achieve "excellence" you have to spend at least 15 minutes twice a day working on your teeth, and another 15 minutes a day massaging your gums. If you don't think you can follow this rigorous a routine, take the ADA's advice.

If you plan to get pregnant, see a dentist for a good cleaning first. Women who have little or no plaque before their pregnancy rarely have the gum problems often associated with elevated hormone levels.

Diabetics and anyone undergoing chemotherapy or radiation treatments should see a dentist several times a year.

People with existing gingivitis or periodontitis should see their dentist every three months, or as needed to keep the condition under proper control and prevent recurrences. ■

HAIR LOSS

SYMPTOMS

- in men, thinning hair on the scalp, a receding hairline, or a horseshoe-shaped pattern that leaves the crown of the head exposed.
- in women, thinning of hair in general, but mainly at the crown; complete balding is rare.
- in children or young adults, sudden loss of patches of hair; known as **alopecia areata.**
- complete loss of all hair on the body; a rare disorder called **alopecia universalis.**
- especially in children, patches of broken hairs and incomplete hair loss, usually on the scalp but sometimes involving the eyebrows; the child is most likely rubbing or pulling out hair, a disorder called **trichotillomania.**
- excessive shedding of hair, but not complete baldness, associated with various illnesses and drug treatments, rapid weight loss, ***anemia, stress,*** or pregnancy; a condition known as **telogen effluvium.**

CALL YOUR DOCTOR IF:

- you suspect that you or your child has **alopecia areata,** or that your child has **trichotillomania;** both conditions should be evaluated by a doctor.
- you suffer an unexplained loss of hair on any part of your body; your doctor may want to check for an underlying disorder that might be responsible.

Human hair varies widely in color and texture, and people differ considerably in the amount of facial and body hair they have, depending on their age, sex, race, and genetic makeup. But in spite of the many differences that are found in hair, it's normal for all of us to have it on the top and back of our heads. When it starts to disappear there, it's considered **alopecia,** or baldness.

Hair grows everywhere on the body except the palms of our hands and the soles of our feet, but many hairs are so fine they're virtually invisible. Hair is made up of a protein called keratin, produced in hair follicles in the outer layer of skin; as follicles produce new hair cells, old cells are being pushed out through the surface of the skin at the rate of about six inches a year. The hair you can see is actually a string of dead keratin cells. The average adult head has about 100,000 hairs, and loses up to 100 of them a day; so finding a few stray hairs on your hairbrush is not necessarily cause for alarm.

Gradual thinning of hair with age is a natural condition known as **involutional alopecia.** More and more hair follicles go into a telogenic, or resting, stage, and the remaining hairs become shorter and fewer in number. **Androgenic alopecia** is a genetically predisposed condition that can affect both men and women. Men can begin suffering hair loss as early as their teens or early twenties, while most women don't experience noticeable thinning until their forties or later. In men, a receding hairline and gradual disappearance of hair from the crown is called **male pattern baldness.** In women, **female pattern baldness** is typically a general thinning over the entire scalp, with the most extensive hair loss at the crown.

Patchy hair loss in children and young adults, often sudden in onset, is known as **alopecia areata.** This disorder may result in complete baldness, but in about 90 percent of cases the hair returns, usually within a few years. With **alopecia universalis,** all body hair falls out and the likelihood of regrowth is slight, especially when it occurs in children. Tearing out one's own hair, a disorder known as **trichotillomania,** is seen most frequently in children.

CAUSES

Doctors do not know why certain hair follicles are programmed to have a shorter growth period than others. Although a person's level of androgens—male hormones normally produced by both men and women—is believed to be a factor, hair loss has nothing to do with virility. For that matter, the presence or absence of ***dandruff*** has no effect on balding either. An individual's genes, however—from both male and female parents—unquestionably influence that person's predisposition to male or female pattern baldness.

Temporary hair loss can occur in conjunction with a high fever, a severe illness, thyroid disorders, iron deficiency, general anesthesia, drug treatments, hormonal imbalance, or extreme ***stress,*** and in women following childbirth. In these conditions, collectively known as **telogen effluvium,** a large number of hair follicles suddenly go into a resting phase, causing hair to thin noticeably. Drugs that can cause temporary hair loss include chemotherapeutic agents used in cancer treatment, ***anticoagulants,*** retinoids used to treat acne and skin problems, ***beta-adrenergic blockers*** used to control blood pressure, and oral contraceptives.

Hair loss can also be caused by burns, x-rays, scalp injuries, and exposure to certain chemicals—including those used to purify swimming pools, and to bleach, dye, and perm hair. In such cases, normal hair growth usually returns once the cause is eliminated.

The causes of **alopecia areata,** a disorder that often strikes children or teenagers, remain unexplained. In most cases the hair grows back, although it may be very fine and possibly white before normal coloration and thickness return.

Although too-frequent washing, permanent waves, bleaching, and dyeing hair do not cause baldness, they can contribute to overall thinning by making hair weak and brittle. Tight braiding and using rollers or hot curlers can damage and break hair, and running hair picks through tight curls can scar hair follicles. In most instances hair grows back normally if the source of stress is removed, but severe damage to the hair or scalp sometimes causes permanent bald patches.

THREE TYPES OF HAIR LOSS

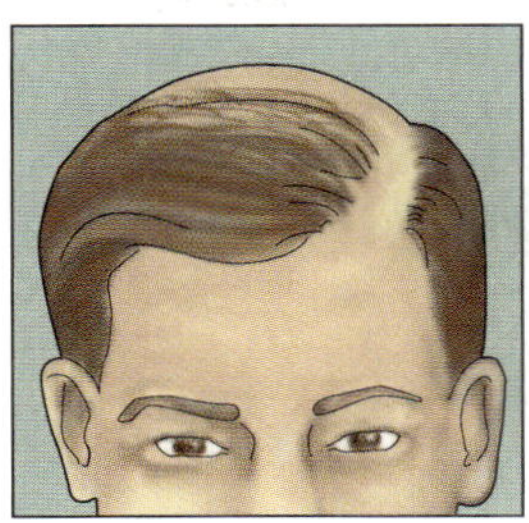

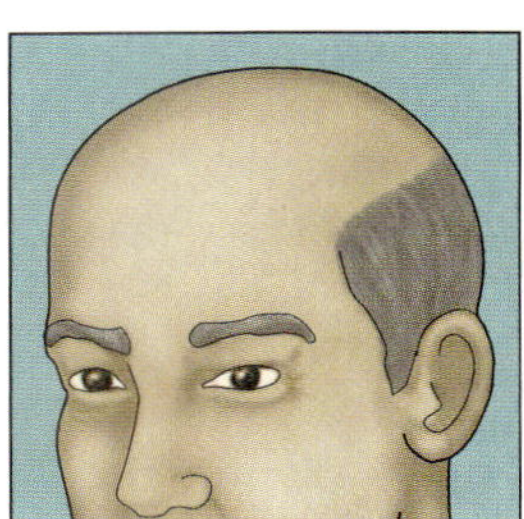

1 Male pattern baldness tends to run in families, affecting some men as early as the midteens. The hair begins to recede from the forehead and temples *(left),* and eventually from the crown, leaving a fringe of hair around the ears and across the back of the head *(right).*

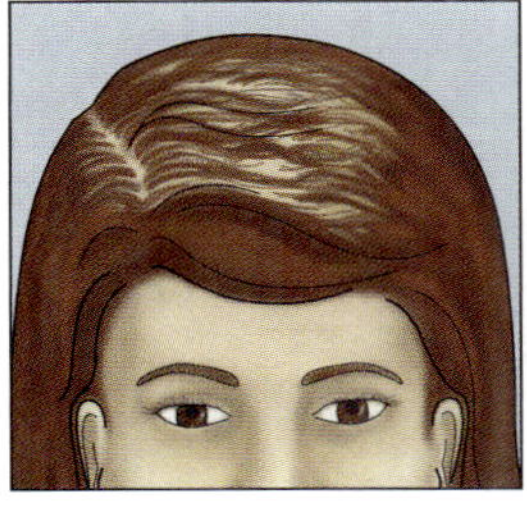

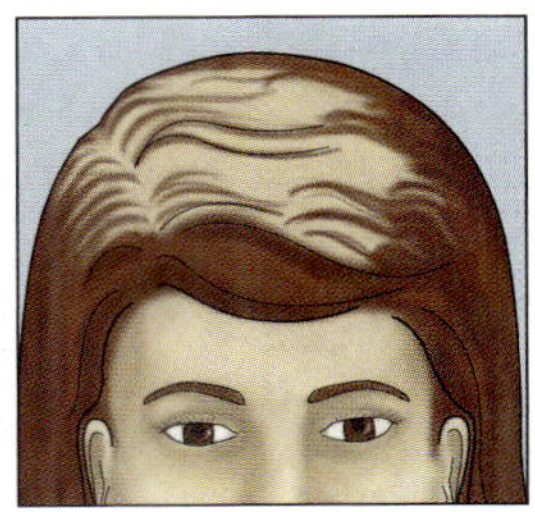

2 Female pattern baldness affects only a small percentage of women, and usually only after menopause. The hair may thin out along the forehead, temples, and crown *(left),* and eventually the crown may become almost completely bald *(right).*

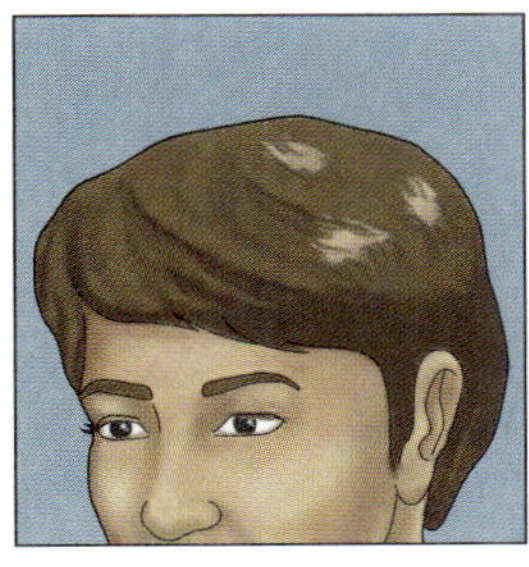

3 Alopecia areata is sudden, spotty balding in children and adults of either sex. Its cause is unknown. The bald spots may occur on the scalp, along the eyebrows, and in the beard, and they may be extensive. In most cases, the hair eventually grows back without treatment.

TREATMENT

Although remedies that promise to restore hair to balding heads have been around since ancient times, most men and women with thinning hair can do little to reverse the process. For cosmetic purposes, or after hair loss from surgical or drug treatments, many people turn to wigs, hairpieces, and hairweaving—even tattooing to simulate lost eyebrows and eyelashes. Some drugs may slow hair loss, and certain alternative treatments can relieve ***stress*** or bolster the health of remaining hair, but until recently no treatment could start hair growth where no hair exists.

CONVENTIONAL MEDICINE

Under certain circumstances, a preparation containing the drug minoxidil appears to provide moderate regrowth of hair on areas of the scalp that have gone bald. The effects are most promising in younger people who are just beginning to show signs of balding or who have small bald patches. The medication is applied to balding spots twice a day and must be continued daily; hair loss will recur if the application is stopped. More than 50 percent of users claim that it can thicken hair and slow hair loss, but it is not considered effective in men who already have extensive male pattern baldness. Side effects appear to be minimal, but in some users the drug may cause skin irritation. Oral minoxidil is reported to affect the heart rate in a small number of patients, so only the topical form should be used by people diagnosed with cardiovascular problems.

Hormone therapy may be prescribed for certain types of hair loss, but not without some risk. Although most cases of **alopecia areata** are resolved naturally, some doctors try to speed recovery with ***corticosteroids*** applied topically or injected in the scalp. The treatment may be painful and may cause permanent scarring in the scalp brought on by skin atrophy. Cortisone taken orally may stimulate new hair growth, but the effect is likely to be temporary. ***Prednisone,*** another orally administered steroid, has proved effective for **alopecia areata** patients, but its potential side effects include weight gain, metabolic abnormalities, ***acne,*** and ***menstrual problems.*** Hormone therapy in the form of birth-control pills may reverse baldness due to hormonal imbalances in young women.

Hair transplantation involves the relocation of plugs of skin from parts of the scalp containing active hair follicles to bald areas. A patient may need several hundred plugs—implanted 10 to 60 at a session. The transplanted hair may drop out, but new hair usually begins to grow from the transplanted follicles within several months.

A form of cosmetic surgery called scalp reduction involves tightening the scalp so that hair-bearing skin from the back and sides of the head is pulled toward the crown. Hair may then be transplanted to the remaining bald area at the top of the head. Like hair transplants, the process is painful and expensive, and it does nothing to retard genetic or age-related hair loss.

USE YOUR HEAD, SPARE YOUR HAIR

Shampoos and conditioners cannot prevent baldness, but overusing them can dry out the hair you have. Virtually all shampoos—even those touted as herbal, hypoallergenic, or vitamin-enhanced—are basically scented detergents with a lathering agent. Most brands are so concentrated that they actually work better when you dilute them. If your hair is very oily, you may want to wash it every day, but shampooing too often can strip your hair of its natural oil, which may lead to brittle, broken strands.

Claims that certain conditioners nourish and revitalize your hair have little merit. Hair—even the thickest, most vibrant-looking hair—is dead keratin. Hair conditioners contain waxes that give your hair a smooth feel, but they cannot alter its actual health. The bottom line: Count on shampoo to keep your hair and scalp clean, nothing more. Proper brushing will do more for the long-term health of your hair and scalp than will spending money on expensive shampoos, conditioners, dyes, and other questionable hair enhancers.

ALTERNATIVE CHOICES

Despite claims to the contrary, no alternative therapies can reverse normal balding, although some may encourage reversal of temporary hair loss and improve damaged hair. Certain relaxation techniques may stem shedding brought on by ***stress.***

CHINESE MEDICINE

In Chinese medicine, hair is thought to be nourished by the blood, which is influenced by the liver and kidneys. Traditional tonics are intended to tone these organs and promote new hair growth; they include such herbs as ***polygonum*** *(Polygonum multiflorum),* ***lycium fruit*** *(Lycium barbarum),* ***Chinese foxglove root*** *(Rehmannia glutinosa),* ***Chinese yam*** *(Dioscorea opposita),* and ***cornus*** *(Cornus officinalis).*

HERBAL THERAPIES

For temporary or partial hair loss from a systemic disease, drug therapy, ***stress,*** or some other known cause, herbalists recommend stimulating hair follicles and improving blood circulation in the scalp to encourage new hair growth. Try massaging your scalp using essential oil of ***rosemary*** *(Rosmarinus officinalis)* or rinsing your hair with tea made from ***sage*** *(Salvia officinalis).* Consult an herbalist for other suggestions.

HOMEOPATHY

More than 20 homeopathic remedies are thought to be effective for hair loss, particularly thinning caused by pregnancy, stress, or emotional trauma. Look in your health food store for over-the-counter preparations, or consult a homeopathic professional for more advice.

MASSAGE

Whether it's visible or not, your scalp needs a steady supply of blood. Massage improves circulation, which in turn improves the health of your hair and scalp. A few drops of ***vitamin E*** oil massaged into the scalp is recommended to strengthen fragile hair and help prevent dry, flaky skin.

MIND/BODY MEDICINE

Emotional or physical ***stress*** may be a factor in some cases of hair loss. A regular exercise program or **relaxation** techniques such as **yoga, guided imagery,** or **meditation** can help relieve stress.

NUTRITION AND DIET

Hair loss can result from poor nutrition or a rapid drop in weight. In such cases, you should get back on a balanced diet and consult your doctor or a professional nutritionist about supplemental ***vitamins A, B complex,*** and ***C,*** as well as ***iron*** and ***zinc.***

PREVENTION

Although you can't reverse natural balding, you can protect your hair from damage that may eventually lead to thinning. Some people, women in particular, put their hair under tremendous stress in the pursuit of beauty. Hair dryers, hot curlers, dyes, bleaches, hair straightening, permanent waves, and chemical-laden cosmetics may eventually result in dry, broken, and thinning hair. People who leave their hair its natural color and texture will end up with healthier hair. Use a basic shampoo designed for your hair type. If you must curl your hair, use sponge rollers and let it air-dry whenever possible.

Proper brushing can do as much for the condition of your hair as any over-the-counter product. Choose a moderately stiff, natural-bristle brush, which will not tear your hair. Use full strokes from the scalp to the tips of your hair, to distribute the hair's natural oil. Begin with 10 to 20 strokes a day and try to work up to 100. Be gentle, and avoid brushing your hair when wet, when it is especially fragile. Remember: Hair is not living tissue, so it cannot repair itself. ■

HAMSTRING INJURY

SYMPTOMS

- sharp pain in the back of the thigh, during or immediately after sports or other strenuous activity.
- swelling and loss of strength in the upper leg.
- difficulty walking or sitting, and inability to bend the leg.

CALL YOUR DOCTOR IF:

- you feel pain shooting down the back of your leg when you cough; you may have ***sciatica.***
- you have chills or fever associated with the muscle pain; these may be symptoms of a bacterial or viral ***infection.***
- your leg hurts when you walk and stops hurting when you are at rest; you may be developing a ***circulatory problem.***

H

As the muscles that flex your knees and bend your legs, the hamstrings are involved in virtually every move you make. Each hamstring is actually a belt of three muscles that run along the back of your thigh from buttock to knee, where they connect to the bones of your lower leg. They are counterparts to the powerful quadriceps muscles at the front of your thighs and can be subject to great stress. Professional athletes and dancers are particularly prone to hamstring pulls, but anyone is susceptible, especially people who push themselves a little too far in weekend sports. The danger in a hamstring pull is giving in to the temptation to "play through the pain," which will aggravate and possibly complicate the injury. Recognizing pain as a warning to stop and let the body heal is the most important step in recovery.

CAUSES

A pulled hamstring is invariably the result of overstressing or tearing the muscle fibers, typically by suddenly twisting, straightening, or overextending the thigh. A minor hamstring pull is simply a case of stretching the muscle too far, but in some cases a crippling muscle spasm can result. Tearing the muscle belt itself, or separating the muscle from the connective tendons, is a much more serious injury.

DIAGNOSTIC AND TEST PROCEDURES

While the signs of a hamstring pull may seem obvious, you may want to confirm the nature and degree of the injury by seeing a family doctor or sports medicine specialist. Aching muscles and joints can sometimes mask more serious ailments such as viral infections, which can be accurately diagnosed only by experts.

TREATMENT

Like other strains, a hamstring pull generally heals itself. You can expect to regain full use of the leg in a few days or weeks, depending on your physical condition and the degree of the injury.

HAMSTRING STRETCH

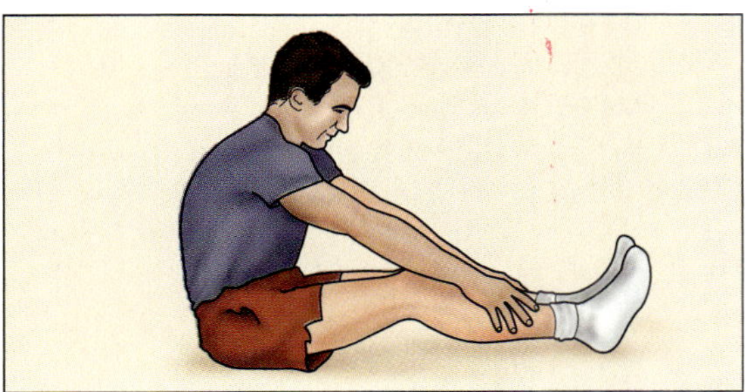

1 Sit on the floor with your legs extended and slightly bent at the knees. Keeping your back as straight as possible, slowly bend from the hips and reach down your legs as far as you can without forcing the stretch. Hold in place for 15 seconds.

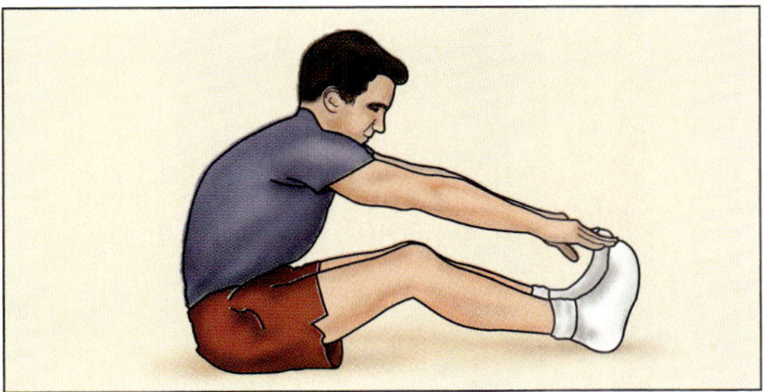

2 Without changing your position, reach toward your feet and try to touch your toes with your fingertips. Hold this position for 15 seconds, then slowly relax the stretch and sit back. Rest for 10 seconds, then repeat the exercise. Do 4 or 5 times.

CONVENTIONAL MEDICINE

The established recovery procedure for muscle strain is RICE: rest, ice, compression, and elevation. *(See* ***Athletic Injuries.****)* Your doctor may also recommend a painkiller such as ***aspirin*** or ***ibuprofen,*** which are also anti-inflammatory agents. Like all painkilling drugs, they should be used to relieve discomfort, not to mask pain in order to continue the activity.

Warm compresses, 10 minutes on and 10 off, will help relax the muscle after the initial pain subsides. Binding your thigh with an elastic bandage will support the injured muscle; you may want to use a crutch to keep weight off the leg.

ALTERNATIVE CHOICES

BODY WORK

If your body is overstressed and your muscles are stiff and contracted, **massage** by a trained therapist will help to relax and tone your muscles. In a typical treatment the therapist uses warm body oil or a cooling gel, sometimes followed by ultrasound to stimulate circulation, before loosening and manipulating the affected muscles.

HOMEOPATHY

Arnica is the homeopath's first-aid remedy for muscle injuries. It can be taken orally and applied as a salve to the painful area. ***Rhus toxicodendron*** and ***Ruta*** are also remedies for muscle strains.

NUTRITION AND DIET

Good natural sources of ***vitamin C,*** essential for tissue building, are citrus fruits and potatoes. ***Potassium*** and ***calcium*** for bones are found in bananas, leafy greens, and low-fat dairy products.

To help your muscles operate at their best, drink plenty of water or a sports beverage before and after every workout.

PREVENTION

The best way to avoid muscle strains is to keep your body in good condition and avoid pushing yourself too hard at work or play.

Before starting your favorite sport or physical activity, particularly those that put heavy demands on your legs, take a few minutes to warm up. Major muscles like your hamstrings work best if you stretch them gradually and let them relax. Once into the activity, don't overstress your muscles. They'll begin to tell you when they have had enough, and it's foolish—even dangerous—to push them past their limits. When the activity is over, stretch the muscles gradually so they don't tighten up and go into a muscle contraction, or cramp, which can be just as painful as a muscle pull—although shorter lived. The exercises above, left are specifically recommended to condition and strengthen your hamstring muscles. ■

H

HAND AND WRIST PAIN

Read down this column to find your symptoms. Then read across.

SYMPTOMS	AILMENT/PROBLEM
◆ painful swelling and stiffness in wrist and/or finger joints; possible chills or fever; wrist or fingers may feel hot.	◆ Inflammation of either the joint itself ***(arthritis*** or ***gout)*** or the bursa, a sac that surrounds the joint and encases it with lubricating fluid ***(bursitis)***
◆ pain in the wrist or fingers when bending your fingers or moving your hand a certain way; no other symptoms.	◆ ***Tendonitis***
◆ numbness, tingling, weakness, or burning in the hands; wrist pain that extends into the forearm and/or the palm; difficulty making a fist; symptoms worsen at night.	◆ ***Carpal tunnel syndrome***
◆ intense pain in the wrist or hand after an injury; the painful area may also be swollen, misshapen, bruised, and/or stiff.	◆ Possibly a sprained ligament, a strained muscle or tendon, or a fractured bone
◆ a wrist or finger joint is painful, red, and swollen; temperature quickly rises to over 100°F; general sick feeling.	◆ A bone ***infection,*** called osteomyelitis, or a joint infection, called infectious ***arthritis***
◆ a few days to six weeks after a streptococcus infection (such as a ***strep throat***), joints (including wrists, fingers, or other joints) are swollen, red, and painful, and may feel warm; temperature is 100.4°F or higher.	◆ ***Rheumatic fever***

H

WHAT TO DO	OTHER INFO
◆ Take ***nonsteroidal anti-inflammatory drugs (NSAIDs)*** or ***aspirin*** to reduce pain and swelling. With rest, bursitis usually heals itself in a few days. See your doctor for treatment of gout, which can cause kidney damage if left untreated.	◆ Gout symptoms may dissipate within a week if you avoid alcohol, caffeine, coffee (regular and decaffeinated), and foods containing purine.
◆ Follow the RICE regimen: rest, ice, compression, and elevation *(see **Tendonitis**)*, and take ***aspirin*** or ***ibuprofen*** as needed for pain. If pain isn't relieved in a week or so, see your doctor.	◆ Usually the inflammation is caused by making repeated, stressful movements or overworking the joint.
◆ Take ***nonsteroidal anti-inflammatory drugs (NSAIDs)*** or ***aspirin*** to reduce pain. When working, take short exercise breaks: For two minutes, slowly move your hand in circles, rotating it around the wrist; then clench both hands into fists and extend your fingers, and repeat 20 times.	◆ Symptoms result when the swollen tendons press on the median nerve, which passes from your wrist into your hand. Wearing a soft wrist splint at night and, if possible, while working can help relieve the pressure and reduce the pain.
◆ For 48 to 72 hours after the injury, follow the RICE regimen: rest, ice, compression, and elevation. See ***Sprains and Strains.*** If the pain is severe, or you cannot move your wrist or hand or lift anything, **call your doctor now.** See ***Emergencies/First Aid: Fractures and Dislocations.***	◆ Homeopaths recommend ***Arnica, Ruta,*** and Symphytum to speed the healing process.
◆ **Call your doctor now.** Without ***antibiotics,*** the stiffness of infectious arthritis can become permanent. For osteomyelitis, the painful joint is immobilized (sometimes with a plaster cast). If an abscess has formed, it may need to be surgically drained.	◆ Osteomyelitis is most common in growing children (under age 12).
◆ **Call your doctor now.** You need bed rest and ***antibiotics*** for at least five weeks. Early treatment is crucial to avoid possibly fatal heart damage.	◆ To prevent a recurrence, your physician may prescribe a daily ***antibiotic*** for a long period of time. You must also be vigilant about receiving treatment for every ***sore throat*** or ***infection*** you get.

HANGOVER

SYMPTOMS

- headache, nausea, dizziness, irritability, thirst, and fatigue—usually on awakening—after drinking excessive amounts of alcohol.
- in some cases, tension, paleness, tremor, vomiting, heartburn, unsteady gait, and loss of appetite.

CALL YOUR DOCTOR IF:

- you are concerned that you have developed or are at risk of developing a dependency on alcohol; this can be triggered by trying to offset a hangover by drinking more alcohol. *(See also **Alcohol Abuse**.)*

H

When you drink to excess, you are likely to suffer the headache, nausea, and other disagreeable symptoms of a hangover. The most intense hangover occurs about 14 to 15 hours after drinking starts—in part, researchers believe, because of the accumulation in your system of products metabolized from alcohol, such as lactic acid.

CAUSES

Alcohol by-products called congeners seem to increase the severity of a hangover. Gin and vodka have few congeners and are thus least likely to produce a hangover, whereas brandy, champagne, and whiskey have the potential to cause the worst hangovers. Red wine can also bring on a hangover because it contains tyramine, a substance that can cause severe headaches.

TREATMENT

Time is the only cure for the occasional hangover. In almost all cases, however, you can ease hangover symptoms through the self-help suggestions offered below. If you suffer frequent hangovers, you may have an ***alcohol abuse*** or dependency problem; seek professional help.

CONVENTIONAL MEDICINE

Most doctors recommend taking ***aspirin, ibuprofen,*** or ***acetaminophen*** for the headache; drinking fluids to offset dehydration; and eating light foods

CAUTION!

Never take aspirin before drinking; when combined with alcohol, aspirin will make you drunker. Never treat a hangover with more alcohol; although you may temporarily offset a hangover's symptoms, you're at risk of developing a dependency on alcohol.

high in carbohydrates and fructose (a natural sugar in fruit juices and honey) to calm nausea.

ALTERNATIVE CHOICES

HERBAL THERAPIES

White willow *(Salix alba)* bark, which contains a natural form of salicylate, the active ingredient in aspirin, may help relieve a headache. Drink hot as a tea (1 cup water simmered with 2 tsp bark for 10 minutes) or chew the bark. ***Ginger*** *(Zingiber officinale)* tea may counter nausea.

HOMEOPATHY

Some homeopathic medicines come in kits that include remedies for the occasional hangover. For nausea, try ***Nux vomica*** (6x to 30c) every hour, for up to three doses.

NUTRITION AND DIET

Nutritionists recommend fruit juices—said to help the body burn alcohol—diluted with water or seltzer and consumed at two times the volume of the amount of alcohol you have drunk; crackers and honey to ease nausea; and bouillon to restore salt and potassium levels. ***Vitamin C,*** taken before and after drinking, is thought to help your body clear the alcohol from your system.

ACUPRESSURE

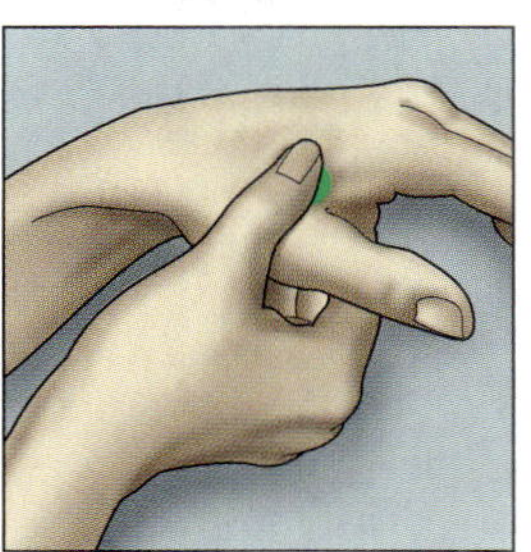

1 Pressing Large Intestine 4 in the web between your thumb and index finger may help relieve hangover headaches. Use the thumb and index finger of your right hand to squeeze the web of your left hand for one minute. Repeat on the right hand. If you are pregnant, do not use LI 4.

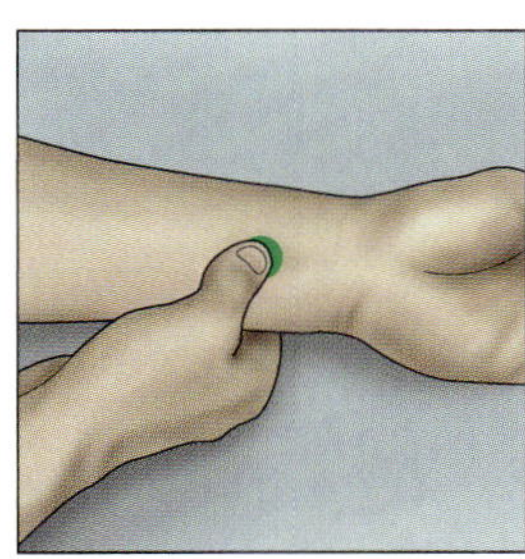

2 To help calm nausea and vomiting, press Pericardium 6. Place your thumb in the center of your inner wrist, two finger widths from the wrist crease and between the two forearm bones. Press firmly for one minute, three to five times; then repeat on the other arm.

HANGOVER MYTHS AND FACTS

MYTH: *Coffee sobers you up or prevents a hangover.*

FACT: *Only time will sober you up. The caffeine in coffee may help get rid of a headache but cannot prevent a hangover. Coffee's stimulating effect might lull you into thinking your judgment or motor control hasn't been impaired.*

MYTH: *If you don't feel hung over, you haven't been impaired by alcohol.*

FACT: *Research shows that drinking affects next-day performance, even if all traces of alcohol are absent from your system. If you are preparing for any activity in which peak performance is required, don't drink the night before.*

AT-HOME REMEDIES

Drink several glasses of water to rehydrate your body. Drink water through the day. Cold compresses on your head or the back of your neck may also bring relief.

PREVENTION

Moderation is the key to preventing a hangover. By drinking slowly, you give your body time to get rid of the alcohol before it enters the blood and your brain. Drink on a full stomach to slow the rate at which alcohol is absorbed. Avoid drinks high in congeners, and avoid mixing alcohol with carbonated beverages: The bubbles speed the alcohol to your bloodstream. The less you weigh, the less alcohol you should consume. ■

H

HAY FEVER

SYMPTOMS

Attacks, often seasonal, of:

- prolonged, sometimes violent sneezing.
- itchy, painful nose, throat, and roof of mouth.
- nasal discharge.
- stuffy, runny nose.
- ***postnasal drip,*** resulting in coughing.
- watery, itchy eyes.
- head and nasal congestion.
- ear pressure or fullness.
- lethargy.

CALL YOUR DOCTOR IF:

- your condition becomes so severe that it interferes with your life and you're unable to control it with over-the-counter medications. Your physician may administer prescription drugs, such as nonsedating ***antihistamines,*** to help.
- a secondary infection develops in congested sinus cavities; signs are fever, pain, a yellow or green discharge, postnasal drip, and sinus or tooth tenderness.

Hay fever is an immune disorder characterized by an allergic response to pollen grains and other substances. Also known as **allergic rhinitis,** there are two types: **seasonal,** which occurs only during the time of year in which certain plants pollinate, and **perennial,** which occurs all year round. (A related problem, **nonallergic rhinitis,** shares symptoms with hay fever but doesn't result from an allergy. See ***Sneezing***.)

Typically, if you suffer from hay fever in the spring, you're probably allergic to tree pollens. Grass and weed pollens may be causing your allergic reaction during the summer. In autumn ragweed may plague you, and fungus spores cause problems from late March through November.

People with **perennial** hay fever are usually allergic to one or more of these outdoor agents. Perennial hay fever can also be brought on by other allergy-causing substances, or allergens. These include house dust mites, feathers, and animal dander (the tiny skin flakes animals shed along with fur), all of which may be found in pillows, down clothing and bedding, shower curtains, heavy draperies, upholstery, and thick carpeting. Another common allergen, mold, is usually found in damp areas such as bathrooms and basements.

A hay fever attack can last between 15 and 20 minutes and may recur several times a day during your hay fever season. Although they can be exhausting, attacks cause no permanent damage.

CAUSES

If you suffer from hay fever, it's because your immune system views harmless inhaled pollen or other allergens as dangerous substances invading your body. Your system overreacts, flooding your bloodstream with a chemical known as histamine, which inflames the lining of your sinuses and eyelids and also sets in motion the other symptoms associated with hay fever, such as sneezing. All of these symptoms are meant to protect your body either by expelling the allergen or by swelling body orifices so it can't enter. As a result of congestion in the veins in the lining of your sinuses, dark circles, commonly known as allergic shiners, may appear under your eyes; if you have perennial allergic rhinitis, they may be present all year round. The swelling of your mucous membranes occasionally results in ***nasal polyps;*** nosebleeds are also common during hay fever attacks.

No one knows why some people's immune systems tend to overreact to pollen and other substances. Evidence points to the likelihood that hay fever is an inherited trait. People under age 40 with ***asthma*** or ***eczema*** are more likely to develop hay fever than those without these ailments.

DIAGNOSTIC AND TEST PROCEDURES

Your doctor may be able to make a diagnosis based on a physical exam and observation of your symptoms. Skin tests may be recommended to determine which pollens cause the most sensitivity. In a scratch or prick test, your physician makes tiny scratches or needle punctures in your back or arm and applies drops containing a small amount of possible allergy-causing substances. If your skin becomes red and itchy after 20 minutes, the test has pinpointed the offending allergens. A radioallergosorbent test, or RAST, may be used to check your blood for elevated levels of the antibodies produced by your immune system to guard against specific allergens. Your doctor may refer you to an allergist for further tests and treatment.

TREATMENT

Many medications are available to deal with the symptoms of hay fever, although the best approach appears to be prevention of attacks, or avoidance of known allergens, or both.

CONVENTIONAL MEDICINE

Medical treatment strategies typically begin with avoidance of allergens, then move on to drug therapy, and may finally resort to immunotherapy. Mild cases of hay fever can be controlled with over-the-counter ***antihistamines,*** such as ***chlorpheniramine*** or ***diphenhydramine,*** which have few side effects. These drugs must be taken regularly and over a long period of time to produce an effect. Phenylephrine and ***pseudoephedrine*** are ***decongestants*** that help unblock nasal passages. They can help during an acute attack but should be taken for a few days only since prolonged use can have the rebound effect of making congestion worse. If you have high blood pressure, are taking medication for a heart condition, or are taking the antibiotic ***erythromycin*** or the antifungal drug ***ketoconazole,*** be sure to check with your doctor before taking a decongestant or an antihistamine. For severe cases your doctor may also prescribe a stronger antihistamine, such as ***loratadine,*** cetirizine, or fexofenadine.

Some over-the-counter nasal sprays contain both a decongestant and an antihistamine. These sprays help with pain and itching by opening clogged nasal passages and reducing inflammation. Regular use of the prescription spray ***cromolyn*** prevents the lining of the nasal passages from reacting to the allergen affecting you. More severe cases may benefit from a ***corticosteroid*** nasal spray such as ***beclomethasone.***

Be aware that over-the-counter nasal sprays and drops may be addictive and should be used sparingly. Medications containing salicylates such as ***aspirin*** should also be avoided as they may worsen symptoms.

Another avenue to try is allergy shots, or immunotherapy. This treatment involves a series of injections of increasingly larger amounts of the allergen until your system becomes desensitized to it and no longer overreacts in response to it. Immunotherapy has shown positive results in up to 75 percent of sufferers with extreme cases of hay fever. Standard treatment lasts from one to three years.

ALTERNATIVE CHOICES

A number of alternative therapies can help with symptom control and as preventive measures.

AROMATHERAPY

Inhalations of ***eucalyptus*** *(Eucalyptus globulus),* ***peppermint*** *(Mentha piperita),* or ***hyssop*** *(Hyssopus officinalis)* may help to ease sinus irritation and pain.

H

CHINESE HERBS

Ephedra *(Ephedra sinica)* has a long history as a hay fever and allergy remedy. Chinese herbalists believe it loses its effectiveness over time and so is best used for short periods in combination with other herbs. An herbalist may combine ephedra with ***licorice*** *(Glycyrrhiza uralensis),* which is thought to have antiallergy and anti-inflammatory properties. In some people, ephedra can produce side effects such as palpitations, insomnia, and high blood pressure. ***Ginseng*** *(Panax ginseng)* is another herb that's compatible with ephedra and may be especially effective when combined with herbal expectorants, which promote the expulsion of mucus. Commonly used expectorants include pinellia *(Pinellia ternata),* cynanchum *(Cynanchum stautoni),* and polygala *(Polygala tenuifolia).* Consult an herbalist specializing in Chinese medicine for more information.

HERBAL THERAPIES

The following mixture may prevent some symptoms. Infuse in 1 cup boiled water for 10 minutes: 2 parts elder *(Sambucus nigra),* 1 part ***ephedra*** *(Ephedra sinica),* 1 part ***eyebright*** *(Euphrasia officinalis),* and 1 part ***goldenseal*** *(Hydrastis canadensis).* Drink 1 cup of this tea three times a day during the two months before hay fever season begins. Be aware that ephedra may be too stimulating for children. Regular doses of ***parsley*** *(Petroselinum crispum)* may help with hay fever; it is thought to work by reducing your body's production of histamine.

You may be able to slow down your body's mucus production with goldenrod *(Solidago virgaurea),* ***garlic*** *(Allium sativum),* ***yarrow*** *(Achillea millefolium),* or agrimony *(Agrimonia eupatoria).* Bathe irritated eyes with compresses soaked in either ***eyebright*** *(Euphrasia officinalis)* or ***chamomile*** *(Matricaria recutita);* make a tea from the leaves and dilute it by 50 percent with water or saline solution before using to soak the compresses.

HOMEOPATHY

For watery, hot eyes, a burning nasal discharge with sneezing, and symptoms that feel worse late at night, try ***Arsenicum album.*** If your eyes feel inflamed and very watery, your nose is blocked at night but has a watery discharge during the day, and you have a headache, consider using *Euphrasia.* ***Pulsatilla*** can help if your symptoms—thick, yellow mucus accompanied by a loss of taste and smell—are made worse by warm rooms but are better outdoors. If your watery, itchy eyes and sneezing, runny nose with a burning discharge become worse in a warm room, try ***Allium cepa.*** Consult a homeopathic practitioner for proper doses of these, and other, remedies.

ACUPRESSURE

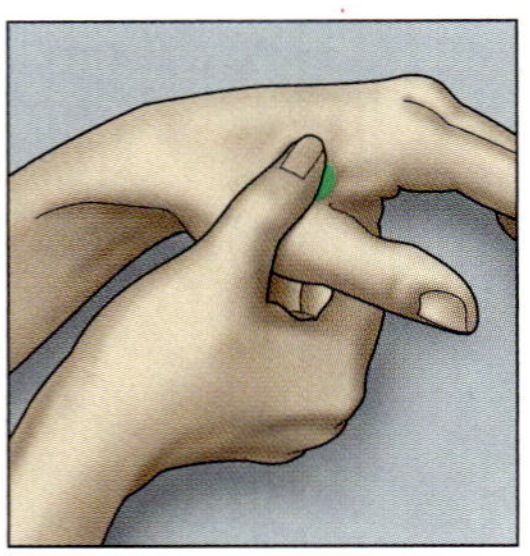

1 Pressing Large Intestine 4 in the web between your thumb and index finger may help ease hay fever. Use the thumb and index finger of your right hand to squeeze the web of your left hand for one minute. Repeat this on the right hand. If pregnant, do not use LI 4.

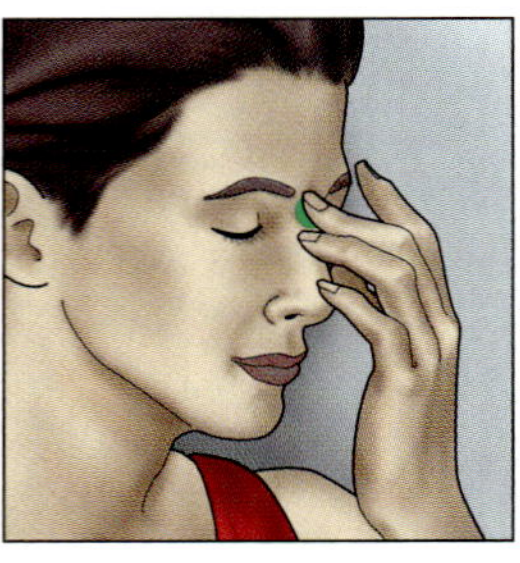

2 Pressure on Governing Vessel 24.5 may also help relieve symptoms of hay fever. Place the tip of your middle finger at the top of the bridge of your nose, between your eyebrows. Press lightly for two minutes and breathe deeply. Do three to five times, at least twice a day.

NUTRITION AND DIET

Nutritionists believe that refined sugar and casein, the protein in dairy products, are mucus-producing substances that are best avoided during hay fever season. Taking a commercial preparation of the mineral dolomite, which contains ***calcium*** and ***magnesium,*** may help regulate histamine production.

Some researchers believe that honey has a desensitizing and antiallergic effect that may relieve some hay fever symptoms. Two months before the season starts, begin eating 2 tsp daily of raw honey that comes from a nearby hive. You can also try chewing a bite-sized piece of honeycomb for 5 to 10 minutes twice a day (but don't

HOMEMADE DECONGESTANT

Make your own decongestant by boiling grapefruit, orange, or lemon peels, including the pith, in water mixed with honey until the peels are spongy, stirring occasionally. Be careful not to overcook—you don't want candied fruit. Eat one piece when symptoms start and one piece each evening at bedtime during hay fever season. Substances in the peel and white rind act as anti-inflammatory agents and will dry mucous membranes. Lemon is considered a stimulant expectorant that may help release mucus from your lungs.

swallow it) or taking five tablets of pollen extract supplements every day beginning several weeks before hay fever season. Check with your doctor first to avoid potential allergic reactions.

Many people with hay fever are also allergic to certain foods and may experience symptoms as a result of eating allergy-triggering substances in such foods as eggs, nuts, fish, shellfish, chocolate, dairy products, wheat, citrus fruits, or food colorings or preservatives. To determine whether food allergies might be at the root of, or perhaps compounding, your hay fever problems, try an elimination diet. Stop eating all the suspected foods, including those mentioned above, as well as prepackaged or prepared foods, for 10 days. If your symptoms disappear or diminish, reintroduce one food at a time and see whether your symptoms recur. If they do, eliminate the offending food and all its by-products from your daily diet.

AT-HOME REMEDIES

The best way to combat the allergens that are assaulting you is to avoid them. Stay indoors between six and ten o'clock in the morning and on days when the pollen count is high. The pollen count drops on rainy days and climbs when it's hot, sunny, and windy outside. If you must go outdoors, wear protective glasses and hold a handkerchief over your nose and mouth or wear a dust mask with a filter for pollen. Resist the temptation to rub your eyes.

Keep windows—in your home and car—closed and the air conditioning turned on. Change ventilation system filters in your home once a month. Remove allergens from the air with ionizing air cleaners. Prevent mold in damp basements by using space heaters and dehumidifiers.

Avoid mowing your lawn or raking leaves since these activities stir up pollens and molds. However, try to keep your grass no more than an inch high in the spring and summer so as not to allow pollination. If you must do yard work yourself, wear a filtered mask and protective glasses. Wash your face, hands, and hair and rinse your eyes when coming in from outdoors to avoid leaving traces of pollen on your pillow.

Mites live in household dust and are impossible to get rid of entirely, but measures can be taken to minimize them: Remove thick carpeting, heavy drapes, and upholstered furniture; put plastic covers on mattresses and pillows; keep floors clean; avoid down (feathers) in comforters, clothing, sleeping bags, and pillows; and wear a mask when vacuuming.

PREVENTION

Although a tendency to develop hay fever could be in your genes, you may be able to avoid symptoms by taking preventive steps and being alert to the signals. If you have eczema or asthma, be aware that you may be more likely to develop hay fever. Consult an allergist or try the elimination or raw honey diets mentioned above. Strengthen your immune system with a healthful lifestyle including wholesome foods, exercise, vitamin supplements, and herbs. Cut down on environmental pollutants and toxins as much as possible by keeping your home clean and your yard neat. ■

HEADACHE

SYMPTOMS

If your headache is:
- a dull, steady pain that feels like a band tightening around your head, you have a **tension headache.**
- throbbing, begins on one side, and causes nausea, you have a **migraine.** Visual disturbances, such as flickering points of light, may precede the headache.
- a throbbing pain around one red, watery eye, with nasal congestion on that side of your face, you have a **cluster headache.**
- a steady pain in the area behind your face that gets worse if you bend forward and is accompanied by congestion, you have a **sinus headache.**

CALL YOUR DOCTOR IF:

- a severe headache is accompanied by vomiting, limb weakness, double vision, slurred speech, or difficulty in swallowing; you may have a cerebral hemorrhage or an ***aneurysm*** **— get medical help now.**
- your headache is of a kind you've never had, occurs first thing in the morning, is persistent, brings on vomiting, and abates during the day; you may have ***high blood pressure*** or in very rare cases a brain tumor. See your doctor without delay.
- you have a high fever, light hurts your eyes, the pain is severe and is accompanied by nausea and a stiff neck; you may have ***meningitis*** **— get medical help now.**
- after a head injury, you are drowsy, with dizziness, vertigo, nausea, or vomiting; you may have a concussion. See your doctor without delay.

Although painful and troublesome, most headaches are minor health concerns and can be easily treated with ***aspirin*** or another ***analgesic.*** But if they are severe, recur frequently, or are attended by other symptoms, you may need to take additional steps, including consultation with your doctor.

Headaches are categorized according to their underlying causes. Muscle contraction, or **tension,** headaches make up one common group. Vascular (blood-vessel) headaches are a second common category; it includes both **migraine** and **cluster headaches.** A third group consists of headaches caused by **sinus** problems. *(See **Sinusitis.**)*

Tension headaches, which afflict almost everyone at one time or another, bring on a dull, persistent, nonthrobbing pain that can make your head feel as if it's gripped in a tight band. The muscles of your neck may seem knotted, and certain areas on your head and neck may be sensitive to touch. Nerve endings in the head and neck that have been irritated by taut muscles are the chief source of pain. Tension headaches can be short-lived and infrequent, or they can be enduring and chronic.

Migraines are the most debilitating of headaches; they can be completely incapacitating. With some sufferers—a minority—a migraine attack is preceded by a warning sign, called an aura; it may include visual disturbances such as flickering points of light, blind spots, or zigzag lines, or more rarely, numbness in a limb or the smelling of strange odors. Whether a warning occurs or not, a migraine will usually begin with an intense, throbbing pain on one side of the head. This pain may spread and is often accompanied by nausea and vomiting. A migraine can last from a few hours to three days and can cause oversensitivity to light, odors, and sound.

All the various symptoms of migraines seem linked to changes in the diameter of blood vessels in the head: The blood vessels constrict during the initial stage and dilate when the headache pain begins. These changes may be due to an imbalance in a brain chemical known as serotonin. Hormones, too, apparently can play a role; there is a strong correlation between changes in estrogen levels and migraines.

Cluster headaches are so named because they tend to come in bunches. Typically they begin several hours after a person falls asleep and are sometimes preceded by a mild aching sensation on one side of the head. The pain—severe, piercing, and usually located in and around one red, watery eye—is generally accompanied by nasal congestion and a flushed face. It lasts from 30 minutes to two hours, then diminishes or disappears altogether, only to recur perhaps a day later. A barrage of four or more attacks may occur in the course of the day, and cluster headaches can strike every day for weeks or months before going into long periods of remission. The vast majority of sufferers are men.

Sinus headaches are characterized by pain in the forehead, nasal area, eyes, and sometimes the top of the head; in some cases, they also produce a feeling of pressure behind the face. Inflammation or infection of the membranes lining the sinus cavities can give rise to such headaches. Also, the headache pain may stem from suction on the sinus walls, which occurs when nasal congestion creates a partial vacuum in the sinuses.

CAUSES

Headaches strike for many reasons. **Sinus headaches** typically result from hay fever and other seasonal allergies, or from a cold or the flu. With **tension headaches,** stress is the most common trigger; it may stem from anxiety about work or family life, or it may derive from some physical factor such as persistent noise. Eyestrain, poor posture, too much caffeine, or the grinding or clenching of teeth at night can also lead to tension headaches.

Migraines are somewhat more mysterious. Although much evidence indicates that constricting and swelling of blood vessels is involved, some researchers believe that the headaches are primarily neurological in origin. Because migraines often run in families, it seems likely that genetics can play a role. In any event, a wide range of factors can trigger an attack; among them are excessive caffeine, various foods or scents, naps, dry winds, changes in altitude or

COMMON SOURCES OF HEADACHE PAIN

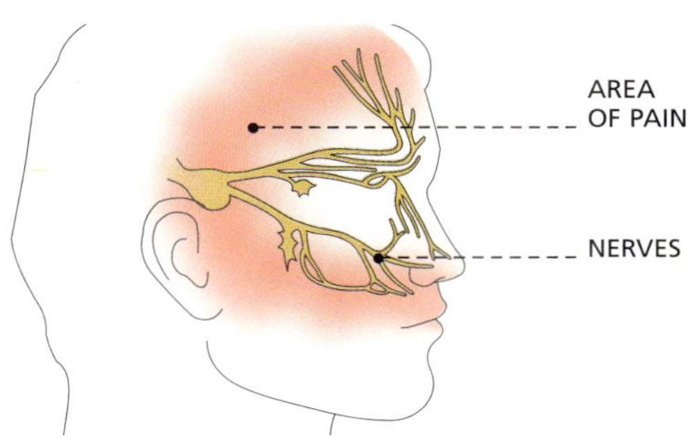

CLUSTER HEADACHE
Although their exact cause is unknown, cluster headaches may arise from pressure on nerves around the eyes. Swollen sinus tissue may press against portions of these nerves, causing these electrical pathways to short-circuit and emit pain signals.

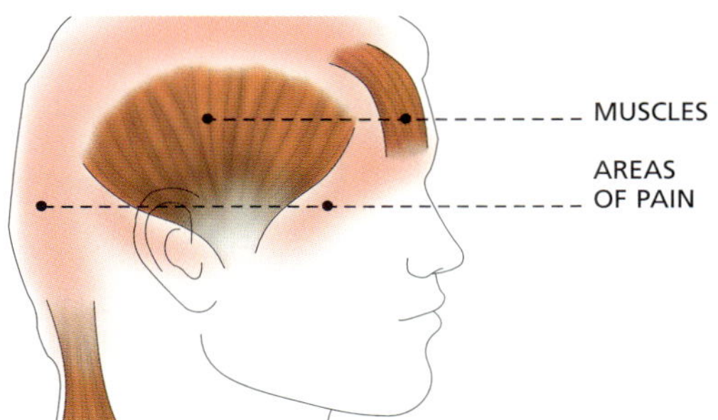

TENSION HEADACHE
Of the various types of tension headaches, one is thought to be linked to disorders in certain muscles in the head and the neck. Pain can be localized around any of these muscles or can spread to affect a broad portion of the scalp.

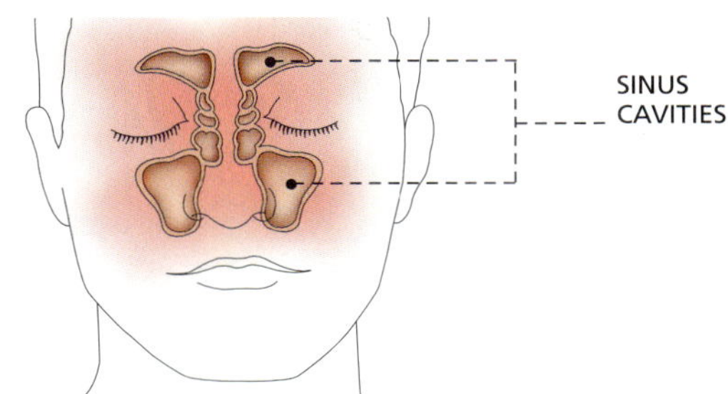

SINUS HEADACHE
With a sinus headache, congestion within the sinus cavities leads to swelling that puts pressure on surrounding tissue and nerves, causing pain to radiate across the face.

ACUPRESSURE

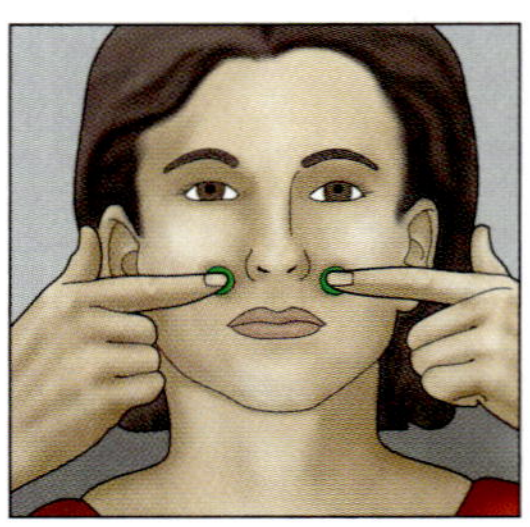

1 Sinus headaches may be relieved by pressing Stomach 3. While looking in a mirror, place the index fingers of both hands at the bottom of your cheekbones, fingertips directly under the pupils of your eyes. Press firmly for one minute. Repeat three times.

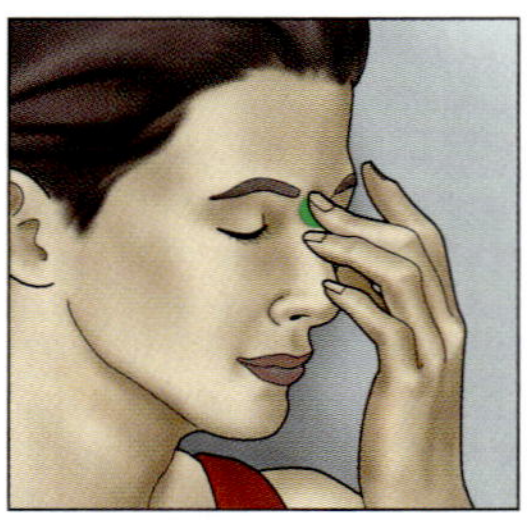

2 Pressure on Governing Vessel 24.5 may help ease headaches. Place the tip of your middle finger at the top of the bridge of your nose, between your eyebrows. Press lightly for two minutes and breathe deeply. Do three to five times, at least twice a day.

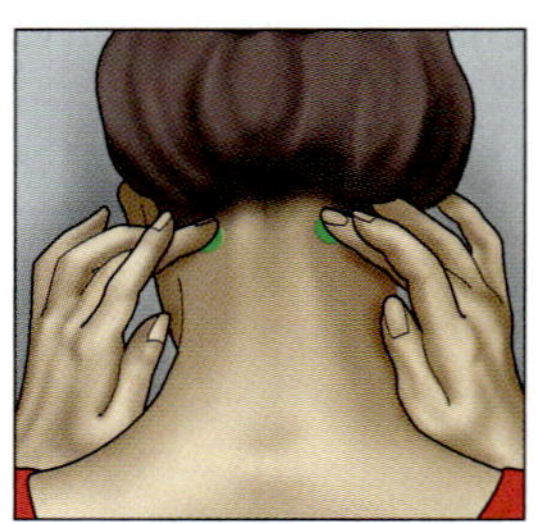

3 To reduce neck muscle stress that may be associated with tension headaches, try pressing Gall Bladder 20. Place the tips of the middle fingers in the hollows at the base of the skull, about two inches apart, on either side of the spine. Press firmly for one minute.

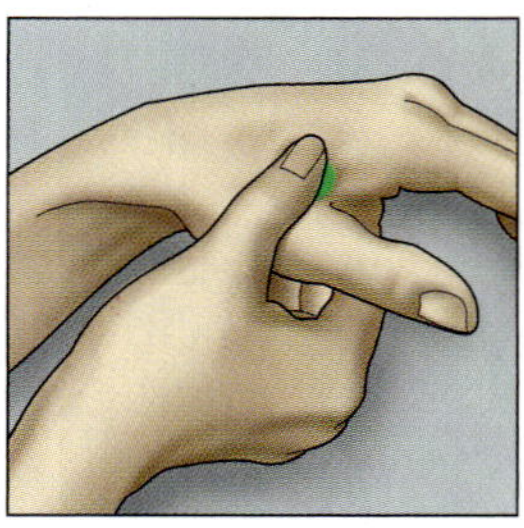

4 Pressing Large Intestine 4 may help relieve sinus headaches. Using the thumb and index finger of your right hand, squeeze the web of your left hand for one minute. Repeat this on the right hand. If pregnant, do not use LI 4.

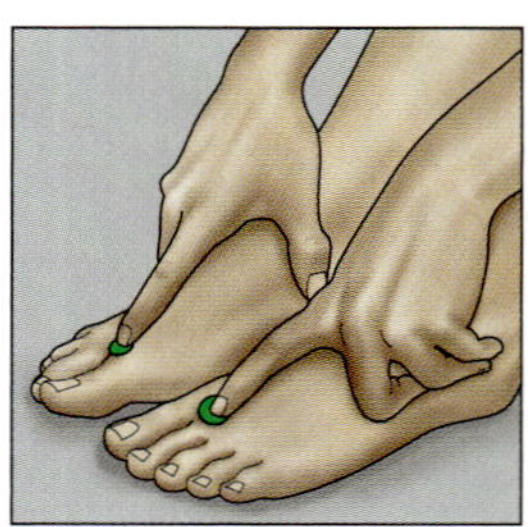

5 Pressure to Liver 3 may provide headache relief. Place the index fingers at the top of each foot, fingertips next to the large knuckle of the big toe, between the big and second toes. Press for one minute, then release. Repeat two or three times, twice daily.

seasons, hormonal fluctuations or birth-control pills, missing a meal, or stuffy rooms. Migraines may also occur in the aftermath of intense emotions such as excitement or anger. Exercise, sexual activity, or very cold foods can also jump-start a migraine.

Cluster headaches are the most baffling of all. They are more common in heavy smokers than in nonsmokers, and alcohol consumption and certain foods seem to be involved in some cases, but the root cause is unknown.

DIAGNOSTIC AND TEST PROCEDURES

To rule out possible organic causes of headaches—for example, an aneurysm, tumor, or structural abnormality—a physician may employ vision tests, x-rays, a CT scan, a lumbar puncture, or an EEG.

TREATMENT

Both conventional and alternative medicine can be effective in dealing with headaches, and the two approaches may be combined. Almost all practitioners consider **relaxation** beneficial for **tension** and **migraine headaches,** for example.

CONVENTIONAL MEDICINE

Most **tension headaches** can be helped by ***analgesics*** such as ***aspirin, acetaminophen,*** or ***ibuprofen; antidepressants*** can help in chronic cases. **Sinus headaches** are relieved by ***antibiotics, antihistamines,*** and ***decongestants.***

A wide range of medications are prescribed for **migraines.** If you have three or more severe, prolonged migraines per month, your doctor may suggest using prophylactic, or preventive, medications on a continual basis. These include ***propranolol,*** a ***beta-adrenergic blocker*** that works by reducing constriction in blood vessels; a ***calcium channel blocker*** such as ***verapamil;*** or ***antidepressants.*** If your migraines are milder and occur less often than three times per month, your doctor may suggest drugs such as an isometheptene-containing combination or ergotamine (available as a suppository if the vomiting caused by your migraines prevents you from keeping a pill down). The drugs ergotamine, noratriptan, ***sumatriptan,*** and zolmitriptan are designed to treat migraines and bring dramatic relief. A therapeutic nasal spray based on the serotonin-inhibiting drug dihydroergotamine (D.H.E. 45) acts quickly to constrict blood vessels and reduce inflammation. Even ***aspirin,*** if taken in effervescent form at the first sign of an attack, can be effective. Drink it 10 minutes after taking metoclopramide, which reduces nausea and improves absorption, to shorten an attack.

Simple analgesics do little for **cluster headaches,** because they do not act quickly enough. However, doctors have found that inhaling pure oxygen can be highly effective in providing relief. *(See **At-Home Remedies, page 441.**)* A short course of ***corticosteroids,*** methysergide maleate, and lithium carbonate can alleviate cluster headaches, as can some of the ***calcium channel blockers*** and vasoconstrictors that are used for migraines.

ALTERNATIVE CHOICES

The vast majority of alternative therapies attempt to address the underlying causes of headaches. Because tension and stress so often figure in headaches, relaxation techniques are a staple of therapeutic programs.

ACUPUNCTURE

Acupuncture can help treat and prevent headaches. Consult an acupuncturist, who will evaluate your particular pattern of headaches and then devise an appropriate treatment.

ACUPRESSURE

Follow the illustrations at far left to locate pressure points associated with headache relief. These techniques are often used in combination with one of the aromatherapy oils below.

AROMATHERAPY

The following herbal oils may aid relaxation, easing the pain of **tension** or **migraine** headaches. Moisten your fingertips with one or two drops of ***lavender*** *(Lavandula officinalis)* essential oil blended with a so-called carrier oil such as sunflower oil, then gently massage your temples with a circular motion; repeat in the hollows at the sides of your eyes, behind your ears, and over your neck. For a **sinus headache,** try the same techniques using ***eucalyptus*** *(Eucalyptus globulus)* or wintergreen *(Gaultheria procumbens).* For any type of headache, inhale a blend of lavender, ***rosemary*** *(Rosmarinus officinalis),* and ***peppermint*** *(Mentha piperita).* Compresses applied to the affected area or a bath using these oils can relax muscles, easing pain.

CHIROPRACTIC

Some **tension headaches** are caused by posture that puts unnecessary strain on muscles. A chiropractor may be able to remove the strain through spinal or cervical manipulation and realignment. In some studies, spinal manipulation has been shown to produce fewer side effects and have longer-lasting results than conventional drug use. Manipulation may also treat **migraine headaches;** consult your chiropractor.

C A U T I O N !

Although they can be effective against headaches when used on a temporary basis, painkillers—especially those containing caffeine or *codeine*—should not be taken over long periods of time. Studies show that the constant use of painkillers may have a rebound effect—actually causing headaches—or can block other medications, such as prophylactic drugs, that you may be taking on a regular basis to prevent migraine headaches. Dependence on painkillers may also hamper the effectiveness of endorphins, the body's natural painkillers. It also seems that dependence on painkillers may permanently alter the pain-control pathways in the brain and spinal cord.

H

HERBAL THERAPIES

Perhaps the most widely recommended herbal remedy for treating and preventing **migraines** is ***feverfew*** *(Chrysanthemum parthenium),* which is thought to work by blocking excessive secretion of serotonin, a neurotransmitter. When blood vessels constrict in the initial stage of a migraine, serotonin is released; feverfew may help counteract this by dilating those blood vessels. Chewing a leaf or two daily is one approach to prevention, but this can occasionally cause mouth ulcers; as a substitute for the leaves, you can use 125-mg capsules. To offset an acute attack, take 3 or 4 capsules right away, then continue this dosage every four hours; but don't exceed 12 capsules in a day. Migraines brought on by stress may benefit from a combination of equal parts of ***hawthorn*** *(Crataegus oxyacantha),* linden (*Tilia* spp.), wood betony *(Pedicularis canadensis),* ***skullcap*** *(Scutellaria lateriflora),* and cramp bark *(Viburnum opulus),* taken three times a day as a tea or tincture. For migraines accompanied by nausea and vomiting, try taking 500 mg of dried ***ginger*** *(Zingiber officinale)* with water at the onset of the warning stage, if your headache pattern includes an aura; repeat every two hours if needed. Three daily doses of ***goldenseal*** *(Hydrastis canadensis),* taken in tincture, tea, or powdered form on a short-term basis, may help reduce acute **sinus headache** pain.

Tension headaches may respond to three daily infusions of ***valerian*** *(Valeriana officinalis)* when combined with skullcap and ***passionflower*** *(Passiflora incarnata).* **Cluster headaches** may get quick relief from several daily applications inside the nostrils of an over-the-counter ointment made from ***cayenne*** *(Capsicum frutescens).* The same ointment applied to the skin is also said to be effective in preventing **migraines.** Because cayenne is hot and can cause painful skin burns, it's best used under a doctor's care.

HOMEOPATHY

A range of homeopathic medicines are available to treat specific types of headaches. For a throbbing headache that is worse on the right side when lying down, try ***Belladonna.*** For severe, "splitting" headaches that feel worse with motion, noise, light, or touch, try ***Bryonia.*** For **sinus** pain with a thick, green nasal discharge, consider ***Kali bichromicum.*** For **migraines** or other chronic headaches, see a homeopathic practitioner.

POURING PAIN AWAY

Your imagination can sometimes be the best medicine for a headache. Try this technique, which relies on your mind's own power to overcome pain. It helps to have a partner talk you through this exercise, but with practice you may be able to do it yourself.

Close your eyes and imagine that your headache is a liquid that fills a certain size of container—the more painful the headache, the bigger the container. Now imagine pouring your headache pain into a slightly smaller container, without letting any of the liquid overflow. Keep pouring the liquid into smaller and smaller containers; bit by bit, you should feel the pain reducing.

LIFESTYLE

Regular **exercise** can release endorphins, the body's natural painkilling agents. Exercise may also help to dilate blood vessels, which increases blood flow and may counteract the constricting action that occurs at the onset of most **migraines.**

To nip a **tension headache** in the bud, try the following exercise while breathing deeply and thinking calm thoughts: While seated, inhale and gently tip your head back until you're looking up at the ceiling (be careful not to tip your head back too far, since this can compress the cervical spine); exhale and bring your head forward until your chin rests on your chest; repeat 4 or 5 times.

Keeping a headache diary can help you pinpoint the factors causing your specific headache patterns. The diary should provide answers to these 10 questions:

1. When did you first develop headaches?
2. How often do you have them?
3. Do you experience symptoms prior to the headaches?
4. Where is the pain exactly?
5. How long does it last?
6. At what time of day do the headaches occur?
7. Does the eating of certain types of food precede your headaches?
8. If you're female, at what time in your monthly cycle do they occur?
9. Are the headaches triggered by physical or environmental factors, such as odor, noise, or certain kinds of weather?
10. What words most accurately describe the pain of your headache: throbbing, stabbing, blinding, piercing . . . ?

MASSAGE

Massage therapy can relieve headache-producing tension in the muscles of your head, neck, shoulders, and face. Try giving yourself a 10-minute scalp massage: Place both middle fingers on your forehead at your hairline; using gentle pressure, gradually work them back to the crown of your head; tracing your hairline, repeat this motion in half-inch increments until you reach your temples; rotate your fingers on both sides for a few minutes; then bring both thumbs to the base of your skull along your hairline and massage both sides of your skull up to your crown to release any tightness.

MIND/BODY MEDICINE

Meditation, yoga, and **progressive relaxation** therapies are effective in reducing ***stress,*** which can cause **tension headaches. Biofeedback** training methods can also be helpful in controlling stress. **Migraine headaches,** too, can be treated through a biofeedback method called thermal biofeedback, in which you learn to increase the temperature of your hands and feet. Warming these extremities involves dilating the vessels that carry blood to them—a process that, in turn, may reduce abnormal blood-vessel constriction in the skull and possibly result in diminished migraine frequency, intensity, and duration.

NUTRITION AND DIET

Among the foods sometimes associated with **migraine headaches** are chocolate, aged cheeses, citrus fruits, processed meats containing sodium nitrates or the food additive MSG, and red wine. Keeping a food diary can help you identify foods to eliminate. White sugar and caffeine can aggravate muscle tension; avoid these substances to decrease **tension headache** occurence.

Magnesium relaxes constricted blood vessels; low levels of magnesium may contribute to **migraine** and **cluster headaches.** Supplemental doses of 200 mg three times a day may be preventive. Taking 50 to 200 mg of ***niacin*** (vitamin B_3) and niacinamide at the first hint of pain may help keep blood vessels dilated, possibly reducing the initial constriction phase of **migraines** and avoiding an attack.

OSTEOPATHY

Osteopaths believe headache pain stemming from pressure on nerves or blood vessels can be eased by neuromuscular manipulation and soft-tissue massage of your head, neck, and upper back.

AT-HOME REMEDIES

- Holding an ice pack or a bag of frozen vegetables against your forehead while soaking your feet in hot water may stop a **migraine** if done right away.
- Placing a warm compress on your head and neck will relax the muscles associated with a **tension headache.**
- At the first sign of a **migraine headache,** drink three glasses of very cold water, then retire with a cold compress to a dark, quiet room to sleep (without a pillow).
- Inhaling pure oxygen from a tank kept near your bed may offset nighttime attacks of a **cluster headache.** But be sure to consult a doctor on how to use the oxygen. ■

H

HEARING PROBLEMS

SYMPTOMS

People often do not recognize a hearing problem until it is brought to their attention by a relative or a friend. Symptoms can include:

- an inability to hear or distinguish some or all sounds in one or both ears.
- difficulty understanding conversation when many people are talking in the background.
- a need to turn up the volume on the television or radio louder than other people find comfortable.

Hearing problems are sometimes accompanied by dizziness, earache, discharge or bleeding from the ear, ringing noise in the ear, or in rare cases, weakness of facial muscles.

CALL YOUR DOCTOR IF:

- you notice any hearing problems; it is important that you receive a timely medical evaluation, because early treatment may enable you to avoid permanent damage and regain full hearing.
- you experience a sudden and total hearing loss in one or both ears; this may indicate a severe reaction to medication, a tumor on the auditory nerve, or a neurological problem. Seek medical care as soon as possible.
- you have some hearing loss and your ear secretes pus or fluid; this may indicate an ear infection or a perforated eardrum.
- your hearing loss is accompanied by dizziness and nausea; these may be signs of ***otitis media, Ménière's disease,*** or another condition that needs medical attention.

Some 28 million people in the United States have a hearing problem significant enough to interfere with their ability to understand conversations and communicate with others. As many as 2 million cannot hear at all and are considered profoundly deaf. Your chances of having a hearing problem increase dramatically with age: More than a third of people over the age of 75 experience difficulty hearing, a problem that often leads to frustration and social isolation.

One form of age-related hearing loss—known as **presbycusia**—usually begins between the ages of 40 and 50 and gets progressively worse. People with presbycusia often have trouble hearing higher frequencies and thus find it particularly difficult to understand women and children, who generally speak at a higher pitch than men. Presbycusia tends to afflict men more frequently and more severely than women.

Hearing problems are less common in children, but if left untreated, they can have a major impact on how well a child learns and makes friends. About 1 in 1,000 infants has a hearing problem severe enough to inhibit the child's ability to learn to speak.

Doctors divide hearing loss into two main categories. **Conductive** hearing loss occurs when something interferes with the transfer of sound waves from the outer to the inner ear. **Sensorineural** hearing loss results from damage to the inner ear or to the nerves that transmit sound impulses from the inner ear to the brain. Sounds may reach the inner ear, but they are not perceived because the necessary messages aren't sent correctly to the brain. Sometimes a person has a mixture of both types of hearing loss.

CAUSES

A hearing loss, whether partial or total, is not in itself an illness, but rather a symptom of an underlying disorder. A wide variety of conditions can lead to hearing problems. Common causes of **conductive** hearing loss include excessive earwax, ear infections, and a ruptured or perforated eardrum. Benign cysts, tumors, and objects lodged in the ear canal, such as an insect or a

H

THE MECHANICS OF HEARING

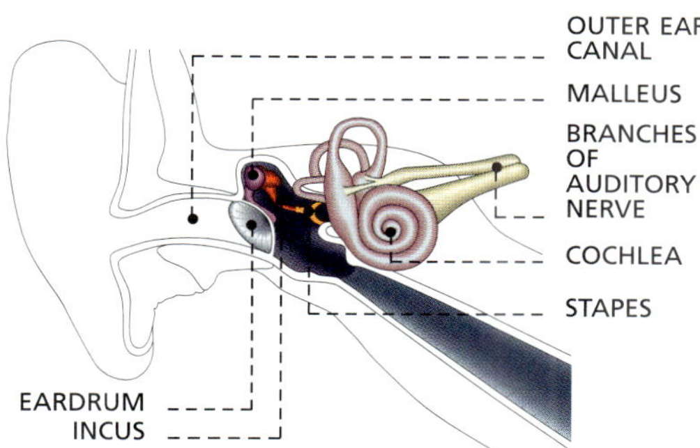

The ear picks up vibrations in the air, or sound waves, which resonate against the eardrum at the end of the outer ear canal. The eardrum transmits the vibrations to three tiny bones—the malleus, incus, and stapes—in the middle ear. The cochlea in the inner ear picks up the vibrations and transmits them as nerve impulses along the auditory nerve to the brain, which interprets the impulses as sound.

piece of a child's toy, can also block the transmission of sounds to the inner ear. In addition, several inherited conditions can cause conductive hearing loss. The most common of these is **otosclerosis,** a degenerative disease of the small bones in the middle ear. About 1 percent of the population is affected by otosclerosis, usually in both ears.

Genetics is also considered a major, if not the major, cause of **sensorineural** hearing loss, particularly in children. Experts estimate that half of the cases of profound deafness in children have a genetic source. A genetic predisposition is also an important factor in the development of **presbycusia.** People with presbycusia experience gradual destruction of the thousands of tiny hair cells that line the cochlea, the spiral-shaped cavity of the inner ear. Without the hairs, which help transfer sound vibrations into nerve signals that travel to the brain, perceiving sounds becomes difficult or impossible.

Prolonged exposure to loud noise, particularly if it is high pitched, can also destroy the sensitive hair cells of the cochlea and lead to partial or total sensorineural hearing loss. Workers whose jobs subject them to high-intensity noise, such as carpenters, construction workers, and rock musicians, are at increased risk, as are people with hobbies such as hunting or snowmobiling.

Several infectious diseases—most notably ***shingles, meningitis, syphilis,*** and cytomegalovirus—have been implicated in sensorineural hearing loss. In addition, if a woman contracts ***German measles*** during pregnancy, her child will be at increased risk of a permanent hearing disability. A child who receives inadequate oxygen during the birth process may also suffer some degree of irreversible damage to the hearing mechanisms of the ears.

Other causes of sensorineural hearing loss include ***Ménière's disease,*** tumors of the brain or auditory nerve, ***diabetes,*** and vascular disorders that lead to ***stroke,*** such as ***high blood pressure*** and ***atherosclerosis.*** High doses of ***aspirin,*** quinine, some types of ***antibiotics,*** and several ***diuretics*** used to treat high blood pressure may also lead to permanent damage of the inner ear. People with ***multiple sclerosis*** or other types of neurological diseases are prone to sensorineural hearing problems as well. In addition, a physical blow or penetrating injury to the ear may cause a permanent loss of hearing.

DIAGNOSTIC AND TEST PROCEDURES

To determine whether the underlying cause of your hearing problem is a medical condition for which you can be treated, your doctor will give you a general physical exam, including a careful examination of your ears. You may also be given some simple hearing tests. If the source of the problem remains unclear, you may be sent to an otologist or an otolaryngologist (both ear specialists) for formal hearing tests.

The most common of these tests is audiometry, which measures first how well you hear sounds conducted through the air (to determine **conductive** hearing loss) and then how well you hear sounds through the bones of your head (to determine **sensorineural** hearing loss). You will be put in a soundproof room and given earphones through which a series of sounds, ranging from low to high frequencies, will be played at increasing or decreasing loudness. You may also be given neurological tests, and the specialist may recommend an MRI or a CT scan to check for possible tumors.

GET THE WAX OUT

One of the most common causes of temporary hearing loss is excessive wax buildup. To remove the wax without damaging your ear, try this simple cleaning method:

Warm 1 tbsp of hydrogen peroxide by setting the jar in a sink full of hot water for a few minutes. Tilt your head to the side and put a dropperful of the warmed liquid in your blocked ear. Let it remain there for three minutes. Then tilt your head the other way and let the hydrogen peroxide run out onto a towel or tissue. The wax should be soft enough to be wiped away with a piece of cotton. Repeat if necessary.

If the wax is particularly stubborn and resists the hydrogen peroxide, try softening it first with several applications of 3 or 4 drops of castor oil or glycerin. If the wax has become firmly impacted, however, you may find it necessary to have the ear cleaned by your doctor.

TREATMENT

In most cases of **conductive** hearing loss, once the underlying cause of the problem has been treated, hearing returns. With **sensorineural** hearing loss, however, the damage tends to be permanent. Treatment can sometimes stop or slow down the progression of the loss, but the quality of hearing seldom returns to what it was before the damage occurred.

CONVENTIONAL MEDICINE

Treatment of your hearing problem will depend on its underlying cause. If it is a simple case of wax buildup, your doctor will clean out your ear with a cotton-tipped probe or a suction device. If your ear is infected, you may be treated with oral ***antibiotics*** or with ear drops containing an antibiotic and ***hydrocortisone*** to help relieve the itching. If fluid created by a middle ear infection does not drain away naturally, your doctor may perform a myringotomy, a procedure in which a small incision is made in the eardrum and the fluid is sucked out.

Repeated attacks of middle ear infections, as well as allergies, recurrent respiratory infections, and enlarged adenoids, can cause the eustachian tubes, which connect the pharnyx with the middle ear, to become blocked. The air pressure within the middle ear then drops, causing fluid to accumulate within the cavity and the eardrum to be sucked inward. This condition is relatively common among young children. Your child's doctor may recommend that a tiny plastic tube be inserted through the eardrum to balance the air pressure in the middle ear for six months or longer while the eustachian tubes recover.

Repeated middle ear infections can lead to other conditions that may require surgery to repair or replace damaged structures within the ear and help return hearing to normal. For example, a middle ear infection in rare cases can spread to an area of the bone behind the ear called the mastoid process, and a special operation known as a mastoidectomy becomes necessary to remove the damaged bone and restore hearing.

If your hearing loss is caused by a ruptured eardrum, your doctor will probably prescribe an ***antibiotic*** to make sure that no infection develops in the middle ear. In some cases, a plastic patch is placed over the eardrum to protect it while it heals. If after a period of three months the eardrum has not responded to this treatment, your doctor may suggest a minor operation in which a tiny piece of tissue, often from a vein, is grafted onto the eardrum. This surgery is usually successful and returns hearing to normal.

If your hearing loss is caused by **otosclerosis,** your doctor will probably recommend a stapedectomy, an operation in which the diseased bones of the ear are replaced with tiny metal substitutes. Studies have shown that stapedectomies improve hearing in 90 percent of cases. However, the operation also has its risks: About 2 percent to 5 percent of people who undergo the surgery become totally deaf in the affected ear.

Because it usually involves damage to nerves or to the inner ear, **sensorineural** hearing loss cannot be treated successfully with either antibiotics or surgery. Some sensorineural losses can be prevented, however, with prompt medical care. A sudden hearing loss caused by a tiny blood clot in the artery that feeds the ear, for example, can be treated with ***anticoagulants.*** Your physician might also prescribe a vasodilator, which causes the blood vessels to expand and allows the clot to pass. If these drugs are taken within 24 hours of the first sign of the hearing loss and if the loss is partial, a full recovery is quite likely.

For **presbycusia** and other kinds of permanent hearing loss, the only method of treatment is a hearing aid, a device that contains a tiny microphone and amplifier to increase the volume of sound electrically. The hearing aid is powered by a tiny battery that lasts several months. Some hearing aids are worn behind the ear, although compact models that fit within the outer ear canal are now more common.

A hearing aid will not make your hearing problem go away, but it will improve your ability to hear. Be sure you are fitted by a qualified professional. Your doctor should be able to recommend a reputable audiologist or hearing-aid dealer, who will give you a hearing-aid evaluation and let you try several different kinds of devices. To ensure an exact fit and good performance, a mold will be made of your ear canal. Give yourself some time to get used to the aid, but if it is uncomfortable or does not seem to improve your hearing, take it back for a refund or an exchange. A reputable hearing-aid dealer should give you a trial period before the sale becomes final.

ACUPRESSURE

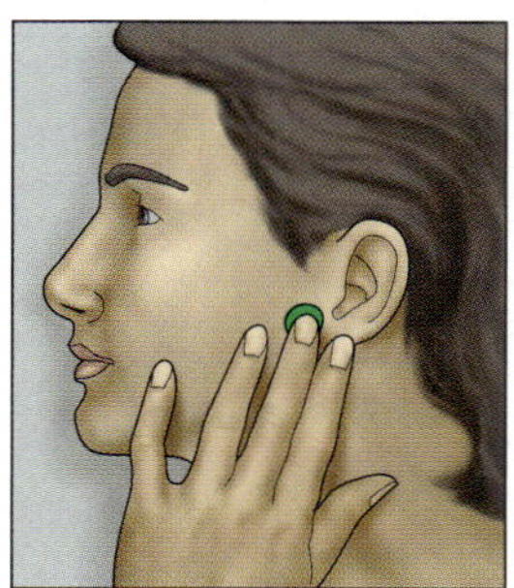

1 Pressing Gall Bladder 2 may help enhance hearing. Open your mouth and find the depression just in front of your ears. Place the tips of your middle fingers at the base of this depression, then slide them down a half-inch and close your mouth; your fingers should be on GB 2. Press for one minute, three to five times.

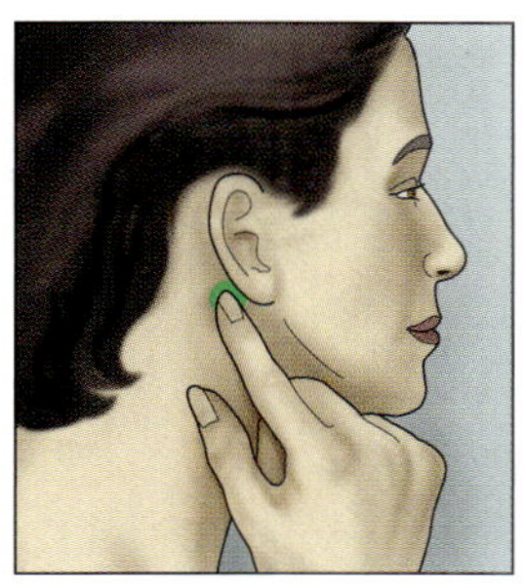

2 Hearing difficulty may also be eased by pressing Triple Warmer 17, located behind your earlobes. Using the tips of your index fingers, find the hollows behind the earlobes where your ears meet your jawbone—the TW 17 point. Press lightly for two minutes while breathing deeply, then release.

A small number of people with profound deafness have benefited from an operation known as a cochlear implant. Very thin wires, called electrodes, are implanted in the cochlea, the spiral-shaped area of the inner ear. One end of each electrode is connected to the auditory nerve, the other end to a small battery-powered speech processor and microphone, which are worn outside the ear. The microphone and processor convert sounds into electrical impulses that travel along the electrodes and stimulate the auditory nerve, which then sends the impulses to the brain. Although promising, cochlear implants have thus far had only limited success. Most people who have had the surgery report that the device improves their lipreading skills but does not enable them to understand speech without lipreading.

ALTERNATIVE CHOICES

As with conventional treatment, alternative therapies primarily address underlying problems that may be causing temporary hearing loss.

YOGA

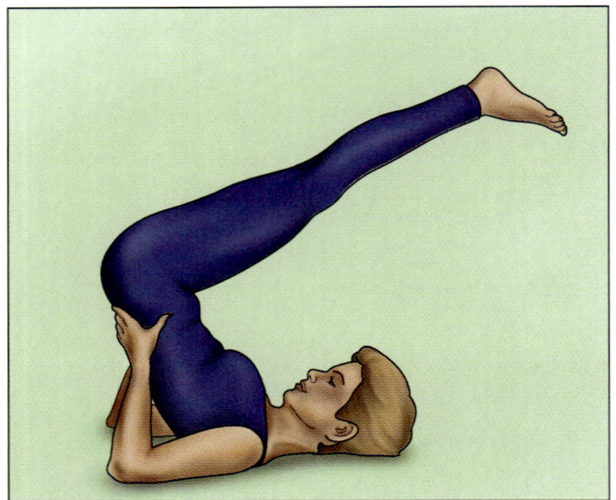

1 For the **Half Shoulder Stand,** lie on your back and bring your knees toward your forehead, supporting your hips with your hands. Inhale and extend your legs, keeping them at a right angle to your back *(above).* Take a few deep breaths, then exhale and lower your legs.

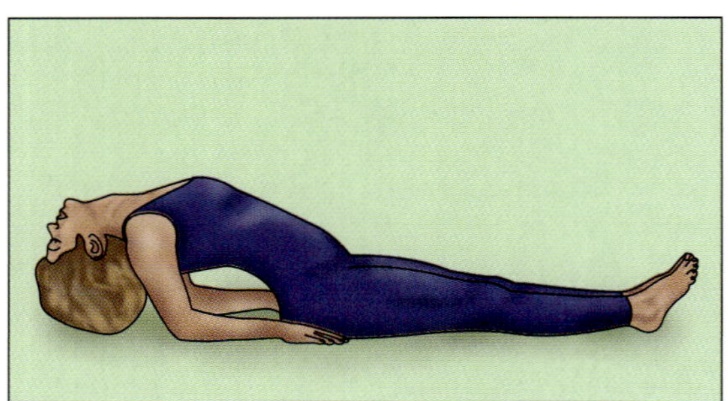

2 To do the **Fish,** lie on your back with your arms along your sides, palms down. Inhale and arch your back and neck, keeping your buttocks on the floor. Support your weight with your hips and elbows *(above).* Hold for 15 seconds, breathing deeply, then exhale and relax.

ACUPUNCTURE

Acupuncture cannot restore hearing lost as a result of permanent damage to the nerves or hearing mechanisms of the ear. However, in some cases it may help patients to discriminate better among the sounds they can hear. Acupuncture may also be used to help treat ear infections that may be causing temporary hearing problems. Consult a professional acupuncturist.

HERBAL THERAPIES

Several herbs may help heal ear infections that might lead to hearing problems. ***Garlic*** *(Allium sativum),* which has been shown to act as a natural antibiotic, is considered very effective. Put 1 to 2 drops of garlic oil in your ear three times daily. You can buy the oil in a health food store or make your own: Slice several garlic cloves and put them in 1 oz of olive oil for up to seven days; strain and store in the refrigerator, being sure to warm the oil before using.

Herbalists also recommend ***ginger*** *(Zingiber officinale),* another natural antibiotic, both in tincture and in tea form. To make ginger tea, put 1 tbsp of the fresh root in 1 cup boiling water; let simmer for 10 minutes. Drink several times a day.

The anti-inflammatory properties of either ***echinacea*** (*Echinacea* spp.) or ***goldenseal*** *(Hydrastis canadensis)* may help heal an ear infection. You can take either herb in tincture form (15 to 20 drops three times a day) or as a tea. To make the tea, pour a cup of boiling water over 1 to 2 tsp of the dried herb; let steep for 10 to 15 minutes. Drink three times a day.

Ginkgo *(Ginkgo biloba),* which has been shown to improve circulation, is sometimes recommended for inner ear disturbances and partial deafness. It is available in herb stores in a variety of forms; the recommended dosage is 40 mg of the dried herb or 1 to 2 tsp of the liquid extract three times a day.

HOMEOPATHY

For acute or chronic hearing problems, homeopaths recommend a variety of medications. Consult an experienced practitioner for specific remedies and dosages.

NUTRITION AND DIET

In some cases, hearing may be improved by reducing salt, which can cause fluids to be retained in the ear, where they can press against the hearing mechanism. If you are prone to repeated ear infections, avoid dairy products, white sugar, and white flour; some alternative practitioners believe these foods create excess, thicker mucus in the body. Some evidence indicates that ***vitamin A*** (5,000 to 10,000 IU a day) and **vitamin B complex** supplements may help hearing loss, particularly if the condition is accompanied by ***tinnitus,*** a ringing or roaring sensation in the ears.

YOGA

The Half Shoulder Stand and Fish positions *(opposite)* may help some forms of hearing loss by increasing the circulation of blood to the ears.

PREVENTION

- ◆ Wear earplugs if you are exposed to noise levels that may be harmful to your ears. Cotton balls are not sufficient, as they do not block enough sound; they can also become lodged deep in the ear canal.
- ◆ Do not listen to loud music with earphones.
- ◆ If you are at a concert and the music hurts your ears, put on earplugs or leave immediately. The overamplified sound may cause permanent damage.
- ◆ Educate your children about the danger of loud recreational noise.
- ◆ If you ride a subway, wear earplugs or cover your ears with your hands as the trains pass. The roar of the trains can damage your ears.
- ◆ To lower the risk of infectious diseases that may lead to permanent hearing loss, make sure your children receive all of their immunizations.
- ◆ If your ears tend to get severely blocked with wax frequently, clean them periodically with hydrogen peroxide *(box, page 444).*
- ◆ Be sure to report any sudden hearing loss to your doctor immediately.

AIR TRAVEL DEAFNESS

If you fly with a stuffy nose, you may experience a condition known as aerotitis media, or barotrauma—a pushing in of the eardrum due to the sudden increase in air pressure in the plane's cabin as the plane descends. Any blockage in the eustachian tubes makes it impossible for air to pass through the tubes into the middle ear, where it would normally balance the air pushing on the eardrum from the outer ear canal. The condition is painful and usually results in some degree of temporary hearing loss. You may also feel dizzy and experience ***tinnitus,*** *a ringing sensation in your ears. The symptoms usually go away completely in a few hours, but sometimes a myringotomy, a procedure that involves a small incision in the eardrum, becomes necessary.*

If you must travel with a cold or sinus infection, take the following preventive steps:

- ◆ *Use a nasal decongestant or antihistamine an hour before takeoff and again an hour before landing.*
- ◆ *Suck on candy or chew gum to promote swallowing and help unblock the eustachian tubes.*
- ◆ *Take a deep breath through your mouth, hold your nose, and then blow out gently while keeping your mouth closed. This can help force air through your eustachian tubes.*
- ◆ *Take the homeopathic remedy* ***Kali bichromicum*** *in 6c or 30c potency at half-hour intervals during your flight, starting a half-hour before boarding the plane. This treatment is especially effective with young children.* ■

H

HEART ARRHYTHMIAS

SYMPTOMS

Keep in mind that occasional, isolated disturbances of the heartbeat are common and usually harmless. Signs of more serious arrhythmias include the following:

For **tachycardia,** or abnormally rapid heartbeat:

- recurrent palpitations, defined as an uncomfortable awareness of your heartbeat. The palpitations may take the form of a strong pulse in the neck, a "flip-flopping" heart, or a fluttering, thumping, pounding, or racing beat in the chest.
- chest discomfort, weakness, fainting, sweating, shortness of breath, confusion, or dizziness.

For **bradycardia,** or abnormally slow heartbeat:

- fatigue, shortness of breath, lightheadedness, or loss of consciousness.

CALL YOUR DOCTOR IF:

- you experience irregular heartbeats that are recurrent or produce discomfort. Any sustained or intense arrhythmia should be investigated to determine its severity.
- while taking drugs to treat one form of arrhythmia, you notice a new pattern of irregular heartbeat. Some antiarrhythmic drugs may actually worsen the original heart condition.
- while taking antiarrhythmic medication, you experience side effects such as dizziness, vomiting, nausea, blurred vision, ringing in the ears, diarrhea, loss of appetite, or loss of consciousness. A new prescription will often correct the problem.

H

The healthy heart is a marvel of efficiency, pumping approximately five quarts of blood through the body every minute by means of regular, forceful contractions of its four chambers. Each perceived thump of the heart actually consists of two beats, one by the upper chambers, or atria, and one by the lower chambers, or ventricles. The contractions are triggered by electrical impulses originating in the sinus node, a specialized group of cells located in the heart's right atrium.

Any disturbance in the normal beating pattern of the heart is called an arrhythmia, or irregular heartbeat. Practically everyone experiences some version of an arrhythmia on occasion, usually in the form of a mild palpitation or a "skipped" heartbeat. (In fact, what feels like a skipped beat is really an early beat, weak enough not to be felt, then a one- or two-second pause, followed by a relatively forceful beat; the delay between beats feels like a skip.) Mild, isolated disturbances of this sort are normally harmless. A recurrent arrhythmia, on the other hand, should be checked by a physician.

There are two main categories of arrhythmia: **tachycardia,** meaning too fast a heartbeat, and **bradycardia,** meaning too slow a heartbeat. (Both conditions refer only to exceptional elevations or depressions of heart rate, not to the normal variance that occurs throughout the day depending on whether you are resting or active.) At rest, the heart beats somewhere between 60 and 100 times per minute. Tachycardia is defined as more than 100 beats per minute, while bradycardia is defined as fewer than 60 beats per minute. Both tachycardia and bradycardia can occur in surges or as persistent conditions.

Most arrhythmias fall into the tachycardia category. Some originate in the atria, some in the ventricles. Ventricular arrhythmias are typically more serious conditions. In fact, most cases of sudden cardiac death are due to ventricular arrhythmias, not ***heart attack,*** as was once thought. Particularly dangerous is **ventricular fibrillation,** in which activity within the ventricles is so uncoordinated that the ventricles are reduced to twitching, and virtually no pumping takes place. Ventricular fibrillation will cause death within a few minutes unless interrupted.

YOUR NATURAL PACEMAKER

Your heartbeat starts with electrical impulses from the sinus node, a group of cells in the right atrium. The impulses travel along pathways in the right and left atria, causing the atria to contract. The impulses continue to the ventricles, slowing briefly in the atrioventricular node. The ventricles contract just after the atria, and the coordinated contractions maintain a constant flow of blood.

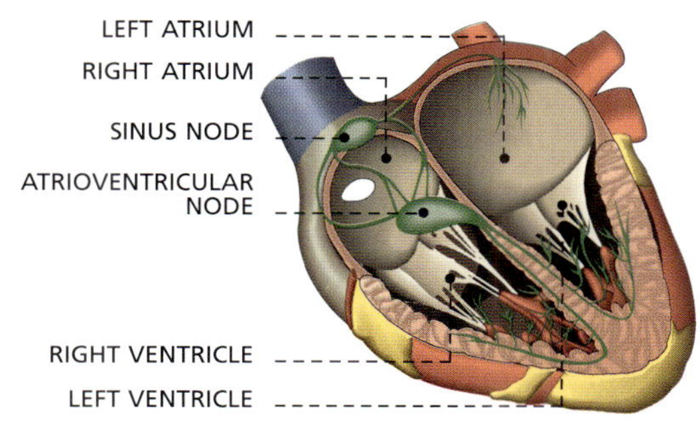

Bradycardias can be due to problems with nerves that control heartbeat, with the sinus node, where the heart's electrical impulses originate, or with actual transmission of those impulses through the heart. In the latter condition, known as **heart block,** electrical signals fail to reach the ventricles from the atria because of some conduction problem. Signals may be blocked continuously or intermittently. In a worst-case scenario, electrical activity within the heart shuts down completely and beating stops.

CAUSES

Any condition that affects the structure of the heart muscle or its valves or that alters electrical activity within the heart is likely to interfere with regular heartbeat. As might be expected, many forms of ***heart disease*** cause arrhythmia. Severe coronary heart disease is a frequent trigger; it produces scar tissue in the heart that can disrupt the transmission of electrical signals. Congenital heart defects, heart muscle disease, heart valve disorders, and other diseases such as lung conditions or hyperthyroidism may also produce arrhythmias. External forces such as electric shock or severe chest injury have also been known to trigger arrhythmias.

Ventricular arrhythmias most often stem from heart disease and are anticipated complications of heart attack. Atrial arrhythmias are also generally associated with heart disease, but may have other causes or no apparent cause. Atrial fibrillation is frequently associated with ***high blood pressure.*** Many bradycardias are associated with heart block.

A dysfunction in the autonomic nervous system (which regulates all involuntary bodily functions, including heartbeat) may also cause arrhythmias. Effective control by the autonomic nervous system depends on a fine balance between sympathetic nerves, which tell functions of the body to speed up, and parasympathetic nerves, which tell them to slow down. Sometimes ***stroke*** upsets the balance, and arrhythmia may result.

A sudden infusion of certain chemicals or hormones into the bloodstream can also disturb heart rate. Many drugs, including caffeine, nicotine, alcohol, cocaine, and inhaled aerosol propellants, can cause heart rate to race or become otherwise irregular. The same may occur in response to conditions that boost adrenaline (also known as ***epinephrine***), such as shock, fright, and anxiety.

DIAGNOSTIC AND TEST PROCEDURES

An ECG reading of the heart's electrical activity provides the most accurate confirmation of arrhythmia. However, the ECG test is useful only when the arrhythmia occurs during testing, which often is not the case. To detect a suspected arrhythmia, a patient may be sent home wearing a Holter monitor. This portable device records the heart's electrical activity over a 24-hour period.

Tests that provoke arrhythmias make diagnosis easier. Exercising on a treadmill, for example, may induce an arrhythmia that is normally triggered by exertion.

Electrophysiologic testing is also useful in the diagnosis of arrhythmia. Tiny electrode catheters—introduced through veins or arteries and positioned at various points in the heart—record the transmission of electrical signals. The "electrical map" produced by the catheter readings diagrams the location, direction, and speed of signals, so that doctors can determine where the problem is originating or where signals may be getting blocked.

TREATMENT

Once an arrhythmia is confirmed, your doctor will decide whether the condition is serious enough to merit medical or surgical treatment. Treatment decisions depend not only on the type of arrhythmia but also on the patient's age, physical condition, and history of heart disease.

H

CONVENTIONAL MEDICINE

For mild conditions, your doctor will suggest some things that you can do to control the arrhythmia *(see **At-Home Remedies**).* If necessary, medication is prescribed. A doctor bases the prescription on the type of arrhythmia, patient medical history, and the presence of other heart disease. Those drugs specifically categorized as antiarrhythmic—including quinidine, amiodarone, and also ***digitalis preparations***—tend to be quite potent and can cause serious side effects. They are often administered in conjunction with electrophysiologic testing to determine whether they will be effective and not cause an adverse reaction.

Application of electric shock to break an arrhythmia and restore normal heart rate is often used in emergencies; patients are then treated with drugs. Electric shock therapy might also be used if a patient fails to respond to medication or if a doctor anticipates an emergency because of another existing heart condition.

Sometimes, implantable devices are used to control arrhythmic conditions for the long term. People with symptomatic bradycardia usually wear implanted pacemakers. Anyone prone to ventricular tachycardias might wear a cardioverter defibrillator, an implantable electrode patch that provides automatic shock therapy when needed. People subject to both tachycardia and bradycardia may be fitted with a pacemaker defibrillator, a device that can both restore normal heart rate by means of electric shock and maintain heart rate at a healthy, steady pace.

More invasive treatments are occasionally necessary. If a region of heart tissue is responsible for an arrhythmia, a technique known as catheter ablation may be used to correct the problem: Radio waves from a device inserted via a vein or artery literally zap the responsible area of heart tissue, putting it out of commission. In some cases, open-heart surgery to remove heart tissue may be called for.

ALTERNATIVE CHOICES

For emergency treatment and long-term prevention of severe arrhythmias, you should see a cardiologist. Alternative therapies may be able to complement, but should not replace, standard treatment of serious heart conditions. You may find that with the added support of alternative medicine, you are able to lessen your dependence on antiarrhythmic drugs. You may also discover that alternative options suffice in controlling mild arrhythmias.

AROMATHERAPY

Citrus oils, added to bathwater, may help quell minor palpitations. Try a few drops of orange flower oil, also called neroli oil.

CHINESE HERBS

Numerous Chinese herbal combinations treat symptoms of arrhythmia, but some herbs—such as ***ephedra*** *(Ephedra sinica)*—can actually worsen the condition. Be sure to consult a qualified herbalist, and tell your doctor of any herbs you may be taking for other problems.

HERBAL THERAPIES

Many herbs contain components that strengthen heartbeat and steady heart rate. Some, such as foxglove *(Digitalis purpurea),* are too potent to be used by the layperson. ***Hawthorn*** *(Crataegus laevigata),* a gentle yet effective herb for treating heart conditions, is most appropriate for home use. Hawthorn dilates vessels and stimulates the heart muscle, which can help stabilize arrhythmias. Take 5 drops of the tincture, 3 or 4 times a day.

HOMEOPATHY

Homeopathic medicine offers remedies for both immediate and long-term treatment of mild arrhythmias. ***Lachesis,*** *Digitalis,* and ***Aconite*** are among the remedies used to control palpitations. Consult a homeopathic physician for dosages.

LIFESTYLE

Heart rate rises in response to exercise, then typically resettles at a lower rate. Nonexercisers tend to have resting heart rates around 80 beats per minute, while exercisers average between 60 and 65 beats per minute. Exercise also helps get rid of excess adrenaline, a hormone that excites the heart along with the rest of the body.

Nicotine from smoking is a stimulant and may provoke arrhythmias in susceptible people. If you have been diagnosed with tachycardia and you smoke, you should quit.

MIND/BODY MEDICINE

Relaxation techniques can help prevent or control some arrhythmias by reducing stress, which elevates heart rate and can trigger certain heartbeat disturbances. Any number of activities, ranging from exercise to **meditation** and **yoga,** might help you relax. Find what works best for you and stick with it; the benefit of relaxation training takes time to be realized.

NUTRITION AND DIET

The minerals ***calcium, magnesium,*** and ***potassium*** play a crucial role in moderating heart activity. Too little of these minerals can cause arrhythmias. (And too much can also be a problem, especially with calcium.) Magnesium administered intravenously can correct tachycardia and many other arrhythmias. You can get magnesium from nuts, beans, soybeans, bran, dark green vegetables, and fish. Many fruits and vegetables supply potassium. Be aware that you can deplete your stores of magnesium and potassium by ingesting too much salt or saturated fat, as well as by overusing diuretics or laxatives.

A COLD SPLASH IN THE FACE

Have you ever wondered how sea lions survive the shock of diving into frozen waters? Like other mammals, they are protected by an automatic nervous response that immediately slows heart rate. Humans also have this nervous response, which may be particularly significant to you if you suffer occasional bouts of tachycardia. Next time an attack occurs, try plunging your face into a basin of cold water. Your heart rate will temporarily plummet, which may serve to break the tachycardia.

AT-HOME REMEDIES

- To control an attack of tachycardia, the best remedy is rest. Take a deep breath and relax.
- Gentle pressure to the prominent carotid artery on the right side of the neck may help break an attack of tachycardia. Ask your doctor to show you how and where to press.
- For atrial arrhythmias, try the "vagal maneuver." Sit down, bend forward at the waist, then hold your breath and strain as if blowing up a balloon. In so doing, you switch control from the sympathetic nervous system, which speeds bodily functions, to the parasympathetic nervous system, which slows them.

PREVENTION

Limit your use of caffeine, nicotine, alcohol, and stimulant drugs, all of which can speed heart rate. If you have a history of tachycardia, you should avoid these substances altogether. Reduce stress through exercise, meditation, or any other technique that works for you. If you have a heart condition, take proper steps to control it; this may also prevent or control arrhythmia. ■

HEART ATTACK

SYMPTOMS

- a prolonged crushing, squeezing, or burning pain in the center of the chest. The pain may radiate to the neck, one or both arms, or the jaw.
- shortness of breath, dizziness, nausea, chills, sweating, weak pulse.
- cold and clammy skin, gray pallor, a severe appearance of illness.
- fainting. (In about 1 case in 10, this is the only indication that a heart attack is in progress.)

H

CALL YOUR DOCTOR IF:

- you or someone you are with manifests signs of a heart attack. **Seek emergency help without delay.**
- you suffer from ***angina*** (chest pain) and begin to experience pain that is similar but does not respond to medication; this may indicate that a heart attack is under way.
- your angina attacks become more frequent, prolonged, and severe; as angina worsens, the risk of heart attack increases.
- you are taking ***aspirin*** to prevent heart attack and your stool appears black and tarry. This could be a sign that aspirin has thinned your blood too much, a problem that can and should be corrected. *(See also **Heart Attack,** page 67,* in ***Emergencies/ First Aid.****)*

In order to keep pumping, day in and day out, the heart requires its own constant supply of oxygen and nutrients. Two large, branching coronary arteries deliver oxygenated blood to the heart muscle. Should one of these arteries or branches shut down, a portion of the heart is starved of oxygen and fuel, a condition called **ischemia.** If an ischemic attack lasts too long, the starved heart tissue dies. This event defines heart attack, otherwise known as myocardial infarction—literally, "death of heart muscle."

Most attacks last for several hours. (But never wait to seek help if you think an attack is beginning.) The signs of the heart attack may be no more than shortness of breath, faintness, or nausea; and in some cases there are no symptoms. But most heart attacks produce some pain. The pain of a severe attack has been likened to a giant fist enclosing and squeezing the heart; if the attack is mild, it may be mistaken for heartburn. The pain may be constant or intermittent.

The majority of heart attack victims are warned of trouble well in advance by episodes of ***angina***—chest pain that, like a heart attack, is provoked by ischemia. The difference is mainly one of degree: With angina, blood flow is quickly restored, pain recedes within minutes, and the heart is not permanently damaged; with heart attack, blood flow is critically reduced or fully blocked, pain lasts, and heart tissue dies.

About a third of all heart attacks occur without any previous warning signs. They are sometimes associated with a phenomenon known as **silent ischemia**—sporadic interruptions of blood flow to the heart that, for unknown reasons, are pain free, although they gradually damage the heart tissue. The condition can be detected by ECG testing. An estimated three to four million Americans may be afflicted with silent ischemia.

A third of all heart attack victims die before reaching a hospital; others suffer life-threatening complications while in the hospital. Serious complications include ***stroke,*** persistent ***heart arrhythmias,*** congestive heart failure, formation of ***blood clots*** in the legs or heart, and aneurysm in a weakened heart chamber. But those who survive the initial attack and are free from major problems a few hours later stand a better chance of full recovery.

Recovery is always a delicate process, because any attack weakens the heart to some degree. But generally, a normal life can be resumed within three months.

Heart disease remains the leading cause of death in the United States, with heart attack as the number one killer. But nothing is inevitable about those figures: Most forms of heart disease, including heart attack, are preventable.

CAUSES

Like earthquakes, many heart attacks occur as sudden catastrophes yet actually represent a culmination of events that have been proceeding beneath the surface for years. Most heart attacks are the end result of coronary heart disease, an atherosclerotic condition that clogs coronary arteries with fatty, calcified plaques. (As blood flow is gradually impeded, the body may compensate by growing a network of collateral arteries to circumvent blockages; the presence of collateral vessels may greatly reduce the amount of heart muscle damaged by a heart attack.) In the early 1980s, researchers confirmed that the precipitating cause of nearly all heart attacks is not the obstructive plaque itself, but the sudden formation of a blood clot on top of plaque that cuts off flow in an already narrowed vessel. Preliminary studies suggest that bacterial or viral infections may also be involved.

WHERE THE PAIN MAY BE

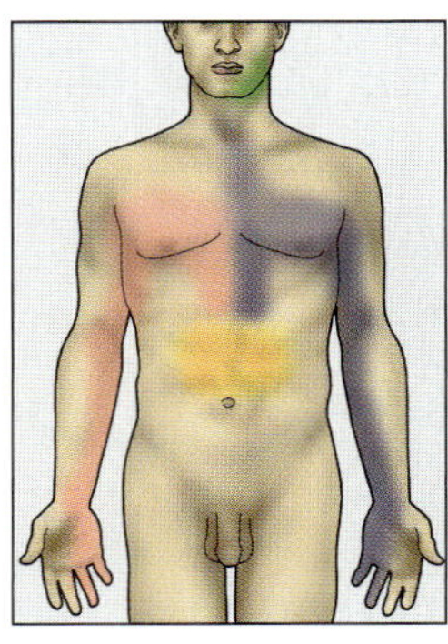

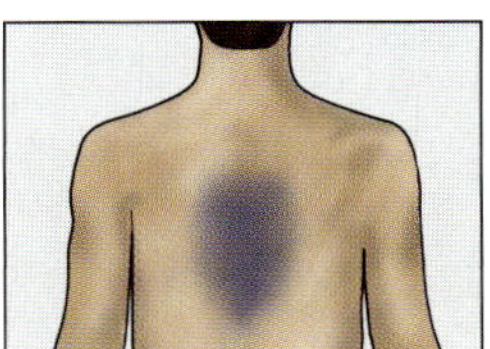

Heart attack pain can strike any of the areas shown at left. On the front of the body *(top),* the most likely sites are the center and left side of the chest, the neck, and the inside of the left arm *(blue).* Pain sometimes develops in the jaws *(green),* in the right chest and arm *(pink),* the shoulders, and in the area between the navel and breastbone *(yellow).* On the back *(bottom),* pain can occur between the shoulder blades *(blue).*

While the step-by-step process leading to heart attack is not fully understood, major risk factors are well-established. Some can be controlled. Of these, the main ones are ***high blood pressure,*** high ***cholesterol,*** obesity, smoking, and a sedentary lifestyle. ***Stress*** is also believed to raise the risk, and exertion and excitement can act as triggers for an attack.

Men over the age of 50 with a family history of heart disease are predisposed to heart attack. High levels of estrogen are thought to protect premenopausal women fairly well from heart attack, but risk increases significantly after menopause. Some women opt for hormone replacement therapy after menopause; the choice should be made with full knowledge that elevated estrogen levels also increase the risk for breast and uterine cancers. *(See **Menopausal Problems.**)*

DIAGNOSTIC AND TEST PROCEDURES

A cardiologist relies on various tests and scans to diagnose a heart attack and to identify sites of arterial blockage and tissue damage. ECG recordings of electrical activity within the heart, supported by blood tests, provide data for an initial assessment of the patient's condition. Images of the heart and coronary arteries supplied by angiograms and radioisotope scans locate specific areas of damage and blockage. With such data, the attending physician can pursue proper treatment and anticipate potential complications.

TREATMENT

Heart attack is a medical emergency that must be quickly addressed by conventional medicine. Alternative medicine cannot compete with standard drug and surgical therapy during the emergency and follow-up phases of heart attack treatment.

However, alternative medicine can make valuable contributions to prevention and recovery.

CONVENTIONAL MEDICINE

Heart attack victims are usually hospitalized in special coronary care units for at least 36 hours. Standard drug therapy includes a painkiller such as morphine, ***beta-adrenergic blocker*** drugs to calm the heart, and ***aspirin*** to reduce clotting activity. In some cases, clot-dissolving drugs like t-PA or streptokinase are also administered. These drugs are most effective if given within a few hours of heart attack onset. Emergency angioplasty, and possibly surgery, might be performed to remove a clot, reopen a clogged artery, or bypass blocked arteries.

Once past the critical phase, patients continue to receive beta blockers to calm the heart, ***pentoxifylline*** or ***nitrates*** to increase heart blood flow, and ***anticoagulants*** such as ***heparin, warfarin,*** or aspirin to prevent further clotting.

While hospitalized, heart attack patients are hooked to ECG machines for constant monitoring, in case heart rhythm abnormalities develop. If the heart starts beating too fast or too slow, various medications may be given. Some patients may be fitted with pacemakers. If a patient experiences a dangerous arrhythmia known as ventricular fibrillation, an electric shock to the chest is administered. Patients who show signs of congestive heart failure are given a variety of medications to decrease strain on the heart and to encourage the heart to beat more forcefully.

People recovering from a heart attack are urged to get back on their feet as quickly as possible, which reduces the chances of blood clots forming in the deep veins of the legs; the clots could travel through the circulatory system and lodge in the lung, creating a blockage. Gentle exercise is recommended, but nothing that requires significant exertion. Long-term recovery from heart attack requires psychological and lifestyle adjustments: Habits such as smoking, heavy drinking, and eating high-fat foods have to go.

As a preventive measure, most heart attack survivors take a daily aspirin tablet to thin the blood. Other drugs may also be prescribed.

TROUBLE FOR TYPE A

In 1964 Dr. Meyer Friedman and Dr. Ray Rosenman published an article in JAMA, the Journal of the American Medical Association, that launched a debate about personality and heart disease. They contended that people with certain traits are more likely to have heart attacks. These people fit a behavior pattern described as Type A: impatient, competitive, driven, achievement oriented, and quick-tempered. Their Type B counterparts are less hurried, more easygoing, and less easily riled.

Over the years, researchers have continued to test the theory. Some studies confirm Type A personality as a major risk factor for heart disease, while others conclude just the opposite. On balance, the data seem to favor a link between Type A personality and heart disease. The task now is to identify those traits that are most responsible for increased risk. Two traits seem particularly significant: the tendency to react with hostility to even minor irritations, and consistently high levels of stress-related hormones.

Some patients require invasive procedures to improve blood flow to the heart over the long term. The two most common procedures are angioplasty—a catheter technique that widens clogged arteries by splitting plaques—and coronary bypass surgery, which diverts blood flow around clogged arteries.

ALTERNATIVE CHOICES

HERBAL THERAPIES

Of the many herbs used to treat chronic heart

conditions, ***hawthorn*** *(Crataegus laevigata)* is perhaps most valuable; it dilates coronary arteries and is said to improve metabolic function within the heart. Hawthorn not only may help prevent heart attacks but also is thought to speed recovery from an attack. Numerous other herbs are used to treat conditions that increase the risk of heart attack. For more information, see ***High Blood Pressure, Blood Clots,*** and ***Cholesterol Problems.***

LIFESTYLE

Regular aerobic exercise greatly enhances efforts to prevent or recover from heart attack. If you already have a heart condition, schedule a stress test before beginning an exercise program in order to determine how much exertion is safe. Heart attack survivors are advised to exercise with other people rather than alone during the first months of recovery. Many community health and recreation centers offer physician-supervised cardiovascular rehabilitation programs.

MIND/BODY MEDICINE

Reducing stress by training the mind and body to relax may help prevent heart attack and can aid in recovery. Many techniques promote relaxation—among them, **meditation, biofeedback,** and **yoga.** Relaxation has also been shown to provide relief from pain, which may be encountered during the recovery period.

State of mind is another important consideration in heart attack recovery. People with a positive attitude about recovery tend to do much better than people who view themselves as "cardiac cripples." You may find that a particular mind/body technique helps you to focus on positive thoughts. You may also find, as many others have, that sharing thoughts and emotions with a support group is extremely beneficial.

NUTRITION AND DIET

The basic goals of a heart-healthy diet are to keep salt, sugar, and saturated fat to a minimum so as to reduce cholesterol, control blood pressure, and hold weight in check. Eating ***magnesium***-rich foods such as nuts, beans, bran, fish, and dark green vegetables may help prevent heart attack. Magnesium protects the heart directly and indirectly, by stabilizing heart rate, reducing coronary artery spasm, and combating such conditions as atherosclerosis and high blood pressure.

Much evidence suggests that unstable chemical compounds known as free radicals make the body more vulnerable to heart attack by striking the heart and coronary arteries and promoting atherosclerosis. Free radicals can be neutralized by antioxidants like ***vitamins A, C,*** and ***E.*** Fruits, vegetables, and grains supply many of the antioxidant vitamins.

Eating root vegetables such as carrots may also help prevent heart attack. These vegetables lower cholesterol over the long term and reduce blood-clotting activity.

AT-HOME REMEDIES

- Remember: Having a heart attack does not make you an invalid. You can best heal your heart by remaining active.
- Do not take birth-control pills if you have had a heart attack; they are linked to increased blood-clotting activity.
- Get a pet. Pet owners recover more quickly from heart attacks—probably because of reduced stress levels—and tend to live longer than people without pets.

PREVENTION

- Stay in touch with friends and family. Research shows that people with poor social support are more vulnerable to heart disease. Also, seek ways to control feelings of anger and hostility; these emotions may add to heart attack risk.
- Assess your heart attack risk profile and make appropriate changes to diet and lifestyle early.
- If you are at high risk for heart attack, have yourself tested regularly for silent ischemia.
- Talk with your doctor about taking an aspirin daily. Studies have shown that this regimen significantly reduces the risk of heart attack. ■

HEARTBURN

SYMPTOMS

- a burning feeling in the chest just behind the breastbone (the sternum) that occurs after eating and lasts a few minutes to several hours.
- ***chest pain,*** especially after bending over or lying down.
- burning in the throat—or hot, sour, or salty-tasting fluid at the back of the throat.
- belching.

H

CALL YOUR DOCTOR IF:

- you experience heartburn along with any of the following: difficulty swallowing, shortness of breath, sweating, dizziness, vomiting, diarrhea, extreme abdominal pain, fever, or black or bloodstained bowel movements. You may have a strangulated ***hiatal hernia, pancreatic problems, gastritis, stomach ulcers,*** or ***cancer.*** Or it could be a ***heart attack;* call for medical help now.**
- you take an ***antacid*** to relieve heartburn and do not feel relief within 15 minutes. This may also be a sign of a ***heart attack;* call for medical help now.**
- your heartburn is aggravated by exercise and relieved by rest. You may have ***heart disease.***
- you have chronic heartburn (daily or almost daily). Your esophagus is being repeatedly burned by stomach acid, which can lead to esophagitis, esophageal scarring, ***stomach ulcers,*** or ***cancer.***

Despite its name, heartburn has nothing to do with the heart. (Some of the symptoms, however, are similar to those of a ***heart attack*** or ***heart disease.***) It is an irritation of the esophagus that is caused by stomach acid. With gravity's help, a muscular valve called the lower esophageal sphincter, or LES, keeps stomach acid in the stomach. The LES is located where the esophagus meets the stomach—below the rib cage and slightly left of center. Normally it opens to allow food into the stomach or to permit belching; then it closes again. But if the LES opens too often or too far, stomach acid can reflux, or seep, into the esophagus and cause a burning sensation.

Occasional heartburn isn't dangerous, but chronic heartburn can indicate serious problems. Heartburn is a daily occurrence for 10 percent of Americans and 50 percent of pregnant women. It's an occasional nuisance for another 30 percent of the population.

CAUSES

The basic cause of heartburn is an underactive LES that doesn't tighten as it should. Two excesses often contribute: too much food in the stomach (overeating) or too much pressure on the stomach (frequently from ***obesity*** or pregnancy). Certain foods commonly relax the LES, including tomatoes, citrus fruits, garlic, onions, chocolate, coffee, alcohol, and peppermint. Dishes high in fats and oils (animal or vegetable) often lead to

CAUTION!

Antacids can mask or aggravate some ailments. Do not take antacids without consulting your doctor if you have high blood pressure, an irregular heartbeat, kidney disease, chronic constipation, diarrhea, colitis, any kind of intestinal bleeding, or any symptoms of appendicitis. Pregnant or nursing mothers should consult a physician before taking any medication, including antacids.

heartburn, as do certain medications, especially some ***antibiotics*** and ***aspirin***. ***Stress,*** which strains the nerves controlling the LES, can cause heartburn. And smoking, which relaxes the LES and stimulates stomach acid, is a major contributor.

DIAGNOSTIC AND TEST PROCEDURES

Your description of your symptoms may be all a doctor requires, but sometimes additional procedures are necessary. The esophagus can be viewed through an endoscope, a long, thin, flexible tube inserted through the mouth, or by x-ray. To determine if your heart is the cause of your symptoms, an electrocardiogram (ECG), a recording of the heart's electrical activity, may be taken.

THE MILK MYTH

Milk is not a remedy for heartburn. The soothing effect felt when drinking milk is deceiving; once in the stomach, milk's fat, calcium, and protein cause increased acid secretion and worsened heartburn. Mints are also often credited with alleviating heartburn, but they don't: Mint actually relaxes the LES, making heartburn more likely.

TREATMENT

Most physicians advocate antacids for occasional heartburn. Alternative practitioners rely on herbal remedies to reduce acid and relaxation therapies to lessen stress.

CONVENTIONAL MEDICINE

The primary objective is to identify the cause of the heartburn, so it can be avoided in the future. Over-the-counter ***antacids*** or ***bismuth subsalicylate*** is commonly prescribed to neutralize stomach acid. If antacids don't quell the symptoms, your doctor may suggest ***cimetidine, ranitidine,*** or ***omeprazole*** to reduce the stomach's production of acid, or cisapride or metoclopramide to make the stomach empty itself faster. When all else fails, surgery may be required to repair the LES, but this is relatively rare.

ALTERNATIVE CHOICES

For additional therapies, see ***Hiatal Hernia,*** a condition often accompanied by heartburn.

CHINESE HERBS

Taken once or twice, a tea made from 10 grams orange peel, 4 slices fresh ***ginger*** *(Zingiber officinale),* 10 grams poria *(Poria cocos),* 10 grams ***agastache*** *(Agastache rugosa),* and 3 grams ***licorice*** *(Glycyrrhiza uralensis)* may alleviate heartburn. If it doesn't, call your physician. This mixture should not be taken daily.

HERBAL THERAPIES

Slippery elm *(Ulmus fulva)* tea can diminish heartburn quickly, and ***chamomile*** *(Matricaria recutita)* tea's calming effects are especially helpful for stress-related heartburn.

HOMEOPATHY

Specific heartburn symptoms often respond well to homeopathic remedies. The dosage is 12x or 12c, taken every 15 minutes; repeat up to three times, then repeat the series once if needed. After eating spicy foods, take ***Nux vomica;*** after rich foods take *Carbo vegetabilis;* and for burning pain, take ***Arsenicum album.***

PREVENTION

Heartburn is often preventable. The keys are maintaining a reasonable weight, avoiding things that cause stomach acid to reflux into your esophagus *(see **Causes,** above),* getting adequate rest and exercise, and minimizing stress.

If you must lie down after eating, lie on your left side; your stomach is lower than your esophagus in this position. ■

H

HEART DISEASE

SYMPTOMS

The symptoms listed below apply to several types of heart condition. Bear in mind, however, that each type of heart disease has its own set of indicators; that most symptoms associated with heart disease could be caused by other conditions; and that some forms of heart disease may have no noticeable effects.

- tight, suffocating chest pain, often associated with ***angina*** and ***heart attack.***
- sharp, piercing chest pain, a common sign of **pericarditis.**
- sensations of fluttering, thumping, pounding, or racing of the heart, known as **palpitations.**
- shortness of breath.
- fluid retention in the legs, ankles, abdomen, lungs, or heart.
- lightheadedness, weakness, dizziness, or fainting spells.

CALL YOUR DOCTOR IF:

- you experience unusual chest pain, particularly if it persists or recurs. It may be heartburn, but it could also indicate a ***heart attack.***
- you experience recurrent disturbances of heartbeat *(**heart arrhythmias**).* If frequent or persistent, irregular heartbeats may signal a serious heart condition.
- you become suddenly dizzy, lightheaded, weak, or faint. Even if the cause is not heart disease, it could be serious.

See also ***Emergencies/First Aid*** entries on ***heart attack*** and ***cardiac and respiratory arrest.***

H

The human heart is built for amazing endurance—billions of beats in an average lifetime—but, like any other part of the body, it is vulnerable to breakdowns. Heart problems vary widely in their nature and severity. They may be transient or chronic, slow-developing or sudden, inconvenient or deadly. Some types of heart disease, closely linked to diet and lifestyle choices, are preventable; others are due to genetic inheritance, infections, or other uncontrollable factors. Two of every five Americans will ultimately die of heart disease; the daily toll is approximately 2,500 people. Fortunately, the death rate is declining steadily, thanks largely to improved medical care and widespread public education about risk factors.

Following is a list of the most common types of heart disease; see also individual entries for more specific information.

HEART ARRHYTHMIAS

Arrhythmias are disturbances in the heart's normal beating pattern. The irregularities occur in many forms, each with its own potential causes and treatments. Serious arrhythmias are a frequent consequence of other heart diseases but may also occur independently. *(See **Heart Arrhythmias.**)*

CORONARY HEART DISEASE

Coronary heart disease, the most common of all heart problems, is characterized by blockages in the coronary arteries that result in a reduction in blood flow to the heart muscle, depriving it of vital oxygen. Usually, the disease stems from ***atherosclerosis,*** an inflammatory condition sometimes called hardening of the arteries.

Severe coronary heart disease can lead to **congestive heart failure,** a general weakness of the heart that results in ineffective pumping action. Coronary heart disease can also result in painful episodes of ***angina*** or a ***heart attack*** or, in the worst case, sudden cardiac death.

While the exact causes of coronary heart disease are imperfectly understood, certain major risk factors have been identified. People with family histories of heart disease are at risk. Men are more apt to be affected than women, although neither sex is immune. Age is important:

PUMPING BLOOD

Oxygen-depleted blood enters the right atrium through the superior and the inferior vena cava and flows through the tricuspid valve to the right ventricle, then through the pulmonary valve and artery into the lungs. Oxygenated blood from the lungs enters the left atrium through the pulmonary veins, enters the left ventricle through the mitral valve, and is pumped back to the body through the aortic valve and aorta.

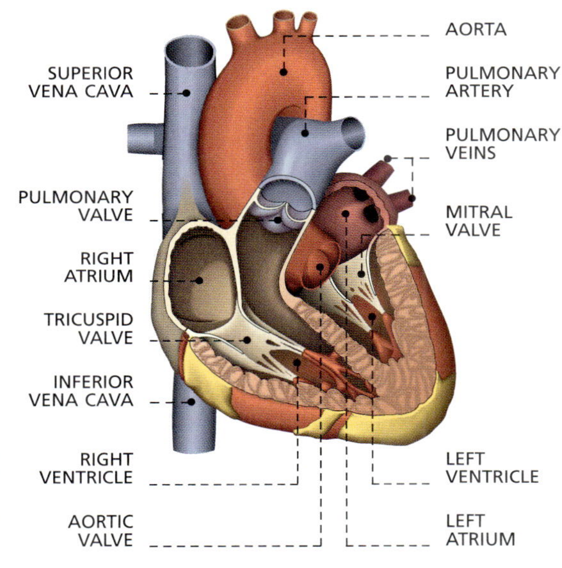

For both men and women, the likelihood of heart disease increases significantly after the age of 65. Diabetics are also more prone to heart disease. *(See **Diabetes.**)*

A number of risk factors can be mitigated or eliminated. People with ***high blood pressure*** and high blood levels of "bad" (LDL, or low-density lipoprotein) cholesterol are inclined to develop atherosclerosis and related conditions; but both blood pressure and cholesterol levels can often be moderated through proper diet and lifestyle choices. Smoking—also obviously a matter of choice—greatly increases the risk of heart disease because of the damaging effect that toxins in the smoke have on blood vessels. Nicotine also boosts heart rate, which takes a direct toll on the heart by forcing it to work harder; additionally, the chemical causes blood vessels to constrict, elevating blood pressure.

Obese people have a greater-than-average likelihood of developing heart disease. Their extra weight places added strain on the heart and blood vessels. In addition, obese people tend to have high cholesterol; this may be due partially to dietary choices, but is also tied to the fact that obesity is associated with abnormal fat metabolism.

Being sedentary increases risk, since exercise has a protective effect on the heart and blood vessels. People who exercise regularly tend to be trimmer and to have lower blood pressure and higher levels of "good" (HDL, or high-density lipoprotein) cholesterol. For many people, exercise also acts to reduce ***stress***—another risk factor.

Medical researchers define stressful situations as those that arouse a fight-or-flight response—the body's physiological preparations to deal with a threat—yet allow for neither, thus generating feelings of anxiety, helplessness, and loss of control. Because stress is intangible, its effect on heart disease is difficult to quantify, but there is much evidence to suggest that persistent internalized stress—no matter what the cause—increases the chances of developing heart disease and may aggravate an existing heart condition.

HEART VALVE DISEASE

The heart has four valves: the pulmonary, mitral, tricuspid, and aortic. The valves open and close to permit blood flow between the heart's four chambers and connected blood vessels. A defective valve may fail either to open properly, obstructing blood flow, or to close properly, allowing blood leakage. Congenital heart disease and various inflammatory conditions are among the causes of valve disorders.

Valve disorders frequently involve the mitral and aortic valves, which control blood flow on the left side of the heart. The most common valve disorder is called **mitral valve prolapse:** Excess valve tissue interferes with the normal closing of the valve, causing leakage. In most people this is not a serious problem, but some individuals require medication or, in rare cases, surgery to prevent infection of the valve or excessive stress on the heart.

Endocarditis is an inflammatory condition that affects heart valves. This disease is an infection or inflammation of the endocardium, the innermost layer of heart tissue that lines the chambers and valves. It is usually caused by bacterial infection, with the staphylococcus and streptococcus bacteria as most likely culprits. Bacteria may enter the blood and take root in the heart during illness, after surgery, or as a result of intravenous drug use. Endocarditis tends to strike people with preexisting valve problems. The disease can be fatal if left untreated, but it can generally be cured with ***antibiotics.*** If heart valves are seriously damaged as a result of endocarditis, valve replacement surgery may be needed.

Rheumatic heart disease, another type of heart disease affecting valves, was very common earlier in this century but is now largely preventable with antibiotic treatment, although it still occurs. The disease stems from damage to the heart muscle and valves caused by ***rheumatic fever,*** which itself is associated with ***strep throat.*** Symptoms of rheumatic heart disease are usually delayed for many years, but if valves were damaged severely enough by the fever, they will eventually leak or impede proper blood flow.

Rheumatic heart disease generates characteristic heart murmurs that can be detected upon examination. Congestive heart failure and atrial fibrillation, a particular type of arrhythmia, are also common complications. In cases of severe rheumatic heart disease, valves must be either reopened or replaced surgically.

PERICARDIAL DISEASE

Any disease of the pericardium, the membranous sac surrounding the heart, is classified as pericardial disease. One of the more common is an inflammatory condition called **pericarditis.** It is usually caused by viral infection, a connective-tissue disease such as ***lupus*** or rheumatoid ***arthritis,*** or trauma to the pericardium. Pericarditis often follows open-heart surgery. Excess fluid buildup within the pericardium is a frequent symptom of the disease. Listening with a stethoscope, a doctor might detect the disease upon hearing a characteristic scratching sound called a pericardial rub. Acute cases are marked by fever and sharp pain in the center of the chest. Pericarditis often subsides on its own, but it also responds to anti-inflammatory drugs such as ***aspirin*** or, in severe cases, ***corticosteroid*** hormones. Occasionally, fluid must be drained from the pericardium.

PRIMARY MYOCARDIAL DISEASE

Diseases of the heart muscle, or myocardium, are collectively referred to as primary myocardial disease, or **cardiomyopathy.** When diseased, the myocardium becomes abnormally stretched, thickened, or stiff. Among the many potential causes of cardiomyopathy are connective-tissue diseases, genetic heart conditions, metabolic disorders, reactions to certain drugs or toxins such as alcohol, and viral infections. Often, the precise cause of cardiomyopathy is unknown. In any event, either the myocardium becomes too weak to pump efficiently, or stiffening prevents filling of the heart. Symptoms can include chest pain, shortness of breath, swelling of the feet and ankles, and lightheadedness. When cardiomyopathy progresses to the point of causing serious arrhythmias or congestive heart failure, the outlook for long-term survival is poor. Sudden death is another outcome associated with some cardiomyopathies, including **idiopathic hypertrophic subaortic stenosis,** which has claimed the lives of a number of prominent young professional athletes. If cardiomyopathy can be detected and treated early enough, either with drugs or with transplant surgery, symptoms can often be controlled and heart failure averted for many years.

CONGENITAL HEART DISEASE

Should anything go awry in the formation of the heart during prenatal development, a baby will be born with one or more congenital heart defects. Such defects are quite common, occurring in about 7 of every 1,000 babies.

The exact causes of defects are generally hard to pin down; genes and environmental factors inside the mother's body may both contribute. Chromosome abnormalities, including the one that causes Down syndrome, have been linked to many congenital heart defects. Infections contracted during pregnancy by the mother, such as ***German measles,*** may also result in congenital heart disease for the child.

Congenital heart defects range widely in their effects. Some are apparent immediately, but others do not produce noticeable symptoms until adulthood. Minor conditions often clear up on their own, while the most severe conditions cannot be corrected and are fatal. Fortunately, many congenital heart defects can be treated surgically, if necessary.

Among the most common types are **septal defects,** or holes in the wall dividing the left and right sides of the heart. If a septal defect is big enough to cause problems, it can be patched surgically. Another frequently seen defect is **pulmonary stenosis,** a condition in which one of the four heart valves—the pulmonary valve—is so narrow that blood flow to the lungs is restricted; with surgery, the valve can be pried open or replaced. In some babies, a small blood vessel known as the ductus arteriosus fails to close at birth as it should. This condition, known as **patent ductus arteriosus,** allows some blood that is headed for the body via the aorta to leak back into the pulmonary artery, placing the heart under added strain. This problem can also be corrected surgically.

Some so-called blue babies are born with a combination of four heart defects, which basically results in oxygen-poor blood flow to body tissues. The excess of deoxygenated blood gives the baby a bluish tinge. Unless treated, most people with this condition would not survive to middle age. However, surgery successfully corrects the condition 90 percent of the time.

THE RISKS FOR WOMEN

A 50-year-old woman arrives in the emergency room complaining of severe chest pain and difficulty breathing. The attending physician orders tests and eventually finds that the patient's coronary arteries are smooth and free of clots. In medical parlance, this patient is said to have Syndrome X—a condition that presents the classic symptoms of angina or heart attack without the classic cause, coronary artery blockage.

Until recently, cardiologists had done little to explain Syndrome X. (It is still under study, but one theory holds that it is caused by circulation problems in small vessels of the heart.) Lack of interest stemmed in part from lack of concern: Nearly two-thirds of Syndrome X patients are women, and traditionally women were thought to get heart disease only rarely. However, statistical evidence is challenging that notion—and changing attitudes about women and heart disease.

Among other things, the evidence indicates that heart disease is the number one killer of American women. Half of all American women eventually die of heart disease, and six times as many die of heart attacks annually as succumb to breast cancer.

Women tend not to display the textbook symptoms of heart disease—most likely a result of the fact that most of the textbooks are based on all-male studies. It also turns out that some traditional diagnostic and treatment tools (such as exercise stress tests) do not work as well for women as for men. And the death rate for women who have undergone coronary bypass surgery is twice as high as that for men, probably because women's blood vessels are smaller. However, the same risk factors (such as smoking and high blood pressure) apply to both sexes.

Syndrome X, then, is but one of the challenges confronting doctors in their efforts to address the special problems women face when it comes to heart disease.

DIAGNOSTIC AND TEST PROCEDURES

In diagnosing heart disease, a doctor first asks a patient for a description of symptoms. The patient's general physical condition is assessed through a standard medical examination and history taking. Listening to the heart for swishing or whooshing sounds, collectively known as **heart murmurs,** may provide important clues about heart trouble. If heart disease is suspected, further tests are done to find out what is actually happening inside the heart. An electrocardiogram, or ECG, is usually the first test to be performed. By recording electrical activity within the heart, the ECG quickly reveals any electrical abnormalities in the heart that may be a source of trouble. Further details can be garnered by imaging the heart, using x-rays, a variety of scans, or angiography, a special technique that allows for x-rays of blood vessels.

TREATMENT

With heart disease, conventional and alternative medicines each have their own strengths. When used as complements to each other, they can provide the best possible prevention and treatment of heart disease.

CONVENTIONAL MEDICINE

Conventional medical care—discussed above and in specific entries elsewhere in this book—is essential once heart disease begins to produce noticeable symptoms. Conventional care aims to stabilize the condition immediately, to control symptoms over the long term, and to provide a cure when possible. While appropriate changes to diet and lifestyle are always recommended, the mainstays of conventional care are drugs and surgery.

ALTERNATIVE CHOICES

The strong suit of alternative medicine is prevention. Natural therapies that focus on diet, nutrition, herbalism, and purification of the body through exercise, stress reduction, and detoxification can significantly reduce the body's vulnerability to certain types of heart disease, although some cannot be prevented. Several alternative therapies are also beneficial complements to the conventional treatment of heart disease.

BODY WORK

Since all forms of body work help the body to relax, any of them might be applicable to prevention and control of heart disease. The reason is simple: Relaxation reduces stress, and stress has been identified as a likely risk factor for coronary heart disease. You can put yourself in the hands of a body work therapist, or you can teach yourself **yoga** or **qigong.** See also **Mind/Body Medicine,** opposite.

YOGA

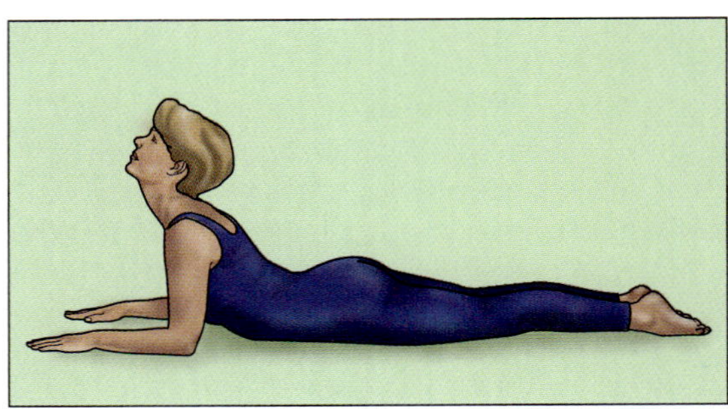

Use the **Sphinx** to reduce stress. Lie on the floor. Place both forearms on the floor with your palms down and your elbows directly under your shoulders. Inhale and push your chest away from the floor as far as comfortably possible without lifting your elbows. Hold for 20 to 30 seconds; then exhale, release, and relax.

CHELATION THERAPY

Chelation therapy is sought annually by thousands of Americans who suffer from angina and atherosclerosis. Advocates claim that it is safer and cheaper than, and as effective as, many conventional drug or surgical treatments. Critics contend that while chelation therapy is useful in treating certain conditions, cardiovascular disease is not necessarily one of them. See ***Atherosclerosis*** for a fuller explanation of chelation therapy.

CHINESE MEDICINE

Practitioners of traditional Chinese medicine generally view heart disease as arising from heart weakness or blocked energy flow. Depending on the symptoms, standard treatment would involve prescribed herbal remedies plus massage, **acupuncture,** and dietary recommendations.

CHIROPRACTIC

While chiropractic medicine is inappropriate for acute care of heart conditions, it shares with conventional medicine many long-term treatment aspects. A chiropractic physician would recommend suitable diet and lifestyle changes, and would also perform skeletal manipulation when appropriate. Some studies indicate that regular chiropractic manipulation can reduce hypertension.

HERBAL THERAPIES

The plant world is full of herbs that can affect the heart. The therapeutic properties of some have been rigorously documented. The effects of others, such as motherwort *(Leonurus cardiaca)* and linden flower (*Tilia* spp.), are not as well researched yet perhaps no less valid. Certain herbs, such as foxglove *(Digitalis purpurea)* and lily of the valley *(Convallaria majalis),* contain compounds called cardiac glycosides that make them particularly potent. Because of their potentially dangerous side effects, they should be administered only by a qualified medical herbalist. Many of the gentler "heart" herbs do not contain cardiac glycosides yet still improve cardiovascular function. The most noteworthy of these is ***hawthorn*** *(Crataegus laevigata).* Any herbal treatment of the heart should be supervised by a medical herbalist and approved by your doctor. For further herbal recommendations, see ***Atherosclerosis, Cholesterol Problems, Circulatory Problems,*** and ***High Blood Pressure.***

HOMEOPATHY

Homeopathic remedies may complement, but should not replace, prescribed medication for chronic heart conditions. A homeopath would provide a constitutional remedy based on the manifest symptoms of heart disease, plus other characteristic symptoms such as food preferences, sleep patterns, mood, and temperament.

LIFESTYLE

If you smoke, quit. You should also get in the habit of exercising, since exercise strengthens the heart and blood vessels, reduces stress, and has been shown to reduce blood pressure while also boosting HDL cholesterol levels. Numerous studies done in recent decades indicate that drinking wine in small amounts may actually reduce the risk of heart disease. But more than one glass a day, or a few glasses per week, is not recommended.

MIND/BODY MEDICINE

For many people, learning to relax can help prevent and treat heart disease. While success varies from person to person, stress-reduction techniques have been shown to moderate high blood pressure, heart arrhythmias, and emotional responses such as anxiety, anger, and hostility that have been linked to coronary heart disease, angina, and heart attack. The choice of relaxation technique is up to you. Some that have proved beneficial are **yoga, meditation,** progressive relaxation, prayer, and **biofeedback** training.

NUTRITION AND DIET

Even modest changes in diet and lifestyle can significantly reduce the risk of heart disease. Most people now know that eating foods low in cholesterol, saturated fat, and salt will help keep blood pressure low and decrease the formation of plaques—calcified fatty deposits—in blood vessels. Less known to the general public are those specific vitamins, minerals, and nutrients, such as ***magnesium, potassium, niacin*** (vitamin B_3), many other ***B-complex vitamins, vitamin E,*** coenzyme Q10, L-carnitine (an amino acid), and the fatty acids in fish oils, that specifically protect against heart and arterial disease. For more information concerning these and other heart-related nutrients, see ***Atherosclerosis, Cholesterol Problems, Heart Attack,*** and ***High Blood Pressure.***

PREVENTION

- To stabilize both blood pressure and cholesterol levels and to keep your weight in check, try to eat more fruits, vegetables, and grains, and fewer foods that are salty, high in fat, or fried.
- Exercise regularly, in order to tone your heart and blood vessels—and to shed excess pounds.
- Drink alcohol in moderation, if you do drink.
- Don't smoke.
- Learn to control, and release, stress rather than letting it control you.
- If you feel you are at risk, ask your doctor about taking an aspirin a day to prevent heart attack. ■

H

HEMORRHOIDS

SYMPTOMS

- bright red ***anal bleeding*** that may streak the bowel movement or the toilet tissue.
- tenderness or pain during bowel movements.
- painful swelling or a lump near the anus.
- anal itching.
- a mucous anal discharge.

H

CALL YOUR DOCTOR IF:

- you experience any anal bleeding for the first time, even if you believe you have hemorrhoids. Colon polyps, ***colitis, Crohn's disease,*** and ***colorectal cancer*** can also cause anal bleeding. An accurate diagnosis is essential.
- you have been diagnosed with hemorrhoids, and you have anal bleeding that is chronic (daily or weekly) or more profuse than the streaking described above. Though rare, excessive hemorrhoidal bleeding can cause ***anemia.***

Hemorrhoids are essentially ***varicose veins*** of the rectum. The hemorrhoidal veins are located in the lowest area of the rectum and the anus. Sometimes they swell, so that the vein walls become stretched, thin, and irritated by passing bowel movements. When these swollen veins bleed, itch, or hurt, they are known as hemorrhoids, or piles. Hemorrhoids are classified into two general categories: internal and external.

Internal hemorrhoids lie far enough inside the rectum that you can't see or feel them. They don't usually hurt, because there are few pain-sensing nerves in the rectum. Bleeding may be the only sign of their presence. Sometimes internal hemorrhoids prolapse, or enlarge and protrude outside the anal sphincter. If so, you may be able to see or feel them as moist, pink pads of skin that are pinker than the surrounding area. Prolapsed hemorrhoids may hurt, because the anus is dense with pain-sensing nerves. They usually recede into the rectum on their own; if they don't, they can be gently pushed back into place.

External hemorrhoids lie within the anus and are usually painful. If an external hemorrhoid prolapses to the outside (usually in the course of passing a stool) you can see and feel it. Blood clots sometimes form within prolapsed external hemorrhoids, causing an extremely painful condition called a thrombosis. If an external hemorrhoid becomes thrombosed, it can look rather frightening, turning purple or blue, and possibly bleeding. Despite their appearance, thrombosed hemorrhoids are usually not serious and will resolve themselves in about a week. If the pain is unbearable, your doctor can remove the thrombosis, which stops the pain, during an office visit.

Anal bleeding and pain of any sort is alarming and should be evaluated; it can indicate a life-threatening condition, such as ***colorectal cancer.*** Hemorrhoids are the most common cause of anal bleeding and are rarely dangerous but a definite diagnosis from your physician is a must.

CAUSES

About half of the people in the U.S. will suffer from hemorrhoids at some point in life; for most,

WHERE HEMORRHOIDS FORM

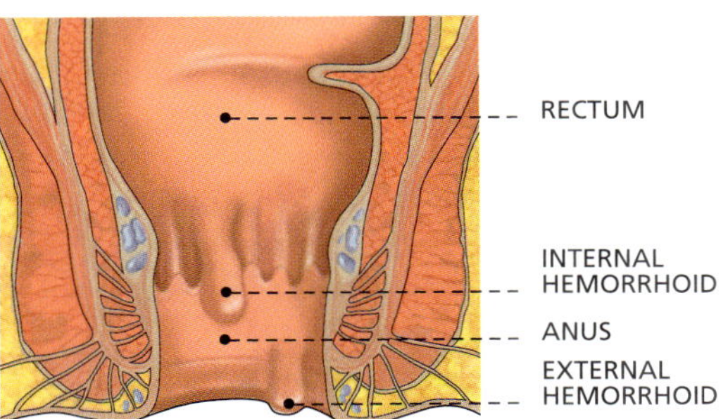

Veins in the rectum and anus are subjected to considerable pressure whenever a stool is passed. Pushing or straining may cause veins in the rectal wall to bulge, creating clusters of swollen, or dilated, veins called hemorrhoids. Internal hemorrhoids can form anywhere inside the anal canal, while external hemorrhoids are visible at, or just below, the opening of the anus.

this will happen between ages 20 and 50. Researchers are not certain what causes hemorrhoids. "Weak" veins—leading to hemorrhoids and other varicose veins—may be inherited. It's likely that extreme abdominal pressure causes the veins to swell and become susceptible to irritation. Sources of this pressure include ***obesity,*** pregnancy, standing or sitting for long periods, liver disease, straining from constipation or diarrhea, coughing, sneezing, vomiting, and holding one's breath while straining to do physical labor.

Diet has a pivotal role in causing—and preventing—hemorrhoids. People who consistently eat a high-fiber diet are unlikely to get hemorrhoids, whereas those who prefer a diet high in refined foods can expect them. A low-fiber diet or inadequate fluid intake causes ***constipation,*** which contributes to hemorrhoids in two ways: It encourages straining to have a bowel movement, and it also aggravates the hemorrhoids by producing hard stools that further irritate the swollen veins.

DIAGNOSTIC AND TEST PROCEDURES

Your doctor will first visually examine the anal area, perhaps by inserting a lubricated gloved finger or an anoscope (a hollow, lighted tube for viewing the lower few inches of the rectum) or a proctoscope (which works like an anoscope but provides a more thorough rectal examination). More procedures may be needed to identify internal hemorrhoids or rule out other ailments that frequently cause anal bleeding, such as ***anal fissure, colitis, Crohn's disease,*** and ***colorectal cancer.*** To see further into the anal canal (into the lower colon, or sigmoid), sigmoidoscopy may be used, or the entire colon may be viewed with colonoscopy. For both procedures, a lighted, flexible viewing tube is inserted into the rectum. A barium x-ray can show the entire colon's interior. First a barium enema is given, then x-rays are taken of the lower gastrointestinal tract.

TREATMENT

Once you have them, hemorrhoids don't usually go away completely unless you undergo one of the procedures below. They can get better, however, so that living with them is tolerable. Both conventional and alternative practitioners consider diet the best tool for treating hemorrhoids. A diet rich in high-fiber foods and low in refined and junk foods is essential. Probably half of all hemorrhoid sufferers find relief with dietary changes alone.

Most hemorrhoid treatments aim to minimize pain and itching. Warm (but not hot) sitz baths are the most time-honored and oft-suggested therapy: Sit in about three inches of warm water for 15 minutes, several times a day, especially after a bowel movement. If you are pregnant, discuss any treatment, including dietary changes, with your doctor before proceeding.

CONVENTIONAL MEDICINE

If you have been diagnosed as having hemorrhoids, a high-fiber diet combined with sitz baths and ***acetaminophen*** should reduce discomfort within two weeks. If symptoms persist, your physician may suggest one of the following procedures. All except laser coagulation and surgery can be performed in your doctor's office.

Injection. An internal hemorrhoid can be injected with ***phenol*** in oil, quinine, and urea, or morrhuate sodium, which creates a scar and closes off the hemorrhoid. The injection hurts only a little, as any injection does. With a success rate of 90 percent, this is many physicians' first choice. Results are not permanent, however; repeat injections may be needed every two or three years.

Banding. Prolapsed hemorrhoids are often removed using rubber-band ligation. A special tool secures a tiny rubber band around the hemorrhoid, shutting off its blood supply almost instantly. Within a week, the hemorrhoid shrivels and falls off. This painless method is successful about 75 percent of the time.

Coagulation or **cauterization.** Using either an electric probe, a laser beam, or an infrared light, a tiny burn painlessly seals the end of the hemorrhoid, causing it to close off and shrink. This is most useful for prolapsed hemorrhoids.

Surgery. For large internal hemorrhoids or extremely uncomfortable external hemorrhoids (such as thrombosed hemorrhoids that are too painful to live with), your physician may elect traditional surgery, called hemorrhoidectomy. In the hospital, under general anesthesia, the hemorrhoid is removed. After the operation, expect a week or so of bed rest, with ***analgesics*** prescribed for discomfort.

The success rate for hemorrhoid removal approaches 95 percent, but unless dietary and lifestyle changes are made, hemorrhoids are likely to recur.

OVER-THE-COUNTER RELIEF

Controversy continues to rage about the efficacy of hemorrhoid medicines. In the United States, we annually spend roughly $200 million on creams, ointments, and suppositories that promise to relieve inflammation and pain.

The basic ingredient in all these medicines is a lubricant, such as lanolin, cocoa butter, vegetable oil, or one of many others. Some also include an ***anesthetic*** *such as* ***benzocaine,*** *lidocaine or pramoxine, or an astringent such as tannic acid or zinc compounds, purported to reduce swelling by constricting capillaries. Hemorrhoids, however, are not capillaries; they're veins, and astringents may have no effect on them. Anesthetics may provide short-term relief, but only in cream or ointment form: Suppositories usually go too far up into the anal canal to help the hemorrhoids below.*

Lubrication is the greatest benefit of most over-the-counter hemorrhoid medications. Plain petroleum jelly works as well and can be applied with your finger. For pain relief, try ***acetaminophen*** *and sitz baths.*

ALTERNATIVE CHOICES

Try one or several of these therapies to alleviate hemorrhoid discomfort. If symptoms persist despite your efforts at relief, contact your physician.

ACUPUNCTURE

The most responsive point for relieving hemorrhoid pain is Governing Vessel 20. Others that may augment it are Stomachs 25 and 36, Governing Vessel 14, and Large Intestine 11. See a licensed practitioner for treatment; see the ***Appendix*** for point locations.

HERBAL THERAPIES

Applied twice daily, pilewort *(Ranunculus ficaria)* ointment can reduce the pain of external hemorrhoids: Simmer 2 tbsp fresh or dried pilewort in 7 oz petroleum jelly for 10 minutes. Allow to cool before using; store leftover ointment in a closed container. Pilewort may also be taken as a tea.

HOMEOPATHY

More than a dozen remedies, each taken at 12x, can help hemorrhoid pain. Choosing the right one requires attention to your symptoms and, usually, a homeopath's help. For a sore, bruised, and perhaps bleeding anus, try *Hamamelis. Aesculus* can ease sharp, spiking rectal pain that is worsened with bowel movements, and ***Sulphur*** can reduce burning and itching aggravated by warmth.

MASSAGE

This technique moves matter through the intestines, helping to prevent the constipation that contributes to hemorrhoids. Lie on your back, and use your fingers or your palm to make long, sweeping strokes. Repeat each stroke three to six times. Begin on your left side. Just below your ribs, stroke toward your feet; then stroke across your abdomen from the right to left just below your rib cage. Finally, point your fingertips toward your feet, and drag your hand up your right side from pelvis to ribs.

NUTRITION AND DIET

Prevent constipation by following a high-fiber diet. Meals and snacks should consist primarily of vegetables, fruit, nuts, and whole grains, and as few refined foods and meats as possible. If this is a big change for you, introduce the new foods slowly, to avoid gas. If you aren't able to eat enough high-fiber food, supplement your diet with ***psyllium*** stool softeners or bulk-forming agents such as wheat bran. (Avoid ***laxatives,*** which cause diarrhea that can further irritate the swollen veins.) Drink six to eight glasses of water each day; if your life is especially active or you live in a hot climate, you will need more.

Monitor your sodium intake. Excess salt in the diet causes fluid retention, which means swelling in all veins, including hemorrhoids.

YOGA

Yoga can encourage blood flow away from hemorrhoids, reducing pain, inflammation, and bleeding. Try the Half Shoulder Stand, Shoulder Stand, Plow, and Bridge, holding each posture for 20 to 30 seconds twice each day. A good complement for these postures is lying on a slant board with your head down for 15 minutes each day. *(See the* ***Appendix*** *for information on yoga exercises.)*

AT-HOME REMEDIES

- Try not to sit (or stand) for hours at a time, but if you must, take breaks: Once every hour, get up and move around for at least five minutes. A doughnut-shaped cushion can make sitting more comfortable and ease hemorrhoid pressure and pain.
- Insert olive or canola oil just inside the anus to make bowel movements less painful.
- Dab witch hazel *(Hamamelis virginiana),* a soothing anti-inflammatory agent, on irritated hemorrhoids to reduce pain and itching.
- Resist the temptation to scratch hemorrhoids, as it makes everything worse: The inflamed veins become more irritated, the skin around them becomes damaged, and the itching itself intensifies. Instead, to help stop the itching, apply witch hazel cream to the hemorrhoid and a cold pack.
- If you need a pain reliever, try ***acetaminophen.*** Avoid ***ibuprofen*** and ***aspirin,*** which foster bleeding.
- Bathe regularly to keep the anal area clean, but be gentle: Excessive scrubbing, especially with soap, can intensify burning and irritation.
- Don't sit on the toilet for more than five minutes at a time, and when wiping, be gentle. If toilet paper is irritating, try dampening it first, or use cotton balls or alcohol-free baby wipes.
- When performing any task that requires exertion, be sure to breathe evenly. It's common to hold your breath during exertion, and if you do, you're straining, and contributing to hemorrhoid pain and bleeding.

PREVENTION

A healthful diet and lifestyle are good insurance for preventing hemorrhoids, whether you already suffer hemorrhoid symptoms or are intent on never experiencing them. Regular exercise is also im-portant, especially if you work a sedentary job. Exercise helps in several ways: keeping weight in check, making constipation less likely, enhancing muscle tone, and stimulating blood circulation. ■

H

HEPATITIS

SYMPTOMS

Many cases of hepatitis go undiagnosed because the disease is mistaken for the ***flu*** or because there are no symptoms at all. The most common symptoms of hepatitis are:

- loss of appetite.
- fatigue.
- mild fever.
- muscle or joint aches.
- nausea and vomiting.
- abdominal pain.

H

Less common symptoms include:

- dark urine.
- light-colored stools.
- ***jaundice.***
- generalized itching.
- altered mental state, stupor, or coma.

CALL YOUR DOCTOR IF:

- your flulike symptoms persist or you notice any of the more serious signs; chronic hepatitis can lead to ***cirrhosis*** and even death.
- a friend or family member comes down with hepatitis; you may be infected with the organism that causes the disease.
- your symptoms follow a visit to a country where hepatitis is common; you may have contracted the disease during your travels.

Hepatitis, a general term that means inflammation of the liver, applies to a group of viral disorders commonly known as hepatitis A, B, C, D, and E. Another type of hepatitis is brought on through alcohol abuse or the use of drugs, or by ingestion of toxins in the environment.

Hepatitis is the most common of all serious contagious diseases. About 70,000 cases are reported to the Centers for Disease Control and Prevention each year, but researchers estimate that the number of people in the United States who actually have the disease is closer to 500,000. Many hepatitis cases go undiagnosed because they are mistaken for the ***flu.*** Hepatitis is serious because it interferes with the liver's many functions. Among other things, the liver produces bile to aid digestion, regulates the chemical composition of the blood, and screens potentially harmful substances from the bloodstream.

The five viruses that cause hepatitis can be transmitted in different ways, but they all have one thing in common: They infect the liver and cause it to become inflamed. Generally, the acute phase of the disease lasts from two to three weeks; complete recovery takes about nine weeks. Although most patients recover with a lifelong immunity to the disease, a few hepatitis victims (less than 1 percent) die in the acute phase. Others may develop chronic hepatitis, in which the liver remains inflamed for six months or more. This condition can lead to ***cirrhosis*** and possibly death.

CAUSES

Although their effects on the liver and the symptoms they produce can be similar, the various forms of hepatitis are contracted in different ways. In the case of viral hepatitis, the severity and duration of the disease are largely determined by the organism that caused it.

Hepatitis A, which is generally contracted orally through fecal contamination of food or water, is considered the least dangerous form of the disease because it does not lead to chronic inflammation of the liver. The hepatitis A virus commonly spreads through improper handling of food, contact with household members, sharing toys at day-care centers, and eating raw shellfish taken from polluted waters.

Hepatitis B, the most widespread of the hepatitis viruses, infects an estimated 300,000 people every year in the United States alone. The virus can pass from mother to child at birth or soon afterward; the disease organism can also travel between adults and children to infect whole families. Hepatitis B can also spread through sexual contact, blood transfusions, and needle sharing by intravenous-drug users. In a third of all hepatitis B cases the source cannot be identified.

The majority of hepatitis B patients recover completely, but a small percentage of them can't shake the disease and may develop chronic hepatitis and possibly ***cirrhosis.*** People with chronic hepatitis become carriers, meaning they can transmit the disease to others even when their own symptoms have vanished. Only 1 or 2 percent of hepatitis B patients die from the disease.

Hepatitis C is usually spread through contact with blood or contaminated needles. Although hepatitis C may cause only mild symptoms or none at all, 20 percent to 30 percent of chronic carriers develop ***cirrhosis*** within 10 years. The disease can be passed on through blood transfusions, but a recently developed test has greatly reduced the number of such cases. In a third of all hepatitis C cases, the source of the disease is unknown.

Hepatitis D occurs only in people infected with hepatitis B and tends to magnify the severity of that disease. It can be transmitted from mother to child and through sexual contact. Rarest among the five hepatitis viruses, hepatitis D is also the most dangerous because it involves two forms of the disease working at once.

Hepatitis E occurs mainly in Asia, Mexico, and Africa; only a few cases are reported in the United States, mostly among people who have returned from a country where the disease is widespread. Like hepatitis A, this type is usually spread through fecal contamination, and it does not lead to chronic hepatitis. This form is considered slightly more dangerous than hepatitis A, especially in pregnant women.

Alcoholic, toxic, and **drug-related hepatitis** can produce the same symptoms and liver inflammation that result from viral hepatitis. This form is caused not by invading microorganisms but by excessive and chronic consumption of alcohol *(see **Alcohol Abuse**)*, ingestion of environmental toxins, or misuse of certain prescription drugs and over-the-counter medications such as ***acetaminophen.***

DIAGNOSTIC AND TEST PROCEDURES

When the patient's symptoms suggest hepatitis, the doctor normally takes blood samples and runs tests to check for the presence of a disease organism. More blood samples may be necessary later—even after the symptoms have vanished—to check for complications and determine if the patient is a carrier of the disease.

The doctor may also require a liver biopsy, or tissue sample, in order to determine the extent of the damage. A biopsy is commonly performed by inserting a needle into the liver and drawing

C A U T I O N !

Beware of Hidden Dangers

Because the liver plays a key role in processing drugs, alcohol, and toxins in the bloodstream, a patient with hepatitis may find that some medications, alcoholic beverages, and herbs that are normally tolerated can aggravate the condition. If you have hepatitis, do not attempt to treat the disease on your own; consult a physician or licensed practitioner. Avoid alcoholic beverages and ask your doctor if it is all right to use birth-control pills, *antibiotics,* or over-the-counter medicines. Be sure to tell your physician or practitioner all the medications that you are taking, including even seemingly innocuous over-the-counter drugs such as *aspirin* or *acetaminophen.*

out a fragment of tissue, which is then sent to a laboratory to be analyzed.

TREATMENT

There are only a few specific remedies for most types of hepatitis. The conventional approach in each case is to treat the disease with rest and proper diet and to make efforts to contain its spread. Some alternative remedies, when administered by a trained professional, can be used to complement a doctor's care and may help relieve symptoms.

CONVENTIONAL MEDICINE

Although your doctor may recommend bed rest, you may find that simply restricting physical activity is enough to make you feel better. The general rule is this: If you feel well, get up; if you don't, take it easy or lie down. Avoid contact with others to keep the virus from spreading.

Good nutrition is an important part of treatment for all types of hepatitis. In most cases, eating properly means a simple regimen of nutritious, well-balanced meals that supply adequate calories. Many hepatitis patients like to eat a hearty breakfast because their appetites wane and nausea intensifies as the day progresses. Patients who have trouble eating larger meals may prefer to eat smaller amounts at each sitting and snack frequently throughout the day.

Treatment for alcoholic, toxic, and drug-related hepatitis is generally the same as that for viral hepatitis, although hospitalization is more common for nonviral hepatitis, and severe cases tend to be more life-threatening. As is often the case, simply removing the offending drink, toxin, or drug goes a long way toward helping patients recover from nonviral hepatitis.

If your hepatitis, either viral or nonviral, is in the acute stage, avoid alcoholic beverages, as the body's efforts to process alcohol put an added strain on the already injured liver. Also be aware that the sexual partner of an infected person, particularly if he or she has hepatitis B, may run the risk of contracting the disease.

A primary-care physician can usually provide adequate care for patients with all types of hepatitis. However, severe cases may require treatment by a hepatologist or gastroenterologist—specialists in diseases of the liver. Hospitalization is normally unnecessary unless the patient cannot eat or drink, or is vomiting.

Most people recover completely from hepatitis. Mild flareups may occur over a period of several months as the disease is subsiding, but each flareup is usually less severe than the one before it, and a relapse doesn't mean you won't make a full recovery.

Hepatitis in pregnant women usually does not increase the risk of birth defects or other pregnancy problems, and infection of the baby in the uterus is rare. If the mother has hepatitis B, however, the baby is likely to contract the disease at birth. A hepatitis B vaccine now available will reduce these chances significantly if adminis-

WHAT'S BEST TO EAT

The right kind of diet can play a very important part in how your body handles a case of hepatitis. If you have acute or chronic hepatitis, you should increase your intake of fiber, including whole-grains, fruits and vegetables, and cooked dried beans and peas. These foods encourage the elimination of bile acids and toxins that can accumulate in the liver and gallbladder.

*Some nutritionists contend that massive doses of **vitamin C,** perhaps taken intravenously, can improve viral hepatitis by reducing inflammation in the liver. Studies also suggest that large doses of **vitamin B_{12}** and **folic acid** may reduce the time that it takes a patient to recover from the disease. Ask your doctor or a licensed nutritionist for the vitamins and dosages that are right for you.*

tered to the infant immediately after delivery. If you are pregnant, your doctor will test you for hepatitis B; if you are infected with the virus, your baby will be given immune serum globulin shots and a hepatitis vaccination.

Doctors sometimes recommend drug therapy for patients with certain types of hepatitis. The drug interferon is commonly used to treat chronic cases of hepatitis B and hepatitis C. Interferon has been shown to help rid the body of the virus and reduce inflammation and liver damage in 15 percent to 20 percent of people with these forms of the disease, thus reducing the risk of ***cirrhosis.*** For some hepatitis cases doctors prescribe ***corticosteroids*** to suppress inflammation. Use of these drugs to control hepatitis is controversial, however, because they may have side effects that harm the immune system.

Almost every known drug has at one time or another been implicated as a cause of liver damage. If you currently have hepatitis, or if you have a history of liver disease or other liver problems, tell your doctor before taking any medication.

Regardless of what kind of hepatitis you have or what treatment you receive, you should continue seeing your doctor for checkups until blood tests indicate the virus is gone. A person can remain a carrier of hepatitis B or hepatitis C as long as the virus is present in the blood, even if all symptoms have disappeared.

ALTERNATIVE CHOICES

Nonconventional therapies, when taken properly, may help reduce inflammation in the liver and alleviate symptoms of hepatitis. Used improperly, however, some of these treatments can inflict further damage on the liver or lead to other complications. In general, hepatitis does not lend itself to self-medication. Don't take chances with this disease. If you want to supplement a doctor's care with an alternative remedy, consult a licensed practitioner for help in choosing the right medications and determining exact dosages.

CHINESE HERBS

A practitioner of Chinese medicine can suggest herbal formulas to treat symptoms such as nausea and fatigue. Other herbal formulas may help improve liver function.

HERBAL THERAPIES

Osha *(Ligusticum porteri)* may help your body fight the hepatitis virus; take 15 to 20 drops of osha tincture twice a day.

HOMEOPATHY

Homeopaths sometimes prescribe ***Phosphorus*** to reduce liver inflammation and relieve the symptoms of hepatitis. Other remedies include *Taraxacum officinale,* ***Lycopodium,*** and *Chelidonium majus,* depending on the individual symptoms. Consult a professional homeopath for exact preparations and dosages.

PREVENTION

The keys to avoiding hepatitis are vaccinations, good hygiene, and informed common sense. Adequate sanitation and clean personal habits will help reduce the spread of hepatitis A and hepatitis E. In areas where sanitation is questionable, boil water. Cook all food well and peel all fruit.

Healthcare workers involved in the treatment of patients with hepatitis B, C, or E should wash their hands, utensils, bedding, and clothing with soap and hot water, especially in the first two weeks of illness, when the patient is most contagious.

People planning to travel to countries where hepatitis is widespread are advised to have immune serum globulin shots or vaccinations before leaving. Immune serum globulin may prevent infection from some types of hepatitis after exposure if administered within 48 hours.

To prevent the spread of hepatitis B, avoid exposure to infectious blood or body fluids. Do not have intimate contact or share razors, scissors, nail files, toothbrushes, or needles with anyone who has the disease. If you suspect that you have been exposed, you should receive immune serum globulin and vaccinations for hepatitis A and hepatitis B as soon as possible. ■

HERNIA

SYMPTOMS

- an obvious swelling beneath the skin in the abdomen or the groin; it may disappear when you lie down and may or may not be tender.
- a heavy feeling in the abdomen that is sometimes accompanied by constipation.
- discomfort in the abdomen or groin when lifting or bending over.

H

CALL YOUR DOCTOR IF:

- you suspect that you have a hernia. Sometimes hernias require urgent medical care; an accurate diagnosis is important.
- you know you have a hernia, and you are nauseated and vomiting or are unable to have a bowel movement or pass gas. You may have a strangulated hernia or an obstruction, which are emergencies. **Seek medical care immediately.**

A hernia occurs when an organ or tissue squeezes through a hole or a weak spot in a surrounding muscle. The most common types are inguinal, incisional, femoral, and umbilical.

In an **inguinal hernia,** the intestine or the bladder protrudes through the abdominal wall or into the inguinal canal, in the groin. About 80 percent of all hernias are inguinal, and most occur in men because of a natural weakness in this area.

In an **incisional hernia,** the intestines push through the abdominal wall at the site of previous abdominal surgery. This type is most common in elderly and overweight people who are inactive after abdominal surgery.

A **femoral hernia** occurs when the bladder or intestine enters the canal carrying the femoral artery into the upper thigh. Femoral hernias are most common in women, especially those who are pregnant or obese.

In an **umbilical hernia,** part of the small intestine passes through the abdominal wall near the navel. Common in newborns, it also afflicts obese women or those who have had many children.

CAUSES

Ultimately, all hernias are caused by a combination of muscle weakness and strain: A weak spot in the muscle tears under the pressure of strain, and an internal organ or tissue then pushes through the tear. Sometimes the muscle weakness is present at birth; more often, it occurs later in life. Poor nutrition, smoking, and overexertion all can weaken muscles and make hernias more likely. Anything that causes muscle strain can then induce hernia, including ***obesity,*** lifting heavy objects, diarrhea or constipation, or persistent coughing.

DIAGNOSTIC AND TEST PROCEDURES

A doctor's physical examination is often enough to diagnose a hernia. Sometimes hernia swelling is visible when you stand upright; usually, the hernia can be felt if you place your hand directly over it and then bear down. Ultrasound may be used to see a femoral hernia, and abdominal x-rays may be ordered to identify a bowel obstruction.

INGUINAL HERNIA

An inguinal hernia occurs in the thin band of muscles at the inguinal canal, where a man's spermatic cord runs from the testicles through the abdominal wall. If the muscle wall is weakened, part of the small intestine can protrude through it, creating a bulge in the groin *(below)*. An inguinal hernia can restrict blood flow or cause a bowel obstruction and is considered a medical emergency.

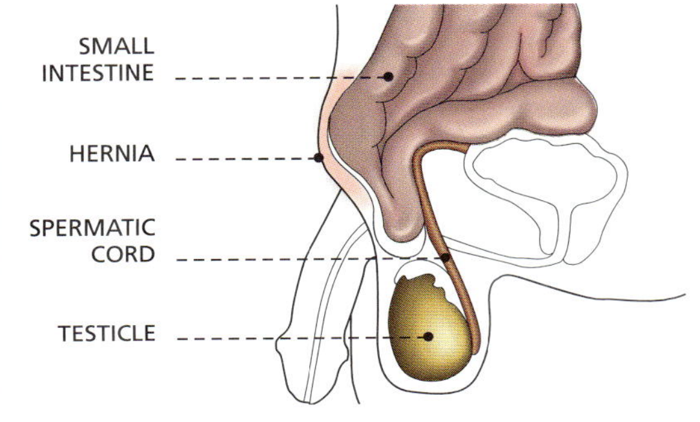

TREATMENT

In babies, umbilical hernias frequently heal themselves within four years, making surgery unnecessary. For all others, the standard treatment is conventional hernia-repair surgery (called herniorrhaphy). If left untreated, the protruding organ may become strangulated (have its blood supply cut off), and infection and tissue death may occur as a result. A strangulated intestinal hernia may result in intestinal obstruction, which can lead to infection, gangrene, intestinal perforation, shock, or even death.

CONVENTIONAL MEDICINE

Your doctor may manually press your hernia back into place and advise you to wear a special belt, known as a truss, that holds a hernia in place until surgery. Over-the-counter ***analgesics*** can help ease discomfort.

Hernia surgery is performed under either local or general anesthesia. The surgeon repositions the herniated tissue and, if strangulation has occurred, removes the oxygen-starved part of the organ. The damaged muscle wall will then be repaired. Increasingly, inguinal herniorrhaphy is performed using a laparoscope, a thin telescope-like instrument that requires a smaller incision and involves a shorter recovery period.

Patients often walk around the day after hernia surgery. There are usually no dietary restrictions, and work and regular activity may be resumed in a week. Complete recovery takes four to six weeks, with no heavy lifting for at least three months. Hernias often return after surgery, so preventive measures are especially important to avoid a recurrence.

ALTERNATIVE CHOICES

If you have—or believe you have—a hernia, you need to be under a doctor's care. Alternative therapies cannot cure hernia; they can, however, relieve the discomfort.

CHINESE HERBS

To make a compress that may help relieve the pain of an umbilical hernia, crush ⅓ tsp wood sorrel *(Oxalis corniculata)* and ¼ tsp Asian pennywort *(Hydrocotyle rotundifolia)* and add to ½ cup warm cooked rice. Place the compress over the navel for three to four hours; repeat two or three times.

LIFESTYLE

Gentle exercise on a regular basis tones and strengthens stomach muscles. One good choice to do daily: Lie on your back with knees bent and feet on the floor. Keeping your shoulders on the floor, lift your buttocks and your lower back; gently lower yourself. Repeat 10 times.

PREVENTION

Avoid obesity and physical strain; practice good nutrition (both to avoid constipation and to enhance muscle strength); and maintain toned abdominal muscles. When lifting heavy objects, always bend from the knees, not the waist. If something is too heavy, don't lift it at all. ■

H

HIATAL HERNIA

SYMPTOMS

The majority of people who have hiatal hernias don't even realize it. Those who do know typically find out when visiting a doctor because of chronic ***heartburn.*** Symptoms may include the following:

- heartburn; regurgitation.
- difficulty swallowing; lump in the throat.
- ***chest pain*** radiating from below the breastbone (the sternum).
- a bloated feeling after eating.
- shortness of breath.

CALL YOUR DOCTOR IF:

- radiating chest pain is not relieved by taking an antacid. You may have ***angina,*** or you may be having a ***heart attack.*** **Get medical care immediately.**
- you are being treated for heartburn or hiatal hernia, and you feel sudden chest or stomach pain, have difficulty swallowing, and are vomiting. You may have a hernia that has strangulated, which is a medical and surgical emergency. **Seek medical help without delay.**
- your hiatal hernia is accompanied by chronic heartburn. Stomach acid is repeatedly burning your esophagus, which can lead to esophagitis (an inflamed and ulcerated esophagus), esophageal scarring, ***stomach ulcer,*** or ***cancer.*** See a physician soon.

The hiatus is an opening in the diaphragm (a muscle separating the abdomen and chest) that the esophagus passes through to reach the stomach. If the hiatus weakens and stretches, part of the stomach and/or the esophagus can squeeze into the chest cavity, producing a hiatal hernia.

Essentially, there are three types of hiatal hernias. In a **sliding hernia,** the lower esophagus and stomach move upward, bringing the top part of the stomach into the chest cavity. In a **paraesophageal hernia,** the stomach moves through the hiatus and rests beside the esophagus. **Mixed hernias** have features of both sliding and paraesophageal hernias.

Although typically small, some hiatal hernias expand until a large portion of the stomach is squeezed through the hiatus. Slow bleeding, from the compressed stomach or from esophagitis, can eventually cause ***anemia.*** Sometimes a hernia will become strangulated, or so tightly constricted that blood flow is cut off to the squeezed part of the stomach and the nearby esophagus. This is unlikely in mixed and sliding hernias but common in paraesophageal hernias. Generally, sliding and mixed hiatal hernias show no symptoms and pose no threat to good health.

CAUSES

All ages are susceptible, but frequency increases with age: More than half of those over age 50 have a hiatal hernia. Sliding hernia is by far the most common type. Like other ***hernias,*** hiatal hernias are probably caused by excessive pressure in the abdomen related to pregnancy, ***obesity,*** injury, or straining to have a bowel movement. Risk factors include constipation, heavy lifting, and persistent coughing or vomiting.

Hiatal hernias may cause no symptoms, but when they do, symptoms are worsened by wearing tight clothing, eating foods that cause heartburn, and bending over or lying down after eating.

DIAGNOSTIC AND TEST PROCEDURES

A physical examination for hiatal hernia is similar to that for heartburn, with two additions:

X-rays may be ordered to show the hernia, and if anemia is a concern, a blood sample may be taken to check your red blood cell count.

TREATMENT

Heartburn or other symptoms that occur with **sliding** or **mixed hernias** may be treated by both conventional and alternative therapies. **Paraesophageal hernias,** however, should be repaired by conventional surgery because the danger of strangulation is high.

CONVENTIONAL MEDICINE

Often, alleviating heartburn is all that is required. Surgery is indicated, however, if a paraesophageal hernia exists, or when sliding or mixed hernias bleed or become large, strangulated, or inflamed. In surgery, the hiatus is reinforced and the stomach is repositioned. This surgery is now commonly done using a laparoscope, a thin telescope-like instrument for viewing inside the abdomen. Typically, a two-night hospital stay is required and regular activity may be resumed in two weeks.

TWO TYPES OF HIATAL HERNIAS

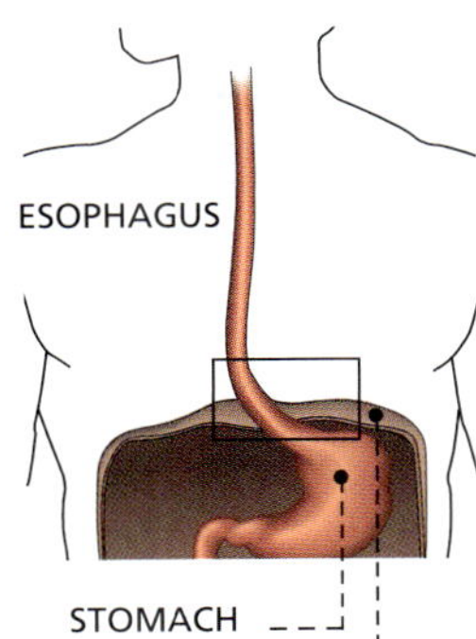

The esophagus passes through the hiatus—a small opening in the diaphragm separating the chest and abdominal cavities *(left)*. A sliding hiatal hernia *(inset, below, left)* occurs when the lower esophagus and a small part of the stomach push through the hiatus into the chest cavity. In a paraesophageal hiatal hernia *(inset, below, right)*, part of the stomach balloons up beside the esophagus.

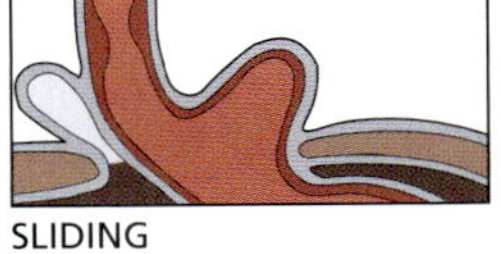

SLIDING HIATAL HERNIA

PARAESOPHAGEAL HIATAL HERNIA

ALTERNATIVE CHOICES

The therapies for hiatal hernia symptoms are similar to those for ***heartburn.***

ACUPRESSURE

To relieve heartburn, use deep thumb pressure to massage these points for at least one minute: Stomach 36, Spleen 6, Pericardium 6, and Liver 14. *(See the **Appendix** for point locations.)*

HERBAL THERAPY

Slippery elm *(Ulmus fulva)* tea is soothing and is reputed to have strong anti-inflammatory qualities. Mix 1 tbsp in 10 oz water, simmer for 10 minutes, and drink ½ cup, three times daily.

LIFESTYLE

Refrain from eating large meals; instead, eat four or five small meals each day and chew your food slowly. This, along with maintaining a weight in proportion to your height, will minimize abdominal pressure—and heartburn. Reducing fat and caffeine in your diet may also substantially reduce symptoms. Smoking is an intense heartburn generator; if you smoke, stop.

PREVENTION

To prevent symptoms:

- ◆ Wear loose clothing. Anything that presses on the stomach can aggravate hiatal hernia symptoms.
- ◆ When your stomach is full, avoid bending over or lying down. This increases abdominal pressure and makes gravity work against you, so heartburn is more likely.
- ◆ Do not eat within three hours of going to sleep.

To prevent hiatal hernia:

- ◆ Maintain a reasonable weight.
- ◆ Don't smoke. ■

HICCUPS

SYMPTOMS

- repeated, involuntary contractions of the diaphragm that cause air to rush suddenly into the lungs and close the glottis—the part of the larynx containing the vocal cords—creating the "hic" sound; hiccups generally are of short duration and often follow a big meal or too much alcohol. Occasionally, a prolonged episode of hiccups can last days or weeks.

H

CALL YOUR DOCTOR IF:

- your hiccups persist for more than a day; prolonged hiccups can result from irritation of the nerves of the diaphragm or of the diaphragm itself from ***pneumonia,*** esophagitis, ***pancreatic problems, alcohol abuse,*** or ***hepatitis.***
- hiccups and fever occur after major surgery in the upper abdomen and lead to a loss of appetite; under these conditions the hiccups may be indicative of an abscess under the diaphragm or over the liver.

Hiccups—involuntary spasms of the diaphragm—are usually a minor annoyance and last only for a short time. They can affect anyone, and most pregnant women will tell you that they have even felt their unborn child hiccup in the womb.

CAUSES

No one knows why the diaphragm sometimes contracts involuntarily, causing hiccups. But the condition can be related to nerves or to having had too much food or drink; rarely is it a secondary complication of a disease, but it has been associated with both ***appendicitis*** and ***diabetes.***

TREATMENT

Most cases of hiccups resolve spontaneously, although sufferers can try to hasten this resolution with various home remedies.

CONVENTIONAL MEDICINE

Medical intervention is rarely needed; but if a case of hiccups fails to stop after a day, a visit to the doctor's office may be warranted to rule out disease-related causes. Drugs that have given relief in cases of prolonged hiccups include baclofen and chlorpromazine. If your hiccups arise from esophagitis, a condition caused by stomach acid backing up into the esophagus, your doctor may suggest ***cimetidine, ranitidine,*** or ***omeprazole,*** drugs that suppress acid production in the stomach at the cellular level. See ***Heartburn*** for more information.

ALTERNATIVE CHOICES

ACUPRESSURE

Acupressure exercises seek to trigger a relaxation response in the throat, lungs, or diaphragm to stop the hiccups. Deep breathing is an important part of the exercise. Try the following exercises in succession to relieve the hiccups. *(See the* ***Ap-***

ACUPRESSURE

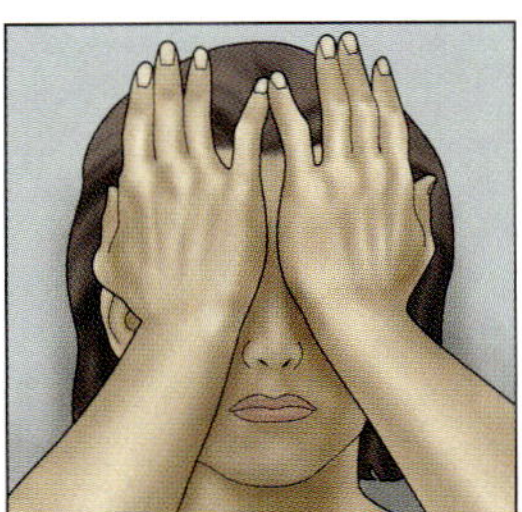

1 To stop an attack of hiccups, try palm pressure. Place the palms of your hands over both eyes, with the heels resting on your cheekbones. Gently massage around your eyes for one minute by pressing the pads below your thumbs inward toward your palms.

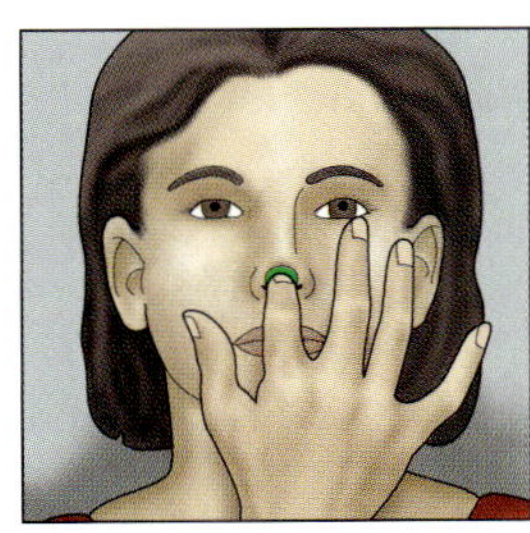

2 Follow the palm treatment with a short series of light presses with the end of your finger to Governing Vessel 25, at the tip of your nose. The combination of palm and finger pressure should make your hiccups go away.

***pendix** and pages 22-23 for more information on point locations.)*

- Lightly press Triple Warmer 17 (in the indentation behind the earlobes) with your middle and index fingers. Hold lightly for one minute.
- Curve your fingers to hold the base of your rib cage directly below your nipples (Spleen 16). Press up, into the indentations at the base of your ribs, and breathe deeply for one minute.
- Place your right middle finger in the hollow at the base of your throat (Conception Vessel 22) and gently direct pressure downward. At the same time, use all the fingers of your left hand to firmly hold the center of your breastbone (Conception Vessel 17). Close your eyes and breathe deeply for one minute.

ACUPUNCTURE

Acupuncturists report effective relief of prolonged hiccups by stimulating points on the hands, feet, and back; seek help from a professional.

HERBAL THERAPIES

To stop the hiccups, herbalists recommend warm ***chamomile*** *(Matricaria recutita)* tea, which is said to act as an antispasmodic agent. Another remedy that might bring relief is a tea that combines ½ tsp of tinctures of ***peppermint*** *(Mentha piperita)* and ***boneset*** *(Eupatorium perfoliatum)* with a few drops of ***cayenne*** *(Capsicum frutescens)* and the juice of a quarter lemon in 1 cup hot water.

HOMEOPATHY

Spasming of the diaphragm may be eased by ***Ignatia,*** *Cuprum metallicum,* or ***Nux vomica.*** Seek help from a practitioner.

OSTEOPATHY

In cases of prolonged hiccups, an osteopath might adjust the painful areas around the vertebrae at the level of the diaphragm to bring relief.

AT-HOME REMEDIES

The goal of any of these cures is either to override or to disrupt the nerve impulses that cause the hiccups. Here are some suggestions that may help you stop the hiccups:

- Place a tsp of sugar under the tongue and let it dissolve slowly; or swallow the sugar dry; or take the sugar with a glass of water.
- Bend forward from the waist and drink water from the opposite side of the glass.
- Tickle the roof of your mouth with a cotton swab at the point where the hard and soft palates meet.
- Hold your breath and swallow at the same time you feel the urge to hiccup. You may need to repeat this two or three times until your hiccups cease.
- Place a brown paper bag over your mouth and breathe forcefully and rapidly into it at least 10 times. Be sure the seal around your mouth is tight so no air gets in.
- Suck on a lemon wedge soaked in angostura bitters or sprinkled with cayenne, or swallow 1 tsp vinegar.
- If your child has the hiccups, tickle him gently while instructing him to hold his breath and not to laugh. ■

H

HIGH BLOOD PRESSURE

SYMPTOMS

In the vast majority of cases, there are no clear warning signs of hypertension (high blood pressure). If symptoms do occur, they may include:

- headaches, chest pain or tightness, nosebleeds, and numbness and tingling; you may have severe hypertension.
- excessive perspiration, muscle cramps, weakness, palpitations, and frequent urination; you may have secondary hypertension, possibly caused by a tumor or an adrenal gland disorder.

CALL YOUR DOCTOR IF:

- while taking ***antihypertensive drugs*** you experience worrisome side effects, such as drowsiness, constipation, dizziness, or loss of sexual function. Your doctor may need to prescribe a different drug.
- you are pregnant and develop hypertension; high blood pressure can affect not only your health but also that of your unborn child.
- you are experiencing severe headaches, nausea, blurred vision, and confusion or memory loss; you may have **malignant hypertension,** which can result in ***stroke*** or ***heart attack*** if left untreated.
- your diastolic pressure—the second number in a blood pressure reading—suddenly shoots above 130; you may have **malignant hypertension.**

If someone were to take your blood pressure immediately after you'd delivered a speech or jogged five miles, the reading would undoubtedly seem high. This is not necessarily cause for alarm: It's natural for blood pressure to rise and fall with changes in activity or emotional state. It's also normal for blood pressure to vary from person to person, even from one area of your body to another. But when blood pressure remains consistently high, corrective steps should be taken.

High blood pressure, or hypertension, is the most common of all cardiovascular diseases in the industrialized world. It is the leading cause of ***stroke*** and a major cause of ***heart attack.*** In the United States alone, approximately 40 million people have high blood pressure. This figure includes more than half of all Americans over the age of 60, and about 64 percent of those over 70.

Blood pressure refers to the force of blood pushing against artery walls as it courses through the body. Like air in a tire, blood fills arteries to a certain capacity. Just as too much air pressure can damage a tire, so can too much blood pressure threaten healthy arteries.

A blood pressure reading appears as two numbers. The first and higher of the two is a measure of systolic pressure, or the peak force of blood as it is actually being pumped by the heart. The second number measures diastolic pressure, or the force of blood when the heart is filling for the next beat. Normal blood pressure rises steadily from about 90/60 at birth to about 120/80 in a healthy adult. People with blood pressure as high as 140/90 on at least two occasions are said to have high blood pressure. If the levels remain high, the doctor will probably begin treatment. Patients with blood pressure readings as high as 200/120 should receive treatment immediately.

Consistently high blood pressure forces the heart to work far beyond its capacity. Besides injuring blood vessels, it can damage the brain, eyes, and kidneys. Even so, many hypertensives do not realize they have the condition. Indeed, hypertension is often called "the silent killer" because it rarely exhibits symptoms even as it inflicts serious damage on the body. Left untreated, high blood pressure can lead to ***vision problems,*** such as swelling of the optic nerve or hemorrhaging in the retina, as well as to ***heart attack, stroke,*** and other potentially fatal conditions, including kidney failure *(see* ***Kidney Disease****).* Hypertension may also lead to congestive heart failure, a common disorder of the elderly that can result in breathing problems. Fortunately, high blood pressure can be controlled effectively. The first step is discovery, so have your blood pressure checked regularly.

CAUSES

In as many as 95 percent of reported hypertension cases in the United States, the underlying cause cannot be determined. This type of high blood pressure is called **essential hypertension.** Patients who suffer organ damage as a result of high blood pressure are said to have **malignant hypertension;** the diastolic pressure in such cases usually exceeds 130. Malignant hypertension is a dangerous condition that develops rapidly and requires immediate medical attention.

When a direct cause can be identified, the condition is described as **secondary hypertension.** Among the known causes of secondary hypertension, ***kidney disease*** ranks highest. The condition can also be triggered by tumors or other abnormalities that cause the adrenal glands to secrete excess amounts of the hormones that elevate blood pressure. Birth-control pills (specifically those containing estrogen) and pregnancy can boost blood pressure, as can medications that constrict blood vessels.

Though **essential hypertension** remains somewhat mysterious, it has been linked to certain risk factors. High blood pressure tends to run in families, for example, and it is more likely to affect men than women. Age and race also play a role. In the United States, African Americans are twice as likely as Caucasians to become hypertensive, although the gap begins to narrow at around age 44. After age 65, African American women have the highest incidence of high blood pressure.

Essential hypertension is also greatly influenced by diet and lifestyle. The link between salt and high blood pressure is also compelling. People living on the northern islands of Japan eat more salt per capita than anyone else in the world and exhibit the highest incidence of essential hypertension. By contrast, people who add no salt to their food show virtually no traces of essential hypertension. Many hypertensives are "salt sensitive," meaning that anything more than the minimal bodily need for salt is too much for them and leads to an increase in blood pressure. Other factors that have been associated with essential hypertension include ***obesity; diabetes; stress;*** insufficient intake of potassium, calcium, and magnesium; lack of physical activity; and chronic alcohol consumption.

TREATMENT

While **essential hypertension** cannot be cured, it can be treated effectively, and **secondary hypertension** can often be cured by addressing the underlying cause. You can do a number of things to control your high blood pressure—but consult a physician before you get started. Together, you and your doctor can design a treatment program that's just right for your condition.

CONVENTIONAL MEDICINE

If you have high blood pressure, you'll probably find out about it during a routine checkup. (You may also have noticed a problem while taking your own blood pressure, but be sure to check with your doctor for a diagnosis.) Take the opportunity to learn what you can do to bring your pressure under control. Most doctors prefer to suggest lifestyle changes before prescribing drugs. A comprehensive lifestyle program will include dietary changes that promote nutrition and lower salt intake, regular aerobic exercise, weight loss, and a ban on smoking. These days, many conventional physicians recommend **yoga, meditation,** or other relaxation techniques to reduce stress.

Some hypertension cases require drug therapy, either because of their severity or because they have failed to respond to self-help measures. A number of drugs have proved effective for high blood pressure—among them ***diuretics,*** which rid the body of salt and excess fluids, and ***beta-***

adrenergic blockers, drugs that make the heart beat more slowly and with less force. Other medications—including ***calcium channel blockers, angiotensin-converting enzyme (ACE) inhibitors, alpha$_1$-adrenergic blockers,*** and centrally acting agents—lower blood pressure by relaxing and dilating arteries. Warning: Do not stop taking prescribed medication until you have consulted your physician; abrupt cessation can be harmful.

ALTERNATIVE CHOICES

Many alternative therapies for high blood pressure focus on relaxation techniques. Others are attempts to get closer to the physiological roots of the problem, either by changing the patient's habits or lifestyle, or by influencing the operation of the heart and blood vessels.

ACUPRESSURE

Applying gentle pressure to several key points on the body *(right)* may help improve circulation and reduce high blood pressure.

ACUPRESSURE

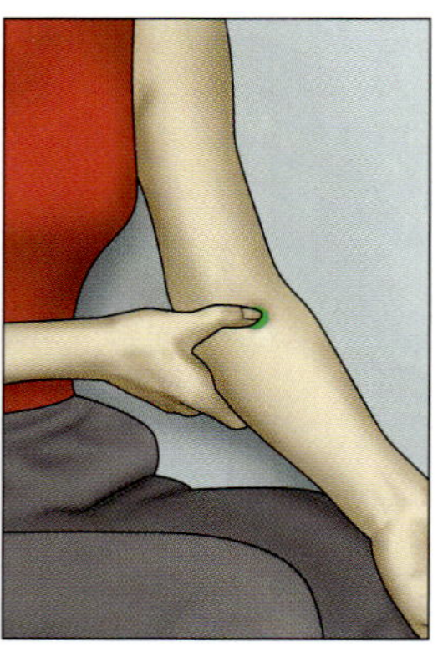

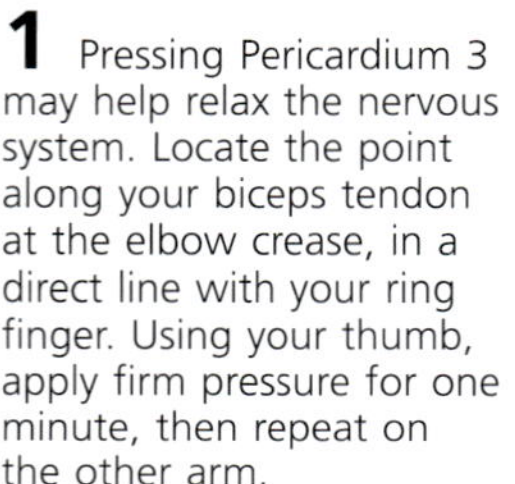

1 Pressing Pericardium 3 may help relax the nervous system. Locate the point along your biceps tendon at the elbow crease, in a direct line with your ring finger. Using your thumb, apply firm pressure for one minute, then repeat on the other arm.

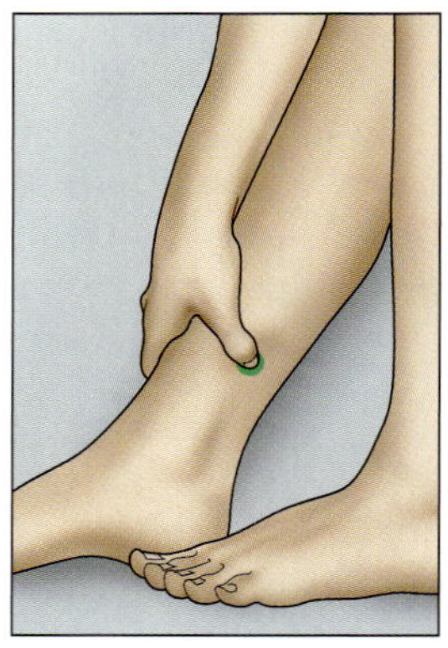

2 Pressure on Spleen 6 may help regulate blood pressure. The point is four finger widths up from the inner anklebone, near the edge of your shinbone. Press gently with your thumb for one minute, then switch legs. Do not use this point if you are pregnant.

BODY WORK

Regular sessions of **massage** or **shiatsu** can help lower blood pressure by promoting relaxation. Both therapies employ touch and manipulation to reduce tension in the body. While massage treats the entire body, shiatsu emphasizes special pressure points, such as those on the backs of the legs and on the inner wrist.

CHINESE MEDICINE

Traditional Chinese healers treat high blood pressure by coupling **acupuncture** with **herbal** and **massage** therapy. Acupuncture may benefit people with moderate hypertension, but it is not recommended for those with severe cases. ***Chrysanthemum flower*** *(Chrysanthemum indicum),* peony *(Paeonia lactiflora)* root, ***eucommia bark*** *(Eucommia ulmoides),* and prunella *(Prunella vulgaris)* are among the many Chinese herbs that might be prescribed for high blood pressure.

HERBAL THERAPIES

Hawthorn *(Crataegus laevigata),* used to treat many circulatory disorders, may help reduce high blood pressure. Over time, the herb may help dilate blood vessels while also moderating heart rate. Hawthorn tea can be prepared at home by steeping the dried flowers and berries in hot water for 10 to 15 minutes. Research indicates that ample consumption of ***garlic*** *(Allium sativum)* and onion *(Allium cepa)* can help reduce blood pressure. ***Valerian*** *(Valeriana officinalis),* used only when needed, may work as a relaxant for people experiencing undue stress. *(See also **Anxiety.**)*

MIND/BODY MEDICINE

A number of methods, including **biofeedback, meditation,** and **hypnotherapy,** call on the mind to relax the body and, practiced over time with guidance from trained professionals, may help lower blood pressure. Positive imagery—picturing yourself floating in calm water, for instance—can also work well for some people.

NUTRITION AND DIET

Adjusting the foods you eat will help keep your blood pressure in check. Your diet should be high

KEEPING A LID ON STRESS

Pets can be a powerful tonic for hypertension. Evidence suggests that just being around animals reduces anxiety and stress for many people.

You may also find calm reassurance in the sound of your own voice. Studies show that speaking softly and slowly, even about the most enraging subjects, keeps blood pressure steady. By contrast, speaking loudly and rapidly, no matter what the topic, can cause blood pressure to rise.

in fiber, low in fat and salt. With these pointers in mind, emphasize fruits, vegetables, and whole grains. Enhance the flavor of your food with seasonings other than salt, and avoid processed foods, which tend to be high in sodium. You should also watch what you drink. Studies suggest that caffeine elevates blood pressure, at least in the short term, while moderate use of alcohol may lower it. Keep cocktails to a minimum, though; more than two ounces of alcohol per day can aggravate hypertension.

Of the vitamins and minerals that help lower blood pressure, ***potassium*** has one of the best track records. To get the 3,000 to 4,000 mg per day that researchers recommend, start eating more fresh vegetables and fruits, especially bananas. (Ask your doctor before taking potassium supplements, as too much of the substance can be dangerous.) Fish is a good source of fatty acids, which help relax arteries and thin the blood. Although it does contain sodium, celery is especially beneficial because it also contains ingredients believed to relax blood vessel walls.

Several studies have demonstrated that hypertensives benefit from daily doses of ***calcium*** (800 mg) or ***magnesium*** (300 mg). Patients sometimes respond better to one than to the other. After checking with your doctor, try calcium supplements for a month. If you do not notice improvement, try magnesium. You can also get calcium naturally from nonfat or low-fat milk, yogurt, and cheese. Many types of seeds, nuts, beans, peas, and dark green leafy vegetables contain both calcium and magnesium.

YOGA

Mainly because of its relaxing effects, yoga is highly recommended for hypertension.

AT-HOME REMEDIES

- Adopt a healthful diet. Eat lots of fruit, vegetables, and whole grains. Give up salty foods and add seasonings other than salt to your meals. Consume alcohol and caffeine sparingly.
- Exercise regularly to shed extra pounds and get your blood flowing. Activities such as walking, jogging, cycling, and swimming lower blood pressure over the long term.
- You can't always avoid stress, but you can learn better ways to cope with it. Researchers believe that stress does not come simply from having too much to do. Rather, it arises from situations that leave you feeling you have no control over matters. Next time you feel stressed, ask yourself why, then concentrate on solving the problem.
- If you smoke, quit.

PREVENTION

You can help keep your blood pressure at a healthful level and reduce your risk of heart disease by making a few changes in your lifestyle.

- Watch what you eat. Stay away from salt and fat, concentrating instead on foods that are high in fiber, ***calcium,*** and ***magnesium.***
- Get plenty of exercise. Regular aerobic workouts condition the heart and keep blood vessels dilated and working properly.
- If you are overweight, try to trim down. Even a small weight reduction can make a big difference.
- If you smoke, now is the time to stop. ■

HIVES

SYMPTOMS

- raised, whitish, usually itchy welts of varying size, surrounded by a red ***rash.*** *(See the **Visual Diagnostic Guide.**)*
- swelling below the surface of the skin that burns rather than itches, often around the eyes and lips, less frequently on the hands and feet, and rarely inside the throat, on mucous membranes, or on the genitals; these symptoms indicate an allergic reaction known as **angioedema.**

CALL YOUR DOCTOR IF:

- burning or itchy welts begin to develop in your throat. You may be at risk of suffocation.
- you develop hives accompanied by dry throat, cough, cold sweats, nausea, dizziness, difficult breathing, or a sharp drop in blood pressure after a ***bee sting*** or ***insect bite.*** This may be a severe allergic reaction known as anaphylaxis. *(See **Emergencies/First Aid: Shock.**)*
- you have recurring bouts of hives lasting a month or more. You may have a chronic condition that needs professional treatment.
- you develop symptoms of **angioedema,** particularly in the head and neck. This requires medical attention before the condition spreads to the throat or tongue and blocks the air passage to the lungs.
- you develop hives after a blood transfusion. You may be having an allergic reaction to donor blood.

Hives, or urticaria, is a common allergic reaction in which a rash or welts appear on the skin. Hives are typically quite itchy and can last just a few minutes or several days before going away. Occasionally, however, these annoying blotches can signal more serious problems, especially when accompanied by symptoms such as difficult breathing.

In **angioedema,** hives develop beneath the skin and can cause disabling swelling of internal organs, life-threatening blockage of air passages, or severe, uncontrollable intestinal contractions. If the swelling occurs in the throat, it can cause suffocation. Chronic cases of hives that do not itch but are accompanied by abdominal pain or diarrhea may be the result of **hereditary angioedema.**

People who simultaneously develop hives and such symptoms as fever, nausea, abdominal cramps, and shortness of breath immediately after a ***bee sting, insect bite,*** or drug injection are in the throes of **anaphylaxis.** This severe shock to the immune system requires prompt medical attention. In rare cases, failure to get help quickly can be fatal.

CAUSES

When an allergen invades or irritates your body, it unleashes chemicals known as histamines. *(See **Allergies.**)* Some people react to a high histamine level by developing the ***rash*** we call hives. Common allergens that can provoke hives include certain milk products, fish, and nuts; drugs such as ***penicillins*** and ***aspirin;*** and various food additives, emulsifiers, flavorings, or preservatives. Extreme cold or heat, ***stress,*** and pressure on the skin may induce an attack of hives, as can ***insect bites,*** infections such as ***strep throat*** in children and ***hepatitis*** B in adults, and—in very rare cases—blood transfusions.

TREATMENT

The first step in controlling hives is to identify the cause, if possible. Once you have identified the source of the problem, try to avoid exposure to it in the future. To relieve itching, apply calamine lotion or a cold compress to the area.

A mild case of hives often disappears on its own after a few hours. A longer-lasting case should respond to the manufacturer's recommended dosage of an over-the-counter oral ***antihistamine*** or ***hydrocortisone*** cream. If your hives don't disappear in a few days, see a doctor. If you develop symptoms of **angioedema** or **anaphylaxis** get medical help immediately. *(See **Emergencies/First Aid: Shock.**)*

CONVENTIONAL MEDICINE

For chronic or especially troublesome outbreaks of hives, your doctor will probably order a course of prescription ***antihistamines.*** Treatment with oral ***corticosteroids*** will reduce swelling faster than antihistamines but is usually reserved for severe cases in which suffocation or other complications are indicated. Ultraviolet light treatments are effective for hives caused by exposure to cold. If you have the subsurface welts of **angioedema,** you may require hospitalization.

ALTERNATIVE CHOICES

Herbal, homeopathic, and other alternative therapies offer various ways to relieve the itching of hives. Relaxation techniques and special diets may provide answers for chronic cases that may be rooted in ***stress*** or ***allergies.***

ACUPRESSURE

Pressure points that may help counteract an attack of hives are Gall Bladder 20, at the back of the head on either side of the spinal column, and Large Intestine 4, in the web between thumb and forefinger. Massage these points firmly for 60 seconds several times a day. CAUTION: Do not press Large Intestine 4 during pregnancy. *(See the **Appendix** for more information on point locations.)*

HERBAL THERAPIES

To combat itchy hives, apply a ***chickweed*** *(Stellaria media)* poultice or add a few teaspoons of the dried herb to your bathwater. A tincture or infusion of **valerian** *(Valeriana officinalis),* ***passionflower*** *(Passiflora incarnata),* or ***peppermint*** *(Mentha piperita)* may help relieve stress-related hives; valerian should be taken in doses up to 10 ml to be effective.

HOMEOPATHY

If your hives sting and itch, try *Urtica urens* (30x). ***Apis*** (30x), derived from the honeybee, is especially good when you have considerable redness and swelling. Either remedy is available over the counter and should be taken every two to three hours up to four doses, or until symptoms ease.

MIND/BODY MEDICINE

Stress can raise histamine levels in some people just as easily as a bee sting. Several relaxation techniques, such as **hypnotherapy, guided imagery,** and **qigong,** may be helpful in relieving chronic hives.

NUTRITION AND DIET

Food additives, as well as natural toxins in certain foods, are prime suspects in tracing the cause of mild to moderate cases of hives. Some of the most likely irritants are found in milk products, nuts, fish, shellfish, eggs, flour, beans, chocolate, strawberries, and tomatoes. You may be able to identify the food responsible for your hives by process of elimination: For a few days eat foods that you think will not make you break out, then gradually start eating suspect foods, keeping a careful record of how your body responds to each one. If your hives persist, consult an allergy specialist for more intensive testing.

AT-HOME REMEDIES

One of the best remedies for hives is a soothing bath. Add 5 or 6 tbsp of oatmeal, 3 tbsp of cornstarch or sodium bicarbonate, or a strong infusion of chickweed to your bathwater. If you are allergic to ***bee stings*** or other ***insect bites,*** ask your doctor about prescribing an emergency kit containing ***epinephrine,*** which is a potent bronchodilator. ■

HYPOGLYCEMIA

SYMPTOMS

- weakness.
- hunger.
- nervousness.
- dizziness.
- trembling.
- heavy or cold perspiration.
- pale or ashen skin.
- tingling in hands and feet.

For diabetics, symptoms might also include:

- headache.
- nausea.
- rapid heartbeat.
- uncooperative behavior, suggesting confusion or drunkenness.
- unconsciousness, coma, or convulsions.

CALL YOUR DOCTOR IF:

- you are diabetic and experience symptoms of hypoglycemia several times within a few days; your doctor may need to adjust your dosages of insulin or oral hypoglycemia medication.
- you feel faint and think you might become unconscious; if you have ***diabetes,*** you need immediate treatment for your blood sugar levels. If you are not diabetic, you should have a professional evaluation of your overall health to pinpoint the underlying cause of your blood sugar imbalance. For diabetics on ***insulin,*** untreated hypoglycemia can result in a coma or irreversible brain damage.

In most cases, hypoglycemia—literally, low blood sugar—can be treated easily without professional intervention when the symptoms are recognized early enough. Although the condition most often occurs in people with ***diabetes,*** nondiabetics can, in some cases, also experience hypoglycemia attacks. Whether you are diabetic or not, if these episodes become frequent, you need to consult a professional about how to keep your blood sugar levels under control.

CAUSES

The body draws on glucose, the sugar circulating in your bloodstream, for energy. When glucose levels fall below normal, the body cannot meet its energy requirements. The symptoms and complications of hypoglycemia develop as your system tries to extract energy from body fat and muscle.

To convert glucose into energy, the body relies on the pancreatic hormone insulin, whose levels normally rise and fall with energy demand. When there is too much insulin in the bloodstream, available supplies of glucose are burned up too quickly, resulting in hypoglycemia.

Insulin levels can rise sharply after a meal, when the sudden rise in blood sugar levels triggers increased production by the pancreas. By the same token, glucose levels may drop as a result of a missed meal or vigorous exercise. Hypoglycemia can also be brought on by stomach surgery, some types of cancer, liver disease, alcohol, high fevers, and reactions to food or drugs.

In some people, excess insulin production is caused by small tumors that develop on the pancreas. Certain foods, especially simple sugars, can also boost insulin production. To avoid bringing on an attack of hypoglycemia, diabetics who administer their own insulin thus need to monitor their dosages and their diet carefully.

DIAGNOSTIC AND TEST PROCEDURES

If you have several attacks of hypoglycemia, you need to find out if diabetes is the underlying cause. Your doctor can determine this through a glucose tolerance test, which measures your body's ability to process glucose, or through a blood test two hours after eating. If you have diabetes, the physician may induce an attack of hypoglycemia to help you learn to recognize and respond to the symptoms.

TREATMENT

Most remedies for hypoglycemia concentrate on regulating the content and timing of your diet to make sure you receive sufficient blood glucose and insulin supplies at appropriate times.

CONVENTIONAL MEDICINE

If you are diabetic and become unconscious during a hypoglycemia attack, it is essential that you receive immediate medical treatment. A doctor can inject glucose directly into your bloodstream, but if that is not possible, a friend or family member trained in the procedure can give you an injection of glucagon, a hormone that helps your body regulate blood sugar levels. Diabetics should always wear a Medic Alert bracelet or tag identifying their condition so that medical personnel can give appropriate treatment if the patient becomes disoriented or unconscious during a hypoglycemia attack. People with diabetes also should always have some hard candy on hand to eat if they start feeling hypoglycemic.

For diabetics, conventional long-term treatment for hypoglycemia aims to regulate blood levels of glucose and insulin to maintain the proper balance between the two. In many cases, this equilibrium can be achieved through diet modification alone. The recommended diet for alleviating hypoglycemia includes small, frequent meals (at least six a day) made up of foods with lots of complex carbohydrates (such as beans, pasta, bread, and potatoes); fiber (vegetables) and fat; and only limited amounts of simple sugars (such as candy or cookies), alcohol, and fruit juices.

If necessary, your doctor may also treat your diabetes with medications such as streptozocin or diazoxide to limit your body's insulin production or to improve your blood glucose levels. If your hypoglycemia is caused by small pancreatic tumors that secrete too much insulin, the doctor may recommend having the tumors removed.

ALTERNATIVE CHOICES

Nonconventional remedies emphasize nutrition and diet, with supplements of vitamins, minerals, and herbs.

HERBAL THERAPIES

A decoction made from ***gentian*** *(Gentiana lutea)* helps improve digestion and the absorption of nutrients. Boil ½ tsp of shredded gentian root in a cup of water for 5 minutes and drink warm, 15 to 30 minutes before a meal. It must taste bitter to be effective.

NUTRITION AND DIET

- Small, frequent meals of whole foods, especially whole grains, fermented dairy products (such as cheese), and lean meat and fish will boost your blood sugar; fruit juice may also help during a hypoglycemia attack.
- Supplements of ***chromium,*** 200 mcg daily—a mineral found in brewer's yeast, whole-grain breads and cereals, molasses, cheese, and lean meats—may help improve blood sugar levels. If you are diabetic, check with your healthcare practitioner before beginning to supplement your diet with ***chromium*** picolinate.
- Avoid alcohol (a simple sugar), caffeine, white sugar, and cigarette smoke, since they can create large swings in your blood sugar levels.

AT-HOME REMEDIES

Whether you are diabetic or not, if you take action immediately in response to the symptoms of hypoglycemia, you can ward off a more serious attack and avoid any lingering aftereffects. Treatment is as easy as drinking orange or apple juice or eating hard candy. Juice, combined with a protein source like a piece of cheese or nuts, may help slow the absorption of glucose into your blood and prevent the disorienting "seesaw" effect caused by rapidly changing blood sugar levels. *(See **Diabetes.**)* ■

IMMUNE PROBLEMS

SYMPTOMS

In general, problems with your immune system manifest themselves as a tendency to catch colds, the flu, and various other infections more frequently than usual; to get easily tired; or to develop allergies. For specific symptoms of immune system disorders, see ***AIDS, Allergies, Arthritis, Asthma, Chronic Fatigue Syndrome, Diabetes, Hay Fever, Lupus,*** and ***Multiple Sclerosis.***

CALL YOUR DOCTOR IF:

- you suspect you have an immune system disorder; you need to be properly diagnosed so that you can be properly treated.

I

The job of the immune system is to seek out, recognize, and destroy pathogens—disease-causing substances or organisms, such as bacteria and viruses. In fighting off these trespassers, your body produces such symptoms of illness as fever and malaise.

When a pathogen enters the bloodstream, a type of immune cell called a macrophage absorbs it, then calls up two other types of immune cells—B cells and T cells. B cells produce antibodies to fight the invader directly. T cells help in various other ways. So-called helper T cells activate the immune response by alerting other immune system cells that an invader is present; killer T cells destroy the intruder; and suppressor T cells regulate and switch off immune activity when the job is done. The immune system then remembers the chemical signature of that particular pathogen and can respond much more rapidly with antibodies should the same pathogen ever attempt another invasion.

In most people, most of the time, the immune system does its job efficiently, but problems in its response to the environment are common. An overactive immune system, for example, results in **autoimmune disorders.** In these cases, for reasons that aren't clear, the immune system mistakes normal, healthy tissues for foreign invaders and attacks them. Examples of autoimmune disorders include rheumatoid ***arthritis, multiple sclerosis, lupus,*** Type 1 ***diabetes,*** scleroderma (skin hardening), and myasthenia gravis (destruction of muscle proteins). Researchers suspect that ***chronic fatigue syndrome*** and ***Lou Gehrig's disease*** may be autoimmune diseases as well.

Another type of immune error occurs when the system overreacts to something harmless, as with ***allergies.*** In the case of ***hay fever,*** for example, the immune system mistakes pollen for a dangerous invader and marshals a powerful and sometimes deadly response.

The opposite occurs when the immune system fails to respond adequately, resulting in **immunodeficiency** diseases. ***AIDS*** is perhaps the best-known example; other immunodeficiency disorders are inherited, extremely rare, and potentially fatal.

For people who are generally healthy, it's

possible for the immune system to become temporarily depressed. When this happens, fighting pathogens becomes more difficult, and as a result, your body becomes more susceptible to infections, which hit you harder and stay with you longer than they would otherwise.

CAUSES

Among the things that can temporarily weaken the immune system are environmental toxins, stress, poor diet, lack of exercise and sleep, and abuse of alcohol and tobacco. Over time, these factors can have a long-lasting debilitating effect on your immunity. Studies have also shown that emotional stress, ranging from such everyday events as a disagreement to such dramatic ones as the death of a spouse, can affect immune functioning. Certain medications (especially ***corticosteroids*** and ***anticancer drugs***), radiation therapy, and—some researchers believe—an overdependence on ***antibiotics*** can also adversely affect your immune system.

Scientists believe that **autoimmune diseases** may result from a combination of genetic, molecular, cellular, and environmental factors. Any enduring illness, but particularly ***cancer, diabetes,*** or ***kidney disease,*** can weaken your body's immune defenses.

People born with inherited defects in their immune systems, such as a decreased number of lymphocytes (a type of white blood cell that produces antibodies), suffer from serious **immunodeficiencies** that make them extremely vulnerable to infection. Diminished immune functioning can also result from such events as having your spleen surgically removed or having to take immune-suppressing medication following organ transplant surgery.

DIAGNOSTIC AND TEST PROCEDURES

To check for impaired immune functioning, your doctor may administer a number of tests. An immunoelectrophoresis test detects lower-than-normal levels of various antibodies. Another test, known as antigenic stimulation, determines whether your body is able to produce certain antibodies. Your doctor may also test for the effects of an impaired immune system: A thyroid function test, for example, will reveal an underactive thyroid, and x-rays can reveal ***pneumonia*** or ***sinusitis.***

TREATMENT

Boosting your immunity may involve altering your eating and exercise habits. Your doctor may refer you to a nutritionist and a physical therapist for specific guidelines.

CONVENTIONAL MEDICINE

Your doctor may discuss with you any stressful events or situations that are adversely affecting your health and suggest making necessary lifestyle changes. The first step your doctor may suggest is to actively stimulate your immune system with vaccines; if that fails, he may try gamma globulin, a blood derivative product that may also work to normalize your immune system.

For people with serious, inherited **immunodeficiencies,** antibody injections, tissue or bone marrow transplantation, and long-term courses of ***antibiotics*** may control the problem.

Medical researchers are uncertain of exactly how the malfunctioning of your immune system known as autoimmunity works. For **autoimmune disorders** your doctor may suggest ***nonsteroidal anti-inflammatory drugs (NSAIDs), corticosteroids,*** or other, more powerful, immunosuppressive medications, depending on your particular ailment and its severity.

If you suffer from allergies, your doctor may suggest a variety of environmental controls to avoid the substances causing your system to overreact. If that proves insufficient to relieve your symptoms, medications such as ***antihistamines, decongestants,*** or inhaled ***corticosteroids*** may be advised. The third step in controlling overactive immunity is a series of allergy shots, or immunotherapy, to desensitize your system so it can react normally.

YOGA

1 The **Child** may help strengthen your immune system. Sit on your heels, thighs together. Exhale slowly while bending forward from your hips. Bring your forehead to the floor. Breathe deeply for 20 seconds, then inhale as you arise. Do once.

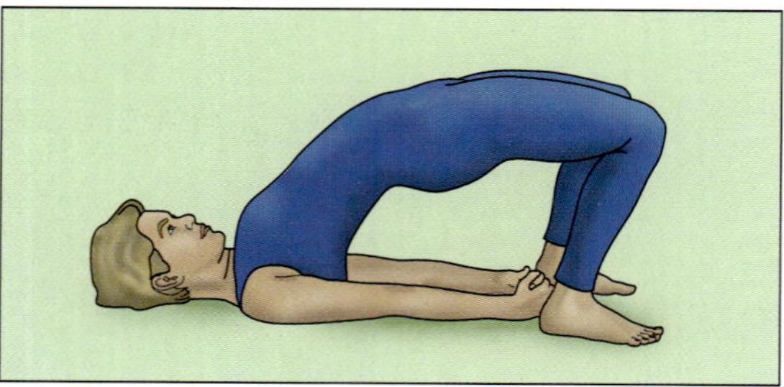

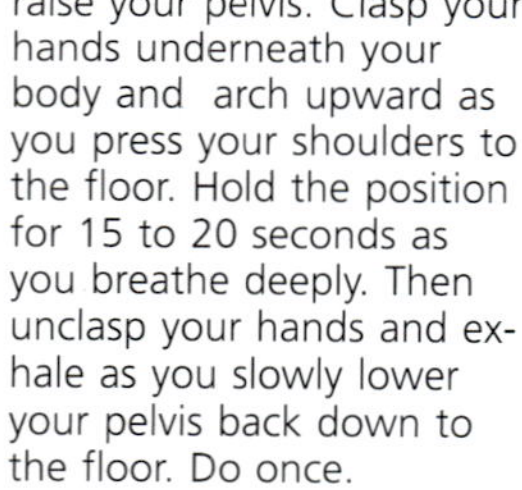

2 For vitality, do the **Bridge.** Lie on your back, knees bent and palms on the floor. Inhale and tense your buttocks, then slowly raise your pelvis. Clasp your hands underneath your body and arch upward as you press your shoulders to the floor. Hold the position for 15 to 20 seconds as you breathe deeply. Then unclasp your hands and exhale as you slowly lower your pelvis back down to the floor. Do once.

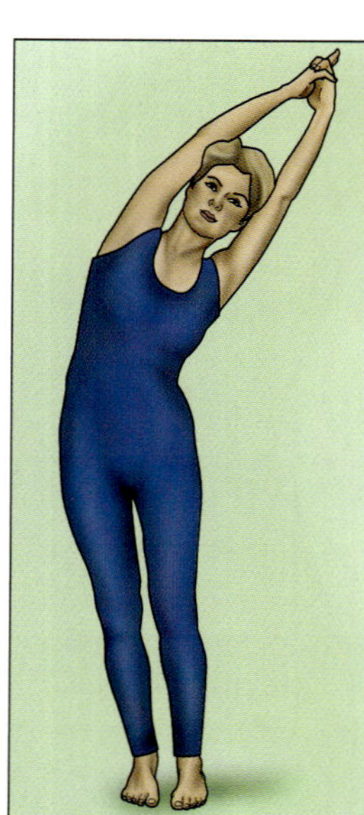

3 For stamina, try the **Half Moon.** Raise your arms as you inhale. Clasp your hands and exhale as you push your right hip out and stretch to the left. Breathe deeply for 20 seconds, keeping your shoulders and hips in line. Inhale as you return to center. Do once on each side.

ALTERNATIVE CHOICES

A number of alternative therapies are available for various autoimmune disorders. Consult the entries on ***multiple sclerosis, arthritis, lupus,*** and ***diabetes*** for possible remedies. The alternative choices suggested in the sections on ***allergies*** and ***hay fever*** may be helpful for those problems. Always consult your healthcare practitioner before embarking on alternative treatments. In addition to the remedies mentioned below, you might want to consider **acupuncture, massage,** or **homeopathy,** which may help with your specific symptoms. For each method, consult a specialist in the field.

CHINESE HERBS

Dried slices of the Chinese remedy known as polyporus, from the mushroom *Polyporus umbellatus,* can be made into a tea and drunk for a tonic effect on the immune system. ***Astragalus*** *(Astragalus membranaceus)* tea or tincture may help combat viral infections and enhance the functioning of immune cells. The traditional Minor Bupleurum Combination, taken as a tea or in tablet form, may strengthen the immune system. ***Ginseng*** *(Panax ginseng)* may improve immune functioning by protecting against the damage caused by free radicals.

HERBAL THERAPIES

Siberian ginseng *(Eleutherococcus senticosus),* long thought to be a potent immunostimulant, helps the body resist disease and improves physical and mental performance. ***Garlic*** *(Allium sativum)* may have anti-infective and immune-enhancing qualities. ***Shiitake*** *(Lentinus edodes),* enokidake *(Flammulina velutipes),* and reishi *(Ganoderma lucidum)* mushrooms may promote production of antibodies.

MIND/BODY MEDICINE

Research into the mind's effect on the immune system, called psychoneuroimmunology, has produced some findings on the relationship between happiness and health. One study has confirmed earlier reports that stress depresses immunity, and feeling good boosts it. Moreover, the data turned up an unexpected discovery: It seems that the impact of positive experiences such as expressions of love or feelings of accomplishment continues for two days, whereas the effects of negative events such as criticism or arguments last only one day. This suggests that the affirming consequences of happiness are more powerful and longer lasting than the negative effects of sadness—by 2 to 1.

Progressive relaxation techniques such as **meditation, yoga,** and **qigong** can promote a deep sense of relaxation and reduce stress. Regular exercise is considered to be another effective way to relieve stress.

Researchers are exploring how **guided imagery** or visualization techniques may help boost immune systems that have become depressed from tension buildup or illness. Athletes have long employed guided imagery to picture themselves winning a race or performing a difficult maneuver. One visualization exercise, called palming, involves summoning up a particular mental image to reduce stress and enhance your mental focusing abilities. To try this technique, close your eyes and cover them with your hands. Concentrate on filling your visual field completely with blackness, then invite yourself to see a color you associate with stress; next, substitute that color in your mind's eye with one you perceive as soothing—replace red with blue, for example. A variation on this technique might be to picture a tense scene, such as a traffic jam, and replace the image with a calmer one, such as a lake or meadow.

NUTRITION AND DIET

Nutritionists may recommend a diet high in fresh vegetables and fruit, whole grains, brown rice, low-fat dairy products, fish, and poultry, and low in refined sugars, white flour, junk foods, red meats, and saturated fats. A daily antioxidant multivitamin containing the U.S. recommended daily allowance of ***vitamins A, B complex, C,*** and ***E,*** with ***zinc, selenium,*** and other trace minerals, can play a role in shoring up immunity. *(See* ***Atherosclerosis*** *for more information on antioxidants.)*

One theory holds that juice or water fasts may release hormones that enhance the immune system. Fasts also cut down on the system's work load, because less energy is expended to process food allergens. Fasts are best attempted under the care of a doctor or nutritionist who will advise you on how to safely begin and end one, as well as about some of the side effects to expect. Don't fast if you're pregnant or diabetic, or if you have a heart condition or an ulcer.

AT-HOME REMEDIES

- Any of the herbal teas mentioned under **Chinese Herbs** or **Herbal Therapies** can easily be made at home and used for self-treatment.
- Identify the stressors in your life and try to avoid them, or else reduce their toll by practicing one of the relaxation therapy techniques mentioned at left under **Mind/Body Medicine.**

I

PREVENTION

Change your habits to include things that actively promote good health.

- Avoid overeating and overindulging in alcohol, caffeine, and tobacco. Get plenty of rest, exercise regularly, and eat a balanced diet.
- Don't assault infections with antibiotics right away unless your physician deems it necessary. The immune system grows stronger with every battle won, so helping it fight with remedies less powerful than antibiotics—such as analgesics, vitamins, and herbal therapies—will allow the immune system to do its job.
- As much as possible, avoid radiation exposure, harmful chemicals, and prolonged use of immunosuppressive drugs such as corticosteroids, all of which can damage immunity. ■

IMPETIGO

SYMPTOMS

- a small patch of blisters that after a few hours breaks into a red, moist area that oozes or weeps fluid; appears mainly on the face, but also on exposed areas of the arms and legs.
- in a few days, formation of a golden or dark-yellow crust resembling grains of brown sugar. The infection may continue to spread at the edges of the affected area.

See also the ***Visual Diagnostic Guide.***

I

CALL YOUR DOCTOR IF:

- you have sores on your face that do not go away in 48 hours after starting treatment. An impetigo ***infection*** needs prompt medical attention.
- small, very itchy, pus-filled ulcers form, with a dark brown crust. This indicates **ecthyma,** an ulcerated form of impetigo that penetrates deep into the skin. If left untreated, it may cause scarring and permanent changes in pigmentation.
- symptoms of impetigo appear on a baby. Any persistent skin disorder in infants requires medical attention.
- a child suffering from impetigo develops nausea, headaches, low urine output, or puffiness around the face and on limbs. These are signs of **glomerulonephritis,** a ***kidney disease*** caused by bacterial toxins.

Note: Sores associated with impetigo may be mistaken for herpes, a viral ***infection.*** Impetigo spreads faster, never develops inside the mouth, and is rarely confined to one area of the body. If in doubt, see a doctor for an accurate diagnosis.

Impetigo is a highly contagious bacterial skin infection. It can appear anywhere on the body but usually attacks exposed areas. Children tend to get it on the face, especially around the nose and mouth, and sometimes on the arms or legs. The infected areas appear in patches ranging from dime- to quarter-sized, starting as tiny blisters that break and expose moist, red skin. After a few days the infected area is covered with a grainy, golden crust that gradually spreads at the edges.

In extreme cases the infection invades a deeper layer of skin and develops into **ecthyma,** an ulcerated form of the disease. Ecthyma forms small, pus-filled ulcers with a crust much darker and thicker than that of ordinary impetigo. Ecthyma can be very itchy, and scratching the irritated area spreads the infection quickly. Left untreated, the ulcers may cause permanent scars and pigment changes.

The gravest potential complication of impetigo is **glomerulonephritis,** a severe ***kidney disease*** that occurs in about 1 percent of cases, mainly in children. With ***antibiotic*** treatment and dietary restrictions, most patients recover from this disease without lasting effect.

CAUSES

Impetigo is an infection caused by either streptococcus or *Staphylococcus aureus* bacteria. These bacteria lurk everywhere—in unclean bathrooms, in spoiled food, and in our own bodies. If a child with an open wound or fresh scratch bathes in an unscrubbed basin or tub, for example, he may contract impetigo. Using a towel or even a bar of soap previously used by a person infected with impetigo can spread the infection. Other skin-related problems, such as body ***lice,*** fungal or strep ***infections, boils,*** or various forms of ***dermatitis,*** can make a person susceptible to impetigo.

Most people get this highly infectious disease through physical contact with someone who has it, or from sharing the same clothes, bedding, towels, or other objects. The very nature of childhood, which includes lots of physical contact and large-group activities, makes children the primary victims and carriers of impetigo. Excessive sweating, malnutrition, and poor hygiene can aggravate the condition.

TREATMENT

The key to treating—and preventing—impetigo is good personal hygiene and a clean environment. Once the infection occurs, prompt attention will keep it under control and prevent its spread.

CONVENTIONAL MEDICINE

Even if only one family member has impetigo, everyone in the household should follow the same sanitary regimen. Regular washing with soap and water can clear up mild forms. If the sores don't clear up in 48 hours, or if the infected person is a small child, see a doctor. To break the chain of contagion, the doctor may prescribe antibacterial baths for the entire household as well as for the infected patient.

A topical ***mupirocin*** ointment, available only by prescription, is highly successful in treating routine cases. Don't try over-the-counter antibacterial ointments; they are too weak to kill strep and ***staph infections,*** and applying the ointment carelessly may actually spread the impetigo. If mupirocin does not help in 48 hours, ask your doctor about an oral ***antibiotic*** such as ***penicillin*** or ***erythromycin.*** Penicillin injections protect against complications of severe infections, shorten healing time, and reduce the chance of recurrence.

ALTERNATIVE CHOICES

As a superficial bacterial infection, impetigo may respond to various alternative treatments, particularly herbal ointments. Be wary of further irritating the skin with products you've never tried before, and see a doctor if the sores do not improve markedly in 12 to 24 hours.

HERBAL THERAPIES

Goldenseal *(Hydrastis canadensis)* is recommended for ***staph infections.*** Mix 1 tsp of goldenseal powder with enough water or egg white to make a paste; apply it to your sores, which should clear in two to three days. Goldenseal may stain the skin, temporarily making the impetigo look worse.

Another recommended herbal remedy is ***myrrh*** *(Commiphora molmol).* Place 5 to 10 drops of tincture directly on the impetigo three times a day. ***Tea tree oil*** (*Melaleuca* spp.) is cited specifically for its antibacterial properties. Diluted, then applied topically, it soothes the itch and promotes healing.

HOMEOPATHY

Treat impetigo with *Mezereum* when there are thick scabs with pus underneath. *Graphites* may be helpful when there is an oozing, honeylike discharge. Try ***Rhus toxicodendron*** to relieve extreme itchiness and ***Arsenicum album*** when burning or rawness is present. Take the suggested remedy in 12x potency every four to six hours, stopping when you see improvement. See a doctor if sores persist after 48 hours of treatment or if they spread.

NUTRITION AND DIET

Since ***vitamin A*** is crucial for skin growth and maintenance, impetigo sufferers should eat plenty of yellow and leafy green vegetables, or add 50,000 IU of beta carotene *(see* ***Vitamin A****)* to their daily diet. ***Zinc,*** said to boost the immune system, is also recommended at up to 45 mg a day. Do not take megasupplements for more than a few weeks, or give them to a child, without medical supervision.

AT-HOME REMEDIES

- If you have only a few small impetigo sores, simply bathing them regularly with soap and warm water, using the medications mentioned above, and exposing them to air will soothe the itchiness and should clear them up. For more severe cases, wash the infected area with antibacterial soap and follow up with an appropriate medical treatment.
- Anyone in a household who develops impetigo should use a clean towel with each washing. Be sure to launder those towels separately. ■

I

IMPOTENCE

SYMPTOMS

Being unable to have or keep an erection is the defining mark of impotence. The problem may manifest itself in several ways. If impotence

- is transient or appearing only occasionally, the problem is not likely to be serious; all men experience impotence at some time.
- develops gradually and persistently, there is probably a physical cause; this is generally the case with chronic impotence.
- develops abruptly but you still have early-morning erections and are able to have an erection while masturbating, the problem is likely to have a psychological cause.

CALL YOUR DOCTOR IF:

- impotence is linked with ***anxiety*** or threatens your sexual relationship. At a minimum, your physician can help clear up misinformation, which commonly exacerbates sexual problems.
- impotence persists. Physical causes of impotence can be harbingers of more-general, potentially dangerous conditions; for example, narrowing of the penile artery may indicate coronary artery disease *(see* ***Atherosclerosis; Heart Disease****)*. For the impotence itself, a physician may be able to suggest a procedure that can alleviate the problem, or might advise the use of a mechanical device if there is no cure.

Impotence—the inability to attain or maintain an erection of the penis adequate for the sexual satisfaction of both partners—can be devastating to the self-esteem of a man and of his partner. It afflicts as many as 20 million American men on a continuing basis, and transient episodes affect nearly all adult males. But nearly all men who seek treatment find some measure of relief.

CAUSES

As recently as two decades ago, physicians tended to blame impotence on psychological problems or, with older men, on the normal aging process. Today, the pendulum of medical opinion has swung away from both notions. While arousal takes longer as a man ages, chronic impotence warrants medical attention. Moreover, the difficulty is often organic in origin. Today, urologists believe that physical factors underlie perhaps 90 percent of cases of persistent impotence in men over age 50.

Because erection is primarily a vascular event, it is not surprising that the most common causes in this age group are conditions that block blood flow to the penis, such as ***atherosclerosis*** or ***diabetes.*** Another vascular cause may be a faulty vein, which lets blood drain too quickly from the penis. Other physical disorders, as well as hormonal imbalances and certain operations, may also result in impotence.

The vascular processes that produce an erection are controlled by the nervous system, and certain prescription drugs may have the side effect of interfering with necessary nerve signals. Among the possible culprits are a variety of stimulants, sedatives, ***diuretics, antihistamines,*** and agents to treat ***high blood pressure, cancer,*** or ***depression.*** In addition, alcohol, tobacco, and illegal drugs, such as marijuana, may contribute to impotence.

With younger men, psychological problems are the likeliest reason for impotence. Tension and anxiety may arise from poor communication with the sexual partner or a difference in sexual preferences. The sexual difficulties may also be linked to depression, feelings of inadequacy, personal sexual fears, rejection by parents or peers, or sexual abuse in childhood.

TREATMENT

If you are troubled by occasional impotence, remember that arousal takes longer as you get older and that satisfaction should not be equated with performance. If your impotence is severe and persistent, you should seek medical help. The number of treatment options has increased in recent years.

CONVENTIONAL MEDICINE

Sildenafil (better known by the brand name Viagra) is the drug most often prescribed to help maintain an erection. However, you should not take sildenafil if you are also taking any ***nitrate*** medications; the interaction of these drugs may cause dangerously low blood pressure.

An erection can be produced by self-injection of papaverine or prostaglandin before sex; these drugs may also improve long-term potency and penile blood flow. Medically administered testosterone shots help some men, but no specific level of the hormone guarantees potency.

For safety and efficacy, and in cases of chronic, severe impotence, many urologists recommend a vacuum inflation device, especially for elderly men.

For blood-vessel problems, vascular surgery to open arteries leading to the penis benefits up to half the patients who opt for this treatment. The effectiveness of such surgery was oversold when it was first developed in the 1970s, but techniques have been improved.

When none of these therapies work, some men choose a penile implant. The least expensive is a semirigid type that produces a permanent erection. More-sophisticated and -expensive implants are inflated by a pump mechanism placed beneath the skin of the scrotum.

If the cause is judged to be psychological, it is crucial to review your relationship with your partner and to examine other possible sources of stress or tension in your life. A trained therapist can aid in these matters and may help unearth problems such as unreasonable guilt, performance anxiety, or inhibiting attitudes toward sex that were learned at an early age.

ALTERNATIVE CHOICES

Many alternative therapies promote the good health and relaxation needed for a satisfying sex life. In addition to trying the choices listed below, you may want to consider consulting a professional, such as an **acupuncturist** or a **homeopath.**

AROMATHERAPY

Essential oils of clary, sandalwood, and ylang-ylang encourage relaxation and feelings of sensuality. Add 2 drops of each to 4 tsp of massage oil or to a warm bath.

CHINESE HERBS

Practitioners believe that too much anxiety can cause energy stagnation in the liver. ***Golden chamber,*** a combination of herbs, sometimes with ***cibot root*** added, is often prescribed.

HERBAL THERAPIES

Ginkgo, damiana, Asian ginseng, and yohimbe are sold in many formulations as sexual stimulants. Keep in mind, however, that claims that they act as aphrodisiacs are misleading at best.

AT-HOME REMEDIES

- Practice different kinds of intimacy and touching; try not to focus only on the erection. Partners who proceed with patience and learn to enjoy each other in a variety of ways often return to full potency. *(See Sensate Focus Exercises in the* ***Sexual Dysfunction*** *entry.)*
- Moderate (not excessive) exercise helps relax the body, boost energy levels, increase physical awareness, and stimulate sexuality.
- Stress or anxiety diverts blood from the sexual organs. Try relaxation techniques, including **yoga, meditation,** and **massage.** Mutual massage slows down lovemaking and opens up communication. ■

I

INCONTINENCE

SYMPTOMS

- inability to control urination.
- involuntary urination when coughing, laughing, sneezing, running, or performing other physical activity.

CALL YOUR DOCTOR IF:

- you have become unable to control your urination after an illness such as a ***bladder infection*** or after taking a new medication. Sudden loss of urinary control may also indicate neurological damage.
- self-help remedies for controlling your urination are not working.

I

Although it is typically age related, incontinence—the involuntary loss of urine—is not, as commonly believed, an inevitable consequence of aging. The condition often reflects an underlying disorder and is usually treatable, even in the elderly. With proper care, about 70 percent of cases can be improved or cured.

If left untreated, however, the condition will not improve and may actually worsen. Incontinence can lead to bladder or urinary tract infections. And the presence of leaked urine on the skin may cause uncomfortable rashes or other skin disorders. In those instances where treatment doesn't work, patients can avoid such complications by using special absorbent pads and other aids designed to help manage the problem.

An estimated 10 million American adults are incontinent. Women are more prone to the condition than men, in part because they have a pelvic floor (a group of tissues and muscles) that weakens and sags with age or after childbirth, making leakage more likely.

CAUSES

Normal urinary control involves the entire urinary system—the kidneys, ureters, bladder, urethra, and pelvic muscles—as well as the central nervous system. When the bladder fills, it sends a message to the nerves in the spinal cord, which then initiates what is known as the voiding reflex, the contraction of the bladder muscles that forces urine into the urethra and out of the body. Incontinence can occur when any part of this complex process is disrupted.

Medical professionals group incontinence into three major categories, although many people—women especially—experience symptoms of more than one. With **stress incontinence,** the muscles surrounding the urethra are so weakened that they can no longer resist a sudden increase in bladder pressure. Coughing, sneezing, laughing, exercising, or otherwise moving in a way that puts sudden pressure on the bladder can cause leakage—but usually only a few drops.

With **urge incontinence,** the bladder, like that of an infant or toddler, simply contracts whenev-

KEGEL EXERCISES

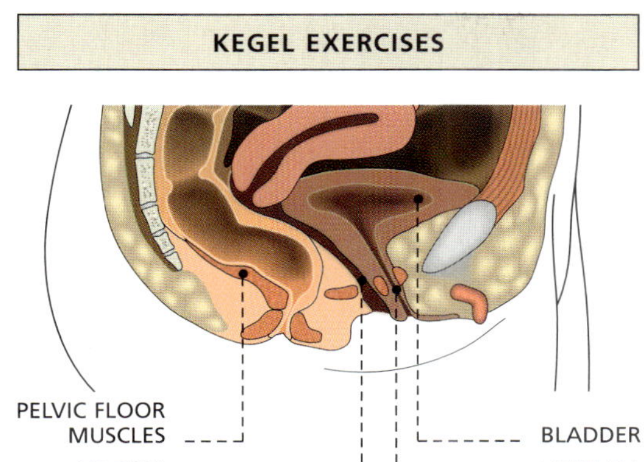

Women with stress incontinence can use Kegel exercises to strengthen the pelvic floor muscles that support the uterus and bladder and control contractions of the vagina and urethra. While urinating, slowly contract the pelvic floor muscles, halting the flow of urine. Hold for up to 10 seconds and repeat several times. You can also do the exercises at other times, while standing, sitting, or lying down.

er it is full; the patient has no control over the sudden urge to void. This is a common type of incontinence among healthy people, but it can also occur in people with illnesses involving the central nervous system, such as ***stroke, Alzheimer's disease, Parkinson's disease,*** and ***multiple sclerosis.*** The leakages typically involve copious amounts of urine, because the bladder empties.

Overflow incontinence occurs when a patient can no longer feel the sensation that signals when it is time to go. The bladder never empties normally and remains at least partially full; excess urine just spills out, usually in relatively small amounts. Overflow incontinence is associated with ***diabetes*** or, in men, with an enlarged prostate that blocks the flow of urine *(see **Prostate Problems**)*; in women, a fibroid or ovarian tumor can be at fault. Medicines or neurological disorders affecting the bladder nerves can be a cause.

Surgery on or near the urinary tract can sometimes leave scars or other damage that causes incontinence. Even a slipped spinal disk can trigger leakages by pressing on the nerves that send messages to and from the bladder.

In women, pregnancy and childbirth, which stretch and weaken many of the muscles that support urinary control, can result in incontinence. Studies have shown that the more vaginal births a woman has had, the more likely she is to leak urine while exercising. After ***menopause,*** falling levels of the hormone estrogen cause the tissues of the urinary tract system to thin, which may weaken the pelvic floor, leading to incontinence.

Incontinence is a potential side effect of many diuretics, sedatives, antidepressants, antihistamines, and other medications. Sometimes curing the condition can be as simple as switching to a different drug. Talk to your doctor.

DIAGNOSTIC AND TEST PROCEDURES

To determine the cause of your condition, your doctor will ask for a detailed medical history, including questions about your symptoms—for example, how frequently you urinate or how much urine you are able to pass each time you urinate. You will then be asked for a urine sample, which will be checked for infection. The doctor will also examine the rectum, genitals, and abdomen to rule out such problems as a tumor or an enlarged prostate. You may be asked to cough to see if that triggers a leakage—a sign of **stress incontinence.** To test for **overflow incontinence,** the doctor may insert a catheter into your bladder after you have urinated to see if any residual urine remains.

If standard treatments have failed to resolve your incontinence, or if your doctor believes surgery may help, you may be referred to a specialist, usually a urologist, for additional tests. A common one is uroflowmetry, in which you will be given fluids to fill your bladder and then be asked to urinate into a special machine that records the rate of flow. Another useful test is cystometry, a somewhat uncomfortable procedure in which narrow tubes are inserted into the bladder and rectum to measure how much pressure the muscles in the bladder exert.

TREATMENT

Most cases of incontinence can be cured or, at the very least, greatly improved with treatment.

Both conventional and alternative medicine have effective strategies for dealing with the problem. Indeed, many conventional practitioners routinely recommend two nonmedical approaches—**Kegel exercises** and **biofeedback**—for patients suffering from stress incontinence. If you wish, you can try alternative methods first. However, if the condition persists or worsens, see a doctor for a full evaluation and diagnosis.

CONVENTIONAL MEDICINE

Many physicians prefer that their patients try behavior modification techniques before taking any medication. Such treatments are safer than drugs and are often just as effective. Two of the most commonly prescribed are the muscle-strengthening exercises known as **Kegels** *(page 495)* and **biofeedback.**

Bladder retraining is another useful technique. For seven days you will keep a written record of how much you drink, how often you urinate, and how much urine you produce. You will then start urinating at scheduled intervals, usually every 30 or 60 minutes. Gradually, over a period of several weeks, you will increase the length of time between visits to the toilet.

If your doctor decides you need medication for your condition, the drug he or she prescribes will depend on the cause of the incontinence. If your urine test reveals signs of an infection, you will be given ***antibiotics.*** If you are a postmenopausal woman, you may be given hormone replacement therapy to increase your estrogen levels (although the benefits of this treatment are unconfirmed). If you have **stress incontinence,** you may receive ***pseudoephedrine, ephedrine,*** or ***phenylpropanolamine,*** drugs that tone the sphincter, the circular muscle around the urethra that helps control urination. To help reduce the involuntary bladder contractions that characterize **urge incontinence,** you may be given propantheline bromide, imipramine, or oxybutynin chloride, drugs that also help muscles involved in urination work properly.

Special devices called pessaries, which are inserted into the vagina to support the pelvic muscles, can help some women with **stress incontinence.** A doctor must fit you for a pessary and give you a prescription for it.

A newer treatment for stress incontinence in women is the use of small, cone-shaped vaginal weights that train weakened pelvic muscles by exercising them in much the same fashion as other muscles are trained using barbells. You insert the lightest cone into your vagina, pointed end down, and contract the muscles for several minutes to keep it from falling out. When you can keep the cone in place for 20 to 30 minutes, you then try a heavier weight—and so on over a period of weeks, progressively toning and conditioning your pelvic muscles until they are working at full strength once more.

If none of these treatments work, your doctor may recommend surgery. In women whose incontinence is the result of pregnancy and childbirth, operations to repair damaged muscles and ligaments or to reposition the bladder can be very effective, particularly in cases of **stress incontinence.** In another procedure an artificial sphincter is implanted; by manually opening and closing this device, you can control the flow of urine and prevent leakages.

If your incontinence cannot be cured or controlled, you can learn to manage the problem with the help of some specially designed aids, including absorbent and odor-neutralizing undergarments and devices that catch urine and drain it into a concealed plastic bag. Talk to your doctor about these options.

ALTERNATIVE CHOICES

Most alternative methods for dealing with incontinence are aimed at building up the pelvic floor to give the bladder more support—and therefore more control.

ACUPUNCTURE

Acupuncturists believe that incontinence results from a deficiency of kidney and spleen chi. To restore the balance of chi in the affected parts, practitioners stimulate the specific points related to these organs and their channels. Consult a professional acupuncturist.

BIOFEEDBACK

Studies have shown that biofeedback techniques can lead to complete bladder control in up to 25 percent of incontinent patients and to substantial improvement in another 30 to 50 percent. Treatment sessions typically involve inserting a catheter through the urethra into the bladder and then slowly filling the bladder with fluid while the patient uses biofeedback techniques to control the urge to urinate.

CHINESE HERBS

Golden lock tea, a mixture of several herbs that traditional Chinese herbalists believe helps the body retain fluids, is sometimes recommended as a treatment for incontinence.

CHIROPRACTIC

Adjustment of the bones and joints around the pelvis can help strengthen the muscles of the urinary system, leading to increased bladder control. An **osteopath** can provide a similar form of this treatment.

HOMEOPATHY

Depending on the cause of the condition, homeopaths have numerous remedies to treat incontinence. Some that are often prescribed include:

- for **stress incontinence,** particularly in the elderly, *Causticum,* which is said to restore vitality to aging tissue.
- for both **stress** and **urge incontinence,** particularly when a person is rising from a prone position, ***Pulsatilla,*** thought to relieve irritation of the lining of the urinary tract system and restore it to proper functioning.

Consult a homeopathic practitioner for additional remedies.

NUTRITION AND DIET

Try to keep your weight down. Excess body weight puts pressure on your bladder muscles, weakening them.

The straining that accompanies constipation can also weaken bladder muscles. Avoid constipation by increasing the amount of fiber in your diet; eat more whole-grain foods and fruits and vegetables.

Avoid alcohol, caffeine, sugar, spicy foods, and acidic fruits and juices—all of which can irritate the bladder and trigger leaks.

REFLEXOLOGY

Reflexologists manipulate those areas on the foot that are said to stimulate the ureters, bladder, kidneys, adrenal glands, and lower spine. *(See **Bladder Infections.**)*

AT-HOME REMEDIES

- Avoid constipation: Eat plenty of whole grains, fruits, and vegetables.
- Do Kegel exercises daily *(page 495).*
- Retrain yourself to urinate at longer intervals. Aim for three to six hours between trips to the bathroom.
- Don't smoke. Nicotine can irritate your bladder.
- Double void: After urinating, wait a few seconds, then try again.
- If you are a woman with **stress incontinence,** try crossing your legs when sneezing or coughing. A recent study showed that this simple practice can be very effective in stopping leakage.
- If all else fails, buy special supplies. A variety of highly absorbent and odor-neutralizing underpants, pads, and shields are available. Try different brands until you find the ones that suit your needs. ■

INDIGESTION

SYMPTOMS

- ***heartburn.***
- ***gas*** or belching.
- abdominal pressure and/or pain, which can radiate toward the chest.
- mild ***nausea.***
- ***vomiting.***

CALL YOUR DOCTOR IF:

- any ***abdominal pain*** continues for more than six hours; this may indicate ***appendicitis, stomach ulcer, gallstones,*** or other disease. You may need emergency care.
- you experience indigestion with any of the following: prolonged vomiting, vomiting of blood, black or bloody bowel movements, severe upper abdominal pain, pain radiating into your neck and shoulder, shortness of breath, or feeling weak or faint. Your indigestion may be part of a larger problem, such as ***gallstones, gastritis, pancreatic problems, stomach ulcer,*** or possibly ***cancer.*** Or you might be having a ***heart attack;* get medical help immediately.**
- you have repeated bouts of indigestion accompanied by abdominal pain, fever, or dark urine. Your discomfort may indicate ***gallstones, stomach ulcer,*** or liver disease.
- your indigestion consistently follows your eating dairy products. You may suffer from ***lactose intolerance.***

Indigestion is a catchall term for assorted stomach discomforts. Symptoms of indigestion are cues that normal digestion has been interrupted for one or more reasons. If stomach acid enters the esophagus, for example, you may feel ***heartburn.*** Swallowing too much air while eating or drinking can induce a distended stomach and cause excessive belching. Stomach infections or inflammation can bring on ***gastritis.*** Sufferers of ***irritable bowel syndrome*** may regularly experience ***abdominal pain,*** bloating, and ***diarrhea.***

Indigestion may be occasional or chronic (daily or almost daily). Though uncomfortable, indigestion itself is not life-threatening. It can accompany serious problems, however, and should not be ignored.

CAUSES

Everyone—all ages, men and women alike—feels occasional indigestion. The likelihood increases with age, as the digestive system gradually becomes less efficient.

Occasional or chronic indigestion may be brought on by overeating; overindulging in alcohol; frequently using ***analgesics***—such as ***aspirin***—and other pain relievers; eating while under ***stress;*** or eating food that does not agree with your system. For a list of common "trigger foods," see ***Heartburn.***

The two most common causes of chronic indigestion are ***obesity,*** which increases pressure in the abdomen, and smoking, which increases production of stomach acid and relaxes the sphincter between the esophagus and stomach. Also, about half of all chronic indigestion sufferers are infected with the bacterium *Helicobacter pylori.* This bacterium is known to cause ***stomach ulcers,*** and researchers are trying to determine if it causes other kinds of indigestion as well.

DIAGNOSTIC AND TEST PROCEDURES

Your own description of your symptoms and a physical examination may be all your doctor requires for a diagnosis. Tests that may be necessary include those used to diagnose heartburn.

Depending on your symptoms, your doctor may order other procedures to identify or rule out more serious disorders.

TREATMENT

Indigestion can result from a number of causes, so no single remedy will help everyone. Fortunately, there are many choices for relief. For indigestion with heartburn, also read the treatment suggestions for ***heartburn*** and ***hiatal hernia.***

CONVENTIONAL MEDICINE

During a physical examination, your doctor will discuss your symptoms and try to determine what caused the indigestion. If there is no serious underlying disorder, the doctor will treat the symptoms and suggest ways to avoid indigestion in the future. Heartburn remedies—***antacids*** and other medications that alter the stomach's production of acid—are often the first line of defense. If excess stomach acid makes ulcer a threat, ***sucralfate,*** which coats and protects the stomach lining, may be prescribed. Extremely painful indigestion may warrant a combination of antacid and the anesthetic lidocaine. If *H. pylori* is detected, ***antibiotics*** will be given to treat the infection.

ALTERNATIVE CHOICES

Because indigestion sufferers may have several disorders at once, healers suggest diverse therapies. With most alternative treatments, patience is essential. Quelling persistent indigestion may take weeks or even months.

ACUPRESSURE

To reduce symptoms of indigestion, massage the following for at least one minute: Large Intestine 4 and Stomach 25, 36, and 37. If gas is also a problem, add Bladder 20 and 60, and Spleen 6. See the ***Appendix*** for information on point locations.

AYURVEDIC MEDICINE

Shatavari *(Asparagus racemosus)* may speed up digestion and alleviate many indigestion symptoms. Ayurvedan bitters may also enhance digestion, including those from *Picrorhiza kurrooa* rhizomes and the trunk wood and bark of the common teak tree *(Tectona grandis).* Visit an Ayurvedic healer to select a remedy and dosage.

HERBAL THERAPIES

Various teas may calm digestive distress. To reduce stomach acidity, drink meadowsweet *(Filipendula ulmaria)* tea once or twice daily, before meals (add 2 tsp to 1 cup boiling water, steep for 10 minutes, then filter). If you also feel stressed, add ***lavender*** *(Lavandula officinalis)* or ***chamomile*** *(Matricaria recutita).* If bloating or gas is a problem, try a tea of ***peppermint*** *(Mentha piperita),* chamomile, or lemon balm *(Melissa officinalis).*

Certain herbs are reputed to soothe and heal the esophagus and stomach, making them particularly appropriate for indigestion with heartburn. About 30 minutes before eating, drink ½ cup of tea made from ***slippery elm*** *(Ulmus fulva)* or ***plantain*** *(Plantago major).*

AT-HOME REMEDIES

- ◆ Refrain from smoking, especially before eating.
- ◆ For occasional indigestion with heartburn, use ***antacids*** or ***bismuth subsalicylate.***
- ◆ Try one or several of the herbal teas above to relieve your specific symptoms.
- ◆ Relax after eating. Exercise diverts blood from the stomach, making digestion less efficient.
- ◆ If you frequently chew gum, stop for a while to see if your symptoms dissipate. It's common to swallow air when chewing gum, which can cause indigestion.

PREVENTION

Indigestion is universal; it's almost impossible to avoid it forever. You can encounter it less often, however, if you watch your weight; avoid overeating (especially foods rich in fat) or overindulging in alcohol; chew your food well; avoid your "trigger" foods; and abstain from smoking.■

INFECTIONS

SYMPTOMS

Fever, chills, sweating, headaches, muscle aches, and fatigue are symptoms common to many infections.

- Diarrhea, vomiting, nausea, abdominal cramps, gas pains, and dehydration may result from an **intestinal infection.**
- Coughing, sneezing, chest pain, sore throat, congestion, and watery eyes are signs of a **respiratory infection.**
- Painful and frequent urination, bloody or foul-smelling urine, or vaginal itching may occur with a ***bladder infection.***
- Rash, sores, inflammation, itching skin, redness, blisters, or pimples may develop because of a **skin infection.**
- Localized pain, irritation, or tenderness may occur with infections of the ears, eyes, mouth, teeth, or gums.
- Intense anal itchiness may accompany a **worm infection** in the lower intestines.
- Arthritic pain and inflammation, often localized, may signal a **joint infection.**

CALL YOUR DOCTOR IF:

- you or your child develops a fever over 101°F or that lasts more than 24 hours. If your ability to breathe, swallow, see, speak, or move is impaired, **get emergency medical help now.**
- diarrhea, vomiting, sore throat, or other symptoms persist or worsen after several days. Your infection needs medical diagnosis and treatment.
- a bite or other injury penetrates the skin. Bite and puncture wounds need immediate medical attention.

The human body is at constant war against disease-causing pathogens, or germs, which can enter the body through inhaled air, ingested food and water, broken skin, insect or animal bites, and sexual contact. Once on or inside the body, pathogens try to survive and reproduce. Most do not succeed. Many succumb to the body's internal heat or chemical environment, or to "friendly" bacteria; others are expelled in mucus, urine, sweat, and feces. Those that survive do so by preying on healthy cells and tissue. Some pathogens can live only in certain types of tissue; others can spread through the body. The three-part process of invasion, growth, and the body's reaction constitutes infection, and though most infections are minor and short-lived, some evolve into serious—even life-threatening—diseases.

Once a pathogen invades, the body's immune system counterattacks. Proteins called antibodies team up with special white blood cells to neutralize and destroy pathogens. The immune system also is able to "remember" contacts with a particular pathogen so it can suppress repeat invasions. This cellular memory—sometimes aided by vaccines—gives the body immunity against countless disease-causing pathogens.

Rapid immune system response stops or weakens most—but not all—infections. Sometimes immune cells fail to recognize and attack pathogens, especially unfamiliar ones. At other times, the body's counterattack isn't enough. People whose immune systems are weakened by fatigue, poor nutrition, certain medical treatments, or illnesses such as ***AIDS*** are more susceptible to infection than are people in good general health.

CAUSES

The pathogens that cause infections are bacteria, fungi, animal parasites, and viruses. **Bacteria, fungi,** and **parasites** generally invade body tissue, steal nutrients from healthy cells, and release toxins; some parasites—which can range in size from single-celled protozoa to visible worms—actually kill healthy cells. **Viruses** are really sub-life forms that survive only by invading living cells and multiplying inside them.

Understandably, the parts of the body that are most accessible to pathogens are those most vulnerable to infection. Pathogens readily infect the eyes, ears, mouth, genitals, and the skin itself. **Skin infections** are extremely common and can be caused by any type of pathogen. Ear infections are usually bacterial; eye infections may be viral or bacterial. Other pathogens can enter the body through broken skin and infect the bloodstream.

Any type of pathogen can invade the gastrointestinal tract, usually through contaminated food or water. Most cases of ***food poisoning*** are caused by bacteria, while giardiasis, an intestinal affliction dreaded by hikers, results from drinking water contaminated by parasitic protozoa.

Most respiratory infections, including ***common colds, flu,*** and mild forms of ***pneumonia,*** are caused by inhaling or ingesting viruses. Severe cases of pneumonia are usually bacterial, as are ***whooping cough*** and ***strep throat.*** Many lesser-known respiratory ailments are fungal infections.

The urinary tract usually flushes out pathogens but is prone to infection when it is swollen, irritated, or obstructed. Ailments ranging from common ***bladder infections*** to serious ***kidney infections*** are usually bacterial.

Although many infections are confined to a body part or system, some infectious diseases spread through the body. ***Malaria,*** for example, is caused by a mosquito-borne parasite; ***tuberculosis*** is bacterial. ***AIDS,*** the deadliest infectious disease of recent times, is a viral disorder.

DIAGNOSTIC AND TEST PROCEDURES

Many common infections are recognizable from their symptoms, but to treat infections that persist or whose potential severity is unknown, a doctor needs to determine the specific cause. Diagnosis usually is accomplished by lab analysis of blood, urine, feces, or infected tissue samples.

TREATMENT

Minor infections are of short duration and usually clear up on their own, but serious infectious diseases require medical treatment.

CONVENTIONAL MEDICINE

Bacterial infections are cured by killing the bacteria with ***antibiotics,*** such as ***penicillin*** and its derivatives. Many fungal and parasitic infections also respond to antibiotics or antimicrobial drugs. The only downside is that overuse or misuse of antibiotics can suppress the body's own natural immune reactions.

Antibiotics are useless against viral infections. Although some ***antiviral drugs*** can reduce symptoms, it's difficult or impossible to develop more effective treatment because viruses mutate, or change forms, so often. Standard therapy for most viral infections is simply to relieve symptoms, prevent secondary bacterial infection, and allow the body to heal itself.

Over-the-counter and prescription medications can relieve typical symptoms and speed recovery from minor infections. Preventive vaccines are by far the best medicine against viral infection, and they are available for many infectious diseases.

ALTERNATIVE CHOICES

Proper nutrition, rest, and ***stress***-reducing activities can help prevent and combat infection. Various herbal, Chinese, and other alternative therapies can relieve symptoms and promote healing. See the entries for specific ailments for more information.

PREVENTION

- Be sure you and your children are vaccinated against infectious diseases, especially before starting school or traveling abroad.
- To prevent the start of infection, refrigerate meat, seafood, and dairy products; wash raw vegetables and fruit thoroughly; keep a clean kitchen; wash your hands before and after handling food.
- Practice good personal hygiene: Bathe regularly; wash your hands after using the toilet; sterilize cuts and wounds with antiseptic soap. ■

INFERTILITY

SYMPTOMS

Infertility is defined as an inability to conceive after a year of regular, unprotected intercourse. The male partner, female partner, or both may account for the condition. It is an impairment; it is not the same as sterility, which means that reproduction is physically impossible.

CALL YOUR DOCTOR IF:

you desire a child but have not conceived after a year of trying ("trying" means unprotected intercourse averaging three times a week). Begin by seeing your regular doctor before approaching a specialized clinic. The cause may be a simple one, such as not having intercourse near the time of ovulation.

For many couples, infertility is a crisis, often accompanied by feelings of guilt or inadequacy. But a diagnosis of infertility is not a verdict of sterility. While about 15 percent of all couples are infertile (that is, they are unable to conceive after a year of trying), only 1 or 2 percent are sterile (meaning that conception is physically ruled out). Of couples who seek help, about half can eventually bear a child, either on their own or with medical assistance.

In cases of infertility, about 40 percent are caused by a problem in the man, and another 40 percent by a problem in the woman. Both the man and the woman are contributors in the remaining 20 percent of cases.

CAUSES

In men, the most common reasons for infertility are sperm disorders, such as a low count (the number of sperm in the ejaculate), low motility (impaired swimming ability of sperm), malformation of the sperm, or blocked sperm ducts. Sperm output can also be temporarily reduced by high temperature in the sperm-manufacturing testicles—a result of spending long periods in a hot tub, for example, or wearing tight underwear. A temperature problem may also have an organic origin: If a vein around a testicle gets twisted—a fairly common condition called a varicocele—cooling of the testicle by blood is diminished.

In women, infertility can often be traced to a lack of ovulation or an impeded journey of the egg from the ovary to the uterus via the fallopian tubes. A failure to ovulate may be caused by hormonal imbalances or by cysts in the ovary. Interruption of an egg's progress through the fallopian tube from ovary to uterus may result from ***endometriosis,*** tumors, adhesions, infection, or prior surgery. In the uterus, implantation of the egg may be prevented by fibroid growths, endometriosis, tumors, ***cervical problems,*** or irregular uterine shape. Fertilization may not take place if the cervical mucus damages sperm or impedes their progress.

Age is a factor: In women, fertility declines after 35, and conception after 45 is rare. Being overweight, or underweight, can also play a role.

In both men and women, fertility can be diminished by psychological factors, such as ***anxiety*** and ***depression,*** and by environmental agents, such as radiation, pesticides, and other chemicals *(see* ***Environmental Poisoning****).*

DIAGNOSTIC AND TEST PROCEDURES

In tracing the cause of infertility, a physician generally begins by interviewing the partners about their health histories, use of medications, and sexual histories and practices. The man undergoes a physical examination first, since male infertility is usually related to sperm health or function, which can be readily tested.

For the woman, testing generally begins with a full physical exam and cervical smear. A physician will then determine whether the ovaries are producing and releasing eggs normally. Blood tests can measure hormone levels.

The ovaries and uterus may be examined by ultrasound, and a specific test can check for tubal blockage or abnormality in the uterus. A postcoital test, done two to five hours after intercourse, can determine whether the man's sperm and woman's cervical mucus are compatible.

TREATMENT

Many couples once pronounced barren can now produce their own child. Some may be helped by common-sense steps that raise the chances of conception *(see* ***At-Home Remedies****).*

Couples are often advised to have intercourse just before ovulation, which occurs 13 to 15 days before menstruation and may be indicated by a slight rise in body temperature or by chemical changes detectable with an over-the-counter urine-testing kit. A new device is able to detect ovulation from a single drop of saliva.

A more aggressive strategy is to induce ovulation with hormones or fertility drugs. Such drugs have a good record of success, but they also increase the chance of multiple births.

In men, disorders of the prostate gland, seminal vesicles, testicles, or urethra can often be treated. A varicocele can be tied off, allowing testicle temperature to return to normal.

The small percentage of couples whose infertility cannot be corrected can try artificial fertilization. In the procedure known as IVF (in vitro fertilization), the egg is fertilized outside the woman's body, then placed in the womb or fallopian tube. In another procedure, called GIFT (gamete intrafallopian transfer), egg and sperm are brought together in a fallopian tube. Both methods are difficult and seldom succeed on the first attempt; they are also costly.

ALTERNATIVE CHOICES

A variety of alternative treatments may enhance fertility. Among professionals you may want to consult are **acupuncturists** and **homeopaths.**

MIND/BODY MEDICINE

Relaxation techniques can reduce psychological stress, which sometimes contributes to infertility. Behavior therapy may help, as can **massage, yoga,** or **meditation.**

NUTRITION AND DIET

Zinc is important for fertility in both sexes; a supplement of 15 mg a day may help (take 2 mg of ***copper*** if taking zinc). ***Vitamin C*** has been shown to aid men whose sperm clump together, and it may improve sperm count. The amino acids arginine and carnitine may be of benefit to men whose sperm count or sperm motility is low.

AT-HOME REMEDIES

For women:

- ◆ Don't douche; it makes the vagina less hospitable to sperm.
- ◆ After intercourse, remain supine for a few minutes; this holds your organs in the best position for sperm to enter the cervix.

For men:

- ◆ Avoid excessive alcohol.
- ◆ Stay healthy; a bad cold or flu can depress sperm count for up to three months.
- ◆ Keep testicles cool; avoid saunas, hot tubs, and close-fitting underwear. ■

I

INFLAMMATION

Read down this column to find your symptoms. Then read across.

SYMPTOMS	AILMENT/PROBLEM
◆ a scratch, cut, or break in the skin anywhere on the body that becomes painful, red, swollen, and/or oozes pus; may be accompanied by fever and swollen lymph nodes.	◆ ***Infection;*** skin abscess
◆ cuticle or nail fold becomes swollen, red, painful; cuticle may lift away from the base of the nail; pus may ooze out if the inflamed area is pressed.	◆ Paronychia (infection of the cuticle or nail fold)
◆ rim of eyelid becomes inflamed and the skin scales; may itch; often seen in people with ***dandruff.***	◆ Blepharitis (inflammation of the eyelids)
◆ redness, burning, and itching in one or both eyes; your eye may become bloodshot and have a sticky discharge.	◆ ***Conjunctivitis***
◆ swollen, red vulva and itching, irritated vagina; may have an unusual, thick, white discharge; sexual intercourse may be painful; urinating may sting and be more frequent.	◆ ***Yeast infection***
◆ in men whose partners use contraceptive jelly or douches, the foreskin or glans (head of the penis) becomes inflamed after sexual intercourse; in women, the area around the vaginal opening (labia, urethra, clitoris) becomes inflamed after using contraceptive foam or gel, douching, spraying deodorant, or washing with soap.	◆ Genital allergic reaction
◆ sore, swollen foreskin; may have difficulty cleaning under the foreskin without pain.	◆ Balanitis (inflammation of the foreskin)

WHAT TO DO	OTHER INFO
◆ See ***Cuts, Scratches, and Wounds; Infections.***	◆ **Call your doctor now** if you develop an infected cut on the palm or web of your hand; such infections spread quickly and can lead to permanent loss of function.
◆ See ***Nail Problems.*** Warm soaks can help cleanse the wound and soothe the pain.	◆ Infection often starts under a hangnail or after some trauma to the nail bed, so keep your nails cut and clean, and avoid polishes and cuticle trimmers.
◆ Bathe eyelids with warm saline solution to remove crusts; your doctor may recommend an ***antibiotic*** or ***sulfonamide***-based ointment.	◆ Your eyelid may invert and lashes may fall out; ***sties*** often develop.
◆ Conjunctivitis usually resolves itself on its own, although in some cases you may need an ***antibiotic*** ointment; consider a boric acid eyewash to soothe the irritation or an eyewash solution of the herbal remedy ***eyebright*** *(Euphrasia officinalis).*	◆ Bacteria, viruses, allergies, stress, eyestrain, and poor nutrition can all cause forms of conjunctivitis.
◆ Use over-the-counter or prescription medications for a vaginal yeast infection. See also ***Vaginal Problems.***	◆ ***Diabetics*** and people who have HIV infection are more prone to all types of yeast infections.
◆ See ***Allergies; Penile Pain; Vaginal Problems.***	◆ Wash your genitals with plain water; harsh or perfumed soaps (especially shampoos) can irritate sensitive tissue.
◆ See ***Penile Pain.***	◆ Young boys may develop balanitis from inadequate washing; see a doctor if the inflammation persists.

I

INGROWN NAIL

SYMPTOMS

- pain, swelling, and redness around a toenail, usually the big toe. The sharp end of the nail will be pressing into the flesh on one or both sides of the nail bed.

CALL YOUR DOCTOR IF:

- the ingrown nail becomes infected (severe pain and pus develop), the pain doesn't go away after attending to the nail, or your nails are so hard or thick that you cannot relieve the condition. Medical intervention is needed, especially in diabetics, who are at risk for complications from foot infections.

I

Ingrown nails—when the nail grows into the flesh instead of over it—usually affect the toenails, particularly the big toe. People with curved or thick nails are most susceptible, although anyone can suffer from ingrown nails as a result of an injury or because of improper grooming of the feet. ***Diabetics*** need to be aggressive in treating and preventing minor foot ailments because they can develop into serious medical problems.

CAUSES

Ingrown nails are most frequently caused by cutting your toenails too short or rounding the nail edges, or by wearing ill-fitting shoes or tight hosiery that presses the nail into your toe. You can also develop an ingrown nail after an injury such as stubbing your toe.

TREATMENT

Most ingrown nail problems can be prevented with proper grooming of the toes and by wearing better-fitting shoes and hosiery *(see **Prevention,** opposite)*. Seek help from a healthcare professional if home management techniques do not relieve your symptoms or if the nail becomes infected.

CONVENTIONAL MEDICINE

If you seek medical help because your ingrown nail has become infected, your doctor will probably prescribe an oral ***antibiotic*** such as ***erythromycin*** or ***cephalexin*** and may prescribe a topical ***corticosteroid*** ointment or inject a corticocosteroid solution into the area around the inflammation. In some cases your doctor may recommend partial removal of a severely ingrown nail. Permanent removal of the entire nail may be advised if ingrowth occurs repeatedly.

ALTERNATIVE CHOICES

Alternative therapies focus on relieving symptoms and healing any infection.

DIGGING IN

SITE OF INFECTION

INGROWN NAIL

A damaged or improperly trimmed nail can become ingrown, burrowing into the skin at the side of the nail bed. The site can become painful and infected and may not heal until the nail is removed. If a nail is ingrown, soften the area with water or lotion; lift the nail away from the skin and trim the ingrown portion. To avoid ingrown nails, always trim nails straight across.

HERBAL THERAPIES

Medical herbalists may suggest soaking the toe in a warm solution of ***calendula*** *(Calendula officinalis)*—1 tbsp tincture to 1 pt water—to soften and cleanse the nail. Dry the foot and insert a thin strand of sterile cotton under the nail to lift it away from the skin until it grows out. Change the cotton daily. Calendula tincture (10 drops) may also be applied directly to the toe as an antiseptic and to encourage new skin growth.

HOMEOPATHY

If home management doesn't bring relief, consult your homeopathic physician. When pus is present and the toe is sensitive, the remedy usually prescribed is ***Hepar sulphuris*** (12c), three times daily for one to two days. For minor pain and inflammation a homeopath may recommend ***Silica*** (12c) three times a day for two or three days.

AT-HOME REMEDIES

Trim the excess nail and put a thin strand of sterile cotton under the corner of the nail to lift it away from the skin until it grows out. Change the cotton daily. If you can't ease the nail out of the skin, try first soaking your foot in warm salt water and then applying an over-the-counter topical solution for ingrown nails or a cream containing 10 percent urea. Lemon is said to act as a natural softening agent. If you want to try a natural remedy, tie a fresh lemon slice around the toe and leave it on overnight. When the nail is pliable enough to ease out of the flesh, trim it, and then apply the cotton as directed above.

PREVENTION

Proper grooming is the first step in preventing ingrown nails. An elderly relative may need assistance, because nails get thicker and wider with age and because older people often have impaired vision and greater difficulty reaching their feet. Parents should groom young children's nails.

Soak the feet first to soften the nails. Always cut the nail straight across using nailclippers, and leave enough nail to cover the toe to protect it. (Do not use scissors, which are difficult to manipulate in the corners of the nail.) Smooth sharp edges with an emery board.

Wear socks and shoes that fit properly. Women especially need to be aware that tight, pointed, high-heeled shoes and tight stockings can cause ingrown nails by putting pressure on the toes.

DON'T TRY IT!

Never try to correct an ingrown nail by cutting a V into the top edge of your toenail. This old wives' tale developed from the mistaken idea that the ingrown nail was caused by the nail being too big and that the sides could be encouraged to grow toward the center by cutting away some of the existing nail. Nails grow only from the base of the nail bed to the top of the toe. ■

INSECT AND SPIDER BITES

SYMPTOMS

Most insect bites produce only minor irritation and such symptoms as:

- swelling at the site of the bite.
- itching or burning.
- local numbness or tingling.

Bites of poisonous spiders and scorpions may produce the following symptoms:

- intense pain.
- stiffness; joint pain.
- muscle spasms.
- abdominal pain.
- fever or chills.
- difficulty breathing or swallowing.
- spreading, ulcerated wound.
- impaired speech, convulsions.

Sometimes, an insect or spider bite causes a potentially fatal allergic reaction known as **anaphylactic shock.** Its symptoms include:

- rapid swelling around the eyes, lips, tongue, or throat.
- difficulty breathing.
- wheezing or hoarseness.
- severe itching or cramping, or numbness.
- dizziness.
- a reddish rash, or ***hives.***
- stomach cramps.
- loss of consciousness.

CALL YOUR DOCTOR IF:

- you think you have been bitten by a poisonous spider or scorpion.
- you experience any of the symptoms of anaphylactic shock. It is a very severe, possibly life-threatening condition. **Call 911 or your emergency number now.**

See ***Emergencies/First Aid: Shock.***

The bites of most spiders and insects, including mosquitoes, fleas, flies, bedbugs, and chiggers, are similar in appearance and pose little danger. Typically, the injection of salivary fluid or venom into the skin provokes a small itchy swelling that lasts a few hours or days. The bites are seldom dangerous; however, mosquitoes in certain areas may transmit diseases such as ***malaria*** and encephalitis.

For people allergic to insect or spider bites, such bites can cause severe trauma and even life-threatening **anaphylactic shock.** Also, the bites of a few spiders, ticks, and insects are poisonous or associated with specific diseases.

Ticks. While most tick bites are harmless, several species can cause life-threatening diseases; see ***Rocky Mountain Spotted Fever*** and ***Lyme Disease.*** Ticks may also transmit tularemia, relapsing fever, and a newly identified and potentially fatal ailment called ehrlichiosis. Rarely, a bite may trigger tick paralysis, which starts with numbness and pain in the legs and can result in respiratory failure.

Spiders. Bites are seldom fatal; infants, the elderly, and people with allergies are at greatest risk. Most dangerous is the **black widow,** found throughout the country and especially in warmer areas. The bite itself often passes unnoticed, but within hours, intense pain and stiffness may begin, occasionally followed by muscle spasms, abdominal pain, chills, fever, and difficulty in swallowing or breathing. About 4 percent of bites end in death.

The bite of the **brown recluse spider** is painless but may cause a spreading, ulcerated wound. Infrequently, reactions include fever, chills, joint pain, and convulsions; death is rare.

Scorpions. Stings cause a sharp, burning pain, followed by numbness. Rarely, scorpion neurotoxin produces shock, or even a life-threatening syndrome of rapid breathing, impaired speech, and muscle spasms. Fewer than 1 percent of stings are fatal, usually to very young and elderly victims.

Fire ants. Recent arrivals from Mexico, fire ants produce small, fluid-filled bites that may ulcerate. The ants bite into the skin, then sting repeatedly in an arc around the bite. The venom is capable of causing severe reactions and even, in some cases, death.

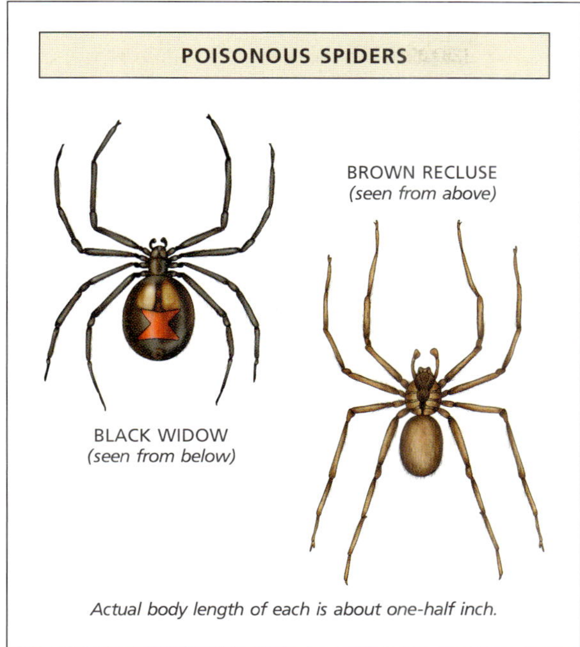

Actual body length of each is about one-half inch.

TREATMENT

For insect bites that aren't serious, the goal of treatment is simply to relieve discomfort. In the rare cases of bites that cause a severe reaction, it is essential to get medical help immediately.

CONVENTIONAL MEDICINE

The discomfort of many insect bites can be soothed by an ice cube, a cold washcloth, calamine lotion, a paste of baking soda, or an over-the-counter ***hydrocortisone*** ointment.

If you think you've been bitten by a **black widow spider,** seek medical help. A doctor may prescribe cold compresses, calcium gluconate for muscle pain, and an ***antianxiety drug*** for spasms. A spreading, ulcerated wound from a **brown recluse spider** bite should be surgically cleaned and repaired; a ***corticosteroid*** injection can ease pain. Do not apply ice. For any spider bite, be sure your ***tetanus*** immunization is current.

If you find a **tick** embedded in your skin, remove it carefully without crushing; grip it near the head with tweezers or gloved fingers and pull gently and steadily. If you think you've been infected, watch for a rash at the site of the bite, which may indicate tularemia, relapsing fever, ehrlichiosis, or other disease.

For a **scorpion** sting, seek medical help if symptoms are severe. You may receive antivenin to neutralize the poison, or calcium gluconate or phenobarbital to relieve muscle spasms.

Some relief for the itchy pustules caused by **fire ants** is provided by anti-itching cream.

For **mosquito** or other minor bites, apply calamine lotion.

ALTERNATIVE CHOICES

For minor bites, herbalists suggest putting ***echinacea*** (*Echinacea* spp.) liquid extract directly on the bite. Others recommend ***calendula*** *(Calendula officinalis)* ointment every four to six hours.

HOMEOPATHY

Pyrethrum tincture may help relieve pain. For allergic reactions, ***Apis*** (6c) every 10 minutes may help before medical care arrives.

NUTRITION AND DIET

Large doses of ***B-complex vitamins,*** including 50 mg ***vitamin*** B_1 (thiamine), taken orally may act as an insect repellent. Use with caution; in some people this approach may cause itching or rash. ***Zinc,*** taken daily (60 mg), is also said to be a natural repellent; because it is a copper antagonist, it should not be taken for more than one month unless copper supplements are included. ***Garlic*** *(Allium sativum)* may also repel insects; try one 400-mg capsule three times a day.

PREVENTION

Essential oils of ***eucalyptus*** *(Eucalyptus globulus)* and pine *(Pinus sylvestris)* are natural insect repellents. Make a solution by adding 5 drops of either oil to a cup of water, and dab on your skin. Essential oil of citronella discourages insects when placed on exposed skin. ■

INSOMNIA

SYMPTOMS

- persistent trouble falling asleep.
- failure to sleep through the night.
- waking up earlier than usual.

CALL YOUR DOCTOR IF:

- you experience disturbed sleep for more than a month without apparent cause. You may need referral to a sleep-disorder specialist to monitor your sleep patterns and test for underlying physical ailments.
- your insomnia is associated with a life-changing event, such as the loss of a job or a loved one. You may need sleep medication for a brief period.
- your sleep medication is no longer effective, or you have been taking medication for more than a few nights without success. You may be at risk of becoming addicted to the medication.
- you never seem to get enough sleep and fall asleep without warning during the day. You may be suffering from **narcolepsy.**

After infancy, humans function the way the world turns—on a natural cycle that repeats itself about every 24 hours. During this daily cycle—known as the circadian rhythm—most adults sleep between 6 and 8 hours, usually at night and without interruption. A few nights of poor sleep do us no harm, but prolonged insomnia can have serious consequences. Insomnia is one of the most commonly reported health problems: About 1 in 3 people encounters sleep problems in a given year, and twice as many women as men. Because sleep patterns change as we age, most sleep disorders are reported by the elderly.

Insomnia can be described in terms of both duration and severity. **Transient insomnia** is associated with a temporary disturbance of one's normal sleeping pattern—caused, perhaps, by travel or relocation—and usually lasts no more than several nights. **Short-term insomnia,** lasting two or three weeks, can accompany worry or ***stress*** and typically disappears when the apparent cause is resolved. **Chronic insomnia** is a more complex disorder with potentially serious effects, including immune disorders: When people are deprived of sleep over long periods, the body's production of natural killer cells—an important part of the immune system—becomes depressed, potentially lowering resistance to disease.

The rare disorder called **narcolepsy** is characterized by attacks of irresistible drowsiness during the day, disrupting the pattern of a person's normal activity. A narcoleptic may not sleep well at night but suffer sleep attacks during the day, while talking, working, and even when driving a vehicle—a potentially life-threatening event.

CAUSES

Insomnia may be caused by physical illness, a stress-filled lifestyle, excessive caffeine consumption, or chronic pain; or it may simply be the result of poor sleeping habits, such as napping during the day and going to bed at irregular hours. It is often linked to ***alcohol*** or ***drug abuse*** and to misuse of certain medications. Psychological factors alone account for about half of all insomnias evaluated by sleep therapists. For example, ***stress*** brought on by situations like a troubled marriage, a chronically ill child, or an unrewarding job can disrupt sleep. ***Depression*** is one of the most common causes of insomnia, and people with ***anxiety, schizophrenia,*** and other psychiatric disorders may also sleep poorly.

Certain physical illnesses interfere with sleep, especially disorders of the heart, lungs, kidneys, liver, pancreas, and digestive system. Other important physical causes include ***heartburn,*** chronic pain, and breathing disorders such as sleep apnea *(see **Snoring**)*. Insomnia often accompanies menopause, when sleep is disrupted by hot flashes or night sweats. Abnormal blood sugar levels can cause people suffering from ***diabetes*** or ***hypoglycemia*** to wake up during the night.

Your own habits and lifestyle may be impeding your sleep pattern. Sedentary behavior and keeping an erratic schedule can contribute to insomnia, as can overconsumption of caffeine and other stimulants, or alcohol and other depressants. Over-the-counter drugs and prescription medications—from ***beta-adrenergic blockers*** to thyroid preparations—can interfere with sleep, as can the accidental or deliberate misuse of sleeping pills, to say nothing of illegal drugs *(see **Drug Abuse**)*. There is even some evidence that using electric blankets can disrupt normal sleep.

Many illnesses are disturbing enough to the body that the normal sleep pattern is disrupted. Among them is the mysterious ailment called ***restless leg syndrome*** (RLS). Sufferers describe an unpleasant, creepy-crawly sensation when they lie still, causing an irresistible urge to move their limbs, even during sleep.

A common cluster of causes known as **circadian rhythm sleep disorders** include jet lag and shift-work sleep disorder. Airplane travel over several time zones disrupts the body's biological clock, which may not adjust itself to the time change for several days. An irregular work schedule or changing from day work to a night shift can also cause insomnia until a person adjusts to the new sleep pattern; some people never adjust completely. Environmental factors such as noise, light, and stale air can cause insomnia or reduce the quality of sleep, even when they don't actually keep you awake.

Transient insomnia, while not physically harmful, can become habitual and very difficult to resolve. The cause of **narcolepsy** is unclear. It may follow an injury to the head or brain, but most cases show no evidence of medical abnormality. The disorder may have its basis in a neurological malfunction of sleep-wake mechanisms in the brain.

TREATMENT

Transient insomnia, which may occur during travel, usually disappears when you return to a regular sleep pattern. **Short-term insomnia,** which may be caused by a family illness or by job stress, may be treated with natural sleep aids *(see **Nutrition and Diet,** page 513)* or, in some cases, with medication. **Chronic insomnia,** which disrupts sleep for extended periods of time, may call for a thorough physical examination, alteration of some life habits, and perhaps psychotherapy to identify a hidden cause.

Treatment for **narcolepsy** is limited by inadequate understanding of its cause. A physician or professional sleep therapist may advise 10-minute naps when you feel drowsy so you will feel rested when you need to be awake. Caffeine, used in moderation, may be helpful, and sometimes medications such as amphetamines are prescribed. For **circadian rhythm sleep disorders,** most people will readjust after a few days on a new schedule. If you have to sleep during the day, keep the bedroom as quiet and dark as possible. If insomnia is due to a physical ailment or condition such as ***diabetes*** or menopause, treating that underlying condition should correct the insomnia.

CONVENTIONAL MEDICINE

Persistent or severe insomnia is something you should discuss with your doctor in order to rule out an underlying ailment and possibly to try an appropriate medication. If you suspect that your sleeplessness is caused by ***depression,*** ongoing ***anxiety,*** or ***stress,*** your doctor may want you to consult a psychiatrist or psychologist. You may be referred to a sleep evaluation center, where experts will conduct physical and psychological tests and monitor your sleep pattern in order to evaluate your situation in depth.

Each year about five million people use sleep medications, but doctors no longer prescribe them as freely as they once did. Barbiturates, in particular, are to be avoided whenever possible because of their addictive power, the danger of overdose, and their toxicity when combined with alcohol. If you take barbiturates, do so only for a day or two at a time and only as prescribed for your particular condition. *(See **Drug Abuse.**)* ***Benzodiazepines*** such as ***triazolam*** and ***temazepam*** are safer than barbiturates, but even they can cause dependence, and they can be fatal if taken with alcohol or other drugs that depress the central nervous system. Benzodiazepines gradually lose their effectiveness and may even worsen insomnia as people develop tolerance to them. It is difficult to stop using benzodiazepines, because abrupt withdrawal may cause distressing symptoms, including renewed insomnia. An anti-insomnia drug called ***zolpidem*** is said to be less addicting than ***benzodiazepines.***

ALTERNATIVE CHOICES

Many poor sleepers simply need help relaxing. If you're a habitual insomniac, and trying to get to sleep just makes you more awake, the following alternative choices may help reduce your worry about sleep while relaxing your body and mind. If the root cause of insomnia is stress, any treatment must address the underlying problem.

AROMATHERAPY

A relaxant effect may be provided by oils of ***chamomile*** *(Matricaria recutita),* ***lavender*** *(Lavandula officinalis),* neroli, rose, and marjoram. Add a few drops to your bathwater or sprinkle a few drops on a handkerchief and inhale.

BODY WORK

Massage can promote relaxation and better sleep. While this may not be possible on a daily basis, it is a good complement to full-body exercises that may have caused stiff, tight muscles.

TIPS FOR A GOOD NIGHT'S SLEEP

- *Go to bed only when you are sleepy.*
- *Get up at about the same time every morning, no matter when you go to bed.*
- *Use relaxing presleep rituals: Try a warm bath with Epsom salt, an excellent muscle relaxant.*
- *Have a light snack—a piece of toast or an apple—or read for 10 minutes before you turn out the light.*
- *Keep a regular schedule for vigorous exercise during the day. If possible, exercise at the time of day that helps you sleep best. For most people, this means in the morning or afternoon, not close to bedtime.*
- *Avoid alcohol and caffeine for several hours before bedtime. Remember that caffeine is present not just in coffee but in chocolate, tea, and many soft drinks and over-the-counter remedies.*
- *For children, avoid overstimulation, such as loud games or exciting TV shows, just before bedtime.*

HERBAL THERAPIES

Half an hour before bedtime, drink a calming herbal tea made with ***chamomile*** *(Matricaria recutita),* ***St.-John's-wort*** *(Hypericum perforatum),* lime blossom, ***passionflower*** *(Passiflora incarnata),* or ***hops*** *(Humulus lupulus);* for insomnia from nervous tension, use vervain or ***skullcap*** *(Scutellaria lateriflora).* **Valerian** *(Valeriana officinalis)* is effective and seldom causes morning sleepiness: Brew valerian tea or take about 20 to 40 drops of tincture in water at bedtime; experiment to find the dosage that suits you best. Note that valerian should not be used in combination with any other sleep medication.

HOMEOPATHY

A homeopathic practitioner may prescribe ***Nux vomica*** for insomnia caused by anxiety or restlessness, ***Ignatia*** for grief, or *Muriaticum acidum* for emotional problems. Other remedies are available, depending on the nature of the insomnia.

LIFESTYLE

Moderate exercise—a 20- to 30-minute routine three or four times a week—will help you sleep better and give you more energy. Tailor the routine to your physical condition, and exercise in the morning or afternoon, not close to bedtime. Breathing exercises can promote relaxation; here's a routine you can do anywhere, anytime:

- Exhale completely through your mouth.
- Inhale through your nose to a count of four.
- Hold your breath for a count of seven.
- Exhale through your mouth for a count of eight. Repeat the cycle three times.

MIND/BODY MEDICINE

Meditation, yoga, and **biofeedback** can reduce tension and promote better sleep. Visualization or **guided imagery** is an effective path to relaxation: Hold a peaceful image in your mind before bedtime. You can learn these techniques from an instructor, a how-to book, or an instructional tape.

NUTRITION AND DIET

Melatonin, a hormone secreted naturally by the pineal gland, is said to induce sleep; try a 0.5-mg capsule nightly for two weeks at bedtime. Because experience with this hormone is limited, consult your doctor.

Calcium and ***magnesium*** taken 45 minutes before bedtime have a tranquilizing effect. Use a 2:1 ratio, such as 500 mg of calcium and 250 mg of magnesium in tablet or capsule form.

High or low blood sugar can disrupt sleep patterns. To help stabilize blood sugar, avoid sweets and fruit juices. To actuate the brain's sedative neurotransmitters, eat starchy food—a plain baked potato, a slice of bread, or an apple—half an hour before bedtime.

Warm milk, a traditional sleep aid, may provide more psychological than physiological benefit. It does contain tryptophan, a sleep-inducing amino acid, but it also contains many other amino acids that compete to enter the brain.

AT-HOME REMEDIES

Be sure your bedroom is quiet and dark. Earplugs and eye shades may help; light comes in even through closed eyelids.

Both children and adults may have trouble sleeping if they are overstimulated by activity or watching television just before bed-time. A quarter hour of quiet conversation, light reading, or soft music may make all the difference.

If you wake up at night and can't go back to sleep, remain quiet and relaxed. Sleep is normally punctuated by periods of restlessness, or even waking. Be patient; sleep usually returns.

Remember, a few nights of poor sleep do no long-term harm. Even if you toss and turn trying to get to sleep, you are probably getting more periods of sleep than you think.

PREVENTION

If your bedroom is too noisy or too bright, do what you can to create a quiet, dark environment with adequate ventilation and humidity; excessively dry air can cause nasal passages to contract and make you uncomfortable. Wearing earplugs and eye shades will help to keep out distractions.

If you're working nights and simply can't sleep well during the day, ask your employer about changing back to a regular daytime job. A strategy that works for some people who must work at night involves installing lights much brighter than normal during the night shift and then wearing dark glasses as they go home and prepare for sleep. This helps to shift their circadian rhythm so they sleep better in the daytime and remain more alert at night.

Try not to be rigid about when and how much you sleep. Worrying about a sleep schedule can just make it harder to fall asleep. If you prefer taking a nap during the day and sleeping less at night, do so. The total amount of sleep you get in a 24-hour period is more important than your daily schedule. ■

IRRITABILITY

Read down this column to find your symptoms. Then read across.

SYMPTOMS	AILMENT/PROBLEM
Persistent irritability, combined with the following symptoms, events, or situations:	
◆ pessimistic attitude; lack of self-esteem; poor appetite; lethargy; insomnia; loss of interest in normal activities, including sexual relations.	◆ ***Depression***
◆ depression alternating with elation, hyperactivity, or continuous talking.	◆ ***Manic-Depression***
◆ inability to sleep; periods of wakefulness at night.	◆ ***Insomnia***
◆ in women, changes in behavior—along with fatigue and anxiety—up to 10 days before a menstrual period, with changes disappearing a few hours after the onset of menstruation.	◆ ***Premenstrual Syndrome***
◆ in women, a noticeable change of behavior at about age 50.	◆ ***Menopausal Problems***
◆ eliminating caffeine or alcohol from your diet, stopping smoking, or discontinuing a drug or medication.	◆ Withdrawal symptoms
◆ a change in family, work, or other routine activity or lifestyle.	◆ ***Stress***
◆ dizziness, headache, fatigue, anxiety, nausea, or shortness of breath not related to any other known ailment.	◆ ***Environmental Poisoning***
◆ during winter months, depression.	◆ ***Seasonal Affective Disorder***

WHAT TO DO	OTHER INFO
◆ See ***Depression.*** Consult a doctor, psychotherapist, member of the clergy, or friend. If symptoms are accompanied by thoughts or threats of suicide, see your doctor immediately.	◆ Depression often goes undiagnosed because symptoms vary among individuals. For example, some people sleep or eat more, not less, than usual when they become depressed.
◆ See ***Manic-Depression.*** Exercise or relaxation activities may help to reduce or counter the symptoms.	◆ Mood swings may occur frequently or years apart. Family or spouse should be involved in any treatment.
◆ See ***Insomnia.*** Try to identify and correct the underlying cause of sleeplessness. Exercise or relaxation activities may be helpful.	◆ Transient insomnia associated with travel or relocation usually lasts only a few nights.
◆ See ***Premenstrual Syndrome.*** When symptoms are present, try to avoid irritating or stressful situations at home and at work.	◆ ***Premenstrual Syndrome*** (PMS) may share symptoms of depression, but the conditions are not the same. No specific cause of PMS has been identified, but some authorities cite hormonal imbalances.
◆ See ***Menopausal Problems.*** Ask your doctor about hormone replacement therapy.	◆ Men also experience more irritability as they age. If behavioral changes seem extreme, or there are other persistent symptoms, consult your physician about an underlying ailment.
◆ See ***Alcohol Abuse, Drug Abuse, Nicotine Withdrawal.***	◆ Severity of withdrawal symptoms is related to the duration of substance abuse. During any withdrawal period, work closely with a therapist.
◆ See ***Stress.*** Try exercise and relaxation techniques. Family dysfunctions are best treated by a family therapist.	◆ Persistent conflict between parents can raise the likelihood of behavioral and emotional problems in children.
◆ See ***Environmental Poisoning.*** Discuss symptoms with your employer or doctor to determine the precise cause.	◆ If you think a chemical, persistent noise, or other environmental agent is making you ill, change surroundings or otherwise avoid contact with it.
◆ See ***Seasonal Affective Disorder.*** Exposure to sunlight or other full-spectrum light.	◆ Seasonal affective disorder is linked to short days and periods of low sunlight.

IRRITABLE BOWEL SYNDROME

SYMPTOMS

- ***constipation*** or ***diarrhea*** shortly after meals, over a period of several months, usually accompanied by abdominal cramps or bloating and increased intestinal gas.
- bowel movements different in frequency or consistency from your normal pattern.

CALL YOUR DOCTOR IF:

- you have pain in the lower left abdomen, fever, and sometimes a change in the frequency of bowel movements; you may have ***diverticulitis.***
- you discover blood in your stools; you could have colon polyps or ***colorectal cancer.***
- you have a fever, or you have been losing weight unexpectedly; such symptoms may signal disorders such as ulcerative ***colitis*** or ***Crohn's disease.***
- your stools are different from their usual frequency and consistency and may be passed with mucus; these may be warning signs of ***colorectal cancer.***

Your digestive system seems totally out of control. Either you can't stay out of the bathroom, or your stomach is tied in knots. Your bowel movements may be loose and runny, or unusually hard. One likely explanation is that you may be having a bout of irritable bowel syndrome, sometimes called **spastic colon** or **spastic colitis.**

Irritable bowel syndrome (IBS) is the most common of all digestive disorders. The most frequently encountered symptom is ***abdominal pain*** with ***diarrhea*** or soft, frequent stools. In other cases, IBS comes with abdominal cramps and painful ***constipation,*** usually following meals. Whatever the specific symptoms, your digestion seems normal but your bowel movements become abnormal and stay that way for several weeks or longer.

Twice as many women as men report IBS symptoms to their physicians, but many people experience IBS without recognizing it and never seek medical assistance. Only a small percentage of the general population has chronic symptoms, yet IBS is estimated to affect 10 to 15 percent of adults at some time in their lives, often during periods of significant change or stress. The onset of IBS is usually in early adulthood, although it can affect children.

CAUSES

As part of the digestive process, the intestines move food through the intestinal tract by synchronized wavelike contractions called peristalsis. Irritable bowel syndrome occurs when peristalsis becomes irregular and uncoordinated, disrupting the normal digestive process. IBS usually strikes without warning, and most sufferers have bowel movements more frequently than normal, although some become constipated.

There is no known cause of IBS. Many authorities consider it a ***stress***-induced illness, while others lean toward food sensitivities, especially as people age. Overeating, or binge eating, is known to aggravate IBS, as is too much fat in the diet. ***Lactose intolerance,*** eating irregularly or too quickly, and smoking may all be factors in IBS. The sugar substitutes sorbitol and aspartame can induce diarrhea in some people. Certain ***antibiotics*** alter the population of bacteria in the intestines, causing diarrhea, fever, and abdominal pain. Morphine and ***codeine,*** the aluminum salts of ***antacids,*** and the prescription drug methotrexate can cause constipation and intestinal upset. ***Tricyclic antidepressants*** may cause constipation, yet newer serotonin uptake inhibitors do not have this effect. Certain ***antihistamines,*** mineral supplements, ***diuretics,*** antipsychotics, and sedatives can also result in constipation in some people.

DIAGNOSTIC AND TEST PROCEDURES

No specific medical test diagnoses IBS, but your doctor will probably send stool samples for lab testing to rule out more serious diseases. Since stress is a potential element in IBS, you may be asked about your personal history, including factors that may be causing emotional or psychological problems. The diagnosis may also include a sigmoidoscopy, in which a flexible tube is inserted into the rectum to allow the doctor to examine the inside of the colon. Other procedures may include a barium enema, which coats the intestinal lining so it can be seen on an x-ray.

TREATMENT

Since irritable bowel syndrome does not have a specific underlying cause, treatment is directed mainly at relieving the symptoms.

CONVENTIONAL MEDICINE

The first line of conventional medical therapy involves an assessment of the quality of your diet—especially your fat and fiber intake. Your doctor may then recommend an appropriately balanced nutritional program. You may be told to cut fat consumption and to take a bulk-forming, soluble fiber dietary product like ***psyllium*** *(Plantago psyllium).* If that doesn't help, your doctor may prescribe ***loperamide*** to slow the movement of food through the intestines, ***dicyclomine*** to calm the gastrointestinal tract, or atropine or belladonna to relieve stomach cramps.

Reassurance that IBS is not a psychosomatic or an imaginary illness may help reduce or alleviate many symptoms and reduce stress. If you appear depressed or under excessive strain, from either past or present experiences, you may be referred to a mental health practitioner for further evaluation. Counseling or psychotherapy may help you relieve concerns that are aggravating your condition.

ALTERNATIVE CHOICES

Various herbal and dietary remedies may be effective in preventing or soothing the discomfort of diarrhea and constipation. Relaxation techniques may be particularly effective in coping with stress-related aspects of the problem.

ACUPUNCTURE

An acupuncturist will determine an appropriate approach by asking you questions about stresses in your life that may be at the root of the problem. Treatment for IBS typically involves 10 to 12 sessions in which needles are inserted along the liver, spleen, and kidney meridians. For symptomatic relief of diarrhea, the acupuncturist will probably insert the needles near the navel and left knee. If you are experiencing a bad bout of diarrhea, the practitioner may employ moxibustion, in which heat is applied near the points, for quick relief.

EXERCISE

Walking at an aerobic pace for 20 to 30 minutes gets the heart pumping, stimulates the digestive process, and relaxes the body. Vigorous exercise is also recognized as an effective way of combating and controlling stress. **Yoga** *(see illustration page 518)* not only conditions the muscles and connective tissue but also is thought to tone the internal organs, including the digestive tract.

HERBAL THERAPIES

For diarrhea, make a carob *(Ceratonia siliqua)* tea: Pour 1 cup of hot water over 1 tsp of roasted carob powder. Drink three times a day.

YOGA

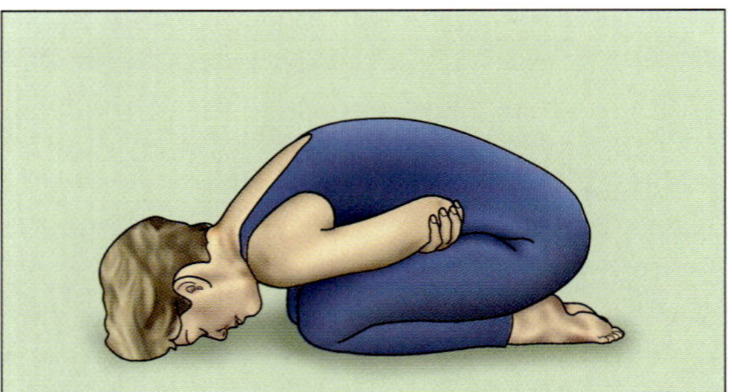

1 To ease bowel spasms, try abdominal massage. Sit on your heels, thighs together. Place your left fist on the right side of your abdomen, press your right elbow over it, and cup your left elbow in your right hand. Exhale, bend forward, and bring your forehead to the floor. Breathe deeply. Relax and gently massage the area with your fist 15 to 20 seconds. Rise and massage your abdomen with your fingers. Repeat on your left side. Do twice daily.

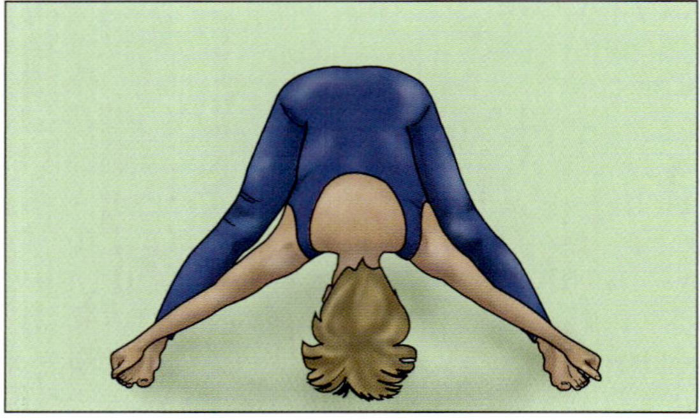

2 **Standing Angle** may help release bowel tension. Inhale and step wide to the right, with your arms outstretched. Exhale, bend forward at the hips, and grasp your feet, ankles, or legs *(above)*. Breathe deeply for 15 to 20 seconds, then inhale and rise slowly. Do once.

To calm an overactive gastrointestinal tract, try a European favorite: Take one or two enteric-coated ***peppermint*** *(Mentha piperita)* oil capsules between meals, three times daily. Reduce the dose if you have a burning sensation when you move your bowels. If you can't locate the capsules, try peppermint tea: Steep 1 tsp of dried peppermint leaves in a cup of boiling water for 30 minutes, and drink three to four cups a day. Infusions of ***chamomile*** *(Matricaria recutita),* ***marsh mallow*** *(Althaea officinalis)* root, ***bayberry*** (*Myrica* spp.), or ***slippery elm*** *(Ulmus fulva)* also are soothing to the intestinal tract and can be made the same way.

Sometimes the bacteria in your digestive tract are killed when you take certain antibiotics, or they become overwhelmed by other types of intestinal flora. To make sure that your digestive tract contains healthy bacteria, eat a cup of plain yogurt daily or ask your doctor about taking *Lactobacillus acidophilus* supplements.

HOMEOPATHY

A homeopathic practitioner will determine which remedy is appropriate to get at the root cause of the IBS. For relief of occasional diarrhea, try prepared remedies available in health food stores. ***Ignatia*** may be helpful if you are having spasms of pain and diarrhea after emotional upsets. If you are passing offensive-smelling gas and mucus in the stools, take ***Mercurius vivus.*** If sudden cramplike pains are relieved by bending over, take *Colocynthis.* If your stools are scanty and you have to strain to pass them, try ***Nux vomica.***

LIFESTYLE

A number of techniques have been found helpful for IBS, including training in muscle **relaxation.** After four to six weeks of daily practice, you will learn how to relax your previously tense muscles and relieve symptoms brought on by stress.

Regular **yoga** practice helps release stress and relax the bowels.

Biofeedback training is another technique that has become accepted by more and more conventional doctors and often is covered by insurance. In one form of biofeedback, painless electrodes are placed on the forehead to monitor muscle tension as an indicator of stress. Patients are taught to relax their muscles by actuating audio or visual signals that indicate the level of tension in the muscle.

Of all the relaxation techniques, the most familiar may be **hypnotherapy.** A practitioner uses the power of suggestion to teach a patient in a hypnotic state how to relax the smooth muscles of the intestines. **Guided imagery,** often taught by yoga instructors and massage therapists, can also teach you new ways to relax yourself.

NUTRITION AND DIET

Certain foods may contribute to IBS by irritating your gastrointestinal tract. Most things that people say taste good—from hamburgers and fries to ice cream and chocolate—are made with lots of fat. Whether it's vegetable oil or animal fat, or saturated or unsaturated, dietary fat overload is something many people simply can't handle, no matter how much they love the taste. Other known irritants to some people's digestive tracts are eggs and dairy products, spicy foods, and coffee—especially decaffeinated. To check for food sensitivities, try an elimination diet: Stop eating a suspected food for 10 to 30 days, then try it again. If you get an adverse reaction, avoid that food in the future.

If you are like most Americans, you are not eating enough fiber. To correct a dietary fiber imbalance:

- gradually increase the amount of fresh fruits and vegetables, whole grains, and bran in your diet, or
- take 1 tbsp of bran stirred into a glass of fruit juice or water every day, or
- take a soluble fiber, like ***psyllium*** *(Plantago psyllium)* seed. Stir 1 tbsp into a glass of cold water and drink once a day, followed by 8 oz of plain water.

When you are taking supplemental fiber, be sure to drink several extra glasses of plain water a day. You may experience a certain amount of intestinal gas at first, but it should subside as your body adjusts.

To stop diarrhea, try two capsules of activated charcoal three or four times a day. Be aware, however, that charcoal can interfere with the body's absorption of any other medications you may be taking.

ACUPRESSURE

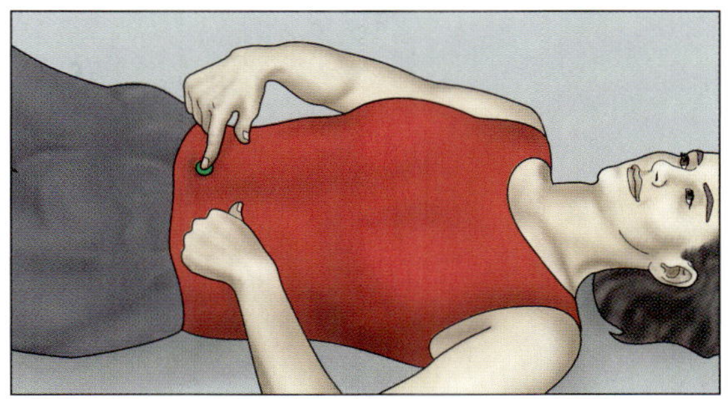

To ease bowel pain caused by IBS, place the index fingers of both hands on points ST 25, two finger widths from your navel on either side. Press down firmly for one minute while breathing deeply, then release. Do three to five times.

PREVENTION

Whether your own case of IBS is characterized by diarrhea or constipation, making sure you have enough fiber in your diet is a must. The average American adult ingests less than 20 grams of fiber a day, although the recommended amount is 30 grams. It makes no difference whether you eat more fiber-rich foods or take dietary supplements, as long as you get your fiber allowance up to par. If you smoke, quit; and avoid excessive amounts of caffeine.

For coping with stress, you have lots of options. If you practice yoga, include Cobra and knee-to-chest postures *(see **Constipation**)*, which help the abdominal organs as well as enhance overall relaxation. Purchase or make a guided imagery tape that you can listen to at home. Get regular exercise—anything from a brisk 20-minute walk, to a round of golf or tennis or a half-hour's worth of swimming laps. Healthy outlets for stress are great preventives to many gastrointestinal problems, including IBS. ■

ITCHING SKIN

Read down this column to find your symptoms. Then read across.

SYMPTOMS	AILMENT/PROBLEM
For itching accompanied by a rash, see also ***Rashes.***	
◆ bloodstains, pain, and itching when you have a bowel movement; most common in middle-aged women.	◆ ***Anal fissure***
◆ intensely itchy, dry, thickened skin that usually appears on the wrist, face, behind the knees, and in the crook of the arm; can be aggravated by food allergies, stress, and weather conditions.	◆ ***Eczema***
◆ itching and a feeling of fullness around the anus, possibly accompanied by a mucus discharge, some pain, and constipation.	◆ ***Hemorrhoids***
◆ an itchy, ring-shaped lesion that extends from the groin to the upper thigh and, possibly, includes the genitals; most common in men. Aggravated by tight clothes, obesity, and warm weather.	◆ ***Jock itch***
◆ severe itching on your head or pubic area; you may see small white specks. General itching, possibly accompanied by lesions on the shoulders, buttocks, and stomach.	◆ ***Lice***
◆ threadlike streaks in your stools, sometimes accompanied by extreme itching around the anus and possible swelling; insomnia and stomach pains.	◆ Pinworms
◆ unexplained localized body itch that precedes an outbreak of extremely painful small blisters, usually on one side of the face or torso.	◆ ***Shingles***
◆ unexplained general body itch.	◆ Any of a number of diseases and conditions, including ***diabetes,*** Hodgkin's disease and non-Hodgkin's ***lymphoma, jaundice*** and other liver problems, kidney failure, ***liver*** or ***pancreatic cancer***

I

WHAT TO DO	OTHER INFO
◆ Use a ***hydrocortisone*** or ***anesthetic*** cream for pain and swelling. See your doctor about any ***anal bleeding.***	◆ Ice compresses will reduce swelling. Two or three warm baths a day can provide relief.
◆ Apply ***corticosteroid*** cream to the affected areas, then cover them with plastic wrap overnight.	◆ Eczema is also called atopic ***dermatitis.***
◆ Take ***acetaminophen*** for pain. Drink at least eight glasses of water a day and eat plenty of fiber. See your doctor for persistent or recurring cases.	◆ Whole-grain breads, vegetables, fruits, and nuts help prevent ***constipation,*** which can lead to hemorrhoids or make them worse.
◆ Use an over-the-counter ***antifungal*** medication or ***tea tree oil*** (*Melaleuca* spp.) cream.	◆ Herbalists recommend swabbing white vinegar on the affected area to soothe and dry up the lesion.
◆ Use over-the-counter shampoo or medication containing a pediculicide (an insecticide for use on the skin to kill mites and lice).	◆ Never use pediculicides around the eyes; rub petroleum jelly onto eyelashes and eyelids and then pluck trapped lice off with tweezers. Combing hair with a fine-toothed comb can work for head lice.
◆ The entire household needs to see a doctor for treatment (even those not infected). Mebendazole is commonly prescribed. See ***Worms.***	◆ Most patients have no symptoms. If you have shared clothes or bedding with someone with pinworms, get treated as a precaution.
◆ See your doctor. Take ***analgesics*** for pain; you may be prescribed an ***antiviral drug.***	◆ Shingles on the face, especially around the eyes, can scar and impair vision. **Call your doctor now.**
◆ Call your doctor without delay if you suspect you have one of these conditions. See ***Kidney Disease*** and entries for the other diseases listed at left.	

JAUNDICE

SYMPTOMS

- a yellowish or greenish tinge to the skin.
- yellowing of the whites of the eyes; this is usually a more reliable sign of jaundice than yellowing of the skin.
- dark-colored urine.
- in some cases, generalized itching.

CALL YOUR DOCTOR IF:

- you notice jaundice in your infant; though jaundice in newborns is common, it may indicate a more serious condition.
- you notice jaundice in yourself, in another adult, or in a school-age child; jaundice may be a sign of ***gallstone***-related problems or liver failure, both of which can be serious if left untreated.

Jaundice, a yellowing of the skin and whites of the eyes, is not a disease itself but a symptom of an underlying disorder. The discoloration occurs when excessive amounts of the body pigment bilirubin accumulate in the bloodstream. Normally bilirubin—a natural by-product of the breakdown of red blood cells in the liver—mixes with the digestive juice bile and passes harmlessly out of the body through the digestive tract. But if the liver is not functioning properly or the passage of bile is obstructed (perhaps by ***gallstones***), bilirubin backs up into the blood. Jaundice in newborns and very young children, in most cases, is relatively benign. But in older children and adults it can be a sign of a more serious ailment.

CAUSES

More than half of all newborn infants experience what is called **physiological jaundice,** the consequence of an inexperienced liver suddenly being required to function on its own. In the womb, a fetus's blood passes through the mother's liver, which disposes of any excess bilirubin. After birth, however, the newborn's liver has to handle the job alone, and sometimes it takes time for the new organ to get up to speed. In rare cases, excessive amounts of bilirubin can damage the child's brain. For this reason, and because it may be a symptom of a serious underlying problem, jaundice should never be ignored.

Premature infants and those with a family history of jaundice stand a slightly higher than normal chance of developing it, as do some breast-fed infants. Physicians can't predict which infants will get jaundice and which will not.

Some cases of jaundice in newborns stem from an incompatibility between the mother's and child's blood types. The mother's immune system attacks blood cells in the fetus, resulting in the development of jaundice in the child after birth. Infant jaundice can also come as a result of some other illness or disorder, such as blocked bile ducts, bowel obstructions, ***hepatitis, mononucleosis,*** herpes infections, or even bruises sustained at birth. *(See also **Bowel Movement Abnormalities** and **Genital Herpes.**)*

Illness-related jaundice is generally a more serious concern in older children and adults. Frequently the underlying cause in such cases is ***cirrhosis,*** caused when liver cells are damaged and replaced by scar tissue. The damaged liver cannot process and dispose of bilirubin effectively, so the pigment backs up into the bloodstream.

Other factors or conditions that can disrupt liver function and lead to jaundice include ***hepatitis,*** certain drugs and toxins, pregnancy, and congestive heart failure. In some cases, ***gallstones*** become lodged in a duct carrying bile from the liver and gallbladder to the small intestine. Its path blocked, the bile backs up and seeps into the bloodstream.

DIAGNOSTIC AND TEST PROCEDURES

You can perform a simple test to check for jaundice in your infant. Using your finger, press gently on the tip of the baby's nose or forehead. If the skin looks white when you pull your finger away, the baby is fine. (This is true regardless of the child's race.) If the spot has a yellowish tinge, the baby is developing jaundice. It's best to perform this test in natural daylight, as artificial light can give the skin a yellow cast. Note: Dark orange or tea-colored urine may indicate jaundice even when the skin appears normal.

If jaundice shows up in school-age children or adults, the doctor may take a blood sample to check for liver damage. The physician may also recommend an examination with ultrasound or x-rays to check for bile duct obstructions.

TREATMENT

Generally, the best way to treat jaundice is to correct the underlying cause; the exact remedy, conventional or alternative, will depend on the nature and severity of the case.

CONVENTIONAL MEDICINE

Most cases of **physiological jaundice** in an infant can be treated through carefully timed exposure to early-morning, late-afternoon, or indirect sunlight. The light will mimic the function of the liver, changing the bilirubin in the child's body to a form that can be excreted through the digestive tract.

If blood tests show that the newborn has high levels of bilirubin, the physician may recommend phototherapy, in which the infant is placed under a special high-intensity lamp until the bilirubin levels drop. Some hospitals rent lamps that are designed to hang over the crib, or fiberoptic blankets that allow light to penetrate to the baby's skin.

Infants whose jaundice is caused by an illness or other disorder may have to be hospitalized while doctors care for the underlying condition. Treatment for illness-related jaundice in older children and adults will depend on the cause. *(See **Cirrhosis, Gallstones,** and **Hepatitis.**)*

ALTERNATIVE CHOICES

Since jaundice is a symptom and not a disease in itself, the underlying disease must be diagnosed before a course of treatment can be established. Alternative remedies should be regarded as complementary care, used to supplement conventional medical treatment.

CHINESE HERBS

A Chinese practitioner may treat jaundice with various combinations of herbs. These remedies must be prepared only by a trained professional.

HERBAL THERAPIES

Various herbs, including ***dandelion*** *(Taraxacum officinale),* vervain *(Verbena officinalis),* and ***milk thistle*** *(Silybum marianum),* are used in the treatment of jaundice. Consult a practitioner for the proper amounts and methods of use.

HOMEOPATHY

A number of homeopathic remedies are appropriate for treating jaundice; the exact prescription will depend on the underlying cause. Consult a professional homeopath for the preparations and dosages that are appropriate for you. ■

J

JOCK ITCH

SYMPTOMS

- itchy red bumps in the groin area and on the external genitalia; the rash may extend to the buttocks and inner thighs.

CALL YOUR DOCTOR IF:

- over-the-counter remedies fail to work after a week or two.
- the rash spreads or gets worse.
- you develop a chronic condition, in which the rash keeps coming back.

J

Jock itch is the common name for a fungal infection of the groin known technically as tinea cruris. If you're a man, you've probably had it at some time in your life. But women can get jock itch too; although the fungus is different, the symptoms are the same. The culprit in women is a ***yeast infection*** called candidiasis, which begins in the vagina and may spread to external skin if left untreated. Men and women who perspire a lot or who are obese and are likely to have folds of skin that rub against each other are particularly prone to developing rashes in the groin area.

CAUSES

Jock itch is caused by a fungus known as *Trichophyton rubrum,* which is from the same family of organisms responsible for ***athlete's foot.*** The fungus thrives in moist, warm areas. Wearing an athletic supporter, or jockstrap, can promote it.

You will probably be able to tell on your own that you have jock itch. If you are in doubt, though, see your doctor, who will almost certainly be able to confirm a diagnosis by visual examination alone.

TREATMENT

You will usually not need to seek professional care for jock itch, unless the rash is severe or widely spread. In the vast majority of cases, you will be able to treat the problem with over-the-counter medications.

With proper treatment, the cure rate for jock itch is very high, but about 20 percent of people develop a chronic condition. If this turns out to be the case for you, seek help from your doctor, who will be able to prescribe stronger medications.

CONVENTIONAL MEDICINE

Most ointments for jock itch contain antifungal agents such as ***miconazole*** and ***clotrimazole***.

BEST TREATMENT TIPS

- ◆ *Keep your groin area clean and dry.*
- ◆ *Change your athletic supporter and underwear every day, and wash them in hot water.*
- ◆ *Wear clean cotton shorts under your jockstrap.*
- ◆ *If you have been prone to jock itch in the past and normally wear briefs, consider switching to boxer shorts, which can help keep the groin area drier by allowing better air circulation.*
- ◆ *Use baby powder to prevent the moisture that can lead to jock itch.*
- ◆ *Shower with antibacterial soaps; rinse well to prevent the buildup of potentially irritating soap remnants.*
- ◆ *Do not use someone else's towel at the gym; jock itch is mildly contagious.*
- ◆ *Dry your groin well with a towel or with a hair dryer on its lowest setting.*
- ◆ *Change your clothes as soon as you finish working out.*

These ointments are available in drugstores without a prescription. If you're not sure what to buy, ask the pharmacist to recommend something.

Apply the medicine to the affected area every day as directed until the rash goes away; keep using it for at least a month longer to make sure you have killed the fungus. Keep the area dry and wear loose-fitting clothing until the rash clears up.

To prevent the rash from getting worse or coming back, change your underwear every day and wash it in hot water. If the rash comes back or if you develop an infection, consult your doctor, who can prescribe an ***antibiotic.***

ALTERNATIVE CHOICES

In addition to prescription and over-the-counter medicines, a number of alternative therapies may help speed the healing process.

AROMATHERAPY

A common aromatherapy treatment for a variety of skin conditions involves applications of ***tea tree oil*** (*Melaleuca* spp.). Dilute it with a carrier oil such as almond oil and apply to your rash several times a day.

Other oils recommended by aromatherapists to relieve itching are cedarwood *(Juniperus virginiana)* and jasmine *(Jasminum officinale).* Apply these oils in a similar fashion, several times a day.

HERBAL THERAPIES

Herbalists say that one of the best remedies for jock itch is to swab your groin area with diluted freshly squeezed lemon juice, though it may be painful. Lemon juice soothes the skin and will help to dry up the rash.

AT-HOME REMEDIES

- ◆ Wash the affected area with an antibacterial soap.
- ◆ Use a hair dryer on the lowest setting after showering to dry the affected area as thoroughly as possible.
- ◆ Apply over-the-counter antifungal creams or drying powder two or three times a day until the rash goes away.
- ◆ Take a warm bath to relieve itching.
- ◆ Apply diluted lemon juice *(see **Herbal Therapies,** above).*
- ◆ Apply oils of tea tree, cedarwood, or jasmine.■

JOINT PAIN

Read down this column to find your symptoms. Then read across.

SYMPTOMS	AILMENT/PROBLEM
◆ joint pain after an injury; the joint is misshapen and can't be moved.	◆ Dislocation
◆ joint and muscle pain; fever, chills, headache, weakness, malaise, nasal congestion, cough; possibly, vomiting and diarrhea.	◆ ***Flu***
◆ chronic joint pain and stiffness; limited joint movement; symptoms worse after sitting or sleeping; more common in people over 50 and those who overexert their bodies.	◆ Osteoarthritis
◆ pain, swelling, redness, warmth, and stiffness in more than one joint.	◆ Rheumatoid ***arthritis***
◆ sharp, intense pain, swelling, redness, warmth, and stiffness in one joint, often affecting the joint at the base of the big toe, or sometimes the ankle or knee.	◆ ***Gout***
◆ pain, warmth, and stiffness in one or more joints, and possibly redness and swelling, especially when stretching or extending the joint; restricted range of movement.	◆ ***Bursitis***
◆ pain, swelling, redness, warmth, and stiffness; possibly, chills, fever, weakness, sore throat, rash.	◆ Infectious ***arthritis***
◆ pain, swelling, redness, and warmth in joints; abdominal pain and diarrhea; cramps or pain after eating; chronic low-grade fever; loss of appetite, fatigue, weight loss.	◆ Inflammatory bowel disease ***(Crohn's disease*** or ulcerative ***colitis)***
◆ joint and muscle pain; headache, fatigue, malaise, fever; several months earlier, circular or oval-red rash with white center, preceded by a tick bite.	◆ ***Lyme disease***

WHAT TO DO	OTHER INFO
◆ **Call your doctor or obtain emergency care now.** See ***Emergencies/First Aid: Fractures and Dislocations.***	◆ If a joint appears misshapen, do not move the patient or the joint unless absolutely necessary.
◆ Rest, drink plenty of fluids, and if needed, take an anti-inflammatory painkiller such as ***ibuprofen.*** Herbalists recommend the anti-viral herb osha *(Ligusticum porteri).*	◆ ***Antibiotics*** are not helpful for flu because it is caused by a virus, but they may be required if there is a secondary bacterial infection, such as ***bronchitis*** or ***pneumonia.***
◆ See ***Arthritis.*** Your doctor may prescribe ***analgesics,*** exercises, heat treatment, and physical therapy.	
◆ See ***Arthritis.*** Take an anti-inflammatory painkiller such as ***ibuprofen.***	◆ Other types of inflammatory arthritis include psoriatic arthritis, which may accompany ***psoriasis;*** reactive arthritis, which may follow a systemic infection; and ankylosing spondylitis (usually inherited).
◆ The usual treatment is a ***nonsteroidal anti-inflammatory drug (NSAID)*** and/or the drug colchicine.	◆ Following a low-purine, vegetarian diet may help prevent attacks. Eating cherries, strawberries, or blueberries may help ease the pain.
◆ Avoid activities that bring on the pain and take an anti-inflammatory painkiller such as ***ibuprofen.*** If pain or swelling persists, your doctor may suggest ***corticosteroid*** treatment or draining fluid from the joint.	◆ Professional deep-heat therapy may relieve symptoms. Extra ***vitamin C, vitamin A,*** and ***zinc*** may be helpful, as may ***vitamin*** B_{12} injections. Homepaths suggest taking ***Rhus toxicodendron*** (30c).
◆ **Call your doctor now.** The usual treatment is anti-inflammatory drugs, intravenous ***antibiotics*** if the cause is bacterial, and drainage of excess fluid from joint.	◆ This type of arthritis is usually a complication of a recent injury or disease.
◆ See ***Crohn's Disease*** and ***Colitis.*** The usual treatment involves dietary changes and medication.	◆ Topical capsaicin ointment may be helpful in relieving the joint pain.
◆ **Call your doctor now.** The usual treatment is with ***antibiotics.***	◆ The disease always starts with the bite of a deer tick. Joint pain may occur in a later stage of the disease, several months or more after the bite.

J

KIDNEY CANCER

SYMPTOMS

- reddish or cloudy urine, although microscopic traces of blood may be evident in routine urine analyses before the urine changes color. While blood in the urine is usually a sign of ***kidney infection,*** it can also be associated with cancer.
- dull pain in the abdomen, lower back, or side.
- a detectable mass in the lower back that feels smooth and firm, but not tender.
- with advanced kidney cancer, fatigue, intermittent low-grade fever, vomiting, appetite and weight loss, and a general sense of ill health.

K

CALL YOUR DOCTOR IF:

- you experience any symptoms of kidney cancer. The most likely symptoms will be discolored urine, pain in the back or side, and sometimes a mass in the kidney region.

The kidneys are a pair of bean-shaped organs located just above the waist on either side of the spine. The outer portion of each kidney is actually a web of nephrons (capillaries and tubules), which cleanse the blood and produce urine. Benign cysts that resemble fluid-filled sacs commonly develop in the nephron web; much less often, a malignant tumor forms.

Renal cell carcinoma, the most common type of adult kidney cancer, starts in a kidney's outer portion. The next most common type, **transitional cell carcinoma,** originates in the interior of the kidney, where urine collects. Cancer cells may eventually spread to blood vessels, lymph nodes, fat, nearby organs such as the liver or adrenal glands, and ultimately the lungs or bones.

Adult kidney cancer accounts for about 2 percent of cancers in the U.S., but its incidence is steadily rising. It is twice as common in men as in women, and it usually begins after age 40. If diagnosed early, patients have a 60 to 80 percent chance of surviving at least five years; the five-year survival rate for advanced cases drops substantially, depending on how far the cancer has spread beyond the kidney. Of children with kidney cancer, 95 percent have **Wilms' tumor;** if treated early enough, almost all cases are curable.

CAUSES

Kidney cancer is strongly associated with a number of other health problems: congenital defects of the kidney or bladder, frequent urinary tract infections, ***kidney disease*** requiring long-term dialysis, and von Hippel-Lindau disease—a rare condition affecting the brain capillaries. A specific genetic defect has been found to cause **Wilms' tumor.**

Smokers are twice as likely to develop kidney cancer as nonsmokers. The disease is also associated with exposure to industrial agents such as asbestos, naphthalenes, aniline dyes, and benzidines, and to phenacetin, a painkiller no longer marketed in the U.S. Diets high in fat and protein may increase risk, as does ***obesity.*** Aflatoxins—molds that grow in milk, grains, nuts, and seeds—have also been linked to kidney cancer.

DIAGNOSTIC AND TEST PROCEDURES

If your doctor detects a mass in the abdominal or kidney region or—using a stethoscope—hears an unusual noise over the renal artery, he will check for kidney cancer. (Less commonly, high blood pressure, abnormal liver function, high red blood cell count, or a high level of calcium in the blood may raise suspicions.) The doctor will use ultrasound, a CT scan, or a special x-ray test called an intravenous pyelogram (IVP) to identify and locate a kidney tumor. If the tumor proves malignant, other imaging tests help to determine whether the cancer has spread.

TREATMENT

If it is caught early, a kidney tumor will be removed surgically. The surgeon tries to remove only the cancerous area but may have to take out the entire kidney along with surrounding fat, lymph nodes, and possibly the adrenal gland. Radiation therapy and chemotherapy can reduce tumor size but are not consistently effective in preventing the spread of kidney cancer. Chemotherapy after surgery cures local **Wilms' tumor** in 9 out of 10 cases.

Neither radiation nor chemotherapy is particularly successful in treating advanced kidney cancer. Hormonal therapy is sometimes prescribed, and new therapies are being tested constantly in the hope of improving cure rates. Immunotherapy using either interferon or interleukin 2 to boost the body's natural cancer-killing powers has shown promise. After remission, patients must be checked regularly for recurrence or delayed complications. *(See **Cancer** for more information about therapies.)*

PREVENTION

If you smoke, quit now. Keep trim, cut back on high-fat foods, and limit your consumption of red meat. Throw out any foods that become moldy or rancid, including nuts, seeds, or rice.

CANCER IN THE KIDNEYS

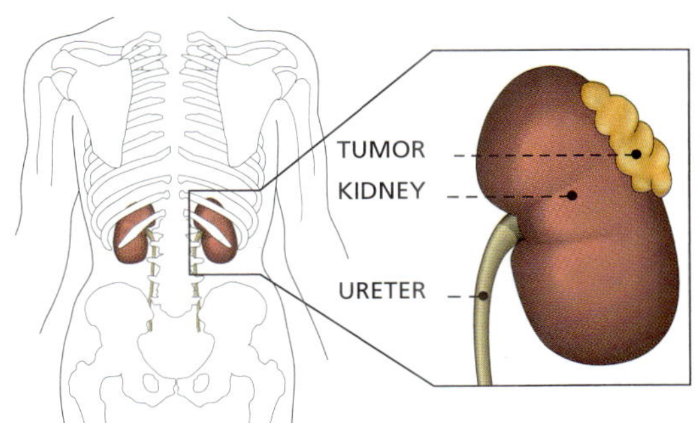

The kidneys are a pair of fist-sized organs that filter waste from the blood at the amazing rate of 1½ qt a minute. Early detection of kidney cancer is difficult, because small kidney tumors produce very few symptoms. The cancer tends to start near the top of the organ *(inset)*. The kidneys' waste-processing efficiency is affected only in the late stages of the disease.

K

PLANTS AND CANCER TREATMENT

Researchers at the National Cancer Institute have tested thousands of plant samples in the hope of isolating specific chemical compounds that may help treat or prevent cancer. Occasionally a promising compound is identified. For example, tests show that a compound called coumarin, found in certain nontoxic herbs, can enhance the effects of the chemotherapy agent ***cimetidine;*** treatment combining coumarin and cimetidine induced significant regression in several kidney cancer patients.

Nevertheless, active plant constituents interact in complex ways that are neither predictable nor fully understood. Herbal specialists warn against taking herbs in the hope of benefiting from one of their constituents; cancer patients should never take any herbal remedy without an oncologist's explicit approval. Taking toxic herbs is dangerous under any circumstances. A knowledgeable physician may be able to recommend herbs that improve overall health by stimulating the immune system, but no herbal remedy has been shown to cure cancer. ■

KIDNEY DISEASE

SYMPTOMS

- frequent thirst and urge to urinate.
- the passing of very small amounts of urine.
- swelling, particularly of the hands and feet, and puffiness around the eyes.
- unpleasant taste in the mouth and urinelike odor to the breath.
- persistent fatigue or shortness of breath.
- loss of appetite.
- increasingly higher blood pressure.
- pale skin.
- excessively dry, persistently itchy skin.
- in children: increased fatigue and sleepiness; decrease in appetite; and eventually, poor growth.

K

CALL YOUR DOCTOR IF:

- you are experiencing any of the symptoms listed above. Although any of them may indicate another disorder, each is one of the warning signs of kidney disease, which is a life-threatening illness. Consult your doctor without delay.

The kidneys, two fist-sized organs located on either side of the spine just above the waist, perform a life-sustaining role. They cleanse the blood by removing waste and excess fluids, maintain a healthful balance of various body chemicals, and help regulate blood pressure.

When the kidneys become diseased or damaged, they can suddenly or gradually lose their ability to perform these vital functions. Waste products and excess fluid then build up inside the body, causing a variety of symptoms, particularly swelling of the hands and feet, shortness of breath, and a frequent urge to urinate. If left untreated, diseased kidneys may eventually stop functioning. Loss of kidney function is a very serious and potentially fatal condition.

CAUSES

Kidney disease is classified as either **acute** (when loss of function occurs suddenly) or **chronic** (when deterioration takes place gradually, perhaps over a period of years). The chronic form can be particularly insidious: It may not show any symptoms until considerable, often irreparable damage has been done.

The causes of **chronic kidney disease** are often difficult to pinpoint. Most are the result of another disease or condition, such as ***diabetes, high blood pressure,*** or ***atherosclerosis***—all of which impede the flow of blood inside the kidneys. ***Lupus*** and other diseases of the immune system that affect blood vessels may also trigger kidney disease by causing the kidneys to become inflamed.

Some chronic kidney diseases, most notably polycystic kidney disease (in which cysts form on the kidneys), are inherited. Others are congenital—the result of some sort of urinary tract obstruction or malformation that the person was born with and that predisposes the victim to kidney infections and diseases.

Chronic kidney disease may also result from long-term exposure to toxic chemicals or to drugs, including certain illegal drugs, such as heroin. Researchers also suspect that excessive amounts of ***vitamin D*** and protein, particularly in the diets of the elderly or the very ill, may harm the kidneys. But in many chronic cases, the precise cause remains unknown.

Acute kidney disease can occur within a matter of days following the onset of any medical condition that suddenly and dramatically reduces the flow of blood to the kidneys. Examples are a ***heart attack,*** a traumatic injury such as one sustained in an automobile accident, a serious infection, or a toxic reaction to a drug.

Inhaling or swallowing certain toxins, including methyl, or wood, alcohol; carbon tetrachloride; antifreeze; and poisonous mushrooms, can also cause the kidneys to suddenly malfunction. Marathon runners and other endurance athletes who do not drink enough liquids while competing in long-distance athletic events may suffer acute kidney failure due to a sudden breakdown of muscle tissue, which releases a chemical called myoglobin that can damage the kidneys.

DIAGNOSTIC AND TEST PROCEDURES

For a diagnosis, your physician will have you undergo blood and urine tests and, if your kidneys can tolerate it, a special x-ray, known as an intravenous pyelogram (IVP), for viewing them. If the diagnosis remains unclear, your doctor may also do a needle biopsy, using a special needle device to remove a small sample of kidney tissue for microscopic examination.

TREATMENT

Kidney disease is a life-threatening condition that requires medical care. Alternative treatments may be used to supplement that care, but before trying them you should discuss them thoroughly with your doctor.

Medications, especially those that control diabetes and high blood pressure, can sometimes help slow the progress of chronic kidney disease. Some medical practitioners have found that certain restrictive diets are useful, particularly if the condition is caught early. But if these measures fail, and the kidneys deteriorate to the point where they can no longer function at all, there are only two treatments: dialysis, in which artificial devices clean the blood of waste products, or a kidney transplant.

CONVENTIONAL MEDICINE

If you are diagnosed with one of the more serious forms of kidney disease, your doctor may prescribe several medications. Because high blood pressure is both a cause and a symptom of the condition, you will probably receive a prescription for ***angiotensin-converting enzyme (ACE) inhibitors*** to slow the rate of injury to the kidneys or a ***diuretic*** to keep your blood pressure down. To balance your body's chemicals, which can be thrown dangerously out of kilter by malfunctioning kidneys, you may also be given drugs such as sodium polystyrene sulfonate, which lowers ***potassium*** levels, and ***calcium*** citrate, which blocks the stomach's absorption of ***phosphorus.***

If a blood test reveals that the level of your red blood cells has fallen, your doctor may prescribe a medication with an ***iron*** supplement to rebuild your body's stores of erythropoietin, a natural blood-building substance. Your doctor may also recommend that you take calcium supplements to keep your bones from weakening, an occasional side effect of chronic kidney disease. Because many drugs are excreted through the kidneys, you will also need to consult with your doctor before taking any over-the-counter medications. You may be told to avoid ***ibuprofen*** and ***acetaminophen,*** which have been implicated as possible contributors to kidney disease.

Although the approach remains controversial in conventional medical circles, a growing number of physicians now encourage dietary changes to help manage chronic kidney disease. *(See **Nutrition and Diet.**)* Some studies have shown that rigid adherence to a diet that severely restricts protein can delay or even prevent continued kidney deterioration. This is especially true of people whose kidney disease is the result of ***diabetes.*** Studies have shown that diabetics who follow a diet that keeps their blood glucose levels within a tight range can help retard the progress of kidney disease.

Dialysis treatment, which uses artificial devices to perform the kidneys' functions, is neces-

K

sary for cases of advanced kidney disease. Two types of dialysis are commonly used today. **Hemodialysis** involves a mechanical filter that cleans the blood. A surgeon implants a shunt, a small tube that connects an artery and a vein in the patient's arm or leg. Several times a week, for three or four hours at a time, another tube is connected to the shunt and the patient's blood is pumped out of the body into the hemodialyzer and then pumped back.

Another method, called **peritoneal dialysis,** makes use of the inner lining of the abdomen, or peritoneal membrane—which has many of the kidneys' filtering characteristics—to help clean the blood. A plastic tube is surgically implanted in the patient's abdomen. Then, during each treatment, a fluid called dialyzate is infused through the tube into the abdomen. Waste products carried by the blood circulating through tiny vessels in the peritoneal membrane filter into the dialyzate, which is drained out after several hours. This process is repeated three to five times a day. While the fluid is in the abdomen, the patient can go about normal daily activities.

Both types of dialysis present possible complications and risks, most notably that of infection. The stress of having to continually do the procedure can also take its toll on a patient's emotional well-being. For these reasons, people with advanced kidney disease often opt for a **kidney transplant.** New antirejection drugs and improved follow-up care have greatly increased the success rate for such surgery. Today, the three-year survival rate for patients who receive a donor kidney from a living relative is about 75 percent; for those whose transplanted kidney comes from an unrelated deceased donor, the rate is about 60 percent.

Not every person with kidney disease is a candidate for a transplant; a patient may have an underlying condition or other medical factor that rules out such an operation.

ALTERNATIVE CHOICES

Because kidney disease is a serious illness, you should try alternative therapies only after talking them over with your physician.

CHINESE HERBS

Traditional Chinese health practitioners use several herbs in the treatment of kidney disorders. However, because many herbs can be harmful to the kidneys, you should always consult your physician before taking the advice of an herbalist or ingesting any herbal remedies.

HOMEOPATHY

Homeopathic remedies are generally safe for the treatment of chronic kidney conditions. However, the remedies should be prescribed by a practitioner skilled in both conventional and alternative medicine, and they should never be used as a substitute for conventional medicine.

NUTRITION AND DIET

A special restricted diet can decrease the workload on diseased kidneys, keep body fluids and chemicals in balance, and fend off a buildup of waste products in the body. Although such diets should be specifically tailored to each patient's individual needs, they all typically incorporate the following general restrictions:

- protein: no more than 1 gram per kilogram of body weight per day.
- ***potassium:*** no more than 2 grams per day.
- ***phosphorus:*** no more than 1 gram per day (usually accomplished by adhering to protein restrictions).
- ***sodium:*** in advanced cases of kidney disease, no more than 2 grams per day.

Calcium supplements (1,500 mg per day) are frequently recommended in order to counteract the bone weakening that frequently accompanies kidney disease.

CHEMICALS THAT CAN DAMAGE THE KIDNEYS

Several of the chemicals found in common household products have been linked to both acute and chronic kidney disease. By reading product labels carefully and taking a few simple precautions, you can limit your exposure to these harmful toxins.

Cadmium. This rare, naturally occurring metal is used in the manufacture of pesticides, rubber tires, plastics, paints, and other products. Because of its industrial uses, it is now widely found in water and food supplies. Some precautions:

- ◆ Limit your intake of foods with high levels of cadmium, most notably liver and kidney products, flounder, mussels, scallops, oysters, and vegetables grown with sewage sludge fertilizers.
- ◆ Be sure any paints, dyes, or ceramic glazes you use for arts and crafts projects are cadmium-free.
- ◆ Do not use antique cookware or serving dishes; they may contain cadmium-based pigments.
- ◆ Avoid tobacco smoke.

Carbon tetrachloride (methane tetrachloride; tetrachloromethane; perchloromethane). A clear, colorless liquid with an etherlike smell, carbon tetrachloride was once a common household solvent until questions were raised about its toxicity. To avoid:

- ◆ Dispose of any old cans or bottles of cleaning products in your home during your community's next hazardous waste roundup program.
- ◆ Use a carbon filter on faucets to remove the chemical from your drinking and cooking water.

Chloroform (trichloromethane; methenyl chloride; methane trichloride; methyl trichloride; formyl trichloride). This sweet-smelling and sweet-tasting chemical is found in drinking water as a by-product of chlorination and found in the air as the result of automobile and industrial pollution. Chloroform is also still used as an ingredient in some cough syrups, toothpaste, liniments, glues, pesticides, and other consumer products. To avoid:

- ◆ Be sure your shower stall is well ventilated. Chloroform evaporates from chlorinated hot water, and levels can rise quickly inside an enclosed shower.
- ◆ To further reduce your exposure to chloroform while showering, put an activated charcoal filter on the cold-water pipe going into your hot-water heater.
- ◆ Read product labels carefully, and exercise extreme caution when using any product listing chloroform among its ingredients.

Ethylene glycol (1,2-dihydroxyethane; 1,2-ethanediol; ethylene alcohol; ethylene dihydrate). This clear, sweet-tasting chemical is found primarily in automobile antifreeze and brake fluid and in cosmetics, particularly those with a creamy texture. To avoid:

- ◆ Read cosmetics labels carefully; avoid those products containing the chemical.
- ◆ Do not allow children, who are sometimes attracted to the sweet taste of products containing ethylene glycol, to play in garages or other areas where cars and their supplies are kept. Promptly clean up any fluids that leak from your car.

Oxalic acid (oxalic acid dihydrate; ethane dioic acid). Used in both powder and liquid form, oxalic acid is found in some heavy-duty household cleaning products. Several freckle-fading and skin-bleaching cosmetics contain this chemical. It is also found in the leaves of some plants. To avoid:

- ◆ Read the labels of heavy-duty household cleaners and polishes carefully; avoid those that contain oxalic acid.
- ◆ Do not use any bleaching agents on your skin that contain the chemical.
- ◆ Never eat rhubarb leaves, which contain high concentrations of oxalic acid.

Tetrachloroethylene (PCE; carbon dichloride; perchloroethylene; PERC; 1,1,2,2-tetrachloroethylene). This colorless, heavy liquid is the most widely used dry-cleaning chemical in the United States. Some precautions:

- ◆ Keep your car windows open when bringing clothes home from the dry cleaner.
- ◆ Air dry-cleaned clothes outside or on a well-ventilated porch for at least six hours before bringing them inside.
- ◆ Air dry-cleaned sleeping bags for several days before using them.
- ◆ Avoid spot removers, rug and upholstery cleaners, and paint strippers that contain tetrachloroethylene. ■

K

KIDNEY INFECTIONS

SYMPTOMS

- continuous pain that usually begins in the back above the waist and spreads down into the groin.
- rapidly rising fever—often to 104°F.
- frequent urge to urinate, even though the bladder is empty.
- cloudy or bloody urine.
- severe nausea or vomiting.

CALL YOUR DOCTOR IF:

- you have symptoms that lead you to think you have a kidney infection, which is a serious ailment requiring immediate medical attention.
- you notice blood in your urine; this may also indicate ***kidney disease,*** a ***kidney stone,*** a bladder or kidney tumor, a ***bladder infection,*** or a prostate infection *(see **Prostate Problems**)*. See your doctor without delay.
- you are experiencing any pain or difficulty with urination; this may also be a sign of a ***sexually transmitted disease,*** a ***vaginal problem,*** a ***kidney stone,*** or a bladder or prostate tumor. See your doctor without delay.

Kidney infections occur when infectious organisms—usually bacteria—enter the body and travel to the kidneys, where they cause swelling and inflammation. A kidney infection can be acute (coming on suddenly) or chronic (recurring periodically over the course of many years).

Kidney infections are very serious. Left untreated, they can lead to permanent kidney damage and result in chronic ***kidney disease***. The infection can also spread into the blood, causing ***blood poisoning***. Anyone can develop a kidney infection, but pregnant women are at increased risk, in part because the pressure of the fetus on the bladder makes it more difficult to empty the bladder completely (urine left in the bladder is a potential medium for bacterial growth).

CAUSES

Like ***bladder infections,*** kidney infections are most often caused by the bacterium *Escherichia coli (E. coli)* or other bacteria that normally reside harmlessly in the intestines. Indeed, the infection typically begins in the bladder—having entered through the urethra—and then spreads to the kidneys.

In addition, the use of catheters—tubes that are inserted into the bladder to empty it—can trigger a kidney infection. Catheters may be inserted during the recovery period after a surgical procedure and are also sometimes used with nursing home residents or for people who have certain types of neurological conditions that affect bladder control.

DIAGNOSTIC AND TEST PROCEDURES

You will need a thorough medical evaluation to find out if you have a kidney infection and to determine the infectious agent causing it. The evaluation will include blood and urine tests. If you have had frequent infections, or if your doctor suspects that an underlying structural abnormality is to blame, more tests may be suggested. Your doctor may order an intravenous pyelogram (IVP), an x-ray technique for viewing the kidneys; a cystoscopy, a procedure in which a lighted tube inserted through the urethra is used to examine the bladder; or an ultrasound scan, which produces a detailed image of the kidneys.

TREATMENT

Kidney infections require immediate medical treatment; delay in clearing the body of infection can lead to serious complications. Advocates of alternative medicine stress that their treatments should be used only as a supplement to conventional medical care.

CONVENTIONAL MEDICINE

Antibiotics and bed rest are often all that is required to bring an acute kidney infection under control within 48 hours. Your physician will also ask you to drink large quantities of water—at least 3 qt a day—to help flush out the bacteria from your urinary tract. Young children, the elderly, or people who are very weakened by the illness are sometimes hospitalized to ensure that they get enough fluids and antibiotics.

Chronic kidney infections are also treated with antibiotics and large quantities of fluids. Because a chronic infection is sometimes caused by urine flowing back from the bladder into the kidneys, surgery to repair this structural problem may also be necessary.

Kidney infections sometimes return without manifesting any overt symptoms, so your doctor may also ask you to come in for follow-up blood tests and checkups.

ALTERNATIVE CHOICES

Because kidney infections are so serious, most alternative practitioners will insist that you seek conventional medical care. If you decide to use alternative treatments in addition to conventional ones, be sure your caregivers are in communication with one another. Once the kidney infection has cleared up, alternative therapies may help prevent a recurrence.

HOMEOPATHY

Homeopaths use treatments known as drainage remedies or European-combination remedies to help rid the body of a kidney infection. Be sure to seek out a practitioner familiar with these remedies. One combination sometimes prescribed includes ***Apis, Phosphorus,*** and *Teribinthina.*

NUTRITION AND DIET

Until you are cured of the infection, avoid foods that might irritate the urinary tract and put undue stress on the kidneys. Alcohol, coffee, salt, black tea, chocolate, carbonated beverages, citrus fruits, tomatoes, spicy foods, vinegar, artificial sweeteners, and sugar are all considered potential irritants.

PREVENTION

Because most kidney infections start in the bladder, prevention begins with keeping bacteria out of the entire urinary tract.

- Practice good bathroom hygiene. Clean yourself thoroughly after using the toilet. Women should wipe from front to back to avoid spreading fecal bacteria to the opening of the urethra.
- Urinate as soon as possible when you feel the urge and empty your bladder completely.
- Wear cotton underwear and loose clothing that does not trap heat and moisture in the crotch.
- Drink plenty of liquids.
- Drink at least 12 fl oz of cranberry juice a day. Research suggests that cranberries have properties that help fight off urinary tract infections. *(See **Bladder Infections**.)*

Women:

- Empty your bladder after intercourse to flush any bacteria that may have been pushed in.
- If you use a diaphragm, make sure that it fits properly and don't leave it in too long.
- Avoid using scented soaps, bubble baths, and vaginal deodorants, all of which have chemicals that can irritate the urinary tract and make it more vulnerable to infection. ■

K

KIDNEY STONES

SYMPTOMS

- waves of sharp pain that start in the side and move toward the groin.
- nausea and vomiting.
- profuse sweating.
- blood in urine.

Sometimes an infection is present and may cause these additional symptoms:

- fever and chills.
- frequent urge to urinate.
- painful or excruciating urination.
- cloudy or foul-smelling urine.

CALL YOUR DOCTOR IF:

- you think you have kidney stones; a medical evaluation is essential to diagnosis and treatment.
- you are experiencing waves of sharp pain in your side or abdomen; such pain may also be a sign of another serious condition, such as ***gallstones, pelvic inflammatory disease,*** or an intestinal obstruction. **Seek immediate medical help.**
- you are experiencing any pain or difficulty with urination; this could also be a sign of a ***bladder infection,*** a ***sexually transmitted disease,*** a ***vaginal problem*** such as vaginitis, an enlargement of the prostate *(see **Prostate Problems**)*, or a bladder or prostate tumor. See your doctor without delay.
- you notice blood in your urine; it may also indicate ***kidney disease,*** a bladder or kidney tumor, or a urinary or prostate infection *(see **Prostate Problems**)*. See your doctor without delay.

K

Kidney stones usually form in the center of the kidney, where urine collects before flowing into the ureter, the tube that leads to the bladder. They are created when certain substances in urine—including ***calcium*** and uric acid—crystallize and the crystals clump together. Small stones are able to pass out of the body in the urine and often go completely unnoticed. But larger stones irritate and stretch the ureter as they move toward the bladder, causing excruciating pain and blocking the flow of urine. Sometimes a stone can be as large as a golf ball, in which case it remains lodged in the kidney, creating a more serious condition.

Kidney stones are more common in young and middle-aged adults than in the elderly, and they are much more prevalent in men than in women. People living in hot climates are sometimes prone to kidney stones because their bodies become dehydrated, concentrating the minerals in their urine.

If you've had a kidney stone once, you are likely to get one again. So it's important to determine as best you can what caused the stone to form and to take steps to prevent a recurrence.

CAUSES

Why some people form kidney stones and others don't is not always clear. In 90 percent of cases, the cause remains unknown. The condition appears to run in families, and people who suffer from ***gout,*** inflammatory bowel diseases, and chronic urinary tract infections also seem to be predisposed to it. Medical evidence suggests that drinking too few fluids can cause stones, as can prolonged bed rest.

Chronic use of antacids containing ***calcium*** has also been linked to kidney stones. Dietary deficiencies, especially of ***vitamin*** $\boldsymbol{B_6}$ and ***magnesium,*** and excessive amounts of ***vitamin D*** also may be factors in the formation of stones. An imbalance of these vitamins and minerals can increase the amount of calcium oxalate in the urine; when the levels become too high, the calcium oxalate does not dissolve, and crystals may begin to form. In genetically susceptible people, eating foods that are themselves rich in calcium oxalate—such as chocolate, grapes, spinach, and strawberries—may also promote stones.

DIAGNOSTIC AND TEST PROCEDURES

Because many of the symptoms of kidney stones also indicate other disorders, a doctor must confirm the presence of a stone. An evaluation will include blood and urine tests and probably an intravenous pyelogram (IVP), a special x-ray technique for viewing the kidneys, or an ultrasound scan to reveal the stone's size and location.

TREATMENT

CONVENTIONAL MEDICINE

Because 90 percent of kidney stones pass out of the body on their own within three to six weeks, your doctor will most likely at first prescribe only plenty of water—at least 3 qt a day—and a pain medication, such as ***aspirin*** or ***acetaminophen*** with ***oxycodone***. A hot-water bottle can also help ease the inevitable discomfort. You may be asked to urinate through a strainer so the stone can be recovered and analyzed. Once the stone's composition is known, your doctor can prescribe drugs or suggest dietary changes to prevent your developing another one. The vast majority of kidney stones consist of calcium oxalate, so doctors often prescribe a thiazide ***diuretic*** to prevent recurrences.

If complications develop, such as an infection or total blockage of the ureter, the stone must be surgically removed. Depending on its size, type, and location, the stone is taken out either by conventional surgery or, more commonly, with a thin telescopic instrument called an endoscope. The surgeon passes the endoscope through the urethra into the bladder or ureter and then either pulls the stone out or bombards it with sound waves or laser beams, breaking it up into tiny pieces. If the stone is lodged in the kidney, the instrument is inserted into the kidney through an incision in the patient's side. A new method, known as extracorporeal shock wave lithotripsy, uses high-energy shock waves to break up kidney stones without surgery.

ALTERNATIVE CHOICES

In addition to the Chinese herbal remedy below, you might want to consider **acupuncture** or **homeopathy;** both therapies may help ease pain, and acupuncture may help facilitate the passing of a stone. In all cases, advocates stress that you should be monitored by a health professional.

CHINESE HERBS

Practitioners of Chinese medicine sometimes prescribe star fruit *(Averrhoa carambola)* to help relieve pain and promote urination. Place three fresh star fruit in a pan with 2 tsp of honey. Boil the fruit until it is soft, then eat the fruit and its juice. Repeat every day until the stone has passed and you are pain free.

K

PREVENTION

You can do many things, mainly dietary, to prevent a recurrence of stones. But always check with your doctor first; the stone's composition will determine which preventive steps you should take.

- Drink at least 3 qt of liquid every day, more in hot weather.
- Avoid or eat sparingly foods containing ***calcium*** oxalate (chocolate, celery, grapes, bell peppers, beans, strawberries, spinach, asparagus, beets, black tea). You may need to limit your overall intake of calcium, but do not do so without your doctor's advice.
- Take daily supplements of ***vitamin*** $\boldsymbol{B_6}$ (10 mg) and ***magnesium*** (300 mg), both of which reduce the formation of oxalates.
- Avoid foods that raise uric acid levels: anchovies, sardines, organ meats, brewer's yeast.
- Reduce uric acid by eating a low-protein diet.
- Avoid antacids; they are often high in calcium.
- Reduce salt to no more than 3 grams per day; higher amounts may raise the level of calcium oxalate in your urine.
- Avoid ***vitamin D*** supplements, which can increase calcium oxalate levels. ■

KNEE PAIN

Read down this column to find your symptoms. Then read across.

SYMPTOMS	AILMENT/PROBLEM
◆ knee pain following an injury; knee is not misshapen.	◆ Soft-tissue injury
◆ knee pain following an injury; possibly, popping and the inability to bear weight or move the knee; knee may "catch" or give way or may be misshapen.	◆ Ligament or cartilage damage
◆ knee pain in athletes or active people, or after you bang or twist your knee; possibly, swelling.	◆ Overuse injury such as runner's or biker's knee; water on the knee (synovitis); or jumper's knee (patellar ***tendonitis***)
◆ pain and swelling below the kneecap in an active adolescent undergoing a growth spurt.	◆ Growing pains (Osgood-Schlatter disease)
◆ pain, swelling, redness, warmth, and stiffness in your knee and other joints.	◆ Rheumatoid ***arthritis***
◆ pain, warmth, and stiffness in your knee, especially if you frequently kneel on a hard surface; pain is felt mainly upon bending your knee.	◆ Housemaid's knee ***(bursitis)***
◆ chronic aching and stiffness in your knee; limited movement; may improve with rest; more common in people over 50 and those who overexert their bodies.	◆ Osteoarthritis
◆ knee pain with redness, warmth, and swelling; fever, general feeling of illness; possibly, recent illness.	◆ Bone or joint ***infection***

WHAT TO DO	OTHER INFO
◆ Try RICE: rest, ice (cubes wrapped in a thin cloth), compression (not-too-tight bandage), elevation (with pillows). *(See **Sprains and Strains.**)* Take an anti-inflammatory painkiller such as ***ibuprofen*** or the homeopathic remedy ***Arnica.***	◆ When swelling subsides, consider taking hot baths with Epsom salt, and choose an exercise that strengthens the muscles near the injured area without stressing the injury.
◆ Call your doctor. Apply ice and take an anti-inflammatory painkiller such as ***ibuprofen*** if needed, or the homeopathic remedies ***Arnica*** or ***Ruta.*** Keep the leg raised to reduce swelling.	◆ Surgery may be recommended, especially in young people; physical therapy is usually needed. Severe knee pain after an injury may also indicate a dislocation or fracture. *(See **Emergencies/First Aid: Fractures and Dislocations.**)*
◆ See ***Athletic Injuries.*** Try RICE: rest, ice (cubes wrapped in a thin cloth), compression (not-too-tight bandage), elevation (with pillows). Call your doctor. Bracing or taping may be needed.	◆ Massage can be especially helpful for tendonitis. Runners should run on soft surfaces and wear quality running shoes to prevent overuse injuries. Start any exercise program gradually.
◆ Have the affected person avoid exercise that strains the knee, such as jumping and squatting, until symptoms are gone (6 to 12 months). Muscle-stretching exercises, ice, and anti-inflammatory painkillers such as ***ibuprofen*** may be helpful.	◆ You may be able to feel a tender bump below your child's kneecap. If pain is severe, your doctor may recommend taping or a knee immobilizer. ◆ Yoga and daily stretching may ease the pain.
◆ See ***Arthritis.*** Take an anti-inflammatory painkiller such as ***ibuprofen.***	
◆ Take an anti-inflammatory painkiller such as ***ibuprofen.*** Your doctor may inject your knee with anti-inflammatory and local ***anesthetic*** drugs.	◆ Pain may be alleviated by acupuncture; chiropractic may help restore active range of motion.
◆ See ***Arthritis.*** Your doctor may prescribe ***analgesics*** and exercises.	◆ The cause may be wear and tear on joint tissue from aging, from being overweight, or possibly, from overuse in work or sports activities.
◆ **Call your doctor now.** The usual treatment is with ***antibiotics.*** *(See **Infections.**)*	◆ Both infectious arthritis and bone infection can result in permanent damage if they are not treated.

K

LACTOSE INTOLERANCE

SYMPTOMS

You may be lactose intolerant if you experience some of the following symptoms after consuming milk products:

- abdominal cramps.
- bloating.
- frothy diarrhea.
- vomiting.
- flatulence.

CALL YOUR DOCTOR IF:

- you have the above symptoms in response to even tiny amounts of high-lactose foods, such as milk, ice cream, or soft cheese. This may indicate **primary lactose intolerance.**
- you develop symptoms after an illness or after taking medication. This may indicate **secondary lactose intolerance.**
- your newborn infant has symptoms from birth. This probably signifies **congenital lactose intolerance.**

In all three cases, you should seek an evaluation and treatment advice from your doctor.

Lactose is the primary sugar found in mammalian milk. Digestion of lactose requires the enzyme lactase, produced in the small intestine, which breaks lactose into two simpler sugars. When the intestine produces little or no lactase, milk sugar is not digested. It moves into the colon, where bacteria ferment it, producing hydrogen, carbon dioxide, and organic acids. The results of this fermentation are diarrhea, flatulence, and abdominal discomfort.

Newborns require high intestinal lactase levels for survival. Later in life, though, about two-thirds of all people lose the ability to produce lactase. Most of the people who keep producing it throughout adulthood are those of northern and middle European ancestry, the major population group that has herded milk animals for thousands of years. In other populations—Mediterranean, African, Asian, and Native American—75 to 100 percent of adults are lactose intolerant. It is believed that more than 30 million Americans have some degree of lactose intolerance.

Primary lactose intolerance may begin at any time but usually develops between the ages of 3 and 13 and continues throughout life. **Secondary lactose intolerance** may occur if the intestinal lining is temporarily damaged by diarrhea or medications such as ***nonsteroidal anti-inflammatory drugs (NSAIDs), aspirin,*** and ***antibiotics,*** which can halt lactase production for several weeks.

More unusual is **congenital lactose intolerance,** in which the small intestine produces no lactase. Consumption of any amount of lactose is intolerable and even dangerous, especially for infants, in whom diarrhea quickly leads to dehydration. This disorder is apparent in the first week of life; the infant must be fed a lactose-free diet.

While lactose intolerance has been investigated as a cause of ***colic*** in infants, the evidence is inconclusive. Often, a child who does not seem to tolerate lactose as an infant can consume dairy products without difficulty by age 10 or 12.

CAUSES

In people with **primary lactose intolerance,** the production of intestinal lactase declines steadily from early childhood until adolescence, when levels are less than 10 percent of those present at birth. This is the norm in areas of Asia, Africa, and the subtropics where people historically consume little or no milk after infancy.

Secondary lactose intolerance is caused by illness, side effects of medication, or other environmental change and is usually temporary.

Congenital lactose intolerance, which is present at birth, is caused by a faulty gene for lactase production.

DIAGNOSTIC AND TEST PROCEDURES

Lactose intolerance is traditionally diagnosed by comparing your health history with the symptoms of lactose intolerance. Diagnosis can also be made by a simple breath test. After lactose enters the large intestine, bacteria in the colon attack it and give off large quantities of hydrogen, which is eliminated by the respiratory system. Your doctor can detect this by means of a breath analyzing device.

If you have some of the symptoms listed above, you can check your own level of lactose tolerance by abstaining from all milk products for two weeks. If your symptoms disappear and then reappear when you try milk again, you are probably lactose intolerant. Even so, you will probably be able to eat or drink small amounts of lactose-containing foods, and there is no harm in doing so. *(See **At-Home Remedies,** right.)*

TREATMENT

There is no treatment for the underlying mechanism of lactose intolerance. For **primary lactose intolerance,** the recommended approach is to reduce or eliminate lactose-containing foods from the diet. Often, however, small amounts of lactose—or the symptoms themselves—can be tolerated. Another option is to use lactose-reduced dairy products or to take lactase tablets with any dairy products you consume. For **secondary lactose intolerance** adults can abstain from dairy products and infants can be given soy formula until the underlying illness or condition passes.

AT-HOME REMEDIES

- If your lactose intolerance is severe, read labels carefully; avoid any product that contains lactose, especially milk (including nonfat milk), soft cheeses, and ice cream. Instead, look for special lactose-reduced cottage and American cheeses. Hard cheeses, such as cheddar, Swiss, and Jarlsberg; buttermilk; and sour cream are also generally low in lactose.
- Yogurt with live and active cultures is a good source of calcium and protein for those who are lactose intolerant. The bacteria found in active cultures help digest the lactose in the yogurt.
- Try slowly increasing the amount of lactose you eat; symptoms may decrease. Or try eating some yogurt before drinking milk or eating ice cream.
- For most people intolerance is not the same as an allergy. Even a lactose-intolerant person can assimilate a cup or so of milk, especially when it is accompanied by foods high in fat, which slows digestion. A low-lactose diet is much easier to achieve than a truly lactose-free diet and may be sufficient.
- Look for milk products that contain the enzyme betagalactosidase. Such lactose-reduced milks are easier to digest.
- Lactase produced from a yeast or fungus is commercially available and may be added to milk or taken in capsule or tablet form before consuming milk products.
- Soy protein formulas are effective milk substitutes for lactose-intolerant infants, and soy products (including milk, yogurt, cheese, and ice cream) can be substituted for milk products in adult diets.
- Acidophilus milk, which contains *Lactobacillus acidophilus* (the bacteria found in yogurt), helps the body break down milk protien and fat and is beneficial for digestion in general.
- If you do have to give up dairy products, be sure to get enough **calcium** from other sources, such as dark-green leafy vegetables, canned fish, tofu, beans, apricots, and sesame seeds. ■

L

LARYNGITIS

SYMPTOMS

- hoarseness and loss of voice.
- pain when speaking.
- tickling and rawness in the throat.
- a constant need to clear the throat.
- loss of voice accompanied by the flu, a cold, or ***pneumonia.***
- fever (occasionally).

CALL YOUR DOCTOR IF:

- hoarseness and discomfort last more than a week; this could signal a bacterial infection or more serious disorder.
- you develop laryngitis after being exposed to environmental toxins, such as poisonous fumes or noxious odors; such exposure might have caused more damage than just a simple inflammation of your vocal cords.
- laryngitis occurs along with or as a result of ***alcohol abuse*** or chronic ***bronchitis,*** which require a doctor's care.
- a child's hoarseness turns into a sharp, barking cough, which could indicate a severely restricted airway or, possibly, ***croup.***

L

If you lose your voice, or the sounds coming out of your mouth sound several notes higher—or lower—than normal, you may have laryngitis. Specifically, this disorder is an inflammation of the mucous membrane of the larynx, or the part of your windpipe that contains the vocal cords. Your vocal cords open and close during the course of normal speech *(right).* If your vocal cords are swollen, the sounds you make become distorted. You'll be hoarse, or you may lose your voice altogether.

CAUSES

Anything that makes your vocal cords swell can result in laryngitis. Viruses are the number one culprit, although bacteria are frequently responsible. Allergies and exposure to certain harsh chemicals or toxins can also cause the vocal cords to swell. Overuse is another common cause, to which many rock stars and overexcited football fans can attest. In rare instances laryngitis comes as a result of growths or tumors (called nodules or nodes) that develop on or around the vocal cords.

TREATMENT

Viral laryngitis usually goes away by itself in a few days without any treatment. For this reason, persistent laryngitis is a warning sign that something other than a pesky virus may be causing your hoarseness and tickly throat.

CONVENTIONAL MEDICINE

If the diagnosis is viral laryngitis, you can alleviate symptoms until your body rids itself of the virus. However, if a physician determines that a bacterial infection has set in, you'll most likely be given ***antibiotics.*** Take the entire course—usually 7 to 10 days—even if you feel better right away. Stopping the treatment prematurely can result in a worse infection later on.

For most allergies, doctors usually prescribe ***antihistamines,*** which reduce swelling and in-

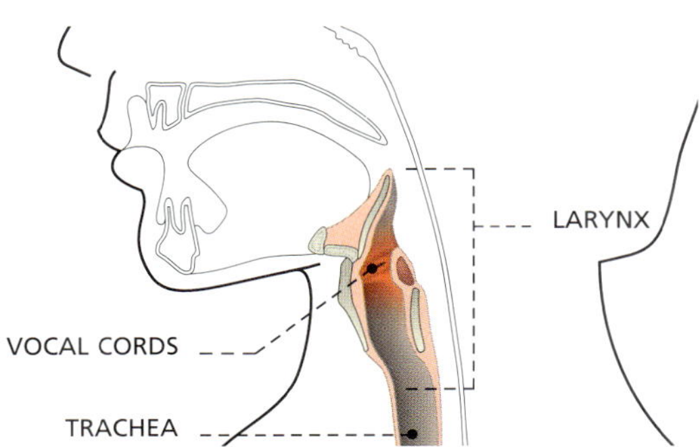

The vocal cords are two taut bands that stretch across the larynx—a boxlike chamber at the upper part of the trachea, or windpipe. Air passing through these bands causes vibrations that produce sounds, which are shaped and modified by the tongue, teeth, and lips into speech. When the vocal cords are inflamed or infected because of laryngitis, the voice typically becomes hoarse or muted.

flammation. For serious allergic reactions, during which you find it hard to breathe, your physician may prescribe a systemic steroid medication. No medication is necessary if your laryngitis is caused by simple overuse; in that case, the best solution is to rest your voice.

ALTERNATIVE CHOICES

To treat laryngitis, alternative practitioners often prescribe methods to soothe the raw throat or boost the immune system, or they encourage rest.

ACUPUNCTURE

A recent study of traditional Chinese remedies found that many patients with laryngitis or ***tonsillitis*** benefited from acupuncture. Consult a licensed acupuncturist for proper treatment.

HERBAL THERAPIES

To help restore the voice, try gargling with a tea made from red sage *(Salvia officinalis* var. *rubia),* ***bayberry*** (*Myrica* spp.), or white oak *(Quercus alba)* bark. A tincture of ***echinacea*** (*Echinacea* spp.) every hour for two days will treat laryngitis caused by an infection. Mix 10 drops of the tincture in a glass of water and swallow.

HOMEOPATHY

If laryngitis is a result of overuse or trauma to the vocal cords, use ***Arnica*** (6x or 12x) every two hours; if you notice no improvement after six hours, try a different remedy recommended by your homeopath. For laryngitis that is accompanied by dryness of the throat and the feeling of a plug in the larynx, use *Spongia tosta* (12x) four times a day. For laryngitis accompanied by a dry, croupy cough that comes on suddenly after exposure to cold weather or with the first signs of a cold, use ***Aconite*** (6x or 12x) every two hours. If these remedies don't work, consult a practitioner.

NUTRITION AND DIET

Drinking plenty of fluids, eating lots of raw fruits and vegetables, and reducing your intake of refined carbohydrates may help speed your recovery from laryngitis. To boost your immune system, supplement your diet with ***vitamin C,*** 20,000 to 50,000 IU a day of beta carotene *(see* ***vitamin A****),* and garlic.

AT-HOME REMEDIES

- Rest your body as well as your voice—completely. If you must speak, whisper; do not engage the vocal cords at all.
- Drink plenty of liquids, such as water or tea mixed with a little honey or lemon.
- Inhale steam from a pot of boiling water.
- Apply warm compresses to your throat.

PREVENTION

The best way to prevent laryngitis is to avoid straining your voice and to give it proper rest after overuse. If you're prone to laryngitis, try to stay away from cigarette smoke or other environmental toxins. If you think your laryngitis stems from an allergic reaction to a certain kind of food, experiment by removing suspected items from your diet, then reintroduce them one by one while monitoring the effect. *(See* ***Allergies.****)* ■

L

LEG PAIN

Read down this column to find your symptoms. Then read across.

SYMPTOMS	AILMENT/PROBLEM
◆ leg pain following an injury, but you can move your leg.	◆ Soft-tissue injury
◆ leg pain following an injury, and you cannot move your leg or walk; severe pain even at rest.	◆ Fracture or dislocation
◆ pain and swelling after excessive athletic or other physical activity.	◆ Overuse injury
◆ aching in your legs with ankle or foot swelling, especially after long periods of standing; possibly, prominent dark blue blood vessels in your legs and feet.	◆ ***Varicose veins***
◆ cramping pain in calves, thighs, feet, or hips when walking or exercising that stops with rest; muscle fatigue.	◆ Peripheral vascular disease (blocked arteries and other venous or arterial problems)
◆ shooting or burning pain in your buttocks and down the back of one leg; worsens with coughing, sneezing, bending, or lifting.	◆ ***Sciatica***
◆ a throbbing or burning sensation beneath the skin of your leg; a red, warm, tender, cordlike vein is visible.	◆ Superficial ***phlebitis***
◆ pain and swelling throughout your leg, especially when your foot is flexed.	◆ Deep ***phlebitis***
◆ persistent, severe pain in one area of your leg; fever above 100°F; general feeling of malaise; tender or red area over a bone in your leg.	◆ Bone ***infection***

L

WHAT TO DO	OTHER INFO
◆ Try RICE: rest, ice (cubes wrapped in a thin cloth), compression (not-too-tight bandage), elevation (with pillows). *(See **Sprains and Strains.**)*	◆ Strenuous use of affected muscles should be avoided until the pain is gone.
◆ **Call your doctor now.** See ***Athletic Injuries*** and ***Emergencies/First Aid: Fractures and Dislocations.***	◆ In addition to conventional treatment the homeopathic remedy ***Arnica*** may be initially helpful to reduce swelling and bruising.
◆ See ***Athletic Injuries.*** Curtail or stop the activity that caused injury.	◆ Overuse injuries of the leg include ***shin splints*** and ***tendonitis.***
◆ Wear elastic support stockings and take an anti-inflammatory painkiller such as ***ibuprofen.*** Medical treatment options include laser therapy, chemical injection, and surgery.	◆ The cause is damage to valves in the veins, resulting in poor circulation in your legs. Deep varicose veins are less common but may cause serious circulatory problems.
◆ Call your doctor. See ***Circulatory Problems, Atherosclerosis,*** and ***Heart Disease.*** Treatment depends on the cause; it may include medication to improve blood flow or bypass surgery.	◆ Stopping smoking, improving your diet, and exercising regularly may be helpful.
◆ See your doctor. Treatment may include muscle relaxants, ***analgesics,*** and/or physical therapy.	◆ Acupuncture treatments may relieve mild or acute sciatica. Chiropractic manipulation may be able to reduce pressure on the nerve.
◆ See ***Phlebitis.*** To ease the pain, lie down and prop your legs up 6 to 12 inches above the level of your heart. Apply a heating pad or moist warm pack to the swollen area.	◆ Your doctor may suggest compression support stockings, ***aspirin*** to reduce inflammation, and if an infection is found, an ***antibiotic.***
◆ **Call your doctor now.** You may need to be hospitalized for tests and anticoagulation treatment. See ***Phlebitis.***	◆ The danger is that a clot in a deep vein can break away and lodge in a lung (pulmonary embolism), a potentially fatal complication.
◆ **Call your doctor now.** See ***Infections.*** Treatment typically includes ***antibiotics.***	◆ Infection may occur after a wound, fracture, or other injury.

L

LEUKEMIA

SYMPTOMS

Many types of leukemia produce no obvious symptoms in early stages. Eventually symptoms may include any of the following:

- ***anemia*** and related symptoms, such as fatigue, pallor, and a general feeling of illness.
- a tendency to bruise or bleed easily, including bleeding from the gums or nose, or blood in the stool or urine.
- susceptibility to infections such as ***sore throat*** or bronchial ***pneumonia,*** which may be accompanied by headache, low-grade fever, mouth sores, or skin rash.
- swollen lymph nodes, typically in the throat, armpits, or groin.
- loss of appetite and weight.
- discomfort under the left lower ribs (caused by a swollen spleen).

In advanced stages, symptoms may include sudden high fever, confusion, seizures, inability to talk or move limbs, and an altered state of consciousness.

CALL YOUR DOCTOR IF:

- you experience any of the symptoms described above and cannot readily explain their occurrence. Your blood cell count should be tested.
- you experience unexplained bleeding, high fever, or a seizure. You may need emergency treatment for **acute leukemia.**
- you are in remission from leukemia and notice signs of recurrence, such as infection or easy bleeding. You should have a follow-up examination.

Leukemia is cancer of the blood. Unlike other cancers, leukemia does not produce tumors but results in rampant overproduction of cancerous white blood cells. Leukemia—the term derives from the Greek words for "white" and "blood"—is often considered a disease of children, yet it actually affects far more adults. It is more common in men than women, and in Caucasians than African Americans; almost 30,000 cases are diagnosed in the United States each year.

The term "life-giving" often applied to blood is no exaggeration. Suspended in its liquid plasma are disease-fighting white cells, wound-stanching platelets, and red cells that carry oxygen to every part of the body. Every day hundreds of billions of new blood cells are produced in the bone marrow—most of them red cells. In people with leukemia, however, the body starts producing more white cells than it needs. Many of the extra white cells do not mature normally, yet they tend to live well beyond their normal life span.

Despite their vast numbers, these leukemic cells are unable to fight infection the way normal white blood cells do. As they accumulate, they interfere with vital organ functions, including the production of healthy blood cells. Eventually the body does not have enough red cells to supply oxygen, enough platelets to ensure proper clotting, or enough normal white cells to fight infection, making people with leukemia anemic and susceptible to bruising, bleeding, and infection.

Cases of leukemia are classified as acute or chronic. Cancer cells in **acute leukemias** start multiplying before they develop beyond their immature stage. **Chronic leukemias** progress more slowly, with cancer cells developing to full maturity. Leukemias are further classified according to the type of white blood cell involved. Under a microscope, two main types of white blood cells are easily distinguishable: Myeloid cells contain tiny particles or granules; lymphoid cells usually do not.

Acute lymphocytic, or **lymphoblastic, leukemia (ALL),** sometimes called childhood leukemia, is the most common type of cancer in children; **acute myelogenic leukemia (AML)** is the most common form of leukemia in adults. Without treatment, acute leukemias are usually fatal within months. Treatment effectiveness varies with the type and stage of the disease, but the younger the patient, the greater the chances of remission. In leukemia, remission means that no more cancerous cells can be detected and bone marrow appears normal. Adult patients treated for **ALL** have an 80 to 90 percent chance of attaining remission; about 40 percent of those who do so survive at least another five years, with a chance of a full cure. Patients treated for **AML** have a 60 to 70 percent chance of remission; about 20 percent of those survive at least three years, with a possibility of a full cure.

Chronic leukemias tend to affect middle-aged adults. **Chronic lymphocytic leukemia (CLL)** is the most benign, slowly progressing type. It can be controlled effectively with medication, and may require no treatment in its early stages. **Chronic myelogenic leukemia (CML)** is more aggressive. Since it is difficult to prevent this disease from escalating to an acute phase even with treatment, average survival time is about four years. Each of these four main types of leukemia can be divided into many subtypes. Other, rare, forms of the disease include **hairy cell, prolymphocytic, megakaryocytic, basophilic,** and **eosinophilic** leukemia.

BLOOD CELL COUNT

NORMAL

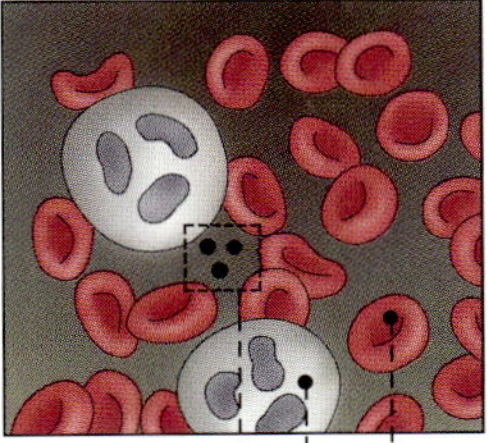

ABNORMAL

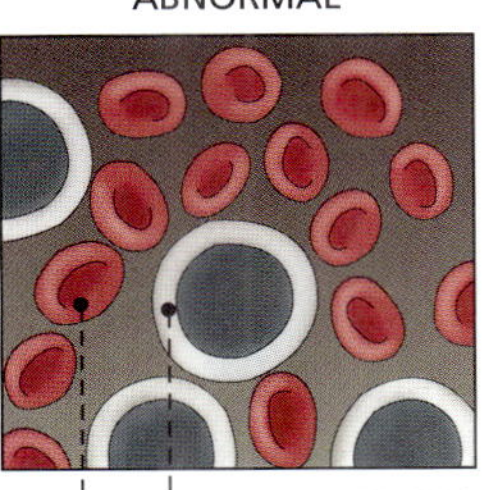

Normal blood *(above, left)* contains mostly red cells and a small percentage of white cells. In the blood of a patient with chronic lymphocytic leukemia *(above, right)*, white cell count is abnormally high. These leukemic white cells live longer than normal, so old cells accumulate as new cells are being produced. The leukemic cells also interfere with production of normal white blood cells that fight infection.

CAUSES

No one knows exactly what causes leukemia, but some people seem genetically predisposed to the disease. Chromosome abnormalities are associated with leukemia and with a preleukemic disease called myelodysplasia. Nine out of ten people with **CML,** for example, have an abnormal chromosome called the Philadelphia chromosome in their blood cells. This chromosome is an acquired abnormality; it is neither inherited nor passed on to one's children. Chromosome abnormalities associated with congenital disorders such as Down syndrome strongly correlate with certain types of leukemia, and at least one virus in the same family as the human immunodeficiency virus (HIV) has been associated with a rare form of the disease.

Environmental factors seem to influence the risk of developing leukemia. Tobacco smokers are more prone to certain leukemias than nonsmokers. Research also suggests that prolonged exposure to radiation, various chemicals in home and work environments, and low-frequency electromagnetic fields may be associated with leukemia—but there is no definitive proof.

DIAGNOSTIC AND TEST PROCEDURES

Because many types of leukemia show no obvious symptoms early on, the disease may be diagnosed incidentally during a physical examination or as a result of routine blood tests. If a patient has enlarged lymph nodes, swollen gums, an enlarged liver or spleen, significant bruising, or a small pinpoint rash, the doctor should suspect leukemia. A blood test showing an abnormal white cell count is usually adequate for a tentative diagnosis. To confirm the diagnosis and identify the specific type, the patient will have a needle biopsy of bone marrow from a pelvic bone and a test for cancer cells. In the case of **CML,** DNA tests will check for the Philadelphia chromosome.

CANCER IN CHILDREN

Having leukemia—or any other cancer—is scary, whether you're a child or an adult. But cancer is

Coping with Chemotherapy

Cancer patients who receive chemotherapy tend to experience unpleasant side effects. This is a particular concern for leukemia sufferers, since chemotherapy is essential to their treatment. Fortunately, medication can help relieve side effects to an encouraging degree, as can various complementary therapies.

The method doesn't matter as long as it works. ***Acupuncture*** *has traditionally been used to relieve the pain and discomfort of many illnesses, including cancer. Any of several* ***relaxation*** *techniques—including* ***massage, yoga, qigong, meditation,*** *or progressive muscle relaxation—may help subdue the pain and nausea frequently experienced after chemotherapy. Others find relief in hobbies, listening to music, or simply reading a good book.*

To control nausea that may occur in anticipation of chemotherapy, adults may find help in ***biofeedback*** *training, while children often respond well to various kinds of distraction or to* ***hypnotherapy.***

not necessarily a death sentence, and all people with cancer deserve to live their lives fully and richly. If your child gets cancer, the best thing you can do is remember he's a child first and a cancer patient second.

Attitudes can be surprisingly contagious. Don't pretend the disease doesn't exist; this won't fool you or your child, and it won't help you face the questions and emotions generated by cancer. Try to have a sense of optimism and good humor. Encourage friends, family, and others in your child's life to act normally and help him live a normal life. This means nurturing without coddling, and empathizing without being either overly protective or overly lenient. If your family needs help coping with cancer, see the ***Appendix*** for a list of organizations to contact.

While you are caring for this special child, don't forget his siblings—they need you, too. And when you're feeling overwhelmed, remember that chances are better than even that your child will recover.

TREATMENT

While the reported incidence of leukemia has not changed much since the 1950s, more people are surviving longer, thanks mainly to advances in chemotherapy. Childhood leukemia **(ALL),** for example, represents one of the most dramatic success stories of cancer treatment: Some 90 percent of children diagnosed with the disease attain remission, and more than half are cured completely. The five-year survival rate for all patients with **ALL** has risen from 4 percent in the 1960s to more than 50 percent in the 1990s.

CONVENTIONAL MEDICINE

For **acute leukemia,** the immediate goal of treatment is remission. The patient undergoes aggressive chemotherapy in a hospital for several weeks and is kept in sterile isolation and cleansed constantly to reduce the chance of infection. Since acute leukemia patients have extremely low counts of healthy blood cells, they are usually given blood and platelet transfusions to boost their natural immune function and to help stop bleeding. They may also receive drugs to combat infection and to reduce nausea and vomiting that may occur as side effects of the chemotherapy.

People with **ALL** are likely to attain satisfactory remission after several weeks of aggressive chemotherapy in a hospital. To keep the disease under control, they will continue receiving low-dose chemotherapy and possibly radiation therapy for a month or more to eliminate residual cancer traces. At home they will receive an on-and-off maintenance protocol for months or even years. Since **AML** does not respond as well to chemotherapy, the best chance of lasting remission or cure depends on successful bone marrow transplantation, which requires a willing donor with compatible tissue type and genetic characteristics—usually a family member.

A bone marrow transplant has three stages: preparation, operation, and recovery. First, the patient's cancerous white blood cell count is brought under control—usually by chemotherapy but possibly by leukopheresis, a mechanical process that separates cancer cells from the blood. During the operation stage, the patient's bone marrow is destroyed by intensive chemotherapy to avoid rejection of new marrow. The patient then receives about one tablespoon of donor marrow. Recovery is the most dangerous stage: Until the donor marrow cells start producing new blood, the patient is left with virtually no white blood cells, making death by infection a strong possibility. Once the donor marrow multiplies sufficiently—usually in two to six weeks—the outlook for long-term remission and sometimes a complete cure is good. Bone marrow transplantation is still both expensive and risky, but it offers the best chance of remission and cure for **AML** and recurring cases of **ALL.**

Since **CLL** generally affects older people and progresses slowly, conventional treatment tends to be conservative. As long as symptoms are absent, the disease requires no treatment. If swelling appears in lymph nodes and other organs, CLL can usually be controlled for years with oral chemotherapy. Many people with CLL lead basically normal lives and die of unrelated causes.

Oral chemotherapy can effectively control symptoms of **CML** for several years before the disease becomes acute. CML sufferers may survive longer if they receive interferon, a naturally occurring protein that can kill or slow the growth of cancerous cells. Because most cases of CML eventually advance to an acute phase despite treatment, some doctors advise bone marrow transplantation during the chronic phase.

In addition to using standard treatments, some doctors are experimenting with immunological ones. The hope is that interferon or other so-called biologic response modifiers will either kill leukemic cells or restore their normal form and function. Scientists are investigating other methods of killing cancer cells without harming normal cells, including use of the experimental drug interleukin and identifying specific antibody proteins that target cancer cells so they can be destroyed by injections of radioactive substances.

For more information on chemotherapy, radiation, and other treatments, see ***Cancer.***

COMPLEMENTARY THERAPIES

Realistically, there is no acceptable substitute for conventional cancer treatment. While many alternative therapies are being incorporated into mainstream medical care, none is a proven cancer cure. Alternative therapies may improve the quality of a cancer patient's life but are best viewed as potential complements to, not replacements for, conventional care.

The best complementary therapies are those that help control the pain, discomfort, and anxiety of cancer and its treatment. Stress-reducing exercises—along with certain vitamins, nutrients, and herbal remedies that may enhance immune function—can be particularly beneficial. For more information on complementary therapies, see ***Cancer.***

AT-HOME CARE

- To lessen the chance of the nausea that may result from chemotherapy, eat light snacks throughout the day rather than large meals.
- To reduce the chance of infection, avoid people who are obviously sick; wash your hands well before eating and before and after going to the toilet; take a warm shower or bath daily, and pat rather than rub yourself dry.
- If you cut or scratch yourself, follow thorough antiseptic procedures. If you develop signs of infection—fever, chills, sore throat, cough, swollen or reddened skin—get medical treatment immediately.
- Leukemia patients prone to bleeding because of a low platelet count should not use medications containing ***aspirin;*** it may inhibit clotting. ■

L

SYMPTOMS

- **head lice:** intense itching on the scalp, especially behind the ears and at the nape of the neck.
- **body lice:** unexplained scratch marks on the body, ***hives, eczema,*** and red pimples on the shoulders or torso.
- **pubic lice:** continual itching around the pubic area, and perhaps a rash.

CALL YOUR DOCTOR IF:

- you need help getting rid of lice or if scratching has led to infection.

Lice are tiny parasites that live on human beings and feed on blood. They seldom cause serious medical problems, but they are both annoying and contagious. Every four hours or so, a louse bites into a tiny blood vessel for a meal. You don't feel the initial bites, because lice inject an anesthetic. However, the bites later begin to itch, and your scratching can lead to infection.

Head lice *(Pediculus humanus capitis)* are about the size of a sesame seed and can be easily seen, although they hide quickly in response to light. Their eggs, called nits, are barely visible, whitish ovals cemented to hair shafts. Head lice are extremely contagious, especially among schoolchildren. They afflict an estimated 6 to 12 million children in the United States. Twice as many girls as boys get head lice, not because of greater hair length, but because girls have more physical contact with one another and share more personal articles (hats, clothing, combs, headphones) that can transmit head lice. Head lice are rare among African Americans, possibly because the shafts of their hair have a shape that lice cannot grasp easily.

Pubic lice *(Phthirius pubis)* are yellow-gray insects found in the pubic region and transmitted by sexual contact. The size of a pinhead, they are slightly translucent and barely visible against light-colored skin. They are also called crab lice, or crabs, because of their shape and the crablike claws with which they cling to hair. Eggs can barely be seen as tiny white particles glued so firmly to hair shafts that they are not removed by normal washing.

Body lice *(Pediculus humanus corporis)* are nearly identical in appearance to head lice but are more difficult to find. When not feeding, they tend to hide in the seams of clothing and folds of bedding. Signs of their presence are scratch marks, ***hives,*** or small red pimples, usually on the shoulders, torso, or buttocks. If the lice are not treated, rashes or welts may develop.

CAUSES

Contrary to common belief, lice are not related to poor hygiene. In fact, head lice are thought to prefer clean hair to dirty hair. Lice live successfully all over the world, wherever people gather in close proximity, as in schools.

TREATMENT

The goal of treatment is to remove all lice and nits. This usually requires repeated efforts, because a few adults may escape by hiding in clothing or bedding, and eggs are difficult to kill.

CONVENTIONAL MEDICINE

To get rid of **head lice,** the most common treatment is to kill the adults with an insecticidal shampoo and to clear out the nits with a special fine-toothed comb. The safest and most effective preparation is permethrin cream rinse, available over the counter. For best results, follow the directions exactly. Other family members should be treated; about 60 percent of infected children have relatives who carry lice.

To avoid spreading the lice, infected children should be kept home from school until they are treated. Wash all clothing, towels, and bed linens in hot, soapy water, and dry in a hot dryer. You can also sterilize bedding or other items by placing them in a plastic bag for 14 days; the nits will hatch in about a week and die of starvation. Combs, brushes, and barrettes can be disinfected by soaking in hot, soapy water for 10 minutes.

For those who prefer to avoid the use of insecticides, try a "combing only" technique. Wash the hair with ordinary shampoo and conditioner and leave wet. With a fine-toothed comb, stroke slowly outward from the roots through one lock of hair at a time. Lice will land on the back of the comb, get caught between the teeth, or fall off. Space at least 30 strokes over the head. Repeat every three days. Because newborn lice do not lay eggs for the first week, all the lice should disappear after about two weeks of combing.

Pubic lice can be treated with over-the-counter medications containing pyrethrins (natural insecticides). Your sexual partners will also have to be treated. Crabs are sometimes found on eyelashes or eyebrows; to remove them, use an ophthalmic ointment such as physostigmine.

To treat **body lice,** wash the entire body with soap and water. If this is not effective, you may have to use an insecticidal preparation, which usually kills all the lice. Wash all clothing and bedding in hot water and dry in a hot dryer. Store clothes for two weeks in plastic bags or place them in dry heat of 140°F for three to five days.

ALTERNATIVE CHOICES

Several alternative treatments may make it easier to get rid of lice.

AROMATHERAPY

For treatment of head lice, wash the hair and rinse slowly with 6 drops each of essential oils of ***rosemary*** *(Rosmarinus officinalis)* and red thyme *(Thymus vulgaris)* mixed in a pint of warm water. You may substitute this combination with 12 drops of essential oil of ***lavender*** *(Lavandula officinalis).* Dry the hair naturally (not with a blow dryer), then comb with a fine-toothed comb. For prevention, soak your comb in water with 10 drops of essential oil of red thyme, and comb hair thoroughly.

HOMEOPATHY

Depending on symptoms, a practitioner may prescribe various remedies, such as *Psorinum* (30c), for children who are afflicted with head lice.

PREVENTION

Preventing reinfestation is as important as initial treatment. This is especially true for **head lice,** which spread quickly from head to head. If you discover lice on your child, notify school or day-care authorities at once, since classmates are likely to be infected. Talk with your children and their friends to be sure they understand the risks. You may be reluctant to talk about this subject with strangers, but head lice are a social ailment that can only be dealt with socially. ■

L

SYMPTOMS

Liver cancer usually has no initial symptoms, but may eventually cause:

- pain, swelling, or tenderness in the upper right section of the abdomen.
- yellowing of the skin and whites of the eyes, as in ***jaundice.***
- itching all over the body.
- swollen legs.

In the advanced stage, symptoms may include fever, appetite and weight loss, nausea, vomiting, fatigue, general weakness, and loss of sexual drive.

CALL YOUR DOCTOR IF:

- you develop symptoms that suggest liver cancer. Although the symptoms may be related to another liver disorder or some other ailment, it's best not to let them go undiagnosed for more than a few weeks. Early detection of cancer ensures better response to treatment.

The liver continuously filters blood that circulates through the body, converting nutrients and drugs absorbed in the digestive tract into ready-to-use chemicals. It also removes toxins and other chemical waste products from the blood and readies them for excretion. Because all the blood in the body must pass through it, the liver is unusually accessible to cancer cells traveling in the bloodstream. Ironically, while the liver can cleanse the body of ingested or internally produced poisons, it cannot cleanse itself of cancer.

Most liver cancer is **secondary,** meaning the malignancy originated elsewhere in the body—usually the colon, lung, or breast. **Primary liver cancer,** which starts in the liver, accounts for about 2 percent of cancers in the United States but up to half of all cancers in some undeveloped countries, mainly because of the prevalence of ***hepatitis,*** a contagious virus that predisposes a person to liver cancer. Worldwide, primary liver cancer strikes twice as many men as women and is most likely to affect people over 50.

CAUSES

Primary liver cancer tends to occur in livers damaged by congenital defects or diseases such as ***hepatitis*** B and C, and ***cirrhosis.*** More than half of all people diagnosed with primary liver cancer have cirrhosis, and those who suffer from hemochromatosis, or iron overload, are at even greater risk. Various carcinogens are associated with primary liver cancer, including some cholesterol-lowering drugs, certain herbicides, and such chemicals as vinyl chloride and arsenic. Male hormones—androgens or steroids—taken by some athletes can cause benign liver tumors and may promote liver cancer. Aflatoxins, a type of plant mold, are also implicated *(box, right).*

DIAGNOSTIC AND TEST PROCEDURES

Screening for early detection of primary liver cancer is not performed routinely but should be considered by people at high risk for the disease. To diagnose liver cancer, a doctor must rule out other causes of the symptoms. Blood studies that

CLEAN OUT YOUR CUPBOARD

Research shows a clear link between aflatoxins in the food supply and the incidence of primary liver cancer. Food grown in some parts of tropical Africa harbors aflatoxins, a potent carcinogen produced by a fungus in the soil. But aflatoxins are not unique to Africa—they may be lurking in the peanut butter that has been on your shelf for the past five years. Aflatoxins develop naturally in many foods—seeds, grains, rice, and nuts—as they age, especially under humid conditions. To avoid contamination, keep dry food in airtight containers and store in a cool place. Discard any food that becomes moldy, soft, rancid, or shriveled, or whose package expiration date has passed.

measure tumor markers—substances elevated in the presence of a particular cancer—can aid diagnosis. Ultrasound and CT scans may reveal existing tumors, but only a biopsy will distinguish a benign tumor from a malignant one.

TREATMENT

Any liver cancer is difficult to cure. **Primary liver cancer** is rarely detectable early, when it is most treatable. **Secondary liver cancer** is hard to treat because it has already spread. Also, the liver's complex network of blood vessels makes surgery difficult. Most therapy concentrates on making patients feel better and perhaps live longer.

CONVENTIONAL MEDICINE

Patients with early-stage tumors that can be removed surgically have the best chance of being cured. Unfortunately, most liver cancers are inoperable at diagnosis, either because the cancer is too advanced or the liver is too diseased to permit surgery. In some patients, radiation or chemotherapy reduces their tumors to operable size. After surgery, chemotherapy or low-dose radiation may help kill remaining cancer cells. Patients in remission must be monitored closely for potential recurrence. A few patients may be eligible for a liver transplant; although the procedure is risky, it offers some chance of cure.

Advanced liver cancer has no standard curative treatment. Chemotherapy and low-dose radiation may control the cancer's spread and ease pain. Most patients receive strong painkilling medication along with drugs to relieve nausea and swelling or to improve appetite. People with advanced liver cancer may choose to join clinical trials testing new approaches to treatment. Such studies include freezing tumor cells to kill them; using biological agents such as interferon or interleukin 2 to stimulate immune cells into attacking cancer more vigorously; and delivering lethal agents directly to cancer cells through synthetic proteins designed to target specific tumors. *(See **Cancer** for more information on treatments.)*

COMPLEMENTARY THERAPIES

Pain is a frequent but manageable consequence of advanced liver cancer. Complementary therapies that may prove beneficial include **massage, yoga, relaxation** techniques, **body work, biofeedback, hypnotherapy,** and **acupuncture.**

PREVENTION

- If you risk exposure to ***hepatitis,*** get immunized against hepatitis B.
- Drink alcohol only in moderation.
- If you work around chemicals linked to liver cancer, follow safety guidelines to avoid unnecessary contact.
- Before taking iron supplements, check with a doctor to make sure you really need them.
- Do not use anabolic steroids unless medically necessary. ■

L

LOU GEHRIG'S DISEASE

SYMPTOMS

- in the early stages, increasing weakness in one limb, especially in a hand.
- difficulty in walking; clumsiness with the hands; impaired speech.
- as the disease progresses, weakening of other limbs, perhaps accompanied by twitching, muscle cramping, and exaggerated, faster reflexes.
- problems with chewing, swallowing, and breathing; drooling may occur.
- rippling of the muscle fibers, called fasciculations, under the skin.
- eventual paralysis.

CALL YOUR DOCTOR IF:

- you have any of the symptoms above; Lou Gehrig's disease requires professional medical care.

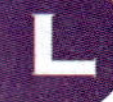

Lou Gehrig's disease—named after the baseball player who died in 1941, and clinically known as amyotrophic lateral sclerosis, or ALS—is an incurable, degenerative neurological disorder. For reasons that are not understood, the nerve cells of the brain and spinal cord that control voluntary muscle movement gradually deteriorate. As a result, muscles waste away, ultimately leading to paralysis and death, usually in two to five years. The only nerve cells affected are the motor neurons; sensory and intellectual functioning remains normal throughout. Pain does not accompany the disease at any stage.

ALS is relatively rare: About 5,000 new cases are diagnosed in the U.S. each year. It almost always strikes after the age of 40, and it afflicts more men than women.

CAUSES

Though the cause of ALS is unknown, genetic inheritance plays a role in 5 to 10 percent of cases. Some researchers believe that so-called familial ALS (that is, inherited ALS) is caused by a defective gene that prevents the body from producing a normal amount of an enzyme called superoxide dismutase (SOD). This enzyme helps neutralize free radicals, highly reactive oxygen molecules produced during metabolism and capable of damaging body tissues. Researchers speculate that defects in protective enzymes may also account for noninherited ALS, and that environmental toxins may be a factor.

Some evidence suggests that the disease may be triggered by exposure to heavy metals, animal hides, or fertilizers. In addition, viral infection and severe physical trauma have been implicated as causative factors. Other theorists link ALS to a phenomenon called excitotoxicity, in which the nerve cells that control movement are so relentlessly stimulated by glutamate, a neurotransmitter, that they eventually die.

DIAGNOSTIC AND TEST PROCEDURES

A neurologist will administer an electromyogram (EMG) to test for nerve damage. Additional tests

A BROKEN LINK

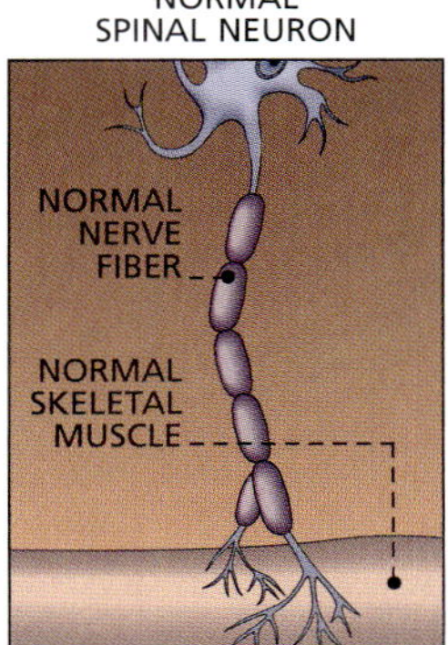

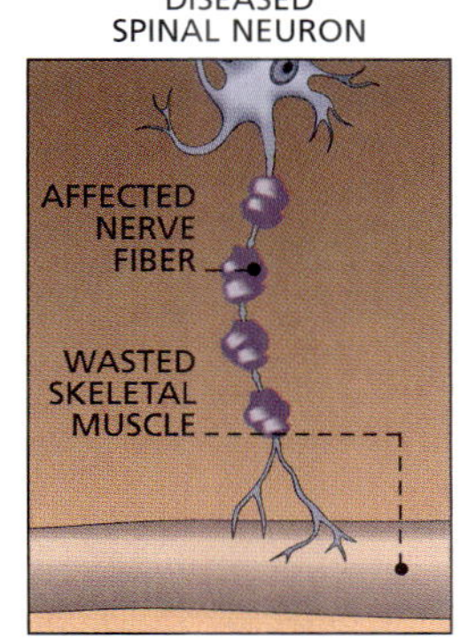

A healthy neuron, or nerve cell *(above, left),* transmits electrical signals from the brain to skeletal muscle, causing contractions that result in movement. But a neuron affected by Lou Gehrig's disease *(above, right)* withers and dies, essentially leaving the muscle stranded without stimulus for motion.

can rule out muscular dystrophy, ***multiple sclerosis,*** spinal cord tumors, or other diseases.

TREATMENT

Although no treatment slows or halts the progression of the disease, various drugs and devices are available to help control symptoms and make living with ALS easier.

CONVENTIONAL MEDICINE

Physical therapy can improve circulation and help prolong muscle use in the early stages of ALS. In addition, various medications may be prescribed as the disease progresses. Baclofen relieves stiffness (spasticity) in the limbs and throat. Muscle decline and weight loss can be slowed with nutritional supplements called branched chain amino acids (BCAAs). Quinine or ***phenytoin*** will ease cramps. ***Tricyclic antidepressants*** can help control excess saliva production—one of the symptoms of ALS.

A highly controversial experimental therapy involves synthetic forms of an insulin-like nerve growth factor called cell-derived neurotrophic factor; it may protect motor neurons and stimulate the regeneration of damaged cells.

ALTERNATIVE CHOICES

ACUPUNCTURE

Acupuncture may temporarily reduce swallowing difficulties and may also alleviate the depression that can come from coping with ALS.

CHIROPRACTIC

Spinal manipulation may relieve back pain for ALS patients who, forced by their condition to remain seated for long periods of time, may experience back and shoulder pain.

NUTRITION AND DIET

Perhaps because of swallowing difficulties, people with ALS are often malnourished and may benefit from vitamin supplements; liquid forms will probably be easier to take than tablets.

Tests indicate that some neuromuscular symptoms may be relieved by 200 to 1,200 IU of ***vitamin E*** with thiamine ***(vitamin B_1)*** each day. Some evidence suggests that supplements of coenzyme Q10, a protein catalyst, may slow the nerve-tissue atrophy that comes with ALS.

In addition, the amino acids leucine, isoleucine, and valine may help ALS patients maintain muscle strength and prolong walking ability.

AT-HOME CARE

As their condition deteriorates, ALS patients will need assistance from a caregiver, but mechanical and electronic devices can prolong mobility and independence. Portable computers and voice amplifiers can make communicating easier. Food processors will reduce hard-to-chew foods into easy-to-swallow portions. A walker or self-propelled wheelchair will enable the patient to get around. A respirator can ease breathing difficulties, and a self-suctioning device can help the patient deal with increased saliva secretions and difficulty in swallowing. ■

L

LUMPS

Read down this column to find your symptoms. Then read across.

SYMPTOMS	AILMENT/PROBLEM
Check with your doctor about any new or unusual lump for which there is no explanation; such lumps may be a sign of ***cancer.***	
◆ one or more red, pus-filled nodules ranging from one-quarter to one inch in diameter on the face, buttocks, neck, or armpits; may last two weeks or sometimes longer.	◆ ***Boil***
◆ a lump that may or may not be painful and that usually is in the upper and outer region of the breast.	◆ Benign cyst (may come and go with hormone fluctuations such as those of the menstrual cycle); possibly, cancerous tumor (may dimple or crease the skin above it or cause the nipple to turn inward or itch)
◆ a lump beneath the skin, especially in the areas of the groin and abdomen; may be tender; you may feel an aching, heavy sensation when you sit down.	◆ ***Hernia***
◆ one or more painless lumps or swellings most likely in the neck, armpits, or groin.	◆ Perhaps swollen lymph nodes caused by the presence of ***infection*** somewhere in your body; potentially a sign of Hodgkin's disease or other ***lymphoma***
◆ swelling, especially in the neck, armpits, or groin, that is accompanied by fatigue, fever, and sore throat.	◆ ***Mononucleosis***
◆ a painful enlargement of the salivary glands (located between the ear and jaw) accompanied by chills, headaches, tiredness, and fever.	◆ ***Mumps***
◆ a small, flesh-colored or whitish lump with enlarged blood vessels, or a firm, wartlike lump that grows gradually, especially in areas exposed to the sun.	◆ Perhaps only a ***wart*** but potentially basal cell carcinoma or squamous cell carcinoma
◆ a painless lump in a testicle; most common in young and middle-aged men.	◆ Perhaps a benign cyst but potentially a cancerous tumor

L

WHAT TO DO	OTHER INFO
◆ Apply hot compresses to bring a boil to a head more quickly . Clean and bandage a ruptured boil until the area heals. Do not squeeze or lance a boil on your own.	◆ Boils are the result of ***staph infection.*** Herbal therapies such as ***echinacea*** (*Echinacea* spp.) and ***goldenseal*** *(Hydrastis canadensis)* may help fight infection.
◆ See ***Breast Cancer; Breast Problems.*** Always check with your doctor about new or unusual lumps.	◆ Milk ducts can become swollen during phases of your menstrual cycle, causing cysts; caffeine can aggravate this condition.
◆ Call your doctor. You will probably need surgery to repair the rupture.	◆ Don't be misled by size. The tinier opening of a small rupture is more apt to cut off circulation to the protruding tissue—a serious condition.
◆ Call your doctor without delay for a diagnosis. An infection may need treatment with ***antibiotics.***	◆ Accompanying symptoms in the case of lymphoma can include fever, loss of appetite, sweats, general feeling of poor health, and sometimes itching.
◆ Call your doctor to confirm the diagnosis. Rest in bed, and return to normal activity gradually.	◆ Certain vitamins and some herbal and homeopathic therapies may speed recovery, possibly by boosting the immune system.
◆ In a child, mumps calls for bed rest and ***acetaminophen*** for pain. In a teenage or adult male, it should be checked by a doctor because of a slight risk of sterility.	◆ The testicles may become swollen in a teenage or adult male with mumps.
◆ See ***Skin Cancer*** and the ***Visual Diagnostic Guide.***	◆ Almost all forms of skin cancer are related to sunlight exposure, so limit sun exposure and wear sunscreen.
◆ See ***Testicle Problems; Testicular Cancer.***	◆ Men should examine their testicles regularly by gently rolling the skin between their fingers to check for lumps. Testicular cancer is highly curable if caught early. A benign cyst may form if the tube that sperm pass through—the epididymis—is clogged.

LUNG CANCER

SYMPTOMS

In its early stages, lung cancer normally has no symptoms. When symptoms start to appear, they are usually caused by blocked breathing passages or the spread of cancer to other parts of the body. Symptoms can include:

- chronic, hacking, raspy coughing, sometimes with blood-streaked sputum—the so-called smoker's cough.
- recurring respiratory infections, including ***bronchitis*** or ***pneumonia.***
- shortness of breath, wheezing, persistent chest pain.
- hoarseness.
- swelling of the neck and face.
- pain and weakness in the shoulder, arm, or hand.
- if cancer has spread beyond the lungs: fatigue, weakness, loss of weight and appetite, intermittent fever, severe headaches, and body pain.

CALL YOUR DOCTOR IF:

- you develop any symptoms that suggest lung cancer, especially chronic cough, blood-streaked sputum, wheezing, hoarseness, or recurrent lung infection. You should have a thorough pulmonary examination.

Although lung cancer is the leading cause of cancer death in the United States, it is also one of the most preventable kinds of cancer. At least 4 out of 5 cases are associated with cigarette smoking, and the cause-and-effect relationship has been documented. During the 1920s, large numbers of men began to smoke cigarettes, presumably in response to increased advertising. Twenty years later, the incidence of lung cancer in men climbed sharply. In the 1940s, significantly more women became smokers. Twenty years later, there was a similar dramatic increase in lung cancer among women.

Lung tumors almost always start in the spongy, pinkish gray walls of the bronchi—the tubular, branching airways of the lungs. More than 20 types of malignant tumors that originate in the lung itself—primary lung cancer—have been identified. The major types are **small cell lung cancer** and **nonsmall cell lung cancer.** The more common nonsmall variety is further divided into **squamous cell carcinoma, adenocarcinoma,** and **large cell carcinoma.**

Squamous cell carcinoma usually starts in cells of the central bronchi, the largest branches of the bronchial tree. It is the most common type of lung cancer in men and in smokers; it is the easiest to detect early, since its distinctive cells are likely to show up in tests of sputum samples. It also tends to be most responsive to treatment because it spreads relatively slowly.

Adenocarcinoma—the most common type of lung cancer in women and nonsmokers—tends to originate along the outer edges of the lungs in the small bronchi or smaller bronchioles. Adenocarcinoma often spreads to spaces between the lungs and the chest wall, and its typical location makes early detection difficult.

Large cell carcinomas are a group of cancers with large, abnormal-looking cells that tend to originate along the outer edges of the lungs. They are the least common of the nonsmall cell lung cancers.

Small cell lung cancer is the most aggressive form of the disease; it is also called oat cell cancer because, under a microscope, its cells resemble oat grains. Like squamous cell carcinoma, this cancer usually originates in the central bronchi.

It spreads quickly, often before symptoms appear, making it particularly threatening.

More than 170,000 people in the U.S. are diagnosed with lung cancer each year, most between the ages of 40 and 70. Only 1 percent of lung cancer patients are younger than 30, and only about 10 percent are older than 70. The overall five-year survival rate for lung cancer is improving and now stands at about 15 percent. An individual cancer sufferer's prognosis will vary according to the type of lung cancer involved, the person's overall health, and the status of the cancer at the time of diagnosis.

CAUSES

As with any cancer, each person's genetic pattern influences susceptibility to lung cancer. The fact that lung cancer runs in some families suggests that a predisposition can be inherited. Additionally, certain genetic traits have been identified that make some people more susceptible than others to carcinogens like those found in tobacco smoke.

TUMORS IN THE LUNGS

Lung cancer is usually not detectable until symptoms appear and a chest x-ray is taken. Squamous cell carcinoma and adenocarcinoma are the two most common forms of the disease. Squamous cell carcinoma is typically found in the central bronchi *(inset, top)*. Adenocarcinoma is found most commonly in the smaller bronchioles *(inset, bottom)*.

Nonetheless, anyone who smokes one pack of cigarettes daily is 20 times more likely than a nonsmoker to develop lung cancer. For people who smoke more than two packs a day, the risk more than triples. Breaking the smoking habit reduces risk significantly, yet former smokers are always slightly more susceptible than nonsmokers. Secondhand tobacco smoke can also cause lung cancer, giving nonsmokers who live or work with smokers a somewhat higher lung cancer risk than those in smoke-free environments.

Carcinogens other than those found in tobacco or tobacco smoke can also cause lung cancer if inhaled in quantity over time. However, experts disagree about how much exposure to specific carcinogens is dangerous. Workers who are exposed on a daily basis to asbestos, silica, mineral dusts, coal dust, arsenic, or the radioactive gas radon *(see the box on page 561)* are much more likely than the average person to develop lung cancer, especially if they are smokers.

Lung tissue that has been scarred by disease or infection, such as scleroderma or ***tuberculosis,*** is most susceptible to tumor growth. Because of a high incidence of lung cancer among people who eat large amounts of dietary fat and cholesterol, some researchers speculate that diet may also influence lung cancer risk.

DIAGNOSTIC AND TEST PROCEDURES

If a routine physical examination reveals swollen lymph nodes above the collarbone, a mass in the abdomen, weak breathing, abnormal sounds in the lungs, or dullness when the chest is tapped, your doctor may suspect a lung tumor. Some lung cancers produce abnormally high blood levels of certain hormones or substances such as calcium. If a person shows such evidence and no other cause is apparent, a doctor should consider lung cancer.

Once a malignant tumor begins to cause symptoms, it is usually visible on an x-ray. Occasionally a tumor that has not yet begun to cause symptoms is spotted on a chest x-ray taken for another purpose. A CT scan of the chest may be ordered for a more detailed examination. While examinations of sputum or lung fluid may reveal fully developed cancer cells, diagnosis is usually confirmed through a biopsy. With the patient lightly anesthetized, the doctor guides a thin, lighted tube through the nose and down the air passages to the site of the tumor, where a tiny tissue sample can be removed. If the biopsy confirms cancer, other tests will determine the type of cancer and how far it has spread. Nearby lymph nodes can be tested for cancer cells, while imaging techniques such as CT scans and bone scans can detect tumors elsewhere in the body.

Because sputum examinations and chest x-rays have not proved particularly effective in detecting small tumors characteristic of early lung cancer, annual chest x-rays for lung cancer screening are not recommended by the American Cancer Society, the National Cancer Institute, or the American College of Radiology.

TREATMENT

If the cancer can be successfully removed surgically, the patient has an excellent chance of surviving at least one year, and usually a better than 50 percent chance of living at least five years. The challenge comes in detecting lung cancer early enough to make surgery possible. See ***Cancer*** for more specific information on treatments such as chemotherapy and radiation therapy.

CONVENTIONAL MEDICINE

The decision to perform surgery is based not only on the type of lung cancer and how far it has spread but also on the patient's overall health. Many patients with lung cancer—especially smokers—have existing pulmonary or cardiovascular problems that rule out surgery. Cancer that has spread to lymph nodes between the lungs was once considered inoperable, but combining surgery with pre- or postoperative chemotherapy and radiation therapy has improved cure rates.

When feasible, the preferred treatment for **nonsmall cell lung cancer** is surgery. Before the procedure, an effort is made to reduce the size of the tumor with radiation therapy or chemotherapy. During the operation, the surgeon removes the tumorous area along with surrounding lung tissue and lymph nodes; often the entire lung must be taken out. After surgery, patients stay in the hospital for several days and receive ***analgesics*** to control postoperative pain. Radiation therapy may be necessary to kill remaining cancer cells, but it is usually delayed for at least a month while the surgical wound heals. Nonsmall cell lung cancers that cannot be treated surgically are usually treated with radiation therapy.

Because of its tendency to spread extensively, **small cell lung cancer** is typically treated with combination chemotherapy—the use of more than one drug—often in conjunction with radiation therapy. For selected patients with small cell lung cancer, some doctors recommend bone-marrow transplant to allow the administration of higher doses of chemotherapy. *(See **Lymphoma.**)*

Patients whose cancers have metastasized, or spread to distant sites, may be treated with either chemotherapy or radiation therapy. Since metastatic lung cancer is very difficult to cure, the main goals of treatment are to provide comfort and prolong life. Current therapies can shrink tumors, which may alleviate pain and other symptoms. Patients with advanced lung cancer commonly take medication to control pain. Morphine and its various derivatives are widely used and extremely effective in the management of cancer pain.

Researchers are constantly looking for better ways to treat lung cancer, to relieve symptoms, and to improve patients' quality of life. New combinations of chemotherapy, new forms of radiation, and the use of drugs that make cancer cells more sensitive to radiation are under study. Experimental laser surgery has successfully reduced or eliminated tumors obstructing bronchi, thereby improving breathing. Trials are also under way to test various forms of immunotherapy and gene therapy against lung cancer. Immunotherapy manipulates the natural immune system in the hope of turning it aggressively against cancer, while gene therapy enlists foreign genetic material injected into tumor cells to slow or stop their spread.

COMPLEMENTARY THERAPIES

Once conventional treatment is under way, much can be done to alleviate the pain, fear, and dis-

Assessing the Risk of Radon

Radon is a colorless, odorless, radioactive gas that seeps constantly from the Earth's crust. Studies of uranium miners working on the Colorado Plateau in the 1950s proved conclusively that prolonged, intense exposure to radon causes lung cancer. The U.S. Environmental Protection Agency (EPA) warns that exposure to radon in the home at a level of 4 or more picocuries may cause lung cancer. (A picocurie is one-trillionth of a curie, the standard unit for measuring radioactivity.) Smokers are believed to be particularly susceptible to radon risk, even at low levels.

The EPA recommends, but does not require, that all American homes be tested for and proofed against radon. Critics of the EPA's campaign contend that the costs of doing so are unwarranted, while supporters insist that the evidence—however indirect it is—justifies EPA policy. In fact, little scientific evidence supports the EPA's contention, and some studies have found that states with the highest household radon levels have a lower-than-average incidence of lung cancer. The EPA's response to the debate: "Better safe than sorry."

comfort of cancer. Most complementary cancer therapies can be pursued safely along with standard treatment but should never be substituted for medical care. While outcomes differ among patients receiving complementary care, many have benefited from support-group therapy, improved **nutrition and diet,** and various **body work** and **mind/body** exercises. For further information on complementary cancer therapies, see ***Cancer.***

NUTRITION AND DIET

Some nutritional studies suggest that certain vitamins and minerals offer protection against lung cancer. Various antioxidants, including ***vitamins C*** and ***E*** as well as beta carotene ***(vitamin A)*** and some other carotenoids, are believed to protect the lungs from the harmful effects of tobacco smoke and other carcinogens. However, enthusiasm for specific nutrients must be tempered by other studies that have either contradicted or failed to support such encouraging results.

Until the full effects of specific nutrients are sorted out, most researchers are reluctant to recommend supplemental vitamins and minerals as potential lung cancer preventives. Instead they advise eating a well-balanced diet that will ensure adequate fiber and nutrients.

AT-HOME CARE

If you've had lung surgery, your nurse or doctor can show you special exercises to improve your breathing and strengthen your chest muscles. You can relieve skin irritation associated with radiation therapy by wearing loose clothes and keeping your chest protected from the sun. Avoid using skin lotions unless approved by your doctor. For other ideas about coping with the difficulties of cancer and its treatment, see ***Cancer.***

PREVENTION

The best defense against lung cancer is not to smoke. Breaking the tobacco habit may be difficult, but it can be done. *(See* ***Nicotine Withdrawal.****)* While preparing yourself to quit, cut back on the number of cigarettes you smoke daily. Many people report that stopping cigarette smoking "cold turkey" is more effective than gradually tapering off. Joining a support group may help you maintain your resolve to quit. See the ***Appendix*** for a listing of substance-abuse support organizations. If you live or work with smokers, encourage them to quit and ask them not to smoke around you. If you are exposed to chemical carcinogens at work, take necessary safety measures to limit inhalation. ■

LUPUS

SYMPTOMS

- profound fatigue, low-grade fever, and severe muscle aches and joint pain.
- skin rash on face or body.
- extreme sun sensitivity.
- weight loss, mental confusion, and chest pain on taking a deep breath.
- nose, mouth, or throat ulcers.
- enlarged lymph nodes.
- poor circulation in fingers and toes.
- bald patches.
- discolored urine, or frequent or blocked urination.

CALL YOUR DOCTOR IF:

- you have several of the above symptoms and suspect you have lupus. This disease is potentially fatal and requires professional medical care. Prognosis improves with early detection and rigorous treatment.
- you have a family history of lupus—especially in your mother or father or an aunt or uncle—and you have experienced several of the above symptoms.

Lupus is a chronic autoimmune disease in which the immune system mistakes the body's connective tissue for a foreign invader and attacks it. One type, **discoid lupus erythematosus (DLE)**, affects only skin that is exposed to sunlight. The other kind, **systemic lupus erythematosus (SLE)**, is more serious. It affects the skin and other vital organs, often causing a raised, scaly butterfly-shaped rash across the bridge of the nose and cheeks that can leave scars if it goes untreated. Systemic lupus may also inflame and damage the connective tissue in the joints, muscles, and skin, as well as the membranes surrounding the lungs, heart, kidneys, and brain. Inflammation of the blood vessels, especially in the fingers, can result in lesions or ulcers. ***Raynaud's syndrome*** appears in 20 percent of patients. SLE can also cause ***kidney disease.***

Lupus is characterized by unpredictable phases of remission and exacerbation that vary in intensity and duration. The course of the disease follows no typical pattern and can range from mildly inconveniencing to debilitating.

Lupus strikes black Americans three times as often as white Americans. Most sufferers are between the ages of 20 and 35, and 90 percent are women.

CAUSES

No single agent has been identified as causing lupus, although some research suggests that a combination of genetic, hormonal, and immunologic factors may be behind it. A predisposition to developing the disease does appear to be an inherited trait.

Environmental elements, ranging from viral and bacterial infections to severe emotional stress or overexposure to sunlight, may play roles in provoking or triggering the disease. Certain drugs such as ***penicillin*** and ***anticonvulsants*** may cause lupuslike symptoms. High estrogen levels resulting from pregnancy, estrogen replacement therapy, and oral contraceptives may aggravate lupus. There may also be a link between lupus and silicone breast implants.

DIAGNOSTIC AND TEST PROCEDURES

Diagnosing lupus can be difficult because symptoms often mimic other diseases and vary from patient to patient. Your doctor will first attempt to rule out ***chronic fatigue syndrome, mononucleosis,*** and autoimmune disorders other than lupus itself. Some of the tests your doctor may perform include a complete blood count, platelet count, and serum electrophoresis to indicate the levels of white blood cells and plasma proteins.

Blood testing for anti-DNA antibodies—which shows whether you have antibodies to the normal genetic material in certain cells—is the most definitive way to identify lupus.

TREATMENT

Due to its unpredictable nature, lupus is a difficult disease to control, but close self-monitoring and proper treatment can help in most cases.

CONVENTIONAL MEDICINE

For milder cases, ***nonsteroidal anti-inflammatory drugs (NSAIDs)*** such as ***aspirin*** or ***ibuprofen*** can be used to relieve joint pain. Stubborn rashes and more severe joint pain may respond to antimalarial medications such as hydroxychloroquine. A short course of ***corticosteroids*** reduces inflammation and fever and is recommended for flareups. Immunosuppressive drugs also decrease inflammation by suppressing abnormal autoimmune activity. ***Antidepressants*** and mild ***antianxiety drugs*** can help with the sleeping problems that frequently accompany the disease. Cyclophosphamides, which subdue the immune system, may be used for severe cases of lupus involving renal damage.

Mild skin rashes can be treated topically with over-the-counter corticosteroid creams; thicker lesions may require prescription fluorinated steroid creams or injections of ***triamcinolone.***

ALTERNATIVE CHOICES

Although they should never be substituted for prescribed medications, a number of alternative therapies may help you control your symptoms. In addition to the remedies mentioned below, you might want to consider **acupuncture, Chinese herbs,** and various forms of **body work.** Consult a specialist for guidance in using these therapies.

NUTRITION AND DIET

People with lupus often have food allergies that can make symptoms worse. Identifying and avoiding problem foods can help.

A change in diet may reduce inflammation and decrease pain. Nutritionists may recommend cutting down on red meat and dairy products, and increasing consumption of fish high in omega-3 fatty acids—such as mackerel, sardines, and salmon—which have anti-inflammatory properties. Alfalfa contains a substance that has been shown in tests to aggravate symptoms, so avoiding alfalfa sprouts is strongly recommended.

The following supplements may benefit lupus patients: ***vitamins*** B_5***, C,*** and ***E;*** and ***selenium.*** Beta carotene *(see* ***Vitamin A****)* may help clear up the lesions of discoid lupus. Consult your doctor or a nutritionist for suggested dosages.

L

AT-HOME REMEDIES

- Avoid sun exposure by wearing protective clothing (hats, sunglasses, long sleeves, and long pants) along with an SPF 15 (or higher) sunscreen containing para-aminobenzoic acid (PABA).
- Pace yourself throughout the day to conserve energy, and get plenty of rest even if it means scheduling naps into your routine.

PREVENTION

Because no one knows what causes lupus, there is no way to prevent it. Flareups can be managed, however, by avoiding known triggers such as sunlight, stress, and lack of sleep. Pay careful attention to your diet and exercise. In addition, keep a record of your symptoms—when they occur, what preceded them, and how long they last—and adjust your routine with them in mind. ■

LYME DISEASE

SYMPTOMS

- a circular, bull's-eye rash, often with a clear center, expanding to eight inches or more and lasting two to four weeks.
- may be accompanied by headache, fatigue, fever, chills, sore throat, and aching muscles and joints.
- if not treated, weeks later the development of a generalized and painful kind of ***arthritis,*** with swelling in one or sometimes both knees.
- paralysis (most often of the face), memory impairment; random areas of tingling or numbness.
- skin sensitivities.
- stiff neck.
- sensitivity to light.
- irregular heartbeat, chest pain, dizziness.
- psychological changes, including ***depression.***

CALL YOUR DOCTOR IF:

- you think you may have contracted Lyme disease, especially if you notice a bull's-eye rash or if you suddenly develop knee pain and swelling without previous injury or arthritis. Delaying treatment can result in the more serious neurological symptoms that can be difficult and sometimes impossible to cure.

Lyme disease is transmitted by tiny ticks of the Ixodidae family and afflicts about 10,000 people yearly. Initially identified in a group of children in Lyme, Connecticut, the disease has now been found in nearly all states and 18 other countries. About 90 percent of cases are reported in three areas: the northeast and mid-Atlantic states (Massachusetts to Maryland), the upper Midwest (Minnesota and Wisconsin), and the Far West (California and Oregon).

The first sign is usually an expanding bull's-eye rash that swells to several inches in diameter before disappearing after a few weeks. But in some cases, the rash may take a different form or may be absent altogether. Other early symptoms—with or without the rash—are flulike feelings of fatigue, headache, fever, sore throat, chills, or body aches.

You may also have vague pains in the joints, without swelling. In about half the patients who are not treated, this joint pain returns in about six months as painful ***arthritis*** with swelling, usually in one knee. In about 10 percent of these cases, Lyme arthritis becomes chronic. Some patients also experience a complex range of other symptoms, including stiff neck, headaches, sensitivity to light, memory loss, mood changes, chronic fatigue, recurring rashes, paralysis of one or both sides of the face, disruption of heart rhythm, and areas of tingling or numbness.

Because the symptoms are random and vague (aside from the bull's-eye rash), Lyme disease can be hard to diagnose. Unfortunately, unless Lyme disease is treated promptly, it can also be difficult to cure. This is one reason the disease has inspired considerable anxiety among residents in areas where it is common, and may be a reason it is also overdiagnosed.

The good news is that a vaccine that appears to prevent Lyme disease has been under testing. Until a vaccine is approved, however, the best protection is vigilance. Because infection does not occur until a tick has been attached for 36 to 48 hours, a thorough daily tick check can be an effective first-line defense. Be aware, however, that the ticks are very small; they are often the size of poppy seeds, although they are larger when engorged with blood.

THE LYMPHATIC SYSTEM

A fluid called lymph protects the body against infection by circulating lymphocytes, a type of white blood cell that attacks infectious organisms. The system's main organ is the spleen, connected by a network of tiny lymphatic vessels to clusters of lymph nodes throughout the body. Lymphocytes passing through body tissues destroy most infections before they can enter the bloodstream.

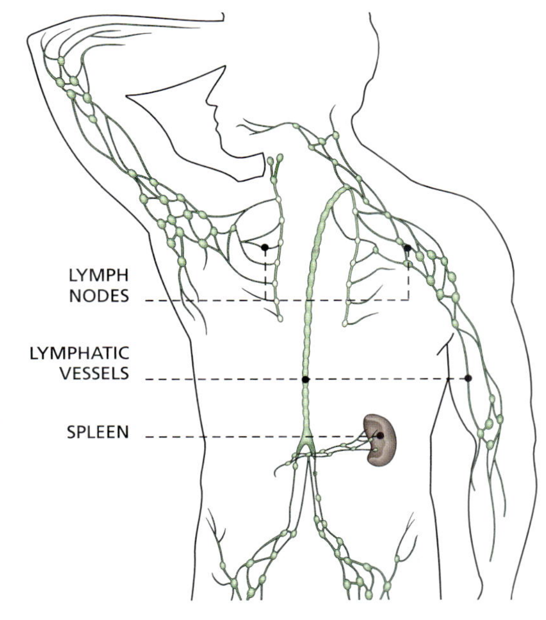

gressively it behaves. Low-grade versions usually progress slowly and tend not to spread beyond the lymphatic system. High-grade versions may spread to distant organs within a few months. Lymphoma is most commonly seen in Caucasian men. Hodgkin's disease usually appears between the ages of 15 and 30, or after 50; non-Hodgkin's lymphomas rarely strike people younger than 45.

Hodgkin's disease is now one of the most curable of all cancers, with an overall five-year survival rate of nearly 80 percent; when the disease is detected and treated early, the rate jumps to 90 percent. Although non-Hodgkin's lymphomas are typically more difficult to cure, the overall five-year survival rate has improved from 30 to more than 50 percent in recent decades. A low-grade case can be controlled for years with treatment but is difficult to eradicate completely. High-grade cases, while more immediately threatening, are potentially curable with aggressive treatment.

CAUSES

The cause of Hodgkin's disease is unknown. Most people diagnosed with this form of lymphoma are in general good health. There may be a hereditary link, as siblings of people with Hodgkin's disease are seven times more likely than average to get the disease.

The causes of non-Hodgkin's lymphoma are also largely unknown. A form called **Burkitt's lymphoma** is strongly associated with infection by the Epstein-Barr virus, a herpesvirus most commonly found in Africa. Other lymphomas have been linked to infection by either HIV—the cause of ***AIDS***—or HTLV, another member of the HIV family. Since the onset of AIDS in the early 1980s, the incidence of non-Hodgkin's lymphoma has increased 65 percent, while the incidence of Hodgkin's disease has decreased. Other conditions that compromise the body's immune function, such as organ transplantation, treatment with radiation or chemotherapy, or such autoimmune disorders as ***lupus*** and rheumatoid ***arthritis,*** also increase a person's risk for non-Hodgkin's lymphoma.

DIAGNOSTIC AND TEST PROCEDURES

Doctors do not know how to detect lymphoma before it starts causing symptoms. Swollen lymph nodes in the neck, armpits, or groin usually offer the first clue. A patient may report the swelling, or it may be detected during a routine checkup. A doctor may also suspect lymphoma when swelling in lymph nodes or the spleen is accompanied by more general symptoms such as fatigue, chills, or night sweats.

Blood and urine studies coupled with imaging tests can reveal abnormalities that help early diagnosis of lymphoma, but the disease must be confirmed by a biopsy—usually of a lymph node but sometimes of affected skin or lung tissue that is removed surgically and studied by a pathologist. The size, shape, and pattern of cells under a microscope can determine whether lymphoma exists and, if so, what type.

If cancer is found, further testing can determine how widespread it is. Doctors can examine the lymphatic system using CT scans or an x-ray procedure called a lymphangiogram. For this procedure, the patient is injected with a dye that highlights the lymphatic system on x-ray. A bone-marrow biopsy is usually performed to check for the presence of cancer cells in the bone marrow. Exploratory surgery may be required to determine the full extent of the affected lymph nodes.

TREATMENT

Lymphomas are among the cancers most responsive to radiation and chemotherapy. As these treatments have become more sophisticated, the survival rates for lymphoma have risen steadily. Most lymphoma patients now survive at least five years with conventional treatment. Success has been especially remarkable with Hodgkin's disease: At least 75 percent of newly diagnosed cases are now considered curable.

CONVENTIONAL MEDICINE

Specifics of treatment vary from case to case, depending on the type of lymphoma involved, the presence or absence of symptoms, and the patient's age and general health. Given the complexity of decision making, lymphoma patients should be encouraged to solicit the opinion of a lymphoma specialist at a major cancer center before starting a particular treatment regimen.

When limited to one or a cluster of lymph nodes, **Hodgkin's disease** can be treated effectively with radiation therapy. To treat large tumors or Hodgkin's disease that has begun to spread, however, chemotherapy—sometimes along with radiation therapy—is the best treatment option. Such treatment pursued aggressively cures up to 40 percent of advanced cases of Hodgkin's disease.

Since success depends on high doses of toxic drugs and radiation, treatment frequently results in unpleasant side effects and can cause residual complications such as infertility. Medication along with various complementary therapies can help control some side effects. Male patients may want to consider banking their sperm before treatment begins. Premenopausal women often stop menstruating during treatment, but menstruation may resume after treatment ends.

Treatment decisions for **non-Hodgkin's lymphoma** depend largely on the grade of the disease. Low-grade disease usually progresses very slowly and—although responsive to chemotherapy—often recurs. Rather than having a patient endure unnecessary treatment, a doctor may choose to monitor a low-grade case closely and act only when it begins to accelerate. By contrast, high-grade cases merit immediate and aggressive radiation therapy, chemotherapy, or both.

Researchers continue to investigate new treatment methods in the hope of improving cure rates for advanced and recurrent lymphoma. The underlying objective is—and always has been—to kill cancer cells, but without harming healthy cells. Various ways to do so are under study. Immunotherapists are experimenting with certain biological agents, such as interferon, to stimulate immune cells into attacking cancer cells more aggressively. Other researchers are synthesizing special proteins called monoclonal antibodies that specifically target cancer cells. When fused with toxic chemicals or radioactive agents, these antibodies are intended to deliver lethal blows to cancer cells without harming the surrounding healthy cells. The anticancer arsenal includes many other techniques for making cancer cells more sensitive to radiation and drug treatment. In some cases, bone-marrow transplantation is used to allow the administration of higher-dose chemotherapy. *(See box at right.)*

Lymphoma patients who achieve remission should have regular cancer-oriented checkups, because lymphoma recurs in a significant percentage of survivors within two or three years. With successful treatment of Hodgkin's disease, relapse after five years of remission is rare.

*(See **Cancer** for further information on chemotherapy, radiation therapy, and other forms of cancer treatment.)*

BONE-MARROW TRANSPLANTATION

A few decades ago, oncologists (cancer specialists) faced a frustrating problem. They knew that heavy doses of chemotherapy or radiation could force some cancers "over the threshold" into remission. They also knew that such treatment could irreparably damage bone marrow, without which a person cannot live. But what if the bone marrow were sacrificed to wipe out the cancer, then resupplied? Bone-marrow transplantation emerged as a potential solution. Today, bone-marrow transplantation is accepted as a risky but appropriate therapy for some types of cancer, curing a significant number of otherwise incurable patients.

Transplantation for lymphoma relies on using the patient's own bone marrow. A small amount of marrow is removed, treated with chemicals to eliminate cancer cells, then placed in cold storage. Meanwhile, the patient receives chemotherapy—sometimes with radiation therapy. As the cancer cells are wiped out, so too are the remaining marrow cells. The stored, cancer-free bone marrow is then returned to the patient's body intravenously.

Gradually, immature blood cells in the replacement bone marrow start to multiply. Until this occurs, a patient's immune system is severely suppressed and the possibility of infection is a constant concern. To minimize this dangerous phase, doctors employ "growth factors" that speed the regrowth of healthy bone marrow. This and other refinements promise to make bone-marrow transplantation an increasingly safe and valuable cancer therapy.

COMPLEMENTARY THERAPIES

Lymphoma and its standard treatment of toxic drugs and radiation contribute to weakening of the immune system. Many therapies that are believed by some researchers to enhance the body's immune function can complement standard treatment safely, may sustain general health, and actually may help the body fight cancer. Rest, relaxation, and sound nutrition are the foundation for restoring good health. Joining a support group may help release emotions that contribute to stress. See ***Cancer*** for more suggestions.

AT-HOME CARE

Chemotherapy and radiation therapy can cause unpleasant side effects, such as nausea, vomiting, diarrhea, fatigue, and vulnerability to infection. Your doctor can prescribe medication to address some of these problems, and you can do a number of things to relieve symptoms: Eat light meals. Avoid dairy products and sweet, fried, or fatty foods. Drink plenty of liquids before and after meals. If the smell of cooked food makes you feel nauseated, try eating foods cold or at room temperature. Wear loose-fitting clothing. Be careful about keeping your skin clean and scratch free, and avoid contact with obviously sick people. Rest whenever you feel the need, but otherwise keep yourself busy with activities that will help take your mind off the immediate discomfort.

PREVENTION

With only limited knowledge of what causes lymphoma, doctors cannot provide detailed preventive guidelines. Staying as healthy as possible may reduce your risk for cancer in general. Standard advice includes eating a well-balanced diet, keeping your weight in check, exercising regularly, and getting adequate sleep. All these measures contribute to healthy immune function. Unless you are absolutely certain that your sexual partner is HIV negative, be sure to use a condom during sexual intercourse to avoid infection. ■

MACULAR DEGENERATION

SYMPTOMS

- dim or distorted vision, especially while reading.
- gradual, painless loss of precise central vision.
- blank spots in your central field of vision; straight lines that appear wavy.

CALL YOUR DOCTOR IF:

- you exhibit any of the symptoms above and have never seen an ophthalmologist. Ask your doctor for a referral.
- you exhibit any of the symptoms above and have hypertension, ***diabetes,*** or ***heart disease.*** You are in the high-risk category for the advanced **wet** form of macular degeneration. Any abnormality in your vision is a sign that you may be developing the disorder.
- you have been diagnosed with **age-related macular degeneration** and then you discover blank spots in your field of vision, printed matter appears distorted, or straight lines appear wavy. You may be developing the advanced **wet** form of macular degeneration.

Macular degeneration is the leading cause of vision loss in the United States, with more than 13 million Americans showing some sign of the disorder. Because the symptoms usually do not appear in people under 55 years of age, the disorder is often referred to as **age-related macular degeneration (ARMD).** If you are over 65, macular degeneration may already affect your central vision, even though most sufferers of the disease maintain functional side, or peripheral, vision throughout life. The disorder occurs in two forms, **dry** and **wet.** The less common **wet** form of ARMD requires immediate medical attention; any delay in treatment may result in loss of your central vision.

CAUSES

Macular degeneration is scarring of the macula, a spot about 1/16 inch in diameter at the center of the retina. The macula enables you to read, watch television, drive, sew—anything that requires focused, straight-ahead vision. Although the rest of the retina can continue to process images at the sides of your field of vision, the scarring distorts or obscures part of the central image that your eye transmits to your brain.

In the **dry** form of ARMD, tiny yellow deposits develop beneath the macula, signaling a degeneration and thinning of nerve tissue. A small number of cases develop into the **wet,** or **neovascular,** form of ARMD, in which abnormal blood vessels grow beneath the macula. As these vessels leak blood and fluid onto the retina, retinal cells die, causing blurs and blank spots in your field of vision.

You are more susceptible to ARMD as you get older, especially if there is a history of the disorder in your family. ***Atherosclerosis, diabetes, heart disease, high blood pressure,*** and nutritional deficiencies are also risk factors.

DIAGNOSTIC AND TEST PROCEDURES

Your ophthalmologist will inspect the macula as part of a routine eye exam. A painless photographic procedure, fluorescein angiography, shows the pattern of your eye's blood vessels and can detect any abnormalities.

TREATMENT

Macular degeneration is not reversible, so people who develop **dry** ARMD typically compensate with large-print publications and magnifying lenses for everyday activities. **Wet** ARMD may be treated with medication or laser surgery.

CONVENTIONAL MEDICINE

The more common **dry macular degeneration** cannot be cured, but it can be kept from getting worse under an ophthalmologist's care. For the **wet** form, your doctor may recommend the drug verteporfin, which slows retinal damage, or laser photocoagulation, a surgical proceedure that destroys leaking blood vessels that have grown under the macula to halt the damaging effects to your vision. This procedure must be done before leakage from abnormal blood vessels causes irreversible damage.

ALTERNATIVE CHOICES

Alternative treatments attempt to restore nutrient deficiencies that can damage the macula.

HERBAL THERAPIES

Collagen, one of the most abundant proteins in the body, plays an integral role in maintaining the strength and function of your eye tissue. The collagen structure of your retina may be strengthened and reinforced by taking 100 mg of ***bilberry*** *(Vaccinium myrtillus)* extract daily.

Dried ***ginkgo*** *(Ginkgo biloba)*—40 mg three times a day—may guard against damage to your macula by free radicals, unstable molecules found in the body that can harm cells.

NUTRITION AND DIET

Many older people exhibit deficiencies in ***zinc,*** which normally appears in high concentrations in the retina, particularly the macula. Ask your doctor about taking a zinc supplement to help protect the macula from damage and improve sharpness of vision. Antioxidants are said to fight the negative effects free radicals have on your retinal blood vessels. To increase your intake of antioxidants, take 1,000 mg of ***vitamin C*** three times a day, 600 IU of ***vitamin E*** a day, 200 mcg of ***selenium*** a day (avoid higher doses), or 20,000 IU of beta carotene *(see* ***Vitamin A****)* a day.

AMSLER GRID

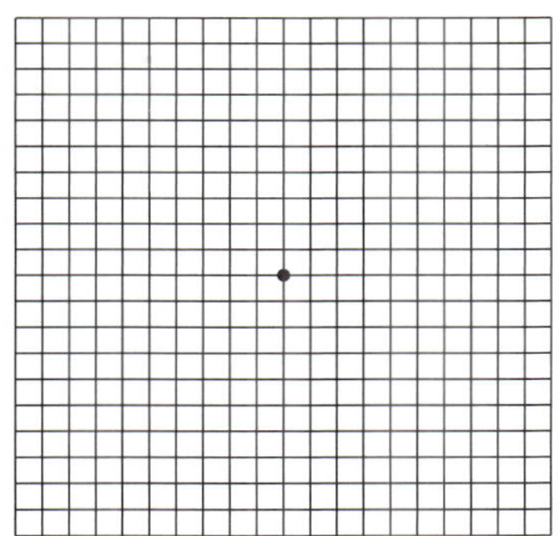

Check yourself for macular degeneration by using this Amsler grid. Place this page on a flat surface in good light. Wearing reading glasses or contact lenses, cover one eye and look at the dot at the center of the grid from a distance of 12 to 15 inches; repeat with your other eye. If any of the lines on the grid appear wavy, distorted, or missing, discuss the condition with your ophthalmologist.

AT-HOME REMEDIES

Your ophthalmologist will suggest large-print reading material, magnifiers, and other aids to enhance your eyesight. You can monitor changes in your eyesight at home with an Amsler grid *(above).*

Eat more fruits and vegetables rich in ***vitamin C,*** such as citrus fruits, cauliflower, and broccoli. Snack on nuts and seeds, which contain ***vitamin E.*** Yellow vegetables containing carotene, as well as cherries, blackberries, and blueberries, all of which contain antioxidant flavonoids, are also said to help stave off degeneration of the macula. Cut back on consumption of alcohol, tobacco, and coffee, all of which may aggravate eye problems.■

MALARIA

SYMPTOMS

- headache, fatigue, low-grade fever, and nausea.
- sudden chills and, sometimes, severe shaking.
- a fever that can be as high as 107°F, accompanied sometimes by rapid breathing.
- profuse sweating.

CALL YOUR DOCTOR IF:

- you experience the symptoms of malaria while in an area of the world where malaria is transmitted or up to several months after returning.
- you will be traveling to an area where malaria is common; your doctor can prescribe a preventive antimalarial medication.

M

Malaria is an infectious disease transmitted by mosquitoes. Worldwide, about 300 million to 500 million people get malaria each year, including about 1,000 people in the United States—all but a handful of whom contract the disease abroad. Almost all tropical and subtropical countries have malaria-transmitting mosquitoes.

Early symptoms of malaria include headache, fatigue, low-grade fever, and nausea. Within about 24 hours, the illness frequently progresses into three distinct stages. First comes the cold stage, characterized by sudden chills and, sometimes, violent shaking, which lasts one to two hours. The second, or hot, stage is marked by a fever, which can go as high as 107°F, at times accompanied by rapid breathing; this lasts three to four hours. The wet stage follows: two to four hours of profuse sweating.

CAUSES

Malaria is caused by a bite from the female *Anopheles* mosquito, which injects the malaria parasites into the bloodstream. Four species of a parasite known as *Plasmodium* cause malaria in humans: *P. vivax, P. ovale, P. malariae,* and *P. falciparum.* Once in the bloodstream, the plasmodia travel to the liver, where they multiply at a tremendous rate. Within a week or so, up to 40,000 of them flow back into the bloodstream, where they continue to multiply and begin to destroy red blood cells. It is this destruction that causes the characteristic symptoms of malaria.

Although all four species can be deadly, *P. falciparum* is particularly dangerous—and more likely to be fatal—because it multiplies much more quickly than the others, destroying many more blood cells. This species is also more resistant to antimalarial drugs.

Forms of both the *P. vivax* and *P. ovale* parasites can remain dormant in the liver without creating any apparent symptoms of malaria for months or, in rare cases, years. Then one day, for reasons as yet unknown to scientists, they leave the liver and return to the bloodstream, causing a malaria attack. So if you have at any time traveled to a part of the world where malaria is prevalent, be sure to report that fact to your doctor if you develop an unexplained illness with a fever.

DIAGNOSTIC AND TEST PROCEDURES

If your doctor suspects that you have malaria, a sample of your blood will be examined for evidence of the parasites. If the first smear is negative but malaria is strongly suspected, samples may be taken and examined every 12 to 24 hours for three consecutive days.

TREATMENT

Left untreated, *P. falciparum* malaria can be fatal. Quick and appropriate conventional treatment, however, can result in a speedy and complete recovery. Other forms of malaria rarely cause death but still require treatment to avoid complications and ease recovery.

CONVENTIONAL MEDICINE

If you are infected with *P. vivax, P. ovale, or P. malariae,* you will receive chloroquine orally for three days. To help avoid later recurrences caused by dormant *P. vivax* or *P. ovale* parasites, you will also be given oral doses of primaquine for 14 more days. Because primaquine can destroy red blood cells and thus threaten the health of a fetus, it is not given to pregnant women; if you are pregnant, you will be kept on chloroquine.

If you became infected with *P. falciparum* in an area of the world where it has not been shown resistant to chloroquine, you will be treated with that drug. Otherwise, you will be given oral doses of either quinine and ***tetracycline,*** or quinine and a combination product of pyrimethamine and sulfadoxine for several days. If you are vomiting or have serious medical complications, you may be given intravenous quinidine until you are well enough to take the other drugs.

ALTERNATIVE CHOICES

Alternative therapies can treat the symptoms of malaria and help your body recover from antimalarial medications, which can cause unpleasant, although temporary, side effects, such as nausea, dizziness, diarrhea, tinnitus, and skin rashes. All remedies should be taken in conjunction with conventional medications and under professional supervision.

HERBAL THERAPIES

Boneset *(Eupatorium perfoliatum),* sometimes called feverwort, was used by Native Americans and early American colonists to treat feverish illnesses, including malaria. Make a tea, using 1 to 2 tsp of the dried herb; drink it as hot as possible and as often as every half hour.

HOMEOPATHY

Remedies prescribed for malaria include ***Arsenicum album*** and ***Sulphur.*** Consult a homeopath for dosages and length of treatment.

PREVENTION

If you are going to an area where malaria exists, tell your doctor several weeks before you leave. Your doctor will put you on a regimen of mefloquine, ***doxycycline*** hyclate, or chloroquine. If you plan to travel in an area where malaria is a problem, take the following precautions:

- Take a preventive antimalarial medication before, during, and after the trip.
- Sleep under mosquito netting treated with an insecticide, such as permethrin or deltamethrin.
- Stay in buildings with air conditioning or screened doors and windows.
- Stay indoors from dusk to dawn, the time when mosquitoes feed.
- If you go out in the evening, wear long pants and a long-sleeved shirt.
- Use a mosquito repellent: a permethrin spray for clothing and a lotion with 35 to 40 percent diethyltoluamide (DEET) for exposed skin.

TIP FOR TRAVELERS

For current information on malaria hot spots in the world, call the Centers for Disease Control and Prevention at 800-311-3435 or 404-639-3534. ■

MANIC-DEPRESSION

SYMPTOMS

Dramatic and unpredictable mood swings are the primary sign of manic-depression. The illness has two strongly contrasting phases.

In the manic phase:

- euphoria or irritability.
- excessive talk; racing thoughts.
- inflated self-esteem.
- unusual energy; less need for sleep.
- impulsiveness, a reckless pursuit of gratification—shopping sprees, impetuous travel, more and sometimes promiscuous sex, high-risk business investments, fast driving.
- hallucinations.

In the depressive phase:

- depressed mood and low self-esteem.
- overwhelming inertia and apathy.
- sadness, loneliness, helplessness, guilt.
- slow speech, fatigue, and poor coordination.
- insomnia.
- suicidal thoughts and feelings.
- use of psychostimulants such as amphetamines to boost energy and spirits.

CALL YOUR DOCTOR IF:

- you notice some of these symptoms in a family member. Note: Manic-depressives often deny anything is wrong, especially in the manic phase. If you are worried about a family member or close friend, a doctor can offer advice on how to handle the situation.
- you notice some of these symptoms in yourself.

M

Manic-depression, known to mental health professionals as bipolar disorder, is a serious, double-edged mental illness. In contrast to the sustained bleakness of generalized ***depression*** (technically described as unipolar disorder), manic-depression is characterized by cyclical swings between elation and despair. The pattern of the mood alternations varies widely among sufferers. In some cases, years of normal functioning can separate manic and depressive episodes. In others, the episodes cycle frequently, three or four times a year, with respites between. For some patients, depression and mania cycle continuously and sometimes rapidly. And for a rare few, an episode of manic-depression may occur only once in a lifetime. (If it occurs twice, it is usually followed by other episodes.) Generally, the depressive phase lasts longer than the manic phase, and it also tends to be more frequent; the cycle can be erratic.

Manic-depression is known to afflict about 1 percent of the U.S. population, although its incidence may be much higher because almost 75 percent of cases go untreated. Men and women are equally susceptible. Much evidence suggests that the illness has a genetic basis, but its origins are still uncertain. The symptoms apparently result from chemical imbalances in the brain, and they lie beyond voluntary control. The disorder is not only life-disrupting but can also be dangerous: About 20 percent of manic-depressives commit suicide, usually when they are passing from one phase to another and feel disoriented. Some 11 percent of sufferers take this drastic action in the first decade after diagnosis.

Fortunately, great strides have recently been made in treating this illness; in most cases, the symptoms can be controlled effectively by medication and other therapies.

The disorder occurs in two main forms, known as **bipolar I** and **bipolar II;** they may have separate genetic origins. In **bipolar I,** both phases of the illness are apt to be very pronounced. In **bipolar II,** mania is often mild (it is termed hypomania), and the depression can be either mild or severe. Bipolar II is more difficult to diagnose and is often mistaken for generalized depression. It has fewer and shorter periods of remission than bipolar I, tends to run in families, and is somewhat less responsive to treatment. It may be the more common form of manic-depression.

The illness is sometimes linked to ***seasonal affective disorder,*** with depression occurring in late fall or winter, giving way to remission in the spring, and progressing to mania or hypomania in the summer.

About 1 case of manic-depression in 5 begins in late childhood or adolescence; adolescents are more likely than adults to have physical and psychotic symptoms such as hallucinations and delusions, and they are more apt to be misdiagnosed *(see* ***Diagnostic and Test Procedures,*** *below).* Usually, however, the illness strikes young adults between the ages of 25 and 35. The first episode in males is likely to be manic; the first episode in females, depressive—and frequently, a woman will experience several episodes of depression before a manic episode occurs. As patients grow older, recurrences of either bipolar I or bipolar II tend to come more frequently and last longer.

CAUSES

Manic-depression is thought to result from chemical imbalances in the brain, caused by a defective gene or genes. Among the neurotransmitters possibly involved are serotonin and norepinephrine, but the neurochemical interplay in manic-depression is complex and not yet completely understood. The likelihood that genes play a role is supported by the fact that usually there is some family history of mood swings, depressive illness, or suicide.

DIAGNOSTIC AND TEST PROCEDURES

Because of the stigma still attached to manic-depression (and to many other mental diseases), patients are frequently reluctant to acknowledge that anything is amiss, and physicians often fail to recognize the disorder. In addition, the symptoms may sometimes seem to be merely exaggerated versions of normal moods. In any event, research suggests that almost 75 percent of all cases go untreated or are treated inappropriately.

The American Psychiatric Association has established a long list of specific criteria for recognizing the disorder. Evaluation involves investigating the patient's history and also any family history of mood swings or suicide. Other disorders must be ruled out—particularly such childhood problems as school phobia and ***attention deficit disorder,*** as well as dementia, ***schizophrenia,*** and psychotic states induced solely by alcohol or drugs. Substance abuse is common in manic-depressives and can mask the symptoms, thus complicating diagnosis and treatment *(see* ***Drug Abuse****).* Recognizing and treating any substance abuse is a priority, since it is a strong predictor of suicide, especially in men.

Before treatment begins, the patient receives a careful physical exam, and blood and urine are tested to detect conditions that could put medical constraints on the choice of treatment. A thyroid analysis is particularly important both because hyperthyroidism *(see* ***Thyroid Problems****)* can look like mania and because lithium—the principal drug treatment for manic-depression—is known to lower thyroid function. During treatment, frequent blood tests are necessary to see that adequate drug levels have been reached and to detect adverse reactions at an early stage.

M

IMPORTANT!

- **Be on the lookout for suicidal tendencies, especially when someone is passing from one phase to another—a time of disorientation.**
- **As a parent or spouse, make sure you understand bipolar disorder and its specific manifestations in your family member.**
- **If you find yourself or a family member consistently taking psychostimulants such as amphetamines to boost spirits and energy, consider the possibility of manic-depressive illness. Untreated bipolar disorder is very serious, and early detection can minimize its lifetime effects.**

TREATMENT

At present, manic-depression is treated most often with a combination of the drug lithium and psychotherapy. While drug therapy is primary, ongoing psychotherapy is important to help patients understand and accept the personal and social disruptions of past episodes and better cope with future ones. In addition, since denial is often a problem, routine psychotherapy helps patients stay on their medications. (Patient compliance is particularly tricky in adolescence.) Almost all forms of psychotherapy can be used—cognitive, behavioral, or psychodynamic; individual, family, or group.

The family or spouse of a patient should be involved with any treatment. Having full information about the disease and its manifestations is important for both the patient and loved ones.

CONVENTIONAL MEDICINE

Lithium carbonate is the principal drug used in treating manic-depression; it can be remarkably effective in reducing mania, although doctors still do not know why. Lithium may also prevent recurrence of depression, but it is often given in conjunction with varying combinations of ***antidepressants.*** The newly developed ***selective serotonin reuptake inhibitors (SSRIs)***—specific to the neurotransmitter serotonin—are usually the antidepressants of choice because they have fewer side effects than older drugs. Among the SSRIs are ***fluoxetine, sertraline,*** and ***paroxetine.*** Other antidepressants include the ***tricyclics***—such as desipramine, imipramine, and ***amitriptyline***—and ***bupropion,*** a class of drug different from but similar to the SSRIs.

Haloperidol is sometimes given to patients who fail to respond to lithium, or to treat acute symptoms of mania before lithium can take effect (7 to 10 days). In severe cases, or when a patient does not respond to lithium, other drugs such as ***carbamazepine*** and ***valproic acid,*** used alone or in combination with lithium, may be prescribed.

Many of these drugs can be toxic and should be closely monitored through blood tests to see that adequate levels have been reached and to detect any adverse reactions early on. When beginning treatment, the psychiatrist will need to experiment with medications. It is almost impossible to predict which patient will react to what drug or what the dosage should be.

Electroconvulsive therapy (ECT) is sometimes used for severely manic or depressed patients and for those who don't respond to medication. Because it acts quickly, it can also help patients who are considered to be at high risk for committing suicide. ECT fell out of favor in the 1960s, but the procedure has been greatly refined since then. The patient is first anesthetized. Then an electric current is passed through the temporal lobe to produce a grand mal seizure of short duration—no more than a few seconds. During the course of ECT treatments—usually two to three weeks—lithium is discontinued to prevent neurotoxic complications.

Light therapy has proved effective when bipolar disorder has a connection to winter depression. For those people who usually become depressed in winter, sitting for 20 to 30 minutes a day in front of a special light box with a full-spectrum light of about 10,000 lux can effectively treat their depression *(see* ***Seasonal Affective Disorder****).*

ALTERNATIVE CHOICES

With severe manic-depression **(bipolar I),** alternative medicines and practices may not be very useful during the episodes themselves. The depressed patient is often too low to initiate any exercise or energizing techniques; the manic, too hyperactive to undertake relaxation practices. However, alternative approaches may be beneficial between episodes and for less severe manic-depression **(bipolar II).**

One research study has suggested that ***magnesium*** may be a possible replacement for lithium in cases that involve frequent shifts from one manic-depressive phase to the other. It has the advantage of being nontoxic and is available in health food stores. Further studies are needed, but researchers believe that the outlook for the use of magnesium is favorable. Talk to your doctor or psychiatrist about this option.

M

ACUPRESSURE FOR MANIC PHASE

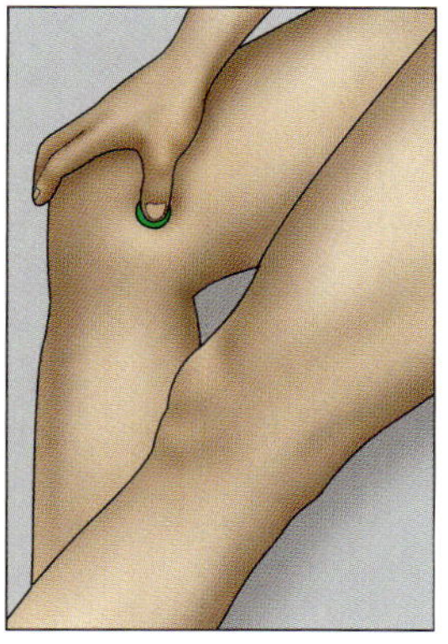

Pressing Liver 8 may help relieve the effects of manic-depression. Bending your right knee, place your thumb above the inside knee crease, just below the joint of the knee (swing your leg a few times to find it). Press for one minute, two or three times, then repeat on your left leg.

YOGA FOR DEPRESSIVE PHASE

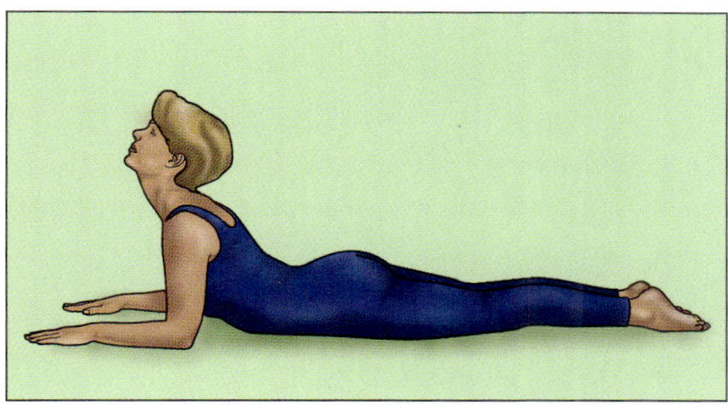

For the **Sphinx,** place both forearms on the floor, palms down and elbows directly under your shoulders. Inhale and push your chest away from the floor as far as comfortably possible. Hold for a few deep breaths, then relax and exhale.

Chinese herbs may soften mood swings, bringing some relaxation to the manic phase and reducing depression in the depressive phase. But be sure to seek a practitioner of Chinese medicine who is experienced in treating depression and knows how to use herbs. (Not all people who practice Chinese medicine are skilled in treating mood states or in using herbs to do so.)

A diet low in ***vanadium*** (a mineral found in meats and other foods) and high in ***vitamin C*** can be similarly helpful, but the diet should be monitored by a nutritional expert or an orthomolecular physician. Fish oil supplements may also be helpful; take 2,000 to 3,000 mg twice a day with food. A skilled **homeopath** may also ameliorate the intensity of mood swings.

Certain **acupuncture** treatments are designed to either energize or relax the body, depending on the acupuncture points used. Oil **massage** can also be relaxing or energizing.

MIND/BODY MEDICINE

Practitioners report that EEG **biofeedback** is effective in training manic-depressives to control some of the brain-wave states underlying hyperactivity, racing thoughts, irritability, lack of sleep, and poor self-control; it also seems to work for brain-wave activity associated with low energy, low self-esteem, and poor motor coordination. If the manic-depression is mild, this form of biofeedback may substitute for lithium and other drugs, although it can be used safely together with lithium. Because EEG biofeedback is new, only a thousand or so practitioners in the U.S. are trained in the technique. See Health Associations and Organizations in the ***Appendix*** for more information.

Yoga, meditation, t'ai chi, gigong, and other relaxation techniques can soften both the manic and depressive phases and help the patient maintain mental balance.

AT-HOME REMEDIES

Maintain a calm environment, particularly when someone is in a manic phase. Keep to regular routines for daily activities—sleeping, eating, and exercise. Adequate sleep is very important in preventing the onset of episodes. Avoid excessive stimulation: Parties, animated conversation, and long periods of watching television or videos can exacerbate manic symptoms.

In the manic phase, patients may engage in risky activities, such as fast driving or certain sports; they should be monitored and prevented from taking chances, especially in a car. Drinks and foods containing caffeine—tea, coffee, cola, and chocolate—should be eliminated in the manic phase. Avoid alcohol at all times. ■

MEASLES

SYMPTOMS

If your child has measles, he will be very sick. Look for the following symptoms:

- Days 1-3: mild to high fever, harsh cough, runny nose, red eyes, and sneezing; tiny white spots on gums near upper molars or inside cheeks.
- Days 4-8: high fever; characteristic rash, spreading from face to trunk, then to arms and legs. Skin starts to peel in 2 to 3 days. Rash fades from the face by the time it reaches the arms and legs.

Your child may also develop inflammation of the eyes ***(conjunctivitis),*** which will make the eyes sensitive to light. *(See also the **Visual Diagnostic Guide.**)*

CALL YOUR DOCTOR IF:

- you think your child has measles; your doctor may have received notice of an epidemic and may be able to confirm your diagnosis over the phone.
- your child has measles and his cough becomes harsher or more productive, which could indicate viral ***pneumonia.***
- your child has measles and is having trouble staying fully awake; is extremely lethargic; or is suffering from irritability, disorientation, or convulsions within a week of the onset of the rash. This could indicate encephalitis.
- your child has measles and develops difficulty hearing or pain in the ears, which may indicate an ear infection *(see **Otitis Media**).*

Measles is one of the most contagious childhood viral infections and one of the most severe, with complications ranging from ear infections to pneumonia and encephalitis (an inflammation of the brain that occurs in 1 out of 1,000 patients). Measles can easily become an epidemic in schools. Preventive immunization is usually recommended, if not required by state law *(see page 33).*

Adults can contract measles if they have not been previously exposed or immunized. People who have once had measles develop a natural immunity and cannot contract it again.

CAUSES

Measles is a virus that is transmitted by direct contact or by droplets from a sneeze or cough. The incubation period—when the virus multiplies in the body and the child is not contagious—is 8 to 12 days. Your child is most contagious 2 days before symptoms appear, although he is still contagious for 4 days after the rash begins.

TREATMENT

If you suspect that your child has measles, you should always consult your child's pediatrician, who will want to notify the schools and will also want to monitor your child's progress so as to be ready to intercede if complications arise. Infected children should not return to school until a week after the rash appears.

CAUTION!

Never give your child *aspirin*—even baby aspirin—or other products containing the salt called salicylate to reduce a fever or to relieve pain. Aspirin has been linked to Reye's syndrome, a rare but very dangerous illness that causes inflammation of the liver and brain.

IDENTIFYING THE RASH

In the first 24 hours, small, pale red spots appear along the hairline and behind the ears, then spread across the face and down the torso *(right);* they later spread onto the arms and legs. The spots typically expand into irregular patches.

By the third day, the rash becomes more profuse and pronounced. As it wanes, it may become scaly and take on a brownish tinge. The rash usually disappears within a week.

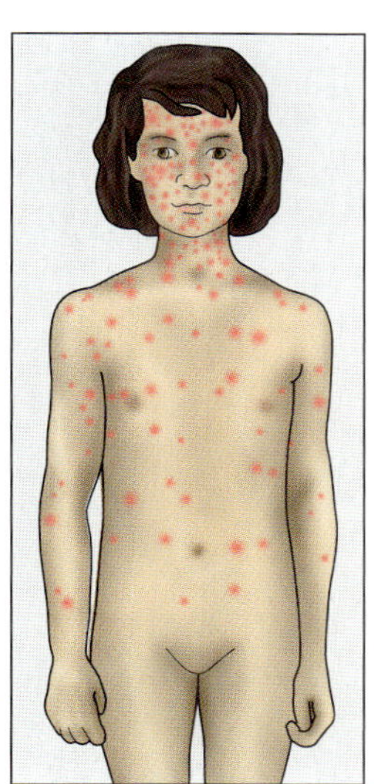

CONVENTIONAL MEDICINE

Your child's pediatrician will prescribe bed rest, a soft-foods diet, and increased liquid intake. The doctor may also give a gamma globulin injection to family members not previously exposed or immunized. While this won't prevent measles from spreading, it may make the course of the illness less severe for at-risk individuals.

ALTERNATIVE CHOICES

Do not rely on home treatment alone; consult the child's primary healthcare practitioner.

HERBAL THERAPIES

No herbs treat measles specifically. However, a number of preparations may help alleviate the symptoms. Teas of ***yarrow*** *(Achillea millefolium),* ***catnip*** *(Nepeta cataria),* and linden (*Tilia* spp.) may help reduce fever. An ***eyebright*** *(Euphrasia officinalis)* eyewash or a ***chamomile*** *(Matricaria recutita)* compress may ease sensitive eyes. You can seek help from a medical herbalist.

HOMEOPATHY

Always consult a homeopath for appropriate dosages for children. In homeopathic medicine, ***Aconite*** is thought to help a child who suffers a sudden onset of fever; has red eyes; is restless, anxious, or fearful, and sensitive to light. ***Belladonna*** is suggested when the child has flushed red hot skin, a hot head and face but cold extremities, and high fever. ***Pulsatilla*** may help if your child has a mild fever, is weepy, is not thirsty, and has a creamy yellow discharge from the eyes or nose.

OSTEOPATHY

Gentle, rhythmic pressure applied over the spleen, a procedure known as spleen pumping, may enhance the release of white blood cells into the blood. Seek help from an osteopath.

AT-HOME CARE

- Children need to be isolated for most of the time they are contagious. A dimmed room may help if their eyes are sensitive to light; in such a case, limit TV viewing and reading.
- Calamine lotion, distilled witch hazel, or cornstarch or baking soda baths alleviate itching. ***Acetaminophen*** may reduce fever.
- A humidifier can ease a bad cough. Be sure to use one with a humidistat for the proper amount of mist in the air. Always clean the humidifier thoroughly before and after use.

PREVENTION

Many alternative practitioners feel it is better for an otherwise healthy child to contract measles than to be vaccinated, because fighting the illness strengthens the immune system. However, immunization is usually required by state law, as measles can cause epidemics in schools. The MMR (measles, mumps, and rubella vaccine) is now given at 12 or 15 months, with a booster at the age of 4 to 6 or 10 to 12. The homeopathic version of immunization is not an accepted equivalent and will not provide adequate protection, but some homeopaths will prescribe remedies to ease the potential side effects of the MMR. ■

M

MÉNIÈRE'S DISEASE

SYMPTOMS

- intermittent dizziness (vertigo), sometimes accompanied by nausea and vomiting, pallor, and exhaustion.
- hearing problems, including increasing hearing loss, ***tinnitus*** (a ringing, roaring, or buzzing sound in the ears), a sensitivity to loud noises, and the sensation of not hearing the same sounds in both ears.
- a feeling of fullness in the ears, sometimes beginning before the attack of dizziness.
- headache.

CALL YOUR DOCTOR IF:

- you suspect you have Ménière's disease, which requires a medical evaluation.
- you have recurrent episodes of dizziness; difficulty in maintaining balance may point to problems in your inner ear that need medical attention.
- you find it more and more difficult to hear; a gradual loss of hearing over time may indicate a problem in any part of your ear (inner, middle, or outer) or in your brain.
- sounds are different to each ear; this may be a sign of other types of inner ear disorder in addition to Ménière's.

M

Approximately 2.4 million Americans have Ménière's disease, a disorder of the inner ear that can worsen over time, often leading to poor job performance, accidents, and psychological distress. First described over a century ago by French physician Prosper Ménière, this disease is characterized by numerous symptoms, all relating to problems in the inner ear, home of the body's sensory organs for hearing and balance.

More than 96 percent of Ménière's disease patients suffer bouts of vertigo, or dizziness. These dizzy spells can last anywhere from less than an hour to two days, striking as infrequently as once a year or as often as several times a year. Following an attack, the patient often feels completely exhausted and falls asleep, waking up later feeling fine.

People with Ménière's disease can also have a variety of hearing complaints with or without vertigo. A person might, for example, experience a gradual loss of hearing, a roaring, buzzing, or ringing in the ears ***(tinnitus),*** or the sensation that tones sound different in one ear than in the other, a phenomenon known as diplacusis.

Ménière's disease usually occurs in people between the ages of 20 and 60, striking on average at the age of 40. However, the disorder has also affected children as young as 4 and seniors as old as 90. The trouble usually starts in one ear and, in many patients, progresses to the other ear. Sometimes, though, the disease simply goes away on its own for reasons that are unclear. Unfortunately, no one knows which patients will get better and which will not.

CAUSES

Attacks of Ménière's disease can be triggered by anxiety, tension, or excessive salt intake. And while scientists are still debating the exact cause of the disorder, they do know that it involves an overabundance of endolymph, the fluid that fills the inner ear, or labyrinth *(above, right).*

The inner ear is actually a pair of sensory organs squeezed into the temporal bone, a tiny compartment in the side of the skull. One component of the inner ear, the spiral-shaped cochlea, converts sound waves into electrical impulses and sends them to the brain. Another part contains a series of rings called semicircular canals. Inside these rings is a fluid that responds to changes in your body's position (lying down, standing up, or leaning to one side, for example). Signals from the canals, together with information streaming in from the eyes and nerve endings in the skin, help the brain figure out if your body is upright or falling down. For some reason, in Ménière's disease the inner ear fills up with too much fluid, throwing off your sense of balance. Occasionally, the fluid can even seep into the cochlea and affect your hearing.

People with an abnormally shaped inner ear or temporal bone, whether by birth or as a result of an injury, are more likely to develop Ménière's disease. The shape and fluid levels of the inner ear can also be altered by certain diseases and conditions including middle ear infections ***(otitis media), syphilis, leukemia,*** otosclerosis (bone hardening in the middle ear), and ***immune problems.***

DIAGNOSTIC AND TEST PROCEDURES

Most of the time, an experienced otolaryngologist (ear, nose, and throat specialist) can tell if you have Ménière's disease simply by examining your medical history and performing some simple tests in the office. However, because dizziness and hearing problems can be caused by a wide variety of disorders—some inconsequential, some quite serious—arriving at a proper diagnosis can sometimes be tricky.

To rule out other problems, your doctor may conduct a thorough examination. Some of the diagnostic procedures your physician may order include audiometry, which tests hearing patterns in the ears; x-rays to determine the shape of your skull or any past injuries; and electrocochleography, in which a probe is inserted through the eardrum to test for electrical characteristics of your inner ear that may indicate the nature of your hearing problems.

INNER EAR DISRUPTION

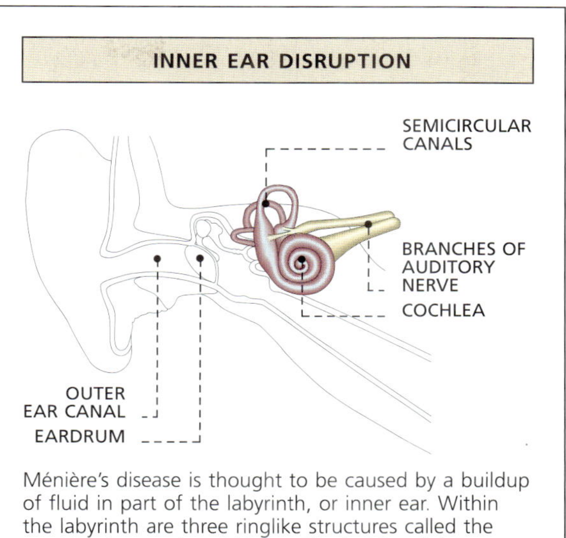

Ménière's disease is thought to be caused by a buildup of fluid in part of the labyrinth, or inner ear. Within the labyrinth are three ringlike structures called the semicircular canals, which are filled with a fluid essential to maintaining the body's sense of balance and motion. An overabundance of this fluid can throw off orientation and lead to vertigo.

TREATMENT

Because scientists haven't yet found a cure for Ménière's disease, most treatment is directed at alleviating the symptoms and dealing with the psychological impact of the disorder. Surgery is reserved as a last resort for patients with extremely serious cases.

CONVENTIONAL MEDICINE

Treatment for Ménière's disease often begins with medications that attempt to reduce the pressure and fluid in the inner ear. Typically prescribed drugs include ***diuretics*** (to increase fluid excretion) and sedatives (to calm the patient and reduce feelings of dizziness). Meclizine and ***diazepam*** are two drugs commonly prescribed to reduce dizziness; some physicians also use ***antihistamines,*** such as ***promethazine*** and dimenhydrinate, to reduce feelings of vertigo. Recently, physicians have also recommended skin patches of scopolamine, used to combat seasickness. Some patients may find these medications helpful, but scientific studies don't uniformly support their use. For one thing, many of these drugs can cause unwanted side effects, and none will cure the disorder.

Some physicians also prescribe "pressure chamber" treatments in an attempt to improve the pressure in the ear by changing the pressure outside it. If a patient is experiencing severe dizziness, a doctor might prescribe a type of drug called an aminoglycoside in an attempt to destroy the balance function of the labyrinth while preserving the patient's ability to hear. This type of drug is usually prescribed when a patient has the disease in both ears.

A number of surgical procedures with a similar aim—intentionally destroying the labyrinth of the inner ear to halt the debilitating dizziness—have also been developed. Surgical techniques include vestibular neurectomy, which involves cutting the nerves going to the balance side of the inner ear, and labyrinthectomy, or removal of the labyrinth. These drastic procedures, which seriously disrupt balance and completely destroy the hearing apparatus, are generally reserved for patients with severe vertigo.

In another operation, called endolymphatic-sac surgery, the physician tries to preserve both hearing and balance by draining the inner ear or installing little valves, or shunts, in the labyrinth to relieve pressure. Results are usually good after the first year, but some people report a return of their dizziness later.

ALTERNATIVE CHOICES

Like most conventional remedies for Ménière's disease, alternative treatments seek to relieve stress and other symptoms.

ACUPUNCTURE

For dizziness, consult an acupuncturist for stimulation at the following ear points: neurogate, sympathetic, kidney, occiput, adrenal, and heart. For chronic cases, an acupuncturist may treat body points on the kidney, triple warmer, and spleen meridians. See the ***Appendix*** for point locations and page 20 for more information about meridians.

AROMATHERAPY

To relieve stress, bathe with essential oils of ***lavender,*** geranium, and sandalwood. Or you might try a gentle massage with blended almond and ***chamomile*** oil.

BODY WORK

For chronic cases of Ménière's disease, consult an **osteopath** or **chiropractor** for adjustments to the head, jaw, neck, and lower back relating to movement restriction that might affect the inner ear. For acute cases of dizziness, a **reflexologist** might suggest massaging the ear area; this and other areas that may prove beneficial are illustrated below.

CHINESE HERBS

Although some practitioners of Chinese medicine distinguish types of dizziness, a general all-purpose remedy includes xanthium *(Xanthium sibiricum),* ***magnolia flower*** *(Magnolia liliflora),* ***licorice*** *(Glycyrrhiza uralensis),* ***honeysuckle flower*** *(Lonicera japonica),* and other herbs. Visit a prac-

REFLEXOLOGY

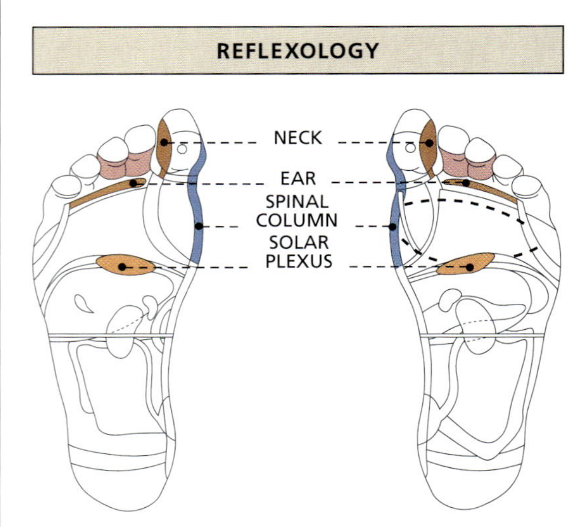

To help relieve symptoms, stimulate the ear area by walking your thumb along the base of the small toes and the shafts of the second and third toes. Walk your thumb up and down the upper portion of the spinal column area, and work the neck area on the big toe. Then stimulate the solar plexus area.

titioner of Chinese medicine for a proper prescription; bear in mind that you may be allergic to some Chinese herbs.

HOMEOPATHY

A patient with Ménière's disease has several homeopathic options. For dizziness during an acute attack that is worse from sensitivity to motion and that is accompanied by a headache and a roaring or buzzing in the ears, try ***Bryonia.*** For dizziness and nausea in an acute attack, use *Cocculus.* And for dizziness that is worse when lying down or turning over and that is accompanied by sensitivity to light, try *Conium.* If you don't feel better in a day or two, or if you have a chronic case of Ménière's disease, you should seek the advice of a professional homeopathic practitioner.

MIND/BODY MEDICINE

In Ménière's disease, patients undergo a vicious cycle of attacks followed by anxiety and stress, which in turn can provoke an attack. A number of communities across the country sponsor Ménière's disease support groups where people can discuss their problems with sympathetic listeners. Various forms of **massage** therapy and **yoga** are also great ways to reduce stress.

NUTRITION AND DIET

Some nutritionists recommend a diet for Ménière's disease that seeks to increase calories, fat, and protein, although there is no evidence that such a regimen can cure the disease. Specialists also recommend a daily intake of the following: 2,000 mg of ***vitamin C;*** 50 mg each of ***vitamins*** B_1, B_2, and B_6; 20 mg of ***zinc;*** and other vitamins and minerals. If you have Ménière's disease, you may want to stay away from salt—which causes your body to retain fluid—and to restrict your intake of liquids. Some experts speculate that lowering fluid levels in your body helps relieve the buildup of pressure in your inner ear, but this has not been proved. A nutritionist or dietitian can help prescribe a diet for any specific problems you may have.

AT-HOME REMEDIES

- During an attack of Ménière's disease, lie still and try to relax.
- Try reducing your intake of liquids and salt; some people believe that lowering fluid levels in the body can help reduce the pressure of fluid buildup in the inner ear.
- Avoid caffeine, smoking, and alcohol, which may increase stress and interfere with a proper resting state.
- Try to get a good night's sleep.
- Avoid driving, swimming, climbing on ladders, and other activities in which an attack of dizziness might lead to a serious injury.

PREVENTION

The best way to prevent an attack of Ménière's disease is to reduce the stress in your life. Seek out enjoyment, perhaps through a hobby or a sport. Give yourself time off to pursue the things that give you pleasure: Listen to music, take a soothing bath, read a magazine, drink a relaxing tea—***chamomile*** *(Matricaria recutita)* is a good choice—or simply take some time to sit and do nothing. If stress and anxiety continue to be problems, you may want to seek the advice of a counselor or a psychotherapist. ■

MENINGITIS

SYMPTOMS

- fever.
- severe headache.
- stiff neck, shoulders, or back.
- severe shooting pain down the back of the neck and sometimes along the spine when bending the neck forward.
- inability to tolerate bright light (photophobia).
- a bumpy and splotchy dark red or purplish rash anywhere on the body.
- drowsiness and mental confusion.
- vomiting.
- seizures and coma.
- in infants, a bulge of the fontanel, the soft spot on the skull.
- in infants, an eerie high-pitched cry.

CALL YOUR DOCTOR IF:

- you develop the symptoms listed above—particularly a combination of severe headache, stiff neck, and painful aversion to light; **seek emergency medical care immediately.**
- your infant develops the symptoms listed above; **seek emergency medical care immediately.**

Meningitis is an infection of the delicate membranes, or meninges, that cover the spinal cord and brain. It is almost always a complication of another bacterial or viral infection that began elsewhere in the body, such as in the ears, sinuses, or upper respiratory tract. The bacterial form is an extremely serious illness, which requires immediate medical care. If not treated quickly, it can lead to death within hours or to permanent neurological damage. Viral meningitis tends to be less severe; most people recover from it fully, with no aftereffects.

Meningitis is relatively rare. In the United States, fewer than 3,000 cases occur each year, mostly in children under the age of two. The illness begins with simple flulike symptoms—fever, headache, and vomiting—followed by progressive drowsiness and often severe neck pain, particularly when the head is bent forward. Very young children often react to the pain by arching their backs uncontrollably. Some forms of meningitis produce a dark red or purplish rash anywhere on the body. In babies, the swelling of the meninges may also cause the fontanel—the soft spot on the top of the skull—to bulge.

Meningitis can be contagious among people living close together—in university dorms, for example. Outbreaks of meningitis, particularly the bacterial form, have been rare in the United States, although since 1991 such outbreaks have been increasing for reasons not yet understood.

CAUSES

Bacterial meningitis is caused by any one of several bacteria. Three types—*Hemophilus influenzae* type b, *Neisseria meningitidis* (meningococcus), and *Streptococcus pneumoniae* (pneumococcus)—account for about 80 percent of bacterial meningitis cases in the United States. These bacteria are often carried harmlessly in the nasal passages or elsewhere on the bodies of a small percentage of healthy people, and are spread from person to person through coughing and sneezing. Some research indicates that people are more vulnerable to bacterial meningitis after a bout of the ***flu*** because inflamed nasal tissues offer bacteria an easy entranceway into the body.

Viral meningitis can be triggered by a variety of viruses, including several that cause ***diarrhea*** and one that can be transmitted to humans from infected hamsters and other rodents. Meningitis can also be caused by a fungus; the most common one is cryptococcus, which is found in pigeon droppings. Fungus-related meningitis is rare in healthy people, but not uncommon in people with HIV, the human immunodeficiency virus that causes ***AIDS.***

DIAGNOSTIC AND TEST PROCEDURES

Confirmation of meningitis requires a lumbar puncture, or spinal tap. This moderately painful procedure is done in a hospital under a local anesthetic. A needle is slipped between two of the bones of the spine to extract a small sample of spinal fluid. If the normally clear fluid appears cloudy and contains pus cells, meningitis is suspected. Further examination will determine which specific organism is involved.

Samples of your blood, urine, and secretions from your nose or ears may also be taken. Because the disease can progress so rapidly, treatment will begin immediately—even before the results of the tests are known.

TREATMENT

The bacterial form of meningitis in particular is life-threatening. It must be treated swiftly by conventional means. Seek emergency medical care at the first sign of symptoms.

CONVENTIONAL MEDICINE

If you have meningitis, you will be admitted to the hospital and remain there until the infection has been eradicated—possibly as long as two weeks. If you have a bacterial form of the disease, you will be given very high doses of ***antibiotics,*** perhaps intravenously. A class of antibiotics called ***cephalosporins*** is widely used to treat bacterial meningitis. Because antibiotics are not effective against viral meningitis, treatment usually involves intravenous fluids and rest.

Meningitis is contagious, so you will probably be put in an isolated room for at least 48 hours. If the meningitis has caused your eyes to be oversensitive to light, your room will be darkened. You will receive plenty of liquids and perhaps ***aspirin*** to relieve fever and headache.

Doctors may need to drain an infected sinus or mastoid (an area of the bone behind the ear) to prevent reinfection.

If you have meningococcal meningitis, your doctor may recommend that people with whom you have been in close contact undergo preventive antibiotic treatment. A vaccine for some types of meningococcal meningitis is sometimes prescribed to larger groups of people when a small epidemic of the disease has broken out, as well as to individuals traveling overseas to a meningitis risk area, such as sub-Saharan Africa. Further, vaccination against the *Hemophilus influenzae* type b bacterium is now a routine part of childhood immunizations.

ALTERNATIVE CHOICES

Because meningitis is a quickly progressing life-threatening illness, you should use alternative treatments only after you have received emergency medical care. Alternative treatments are designed to help your body recover and to build up your resistance to a recurrence. Consult a **homeopath,** for a constitutional remedy, or a practitioner of Chinese medicine, who might advise **acupuncture, acupressure,** or a combination of **Chinese herbs** to strengthen your immune system. A **chiropractor** or **osteopath** may also prescribe treatments to help you regain strength.

NUTRITION AND DIET

To maintain a healthy immune system and prevent recurrences of infections that can lead to meningitis, eat a low-fat, high-fiber, nutrient-dense diet; avoid sugar and processed foods. Vitamin supplements can also be helpful. Take ***vitamin A*** (2,500 to 10,000 IU once a day), ***vitamin B complex,*** and ***vitamin C*** (500 to 2,000 mg once a day). ■

M

MENOPAUSAL PROBLEMS

SYMPTOMS

Not all women experience symptoms with the onset of menopause. If symptoms occur, they may include:

- hot flashes—sudden reddening or heating of the face, neck, and upper back, which may produce sweating. Flashes typically last only a few minutes.
- night sweats, which may disrupt sleep and lead to ***insomnia.***
- pain during intercourse, caused by thinning of vaginal tissues and loss of lubrication.
- increased nervousness, anxiety, or irritability.
- the need to urinate more often than before, especially during the night.

CALL YOUR DOCTOR IF:

- you experience bleeding after menopause; among other possibilities, it may be a sign of ***uterine cancer,*** so you should be checked by your doctor.

Menopause simply means the end of menstruation, but the term is also used to refer to the months and years in a woman's life before and after her final period—a time that may or may not bring with it some physical or emotional changes.

Most women menstruate for the last time at about 50 years of age; a few do so as early as 40, and a very small percentage as late as 60. Most women notice some menstrual changes—such as irregular periods and light menstrual flow—up to a few years before menstruation ceases.

Some symptoms—including hot flashes and mood swings—are temporary and will pass as your body adjusts. But more-permanent problems can also result. Decreased levels of estrogen, for example, affect the way bones absorb calcium and can raise cholesterol levels in the blood; postmenopausal women thus face increased risk for developing both ***osteoporosis*** and cardiovascular diseases such as ***atherosclerosis.***

CAUSES

Typically during a woman's forties, her ovaries slow and then cease their normal functions, including the production of eggs. Even more significant, they decrease their production of estrogen and progesterone. As levels of these hormones—especially estrogen—decline, they cause changes throughout the body and particularly in the reproductive system, the most notable change being the end of menstruation. Decreased estrogen levels may also be responsible for the various symptoms associated with menopause.

TREATMENT

In both conventional and alternative medicine, the most common approach to treating menopausal problems is to resupply the body with the estrogen it no longer produces in sufficient quantities. Known in conventional medicine as **hormone replacement therapy,** this technique is somewhat controversial because of certain side effects, so you should carefully consider the risks and the benefits in consultation with your doctor.

CONVENTIONAL MEDICINE

Hormone replacement therapy (HRT) consists of ***estrogen and progestin*** supplements—usually given orally or through a skin patch. Most HRT patients take a combination of estrogen and progestin because estrogen alone has potentially serious side effects, such as endometrial cancer and ***uterine cancer.*** Progestin can cause side effects such as irregular bleeding, headaches, bloatedness, and breast swelling and pain. You may even develop an artificial monthly period, depending on the dosage regimen you're on. If you have had a hysterectomy and have no uterus, you do not need progestin.

MENOPAUSAL MYTHS AND FACTS

MYTH: *Menopause makes women emotionally unstable.*
FACT: *Most women experience no emotional problems; those that occur can be treated.*

MYTH: *Menopause puts an end to sexual desire.*
FACT: *Vaginal dryness can make intercourse painful, reducing desire, but this is readily treated with vaginal lubricants or estrogen creams. Menopause itself can affect libido either positively or negatively; some women actually have increased libido with menopause.*

MYTH: *Menopause disrupts a woman's life.*
FACT: *Most women experience few or no menopausal problems; 25 percent have moderate, treatable symptoms. In countries where age is respected, women report the fewest symptoms during menopause.*

Your doctor may recommend HRT to help prevent cardiovascular disease and ***osteoporosis,*** particularly if these diseases run in your family.

Your doctor may prescribe a vaginal estrogen cream to help stop the thinning of vaginal tissues and improve lubrication.

If you have had ***breast cancer,*** endometrial cancer, liver disease, or ***blood clots,*** you should not take estrogen; it increases your chance of recurrence. Progestin alone may relieve hot flashes.

ALTERNATIVE CHOICES

CHINESE HERBS

Some Chinese herbs—including ***dong quai*** *(Angelica sinensis)* and ***Asian ginseng*** *(Panax ginseng)*—contain a form of estrogen known as phytoestrogen, or plant estrogen. Exact proportions are important, and some dosages are toxic; consult an herbalist.

HERBAL THERAPIES

Phytoestrogen is found in a variety of herbs and foods. Extracts and teas made from ***black cohosh*** *(Cimicifuga racemosa)* may supply beneficial amounts of phytoestrogen. Estrogenic herbal creams may help relieve vaginal dryness and dry skin. Combinations of motherwort *(Leonurus cardiaca),* ***chaste tree*** *(Vitex agnus-castus),* ***hawthorne*** *(Craetegus oxyacantha),* and other herbs may help with the rapid heartbeat that comes with hot flashes.

NUTRITION AND DIET

Eating foods high in plant estrogens, such as soy beans and lima beans, may alleviate symptoms; other sources include nuts and seeds, ***fennel,*** celery, ***parsley,*** and flaxseed oil.

AT-HOME REMEDIES

- Raise your ***calcium*** intake and engage in weight-bearing exercises to avoid osteoporosis and maintain general good health.
- Take 400 to 800 IU of ***vitamin E*** daily to treat hot flashes and reduce the risk of cardiovascular disease. ■

M

MENSTRUAL PROBLEMS

SYMPTOMS

- Menstruation does not occur. Called **amenorrhea,** this can come from pregnancy, overexercise, or ***anorexia nervosa.***
- Menstruation is painful and produces clots. Called **dysmenorrhea,** this may be entirely normal, but it may also be caused by ***endometriosis;*** polyps, fibroids, or other lesions of the uterus; or an intrauterine device (IUD).
- Menstrual flow is heavy. Called **menorrhagia,** this condition can be a result of ***stress, endometriosis*** or other pelvic lesions, pelvic infection, or an IUD.

CALL YOUR DOCTOR IF:

- you have heavy menstrual flow that fills a tampon or sanitary napkin within an hour; heavy flow can cause ***anemia.***
- you have missed a period and think you may be pregnant; a late flow that is unusually heavy could indicate a miscarriage.
- you experience sharp abdominal pain before periods or during intercourse; you could have ***endometriosis.***
- you get your period after menopause.

M

Menstruation is a normal part of a woman's reproductive cycle. When an ovary releases an egg, it also releases the hormone estrogen, which stimulates the lining of the uterus to grow and engorge with blood. If the egg is not fertilized, the ovary releases progesterone, which makes the uterus shed its lining; the resulting menstrual flow typically consists of a few tablespoonfuls of blood and tissue fragments. This series of events repeats on a cycle of approximately 28 days until interrupted by pregnancy or ended by ***menopause.***

The degree of discomfort or pain a period causes, as well as the amount of menstrual flow, varies widely among individuals. Also, your own period may occasionally be heavier or more painful than usual. Such problems, while unpleasant, generally do not signal underlying disease. But you should be aware that the same complaints can sometimes indicate more serious conditions, such as ***endometriosis*** or an ovarian cyst.

The three main categories of menstrual irregularities are **lack of period** (amenorrhea), **painful periods** (dysmenorrhea), and **heavy periods** (menorrhagia). The following text explains these problems and what you can do about them.

LACK OF PERIOD

Although often no cause for concern, amenorrhea can be a sign of an underlying problem. It might indicate, for example, that you have low levels of estrogen in your system and are therefore at a greater risk of developing ***osteoporosis.*** Or it may signal a lack of progesterone and that you are at a greater risk for endometrial problems, including endometrial cancer *(see **Uterine Problems**).* Also, of course, if you do not menstruate, you cannot become pregnant.

CAUSES

The lack of a period in a woman who has not yet begun to menstruate is known as primary amenorrhea; in a woman who has temporarily stopped menstruating, it is known as secondary amenorrhea. Primary amenorrhea has several causes, the most likely of which is that a girl has simply not yet reached puberty. (It is perfectly normal for puberty to occur as late as the age of 17.) But delayed puberty in a girl who is very thin or who exercises excessively is worrisome, because it could indicate ***anorexia nervosa;*** women with very low body fat do not menstruate.

Primary amenorrhea can also point to other problems. In rare cases, for example, a girl might actually lack ovaries or a uterus and therefore not be able to menstruate. Or a tumor, an injury or trauma, or a structural defect might be interfering with some aspect of the menstrual cycle, from the production of hormones to the actions of the organs and tissues that the hormones affect.

Secondary amenorrhea can also be traced to injuries or structural abnormalities; one common cause is ovarian cysts. But factors such as stress can also disrupt the balance of hormones and thereby interrupt the normal cycle. Also, as in adolescence, extreme underweight can stop menstruation; if your period stops while you are dieting or in athletic training, you may be overdoing it. And, of course, amenorrhea could signal the onset of ***menopause*** or pregnancy.

MENSTRUAL MYTHS AND FACTS

MYTH: *A bath causes or worsens menstrual cramps.*
FACT: *Soaking in a warm bath can soothe and relax muscles, thereby reducing pain.*

MYTH: *Menstruating women should restrict their activities, and even stay in bed and rest.*
FACT: *Women can carry on normal activities during their period. Exercise may actually help lessen pain by stimulating muscles to release endorphins.*

TREATMENT

CONVENTIONAL MEDICINE

Treatment for primary amenorrhea may involve no more than waiting to see if nature takes its course. For a girl who exercises strenuously or who is very thin, a doctor might advise a lighter training regimen or an effort to gain weight. Treatment for ***anorexia nervosa*** might also be necessary. If the doctor suspects a hormonal irregularity, drug treatment to replace missing hormones might be prescribed. In rare circumstances, surgery to remove a cancerous or noncancerous growth—or to correct a structural problem—might be called for.

For secondary amenorrhea, if you think ***stress*** may be to blame, take steps to reduce stress in your life; this alone may restore your cycle. If you are underweight, your doctor will advise you to gain some weight and try to maintain it. If you have been diagnosed with some other condition that may be causing amenorrhea—such as ***endometriosis*** or an ovarian cyst—seek treatment for that problem, and ask your doctor whether your periods will return. If not, or if your amenorrhea is related to the onset of menopause, your doctor may prescribe ***estrogen*** or ask you to take ***calcium*** to lower your risk of ***osteoporosis.*** *(See also **Menopausal Problems** and **Ovary Problems.**)*

ALTERNATIVE CHOICES

HERBAL THERAPIES

To help initiate menstrual flow, make a tincture of one part ***chaste tree*** *(Vitex agnus-castus),* two parts blue cohosh *(Caulophyllum thalictroides),* and two parts ***mugwort leaf*** *(Artemisia argyi);* take 2 ml three times daily until menstrual flow begins.

NUTRITION AND DIET

To address nutrient deficiencies that may be causing amenorrhea, take supplements of or eat foods rich in ***zinc*** (fish, poultry, lean meats) and ***vitamin B complex*** (brewer's yeast, wheat germ).

M

YOGA

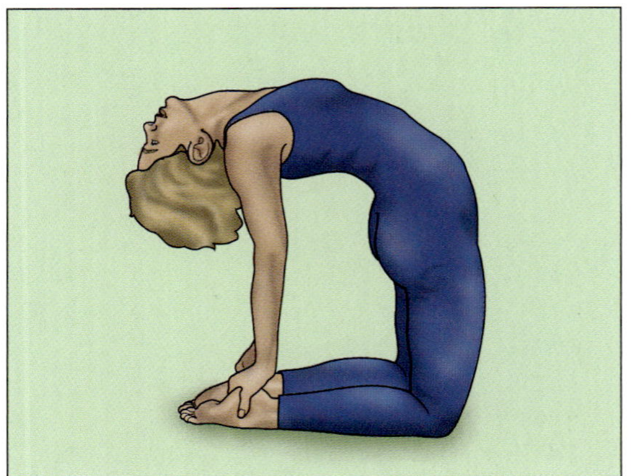

1 Regular use of the **Camel** may help amenorrhea. First, kneel down. Lean backward as you exhale, placing your palms on your heels and tilting your head back. Inhale as you squeeze your buttocks and press your pelvis forward *(above)*. Breathe slowly as you hold for 20 seconds.

To release, exhale as you sit back on your heels. Then inhale as you bring your body up, raising your head last. Breathe slowly and relax for 20 seconds. Do once or twice a day.

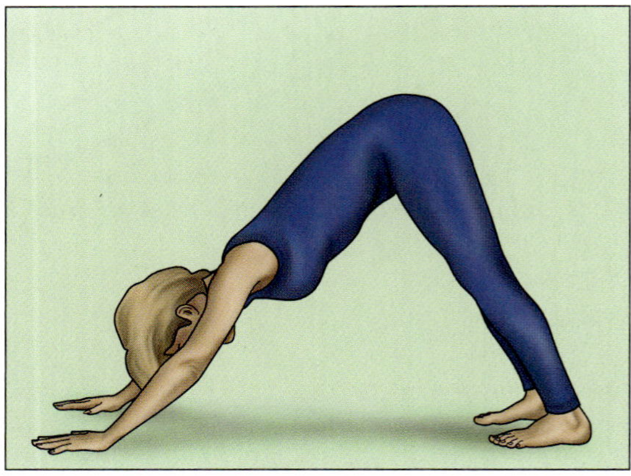

2 The **Downward Dog** pose helps release pelvic tension. From the Table position on your hands and knees, inhale and raise your pelvis to form an inverted V with your knees slightly bent.

Press your palms and heels toward the floor as you breathe deeply, keeping your arms and shoulders open and your back and legs straight *(above)*. Hold for 20 to 30 seconds.

To release, exhale as you resume the Table position. Sit back on your heels, bring your head up, and relax before attempting to stand up again.

PAINFUL PERIODS

Menstrual pain, or dysmenorrhea, is hardly unusual and in most cases is completely normal, even if troublesome. But there are situations in which painful periods may signal a condition that requires further evaluation by your doctor. And if your pain interferes with your normal activities, you should consider some of the treatments listed here, which may help bring you relief.

CAUSES

If you have always had painful periods, they are probably the result of hormonal changes during your menstrual cycle. The factor most likely to be causing pain is that your body is producing an excess of prostaglandins—hormonelike substances that cause contractions of the uterus during menstruation and when a woman goes into labor. During menstruation, these contractions ensure that all the menstrual blood and tissue are expelled from the body, but excess prostaglandins can cause repeated contractions—and perhaps even spasms—which are experienced as cramping. It is common for these pains to persist throughout your reproductive years, but many women find that menstrual cramps become milder after they have had a baby.

Dysmenorrhea may, however, also be caused by an underlying condition, such as ***endometriosis,*** an infection, or growths in the uterus *(see **Uterine Problems** and **Uterine Cancer**).*

TREATMENT

In addition to the suggestions listed below, see the appropriate entries for treatment advice related to an underlying condition.

CONVENTIONAL MEDICINE

Analgesics such as ***aspirin*** and ***acetaminophen*** can relieve mild discomfort, but if your pain is more intense, try an analgesic such as ***ibuprofen,***

mefenamic acid, or ***naproxen,*** all of which inhibit the release of prostaglandins. Your doctor may also prescribe birth-control pills or progesterone, which may affect your balance of hormones in ways that will help relieve pain.

ALTERNATIVE CHOICES

Most of the alternative therapies for menstrual cramps focus on promoting the relaxation of tense muscles or on reducing tension in general. In addition to the treatments listed below, a practitioner of Chinese medicine might advise **acupuncture** or **Chinese herbs** to relieve menstrual cramps.

ACUPRESSURE

An acupressure technique that may prove effective in relieving menstrual pains is illustrated on the following page.

AROMATHERAPY

Massage the lower abdomen, back, and legs with oil or lotion containing ***chamomile*** *(Matricaria recutita).*

CHIROPRACTIC

Chiropractic techniques can sometimes help relieve menstrual cramps; see a chiropractor for treatment.

HERBAL THERAPIES

To relieve cramps, drink a hot tea of 2 tsp cramp bark *(Viburnum opulus)* simmered for 15 minutes in 1 cup water; use this three times a day. ***Dong quai*** *(Angelica sinensis)* and ***feverfew*** *(Chrysanthemum parthenium)* can relax uterine muscles; feverfew may work by inhibiting prostaglandin synthesis. ***Valerian*** *(Valeriana officinalis)* helps relax cramping muscles. Consult an herbalist for appropriate dosages.

Evening primrose oil *(Oenothera biennis)* applied over painful areas can also bring relief, but don't use it if there's a chance you may get pregnant. In addition, a castor-oil pack placed over painful areas can be helpful.

Tension, anxiety, and painful spasms may be relieved with treatments of black haw *(Viburnum lentago),* ***skullcap*** *(Scutellaria baicalensis),* and ***black cohosh*** *(Cimicifuga racemosa).* Take equal parts of these herbs in 1-ml doses up to 4 times each day.

NUTRITION AND DIET

Eating a balanced diet consisting of small meals throughout the day rather than three larger meals and avoiding sugar, salt, and caffeine may help relieve or prevent cramping. You may get relief from a multivitamin, multimineral supplement containing ***vitamin B complex, calcium,*** and ***magnesium.*** You can also try taking 50 mg of ***vitamin*** $\boldsymbol{B_6}$ twice a day. Because your overall goal is to keep your body relaxed, avoid caffeine and other stimulants.

YOGA

Poses for relaxation and relief of cramps are illustrated opposite.

MENSTRUAL SYNCHRONY

Women who live or work together in close quarters may notice that they're all getting their periods at the same time. This is known as menstrual synchrony, and it often happens in closed communities such as convents, prisons, and dormitories. What causes this phenomenon is not clear, but it may be linked to pheromones—chemical messengers that are carried in the air from person to person (or from animal to animal) and that have powerful effects on body functions and behaviors, even though people are not consciously aware of them.

M

ACUPRESSURE

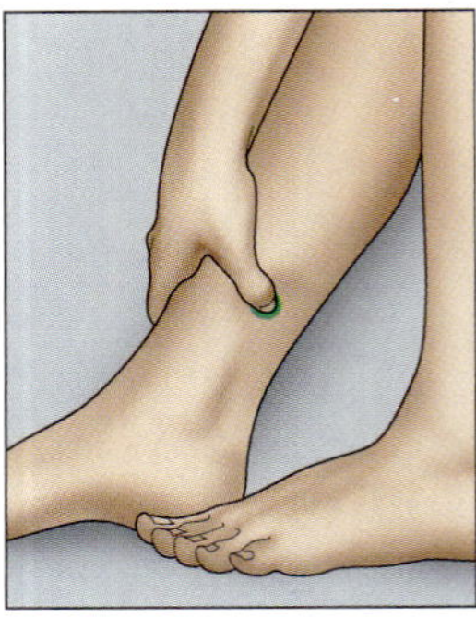

1 Water retention during menstruation may make you uncomfortable. Find SP 6 on the inside of your leg, four finger widths above the anklebone, near the inner edge of your shinbone. Hold for one minute. Repeat on the other leg. Do not use this point if you are pregnant.

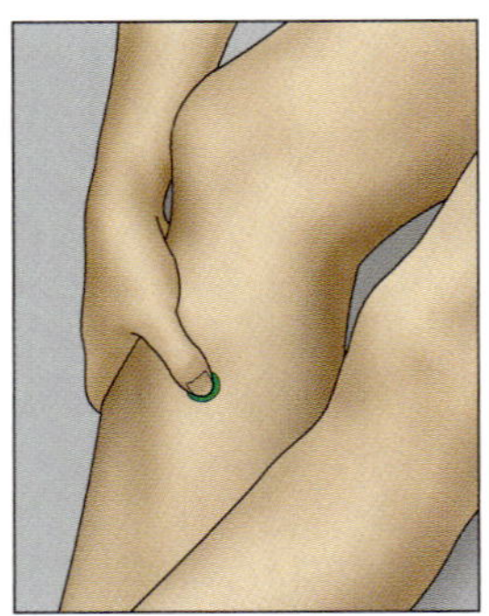

2 To help improve your overall circulation during menstruation, apply pressure to SP 8, four finger widths below the knee on the inside of your leg. Press firmly between your calf muscle and your leg bone, and hold for one minute. Repeat on the other leg.

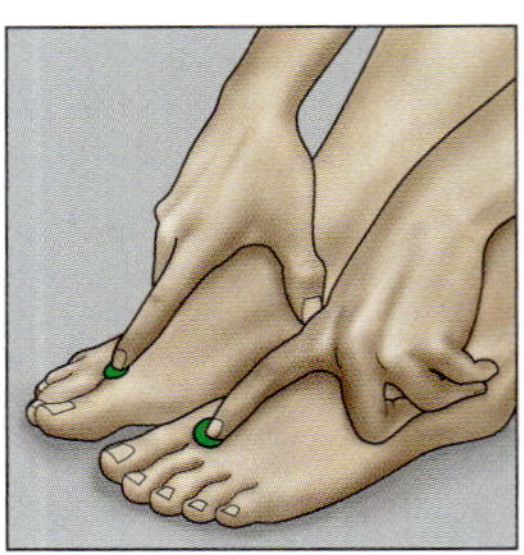

3 Working LV 3 may help relieve cramps and spasms. Place your index fingers in the spaces between the bones of your big toes and second toes as shown. Angle the pressure toward the bones of your second toes and rub firmly. Hold for one minute.

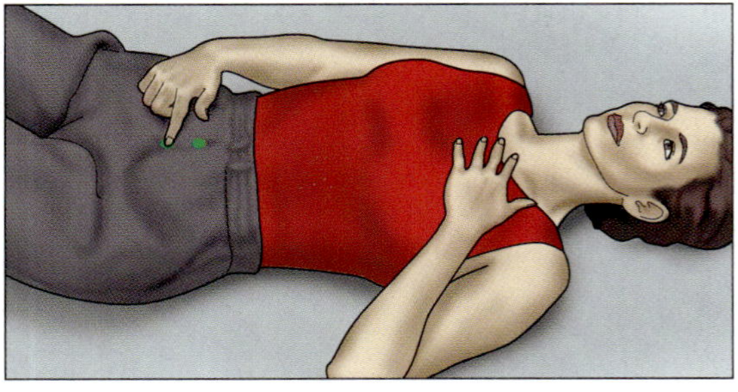

4 You may be able to correct irregular menstrual periods by working point CV 4. Measure four finger widths down from your navel. Press your index finger firmly into your abdomen and hold for one to two minutes. Do this twice a day every day.

HEAVY PERIODS

A heavy period (menorrhagia) is a menstrual flow that lasts longer than eight days, saturates tampons or napkins within an hour, or includes large clots of blood.

CAUSES

Heavy periods may be caused by a hormonal imbalance, ***endometriosis,*** a pelvic infection *(see **Pelvic Inflammatory Disease**),* use of an IUD, or uterine growths such as fibroids *(see **Uterine Problems**).* Excessive bleeding may signal other irregularities in your cycle: lack of ovulation, low levels of progesterone, or an excess of prostaglandins. Heavy periods can cause iron deficiency ***anemia.***

TREATMENT

CONVENTIONAL MEDICINE

Treatment for menorrhagia may include ***iron*** and ***folic acid*** supplements to treat and prevent ***anemia,*** antiprostaglandin analgesics such as ***ibuprofen*** and ***naproxen,*** and hormones to correct any imbalance in your hormone levels. Your doctor may suggest that you reduce your level of physical activity and see whether this has an effect.

Danazol, a male hormone, temporarily stops the menstrual cycle; its side effects include menopausal symptoms such as hot flashes, as well as acne, weight gain, and increased hairiness. Your doctor may prescribe other hormones, such as progesterone and birth-control pills, to balance your hormones.

The minor surgical procedure of dilation and curettage (often called a D and C) may bring relief from menorrhagia; in this operation, the doctor widens the cervical opening, then uses a spoonlike instrument or gentle suction to clean the inside of the uterus. In some cases, your doctor may suggest a hysterectomy—removal of the uterus and perhaps other reproductive organs. Seek a second opinion before deciding to undergo this surgery.

ALTERNATIVE CHOICES

ACUPRESSURE AND ACUPUNCTURE

Both these disciplines use techniques that rely on spleen points to help control blood flow. See a practitioner for points and techniques to relieve excessive menstrual flow.

AROMATHERAPY

Practitioners of aromatherapy find that oils of geranium, ***juniper*** *(Juniperus communis),* and cypress, rubbed on the abdomen, may bring relief for sufferers of heavy menstrual flow.

HERBAL THERAPIES

Tea made from ***yarrow*** *(Achillea millefolium)* may help control bleeding. You may also benefit from taking a tincture made of equal parts life root *(Senecio aureus),* shepherd's purse *(Capsella bursa-pastoris),* and wild cranesbill *(Geranium maculatum);* take 1- to 4- ml doses daily during menstual bleeding.

AT-HOME REMEDIES

- Take extra ***calcium*** and ***magnesium*** to stop uterine muscle cramps and to lessen the flow.
- Take a warm, relaxing bath.
- Take antiprostaglandin analgesics, such as ***ibuprofen*** and ***naproxen.***
- Drink herbal teas containing ***yarrow*** to help control bleeding.
- Apply a castor-oil pack to the abdomen to relax the muscles and lessen the flow.

REFLEXOLOGY

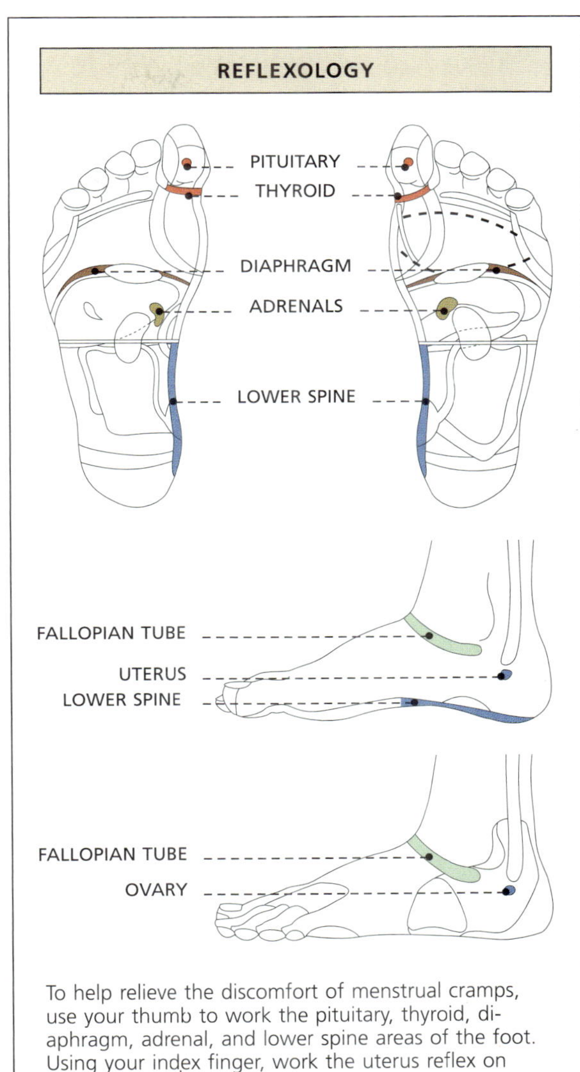

To help relieve the discomfort of menstrual cramps, use your thumb to work the pituitary, thyroid, diaphragm, adrenal, and lower spine areas of the foot. Using your index finger, work the uterus reflex on the inside of the ankle, then across the fallopian tube area to the ovary reflex on the outside of the ankle.

PREVENTION

Maintain normal weight for your build, which helps prevent excess fat and estrogens in the body. Overweight women tend to have abnormal menstrual periods, perhaps because of an increase in estrogen-secreting cells.

Take a multivitamin, multimineral supplement including ***vitamins A, B complex, C,*** and ***E,*** as well as ***calcium*** and ***iron.*** ■

M

MONONUCLEOSIS

SYMPTOMS

The early symptoms of mononucleosis resemble those of the ***flu,*** including:

- severe fatigue.
- headache.
- sore throat, sometimes very severe.
- chills, followed by a fever.
- muscle aches.

After a day or two, the following additional symptoms may occur:

- swollen lymph nodes, especially in the neck, armpits, or groin.
- ***jaundice*** (a yellow tinge to the skin and eyes).
- a ***measles***-like skin rash anywhere on the face or body; sometimes the rash develops suddenly after taking ***amoxicillin*** for a severe sore throat.
- bruiselike areas inside the mouth.
- soreness in the upper left abdomen (from an enlarged spleen).

M

CALL YOUR DOCTOR IF:

- you have these symptoms, particularly for longer than 10 days, or if you have a severe ***sore throat*** for more than a day or two; you need to be examined by a doctor to rule out other illnesses, such as ***strep throat*** or—less likely—***leukemia*** or infectious ***hepatitis.***
- you develop swollen lymph nodes all over your body, which may be a sign of ***tuberculosis, cancer,*** or human immunodeficiency virus *(see* ***AIDS****).*
- you develop abdominal pain, which may indicate a ruptured spleen. Seek emergency medical treatment immediately.

Mononucleosis, often referred to as "mono," is a very common viral illness. About 90 percent of people over age 35 have antibodies to mono in their blood, which means that they have been infected with it, probably during early childhood. When mono strikes young children, the illness is usually so mild that it passes as a common cold or the flu. When it occurs during adolescence or adulthood, however, the disease can be much more serious.

Mono comes on gradually. It begins with ***flu***-like symptoms—fever, headache, and a general malaise and lethargy. After a few days, the lymph glands—especially those in the neck, armpits, and groin—begin to swell, although this symptom is not noticeable in everyone. Most people develop a sore throat, which can be very severe, with inflamed tonsils. A fever—usually no higher than 104°F—can also develop and may last up to three weeks. About 10 percent of people with mono develop a generalized red rash all over the body or darkened areas in the mouth that resemble bruises. In about half of all cases, the spleen may also enlarge, causing an area in the upper left abdomen to become tender to the touch.

In 95 percent of cases, the illness affects the liver. However, only about 5 percent of individuals with mono develop ***jaundice,*** a yellowing of the skin and eyes caused by an increase of bile pigment in the blood. In rare cases of mono, the liver fails. Other major complications that can develop from mono include rupturing of the spleen, ***meningitis,*** and encephalitis, an inflammation of the brain; but these, too, are extremely rare.

Most people who come down with mono feel much better within two or three weeks, although fatigue may last for two months or longer. Sometimes the disease lingers for a year or so, causing recurrent, but successively milder, attacks. In the past, some research suggested that the virus causing mono might be linked to a persistent and debilitating form of the illness known as ***chronic fatigue syndrome,*** which can last for years. Most recent research has shown no such link, however, and the cause of chronic fatigue syndrome remains unknown.

CAUSES

Mono is caused by the Epstein-Barr virus, named after the two British researchers who first identified it in 1964, although the disease itself had been recognized many years earlier. A common member of the herpes family of viruses, Epstein-Barr is spread primarily through the exchange of saliva, which is why mono is sometimes known as the "kissing disease." However, coughing or other contact with infected saliva can also pass it from one person to another.

The mono virus can stay active in a person weeks or months after all overt symptoms are gone, so close contact with someone who shows no sign of the disease can still put a person at risk. On the other hand, not everyone who lives in proximity to an individual infected with mono comes down with the illness. Scientists believe that a healthy immune system may make it possible to fight off the infection successfully.

DIAGNOSTIC AND TEST PROCEDURES

The wide range of symptoms associated with mono can make diagnosis difficult. Your doctor will begin by giving you a complete physical exam. A throat culture may be taken to rule out ***strep throat.*** The doctor may take a blood sample to look for the presence of abnormal white blood cells. A monospot test, in which your blood is examined for special antibodies to mono, will probably be done also. The results of these tests are not always clear, however, and additional ones may be needed.

TREATMENT

Mononucleosis is usually a self-limiting illness. Most people recover on their own without any treatment within two weeks. Thus, the primary prescription for mono by both conventional and alternative practitioners is complete bed rest with a gradual return to normal activity.

CONVENTIONAL MEDICINE

In addition to bed rest, your doctor may prescribe ***aspirin*** or ***acetaminophen*** for the fever, sore throat, and other discomforts of the illness. If your sore throat is so severe that you have trouble breathing or eating, your doctor may give you ***prednisone,*** a steroid drug.

ALTERNATIVE CHOICES

Like their conventional counterparts, practitioners of alternative medicine recommend rest and various medications and treatments to help relieve the symptoms of mono. They also offer treatments to help strengthen your body's immune system and thus ensure a quick and complete recovery.

AROMATHERAPY

Lavender *(Lavandula officinalis),* ***peppermint*** *(Mentha piperita),* bergamot *(Citrus bergamia),* and ***eucalyptus*** *(Eucalyptus globulus)* are sometimes recommended to relieve fatigue and other symptoms of mono. Add a few drops of the essential oils of one or more of these herbs to a warm bath.

CHINESE HERBS

Teas made from ***ginseng***—either the ***Asian*** *(Panax ginseng)* or the ***American*** *(Panax quinquefolius)* form—are sometimes recommended to help relieve the tiredness associated with mono. Drink three times a day.

HERBAL THERAPIES

To help fight the infection, take 2- to 4- ml daily of the tincture of ***echinacea*** (*Echinacea* spp.), ***milk thistle*** *(Silybum maranum),* or ***astragalus*** *(Astragalus membranaceus).*

CAUTION!

To protect your spleen from rupturing, do not participate in any strenuous exercise until you have fully recovered.

M

To reduce the fever associated with mono, try drinking a tea made from elder *(Sambucus nigra)* flowers or ***yarrow*** *(Achillea millefolium).* Drink either tea three times a day. Or, if you prefer, take 2 to 4 ml of the tincture of either herb three times a day.

To help cleanse the lymphatic system, try teas made from cleavers (*Galium* spp.) or wild indigo *(Baptisia tinctoria).* Drink either tea three times a day. Alternatively, take 2 to 4 ml of tincture of cleavers or 1 ml of tincture of wild indigo three times daily.

To help with the anxiety and depression that sometimes accompany long-term bouts with mono, try ***St.-John's-wort*** *(Hypericum perforatum)* or vervain *(Verbena officinalis).* Both herbs, when taken internally, appear to act as mild sedatives. Vervain is also recommended for ***jaundice,*** one of the symptoms of mono. Make a tea out of either herb and drink three times daily. Or take in tincture form: 1 to 4 ml of St.-John's-wort or 2 to 4 ml of vervain three times a day.

HOMEOPATHY

Mononucleosis calls for a constitutional treatment—a set of remedies prescribed specifically for you, based on your symptoms and medical history. You will need to consult an experienced homeopath for such a treatment.

MIND/BODY MEDICINE

Stress can exacerbate the fatigue associated with mononucleosis. It can also weaken the immune system, thus making it more difficult for your body to recover from the illness. Various relaxation techniques, such as **meditation, biofeedback,** and **guided imagery,** can be helpful in reducing the stress.

NUTRITION AND DIET

To strengthen your immune system and help speed your recovery, eat plenty of whole (not processed) foods, especially fresh fruits and vegetables. Avoid foods that are high in saturated fats, animal proteins, and sugar, as they are difficult to digest and put stress on your body.

To maintain a better balance of blood sugar, and thus a more even energy level, eat four to six

ACUPRESSURE

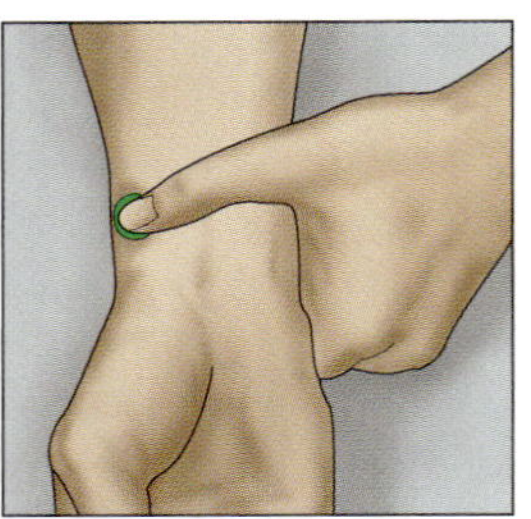

Pressing Lung 7 may bolster immunity and lung function. The point is located on the thumb side of the inner forearm, two finger widths above the crease in the wrist. Apply steady, firm pressure for one minute, then repeat on the other arm.

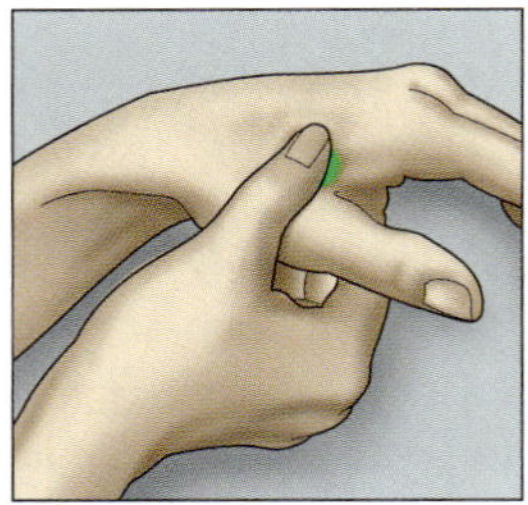

To help relieve muscle aches, use Large Intestine 4, located in the web between the thumb and index finger. Using the thumb and index finger of the right hand, press the web of the left hand for one minute; then repeat on the right hand. Do not use LI 4 if you are pregnant.

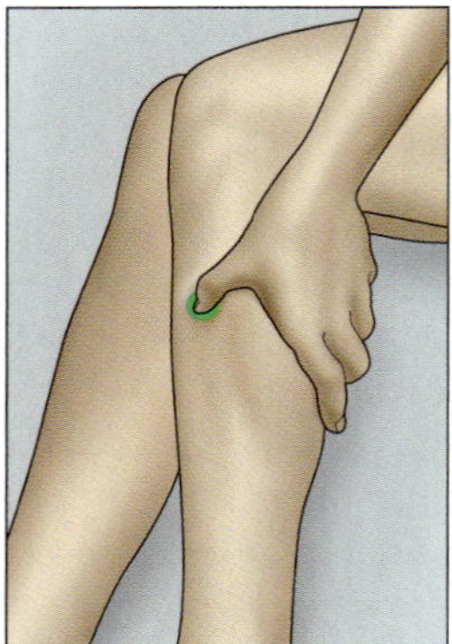

Pressing Stomach 36 may enhance immunity and increase overall vitality. The point can be found four finger widths below the kneecap, just outside the shinbone. You can verify the location by flexing your foot; a muscle should bulge at the point site. Press with your thumb for one minute.

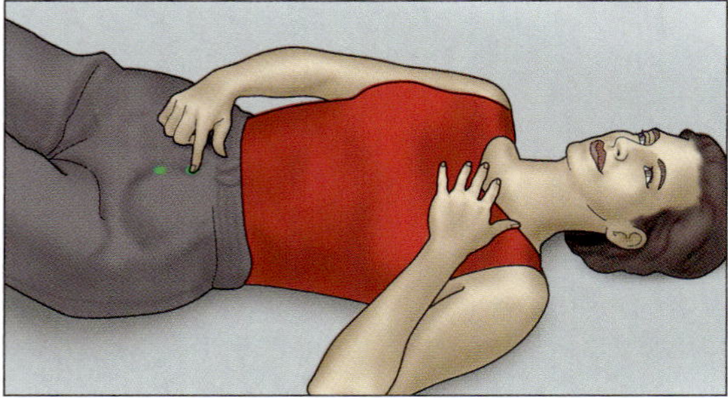

The body's energy reserve may be increased by pressing Conception Vessel 6. The point is three finger widths below the navel, midway to the pubic bone. Gradually apply deep pressure with your index finger until you feel resistance, then hold for one minute.

small meals throughout the day; try not to overeat at any one meal. Some people also find that eating a small portion of low-fat protein immediately on awakening in the morning and again in the evening before going to bed can help raise energy levels. Good choices of protein for this purpose include low-fat cheese as well as tofu, lentils, and other legumes.

Vitamin supplements may also enhance your immune system. Take ***vitamin A*** (2,500 to 10,000 IU daily), ***vitamin C*** (500 to 2,000 mg daily), and ***vitamin B complex*** (50 mg three times a day). You may also wish to try daily ***magnesium*** (200 to 700 mg) and ***potassium*** aspartate (50 to 200 mg) supplements. Research has shown that these supplements can dramatically improve energy levels after six weeks of constant use.

YOGA

Yoga can help reduce the fatigue associated with mononucleosis. The exercises are gentle enough to be done even by someone with the illness. One recommended pose is the **Bow** *(see the **Appendix** for more information on yoga positions).*

AT-HOME REMEDIES

- Rest your body. Do not plan to return to your normal activity level for at least a month.
- Drink plenty of liquids to prevent dehydration.
- Watch what you eat. Enrich your diet with whole foods, especially fresh fruits and vegetables. Avoid foods high in saturated fats, sugar, caffeine, and alcohol; these ingredients can diminish your energy reserves and weaken your immune system. To keep your blood sugar—and energy—level steady throughout the day, eat small but frequent meals.
- Take aspirin or an aspirin substitute to treat headache and sore throat.
- For sore throat, use a saline gargle—½ tsp salt in a glass of warm water.
- To help ease the fatigue associated with mononucleosis, massage your kidneys daily. With loose fists, rub your lower back for three to five minutes. A good occasion to do this is in the shower with warm water running down your back.

REDUCING STRESS, STRENGTHENING IMMUNITY

Early in the 20th century, scientists began studying how humans adapt to stress. They soon discovered that humans have a biochemical reaction to danger—the fight-or-flight response. When a person experiences feelings of fear or anger, the brain releases a stream of stress hormones. One of these is epinephrine (more commonly known as adrenaline). Its release causes the heart to pump faster, blood pressure to shoot up, and blood vessels to redirect blood from the body's extremities to the muscles for greater strength. To ensure further that all the body's resources go toward either fighting or fleeing the danger, the epinephrine inhibits the digestive system and—as researchers have learned more recently—the immune system. Specifically, the stress leads to a lowering of the body's supplies of interferon and natural killer cells, which are needed to help fight disease.

The fight-or-flight response enabled our ancestors to deal with the immediate physical dangers of their frequently hazardous environment. In today's world, however, stressors tend to be more emotional than physical, and they generally occur continually over a long period of time. As a result, our immune systems often suffer from chronic suppression, making it more difficult to fight off and recover from disease.

Studies indicate that several stress-reduction techniques—including **biofeedback, hypnotherapy, meditation, yoga,** and **guided imagery**—can be effective in decreasing the fight-or-flight response and restoring the body's immune system to full strength. Practicing these techniques may therefore help you recover more quickly from mononucleosis. Research has shown that they may also protect you from other illnesses, including ***heart disease, diabetes,*** and ***cancer.*** ■

MOTION SICKNESS

SYMPTOMS

- sweating, dizziness, pallor, and nausea—sometimes leading to vomiting—while traveling by car, bus, train, ship, or airplane.

CALL YOUR DOCTOR IF:

- you are planning a trip and are concerned that you will be bothered by motion sickness; your doctor may prescribe ***antinausea drugs.***

The nausea and dizziness that afflict some people when they are traveling in a vehicle certainly cause discomfort—especially if they lead to vomiting—but they do not represent a serious illness. The symptoms of motion sickness usually subside either once your body adjusts to your mode of travel or shortly after the trip ends.

Nearly 80 percent of the population has suffered at some time from motion sickness. Fortunately, ways to prevent it abound.

CAUSES

Motion sickness may occur because your brain is receiving conflicting information from your sensory organs: Your eyes may not detect motion to the same degree as the balance mechanism in your inner ear registers the movement of the vehicle. Your central nervous system reacts to this stress-producing phenomenon by activating the nausea center in your brain.

TREATMENT

The surest way to cure motion sickness is to stop the activity that's causing your discomfort, but that's not always practicable. If you are prone to motion sickness, preparations for any trip should include measures to prevent the disorder or mechanisms to cope with it.

CONVENTIONAL MEDICINE

Your doctor may recommend over-the-counter ***antinausea*** pills, such as dimenhydrinate, which counter nausea by reducing the sensitivity of the motion-detecting nerves in the ear. If you need something stronger, your doctor may prescribe the same medication in a higher potency. In order to be effective, oral antinausea medications need to be started well before your departure (up to a day ahead).

If you are going on a long trip, your doctor may prescribe scopolamine, in the form of a timed-release skin patch, to reduce the muscle spasms and contractions that trigger vomiting.

Worn behind your ear, the patch releases scopolamine into your bloodstream over a three-day period. If you are especially prone to motion sickness, your doctor may encourage you to take antinausea pills in addition to wearing the patch.

ALTERNATIVE CHOICES

Many alternative treatments rely on similar remedies to prevent or relieve motion sickness. ***Ginger*** *(Zingiber officinale)* is a favorite motion sickness remedy of naturopaths. It causes none of the side effects of antinausea drugs and can be drunk as a tea, eaten candied, or taken in capsule form (two capsules every four hours the day before and as needed during travel); it should be taken on an empty stomach.

ACUPRESSURE

Much scientific research exists to substantiate the use of wrist point Pericardium 6 in relieving nausea. You might want to purchase acupressure wristbands to place over this point when you travel. When worn as directed, the nodules on the bands put pressure on points acupressure proponents say reduce nausea. The bands are often recommended by conventional physicians and alternative practitioners alike, and are sold in many pharmacies and travel-goods stores.

Acupressure applied at the base of the rib cage (Spleen 16) is also said to be especially effective in relieving nausea.

See the illustrations *(below, left)*, the ***Appendix,*** and pages 22-23 for information on point locations.

ACUPRESSURE

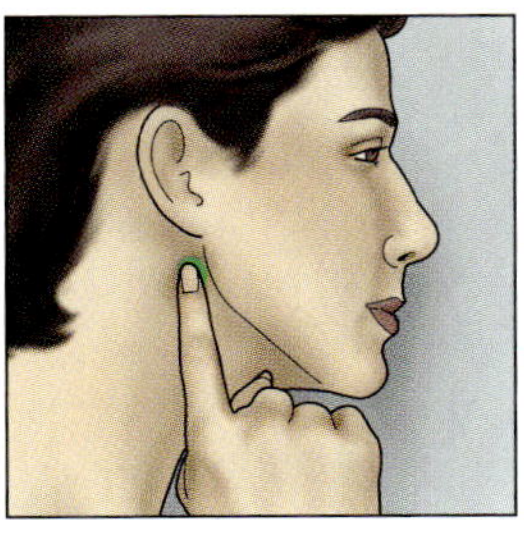

1 Pressing Small Intestine 17 may aid the ear's balancing mechanism. Place your index fingers just below your earlobes in the indentations at the back of the jawbone. Apply light pressure while breathing deeply for one minute. Repeat one to two times.

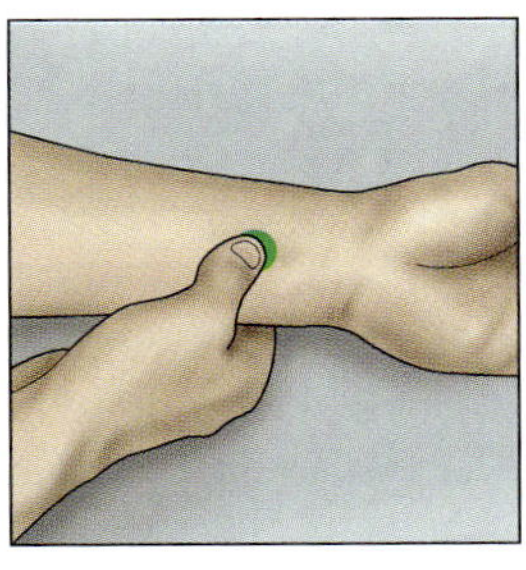

2 To help calm nerves and reduce nausea, press Pericardium 6. Place your thumb in the center of your inner wrist between the two forearm bones, two finger widths from the wrist crease. Press firmly for one minute, three to five times; then repeat on the other arm.

HOMEOPATHY

Homeopathic remedies sometimes come in kits that contain motion sickness remedies, which can be taken before and during travel as directed. Your homeopathic physician may prescribe remedies such as *Cocculus, Petroleum,* ***Ipecac,*** or ***Nux vomica*** to take before or during travel to relieve nausea.

PREVENTION

There are many strategies you can use to lower your vulnerability to motion sickness. In addition to the suggestions above, the following may help:

- Get plenty of fresh air. Open a car window, get on the ship's top deck, or open the overhead air vent in a plane.
- Keep your head as still as possible, close your eyes or focus on the horizon or another stationary object, and sit where motion is felt the least—in the front seat of the car, amidships or in a forward cabin of the ship, or over the wings of the plane. Avoid sitting facing backward on a bus, train, or plane. Don't read while in motion.
- Eat light meals of low-fat, starchy foods and avoid strong-smelling or -tasting foods.
- Don't drink or smoke, which can increase nausea.
- If nausea does set in, try eating olives or sucking on a lemon; these foods make your mouth dry and help diminish nausea. Soda crackers may help absorb excess saliva and acid in your stomach. If you feel too sick to eat, try a drink of ginger ale (made from real ginger) or any carbonated cola drink. ■

MULTIPLE SCLEROSIS

SYMPTOMS

The first attack is generally mild, lasts only a few days, and is followed by a long period of remission—perhaps years—before the next episode. Symptoms vary considerably. They include:

- weakness, stiffness (spasticity), or numbness in one or more limbs.
- sensations of tingling, pins and needles, heaviness, a bandlike tightness around one or more limbs or the trunk of the body.
- tremors, instability, or a lack of balance or coordination.
- blurred or double vision, or rapid, involuntary eye movement.
- bladder or bowel incontinence.
- fatigue: either a feeling of general tiredness or extreme exhaustion.

CALL YOUR DOCTOR IF:

- you or someone you know has symptoms associated with multiple sclerosis. Because other diseases share some of the same symptoms, a proper diagnosis is essential to your treatment.
- you are suffering from an acute attack; steroid injections can help relieve pain.

Multiple sclerosis is a disease of the central nervous system, typically slow and fitful in its progress, with effects that can range from relatively minor physical annoyances to major disabilities. The root problem is electrical. Normally, most nerves in the body are insulated by a fatty substance called myelin, which permits the efficient transmission of electrical impulses—the nerve signals. Multiple sclerosis, or MS, occurs when this protective sheath becomes inflamed and ultimately destroyed in places, short-circuiting the electrical flow. Among the possible consequences of the disruption are loss of muscular coordination, impaired vision, and incontinence.

The initial attack—occurring as early as the teenage years—may be brief and mild, and may not even be recognized. The symptoms temporarily abate or disappear for reasons that are not known, but recurrence is highly likely—although usually after a long latency period. Generally the first full-fledged bout, lasting weeks or months, takes place between the ages of 20 and 40, and further attacks follow at erratic intervals. The repeated inflammation of the nerves produces scarring (sclerosis), and although myelin can normally repair itself, the scarring happens too rapidly for healing to take place; the effects of the lesions become permanent. As a result of such lasting damage, 77 percent of MS sufferers are limited to some degree in their activities, and about 25 percent become wheelchair-bound.

Doctors recognize four basic categories of MS:

- **Benign.** Cases of this kind are typically limited to one attack, and there is no permanent disability. The most common symptoms are limb numbness and temporary vision problems caused by inflammation of the optic nerve. About 20 percent of MS cases are of the benign type.
- **Relapse-remitting.** This and the next category refer to on-again, off-again cycles of attacks and remissions. Cases of this type involve sudden and strong debilitating attacks followed by periods of almost total remission. About 25 percent of MS cases are of this kind.
- **Relapse-progressive.** In this type, attacks are less severe, but the recovery is less complete.

The cumulative effect of many cycles of attacks slowly leads to some degree of disability. This is the most common form of MS, accounting for about 40 percent of all cases.

- **Chronic-progressive.** This form of MS quickly becomes disabling and has no periods of remission. It accounts for about 15 percent of cases.

Multiple sclerosis not only is unpredictable in its on-again, off-again patterns and its broad spectrum of symptoms, it also strikes the population in mystifyingly uneven ways. Women are twice as susceptible as men, and the disease is twice as common among Caucasians as among African Americans. Moreover, the incidence is higher in northerly regions: The rate of MS in Canada is twice that of the United States.

MYELIN LOSS

NERVE CELL

MYELIN SHEATH

ABSENCE OF MYELIN

Myelin, a fatty substance that sheathes and protects the fiberlike axons of cells in the central nervous system, also speeds electrical signals as they travel along nerve pathways to carry out movement and other vital processes. Multiple sclerosis causes myelin to disintegrate, thereby obstructing signal flow and potentially leading to progressive loss of motor coordination and other functions.

CAUSES

No one is sure what causes MS, but most researchers think the immune system plays a major role. Perhaps the disease arises from an inherited problem in the immune system. Perhaps a virus provokes an autoimmune response—a situation in which the immune system attacks the body's own tissue, mistaking it for a foreign invader. It has also been proposed that MS can be triggered by a profound emotional shock or physical trauma, which could affect the immune system.

Dietary factors have also been cited as possible causes. In attempting to explain the higher incidence of MS in northern regions, some researchers note that people there tend to eat more red meat, milk products, and other foods high in saturated fat. MS patients have a lower-than-normal ability to absorb polyunsaturated fatty acids, which are essential to the body's processing of all foods, especially saturated fat. The result is an excess of saturated fats in their systems. Many remedial diets have been devised to correct this imbalance, and some have met with sustained success—but none can be considered a cure *(see **Nutrition and Diet** below).*

Some researchers suspect environmental factors. The list of possible culprits includes lead, pesticides, diesel fumes, chemicals in tap water, solvents, fumes from domestic gas water heaters, and carbon monoxide pollution.

DIAGNOSTIC AND TEST PROCEDURES

A common test for MS is the visual evoked response, in which electrodes attached to the back of the head detect electrical activity in response to visual tracking of a changing checkerboard pattern. Other tests include magnetic resonance imaging (MRI) and lumbar puncture.

TREATMENT

Multiple sclerosis is difficult to treat—and to study, for that matter—for two reasons: Its diverse symptoms vary greatly, and the cycling of attacks and remissions makes tracking the course of the disease and determining the effectiveness of a given treatment especially problematic. (A remission, for example, could be due to medication or might have occurred on its own.)

In general, medicines are effective only in

treating the symptoms of MS, and then only to a limited degree. MS sufferers have thus vigorously explored a wide variety of alternative treatments as well.

CONVENTIONAL MEDICINE

Although the unpredictable nature of MS makes treatments difficult to evaluate, a number of medications are regarded as effective. Among them: interferon beta , which can cut the frequency and severity of relapses; ***corticosteroids,*** which can shorten attacks and reduce inflammation; baclofen and dantrolene, which act to suppress spasticity; and ***muscle relaxants,*** which relieve stiffness and pain. A ***corticosteroid*** is frequently recommended to treat inflammation of the optic nerve, the cause of the double vision or involuntary rapid eye movement that sometimes occurs with MS. Amantadine, an antiviral drug, may promote stamina.

Some medications specifically target muscle stiffness, bladder and bowel problems, tremors, fatigue, and the pins-and-needles sensation. Others are directed at the immune system. In several trials run in 1994, cladribine, a drug used to treat leukemia, either stabilized or improved the conditions of MS patients; it apparently works by killing lymphocytes that may be attacking the central nervous system.

Researchers are exploring various other treatments. In one study, replacement myelin from cows seemed to greatly reduce the number of attacks. Physical therapy has proved effective in relaxing stiff limbs, maintaining motion in the joints, and improving circulation. A physical therapist can also help design an exercise program tailored to the individual's particular limitations.

ALTERNATIVE CHOICES

You'll need professional guidance for some of the alternative therapies described below, but you can learn to do many yourself at home.

ACUPUNCTURE

With MS patients, the goal of acupuncture is to reduce limb stiffness and relax muscles. Acupuncture, which stimulates nerve pathways, may enable messages to bypass damaged nerve fibers.

APITHERAPY

The administering of stings from honeybees *(Apis mellifica)* has been used to treat arthritis for centuries—and recently, MS sufferers, too, have found relief with apitherapy, also known as bee venom therapy (BVT). The recommended treatment involves three weekly sessions of painful stings (from a live bee) for six months. Apitherapy stimulates the immune system. When an already inflamed area is stung and becomes swollen, the body's natural anti-inflammatory agents act to shrink swelling, reducing the inflammation of the original condition in the process.

Bee venom may be beneficial in other ways. It is rich in polyunsaturated fatty acids, which MS patients lack.

BVT has short-lived side effects: itching, swelling, and skin reddening. It has been known to cause fatal shock in some people and severe allergic reactions in others. Be sure to check with your doctor before embarking on a series of treatments. Some doctors will administer the stings themselves, or they may refer you to someone more experienced. You can contact the American Apitherapy Society or your state chapter of the Multiple Sclerosis Foundation for qualified practitioners, who may also help you learn how to administer treatments yourself.

BODY WORK

Although multiple sclerosis cannot be cured through physical movement or exercise, regularly working your muscles is advised in order to keep them from atrophying.

The **Feldenkrais method** involves a series of lessons designed to retrain your neuromuscular system and expand your range of motion. More than a thousand different exercises are covered in the lessons, which you can take either in a group session or in a one-on-one meeting with a practitioner. Movements are performed lightly, slowly, and without strain.

Proprioceptive Neuromuscular Facilitation, or PNF Stretching, is another body-work technique that operates on the principle of reeducating the body. Proprioceptors are sensory receptors—concentrated in muscle tissue around the joints—that monitor physical movements and enable the brain to coordinate the body's motions. In PNF Stretching, a therapist arranges your body in a stretched position and holds you stationary while urging you to move; as you try to respond, your muscles stretch farther. With repetition, the muscles' flexibility increases and, in effect, the proprioceptors "learn" how to achieve a fuller range of motion.

LIFESTYLE

Exercise is highly recommended for MS patients—although it should not be performed during an attack, nor too strenuously at other times, since overexertion can bring on an attack. Because muscle contractions are stimulated by nerve impulses, the exercise of muscles where nerves have been damaged can be difficult. Nonetheless, swimming, stretching, and low-impact aerobics are all within the capabilities of many people with MS, and even patients in wheelchairs can exercise to some degree.

Gentle stretching is particularly helpful for the spasticity, stiff gait, and foot and toe dragging that can accompany the disease. Performing gentle stretches in cool water, a form of **hydrotherapy,** can also help relax spastic limbs.

Studies have demonstrated that regular **yoga** exercises increase secretions of the adrenal medulla, a nervous-system stimulator, which can help to slow degeneration. Yoga exercises can also strengthen muscles and help you keep your balance.

NUTRITION AND DIET

Certain foods can bring on attacks in some MS sufferers. Among problem foods are milk and dairy products, caffeine, yeast, and gluten (found in wheat, barley, oats, and rye). Ketchup, vinegar, wine, and corn can also prove problematic. The best way to isolate sensitivity to a particular food is to stop eating it for a month, then reintroduce it into your diet to see if it provokes a reaction.

A number of special diets attempt to correct the fatty imbalance in MS sufferers. Two approaches (sometimes used together) appear to have the greatest impact in managing the disease: One is to increase the intake of fatty acids; the other, to decrease the intake of saturated fats. The latter tactic is the more common, although in many recommended diets, saturated fats are not the only targets for reduction or elimination. For example, allergen-free diets forbid foods known to produce allergic reactions such as hives, hay fever, and asthma attacks. Diets that are gluten-free eliminate wheat, rye, barley, and oats. Pectin- and fructose-free diets ban fruits and fruit juices. The **Evers Diet** consists primarily of raw food. The **MacDougal Diet** is gluten- and fructose-free and includes megadoses of vitamins. The **Cambridge Liquid Diet** is a balanced, very low-calorie diet usually used for obese MS patients.

The best-known diet for MS sufferers is the **Swank Diet,** devised by Dr. Roy Swank of the Oregon Health Sciences University. In many cases, it has apparently slowed the course of the disease and reduced attacks. Very low in saturated fats, it calls for specific amounts of polyunsaturated oils—sunflower, safflower, olive, and sesame oils, for example, as well as oils in beans, leafy green vegetables such as spinach and kale, and most fish. The diet also includes proteins, supplements of cod-liver oil, and high doses of vitamins. Butter, margarine, shortening, and hydrogenated oils (such as coconut and palm oil) are strictly forbidden. In the first year, you are advised to avoid red meat entirely, as well as peanut butter, cheese, sour cream, sauces, gravies, pastries, whole milk, and snack foods—all of which are high in saturated fats.

Supplements figure in many diets recommended for MS sufferers. Linoleic acid, found in sunflower oil and known for its role in regulating the immune system, is said to reduce the severity of MS attacks and to produce longer remissions. ***Evening primrose oil*** *(Oenothera biennis)* is beneficial because of its specialized fatty-acid content. Nerve sheaths may be strengthened with 5 daily grams of lecithin (kept refrigerated). Coenzyme Q, or CoQ10, in 30 mg doses two or three times a day, may help cells utilize more oxygen. ***Niacin*** may help with tingling and numbness. ■

M

MUMPS

SYMPTOMS

- swollen, inflamed salivary glands located above the angle of the jaw, on one or both sides of the face.
- fever and fatigue.
- in some cases, swelling of the salivary glands under the tongue.
- especially in teens and adults, secondary inflammation of the testes, which is visible, or of the ovaries or pancreas, which is felt as abdominal pain.

CALL YOUR DOCTOR IF:

- you suspect your child has the mumps, to confirm your diagnosis.
- your child has the mumps and has a severe headache and neck pain; these could be signs of ***meningitis.***
- your child has the mumps and has severe abdominal pain and vomiting—symptoms of an inflamed pancreas.
- any teenage or adult male family member with the mumps has swollen testes, which in extremely rare cases can lead to sterility.

M

You will have little trouble recognizing a child with the mumps, a mild viral infection that occurs most frequently between the ages of 3 and 10. The telltale sign: swelling on one or both sides of your child's face, above the angle of the jaw. Once your child has had the mumps, the child will never get it again, having developed what is known as natural immunity. Most states require a child to be immunized against mumps before starting school if not already naturally immune *(see page 33).*

Mumps is only mildly contagious; there is little risk that other family members will get sick at the same time. Though mumps is usually a childhood illness, teens and adults can also contract it. The case is likely to be no more severe for an older individual, but swelling of the testes in a teenage or adult male should be checked out by your doctor because of a very slight risk of its causing sterility.

CAUSES

Mumps is a virus and is transmitted through the air in droplets from a sneeze or cough, or by direct contact. The incubation period—when the virus multiplies in the body and the person is not contagious—is 16 to 18 days from exposure. A person is contagious 2 days before symptoms appear and for 9 days while symptoms are present.

TREATMENT

Call your child's pediatrician to confirm your diagnosis of mumps, as well as to ensure that the physician can intercede if complications arise and to keep your child's health history current. Children with the mumps should stay home from school until all symptoms are gone.

CONVENTIONAL MEDICINE

Your pediatrician will prescribe rest, a soft-foods diet, increased liquids, and heat or ice on the glands to relieve pain. The doctor may also recommend an ***acetaminophen***-based pain reliever.

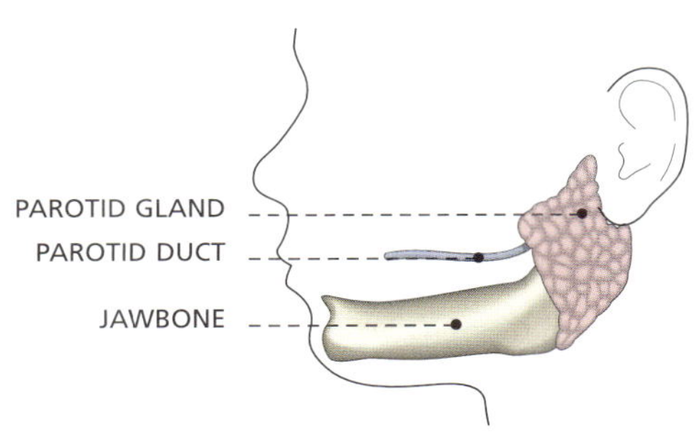

The parotid glands, one of three sets of salivary glands, are located below the ears along the curve of the jaw. They continuously secrete saliva into the mouth through the parotid ducts on the inside of the cheek. When infected with mumps, the parotid glands may swell and become tender to the touch; the openings of the parotid ducts may also contract and prevent the normal flow of saliva.

ALTERNATIVE CHOICES

ACUPRESSURE

To relieve pain caused by swollen glands, place your middle fingers in the hollows just behind your child's earlobes, and hold lightly for two minutes. Encourage your child to breathe deeply.

HERBAL THERAPIES

To reduce swelling, try cleavers *(Galium aparine)* or ***fenugreek*** *(Trigonella foenum-gracum)*. Consult a medical herbalist for dosages.

HOMEOPATHY

Always consult a homeopathic physician for appropriate dosages for children. The homeopath may recommend ***Belladonna*** when a child is flushed, red, and has swelling on the right side; ***Bryonia*** when a child is irritable, thirsty, and doesn't want to move; or *Phytolacca* for extremely swollen glands. Stop treatments that don't help within 24 hours; you need to try another remedy.

NUTRITION AND DIET

Offer your child light foods such as soups, vegetables, and fruits. Avoid dairy products, which are hard to digest, and citrus fruits or juices, which can aggravate the swollen salivary glands.

OSTEOPATHY

Gentle, rhythmic pressure applied over the spleen may enhance the release of white blood cells. Consult an osteopath.

AT-HOME CARE

- Keep your child quiet, especially if he's feverish; confinement to bed is not required.
- An ice pack or a heating pad applied to the swelling may relieve pain. An ***acetaminophen***-based pain reliever may also help.
- A tea made from apple juice and cloves can help relieve painful swallowing. Gently boil eight whole cloves in 1 qt apple juice. Strain and stir, and cool to room temperature.

PREVENTION

Because fighting the illness strengthens the immune system, many practitioners of alternative medicine believe it is better for an otherwise healthy child to contract mumps than to be vaccinated. You should discuss immunization with your child's doctor. The MMR (measles, mumps, and rubella vaccine) is now given at 12 or 15 months, with a booster between the ages of 4 and 6 or 10 and 12. The homeopathic version of immunization is not an accepted equivalent and will not provide the same protection, but some homeopaths will prescribe remedies to decrease the potential side effects of the MMR.

CAUTION!

Never give a child *aspirin*—even baby aspirin—or other products containing the salt called salicylate to reduce a fever or to relieve pain. Aspirin has been linked to Reye's syndrome, a rare but very dangerous illness that causes inflammation of the liver and brain. ■

M

MUSCLE CRAMPS

SYMPTOMS

Once you've experienced a muscle cramp, you'll probably recognize any future ones by the nature of the pain they inflict. Common symptoms include:

- a sharp, sudden, painful spasm—or tightening—of a muscle, especially in the legs.
- the affected muscle's hardness to the touch.
- in some cases, visible distortion or twitching of the muscle beneath the skin.
- in other cases, extremely severe cramps in the arms and legs, beginning without warning, and sometimes affecting the abdominal muscles as well. These symptoms are typical of heat cramps.
- persistent cramping pains in lower abdominal muscles, which may occur with ***back problems*** or during menstruation.

M

CALL YOUR DOCTOR IF:

- you experience frequent muscle cramps.
- your muscle cramp lasts more than an hour.
- your cramp is in your chest or arms; this may indicate a serious heart or abdominal problem. **Seek immediate medical help.** *(See also **Heart Attack.**)*

From a stitch that grabs your side while you're running to a charley horse in your calf awakening you in the dead of night, muscle cramps can be an all-too-common source of discomfort. Normally, a muscle at work contracts—tightening to exert a pulling force—then stretches out when the movement is finished or when another muscle exerts force in the opposite direction. But sometimes a muscle contracts with great intensity and stays contracted, refusing to stretch out again; this is a muscle cramp.

CAUSES

Muscles contract or lengthen in response to electrical signals from nerves; minerals such as sodium, calcium, and magnesium, which surround and permeate muscle cells, play a key role in the transmission of these signals. Imbalances in those minerals—as well as in certain hormones, body fluids, and chemicals—or malfunctions in the nervous system itself can foul up the flow of electrical signals and cause a muscle to cramp.

Physical overexertion depletes fluids and minerals and can lead to cramping, particularly in people who work or exercise in conditions that overheat their bodies. Activities like working in the garden on a hot summer day, if you are not careful to drink plenty of fluids, may cause heat cramps. And if you do not take steps to alleviate them, heat cramps can progress to much more serious **heatstroke** and **heat exhaustion** *(see **Emergencies/First Aid,** page 68).*

CAUTION!

Cramping pain in your chest and arm muscles may indicate a heart problem. Call your doctor or get medical help immediately. If you suffer from *circulatory problems, diabetes, heart disease,* or *varicose veins,* or if you have had a *stroke* or been warned that you might be susceptible to one, avoid massage until you talk to your doctor.

Hormone imbalances caused by ***diabetes*** and ***thyroid problems*** can also cause cramps, as can a reduced supply of blood-borne oxygen to muscles. Blood oxygen levels often fall in smokers, for instance, causing muscles to cramp—especially when smokers engage in hard physical labor. If you move in your sleep, you may pinch a nerve, signaling a muscle to contract and perhaps leading to a cramp. If you're prone to night cramps, do stretching exercises before you go to bed.

TREATMENT

There are simple techniques for easing common, occasional muscle cramps *(see* ***At-Home Remedies,*** *right),* but if you suffer from frequent or severe cramps, see your doctor. Frequent cramps might indicate a more serious illness. And severe cramps in your chest, shoulders, or arms can be symptoms of a ***heart attack;*** call immediately for medical help.

CONVENTIONAL MEDICINE

No medicinal treatment of common muscle cramps is required. Massaging a cramping muscle or drinking water to relieve heat cramps is usually sufficient remedy. For frequent or severe cramps, your doctor will diagnose and treat the underlying cause.

ALTERNATIVE CHOICES

ACUPRESSURE

If the cramp is in your calf, acupressurists recommend applying pressure for two to three minutes at the lower end of the calf muscle bulge.

HOMEOPATHY

Over-the-counter homeopathic preparations (in tablet form) of *Cuprum metallicum* (6c), sucked slowly, are said to relieve the spasm and ache.

NUTRITION AND DIET

Nutritionists recommend taking ***vitamin E*** supplements (300 IU daily) to prevent night cramps. You may also find relief by increasing your intake of ***calcium, magnesium,*** and ***potassium.*** Good sources include milk, cheese, yogurt, dark green leafy vegetables, and canned fish.

AT-HOME REMEDIES

To relieve a typical cramp, you need to make the muscle stop contracting—by physically either stretching it or massaging it, or both. You can stretch a calf muscle simply by standing on your toes and then slowly lowering your heels. For a greater stretch, put your hands or forearms against a wall, and keeping your feet flat on the floor, slide backward until you are leaning against the wall from several feet away. For even more stretch, keep edging your feet backward.

To massage away a cramp, from a sitting position stretch your heel down, pointing your toes up—toward your head—and firmly squeeze your calf with your hand. Begin at the edges of the cramp and move in toward the center with gentle pressure. For an obstinate cramp, immerse the muscle in a hot bath, perhaps while stretching and massaging it. To treat heat cramps, drink plenty of cool water. This is also the best way to prevent heat cramps: Drink a cup of cool water before and after exercise, and every 15 minutes during exercise. If you use a sports beverage instead, drink one low in sugar; sugar in an overheated body can bring on stomach cramps. Dilute juices with 3 parts water.

PREVENTION

Drink 6 to 8 cups of water every day. Be sure to acclimate yourself to exercise routines and sports, especially in early summer. Do stretching exercises regularly, particularly before bed. Practicing **yoga** daily can prevent cramping; yoga helps relax and lengthen your muscles. If you smoke, enroll in a program to help you quit. ■

MUSCLE PAIN

Read down this column to find your symptoms. Then read across.

SYMPTOMS	AILMENT/PROBLEM
◆ muscle and joint pain after excessive or strenuous activity.	◆ Overexertion
◆ cramping muscle pain, often in your calf; may awake you from sleep.	◆ ***Muscle cramp***
◆ muscle pain following vigorous activity or an injury; possibly, swelling.	◆ Strained muscle or muscles
◆ pain in your neck muscles after a jolt.	◆ Whiplash
◆ muscle and joint aches; fever, chills, headache, weakness, runny nose, cough, sore throat; possibly, vomiting or diarrhea.	◆ ***Flu***
◆ muscle pain after taking medication.	◆ Drug reaction
◆ chronic burning or radiating muscle pain, especially in your shoulders, neck, and hips; fatigue; often, a sleep disorder such as ***insomnia;*** typically affecting people in their late forties or older.	◆ Fibromyalgia
◆ pain and stiffness in the muscles of your neck, shoulders, and arms, or your lower back, thighs, and hips.	◆ Polymyalgia rheumatica

WHAT TO DO	OTHER INFO
◆ Use ice packs for swelling. Consider heat rubs, warm baths, a heating pad, or massage when swelling is gone. Take an anti-inflammatory painkiller such as ***ibuprofen.***	◆ A cream containing ***aspirin*** or the homeopathic remedy ***Arnica*** may help relieve pain. Because muscles require 48 hours to recover from exertion, try exercising only every other day. Stretching before and after exercise may prevent pain and strain.
◆ Massage the muscle, rubbing upward and toward the heart. For recurrent cramps avoid heavy blankets and tight pajamas when sleeping.	◆ Extra ***calcium, magnesium,*** or ***vitamin E,*** or a 12-oz glass of tonic water (which contains quinine) taken at night, may reduce the frequency of cramps.
◆ Try RICE: rest, ice (wrapped in a thin cloth), compression (with an elastic wrap), and elevation of the affected area. Take an anti-inflammatory painkiller such as ***ibuprofen.*** *(See **Sprains and Strains.**)*	◆ The homeopathic remedy ***Arnica*** reduces swelling; ***Ruta*** may help you heal the strain. ◆ Yoga can help prevent injury by keeping muscles relaxed.
◆ Rest on a firm bed without a pillow. Take an anti-inflammatory painkiller such as ***ibuprofen.*** Call your doctor if you are no better in 24 hours.	◆ Your doctor may recommend that you wear a supportive collar.
◆ Rest, drink plenty of fluids, and if needed, take an anti-inflammatory painkiller such as ***ibuprofen.***	◆ Flu shots are often recommended for prevention in people over the age of 65 and in those with chronic diseases.
◆ If the drug is by prescription, call your doctor. If the drug is over-the-counter, stop taking it and seek your doctor's advice.	◆ Clofibrate, a lipid-lowering drug, often causes muscle pain. ***Corticosteroids*** may cause such pain indirectly by depleting ***potassium.***
◆ Call your doctor. Take pain relievers recommended by your doctor; a muscle relaxant or a low dose of an ***antidepressant*** may be recommended for pain relief or sleep improvement.	◆ Women are affected by this illness 10 times more frequently than men. Physical therapy, aerobic exercise, biofeedback, yoga, acupuncture, and improved sleeping habits may be helpful.
◆ Call your doctor. The usual treatment is with ***corticosteroids*** and, possibly, anti-inflammatories.	◆ Patients with this disease typically are over 50 years old, and it occurs more often in women than in men.

M

MUSCLE WEAKNESS

Read down this column to find your symptoms. Then read across.

SYMPTOMS	AILMENT/PROBLEM
◆ muscle weakness (inability to exert or sustain much pressure, weight, or strain, or to grasp objects or resist force; lacking vigor; weakness may be actual or perceived) after excessive or strenuous activity or exercise.	◆ Overexertion
◆ muscle weakness and aching; fever, chills, headache, malaise, runny nose, cough, sore throat; possibly, vomiting or diarrhea.	◆ ***Flu*** or other ***infection***
◆ muscle weakness after sweating, vomiting, or diarrhea; possibly, muscle cramps.	◆ Dehydration and/or electrolyte abnormality
◆ muscle weakness with fatigue; bluish lips, pasty skin, slick-feeling tongue; shortness of breath, faintness, dizziness.	◆ ***Anemia***
◆ muscle weakness, trembling hands, nervousness; weight loss despite increased appetite; increased heart rate and blood pressure; excessive perspiration.	◆ Hyperthyroidism
◆ muscle weakness and aching; joint pain; fatigue; low-grade fever; skin rash; sun sensitivity; weight loss; mental confusion; chest pain on taking deep breaths; poor circulation in fingers and toes.	◆ ***Lupus***
◆ unexplained muscle weakness that spreads throughout the body; possibly, tingling, numbness, paralysis.	◆ Neurological disease such as Guillain-Barré syndrome, ***Lou Gehrig's disease, multiple sclerosis,*** or myasthenia gravis
◆ weakness in hip or shoulder muscles; pain, swelling, warmth, and redness in small joints.	◆ Polymyositis or dermatomyositis (inflammation of muscles caused by immune system dysfunction)
◆ muscle weakness that progresses in severity; coordination and gait difficulties; patient always male and usually younger than five years at onset.	◆ Muscular dystrophy

M

WHAT TO DO	OTHER INFO
◆ Slow down for a few days, but continue light activity.	◆ Overexertion may cause weakness from fatigue or fluid losses.
◆ Rest, drink plenty of fluids, and if needed, take an anti-inflammatory painkiller such as ***ibuprofen.***	◆ The flu virus can cause inflammation of the muscle fibers, interfering with their contraction. It is best to return to exercise slowly.
◆ Drink fluids, especially a carbohydrate-electrolyte drink (sports drink). Call your doctor if symptoms persist.	◆ An imbalance of the group of minerals called electrolytes, which give signals to the muscles to contract, may be caused by loss of fluid or other factors, such as medications, alcohol abuse, or various diseases.
◆ If the cause is a deficiency of ***iron, folic acid,*** or ***vitamin B_{12},*** you may need a dietary change or supplement.	◆ Weakness may occur because tissues are deprived of oxygen from blood loss or from a lack of red blood cells.
◆ See ***Thyroid Problems.*** Your doctor may suggest antithyroid medication, surgery, or other treatment.	◆ Muscle weakness can also be caused by an underactive thyroid gland (hypothyroidism) or by a deficiency of another endocrine gland, the adrenal gland.
◆ Call your doctor. Treatment may involve anti-inflammatory painkillers, ***corticosteroids,*** immunosuppressive drugs, and/or ***antidepressants*** or mild ***antianxiety drugs.***	◆ In this autoimmune disease the immune system attacks the body's connective tissue as if it were foreign matter.
◆ Call your doctor. You may be referred to a neurologist for testing and treatment; treatment depends on the specific disease.	◆ Physical therapy is commonly used to increase function in these disabling disorders.
◆ Call your doctor. The usual treatment is with the corticosteroid ***prednisone.***	◆ Although these disorders may disappear within a few months, they can be serious if lung problems develop.
◆ Call your doctor. The only treatment is to lessen deformities through physical therapy.	◆ The muscles in people with this rare, inherited disease lack a protein needed for proper functioning.

NAIL PROBLEMS

Read down this column to find your symptoms. Then read across.

SYMPTOMS	AILMENT/PROBLEM
◆ split, brittle, and/or bent nails following extensive hand washing or a visit to a manicurist.	◆ Possibly, an allergic reaction to a soap, nail polish, or other substance
◆ nails that become pale and spoon-shaped or develop a temporary groove.	◆ ***Anemia;*** damaged nail matrix (the nail-forming region underlying the cuticle)
◆ cracked, thickened, and discolored nails accompanied by an itchy, scaly rash that usually starts between the fourth and fifth toes.	◆ ***Athlete's foot***
◆ greenish black spots under the nail.	◆ Potentially serious bacterial ***infection***
◆ black specks, especially on fingernails; bluish gray spots on the nail bed, and nails that curve over the ends of fingers or toes (also called clubbed nails).	◆ Possibly, heart valve or other heart problems
◆ a nail that grows into the side of the nail bed, causing inflammation; most common in the big toe, especially in women who wear narrow, tight shoes.	◆ ***Ingrown nail***
◆ swollen, red, painful cuticle or nail fold (at the side of the nail); the cuticle may lift away from the base and ooze pus when pressed.	◆ Paronychia (***infection*** of tissue near a nail)
◆ white spots on a nail, usually following a slight blow; similar patches on one or more nails.	◆ Minor physical trauma; vitamin or mineral deficiency
◆ thickened nails, which may be difficult to cut.	◆ ***Circulatory problems,*** possibly related to ***atherosclerosis*** or ***diabetes***

WHAT TO DO	OTHER INFO
◆ See ***Allergies.*** Stop using nail lacquers, polishes, or adhesives (for false nails) and see if the problem clears up.	◆ Acetate-based nail polish removers are less irritating to the skin than acetone-based nail polish removers.
◆ Consult with your doctor. You may only need to increase your ***iron*** intake, but you may need other medical treatment.	◆ Be sure your doctor tests for a ***vitamin B_{12}*** deficiency as well as an iron deficiency.
◆ Use over-the-counter ***antifungal*** medications. Dry your feet thoroughly after washing, and change your socks and shoes regularly.	◆ A persistent or recurring case may require a trip to the doctor for more aggressive treatment.
◆ **Call your doctor now.** See also ***Staph Infections.***	
◆ See ***Heart Disease.*** Call your doctor without delay if you suspect a heart condition.	◆ Clubbed nails are a late—not an early—sign of heart problems.
◆ Trim the excess nail and put a thin strand of sterile cotton under the corner of the nail to lift it away from the skin until it grows out.	◆ Soak the affected foot in warm salt water or a ***calendula*** *(Calendula officinalis)* solution to soften the nail and help in easing it out from the nail fold.
◆ See your doctor for ***antibiotic*** or ***antifungal*** treatment.	◆ Occasionally a case of paronychia is caused by *Candida albicans,* so women should get checked for ***vaginitis*** or ***yeast infections.***
◆ No treatment is necessary for minor nail bruising. Take vitamin and mineral supplements if there was no trauma to the affected nail or nails.	◆ The most likely deficiency is of ***zinc*** or ***vitamin B_6.***
◆ See the entries listed at left.	

N

NASAL POLYPS

SYMPTOMS

- chronic blockage of nasal passages.
- difficulty breathing through nose.
- difficulty smelling.
- headaches.
- nosebleeds.

CALL YOUR DOCTOR IF:

- you suspect you have nasal polyps. (You may be able to see them by looking in a mirror while shining a light up your nostrils; they look like pearly gray lumps.)
- you have a stuffy nose for more than two weeks; this may be a sign of an ***allergy*** or a sinus infection *(see **Sinusitis**),* which may require medical care.
- you have a fever along with your stuffy nose; this could be a sign of an infection, which may require medical care.
- the drainage from your nose is thick and colored; this could indicate a nasal infection, which may require medical care.

When the mucous membrane lining the inside of the nose becomes swollen, it can sometimes distend into the nasal cavity, creating protuberances known as nasal polyps. The polyps look something like small, pearly grapes and can appear singly or in clusters. Although harmless, they often obstruct the nasal passages, making breathing difficult and sometimes affecting the sense of smell. If the polyps block the opening between the nasal cavity and one of the sinuses, headaches can occur.

CAUSES

Nasal polyps are caused by an overproduction of fluid in the mucous membrane lining the nose. People with chronic ***allergies*** and sinus infections are at greatest risk of developing them. Children with cystic fibrosis also tend to develop nasal polyps. In addition, the overuse of ***aspirin*** or other salicylate medications can cause polyps to form in some susceptible people.

DIAGNOSTIC AND TEST PROCEDURES

If you think you have polyps, your doctor will examine the inside of your nose with a special medical instrument called a nasal speculum. If polyps are diagnosed in a child, further tests to rule out cystic fibrosis may be performed.

TREATMENT

The only way to completely rid yourself of nasal polyps is to have them surgically removed. The polyps often recur, however, so it is important that you take preventive steps to manage or control the chronic allergies or sinus infections that usually cause them to form.

CONVENTIONAL MEDICINE

To temporarily reduce the polyps, your doctor may treat them with a ***corticosteroid,*** either by directly injecting the medication into the polyps or by spraying it into your nostrils. You may also be given medications to treat the underlying cause of the polyps: an ***antihistamine*** for allergies or an ***antibiotic*** for a sinus infection.

If the polyps are causing serious discomfort or breathing problems, your doctor may recommend that you have them surgically removed. The operation, which uses a wire snare to clip off the polyps, is considered minor surgery and is usually performed under local anesthesia. Because the polyps often reappear, the surgery may need to be repeated. In very persistent cases, the lining of the sinuses where the polyps originate must be removed as well. This operation requires general anesthesia.

ALTERNATIVE CHOICES

Many of the alternative treatments for nasal polyps are aimed at managing or controlling their underlying causes—the allergies and infections that make the nasal membranes swell with fluid.

AROMATHERAPY

Tea tree oil (*Melaleuca* spp.), ***eucalyptus*** *(Eucalyptus globulus)*, and ***peppermint*** *(Mentha piperita)* are often recommended for clearing stuffy noses. Add 2 drops of each to a warm bath, and soak for 15 minutes or so. Or you can place a drop of each on a tissue and inhale deeply whenever necessary.

HOMEOPATHY

Homeopaths believe that an appropriately chosen medication may help decrease some of the discomfort and problems caused by polyps. Consult a homeopath for a prescription, which might include the following remedies:

- If the polyps are accompanied by loss of smell, swelling around the bridge of the nose, and yellow mucus, ***Calcarea carbonica.***
- If the polyps bleed easily, ***Phosphorus.***
- If mucus drips down the back of the throat and you feel weak and chilled, *Psorinum* or *Thuja.*
- If the polyps are accompanied by sneezing and a crawling sensation in the nose, and mucus forms into large dry pieces, *Teucrium.*

Treatments can be lengthy—up to six months—and require many follow-up visits.

AT-HOME REMEDIES

- To help decongest a stuffy nose and keep the mucous membranes from swelling and forming polyps, try hot baths or showers. Or try steam inhalations: Run very hot water in a sink until steam builds up. With the water running, lean over the sink, and drape a towel over your head to trap the steam. Breathe deeply through your mouth and nose for 5 to 10 minutes. Repeat several times a day.
- You can also decongest your nose with a homemade saline nasal spray: Mix 1 tsp table salt and 1 tsp baking soda in 1 qt boiled water that has been cooled. Fill a sprayer from the drugstore with the solution and use as many times during the day as necessary.

PREVENTION

- If you have ***allergies,*** limit your exposure to whatever is causing them and take an ***antihistamine*** at the first sign of an allergic reaction.
- Avoid ***aspirin,*** which can stimulate the formation of nasal polyps.
- Drink plenty of fluids to keep your nasal membranes moist and healthy.
- Avoid beer, wine, and cordials, which contain tyramine and tannin, ingredients that can cause the nasal membrane to swell.

CAUTION!

Follow directions carefully when using over-the-counter nose drops or spray to clear up a stuffy nose. Overuse of these products can cause your mucous membranes to produce more fluid, making the congestion even worse than it was before. Never use one of these products more frequently or longer than directed on the label. ■

N

NAUSEA

Read down this column to find your symptoms. Then read across.

SYMPTOMS	AILMENT/PROBLEM
For other conditions that may involve nausea, see also ***Vomiting.***	
◆ You feel nauseated (sick to your stomach) after a specific event or stimulus, such as a ride on a roller coaster, an unpleasant odor, or a stressful encounter.	◆ ***Anxiety, motion sickness, stress,*** or merely a natural reaction to an unpleasant stimulus
◆ frequent, burning pain in your upper middle abdomen, usually relieved by eating; possibly, nausea.	◆ ***Gastritis; stomach ulcer***
◆ nausea; severe headache, possibly with vomiting; symptoms may worsen with exposure to bright light.	◆ Migraine ***headache;*** possibly, ***meningitis***
◆ nausea while you are undergoing chemotherapy to treat cancer.	◆ Common side effect of ***cancer*** treatment
◆ sudden attacks of nausea accompanied by bouts of vomiting, extreme dizziness, and severe earache, sometimes with ringing or buzzing in your ears.	◆ ***Ménière's disease***
◆ nausea, diarrhea, vomiting, and fever lasting 48 hours or less; may occur after eating rich, spicy, or possibly spoiled foods, drinking an excessive amount of alcohol, or ingesting a drug you have never taken before.	◆ ***Gastroenteritis*** (also called stomach or intestinal flu)
◆ nausea lasting one to two weeks, headache, malaise, and fatigue; sometimes sore throat, fever, and rash.	◆ ***Mononucleosis; scarlet fever,*** which may follow ***strep throat***
◆ severe nausea with pain starting in the upper abdomen and moving to the right shoulder blade.	◆ ***Gallstones;*** gallbladder ***infection***

WHAT TO DO	OTHER INFO
◆ If you have become nauseated at a sight, sound, or smell, close your eyes or plug your ears or nose, and focus on something pleasurable.	◆ Mind/body medicine, including meditation and biofeedback, can help you lower your stress levels. ***Ginger*** *(Zingiber officinale)* capsules often alleviate motion sickness, as do acupressure wristbands.
◆ If symptoms are constant or recurrent, see a doctor. Avoid irritating substances such as alcohol, tobacco, and caffeine; ***antacids*** may help alleviate symptoms.	◆ Herbal teas of ***chamomile*** *(Matricaria recutita)* or lemon balm *(Melissa officinalis)* may reduce symptoms.
◆ If you suspect meningitis, **call 911 or your emergency number now.** Migraines may respond to various ***analgesics*** (over-the-counter and prescription varieties).	◆ Migraines often have specific triggers, such as red wine or chocolate. Identifying and avoiding your triggers is the best way to control the headaches.
◆ Ask your doctor about specific ways to counteract this effect of your treatment.	◆ Discuss any alternative therapies with your doctor before trying them. See ***Cancer*** for suggestions.
◆ See your doctor. The regimen for minimizing symptoms may include keeping your sodium intake low and taking daily prescription medications to counteract fluid retention and dizziness.	◆ Mind/body medicine, yoga, and massage therapy can help you learn to deal effectively with ***stress,*** which can trigger attacks. When Ménière's flares, avoid reading and bright lights to reduce dizziness.
◆ Rest, drink plenty of fluids, and eat bland foods. You may need an ***antibiotic*** if your stomach bug is the result of a bacterial infection.	◆ Gastroenteritis can be caused by a bacterial or viral infection, food poisoning, overindulgence in alcohol or rich foods, or some medications (including antibiotics). If you suspect that a prescription drug is causing the problem, see your doctor.
◆ See your doctor. For mononucleosis, complete bed rest is essential, with a gradual return to normal activity; scarlet fever requires treatment with ***antibiotics.***	◆ Scarlet fever, though once a common childhood disease, is now quite rare.
◆ Call your doctor today for an evaluation; gallstone attacks may require prompt treatment.	◆ A doctor's care is required, but some alternative therapies, including Chinese herbs (which may help dissolve gallstones), can augment conventional treatment.

SYMPTOMS	AILMENT/PROBLEM
◆ recurrent attacks of nausea, heartburn, and indigestion, particularly after meals; possibly, reduced appetite and weight loss.	◆ ***Stomach ulcer;*** possibly, ***colorectal cancer***
◆ You are addicted to alcohol, have recently quit "cold turkey," and experience nausea, anxiety, insomnia, or delirium tremens (DT).	◆ Common effect of recovering from ***alcohol abuse***
◆ nausea accompanied by increased thirst and urination; dehydration; drowsiness; confusion; possibly, a fruity odor on your breath.	◆ ***Diabetes;*** possibly, diabetic shock
◆ nausea coming in attacks once or twice every several months, accompanied by intense, steady abdominal pain and, in some cases, fever, diarrhea, and vomiting.	◆ ***Crohn's disease; pancreatic problems***
◆ nausea and vomiting that persist after a viral infection; alternating periods of hyperactivity and fatigue.	◆ Reye's syndrome (a neurological disorder typically in children, which may follow an upper respiratory tract infection or ***chickenpox,*** especially if ***aspirin*** has been given during treatment)
◆ nausea with shortness of breath, chest pain, and sweating.	◆ ***Heart attack***
◆ You are allergic to a specific food, drug, or insect sting, and experience nausea, vomiting, and difficulty breathing after encountering the allergen.	◆ ***Allergies;*** possibly, anaphylactic shock (a severe allergic reaction that causes tissues to swell, preventing blood from traveling properly; tissues then become starved for oxygen)
◆ You are or could be pregnant; you have nausea, a bloated feeling in the pelvic area and breasts, and possibly, vomiting.	◆ Normal effects (sometimes called morning sickness, though it can occur any time of day) often felt during the first three months of pregnancy

WHAT TO DO	OTHER INFO
◆ Call your doctor today for diagnosis.	◆ Early detection is crucial for successfully treating colorectal cancer.
◆ Consult with your doctor; some withdrawal symptoms may require immediate medical treatment.	◆ Prescription medications are available that make alcohol withdrawal a much easier process.
◆ Call your doctor. If you suspect diabetic shock, **call 911 or your emergency number now.**	◆ Ketoacidosis, a potentially fatal condition of extremely high blood sugar levels, requires an immediate ***insulin*** injection.
◆ Call your doctor today; a combination of medications may be necessary to control Crohn's disease.	◆ Conventional medical treatment is essential, but discomfort can be lessened with acupuncture, herbal therapies, homeopathy, and mind/body medicine.
◆ **Call 911 or your emergency number now.** Reye's syndrome progresses quickly, and immediate treatment is essential.	◆ Never give ***aspirin*** to a child with a fever or an infection; use ***acetaminophen*** or other nonaspirin pain relievers when needed.
◆ **Call 911 or your emergency number now.**	
◆ If you suspect anaphylactic shock, **get emergency medical treatment.** See ***Emergencies/First Aid: Shock.*** While waiting for emergency care, monitor the patient's breathing and pulse, and give nothing to eat or drink.	◆ Particularly if you have allergies, ask your doctor about preparing an anti-anaphylactic shock kit.
◆ Avoid extremely salty foods, get plenty of rest, and eat small meals several times a day instead of three large meals. See ***Pregnancy Problems.***	◆ ***Ginger*** *(Zingiber officinale)* tea is helpful in relieving nausea due to morning sickness, but check with your doctor before trying any remedy.

N

NECK PAIN

Read down this column to find your symptoms. Then read across.

SYMPTOMS	AILMENT/PROBLEM
◆ neck stiffness or pain upon awakening that wasn't there when you went to bed.	◆ A stiff neck, from sleeping in a position that strained your neck muscles or joints
◆ swelling or a lump on the side or back of your neck; possibly accompanied by neck pain.	◆ Swollen lymph nodes, in response to an ***infection*** somewhere in your body
◆ neck stiffness that progressively worsens.	◆ Osteoarthritis
◆ intense neck pain that shoots into your arms or shoulders, especially when you move your head.	◆ A ruptured or slipped vertebral disk, which is pressing against a nerve
◆ severe neck pain that started in the last 24 hours after some sort of jolt (as when a car stops suddenly); may be accompanied by dizziness, difficulty walking, vomiting, difficulty controlling arms or legs, or loss of bladder or bowel control.	◆ Whiplash
◆ dull, throbbing pain on one side of your neck that may radiate into your cheek, eye, or ear; pain is worse when you chew, yawn, or move your head; symptoms may follow another illness (such as sore throat), or may be associated with migraine headache.	◆ Carotidynia (dilation of the carotid artery, which carries blood to the brain; possibly caused by a virus or bacteria)
◆ pain at the front of your neck when you swallow; possibly, pain along the jaw and below the ear; mild fever; neck may be red and tender.	◆ Thyroiditis (inflammation of the thyroid, possibly the result of ***infection*** or an autoimmune disorder)
◆ severe headache followed by neck pain that is worse when the head is bent forward; any one of the following: nausea, vomiting, confusion, drowsiness, sensitivity to bright light.	◆ ***Meningitis***

WHAT TO DO	OTHER INFO
◆ If the stiffness or pain does not go away within 24 hours, call your doctor.	◆ See the ***Appendix*** for yoga exercises that may help to gently loosen a stiff neck.
◆ See your doctor to identify the infection; you may need an ***antibiotic.***	
◆ See ***Arthritis.*** Pain is often relieved by a daily regimen of over-the-counter ***nonsteroidal anti-inflammatory drugs (NSAIDs).***	◆ Osteoarthritis most commonly affects people over the age of 50. ◆ Chiropractic manipulation may help alleviate pain.
◆ See ***Disk Problems.*** Take ***aspirin*** or ***nonsteroidal anti-inflammatory drugs (NSAIDs)*** to relieve pain. Your doctor may suggest wearing a soft collar to limit movement until the disk returns to position, and possibly stronger pain relievers as well.	◆ Chiropractors, massage therapists, and yoga instructors often have success treating these problems.
◆ **Call your doctor now,** and apply ice to your neck until you can get medical care. If the pain is mild and unaccompanied by other symptoms, you may only need to take ***aspirin*** or ***nonsteroidal anti-inflammatory drugs (NSAIDs),*** but call your doctor if you feel no better after 24 hours.	◆ Wearing a soft padded collar will immobilize and stabilize your neck, but don't use it for more than a week or so or your healing will actually take longer. For more comfortable sleeping, lie on a firm bed and don't use a pillow.
◆ Call your doctor. Pain may be relieved with rest, ***nonsteroidal anti-inflammatory drugs (NSAIDs),*** and a cold or hot compress; prescription ***antimigraine drugs*** sometimes help.	◆ Differentiating between carotidynia and ***sore throat,*** sinus infection, an abscessed tooth, or ***oral cancer*** can be difficult.
◆ Call your doctor to differentiate between thyroiditis and ***sore throat.*** See ***Thyroid Problems; Immune Problems.***	◆ After a bout of thyroiditis, expect frequent checks by your doctor to ensure your thyroid is working properly.
◆ **Get medical care immediately.** You will need two weeks of aggressive ***antibiotic*** therapy, and you may need to stay in the hospital.	◆ Without treatment, bacterial meningitis can be fatal; viral meningitis is rarely fatal.

N

Cross references are indicated by ***bold italics.***

NEURALGIA

SYMPTOMS

Neuralgia, or nerve pain, comes in many different forms: It may be sudden, shooting, sharp, burning, or stabbing, and is sometimes accompanied by a background sensation of burning, itching, or aching, or by hypersensitivity to touch. It occurs in one part of your body, typically on one side. The pain may be intermittent or continuous; it can last for a few seconds or a few minutes, and may recur, on and off, for days or weeks.

CALL YOUR DOCTOR IF:

- you suspect that the pain is caused by a spinal problem, a herniated disk, or a ***pinched nerve.***
- the symptoms include impaired bladder or bowel control or a dragging foot—signs of nerve damage; **call your doctor immediately.**
- facial neuralgia spreads to an eye after a herpes attack; this could lead to blindness if untreated.
- the pain becomes too great to bear; nerve damage could result.

N

Neuralgia, as the name suggests, is nerve pain, occurring when a nerve is irritated or inflamed. The pain, spreading along neural pathways, may be fleeting or chronic and can range from mild to outright unbearable.

Only a few types of neuralgia are common. One, characterized by flashes of facial pain, is called trigeminal neuralgia, after the multibranched cranial nerve that is affected; the condition occurs mostly in people over 50 and afflicts three times as many women as men. Nerves of the buttocks and legs are also vulnerable; irritation of the large sciatic nerve, for example, produces the neuralgia called ***sciatica.*** Another relatively common type is postherpetic neuralgia, which strikes after the type of herpes infection known as ***shingles*** and typically manifests itself as a continuous burning sensation.

CAUSES

Generally, the likeliest source of neuralgias is irritation or inflammation of a nerve or pressure on a nerve from bones or connective tissue. Such pressure may be due to a muscle or spinal injury, a prolapsed disk, or years of poor posture. Trigeminal neuralgia may stem from the pressure of a blood vessel. In postherpetic neuralgia, the nerve inflammation is caused by a viral infection. In many cases of neuralgia, however, the reason for the nerve's irritated state cannot be discovered.

TREATMENT

CONVENTIONAL MEDICINE

Physicians often prescribe ***analgesics*** for mild neuralgia and ***opioid analgesics*** for severe cases. Trigeminal neuralgia pain can be relieved with the anticonvulsants ***carbamazepine*** and ***phenytoin.*** Capsaicin (the active ingredient in cayenne pepper) in ointment form can be an effective over-the-counter remedy for postherpetic neuralgia. ***Corticosteroids*** reduce nerve inflammation, and sedatives help with pain indirectly.

ALTERNATIVE CHOICES

In addition to the therapies listed below, consider seeing a **chiropractor** or an **osteopath;** manipulations of the spine and of soft tissue have proved helpful in relieving several types of neuralgia.

ACUPUNCTURE

Acupuncture has been shown to be extremely effective in treating neuralgia. If the pain is severe, 5 to 10 acupuncture sessions may be required.

BODY WORK

In a series of lessons, an **Alexander technique** instructor can train you to adjust your body posture and movements to prevent future attacks. Deep-tissue **massage** reduces pain by probing into successively deeper layers of muscle and connective tissue, and concentrates on "clearing out" a particular area of the body. When inflammation causes the connective tissue, or fascia, that covers muscles to have an abnormally tight grip on a muscle, myofascial release therapy loosens that grip through gentle stretching, reducing pain.

HERBAL THERAPIES

A cup of boiling water poured over 2 tsp ***St.-John's-wort*** *(Hypericum perforatum)* and steeped for 10 minutes has painkilling properties when drunk three times daily. Recent experiments on extracts from ***black cohosh*** *(Cimicifuga racemosa)* suggest it may have anti-inflammatory qualities.

HOMEOPATHY

For sharp, shooting pain with tingling and burning, try ***Hypericum*** (6x) once an hour for three to four doses. Consult a homeopath for other remedies specific to your symptoms.

NUTRITION AND DIET

When an attack begins, a maximum dose of 50 mg ***vitamin*** B_6 three times a day and ***vitamin B complex*** once a day may help; continue for one week only. For postherpetic neuralgia, add 400 IU ***vitamin E*** twice a day.

Making oats *(Avena sativa)* a regular part of your diet can improve the overall condition of nerves. A drink made from minced oat straw or oat grass steeped for two minutes in warm water and strained is thought to be a valuable tonic; drink 1 to 4 cups daily. To soothe itching skin, bathe in water that has been run over oatmeal in a muslin bag hung under the bathtub tap.

AREAS OF PAIN

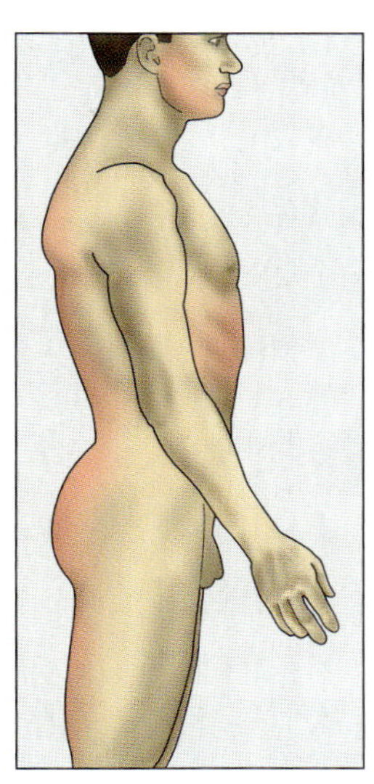

Neuralgia, or pain that results from an irritated or damaged nerve, occurs in various forms in different parts of the body. Trigeminal neuralgia, for example, affects the face. Intercostal neuralgia causes pain between the ribs, and sciatica strikes the lower back and legs. These locations are not exclusive, however; neuralgia can develop in any part of the body where a nerve has been damaged.

AT-HOME REMEDIES

- ◆ A man suffering from trigeminal neuralgia can grow a beard to shield his face from the cold, which sometimes leads to an attack.
- ◆ An old folk remedy calls for cutting a baked potato in half and applying the cooled halves to an afflicted area to draw out the pain.

PREVENTION

Learning how to sit, stand, and lift for proper back support is the best way to forestall some types of neuralgia. Several different **body work** therapies *(above, left)* can teach you how to move properly to avoid attacks. Consult a trained therapist. ■

NICOTINE WITHDRAWAL

SYMPTOMS

In active tobacco users, a lack of nicotine produces a wide range of withdrawal symptoms, including any or all of the following:

- headache.
- nausea.
- constipation or diarrhea.
- falling heart rate and blood pressure.
- fatigue, drowsiness, and insomnia.
- irritability.
- difficulty concentrating.
- anxiety.
- depression.
- increased hunger and caloric intake.
- increased pleasantness of the taste of sweets.
- tobacco cravings.

CALL YOUR DOCTOR IF:

- you are a tobacco user concerned about your health for any reason; tobacco users are more susceptible to ***respiratory problems; circulatory problems*** such as ***stroke, heart attack,*** and occlusive vascular disorder; and many forms of ***cancer.***
- you want to stop using tobacco; your doctor can prescribe nicotine-based aids and refer you to counseling or to other cessation programs to get you through the withdrawal stage.

Withdrawal from nicotine, an addictive drug found in tobacco, is characterized by symptoms that include headache, anxiety, nausea, and a craving for more tobacco. Nicotine creates a chemical dependency, so that the body develops a need for a certain level of nicotine at all times. Unless that level is maintained, the body will begin to go through withdrawal.

For tobacco users trying to quit, symptoms of withdrawal from nicotine are unpleasant and stressful but temporary. Most withdrawal symptoms peak 48 hours after you quit and are completely gone in six months. But even after that you may still have to deal with the fact that you are probably eating more than you did as a smoker and may need to lose some weight.

CAUSES

The symptoms of nicotine withdrawal are physiological responses to the removal of a substance on which the body has become dependent.

TREATMENT

CONVENTIONAL MEDICINE

A combination of ***smoking cessation drugs*** and behavior modification appears to be the most effective treatment in helping tobacco users, especially smokers, quit.

Your doctor may recommend a smoking (or other tobacco-use) cessation program and may also prescribe nicotine-based chewing gum or a skin patch to help you through withdrawal. Most doctors recommend that patients stop using the gum or patch after a month or two. These aids are meant to help you modify your behavior, not to allow you to maintain your nicotine habit.

ALTERNATIVE CHOICES

Alternative therapies can offer support to tobacco users trying to quit their habit. Behavior modification techniques that may help include **meditation, guided imagery, biofeedback,** and **hypnotherapy.**

ACUPRESSURE

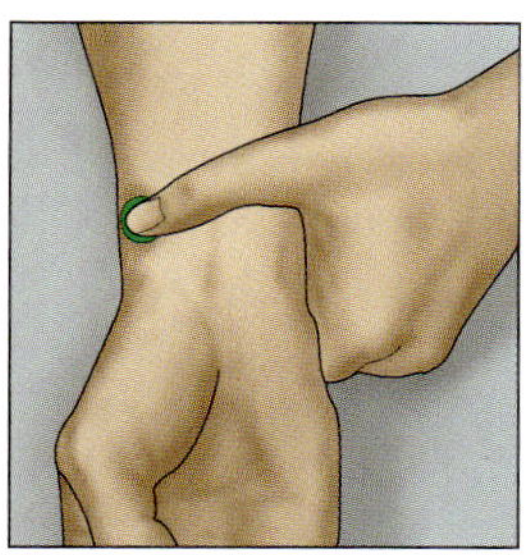

1 To improve lung function after you quit smoking, press Lung 7. Place your left thumb two finger widths above the right wrist crease, along the radius bone, in line with the index finger. Press firmly for one minute, then repeat on the other arm. Do three times.

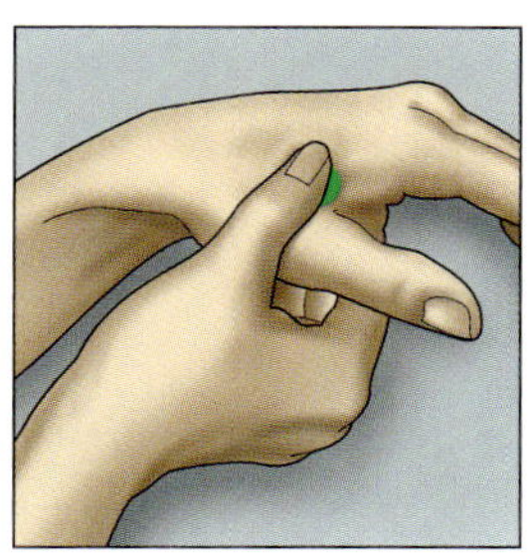

2 Pressing Large Intestine 4, in the web between your thumb and index finger, may ease withdrawal symptoms. Use the thumb and index finger of your right hand to squeeze the web of your left hand for one minute. Repeat on the right hand. Do not use this point if you are pregnant.

ACUPUNCTURE

Acupuncture has been shown to help relieve withdrawal symptoms. Treatment usually involves one to three sessions using points on the ear or the body. Acupuncture may be combined with herbal medicine or other nutritional support but is not appropriate when using the nicotine gum or patch.

Consult a Chinese herbalist or an acupuncturist trained in Chinese herbs for an appropriate course of therapeutic treatment.

HERBAL THERAPIES

Lobelia *(Lobelia inflata)* has actions similar to nicotine but is gentler and longer lasting. It is often used by medical herbalists in conjunction with ***ephedra*** *(Ephedra sinica),* a stimulant, to help tobacco users quit. See a professional; too much of these herbs can cause serious side effects. Herbalists also often recommend herbs to calm the nervous system during withdrawal, including oat *(Avena sativa)* straw, ***chamomile*** *(Matricaria recutita),* ***hops*** *(Humulus lupulus),* and ***valerian*** *(Valeriana officinalis).*

AT-HOME REMEDIES

Most tobacco-use cessation programs offer the following steps to help you quit:

- Analyze your habit for a few weeks; keep a log of when, where, and why you use tobacco.
- List the reasons you want to quit.
- Set a "quit" date and stick to it.
- Find substitutes—sugarless gum to chew or a pen or pencil to hold—and change your routines to avoid triggering a desire for tobacco.
- Reward your resolve. Treat yourself with the money you would have spent on your habit.
- Enjoy your food and eat as much low-calorie food as you want during withdrawal.
- Never let a relapse deter you from continuing your efforts to quit. Former smokers try an average of six times before they quit for good.

PREVENTION

The best preventive step is not to start using tobacco and to educate your children to its dangers. Most tobacco users start in their teens because of peer pressure, a need to rebel, or a desire to appear more mature. Children of tobacco users are more likely to be users because they view tobacco use as acceptable. If you use tobacco and you're serious about preventing your children from doing so, you can provide the best example by quitting.

DON'T SWITCH!

Cigar and pipe smoke have even higher levels of nicotine and carcinogens than cigarette smoke. While most pipe or cigar smokers don't inhale this smoke, research shows that cigarette smokers who switch to cigars and pipes retain their smoking habits, so they inhale even more harmful smoke than before. ■

N

NUMBNESS AND TINGLING

Read down this column to find your symptoms. Then read across.

SYMPTOMS	AILMENT/PROBLEM
◆ numbness or tingling on one side of your body, and one or more of the following: weakness in hands or feet, dizziness, confusion, blurred vision, difficulty speaking.	◆ ***Stroke*** or transient ischemic attack
◆ numbness, tingling, or pain in one arm or one leg, with weakness on that side.	◆ Possible herniated or prolapsed disk
◆ numbness, tingling, or pain in the fingers, hand, or wrist; pain may shoot into the fingers from the wrist.	◆ ***Carpal tunnel syndrome***
◆ tingling in any part of the body; may be accompanied by vision problems, loss of coordination and trembling of one hand, difficulty walking, or loss of bladder control.	◆ ***Multiple sclerosis*** or other neurological ailment
◆ tingling or numbness of the hands or feet, perhaps accompanied by nausea, headache, or dizziness, without underlying disease.	◆ Environmental poisoning/illness
◆ numbness or tingling that you experience in any part of your body while you are taking certain medications or vitamins.	◆ Adverse side effect of a drug
◆ numbness and a bluish color in one or more fingers or toes, quite often triggered by cold.	◆ ***Raynaud's syndrome***
◆ numbness or tingling in your hands and face, especially around your lips, accompanied by shaking, fear, or heart palpitations.	◆ ***Panic attack***
◆ numbness or tingling in a hand, foot, arm, or leg after sitting or sleeping in one position.	◆ Stretching or pressing on a nerve, or decreasing the blood supply to a nerve

WHAT TO DO	OTHER INFO
◆ **Call your doctor now.** Prompt treatment may prevent a full-blown stroke and damage to brain tissue. See also ***Angina; Heart Attack.***	◆ You may be able to prevent a full-blown stroke by lowering your blood pressure, using ***aspirin*** or other drugs to prevent the formation of clots, or having surgery.
◆ See your doctor. Pain may subside when you lie down. See ***Disk Problems.***	◆ Many herniated, or ruptured, disks can be treated with bed rest; sometimes surgery is necessary.
◆ See your doctor. For mild symptoms, a wrist splint may help. Severe symptoms may be corrected surgically.	◆ This syndrome can be caused by repetitive manual tasks. Taking regular breaks and gently rotating the hands help prevent it. Acupuncture may help relieve symptoms; consult a practitioner.
◆ See your doctor. Symptoms may be intermittent in early stages of the disease and hard to diagnose.	◆ Multiple sclerosis destroys the thick myelin sheath that surrounds nerve fibers. Because almost any part of the nervous system may be affected, symptoms may be diverse.
◆ See your doctor, who may suggest tests to check for neurological damage. See ***Environmental Poisoning.***	◆ People most at risk include farmers, environmental and chemical workers, pest exterminators, and people living near industrial plants.
◆ Discuss any medications you are taking with your doctor, who may suggest alternatives.	◆ Such symptoms may be caused by fluoride, ***anesthetics, niacin,*** nitrous oxide, the cancer drug taxol, and ***vitamin*** $\boldsymbol{B_6}$.
◆ Numbness can usually be relieved by warming or rubbing, and normally resolves itself without serious consequences.	◆ Raynaud's may afflict people who work with their hands or are exposed to the cold, or it may have no known cause.
◆ Practice relaxation techniques, including slow, deep breathing; consult your doctor or a psychotherapist for persistent attacks.	◆ The physical effects of panic attacks may be triggered by rapid breathing. Attacks usually subside in a quarter of an hour or less.
◆ Move your limbs around or stand up. Feeling should return to normal in a few moments.	◆ This temporary pins-and-needles feeling is normal and does not indicate an underlying disorder. Daily yoga exercises may release muscle tension and prevent this problem.

OBESITY

SYMPTOMS

- a body-fat percentage greater than 30 percent for women and 25 percent for men. (Your doctor can measure this percentage for you.)
- weighing 20 percent more than your ideal body weight. Your ideal weight is based on your gender, age, and typical activity level (whether you tend to be sedentary or active). Consult your doctor or a nutritionist for an accurate determination of your ideal weight.

CALL YOUR DOCTOR IF:

- you suspect you weigh 20 percent more than your ideal body weight; obesity places you at much greater risk for ***high blood pressure, heart disease, diabetes,*** gallbladder problems, ***respiratory problems,*** and various cancers, including ***breast cancer*** and ***colorectal cancer.***
- you've lost weight many times but always gain it back; you may need professional guidance to develop a long-term, permanent weight-loss program.
- you are overweight and experience a drop in your sex drive, have problems menstruating, or become noticeably hairier; you may suffer from a hormone problem or a tumor on a hormone-secreting gland.

If you consume more calories than you burn, you will gain weight. The tricky part of the equation is that some people metabolize food differently from others. Why this happens is complex and not entirely clear to researchers, who continue to be surprised by each new finding. For example, one recent study concluded that heavy people actually burn calories faster than underweight people because their metabolism speeds up as they put on pounds, and slows if they try to take them off. For obese people—generally defined as those weighing 20 percent more than their ideal weight, or "set point"—the average-sized meal really isn't very filling. Not only do these people have more fat cells sending out signals for food, but their faster metabolism burns more calories as well.

Despite such obstacles, if you are obese, you should make every effort to lose weight. If left unchecked, obesity places you at much greater risk for developing a variety of extremely serious, often life-threatening conditions, from cancer to heart disease. Be particularly concerned if your body tends to store fat around your waist (most common in men). Unlike fat around the thighs, which is more common in women and is more likely to serve as an energy reservoir, abdominal deposits deliver fatty acids directly into the bloodstream for immediate short-term energy; doctors remain uncertain why this can prove to be detrimental to your health.

Unfortunately, many people never take off—and keep off—the extra pounds. According to charts developed by the Metropolitan Life Insurance Company *(see page 37),* which many doctors consider too forgiving, anywhere from a quarter to a third of the adults in the United States are overweight.

A more reliable measuring system, the body mass index (BMI), determines obesity based on body-fat content rather than weight. Determining your body-fat level (something your healthcare practitioner can do for you) is the best way to assess your weight status. For example, you may be the same height and weight as someone considered to be obese, but if you have relatively thick bones and a lot of muscle—and therefore less body fat—you will not merit the same diagnosis.

If you are overweight, you need to realize that you have a lifelong condition that requires not only a special diet and exercise but possibly some counseling and medications to bring under control. Keeping obesity in check requires constant vigilance—no easy task in the high-fat, high-sugar, high-volume nutritional landscape of the United States.

CAUSES

There are many reasons for a person's being obese, including ***diabetes, thyroid problems,*** poor diet, insufficient exercise, and heredity. People with a predisposition to gain weight often aggravate their condition by smoking, drinking alcohol, and leading a sedentary lifestyle. Indeed, watching TV is one of the strongest predictors of obesity. If you are obese, the key is to recognize that you have a disease and to avoid habits that aggravate it.

While most cases of obesity are related to family history, social environment, diet, and other lifestyle habits, there are rare instances in which something specific, such as a thyroid condition, is the cause. Certain drugs, in particular ***estrogens and progestins, insulin,*** and steroids, can also cause weight gain.

In addition to all these factors, a recent study showed that muscles as well as fat cells play a role in obesity. Doctors have long recognized that fat cells in your body increase in size and mass when you put on weight. What they have just learned is that your muscles become more efficient and burn fewer calories when you try to lose that weight, which helps account for your slowed metabolism.

TREATMENT

Weight-loss programs are a billion-dollar business in the U.S., with more overweight people signing up to drop pounds (only to regain them later) every day. Unfortunately, many of these commercial enterprises follow the cultural view that obesity results from some moral inadequacy, that fat people could lose weight if they would just exercise a little will power; but research shows that the answer is nowhere near that simple. Strong biochemical and genetic forces come into play every time any of us approaches a plate of food. Lack of will power has little to do with how your body will eventually process what you eat or how it will respond when you are full.

As knowledge of obesity's causes changes, so do the treatments. For now, most conventional and alternative therapies focus on diet, exercise, and possible psychological complications.

THE DANGERS OF HIGH BODY FAT

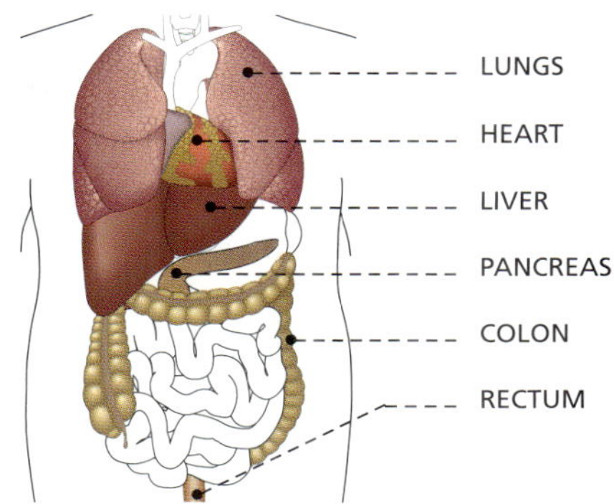

Substantial excess body fat may cause serious health problems. Extra pounds put great strain on the cardiovascular system, contributing to high blood pressure and heart disease, while high fat concentrations can enlarge the liver. Even moderate weight gain can trigger Type 2 diabetes, in which body tissues become resistant to insulin produced by the pancreas. Obesity also increases the risk of colorectal cancer.

CONVENTIONAL MEDICINE

When it comes to obesity, the only thing everyone agrees on is that exercise is crucial to any weight-loss program. One study found that 95 percent of patients on a weight-loss diet regained the pounds they had lost if they did not include exercise as part of their overall program. Other factors, such as the fat and fiber content of your diet, also play a major role, but nothing is as important as exercise.

Indeed, you can conscientiously shun calories but never lose the fat. A key reason for the uphill battle: As you reduce the number of calories you consume, your body reacts in ways that evolved hundreds of thousands of years ago as defense mechanisms. It assumes that you are starving and as a result raises all sorts of barriers to protect against weight loss, including slowing down metabolism and storing energy more efficiently. As you try to lose weight, then, your body does all it can to keep the weight on.

If you are obese, you must think in terms of permanent change rather than short-term dieting, because you have a permanent problem. Consult your doctor about determining a good general target for your caloric intake and then maintain that level; a low-fat, low-sugar, high-fiber diet will help you achieve your goal. Artificial sweeteners such as aspartame decrease the amount of calories in food, and olestra reduces the fat intake of certain foods. However, these food supplements may cause immune related illness; consult with your doctor about the risks. Add an exercise program to your weekly routine; something as simple as a 30-minute walk at lunch can be very effective. There is some evidence that a long-term, strict regimen of regular exercise and a moderate, low-fat diet can permanently lower your set point, making it easier for you to sustain a lower weight.

In some instances your doctor may recommend that you supplement your lifestyle and dietary changes with a drug that suppresses appetite. The most popular options include ***ephedrine,*** which affects metabolism by stimulating the nervous system; sibutramine, which suppresses appetite; orlistat, which blocks fat absorption; and ***fluoxetine,*** an antidepressant that has also been found to suppress appetite.

People desperate to lose weight are easy targets for hucksters who plug a whole host of useless remedies, from amphetamines and thyroid supplements to topical creams that purport to melt away fat. To be on the safe side, always consult with your doctor before you try any over-the-counter or mail-order weight-loss medication.

On rare occasions a doctor may suggest a surgical procedure that essentially shrinks the stomach. Only motivated, healthy patients benefit from this therapy, which has many critics. It does remove the need for appetite suppressants, but research has yet to show whether patients manage to keep weight off for the long term.

Two much simpler techniques, liposuction and jaw wiring, also have many drawbacks and should rarely if ever be considered. To perform liposuction, the surgeon makes a small incision near fatty deposits and then suctions the fat out. Very little fat can be removed, however, because of potential risks to blood vessels and nerves.

Jaw wiring can damage gums and teeth and cause muscle spasms in the jaw joint. The liquid diet that such patients must eat does result in weight loss, but as soon as the wires are removed patients almost always put back on what they lost.

The best treatment skirts these more extreme approaches and attacks obesity on several levels, including a psychological one. Learning to control what you eat, how you react to food in general, and what you do in your free time (watching television versus taking a walk) will do more for you than any surgeon's knife. Consider seeing a professional nutritionist, an exercise therapist, and possibly, a counselor if you believe you have an unhealthy attitude toward food.

ALTERNATIVE CHOICES

Most alternative therapies work well when used to complement an existing program of proper diet and exercise.

ACUPRESSURE

Some food addicts have found that use of a press needle or a plastic device placed over certain acupressure points on the ear helps alleviate cravings. Consult a practitioner familiar with treating eating disorders.

CHINESE MEDICINE

The Chinese herb ***ephedra*** *(Ephedra sinica)* contains ephedrine, which increases the metabolic rate in fat tissue. Be aware that this treatment can have potent side effects, including insomnia, anxiety, heart arrhythmias, and hypertension. Do not use it if you have diabetes, thyroid problems, or heart disease, and do not take this herb for a long period of time. For best results see a practitioner of Chinese medicine, who will work on regulating all of your organs, especially the spleen.

HERBAL THERAPIES

To stimulate your metabolic rate, try ***kelp*** (*Fucus* spp.) in tablet form three to four times a day; it is thought to be especially good for thyroid-related obesity, though you should consult your physician first. ***Dandelion*** *(Taraxacum officinale)* may flush out the kidneys, boost metabolism, and offset a craving for sweets. Eat the leaves raw in a salad or make a tea by boiling 2 to 3 tsp of the root in a cup of water for 10 to 15 minutes. Drink three times a day.

HOMEOPATHY

Homeopathy offers treatments for various aspects of obesity. For example, many over-the-counter mixtures contain *Argentum nitricum,* which may cure intense sugar cravings. If your weight does not improve in one to two months after beginning at-home homeopathic treatment, see a professional.

LIFESTYLE

Smoking provides an excellent example of how a predisposition toward obesity can lure a person into an unhealthy lifestyle. Studies show that overweight teenage girls are more apt to smoke and are less responsive to programs designed to help them quit because they think cigarettes keep their weight down. While smoking does suppress appetite, it also adversely affects fat storage, leading to more deposits in the waist area. Overweight people also tend to drink alcohol more, adding to their caloric intake; alcohol is processed in the body much like fatty foods.

MIND/BODY MEDICINE

Hypnotherapy, guided imagery, and **yoga** may help with weight loss by altering the way you relate to food. Check with a specialist in these techniques.

NUTRITION AND DIET

A diet of complex carbohydrates, such as potatoes and pasta, as well as chicken, fish, and plenty of vegetables, should fill you up without filling you out.

Consider eating your main meal in the middle of the day, when you will burn off more of the calories you take in; a large meal eaten at night, when you are more sedentary, is less easily digested and absorbed.

Replace daily consumption of soft drinks, fruit juices, and milk with six to eight glasses of water.

Avoid diets that count calories. The grueling routine of such a diet increases your risk for developing eating disorders such as ***anorexia nervosa*** and ***bulimia.***

Always keep in mind that you cannot shed pounds unless your energy output exceeds your energy input.

AT-HOME REMEDIES

Certain at-home remedies can help with some side effects associated with obesity, such as constipation.

- 1 to 2 tsp a day of brewer's yeast or some ***dandelion*** will reduce a craving for sweets. Bee pollen or a dash of ***cayenne*** *(Capsicum frutescens)* may increase your metabolism.
- A tea made from rhubarb root may alleviate constipation.

PREVENTION

If you stick to a moderate, low-fat diet and an exercise routine for several years, you may actually lower your set point. Once your body accepts the lower weight as your natural state, it will be much easier for you to sustain it without dieting. Some helpful tips to avoid obesity:

- Eat three or four moderate meals a day, with your main meal in the middle of the day.
- Eat a high-fiber, low-fat diet.
- Avoid sedentary activities, such as watching television, and get into a regular exercise routine.
- Don't turn to calorie-counting diets or diets that require you to fast or deprive yourself of normal helpings of food for extended periods of time.
- Avoid using food as a reward for yourself. ■

OBSESSIVE-COMPULSIVE DISORDER

SYMPTOMS

You may have obsessive thoughts or compulsive behavior or both.

For obsession:

- involuntary and persistent thoughts that appear to be senseless, such as an overwhelming fear of dirt; persistent worry about a past event.
- attempts to suppress such thoughts.
- recognition that these thoughts come from one's own imagination, not from outside factors (not true for children).

For compulsions:

- repetitive acts such as hand washing, checking and rechecking locks, tidying, repeating words.
- recognition that the repetitive behavior is excessive or unreasonable (may not be true for children).
- feverish levels of thought or activity.
- ***depression*** and distress as attempts to deal with compulsions fail.

For children:

- mute behavior with agitated depression.
- withdrawal and social isolation accompanied by delusional thinking.
- mood swings from anxiety to despair.
- exemplary functioning in sports or schoolwork accompanied by compulsive behavior.

CALL YOUR DOCTOR IF:

- you or your child is experiencing some of the symptoms listed above.
- your child is anxious or depressed and has fears of aggression, sexual behavior, contamination, or disorderliness.

Obsessive-compulsive disorder (OCD) is not the ordinary "double-checking" that all of us do from time to time—making sure the doors are locked or the oven is off. For OCD patients these thoughts are so magnified that they interfere with everyday routines, jobs, and relationships. Sufferers have been known to wash their hands for eight hours or to reorganize their entire household daily. Obsessive-compulsive disorder is chronic and cannot be controlled voluntarily. Even after long periods of relative normality, sufferers may have another attack without apparent cause.

Because obsession takes hold gradually—moving slowly from simple interest to brooding to complete preoccupation—people often fail to recognize that they are suffering from a disorder. When OCD eventually produces symptoms that interfere with daily life, patients may try to hide their compulsions from others and attempt to deal with them by using will power.

Although OCD can appear in childhood, onset most often occurs in adolescence; half of adult sufferers show some symptoms by the age of 15. In the United States, between 2 percent and 3 percent of the population experiences some form of OCD during their lives. Obsessive-compulsive features are also found in Tourette's syndrome *(see* ***Tics and Twitches****)*, ***depression,*** and ***schizophrenia.***

CAUSES

At one time, obsessive or compulsive behavior was thought to indicate demonic possession, with exorcism one of the earliest forms of treatment. Currently, some 20 different theories exist on what might cause obsessive-compulsive disorder. The traditional hypothesis from Freudian thought holds that obsessions reflect unconscious desires from an earlier stage of development (anal stage). Although some experts in psychology still support the Freudian hypothesis, the most widely held theory today suggests that there is a genetic predisposition to OCD and that it is triggered by low levels of one of the brain's neurotransmitters, serotonin.

DIAGNOSTIC AND TEST PROCEDURES

Often, the patients' own descriptions of their behavior offer the best clues. A family history is also important, to evaluate whether there is any genetic predisposition. Your doctor will also want to rule out other psychological disorders, such as schizophrenia, that can produce similar patterns of behavior.

TREATMENT

The goal of treatment is to reduce ***anxiety,*** resolve inner conflicts, and help you learn more effective ways of dealing with anxiety. Conventional treatment may include psychotherapy or behavior therapy, ***antidepressants,*** and stress-reduction techniques. Drugs combined with behavior therapy seem to bring the best results.

CONVENTIONAL MEDICINE

An effective antiobsessional drug is the ***tricyclic antidepressant*** clomipramine. Studies have shown that clomipramine, which increases serotonin levels in the brain, produces a 30 to 60 percent reduction in symptoms in adults and a 70 to 80 percent reduction in children. Other ***antidepressants*** that have demonstrated good results with fewer side effects are the ***selective serotonin reuptake inhibitors (SSRIs),*** such as ***fluoxetine,*** fluvoxamine, ***paroxetine,*** and ***sertraline.*** For proper drug choices and dosages, consult a psychiatrist trained in anxiety disorders.

Behavior therapy emphasizes changing a specific behavior—such as compulsive cleaning—by stopping what has been triggering it or by replacing it with a more desirable response. According to some anecdotal evidence, 60 to 70 percent of OCD patients are "much improved" after brief treatment with behavior therapy. For children, family therapy is important.

ALTERNATIVE CHOICES

Alternative therapies are helpful both for relieving the anxiety of OCD and for diminishing the compulsions themselves. **Massage** is useful for reducing the physical rigidity in the neck, shoulders, and back that many OCD patients suffer. By loosening the musculature, massage relieves anxiety and reduces the urgency of compulsions. Exercises of all kinds, particularly those such as **yoga** that stretch and flex many of the body's muscles, do much the same thing.

BIOFEEDBACK

Because obsession and compulsion are often the mind's way of controlling such feelings as anxiety, anger, or sadness, helping the brain reduce the intensity of these feelings reduces the OCD itself. Studies have shown that EEG (brain-wave) biofeedback (also known as neurotherapy) is a good tool for reducing the intensity of unwanted feelings. Between 30 and 60 EEG-biofeedback training sessions are needed to treat OCD effectively, but the sessions may bring about permanent change, and this technique has the advantage of giving patients control over their treatment. *(See **Health Associations and Organizations** in the **Appendix** for more information.)*

HOMEOPATHY

Homeopathic practitioners have specific prescriptions for OCD, which can be tailored to the individual. Among the remedies that may be used by an experienced homeopath are ***Arsenicum album,*** *Hyoscyamus, Medorrhinum,* ***Nux vomica,*** and ***Pulsatilla.***

MIND/BODY MEDICINE

Many mind/body practices may help relieve the anxiety associated with OCD. **Meditation** and other **relaxation** techniques such as progressive muscle relaxation, **yoga, t'ai chi,** and **qigong** all may be helpful. Find one or two you prefer and use them daily.

Since anxiety is almost always accompanied by shallow breathing, deep-breathing exercises are very helpful. *(See **Anxiety** for yoga breathing.)* Alternate nostril breathing, which specifically is thought to stimulate different areas of the brain, is also good for relieving anxiety. ■

O

ORAL CANCER

SYMPTOMS

A whitish or velvety red patch of tissue instead of normal pink membrane in the oral cavity may signal a potential precancerous condition. If left untreated, the discolored patch may grow and begin to feel like a ***canker sore.*** The symptoms of oral cancer may include:

- a persistent lump, sore, or thickening along the side or bottom of the tongue, on the floor of the mouth, inside the cheeks, or on the gums, palate, or roof of the mouth; the lump may eventually bleed or become ulcerated.
- discomfort while eating, drinking, or swallowing.
- loose teeth, or ***toothache*** or ***earache*** that does not respond to conventional treatment.
- a swollen lymph node in the neck.

Symptoms associated with advanced oral cancer include pain in the ear or roof of the mouth, unexplained spasms in facial or neck muscles, or persistent bad breath.

CALL YOUR DOCTOR IF:

- you have persistent hoarseness, soreness, or a sensation of something lodged in your throat. You may have ***throat cancer.***
- you feel persistent and inexplicable discomfort in your mouth or ear. The pain may very well stem from something other than cancer, but the cause should be determined in any event.

Oral cancer refers to all cancers of the oral cavity—the lips, tongue, cheeks, mouth, gums, and oropharynx, or upper part of the throat. These tumors almost always arise in the flat, squamous cells that line the pink membrane of the oral cavity and throat. Although oral cancer may spread through the head and neck, it seldom spreads farther.

Oral cancer sometimes evolves from other oral conditions: **Erythroplakia,** which is signaled by a velvety red patch of tissue inside the mouth, is always considered precancerous. **Leukoplakia,** characterized by whitish tissue, is sometimes precancerous. Both erythroplakia and leukoplakia are strongly associated with alcohol and tobacco use—as are the overwhelming majority of oral cancers.

Like any cancer, oral cancer is most treatable if detected early. Fortunately, you can often feel suspicious tissue changes that may signal oral cancer. The overall five-year survival rate for oral cancer is more than 50 percent; when treated early, 9 out of 10 patients survive more than five years, and most are cured permanently.

CAUSES

The role of alcohol and tobacco—including chewing tobacco—in causing oral cancer cannot be overemphasized. People who use both substances regularly are 35 times more likely to get oral cancer than people who use neither. The disease usually affects tissue that is already irritated by jagged teeth, ill-fitting dentures, or habitual chewing on the inside of the cheek. Iron deficiency has been linked to tongue cancer in women, while excessive exposure to sunlight causes some types of lip cancer. People treated for oral cancer who continue to smoke and drink are very likely to develop the disease again.

DIAGNOSTIC AND TEST PROCEDURES

Routine examination of the mouth by you, your dentist, or your doctor will improve the chance of detecting oral cancer early. In the event of a suspicious abnormality, a doctor will do a biopsy

CANCER IN THE ORAL CAVITY

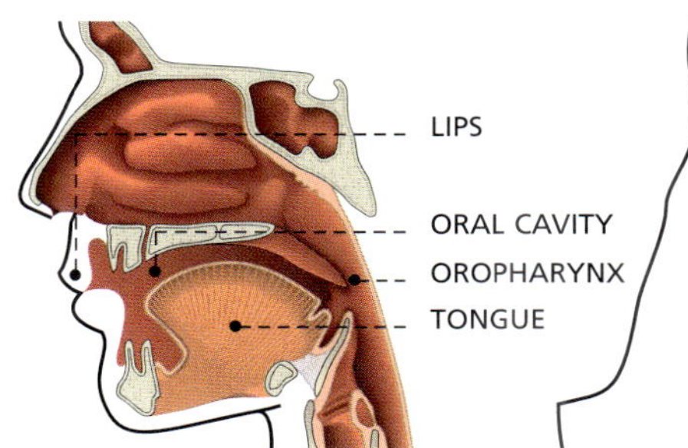

Cancerous cells can develop on the lips and anywhere in the mouth—on the gums, cheeks, tongue, or oropharynx, directly behind the mouth. Most oral cancers emerge from squamous cells that line the inside of the mouth, and usually the cancer does not spread beyond the head and neck. You should have a doctor check any small, pale bump or thickened, discolored tissue that doesn't go away or recurs after other treatment.

by taking a small tissue sample from your mouth, or fluid from swollen lymph nodes in your neck, to examine under a microscope. X-rays or other imaging tests may be needed to identify a primary tumor that is not readily apparent or to establish the extent of spread in an existing cancer.

TREATMENT

CONVENTIONAL MEDICINE

Small oral cancers respond equally well to either surgery or radiation therapy; advanced cancers are treated with both and sometimes with chemotherapy to relieve symptoms. For recurrent cancer, radiation therapy is the primary treatment. Laser surgery or cryosurgery—freezing cells with liquid nitrogen—can kill small tumors without affecting mouth function or the patient's looks. If significant amounts of tissue or bone are removed, reconstructive surgery may be needed. In such cases, patients must adjust to their new appearance and relearn basic chewing, swallowing, and speaking skills. Since postoperative radiation and chemotherapy typically suppress normal saliva production and may injure healthy mouth tissue, most patients must take extra measures to deter gum and tooth decay during and after treatment. *(See **Cancer** for more information about therapies.)*

COMPLEMENTARY THERAPIES

For cancer, there is no acceptable alternative to conventional medical care. Other approaches can complement, but not replace, standard treatment.

NUTRITION AND DIET

High doses of ***vitamin A*** may protect against onset and recurrence of oral cancer. Vitamin A is toxic in high doses, so take supplements only under a doctor's supervision. You can also eat plenty of fresh fruits and vegetables as healthy sources of carotenoids—dietary precursors of vitamin A—and ***vitamin E,*** which also may be protective.

AT-HOME CARE

During radiation therapy, you may have difficulty opening your mouth, keeping your mouth moist with saliva, and brushing your teeth. Try gentle stretching exercises, drinking iced beverages, rinsing frequently, and using a soft toothbrush. For a gentle, effective mouthwash, try ***aloe*** *(Aloe barbadensis)* juice or cool ***chamomile*** *(Matricaria recutita)* tea. To combat dry mouth and restore natural saliva, rinse your mouth with an acidophilus solution, available at most health food stores. Swish the solution in your mouth, then swallow it, several times a day.

PREVENTION

Don't smoke or chew tobacco. Drink alcohol only moderately. If you wear dentures, be sure they fit properly. Use sunscreen to protect your lips. Eat fresh fruits and vegetables daily. If you are diagnosed with a potentially precancerous oral condition, have your doctor monitor it carefully. ■

O

OSTEOPOROSIS

SYMPTOMS

Osteoporosis is usually asymptomatic until a fracture occurs.

- backache.
- a gradual loss of height and an accompanying stooped posture.
- fractures of the spine, wrists, or hips.
- loss of bone in the jaw *(see below).*

CALL YOUR DOCTOR IF:

- you develop a backache or a sudden severe back pain, which can indicate a spinal compression fracture caused by osteoporosis.
- dental x-rays reveal a loss of bone in the jaw, which can be an early sign of osteoporosis.

Osteoporosis, which means "porous bones," is a condition that causes formerly strong bones to gradually thin and weaken, leaving them susceptible to fractures. In the United States about 1.3 million fractures are attributed to osteoporosis each year. Although all bones are affected by the disease, those of the spine, hip, and wrist are most likely to break. In elderly people hip fractures can be particularly dangerous, because the prolonged immobility required during the healing process often leads to ***blood clots*** or ***pneumonia.*** About a third of elderly women with hip fractures die within six months.

Of the estimated 24 million Americans afflicted with osteoporosis, at least 80 percent are women. Experts believe women are more susceptible because their bones tend to be lighter and thinner, and because their bodies experience hormonal changes after menopause that appear to accelerate the loss of bone mass. In men osteoporosis is uncommon until after the age of 70.

CAUSES

Although the exact cause of osteoporosis is unknown, the process by which the bone becomes porous is well understood. Normally, 6 to 12 percent of an adult's total skeleton is replaced each year, a process known as bone remodeling. After skeletal mass peaks—usually around the age of 35—bones begin to lose calcium, the mineral that makes them hard, faster than they can replace it. Less remodeling takes place and the bones begin to thin. For women the loss of bone density speeds up during the first three to seven years after menopause and then slows down again. Scientists believe that this rapid postmenopausal increase in bone loss is caused by a sharp decline in the body's production of estrogen, which appears to help keep calcium in the bones.

Although some loss of bone density is a natural part of aging, certain women are at higher risk than others for developing the very porous bones and the fractures associated with osteoporosis. Women who are small boned, thin, and fair haired, for example, are at higher risk, as are those who smoke, drink more than moderately, or

AT-HOME CALCIUM ABSORPTION TEST

To determine whether the calcium in your supplement tablets is easily absorbed by your body, try this test: Drop a tablet into 6 ounces of vinegar at room temperature. Stir every 2 to 3 minutes. The tablet should disintegrate within 30 minutes. If it does not, try another supplement.

live a sedentary lifestyle. Women with a family history of osteoporosis and those who have had their ovaries removed, especially before age 40, are also more prone to the condition. White and Asian women are more frequently affected than black women. Research has also indicated that women whose hair turns more than 50 percent gray before age 40 are four times as likely to develop osteoporosis as those whose hair doesn't.

Certain conditions that impair the body's ability to absorb calcium, such as ***kidney disease,*** Cushing's syndrome, and hyperthyroidism *(see **Thyroid Problems**)*, can also lead to osteoporosis, as can surgical removal of part of the stomach or intestine and excessive use of glucocorticoids, other steroids, or ***anticonvulsant drugs.*** Prolonged immobility because of paralysis or illness can cause calcium loss and thus, eventually, bone loss.

DIAGNOSTIC AND TEST PROCEDURES

If your doctor suspects you have osteoporosis, he may measure you to check for a loss of height. The vertebrae are often the first bones affected, causing a loss in height of half an inch or more.

Your doctor may also recommend that your bone density be measured. Although osteoporosis is sometimes diagnosed incidentally after an x-ray has been taken for a fracture or an illness, an ordinary x-ray does not reveal bone loss until at least 20 to 30 percent of the bone mass has disappeared, limiting its usefulness for early screening of the condition. Diagnostic tools more likely to catch osteoporosis at an early stage include various forms of a technique called absorptiometry, which is specifically designed to measure bone density. A relatively new diagnostic tool known as quantitative computerized tomography is also an accurate method of measuring bone density anywhere in the body, but it uses higher levels of radiation than the other methods.

In addition to these bone measurement tests, you may be asked to supply blood or urine samples for analysis so that disease-related causes for the bone loss can be ruled out.

TREATMENT

Because osteoporosis is difficult to reverse, prevention is the key to treatment. Both conventional and alternative medicine offer effective preventive measures for the condition.

CONVENTIONAL MEDICINE

To prevent osteoporosis or to slow its progression, many doctors recommend hormone replacement therapy (HRT)—either ***estrogen*** alone or a combination of estrogen and progesterone—to postmenopausal women. Studies have shown that women who take long-term HRT within a few years of menopause keep their bone density and have fewer hip and wrist fractures while they are taking it than women who do not. HRT does not build new bone; it only slows the loss of existing bone, and this effect disappears after age 75, when most dangerous fractures occur. Once the hormone treatment is discontinued, the bone begins to thin again—at the same pace as at menopause. Women who take HRT for osteoporosis, therefore, must continue it indefinitely to help keep their bones from thinning. Because HRT has been associated with an increased risk of serious health problems, most notably ***uterine*** and ***breast cancers,*** many doctors recommend the treatment only for women at high risk of osteoporosis.

An alternative to HRT are the osteoporosis treatment drugs raloxifine, alendronate, and cal-

O

citonin. Raloxifine has estrogen's beneficial effects on bone, without the increased risk of breast and uterine cancer associated with estrogen. Alendronate increases bone mass and may help prevent osteoporosis; however, this drug may also cause heartburn. Calcitonin, available as a nasal spray, treats osteoporosis and vertebral fractures, though it is not as effective in treating the long bones of your arms and legs. Consult with your doctor about which regimen is best for you.

As a preventive measure your doctor may suggest that you increase the amount of calcium in your diet or perhaps take ***calcium*** supplements. To help with the absorption of the calcium, ***vitamin D*** supplements may also be recommended unless you live in a sunny climate. Your doctor may also encourage you to begin a regular exercise program to keep your bones strong and free of fractures. *(For more information, see **Nutrition and Diet,** right, and **Exercise,** below.)*

ALTERNATIVE CHOICES

Like conventional techniques, alternative therapies focus on building and retaining strong bones.

CHINESE HERBS

Chinese practitioners recommend several herbs for preventing bone loss, most notably ***dong quai*** *(Angelica sinensis)* and ***Asian ginseng*** *(Panax ginseng),* which appear to have estrogen-like effects in the body. Consult a practitioner experienced in Chinese herbal medicine for appropriate dosages.

EXERCISE

Studies have shown that weight-bearing exercises—those that put stress on bones, such as running, walking, tennis, ballet, stair climbing, **yoga,** aerobics, and weightlifting—reduce bone loss and help prevent osteoporosis. To benefit from the exercise, you must do it at least three times per week for 30 to 45 minutes. Swimming and bicycle riding, although good cardiovascular exercises, do not appear to prevent osteoporosis because they do not put enough stress on bones.

HERBAL THERAPIES

Although acknowledging that herbal therapies cannot cure osteoporosis, herbalists believe that the use of some herbs can help slow the progression of the condition. Herbs traditionally used for the prevention of osteoporosis include ***horsetail*** *(Equisetum arvense),* ***alfalfa*** *(Medicago sativa),* ***licorice*** *(Glycyrrhiza glabra),* ***marsh mallow*** *(Althaea officinalis),* and sourdock *(Rumex crispus).* Take daily in tea or tincture form. Ask an herbalist about progesterone creams made from the wild Mexican yam; they may stimulate bone formation.

HOMEOPATHY

In addition to a calcium-rich diet and exercise, homeopaths recommend treatments they believe help the body absorb calcium. Remedies are likely to include ***Calcarea carbonica,*** *Calcarea phosphorica, Calcarea fluorica,* and ***Silica.*** Consult a homeopath for remedies and dosages.

NUTRITION AND DIET

To ensure that women get enough calcium to build and maintain strong bones, both alternative and conventional practitioners recommend eating plenty of calcium-rich foods, such as nonfat milk, low-fat yogurt, broccoli, cauliflower, salmon, tofu, and leafy green vegetables. According to a panel convened by the National Institutes of Health, women who are still menstruating or who are postmenopausal but taking hormone replacement therapy should consume 1,000 mg of calcium each day. Postmenopausal women who are not being treated with estrogen should get 1,500 mg daily. (One glass of nonfat milk provides only 300 mg of calcium.)

Because most women take in through their diet only half or a third as much calcium as they need, some practitioners recommend calcium supplements to make up the difference. Calcium supplements are available in many forms, but chelated forms, such as calcium citrate and calcium gluconate, appear to be more effective at reducing bone loss. *(See **At-Home Calcium Absorption Test** on page 637.)* Avoid using dolomite or bone meal as calcium supplements or calcium carbonate supplements labeled "oyster shell," as they may contain lead and other toxic metals.

To help the body absorb calcium, some practitioners suggest taking ***vitamin D*** (400 to 800 IU) and ***magnesium*** (250 to 350 mg) supplements. A veal bone supplement that provides calcium and trace minerals is sometimes prescribed as well.

CAUTION: Calcium supplements can inhibit the absorption of salicylates, ***tetracycline,*** and other medications. Check with your practitioner before beginning a supplementation program.

In addition to eating calcium-rich foods you should also avoid phosphorus-rich ones, which can promote bone loss. High-phosphorus foods include red meats, soft drinks, and those with phosphate food additives. Indeed, several studies have indicated that vegetarians tend to have denser bones later in life than meat eaters, although other studies have shown no such difference. Excessive amounts of alcohol and caffeine are also thought to reduce the amount of calcium absorbed by the body and should be avoided.

To help keep estrogen levels from dropping precipitously after menopause and thus help prevent osteoporosis, some alternative practitioners advise postmenopausal women to consume more foods containing plant estrogens, especially tofu, soybean milk, and other soy products.

AT-HOME REMEDIES

Here are two easy ways of increasing the amount of calcium in your diet:

- Add nonfat dry milk to everyday foods and beverages, including soups, stews, and casseroles. Each teaspoon of dry milk adds about 20 mg of calcium to your diet.
- Add a little vinegar to the water you use to make soup stock from bones. The vinegar will dissolve some of the calcium out of the bones, for a calcium-fortified soup. A pint can contain as much as 1,000 mg of calcium.

PREVENTION

- Eat foods rich in calcium, such as nonfat milk, low-fat yogurt, broccoli, cauliflower, salmon, tofu, sesame seeds, almonds, and leafy green vegetables.
- Eat foods that contain plant estrogens, especially tofu and other soy products.
- Avoid high fat, high protein foods that can interfere with your body's absorption of calcium, such as red meats, carbonated drinks, and excessive amounts of alcohol and caffeine.
- Do weight-bearing exercises for 30 to 45 minutes at least three times a week.
- Do not smoke. Some studies have shown that women who smoke increase their risk of developing osteoporosis by 50 percent.
- Avoid ***antacids*** containing aluminum, as they can prevent calcium absorption by binding with phosphorus in the intestines.

ASSESS YOUR RISK

To help determine whether you are at risk for osteoporosis, ask yourself the following questions. The more "yes" answers, the greater your risk.

- *Is there a history in your family of osteoporosis and hip fractures?*
- *Have you had both of your ovaries removed, especially before age 40?*
- *Are you small boned or slender?*
- *Are you light complexioned?*
- *Did your hair turn 50 percent or more gray before you turned 40?*
- *Do you lead a sedentary lifestyle?*
- *Do you smoke?*
- *Has your diet been low in calcium-rich foods?*
- *Do you drink two or more alcoholic beverages a day?*
- *Do you drink more than 24 ounces of carbonated soft drinks a day?*
- *Do you drink more than two cups of caffeinated coffee a day?*
- *Do you eat red meat and other high-protein foods frequently?*
- *Are you taking* ***corticosteroids?***
- *Have you been on long-term thyroid medications?* ■

O

OTITIS MEDIA

SYMPTOMS

In adults:

- ***earache*** (either a sharp, sudden pain or a dull, continuous pain).
- fever and chills.
- nasal congestion.
- feeling of fullness in the ear.
- nausea and diarrhea accompanying earache.
- muffled hearing.

In children:

- tugging at the ear.
- fever.
- irritability, restlessness.
- nasal discharge.
- diminished appetite.
- crying at night when lying down.

CALL YOUR DOCTOR IF:

- body temperature rises above 101°F or 102°F; a fever signals the possibility of a more serious infection.
- you or your child frequently develops otitis media; repeated bouts with the disorder can lead to hearing loss or more serious infections.
- you or your child has hearing problems; the infection may be affecting the ability to hear.
- you suspect that your young child has otitis media; it's often difficult for a parent to tell if a child has trouble hearing.

Otitis media, sometimes referred to simply as an ear infection or inflammation, is the most common cause of ***earaches.*** Although this condition is a frequent cause of infant distress and is often associated with children, it can also affect adults. Otitis media is an infection of the middle ear, whose tiny bones pick up vibrations from the eardrum and pass them along to the inner ear. But very often, otitis media accompanies a ***common cold,*** the ***flu,*** or another type of respiratory infection. This is because the middle ear is connected to the upper respiratory tract by a pair of tiny conduits known as Eustachian tubes.

Most parents are frustratingly familiar with otitis media. Except for wellness baby visits, ear infections are the most common reason for trips to the pediatrician, accounting for 30 million doctor visits a year in the United States. Today, almost half of all ***antibiotic*** prescriptions written for children are for otitis media, and the cost of treating middle ear infections in the U.S. is estimated at $2 billion a year. Untreated, otitis media can lead to more serious complications, including mastoiditis (a rare inflammation of a bone adjacent to the ear), hearing loss, perforation of the eardrum, ***meningitis,*** facial nerve paralysis, and possibly ***Ménière's disease.***

CAUSES

Cells in the middle ear manufacture a fluid that, among other things, helps keep out invading organisms. Normally, the fluid drains out through the Eustachian tube and into the throat. But if the Eustachian tube becomes swollen, the fluid can become trapped in the middle ear, causing the area to become inflamed and infected. This tube lies in a more horizontal position and is shorter in children, which may put them at even greater risk of infection. To the physician, the eardrum of an infected patient appears red and bulging.

The most common cause of otitis media is an upper respiratory viral infection, such as a cold or the flu. These disorders can make the Eustachian tube so swollen that middle ear fluid cannot escape. Allergies—to pollen, dust, animal dander, or food—can produce the same effect, as can smoke, fumes, as well as other environmental toxins.

Bacteria can cause otitis media directly, but usually these organisms come on the heels of a viral infection or an allergic reaction, quickly finding their way into the warm, moist environment of the middle ear. Invading bacteria can wreak major havoc, turning inflammation into infection and provoking fevers. Among the bacteria most often found in infected middle ears are the same varieties responsible for ***sinusitis, pneumonia,*** and other upper respiratory infections. (Note: Flu shots do not offer protection from otitis media.)

Otitis media occurs in various degrees of severity. A single, isolated case that is easily cured is called acute otitis media. If the condition clears up but comes back as many as three times in a six-month period (or four times in a single year), it is known as recurrent otitis media. If it continues for weeks without clearing up, it is called chronic otitis media. A fluid buildup in the ear without infection is termed serous otitis media.

In recent years, scientists have identified the characteristics of people most likely to suffer recurrent middle ear infections: males, individuals with a family history of ear infections, babies who are bottle-fed (breast-fed babies get fewer ear infections), children in day-care centers; Native Americans and Australian Aborigines, people living in households with tobacco smokers, and people with poor or damaged immune systems.

MIDDLE EAR INFECTION

Excess fluid in the middle ear normally drains harmlessly into the throat via the Eustachian tube. But if this tiny conduit becomes infected—perhaps by the same organisms that bring on a cold or the flu—it can swell shut, trapping fluid in the middle ear and promoting further infection. This fluid buildup causes painful pressure that, without proper treatment, can eventually burst the eardrum.

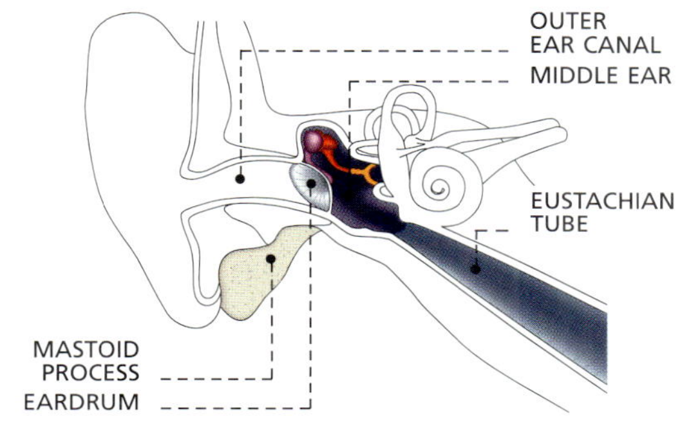

DIAGNOSTIC AND TEST PROCEDURES

If you or your child has an earache accompanied by a stuffy or runny nose, sore throat, and fever, chances are good that the problem is otitis media. Your doctor will most likely examine the eardrum with an instrument called an otoscope for signs of infection—not an easy task if the patient is a fussy infant.

To check for a bacterial infection, the doctor may make an opening in the eardrum, draw out a sample of fluid from the affected middle ear, then culture the sample in a laboratory dish. This more extreme measure is usually used only for serious or particularly stubborn infections.

TREATMENT

The goal of most doctors and therapists is to rid the middle ear of infection before more serious complications set in. Treatment usually involves eliminating the causes of otitis media, killing any invading bacteria, boosting the immune system, and reducing swelling in the Eustachian tubes.

CONVENTIONAL MEDICINE

Otitis media is typically caused by a viral infection, in which case the only relief doctors can offer is treatment of the symptoms. This may involve trying to reduce swelling in the Eustachian tubes with a ***decongestant,*** such as ***pseudoephedrine,*** and an ***antihistamine,*** possibly ***diphenhydramine.*** (Note: Antihistamines will not cure otitis media, and they may cause minor side effects, including drowsiness and nervousness.) To ease the pain, your doctor may recommend an ***analgesic,*** typically ***acetaminophen,*** which also helps reduce a fever. (***Aspirin*** should be avoided in children because of the threat of Reye's syndrome.)

A controversy surrounds the use of ***antibiotics*** in treating bacterial middle ear infections. In England, most physicians treat only the symptoms of otitis media, without the help of bacteria-killing drugs. Studies have shown that up to 88 percent of otitis media cases got better when treated this way. Other research, in fact, suggests that 80 percent of otitis media cases are viral in origin and therefore will not respond to antibiotics.

But many doctors, particularly in the U.S., are concerned that without antibiotics, bacteria lurking inside the middle ear can grow out of control, possibly causing a serious complication such as hearing loss or mastoiditis. After all, they point out, these complications have become rare, largely as a result of antibiotic therapy. To be on the safe side, many American physicians treat all otitis media cases as if bacteria were present.

Amoxicillin is the antibiotic of choice for treating bacterial otitis media. The drug is generally considered safe because it is less likely to cause allergic reactions than ***penicillin,*** from which it is derived. The drug is highly effective: A single course of amoxicillin can knock out an ear infection in 7 to 10 days, at little cost.

Lately, however, doctors have noticed trouble with this wonder drug. As it turns out, some types of bacteria have learned to make a defensive protein that renders amoxicillin useless. Critics of routine antibiotic use in the U.S. charge that the millions of prescriptions of amoxicillin written for otitis media that had no bacterial element helped to create these resistant strains.

Whatever their origin, amoxicillin-resistant bacteria have shown up in a number of communities, prompting many doctors to prescribe other antibiotics for otitis media. Some of these substitutes, which tend to be more expensive than amoxicillin, are taken from a class of medications called ***cephalosporins.*** Others are combination drugs—***amoxicillin and clavulanate,*** for instance. For those allergic to amoxicillin, doctors may prescribe ***sulfamethoxazole and trimethoprim,*** or ***erythromycin*** mixed with a sulfa drug like sulfisoxazole. For patients at least two years of age with severe, recurrent otitis media, doctors can stimulate the immune system by using a special vaccine that causes the body's immune system to recognize and attack certain bacteria.

If a case of otitis media develops serious complications, physicians may suggest surgery to eliminate infection or drain the middle ear. One technique, called myringotomy, involves piercing the eardrum to release fluid from the middle ear. If the Eustachian tubes become completely closed off due to swelling, a surgeon may insert a ventilation tube inside to keep them open. However, this procedure—called tympanostomy—is often expensive and may lead to infection and scarring. If recurring infections in the adenoids or tonsils cause repeated episodes of otitis media, a physician may suggest having the glands removed. *(See **Adenoid Problems** and **Tonsillitis.**)*

ALTERNATIVE CHOICES

Some alternative treatments for otitis media attempt to fight the viruses or bacteria responsible for the infection, while others try to relieve the symptoms or boost the immune system.

AROMATHERAPY

Lavender *(Lavandula officinalis)* essence may sometimes help to reduce the inflammation and pain of ear infections. Other oils used include ***chamomile*** *(Matricaria recutita),* cajuput, ***evening primrose oil*** *(Oenothera biennis),* fatty acid, flax oil, and borage.

AYURVEDIC MEDICINE

To open and drain the Eustachian tubes, Ayurvedic physicians massage the lymph nodes outside the ears. The massage is complemented with a drink made with the herb amala, a source of vitamin C that also has antiviral and antibacterial properties. Amala is often given with raw honey. (CAUTION: Raw honey may contain the organism responsible for botulism and should not be given to infants or people with weak immune systems.)

CHINESE HERBS

Practitioners use certain herbs to help fight infection and open up ear passages. Mixtures might include ***skullcap*** *(Scutellaria baicalensis),* ***alisma*** *(Alisma plantago-aquatica),* ***plantain*** *(Plantago major),* ***bupleurum*** *(Bupleurum chinense),* and

licorice *(Glycyrrhiza uralensis).* Contact a practitioner for exact recipes.

HERBAL THERAPIES

A number of herbs that help the body fight infection—including ***echinacea*** (*Echinacea* spp.), ***chamomile*** *(Matricaria recutita),* and ***goldenseal*** *(Hydrastis canadensis)*—are available in oral tablets. Ear-drop solutions cannot penetrate the middle ear and should be reserved for outer ear infections. *(See* ***Swimmer's Ear.****)*

HOMEOPATHY

In the early stages of an ear infection with sudden onset and feverish restlessness, use ***Aconite*** (30c every four to six hours). For throbbing and sharp pain accompanied by fever, intense heat, and flushing in the outer ear and along the side of the face, use ***Belladonna*** (30c every four to six hours). WARNING: Use extreme caution when treating with *Belladonna,* an extract from a poisonous plant of the nightshade family. Check dosages with your practitioner and follow label directions carefully. For children with otitis media who are very irritable, in great pain, and can't be consoled, try ***Chamomilla*** (30c every four to six hours). When a child is weepy, clingy, feels better in the open air, and has a yellowish green discharge coming from the nose, use ***Pulsatilla*** (30c every four to six hours). For ear congestion without infection, try *Kali muriaticum* (30c every four to six hours). If there is no improvement after two days, try a different remedy or consult a homeopathic practitioner.

NUTRITION AND DIET

Although diet alone won't cure an ear infection, nutritionists suggest using the following vitamins and supplements to fight a viral infection:

- Beta carotene (see ***vitamin A***). Multiply your child's age times 20,000 IU for the daily dosage, with 200,000 as the maximum.
- ***Vitamin C.*** Daily dosage: Your child's age times 250 mg. (WARNING: High doses of vitamin C can cause diarrhea; it is important to spread the dose out evenly over the course of a day. Although for adults and adolescents there is no strict daily maximum, many people cannot tolerate more than 1,000 mg daily.)
- ***Zinc.*** Daily dosage: Your age times 2.5 mg. Do not take more than 50 mg per day without consulting a nutritionist.
- Bioflavonoids. Daily dosage: Your child's age times 50 mg, with 250 mg as the maximum.

OSTEOPATHY

Consult an osteopathic practitioner for therapies that may help drainage of the Eustachian tubes.

AT-HOME REMEDIES

- You can provide a great deal of symptomatic relief for an infected ear at home. Many find that warmth, perhaps from a warm compress, brings comfort. Steam inhalations and hot footbaths may also help.
- If you take antihistamines, which may rob your body of moisture and dry out your throat and respiratory passages, try to replace lost fluids by drinking lots of water.
- Gargling with salt water helps soothe an aggravated throat and clear the Eustachian tubes.
- Holding your head erect also helps drain your middle ear.
- Some people find relief with over-the-counter nasal sprays, which act as decongestants. Used for more than three days, however, sprays can become habit-forming and lead to rebound congestion, or a worsening of your condition.

O

PREVENTION

Because bottle-fed babies are more likely to get otitis media, it is better to breast-feed your infant, if possible, to prevent ear infections. (If you must bottle-feed, never lay your baby down and prop the bottle up.) Also, remove as many environmental pollutants from your home as you can, including dust, cleaning fluid and solvents, and tobacco smoke. Food allergies may play a role in otitis media, so if you or your child is susceptible to the disease, try cutting back on wheat products, corn products, and food additives, as these tend to be more allergenic than other foods. ■

OVARIAN CANCER

SYMPTOMS

Although ovarian cancer rarely produces symptoms in its earliest stages, eventual warning signs may include:

- vague digestive disturbances, such as mild indigestion, bloating, feeling of fullness, or loss of appetite.
- diarrhea, constipation, or a frequent need to urinate.
- pain or swelling in the abdomen, or pain in the lower back.
- vaginal bleeding between menstrual periods or after menopause.

Symptoms associated with advanced ovarian cancer include severe nausea, vomiting, pain, and weight loss.

CALL YOUR DOCTOR IF:

- you have otherwise unexplained abdominal pain or vaginal bleeding, particularly if these conditions accompany the more general symptoms listed above. Do not allow such symptoms to continue undiagnosed for more than two weeks.

Flanking the uterus are the two ovaries, each about the size of an almond, which produce eggs and female hormones. Over a lifetime, the ovaries may develop abnormal but noncancerous growths; for example, fluid-filled ovarian cysts are always benign—or noncancerous—as are 3 out of 4 ovarian tumors. Yet despite those odds, about 1 in 70 women in the United States will develop ovarian cancer. It can occur at any age, even in childhood, but is most common after menopause. The disease accounts for about 20,000 new cases and 12,500 deaths in the United States annually.

If ovarian cancer could be readily detected in its earliest stages, more women would be cured. But like many cancers, it usually has spread by the time it is diagnosed. The importance of early detection is clear: The five-year survival rate for ovarian cancer detected early is 88 percent; the rate for all cases is only about 40 percent.

CAUSES

Most women with ovarian cancer have no family history of the disease, yet a woman is more likely to get the disease if her mother or sister has had ovarian, ***breast,*** or ***uterine cancer;*** the more relatives affected, the greater the risk. Women who have had few or no children, who delay childbearing until their thirties, or who have trouble conceiving are also at greater risk for ovarian cancer. Those who have several children, who breast-feed their infants, or who use birth-control pills are at reduced risk. The difference may be linked to less-frequent ovulation. Evidence suggests that the more saturated fat a woman consumes, the greater her ovarian cancer risk. Many high-fat foods contain estrogen, and all stimulate natural estrogen production. Because most ovarian cancers grow more rapidly in the presence of estrogen, some experts believe that abnormally elevated estrogen in a woman's body promotes the onset of ovarian cancer. Exposure to asbestos is also believed to be a factor in some cases.

DIAGNOSTIC AND TEST PROCEDURES

Annual pelvic examinations help detect ovarian

CANCER IN THE OVARIES

UTERUS
FALLOPIAN TUBE
OVARY
TUMOR

During her childbearing years, a woman's ovaries deliver eggs to the uterus through the fallopian tubes. The ovaries are susceptible to several types of growths *(see inset)*, which are often benign cysts but are sometimes cancerous. The cancer typically has no obvious symptoms until it is well advanced. Early growths can sometimes be detected during a routine pelvic exam.

cancer early. Researchers are developing special blood tests that may help early diagnosis, but the tests are not yet reliable enough for general screening. If an ovarian growth is suspected, a sonogram of the ovaries is made; any visible abnormality justifies further testing in a hospital. Blood studies and other imaging tests may be done, and ultimately a tissue biopsy is necessary to confirm or rule out the diagnosis.

TREATMENT

See ***Cancer*** for further information about some of the conventional treatment options below.

CONVENTIONAL MEDICINE

Surgery is standard treatment for ovarian cancer. Ordinarily, the two ovaries and the other reproductive organs are removed. Young women who have only a small tumor in one ovary and who still want to have children may have just the diseased ovary removed; the second can be removed later to prevent cancer recurrence. In most patients, some cancer remains after surgery. A patient's prognosis depends on how much cancer remains and how well it responds to follow-up treatment. Most patients receive chemotherapy, which can prolong survival and may result in cure. Radiation therapy may be used after surgery to prevent recurrence or to help treat advanced or recurrent cases. Once remission occurs, follow-up examinations are essential; women who have had the disease may be at greater risk for breast and ***colorectal cancer.***

New chemotherapeutic agents, new biological agents designed to stimulate the immune system, and new methods of delivering treatment with fewer adverse effects are under study. One of the more promising new drugs for treating advanced and recurrent ovarian cancer is taxol, originally extracted from the Pacific yew tree but now manufactured in the laboratory.

COMPLEMENTARY THERAPIES

Maintaining a healthy immune system is important for people with cancer. Get regular exercise, adequate sleep, and essential vitamins and minerals by eating fresh fruits and vegetables. Cut down on dairy products, meats, and other high-fat foods. Various herbs with demonstrated immune-enhancing properties may complement standard treatment, but check with your doctor before using them.

PREVENTION

Depending on your stage of life, you should discuss with your doctor the pros and cons of using birth-control pills or hormone replacement pills. Low-dose birth-control pills are considered protective, but hormone replacement therapy may heighten the risk of ovarian cancer; neither practice may be appropriate for women with a family history of the disease. If you are considered high-risk for ovarian cancer, ask your doctor about current recommendations for routine blood screening. For women at extremely high risk, a doctor may recommend having the ovaries removed as a preventive measure. ■

OVARY PROBLEMS

SYMPTOMS

- feeling of fullness or pressure on one side of the abdomen.
- abdominal pain during intercourse.
- sharp abdominal pain.
- irregular vaginal bleeding or absent menstrual periods.
- increase in facial or body hair.
- irregularities in bowel movements or urination.

Many small benign ovarian cysts and tumors produce no symptoms.

CALL YOUR DOCTOR IF:

- you experience sudden sharp or severe abdominal pain, with or without fever; it may be a ruptured or twisted **ovarian cyst** or another problem, such as ***appendicitis,*** that requires immediate medical attention.
- you notice any significant increase in facial or body hair; you may have an ovarian problem that is altering your body's hormonal balance. See your doctor as soon as possible for treatment.
- your menstrual periods become irregular or stop altogether; you may have an ovarian problem that has altered your body's production of hormones or another disease or condition that requires medical treatment, such as ***diabetes.*** See your doctor as soon as possible.

The ovaries are a pair of almond-shaped organs located deep within the pelvis, on each side of the uterus. Each ovary contains thousands of eggs. Once a month during the years a woman is menstruating, one egg (or sometimes more) begins to grow in a small cystlike structure known as a follicle. When the egg is mature, the follicle ruptures and releases the egg, a process called ovulation. The egg then floats down to the uterus through the fallopian tube, propelled by hairlike cilia within the tube. The journey from the ovary to the uterus takes about three days.

The ovaries also produce the hormones estrogen and progesterone. While the egg is maturing, the follicle releases estrogen to help thicken the lining of the uterus in case the egg is fertilized and grows into an embryo. After the follicle ruptures it develops into a structure known as the corpus luteum, which produces progesterone to help the uterus prepare for a fertilized egg. If no pregnancy occurs, the level of progesterone decreases, menstruation occurs, and the cycle repeats itself.

Several problems can develop in the ovary. It can become infected, sometimes alone but more often as part of an infection that involves other pelvic organs *(see **Pelvic Inflammatory Disease**).* Cysts and tumors can also form on the ovaries. Most often these are benign—or noncancerous—and produce no symptoms. They are discovered only through a routine pelvic examination. Sometimes many small cysts form on the ovaries, a

STEPPING ON A NEW OLD WIVES' TALE

MYTH: *Wearing high-heeled shoes contributes to ovarian cysts by blocking circulation to the pelvic area.*

FACT: *Absolutely no evidence supports the notion that footwear has any effect on circulation to the pelvic area, including the ovaries.*

condition known as polycystic ovary syndrome.

Although most benign **ovarian cysts** and tumors disappear after a few menstrual cycles, some grow large enough to cause discomfort. Sometimes the growths disrupt the production of ovarian hormones, causing irregular bleeding or an increase in body hair, or they press on the bladder, leading to more frequent urination. A cyst or tumor that has ruptured or become twisted on its attachment to the ovary can cause significant abdominal pain and may lead to an infection.

CAUSES

Ovarian infections are most frequently caused by ***sexually transmitted diseases.*** Some **ovarian cysts** are the result of a follicle or corpus luteum that continues to grow and fill with fluid long after the egg has been released. **Polycystic ovary syndrome** occurs when egg follicles get trapped just under the surface of the ovary, unable to release their eggs, and form into multiple small cysts.

DIAGNOSTIC AND TEST PROCEDURES

Your doctor will give you a complete physical and pelvic exam. If he or she suspects you have an ovarian cyst or tumor, you may need to undergo an ultrasound scan, which uses sound waves to produce a detailed image of the pelvic organs. The organs can be visualized directly by means of laparoscopy, a surgical procedure in which a special viewing instrument is inserted into the abdominal cavity under general anesthesia.

TREATMENT

Treatment for an ovarian problem depends on the nature of the disorder. Treating **ovarian cysts** is often unnecessary; they tend to disappear on their own. Because of the possibility that a growth on an ovary may be cancerous, you should always seek out a conventional practitioner for the diagnosis of an ovary problem. Alternative treatments should be used only to help ease any discomfort associated with the condition.

CONVENTIONAL MEDICINE

If diagnostic tests reveal an ovarian infection, your doctor will prescribe an ***antibiotic.*** If an **ovarian cyst** or tumor is diagnosed, he or she may recommend prompt surgery to rule out the possibility of cancer. If you are under age 40 and your cyst is soft and smaller than two inches in diameter, your doctor may suggest that you delay surgery for one or two menstrual cycles to see whether the cyst will disappear spontaneously.

Some doctors prescribe birth-control pills to women with a suspected ovarian cyst in the belief that hormones in the pills will help the cyst regress, thus eliminating the need for surgery.

For **polycystic ovary syndrome** doctors prescribe hormonal treatment to reestablish regular menstrual cycles. Either progesterone or birth-control pills, which contain both progesterone and ***estrogen,*** are used. Fertility drugs are also sometimes prescribed for women with polycystic ovaries to induce ovulation.

ALTERNATIVE CHOICES

Alternative treatments for ovary problems should be used only as supplements to conventional treatment methods.

HERBAL THERAPIES

Herbalists recommend blue cohosh *(Caulophyllum thalictroides)* and false unicorn root *(Chamaelirium luteum)* as general tonics for the female reproductive organs. You may take these herbs in either tea or tincture form.

NUTRITION AND DIET

To help prevent and treat **ovarian cysts,** some alternative practitioners recommend a vegetarian diet rich in foods believed to nourish the liver, especially beets, carrots, dark-green leafy vegetables, and lemons. Others prescribe supplements of ***zinc*** and ***vitamins A, E,*** and ***C.*** Supplements of black currant oil, borage oil, and ***evening primrose oil*** *(Oenothera biennis)* may also be recommended because they are believed to help regulate the body's hormone levels. Consult your alternative practitioner for specific dosages. ■

O

PAIN, CHRONIC

SYMPTOMS

Any pain that lasts longer than six months is defined as chronic. The condition may include weakness, numbness, tingling, or other sensations, along with sleeping difficulties, a lack of energy, and ***depression.*** Some common forms of chronic pain are:

- continuing muscle pain, accompanied by cramping, soreness, swelling, and muscle spasms or stiffness.
- lingering back pain, which may be sharp or aching, constant or intermittent, localized, radiating, or diffuse.
- enduring joint pain, with tenderness and a sensation of heat in the affected area as well as radiating pain and a restricted range of motion.

CALL YOUR DOCTOR IF:

- your pain continues for several weeks and doesn't respond to over-the-counter ***analgesics*** and rest; early care may keep acute pain from becoming chronic.
- your pain is unrelenting and unresponsive to prescription medications; your doctor may administer tests to rule out cancer or other possible causes.
- the symptoms of your chronic pain change abruptly. You may be at risk of complications, or you may have developed a different, unrelated problem.

Tens of millions of Americans suffer from chronic pain, the medical term used to describe any pain that, despite treatment, persists for longer than six months. Chronic pain can be mild or excruciating, episodic or continuous, merely inconvenient or totally incapacitating. The most common versions are ***headaches, arthritis, joint pain,*** pain from injury, and ***backaches.*** Other kinds of chronic pain include Achilles ***tendonitis, sinusitis,*** other forms of degenerative joint disease besides arthritis, ***carpal tunnel syndrome,*** and pain affecting specific parts of the body, such as the shoulders, pelvis, and neck. Generalized muscle or nerve pain can also develop into a chronic condition. *(See separate entries for more specific information about these ailments.)*

In some cases, chronic pain is self-perpetuating. For example, although rubbing a tender area may offer temporary relief, it can also inhibit healing; similarly, favoring an injured limb may set up musculoskeletal stresses that create new problems. The emotional toll of chronic pain also can become part of a vicious cycle. Anxiety, stress, depression, anger, and fatigue interact in complex ways with chronic pain and may decrease the body's production of natural painkillers; moreover, such negative feelings may increase the level of substances that amplify sensations of pain, worsening the spiral. Even the body's most basic defenses may be compromised: There is considerable evidence that unrelenting pain can suppress the immune system.

Because of the mind/body links associated with chronic pain, effective treatment may require addressing psychological as well as physical aspects of the condition.

CAUSES

The causes of chronic pain are exceedingly diverse. One frequent factor is the development of any of a number of conditions that can accompany aging and may affect bones and joints in ways that cause chronic pain. Other common reasons for persistent pain are nerve damage and injuries that fail to heal properly. Some kinds of chronic pain have numerous possible causes: Back pain, for example, may be traceable to years of poor posture; to improper lifting and carrying of heavy objects; to being overweight, which puts excess strain on the back and knees; to a congenital condition such as curvature of the spine; to a traumatic injury; to wearing high heels; to sleeping on a poor mattress; or to no obvious physical cause.

Disease can also be the underlying cause of chronic pain. Rheumatoid arthritis and osteoarthritis are well-known culprits, but persistent pain may also be due to such ailments as ***cancer, multiple sclerosis, stomach ulcers, AIDS,*** and gallbladder disease.

In many cases, however, just what the source of chronic pain is can be a very complex and even mysterious issue to untangle. Although it may begin with an injury or illness, continuing pain can develop a psychological dimension after the physical problem has healed. This fact alone makes pinning down a single course of treatment tricky, and it is why doctors and other healers often find they have to try a number of different types of curative steps.

TREATMENT

Many people suffering from chronic pain are able to gain some measure of control over it by practicing mind/body techniques on their own *(see **Mind/Body Medicine,** page 652)*. But others may need professional help. For them, pain clinics—special care centers devoted exclusively to dealing with intractable pain—are often the answer. Some pain clinics are associated with hospitals and others are private; in either case, both inpatient and outpatient treatment are usually available. The length of a full treatment program can vary from several weeks to several months.

Pain clinics generally employ a multidisciplinary approach, involving physicians, psychologists, physical therapists, and alternative health-care practitioners; the patient as well will take an active role in his or her own treatment. The aim in many cases is not only to alleviate pain but also to teach the chronic sufferer how to come to terms with pain and function in spite of it. The first step in many cases is to wean the patient from a dependence on painkilling medications. Other methods used by pain specialists include **biofeedback** and **relaxation** techniques to control brain-wave activity, behavior-modification therapy to revise the way pain is perceived, **acupuncture, hypnotherapy, meditation,** and other forms of alternative therapy. One high-tech method involves a miniature device controlled by the patient or an implanted electronic nerve stimulator that transmits tiny pulses of electric current to block pain signals.

Various studies have shown as much as 50 percent improvement in pain reduction for chronic pain sufferers after visiting a pain clinic, and most people learn to cope better and can resume normal activities.

CONVENTIONAL MEDICINE

Over-the-counter painkillers such as ***aspirin*** and ***ibuprofen*** can control milder cases of musculoskeletal pain and reduce inflammation. Your doctor may prescribe stronger drugs, such as ***muscle relaxants, antianxiety drugs*** (such as ***diazepam***), ***antidepressants,*** prescription ***nonsteroidal anti-inflammatory drugs (NSAIDs),*** or a short course of stronger painkillers (such as ***opioid analgesics***). A limited number of ***corticosteroid*** injections at the site of an injury can reduce swelling and inflammation. Oral doses of the amino acid D-phenylalanine appear to release endorphins, the brain's natural painkillers, which can relieve all types of pain. For injuries that require immobilization to heal, a doctor may also advise wearing a brace, collar, splint, or surgical corset that binds your torso for short periods of time only. Extreme cases of injuries requiring immobilization might call for traction or surgery.

ALTERNATIVE CHOICES

A broad array of alternative options exists to address chronic pain. Some focus on physical aspects of the condition, others on psychological factors, and still others on where physiological and psychological factors overlap.

P

UPPER-BODY ACUPRESSURE

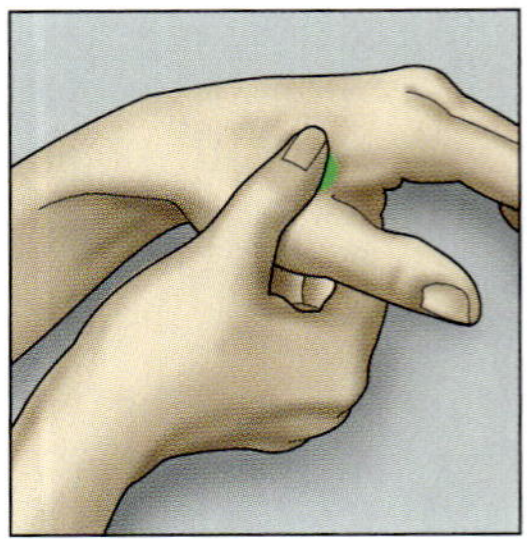

1 Pressing Large Intestine 4, in the web between your thumb and index finger, may help relieve facial pain. Use the thumb and index finger of your right hand to squeeze the web of your left hand for one minute. Repeat on the right hand. Do not use this point if you are pregnant.

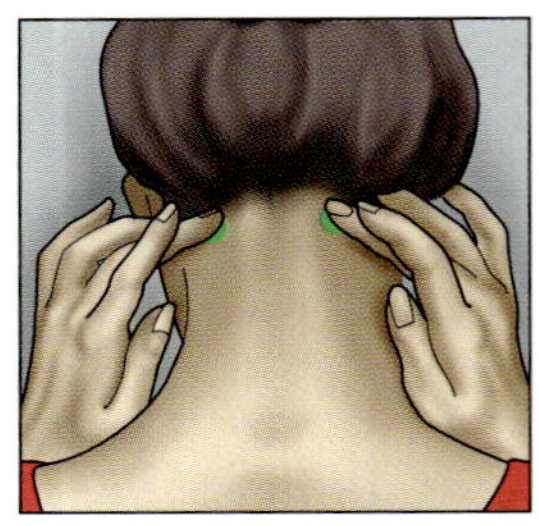

2 To reduce neck muscle stress that may cause head or back pain, try pressing Gall Bladder 20. Place the tips of both middle fingers in the hollows at the base of your skull, about two inches apart, on either side of the spine. Press firmly for one minute.

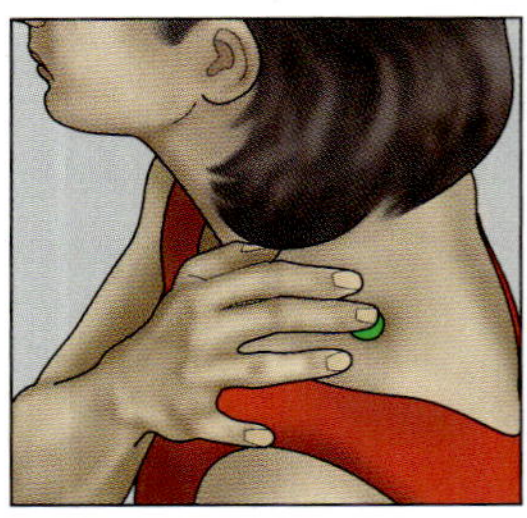

3 Pressing Gall Bladder 21 may help release tension in the shoulders. Place your right middle finger on the highest point of your left shoulder muscle, one or two inches from your lower neck. Press two or three times, then repeat on the other side.

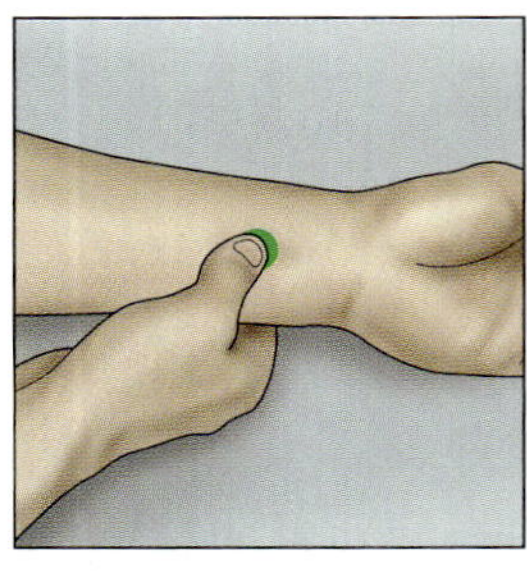

4 To help ease pain in the chest and upper abdomen, press Pericardium 6. Place your thumb in the center of your inner wrist, two finger widths from the wrist crease and between the two bones of the forearm. Press firmly for one minute, three to five times, then repeat on the other arm.

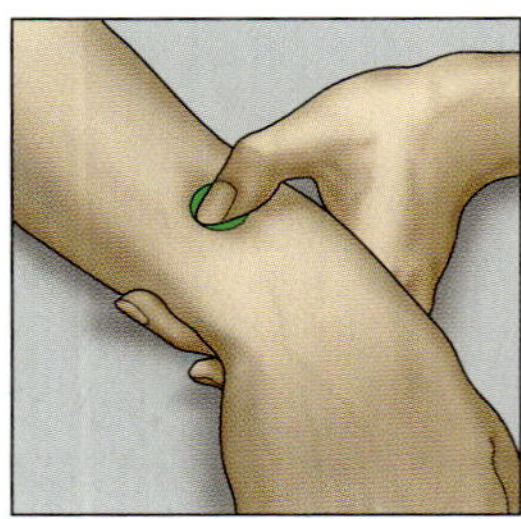

5 Pressing Triple Warmer 5 may help soothe areas of pain in the upper body. Center your thumb on the top of your forearm, two thumb widths from the wrist joint. Press firmly for one minute, then repeat on the other arm. Do two or three times.

LOWER-BODY ACUPRESSURE

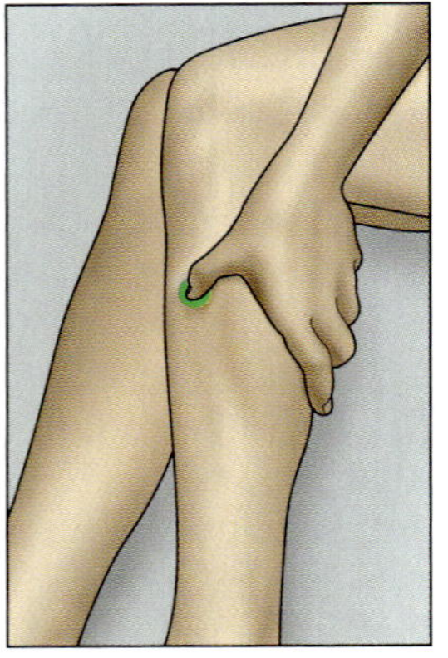

1 Abdominal pain may be eased by steady finger pressure on Stomach 36, four finger widths below the kneecap just outside the shinbone. Maintain pressure for one minute, then switch legs. To verify the location, flex your foot; you should feel a muscle bulge at the point site.

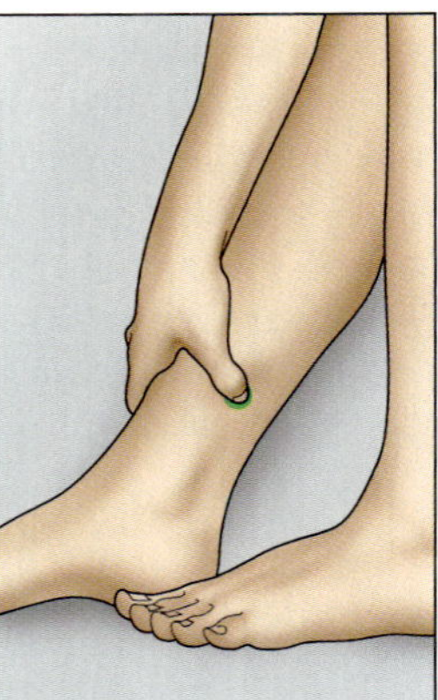

2 Abdominal cramping may be relieved by pressing Spleen 6. Place your thumb four finger widths from your right inside anklebone, near the edge of the shinbone. Press for one minute, then switch legs. Do two or three times. Do not use this point if you are pregnant.

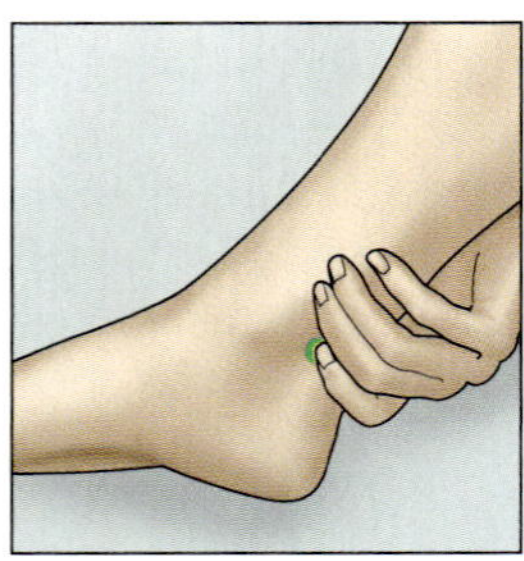

3 Kidney 3, located on the inside of the ankle between the anklebone and the Achilles tendon, may ease back pain. Press firmly with your index finger and hold for one to two minutes, then repeat on the other foot. Do not use this point after the third month of pregnancy.

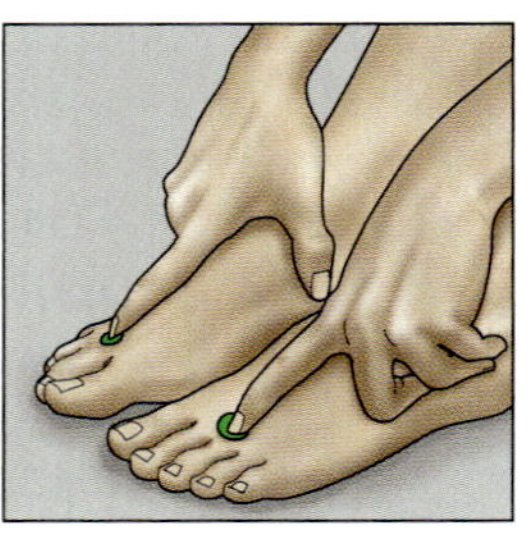

4 Ankle and foot pain may be relieved by pressure on Stomach 44, located on the top of the foot in the web between the second and third toes. Press lightly on both feet with your index fingers for one minute, two or three times.

P

ACUPRESSURE

Acupressure therapy is based on the belief that specific points on your hands, feet, and limbs correspond to various parts of your body where you may be feeling chronic pain. Self-administered, it generally involves pushing straight down with a bent thumb or finger (but not your fingernails) on the indicated point for about a minute, removing the pressure, then pressing deeply again. For techniques targeting specific instances of chronic pain, see the illustrations at left.

ACUPUNCTURE

Acupuncture may be used to reduce swelling and inflammation associated with chronic pain. The treatment may include placing needles along the large-intestine meridian, considered the most effective of pain-relieving channels. One theory holds that acupuncture works by stimulating the release of endorphins, the body's natural painkillers. Because this therapy is thought to have a cumulative effect, it is most beneficial if done on a regular basis. For the best results, consult an acupuncturist who has experience treating a wide range of types of chronic pain.

AROMATHERAPY

Mix together the following essential oils with a carrier oil such as sweet almond, apricot kernel, or jojoba oil, and massage the blend into your skin at the site of the pain: ***lavender*** *(Lavandula officinalis)* to reduce inflammation and relax muscles; ***eucalyptus*** *(Eucalyptus globulus)* to bring down swelling and accelerate healing; ***ginger*** *(Zingiber officinale)* to relieve pain and stiffness associated with ***arthritis*** and other types of degenerative joint disease.

BODY WORK

The **Alexander technique** reeducates you in the way you move to avoid adding unnecessary tension to skeleton-supporting muscles, thus preventing neck and back problems. This therapy has been shown to be especially helpful for correcting poor posture that can cause backaches.

Massage therapy may provide temporary relief of muscle tension, stiffness, and spasms. Its muscular manipulation may break the pain-spasm-pain cycle of many types of chronic pain by reducing muscle tension, which can produce sudden, involuntary contractions and lead to more pain.

Massage with ice packs may interrupt pain messages sent along nerve pathways, replacing those messages with signals about temperature and, in this way, providing relief.

CHIROPRACTIC

Chiropractic manipulation seeks to restore joint mobility in cases of ***bursitis*** and ***tennis elbow.*** It is also used as a means of reducing back or neck pain or muscle spasms.

HERBAL THERAPIES

Capsicum, the active ingredient in ***cayenne*** *(Capsicum frutescens),* is believed to increase blood flow to joint tissues, thereby reducing inflammation. An over-the-counter ointment made with cayenne may bring temporary relief of osteoarthritis and rheumatoid ***arthritis,*** although it is very hot and should be used for only short periods. Infusions of ***black cohosh*** *(Cimicifuga racemosa)* or six 500-mg capsules of ***evening primrose oil*** *(Oenothera biennis)* taken daily may also lessen inflammation. Rubbing a dilution of ***peppermint*** *(Mentha piperita)* oil on the affected area may have a temporary numbing effect.

Topically applied dilutions of wintergreen *(Gaultheria procumbens)* oil—which contains ***methyl salicylate,*** an ingredient similar to those found in ***aspirin***—may have an analgesic effect. Geranium *(Pelargonium odoratissimum)* and ***white willow*** *(Salix alba)* bark are natural painkillers. ***Chamomile*** *(Matricaria recutita)* is an antispasmodic and anti-inflammatory agent. Consult an herbalist to determine the best treatment for your specific condition. You must also take special precautions if you are pregnant.

HOMEOPATHY

Try ***Rhus toxicodendron*** for joint, back, and arthritic problems that feel worse when first rising in the morning and become better with warmth. Persistent pain may be relieved by ***Kali bichromicum.*** If you eat a lot of salt and have severe low-back pain that abates when firm pressure is applied, try ***Natrum muriaticum.*** For burning lower-back pain that improves with movement and grows worse after rest, take *Calcarea fluorica.* ***Sepia*** may be good for lower-back pain that is worsened by sitting. Consult a homeopathic practitioner for the appropriate remedies and dosages.

Topical homeopathic creams that have ***Arnica*** as a main ingredient can help with muscle pain and other kinds of pain that are not associated with your joints.

LIFESTYLE

Although resting for short periods can alleviate pain, too much rest can make muscles shorter, tighter, and weaker, actually increasing pain and putting you at greater risk of injury when you again attempt movement. If chronic pain has sidelined you for a long period, try a technique called "shaping" to get moving again: Determine the length of time you can painlessly perform an activity and establish a regular schedule for doing it; if your pain threshold is 10 minutes of stretching or walking, cut that time in half, but instead of stretching for only five minutes per day, stretch twice a day for five minutes each. You'll achieve the same benefits without feeling the pain. Gradually, you'll be able to increase your exercise time while increasing your pain threshold.

Research has shown that regular exercise can diminish pain in the long run by improving muscle tone, strength, and flexibility. Exercise may also release endorphins, the body's natural painkillers. Some exercises are easier for certain chronic pain sufferers to perform than others; try swimming, biking, walking, or rowing.

MIND/BODY MEDICINE

Some healthcare practitioners propose that, instead of resisting chronic pain, you should find ways to accept it and adjust to it. They suggest that this attitude, far from being defeatist, can enable you to escape a victim mentality. The pain may dissipate as a result, since psychological factors can play a major role in its perception.

The psychotherapeutic method called cognitive restructuring teaches you to replace negative, self-destructive beliefs with positive affirmations to "solve" pain problems. Your internal monologue is changed from "I can't do this; I'll never be better" to "I don't know what the future holds, but this is what I can do now."

REFLEXOLOGY

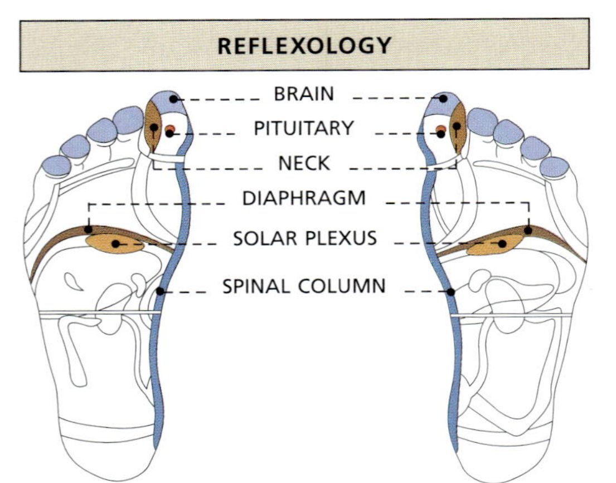

Symptoms of chronic pain may be alleviated by walking your thumb across the solar plexus and diaphragm areas, working from inside to outside. Next, work the neck and pituitary areas on the big toe and the brain area on the tip of each toe with your thumb. Stimulate the spinal column area by walking your thumb up and down the inside of the foot.

Visualization may be another worthwhile pain-controlling technique. Try the following exercise: Close your eyes and try to call up a visual image of the pain, giving it shape, color, size, motion. Now try slowly altering this image, replacing it with a more harmonious, pleasing—and smaller—image. Don't expect this imaging technique to work right away; it takes practice.

Another approach is to keep a diary of your pain episodes and the causative and corrective factors surrounding them. Review your diary regularly to explore avenues of possible change. Strive to view pain as part of life, not all of it.

Electromyographic (EMG) **biofeedback** may alert you to the ways in which muscle tension is contributing to your pain and help you learn to control it.

Hypnotherapy and self-hypnosis may help you block or transform pain through refocusing techniques. One self-hypnosis strategy, known as glove anesthesia, involves putting yourself in a trance, placing a hand over the painful area, imagining that the hand is relaxed, heavy, and numb, and envisioning these sensations as replacing other, painful feelings in the affected area.

Relaxation techniques such as **meditation** or **yoga** have been shown to reduce stress-related pain when they are practiced regularly. The gentle stretching of yoga is particularly good for strengthening muscles without putting additional strain on the body. Try the following so-called Corpse pose for 10 minutes of relaxation: Find a quiet place where you won't be disturbed and lie on your back, with small pillows under your neck and the small of your back if you like; consciously attempt to relax every part of your body, beginning with your toes and working upward to your face; let your breathing slow and deepen, and pay attention to how your body feels.

If you can't get your mind off your concerns, visualize two lists; in one column, list the concerns in order of priority, and in the other, visualize potential solutions to them. Place an imaginary check mark by each one after you've found a solution for it, then put both lists out of your mind and do the relaxation exercise again.

NUTRITION AND DIET

To reduce inflammation, try the following supplements (taken in increments throughout the day): 500 mg daily of ***calcium*** pantothenate, or pantothenic acid ***(vitamin*** B_5***);*** 800 to1,000 mg daily of calcium citrate-malate; and 600 mg daily of the enzyme bromelain. For chronic back pain, a beneficial regimen may be 500 mg of ***vitamin C*** three times a day with meals, 1,200 mg daily of ***calcium,*** and 400 IU daily of ***vitamin E.*** CAUTION: Be sure to check with your doctor or a nutritionist before taking large doses of vitamin supplements. Foods high in calcium and ***magnesium*** relax muscles and may help reduce muscle-related pain.

For rheumatoid ***arthritis*** and other musculoskeletal pain, you may want to avoid dairy products, meat, and other foods that are high in saturated fats; they boost the body's production of prostaglandins, hormonelike fatty acids in the body that may contribute to inflammation.

Food has occasionally been implicated as a cause in some diseases that result in chronic pain. This type of food intolerance is then manifested as symptoms of the disease. Allergies to wheat, corn, citrus fruits, tomatoes, or potatoes, for example, can be expressed as rheumatoid arthritis. Consult your doctor or a recommended specialist to address this type of problem. You will probably be advised to try eliminating certain types of food from your diet to see if they are the source of your trouble.

OTHER THERAPIES

A transcutaneous electrical nerve stimulator, or TENS, is a small battery-powered device that is attached to painful areas by electrodes; the device stimulates nerves, which may block transmission of pain impulses to the brain. With training, this technique can be self-administered.

Hot and cold **hydrotherapy** treatments can relieve aches. Pour hot water into one container and ice water into another. Dip a rolled-up towel in the hot water, wring it out, and place it on the affected area for three minutes; then dip another rolled-up towel in the cold water and apply it for one minute. Repeat these alternating applications for 20 minutes three times a day.

AT-HOME REMEDIES

- Treat the acute pain of an injury to a muscle, ligament, or cartilage with immediate rest, ice, compression, and elevation—acronymically known as RICE. Rest the injured body part, apply ice (a pack of frozen vegetables or ice pack) alternately for 20 minutes on, 20 off, compress the area with an elastic bandage, and keep the injury elevated to reduce swelling. Once swelling has subsided, apply heat (a hot-water bottle or heating pad). Finally, ***aspirin***-based creams can help reduce pain and inflammation. It's important to treat acute pain before it has the chance to become chronic.
- Take capsules or drink infusions of one of the herbal remedies suggested above on a regular basis or as directed by an herbalist.
- A **yoga** class or bicycle-riding club has the benefit of stimulating endorphins—your body's natural painkillers. ■

P

PANCREATIC CANCER

SYMPTOMS

Pancreatic cancer usually produces no symptoms until it reaches an advanced stage. Symptoms that may arise, in typical order of occurrence, include:

- significant weight loss accompanied by ***abdominal pain***—the most likely warning signs.
- vague but gradually worsening abdominal pain, often severe at night, which may radiate to the lower back.
- digestive or bowel complaints such as diarrhea, constipation, gas pains, bloating, or belching.
- nausea, vomiting, loss of appetite, and weight loss.
- ***jaundice,*** indicated by yellowish discoloration of the skin or eye whites.
- sudden onset of ***diabetes.***
- black or bloody stool, indicating bleeding from the digestive tract.

A few rare types of pancreatic cancer cause hormonal imbalances that produce their own symptoms, which might include:

- episodes of weakness, sweating, rapid heartbeat, irritability, or skin flushing related to low blood sugar.
- severe ulcer symptoms, such as stomach pain and watery diarrhea, which do not respond to ulcer medication.

CALL YOUR DOCTOR IF:

- any symptoms listed above endure longer than two weeks. You should have a full physical examination.

P

The pancreas, a small gland located deep in the abdomen, has two vital functions: It supplies the intestines with digestive juices, and it secretes hormones—including insulin—that regulate the body's use of sugars and starches. Endocrine cells in the pancreas are devoted to hormone regulation; they form clusters called islets and are found mostly in the tail and body sections of the gland. Exocrine cells, which outnumber endocrine cells 99 to 1, are spread throughout the gland and perform the digestive functions.

At least 90 percent of pancreatic cancers are **exocrine cell cancers,** usually originating in the head of the gland. **Endocrine cell cancers**—or **islet cell carcinomas**—are slower growing, generally more treatable, and quite rare. Because early pancreatic cancers cause few symptoms, and because indicators of most pancreatic cancer may be misattributed to more benign digestive disorders, the disease is rarely detected before it has spread to nearby tissues or distant organs through the bloodstream or lymphatic system. A few rare types of endocrine cell cancer are likely to be detected early, because they produce abnormal quantities of hormones that cause telltale hormonal imbalances.

Like many other cancers, pancreatic cancer is characteristically a disease of the elderly, usually striking after age 60. It is more commonly diagnosed in men than in women, and most cases are incurable. The incidence of pancreatic cancer has risen with an increase in the average life span, causing some 27,000 new cases and about the same number of deaths annually in the U.S., making it one of the leading cancer killers.

CAUSES

Aside from advanced age, smoking is the main risk factor for pancreatic cancer; a smoker is three times more likely than a nonsmoker to acquire the disease. People frequently exposed to certain petroleum products may also be at increased risk. Excessive dietary fat and protein may promote the disease. ***Diabetes*** is also linked to pancreatic cancer: 10 to 20 percent of patients diagnosed with pancreatic cancer also have dia-

TUMORS IN THE PANCREAS

COMMON BILE DUCT

TUMOR

PANCREAS

Cancer develops most frequently at the head of the pancreas, where it can affect the digestive process. If the common bile duct that connects the liver and gall-bladder to the pancreas is blocked by a cancerous growth *(inset, above),* bile cannot be delivered to the small intestine, impairing digestion. A secondary effect is jaundice, often a symptom of pancreatic cancer.

betes. Other diseases associated with pancreatic cancer include hereditary pancreatitis, an inflammatory ***pancreatic problem;*** Gardner's syndrome, characterized by growths within and outside the colon; neurofibromatosis, or elephant man's disease; and multiple endocrine neoplasia, a condition that promotes growth of benign islet cell tumors; all these conditions are hereditary.

DIAGNOSTIC AND TEST PROCEDURES

To check for tumors in the pancreas, a doctor relies on imaging studies of the gland. The most common tests are sonograms and CT scans of the abdomen. If necessary, detailed images are obtained by inserting an endoscope through the mouth to the pancreas, injecting dye, then taking x-rays. A tissue sample for biopsy can also be extracted through the scope. If a biopsy confirms cancer, further tests are done to determine how far the disease has advanced. Sometimes exploratory surgery is necessary so the surgeon can study the tumor directly, determine if nearby lymph nodes are cancerous, and take tissue samples for microscopic examination.

TREATMENT

See ***Cancer*** for more information about the conventional treatments described below.

CONVENTIONAL MEDICINE

Because most cases of pancreatic cancer are advanced when diagnosed, cure is rarely a realistic goal. Instead, treatment usually aims to extend survival and relieve uncomfortable symptoms. Surgery may cure the cancer, but only if it has not spread beyond the pancreas. If possible the surgeon removes the malignant tumor, leaving as much of the pancreas as possible to allow continued function. More often, however, the entire pancreas must be removed. Then the patient must have a lifelong regimen of replacement enzymes and hormones, including ***insulin.***

Depending on the type of cancer, patients may also be administered radiation or chemotherapy treatments, either after surgery in an effort to extend survival time, or as a means of relieving symptoms. **Exocrine cell cancer** responds best to radiation, sometimes in combination with chemotherapy, while **endocrine cell cancer** responds best to chemotherapy. Prescription medication, usually including narcotics, is given to help manage the pain that is common with advanced pancreatic cancer.

COMPLEMENTARY THERAPIES

For many advanced pancreatic cancer sufferers, pain is significant. Besides taking prescription medication, patients can try pain control through **massage, acupuncture,** and **biofeedback** training, as well as such **relaxation** techniques as **guided imagery** and self-hypnosis.

PREVENTION

Pancreatic cancer is not easily prevented, but you can take measures to reduce your risk. If you work around petroleum products, take precautions to avoid unnecessary exposure to both materials and fumes. And if you smoke, quit now. ■

P

PANCREATIC PROBLEMS

SYMPTOMS

For **acute pancreatitis:**
- sudden, intense pains in the middle of the abdomen, often beginning 12 to 24 hours after a large meal or a bout of heavy drinking. The pain may radiate to your back.
- fever.
- nausea or vomiting.
- clammy skin.
- abdominal distention and tenderness.
- rapid pulse.

For **chronic pancreatitis:**
- intense, long-lasting abdominal pain that may radiate to the back and chest; the pain may be persistent or intermittent.
- excessively foul, bulky stools.
- nausea or vomiting.
- weight loss.
- abdominal distention.

CALL YOUR DOCTOR IF:

- you think you may have pancreatitis. Patients with acute pancreatitis must have professional care to avoid serious, possibly life-threatening complications. Chronic pancreatitis also requires professional evaluation and treatment.
- you continue to lose weight after treatment for pancreatitis; you may have a complication that prevents the body from digesting food properly.
- you are pale, cold, clammy, have a rapid heartbeat, or are breathing rapidly; you may be in **shock** and need emergency care. *(See page 75 in **Emergencies/First Aid.**)*

P

Chronic pancreatitis and **acute pancreatitis** are inflammations of the pancreas, a gland that produces both digestive enzymes and the hormone insulin, which your body uses to metabolize carbohydrates and fats. The symptoms of acute pancreatitis are typically severe and need to be treated. If they aren't, you may develop pancreatic cysts, abscesses, and leaks of pancreatic fluid into the abdomen, which can lead to other long-term problems. Shock is a possibly fatal complication of acute pancreatitis.

Chronic pancreatitis develops over a number of years, usually after a history of recurrent attacks of acute pancreatitis. Chronic pancreatitis may cause you to lose the ability to secrete the enzymes your body needs to digest foods. The resulting condition, known as exocrine insufficiency, is a principal characteristic of chronic pancreatitis and is signaled by weight loss—either gradual or sudden—and foul-smelling stools. Chronic pancreatitis can also lead to ***diabetes*** mellitus and pancreatic calcification, in which small, hard deposits develop in the pancreas.

CAUSES

Acute pancreatitis is associated with excessive alcohol drinking, ***gallstones,*** viral and bacterial infections, drugs, and blockage of the pancreatic duct. These factors appear to encourage pancreatic digestive enzymes to act on the pancreas itself, causing swelling, hemorrhage, and damage to blood vessels in the pancreas. More than half the people who develop **chronic pancreatitis** are heavy drinkers; heavy consumption of alcohol is the most frequent cause of exocrine insufficiency in adults. (The leading cause of exocrine insufficiency in children is cystic fibrosis.)

DIAGNOSTIC AND TEST PROCEDURES

Your doctor will probably press on your abdominal area to see if it is tender, and check you for low blood pressure, low-grade fever, and rapid pulse. Your blood will be tested for abnormal levels of pancreatic enzymes, white blood cells, blood sugar, and calcium. Abdominal x-rays will show if your pancreas is calcified. Ultrasound tests or CT scans will show bile duct problems.

To diagnose **chronic pancreatitis,** your doctor will take blood samples and check your stool for excess fat, a sign that the pancreas is no longer producing enough enzymes to process fat. You may be given a stimulation test to see how well your pancreas releases its digestive enzymes into the duodenum. You may also be screened for diabetes mellitus.

TREATMENT

Conventional medicine treats pancreatitis with drugs, diet, and surgery. Alternative choices focus on alleviating symptoms of pancreatitis and bolstering your overall health.

CONVENTIONAL MEDICINE

If you have an attack of **acute pancreatitis,** your doctor will try to stem the flow of pancreatic enzymes by feeding you intravenously. You may receive meperidine—a strong analgesic—for pain. You may have to have your stomach drained with a tube placed through your nose. If your pancreatitis is caused by gallstones or an obstructed pancreatic duct, you may need surgery once your symptoms have subsided.

If you have **chronic pancreatitis,** your doctor will focus on treating you for pain—guarding against your possible addiction to prescription ***analgesics***—and for complications that affect your digestive abilities. You may be placed on an enzyme replacement therapy to restore your digestive tract's ability to digest nutrients; this will also likely reduce the frequency of new attacks. You may have to avoid fatty foods, and will have to abstain from drinking alcohol. If your pain does not respond to medication, the damaged pancreatic tissue may be surgically removed, but only as a last resort.

ALTERNATIVE CHOICES

Alternative treatments can be used in conjunction with conventional treatment to help improve your overall responsiveness to medical therapy. Because both acute and chronic pancreatitis require conventional treatment, you should discuss any other approaches with your doctor before proceeding with them.

CHINESE MEDICINE

A practitioner will treat pancreatitis in the context of a complete body system imbalance.

HERBAL THERAPIES

A combination of equal parts of glycerates of fringe-tree bark *(Chionanthus virginicus),* balmony *(Chelone glabra),* and ***milk thistle*** *(Silybum marianum)* may help promote fat digestion; take 1 tsp of the mixture three times daily.

NUTRITION AND DIET

Take ***chromium*** supplements, 300 mcg daily, to help maintain normal blood sugar levels. Supplements of buffered ***vitamin C*** as well as ***vitamin B complex*** with extra ***niacin*** (B_3) and pantothenic acid ***(B_5)*** may help reduce stress and fight infection. Do not drink alcohol.

REFLEXOLOGY

Press the adrenal gland areas to help your body fight infection, the stomach and pancreas areas to improve digestion, and the solar plexus areas to relieve stress. *(See page 25 for area locations.)*

PREVENTION

- Limiting yourself to one or two alcoholic drinks per day may significantly lessen your chances of developing pancreatitis. Once you have had pancreatitis, though, you should not drink at all; any drinking carries the risk of new attacks.
- Controlling your weight and maintaining a healthful diet and lifestyle may prevent gallstones. ■

P

PANIC ATTACK

SYMPTOMS

If you have four or more of the following, you are having a panic attack:

- heart palpitations.
- sweating.
- shaking.
- a "smothering" sensation.
- a feeling of choking.
- chest pain or discomfort.
- nausea.
- dizziness or faintness.
- a sense of unreality.
- a fear of going crazy.
- a fear of dying.
- numbness or tingling.
- chills or hot flashes.

If you have recurrent panic attacks and persistent fear of subsequent attacks or change your behavior significantly because of such attacks, you have **panic disorder.**

CALL YOUR DOCTOR IF:

- you think you have **panic disorder.** An isolated panic attack, while extremely unpleasant, is not uncommon or life-threatening.
- you think you may be having an actual ***heart attack,*** whose symptoms can be similar. However, most people having a panic attack have had one before, triggered by a similar event or situation.

You are engaged in some ordinary aspect of life when suddenly your heart begins to pound, and you hyperventilate, sweat, and tremble. You fear you are having a heart attack, going crazy, or even dying. Then, 10 or so minutes later, it's gone. Where did that feeling come from?

Unfortunately, there is no clear answer. You have had a panic attack, and for a small minority of sufferers, they recur again and again in a pattern known as **panic disorder.** Between attacks, sufferers live in dread of the next one.

Many people with panic disorder relate an attack to what they were doing when it occurred. They may assume that the restaurant, elevator, or classroom caused the attack, and decide to avoid that situation. In this case, panic disorder may lead to **agoraphobia**—the fear of leaving home or being in public places—though the relationship between the two conditions is unclear. *(See **Phobias.**)*

Panic attacks are fairly common, afflicting about 35 percent of the population each year. About 1 to 2 percent will develop panic disorder. Attacks usually begin between ages 15 and 25.

CAUSES

The underlying cause of panic disorder is not clear. There is evidence of both a genetic and a biochemical basis. There is also an association with ***phobias,*** such as school phobia or agoraphobia, and with ***depression, alcohol abuse,*** suicide risk, and ***seasonal affective disorder.*** The sudden feeling of terror or doom often brings on hyperventilation—uncontrollable, rapid, shallow breathing. This in itself can cause many of the other physical symptoms by upsetting the balance of oxygen and carbon dioxide in the bloodstream.

Panic disorder may begin after a serious illness or accident, the death of a close friend, separation from the family, or the birth of a baby. Attacks may also accompany the use of mind-altering drugs. Most often, however, a panic attack comes "out of the blue"; it may even begin during sleep.

Some medical problems and medications can cause panic attacks, including ***antidepressants*** at high dosage. Panic disorder that begins after age 40 suggests depression or another underlying medical disorder.

TREATMENT

Because the cause of most panic attacks is not clear, treatment must be based on particular cases and may involve psychotherapy, cognitive-behavioral therapy, or medication. Alternative treatments fight anxiety and relax the body.

CONVENTIONAL MEDICINE

Psychotherapy offers support and helps to minimize the fearfulness of symptoms; sometimes this is sufficient to clear up the disorder. Recurrent attacks, however, require additional measures.

Cognitive-behavioral therapy, which exposes patients to the bodily sensations of panic in a safe setting, is often helpful. These sensations may be induced by rapid breathing, head rolling, or running up stairs. Patients are taught coping skills such as muscle relaxation and breathing techniques. This therapy also helps them learn that panic does not lead to the catastrophic events they fear, such as having a heart attack.

Antidepressants, such as imipramine, often help reduce anxiety and the frequency and severity of panic attacks. ***Antianxiety drugs*** (such as ***alprazolam***) work faster than antidepressants but carry the risk of dependence. Halting the medicine, however, often leads to relapse. Medication is most successful when used with cognitive-behavioral therapy.

ALTERNATIVE CHOICES

A number of alternative techniques may help reduce the anxiety that underlies panic disorder.

AROMATHERAPY

Studies have shown that essential oil of ***lavender*** *(Lavandula officinalis)* can relieve anxiety and stress. Try carrying a small bottle with you and sprinkling a few drops on a handkerchief to inhale at stressful moments.

BODY WORK

Both **qigong** and **yoga** can relax the body and help with the anxiety that patients experience between panic attacks. Either can be learned from a teacher and then practiced at home.

HERBAL THERAPIES

A number of herbs function as relaxants and tranquilizers and may soothe anxiety. Try a tea made from ***skullcap*** *(Scutellaria lateriflora),* ***valerian*** *(Valeriana officinalis),* vervain, or lemon balm.

HYPNOTHERAPY

Hypnosis is effective for many patients with anxiety or phobias, partly because the therapy itself brings deep relaxation. This may be combined with other therapies to enable patients to discover and overcome the cause of the panic.

MIND/BODY MEDICINE

Because hyperventilation is a central feature of panic attacks, the practice of slow and deep breathing can help reduce the severity and perhaps even the frequency of attacks. **Meditation** and other relaxation exercises, such as taking two minutes each hour to breathe slowly, are helpful in both calming the rhythm of breathing and reducing anxiety.

NUTRITION AND DIET

Magnesium has a tranquilizing action; try a 250-mg tablet twice a day. Avoid caffeine and other stimulants, alcohol, and sugar.

PREVENTION

You can take steps to lessen the chance of attacks and learn to manage them better.

- Learn to recognize a panic attack. When you sense the first symptoms, know that others may come. You have survived them before and can do so again. Try slow, deep breaths.
- Take your time. It's important not to hope for a quick cure. Therapy takes time, and improvement comes in small steps.
- Go easy on yourself. People who feel panic tend to be overly critical of themselves. ■

P

PARKINSON'S DISEASE

SYMPTOMS

The disease takes hold slowly, beginning with a sense of weakness and a slight tremor of the head or hands, then gradually progressing to more generalized symptoms. These can include:

- slow, jerky movements; a shuffling gait; and stooped posture.
- unsteady balance; difficulty rising from a sitting position.
- continuous "pill-rolling" motion of the thumb and forefinger.
- indistinct speech; voice weakened to a monotone.
- swallowing problems in later stages.
- in severe cases, rigid trunk and limbs; fixed facial expression and unblinking, staring eyes.

CALL YOUR DOCTOR IF:

- you suspect Parkinson's disease might be at the root of any of the above symptoms. In the disease's early stages, drugs can be very beneficial.

Parkinson's disease, which mostly afflicts older people, results from gradual degeneration of nerve cells in the portion of the midbrain that controls body movements. The first signs are likely to be barely noticeable—a feeling of weakness or stiffness in one limb, perhaps, or a fine trembling of one hand when it is at rest (activity causes the tremor to disappear). Eventually, the shaking will worsen and spread, muscles will tend to stiffen, and balance and coordination will deteriorate. Depression and other mental or emotional problems are common.

Usually the disorder begins between the ages of 50 and 65, striking about 1 percent of the population in that age group; it is slightly more common in men than in women. Medication can treat its symptoms, and the disorder is not directly life-threatening. About half of all patients treated with drugs have no major disabilities 10 years after the onset of the disease.

CAUSES

Bodily movements are regulated by a portion of the brain called the basal ganglia, whose cells require a proper balance of two substances called dopamine and acetylcholine, both involved in the transmission of nerve impulses. In Parkinson's, cells that produce dopamine begin to degenerate, throwing off the balance of these two neurotransmitters. Researchers believe that genetics sometimes plays a role in the cellular breakdown, and in rare instances, Parkinson's may be caused by a viral infection or by exposure to environmental toxins such as pesticides, carbon monoxide, or the metal manganese. But in the great majority of Parkinson's cases, the cause is unknown.

DIAGNOSTIC AND TEST PROCEDURES

Usually, the outward symptoms of Parkinson's are distinctive enough for a diagnosis to be made. The metabolic changes in the brain can be traced with imaging tests such as PET—positron emission tomography.

P

TREATMENT

Most treatments aim at restoring the proper balance of the neurotransmitters acetylcholine and dopamine by increasing dopamine levels. Drugs are the standard way of doing this, but neurosurgeons have had some success with experiments involving operative procedures.

CONVENTIONAL MEDICINE

Symptoms can be effectively controlled for years with medication. The drug most often prescribed is ***levodopa***—also called L-dopa—which the body metabolizes to produce dopamine. (Direct administration of dopamine is ineffective; the brain's natural protections block its uptake.) To suppress nausea and other possible side effects, levodopa is often used in conjunction with a related drug called carbidopa.

But some patients cannot tolerate carbidopa and so take levodopa alone. If you take only levodopa, it's important not to take it at the same time as food or vitamins containing ***vitamin B_6,*** which interferes with its effectiveness.

Most doctors try to postpone starting patients on levodopa as long as possible, because the medication tends to lose effectiveness over time. However, there is some controversy about waiting to begin treatment with levodopa because it can be so beneficial. Researchers have thus investigated ways to offset the loss of effectiveness. Some studies have found that, when used in conjunction with levodopa and carbidopa, the antioxidant selegiline hydrochloride reduces many of the adverse effects associated with long-term drug use.

A class of dopamine-like drugs, including bromocriptine, pergolide, pranipexole, and ropinirole, imitates dopamine's activity rather than adding to the amount of it in the brain. Other medications prescribed for Parkinson's disease include apomorphine, benztropine, amantadine, and anticholinergic drugs; all can help control various symptoms—in some cases by releasing dopamine from nerve cells, in others by reducing the effects of acetylcholine rather than increasing the amount of dopamine.

Neurosurgeons have explored various ways of grafting dopamine-producing cells in the brain rather than trying to correct the neurotransmitter imbalance with drugs. One promising approach uses fetal-tissue implants. Some improvements have been observed, but because of the source of the cells, the technique is highly controversial.

Another experimental technique, stereotactic surgery, creates lesions in the thalamus, the brain's inner chamber. In some studies, this procedure appears to eliminate tremor in 80 percent of patients and to relieve rigidity in almost all. A similar form of surgery—using electrical stimulation instead of lesions—also shows promise.

Scientists are also investigating the use of glial cell-derived nerve growth factor to treat Parkinson's and other neurodegenerative diseases. This substance is produced naturally by tissues throughout the body; some experiments indicate that injections of this nerve growth factor may help preserve and even restore nerve cells in the brain and spinal cord—specifically those that produce dopamine and that help initiate muscle movement.

Some treatments focus on the effects of the disorder rather than the causes. Your doctor might refer you to a physical therapist to restore normal body alignment, enhance your balance and motor responses, and improve your ability to initiate motion. A physical therapist may also give you muscle-strengthening exercises to help with speaking or swallowing.

In many Parkinson's patients, a weakening of social ties because of physical difficulties can lead to depression. ***Antidepressants*** can help. In addition, the American Parkinson Disease Association *(see the **Appendix**)* can provide information about support groups and exercise classes in your area—valuable sources of companionship.

ALTERNATIVE CHOICES

Conventional medicines such as levodopa are widely acknowledged as the best treatments for Parkinson's disease. However, many of the alternative therapies mentioned below can be very helpful for relieving symptoms or easing tight muscles. Some of the herbal and dietary therapies

P

can be applied in conjunction with conventional medicines, but be sure to consult your doctor about possible adverse interactions.

ACUPUNCTURE

According to some studies by acupuncturists, Parkinson's disease may be accompanied by an imbalance of energy along one or more meridians *(see page 20)*. The muscle stiffness, soreness, and imbalance of Parkinson's may be alleviated by a series of treatments.

BODY WORK

Deep-muscle **massage** stretches the connective tissue around tight muscles, ridding them of cramping and allowing greater freedom of movement. Massage can also improve motion in your joints, soften hardened muscle tissue, and stimulate your lymphatic system.

Reflexology practitioners say that the brain, head, and spine all respond to indirect massage. See the illustration below for reflexology techniques that may help relieve some Parkinson's symptoms.

REFLEXOLOGY

To help ease the tremors of Parkinson's, walk your thumb across the reflexology area for the diaphragm and solar plexus. Working areas for the brain and spinal column may help stabilize the nervous system.

Chi yi, a Chinese deep-breathing exercise, increases the oxygen supply in the blood and may thereby help alleviate depression. Sit with your back against the back of a chair and your feet flat on the floor. Reach toward the ceiling with both arms, inhaling deeply through your nose as you do so. Hold your breath as you ball your hands into fists, squeezing your arm muscles. Exhale slowly through your nose to a count of six as you bring your tensed arms down, crossing them on your chest over your heart. Lower your chin to your chest. Take four short breaths, completely filling your lungs, and feel your chest expand. Hold for a few seconds, then exhale slowly. Repeat this exercise several times each day, concentrating on the rhythm and depth of each breath. If tremor prohibits arm or head movements, concentrate on the breathing, working toward a rate of only four or five breaths per minute. Limit practice to five minutes per day.

Yoga is an ideal form of exercise for Parkinson's patients because of its slow movements. Regular exercise is important to avoid the atrophying of muscles and shrinking of tissues from disuse. See the illustration opposite for one useful type of yoga exercise.

CHINESE HERBS

Taken several times a day, combinations that include rhubarb *(Rheum palmatum)*, peony *(Paeonia officinalis)*, **licorice** *(Glycyrrhiza uralensis)*, and magnolia bark *(Magnolia officinalis)* are said to stop tremors and relax stiff muscles. Because using Chinese herbs is complicated, consult an expert in the field for correct dosages.

HERBAL THERAPIES

Passionflower *(Passiflora incarnata)* acts as an antispasmodic when 1/4 tsp of tincture is taken three times a day. Or take it twice daily as a tea: Pour one cup boiling water over 2 tsp dried leaves; steep for 15 minutes. Passionflower has been shown to reduce passive tremor when taken in combination with levodopa better than when either remedy is taken alone. But be sure to check with your doctor first if you are already taking levodopa.

Daily doses of 500 mg of ***evening primrose oil*** *(Oenothera biennis)* may reduce tremors.

P

YOGA

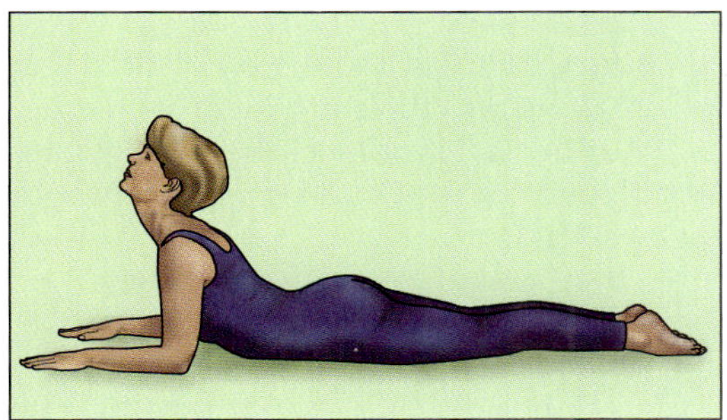

Practice the **Sphinx** for muscle control. Place both forearms on the floor with your palms down and elbows under your shoulders. Inhale and push your chest away from the floor as far as comfortably possible. Hold for a few deep breaths, then relax and exhale.

HOMEOPATHY

A trained homeopath might prescribe a single remedy, a series, or a combination of remedies for the many different symptoms of Parkinson's.

MIND/BODY MEDICINE

The **Feldenkrais method,** which consists of a large number of exercises performed either in group classes or solo with a practitioner, aims at improving autonomic motor responses. While lying down, you are guided through a series of light, slow movements designed to support your neuromuscular system and alter habitual patterns of movement.

NUTRITION AND DIET

Parkinson's patients should pay close attention to diet; weight loss—possibly caused by persistent involuntary movements—is a common problem.

A diet called the 7:1 plan—for the ratio of carbohydrates to proteins—is designed for patients taking levodopa (proteins reduce the drug's effectiveness). Researchers disagree as to whether the proteins should be eaten throughout the day or restricted to the evening meal, when interference with levodopa might be less of a problem. Consult your doctor to determine which method works best for you. Either way, a low-protein diet can lead to deficiencies in ***calcium, iron,*** and ***B vitamins;*** supplements are therefore advised. (If you are taking levodopa without carbidopa, however, avoid ***vitamin*** B_6***;*** the vitamin will interfere with the levodopa.)

Fava beans, also called broad beans, are a natural source of levodopa. One-half cup contains 250 mg, or the same amount as one pill. But don't substitute beans for pills without first consulting your doctor.

Patients attempt to relieve the constipation that often accompanies Parkinson's by eating bran. But recent research shows that bran is high in vitamin B_6, which interferes with the effectiveness of levodopa when the drug is taken alone. Prune juice, grains, and fiber laxatives should be substituted instead.

Foods seasoned with hot spices have been known to cause uncontrollable physical movement in some people with Parkinson's. Avoid such foods.

AT-HOME CARE

- Adding banisters in hallways and along walls can make it easier for a Parkinson's patient to get around.
- Chairs and sofas that are equipped with higher arms make sitting down and rising more manageable.
- Thick carpeting offers protection in falls, common with Parkinson's patients. ■

PELVIC INFLAMMATORY DISEASE

SYMPTOMS

With acute pelvic inflammatory disease (PID):

- severe pain and tenderness in the lower abdomen with vaginal discharge, often accompanied by fever.

With chronic PID:

- mild, recurrent pain in the lower abdomen, sometimes accompanied by backache or irregular menstrual periods.
- pain during intercourse.
- infertility.
- irregular menstrual periods.
- heavy, unpleasant-smelling vaginal discharge.

CALL YOUR DOCTOR IF:

- you experience sudden abdominal pain with or without fever; it may indicate acute pelvic inflammatory disease or another serious condition that requires immediate medical attention, such as ***appendicitis, endometriosis,*** a ruptured ovarian cyst *(see **Ovary Problems**),* or an ectopic pregnancy.
- you experience any abnormal menstrual bleeding; you may have pelvic inflammatory disease or another serious condition, such as ***endometriosis*** or ***cervical cancer.***
- you experience a vaginal discharge that is foul-smelling or unusually heavy; you may have pelvic inflammatory disease or another condition that requires medical treatment, such as ***vaginal, uterine,*** or ***cervical problems,*** or a ***sexually transmitted disease.***

P

Pelvic inflammatory disease (PID) is the term used to describe an infection of any of a woman's pelvic organs, including the uterus, ovaries, or fallopian tubes. The disease has become increasingly common in the United States, affecting an estimated one million women each year. If not treated promptly, PID can lead to serious complications, including ***infertility*** and, in rare cases, death.

PID can be either acute or chronic. Acute PID comes on suddenly and is apt to be more severe. Chronic PID is a low-grade infection that may cause only recurrent mild pain and sometimes backache. Some women with PID have no discernible symptoms and discover they have had the infection only when they later attempt to get pregnant and discover that they are infertile.

CAUSES

PID is caused by bacteria from contaminated semen that ascend from the vagina into the normally sterile uterus. Most cases of PID used to be caused by gonococcus, the organism responsible for the sexually transmitted disease ***gonorrhea,*** or by ***chlamydia.*** Recently, researchers have linked other organisms to PID, including some commonly found in the vagina and elsewhere in the body.

The risk of PID increases after childbirth, miscarriage, abortion, the insertion of an intrauterine device (IUD) for contraception, or certain operations, such as a dilation and curettage (D and C), all of which cause the cervix, or opening to the uterus, to widen temporarily. Douching also increases the risk of PID.

DIAGNOSTIC AND TEST PROCEDURES

Your doctor will give you a pelvic examination. If there is evidence of an infection, he or she will use a cotton swab to obtain a sample of pus from inside your vagina. The sample will be analyzed to determine which organism is causing the infection. Sometimes a laparoscopic exam—a surgical procedure in which a special viewing instrument is inserted into the abdominal cavity—is necessary for an accurate diagnosis. Your doctor may also use ultrasound to help with the diagnosis.

TREATMENT

Because PID can lead to serious complications, such as infertility, it must be treated with conventional ***antibiotics.*** Alternative therapies may be used, however, to complement the antibiotics and to help with recovery and prevention.

CONVENTIONAL MEDICINE

Your doctor will prescribe one or more oral ***antibiotics,*** such as ***tetracycline, erythromycin,*** or ***doxycycline,*** to clear up the infection. You may be treated on an outpatient basis, but if you are pregnant or have severe symptoms or if your case presents other complicating factors, you may be hospitalized and given the antibiotics intravenously.

If you have an IUD, your doctor will remove it. Until the PID is eradicated, you should avoid intercourse, which can cause the pelvic organs to move, spreading infected pus.

If your infection is chronic or recurrent and does not respond to oral antibiotics, your doctor may order intravenous antibiotics. When pelvic abscesses have developed, even intravenous antibiotics may not work; it may then be necessary to operate and drain the abscesses. If your pain is persistent and does not respond to other treatments, your doctor may recommend pelvic surgery to remove or repair infected tissue. Sometimes it is possible to spare one ovary, thus preventing premature menopause, and still get relief from the pain. Discuss this possibility with your doctor.

ALTERNATIVE CHOICES

Use alternative methods during or after conventional antibiotic treatment to speed recovery and help prevent recurrences. To relieve the pain of a PID infection, for example, use castor-oil packs or get **acupressure** or **acupuncture** treatments from an experienced practitioner.

HERBAL THERAPIES

To help fight PID infection, herbalists recommend ***echinacea*** (*Echinacea* spp.) or ***oregon grape*** *(Mahonia aquifolium)* root. Both these herbs are believed to have antimicrobial properties. Blue cohosh *(Caulophyllum thalictroides)* and false unicorn root *(Chamaelirium luteum),* which are prescribed as general tonics for the female reproductive organs, are also recommended. You may take these herbs in either tea or tincture form.

NUTRITION AND DIET

To strengthen your immune system and help speed your recovery, eat plenty of whole (unprocessed) foods, especially fresh fruits and vegetables.

Vitamin and mineral supplements may also enhance your immune system. Take ***vitamin A*** (10,000 IU daily), ***vitamin C*** (500 to 2,000 mg daily), and ***vitamin B complex*** (50 mg three times a day); take ***zinc*** (25 to 50 mg daily).

PREVENTION

- Use barrier contraception (condoms, diaphragm, or a cervical cap with spermicides).
- Avoid putting anything in your vagina for two to three weeks after an abortion, a miscarriage, or a D and C and for six weeks after childbirth. This means no intercourse, no douching, and no tampons. You should also avoid bathing and swimming during this period; take showers or sponge baths instead.
- Do not use an IUD. Women wearing an IUD are three to five times more likely to get PID than those not wearing one, especially if they have more than one partner.
- If you have a history of pelvic infections or have several sexual partners, use barrier methods of contraception and avoid intercourse during your menstrual period. The cervix—the opening to the uterus—widens during menstruation to allow blood and uterine tissue to flow out.
- Get prompt treatment for any ***sexually transmitted disease.*** ■

PENILE PAIN

Read down this column to find your symptoms. Then read across.

SYMPTOMS	AILMENT/PROBLEM
◆ a bend in the penis that may be painful during erection.	◆ Peyronie's disease—a fibrous thickening along the shaft of the penis.
◆ persistent, painful erection unrelated to sexual desire.	◆ Priapism—a state of continuous erection, usually traceable to a disease or other disorder.
◆ painful urination and a clear, thin discharge from the penis.	◆ ***Chlamydia***—a sexually transmitted infection caused by a microscopic organism.
◆ painful urination and a cloudy, thick, pus-like discharge from the penis.	◆ ***Gonorrhea***—a sexually transmitted bacterial infection.
◆ painful blisters along the penis that break and expose raw skin.	◆ ***Genital herpes***—a sexually transmitted viral infection.
◆ itchy, hard, flesh-colored warts along the penis, which may bleed and be mildly painful.	◆ ***Genital warts***—a sexually transmitted viral infection.
◆ pain, redness, and swelling on the foreskin or head (glans) of the penis.	◆ Balanitis—an infection or inflammation of the penis.
◆ pain occurring after injections for erectile dysfunction, or impotence.	◆ Drug-induced pain.
◆ pain and difficulty retracting the foreskin.	◆ Phimosis—an overly tight foreskin.
◆ a lump, swelling, or open sore on the penis.	◆ Possibly a sign of cancer of the penis.

WHAT TO DO	OTHER INFO
◆ See your doctor. Although many cases need no treatment, others require surgery. Taking 200 IU of ***vitamin E*** with each meal may help.	◆ Most common in middle-aged men. Scar tissue from repeated vascular injuries prevents penile skin from sliding normally during intercourse.
◆ See your doctor. Untreated priapism can cause impotence; you need to be evaluated for the existence of another health problem. For temporary relief, take ***acetaminophen*** and apply an ice pack to the penis.	◆ Priapism has various causes—including ***sickle cell anemia.*** Treating the condition promptly should restore normal erections.
◆ See your doctor or a clinic for a blood test. Chlamydia can be successfully treated with ***antibiotics.***	◆ Sexual partners must also be treated for the infection.
◆ See your doctor. Discontinue sexual relations until you are analyzed and treated.	◆ This infection may be transmitted by vaginal, anal, or oral sex, and may spread to other parts of the body.
◆ See your doctor. Wash and dry the area regularly. Avoid sexual intercourse for two weeks after an outbreak.	◆ Herpes usually spreads only during the active phase of the disease. ***Acyclovir*** may relieve pain and reduce the length of the active phase.
◆ See your doctor. Avoid sexual contact until warts disappear. Never treat genital warts with over-the-counter wart preparations.	◆ Genital warts may disappear on their own but often recur, though less often and less severely over time.
◆ Wash beneath the foreskin when bathing. If infection is chronic, circumcision—surgical removal of the foreskin—may be necessary.	◆ May be caused by irritating clothing or by secretions that collect under an uncircumcised foreskin.
◆ See your doctor, who may add ***sodium bicarbonate*** or the painkiller procaine to the medication.	◆ Sodium bicarbonate neutralizes the acidity of injected medications used to treat erectile dysfunction.
◆ See your doctor. If you have persistent pain, circumcision may be necessary.	◆ The cause may be inflammation or a genetic condition. Contrary to myth, circumcision has no noticeable effect on sexual function or satisfaction.
◆ See your doctor immediately, even if there is no pain. Prompt diagnosis increases the chance of successful treatment.	◆ Cancer may begin as small growths beneath the foreskin. Circumcised men rarely develop this cancer.

PHLEBITIS

SYMPTOMS

For **superficial phlebitis:**

- a red, cordlike vein visible in your leg; the vein will feel hard, warm, and tender, and surrounding tissue may become itchy and swollen.
- a throbbing or burning sensation beneath the skin's surface.
- pain and heaviness when lowering your leg.

For **deep phlebitis:**

- potentially no symptoms.
- pain and swelling throughout the entire affected limb.
- fever, skin ulcers, or swellings in your leg that stay indented when pressed.

CALL YOUR DOCTOR IF:

- you suspect you have phlebitis; you need proper diagnosis and treatment.
- symptoms of **superficial phlebitis** do not dissipate within 7 to 10 days; you may have developed a more serious condition.
- you experience unusual bleeding when taking anticoagulant drugs; your doctor may have to adjust the dosage.
- you notice lumps, high fever, or pervasive pain or swelling throughout a limb. All are signs of **deep phlebitis,** possibly accompanied by infection, that requires immediate medical care.
- you have phlebitis and develop an associated infection (which may occur after childbirth or a wound or trauma to a vein, or if you have a heart valve infection). Even in mild cases, infection introduces a risk of blood poisoning.

Doctors often use the general term "phlebitis" (meaning inflammation of a vein) to refer to a more specific condition known as thrombophlebitis, which involves the formation of blood clots, or thrombi, where inflammation occurs. These clots cause pain and irritation, and may also partially or fully block blood flow in affected veins.

The most common form of phlebitis, called **superficial phlebitis,** occurs in veins near the skin's surface, typically in the legs. Though annoying, it is relatively harmless, usually resolving itself in a matter of days. **Deep phlebitis,** which affects interior veins of the legs, is less common and more dangerous: Because interior veins are larger, blood clots tend to be bigger and are more likely to break free and travel to the lungs. Also, people with deep phlebitis often are not aware that they have it and don't seek proper care.

CAUSES

People with ***varicose veins*** are prone to phlebitis. Anyone immobilized for any length of time, such as after surgery, is also vulnerable because blood is not flowing as strongly and clots form more easily. The elderly are also susceptible, because circulatory problems and vascular diseases that can trigger phlebitis tend to worsen with age.

Phlebitis can also develop in response to infection or trauma of some kind. It may occur at the site of an intravenous injection, particularly when that site has been prodded repeatedly.

Researchers have identified several other risk factors. About 70 percent of phlebitis sufferers are women. Pregnant women and those on birth-control pills are more likely to develop the condition. People whose blood tends to clot too readily are at higher risk. Obesity, a sedentary lifestyle, and smoking have also been linked to phlebitis.

TREATMENT

Treatment depends on the type of phlebitis. **Superficial phlebitis** usually responds to simple at-home measures. **Deep phlebitis,** however, often requires a short stay in the hospital. In either

RISK IN DIFFERENT VEINS

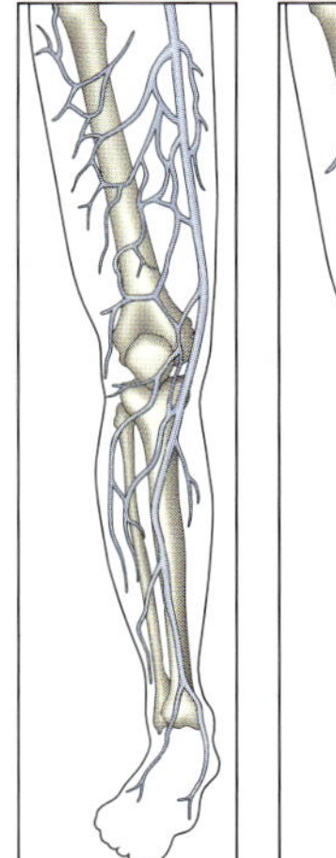

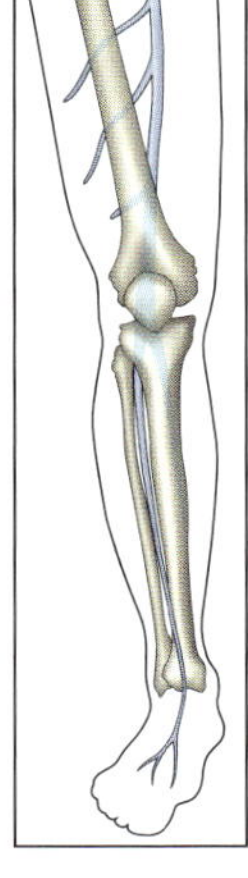

SUPERFICIAL VEINS DEEP VEINS

Phlebitis can strike any vein but typically strikes those in the legs; its severity usually depends on the depth of the affected vessel. Superficial phlebitis, or inflammation and clotting of a vein close to the skin, may produce swelling, redness, and pain, but the condition is rarely serious. Deep phlebitis, which attacks large interior veins, often occurs without symptoms but can have fatal complications.

case, if you smoke, stop; smoking greatly aggravates all circulatory problems. Also, switching from birth-control pills to another form of contraception may help prevent a recurrence.

CONVENTIONAL MEDICINE

If you think you have phlebitis, your doctor may order x-rays to confirm the diagnosis and to determine whether deep veins are involved.

To help relieve the symptoms of **superficial phlebitis,** your doctor may recommend ***aspirin*** to reduce inflammation. You may be given an ***antibiotic*** if your doctor thinks there is an infection. If you're bothered by pain and swelling, inquire about elastic support stockings. Although pantyhose often constrict circulation, specially prescribed compression stockings can greatly improve blood flow; for many, they bring immediate and lasting relief. See also **At-Home Remedies.**

If you're diagnosed with **deep phlebitis,** you will be hospitalized. Doctors routinely prescribe a one-week treatment of ***heparin,*** an ***anticoagulant*** usually given intravenously. You will rest in bed with your legs elevated and be evaluated for signs of lung clots. Your doctor will probably also start you on a 90-day course of another anticoagulant known as ***warfarin,*** taken orally. Warfarin is a powerful drug, so you'll need to watch for side effects your doctor will tell you about.

ALTERNATIVE CHOICES

Some alternative therapies may help with **superficial phlebitis.** Consult a **homeopath,** or a practitioner of Chinese medicine, who might advise **acupressure, acupuncture,** or a combination of **Chinese herbs** designed to reduce inflammation. You might also try increasing your intake of ***vitamin E,*** a natural blood thinner, and ***vitamin C;*** both help keep blood vessels in good shape.

AT-HOME REMEDIES

For **superficial phlebitis,** there are several things you can do at home to ease discomfort and speed your recovery:

- Get plenty of rest.
- When you lie down, prop up your legs so they are 6 to 12 inches above your heart level. This encourages blood to drain from your legs, easing the burden on veins affected by phlebitis.
- Use a heating pad or apply a moist, warm pack to swollen areas for relief. If surrounding skin itches, try a dab of zinc oxide.

P

CAUTION!

It's quite natural to rub an aching muscle to relieve pain, but be careful if you have phlebitis. Though the risk is slight, massage—particularly vigorous massage—might dislodge a blood clot, which could potentially travel to your lungs and cause a life-threatening pulmonary embolism. Don't worry if you forget and find yourself rubbing a sore area without thinking, but try to resist the urge. ■

PHOBIAS

SYMPTOMS

Phobias are ***anxiety*** disorders. Three main types of phobias exist:

- If you have a persistent, irrational fear of particular objects or situations, such as snakes, spiders, heights, blood, flying, or elevators, you have a **specific phobia.**
- If you have a persistent, irrational fear of situations where you may be scrutinized or criticized or embarrassed by other people, you have **social phobia.**
- If you fear leaving home, being alone, or being away from home in a situation where you feel trapped or helpless, you have **agoraphobia.**

CALL YOUR DOCTOR IF:

- you have a phobia that interferes with a normal social or working life. Treatment can often lessen your anxiety and may diminish or even remove the phobia.

P

Phobias (from the Greek *phobos,* meaning fear or flight) are irrational and disabling fears that produce a compelling desire to avoid the dreaded object or situation. A phobic person understands that the fear is excessive or groundless, but the effort to resist it only brings more anxiety. Phobias affect about 7 percent of the population, often beginning in childhood.

Specific phobias are the most common; they involve things such as school, dentists, driving, water, balloons, snakes, fat, age, high places (acrophobia), and enclosed spaces (claustrophobia). The fear is usually not of the object itself but of some dire outcome, such as falling from an airplane. Even though phobics acknowledge that their fear is excessive, this knowledge does not diminish their fear.

A victim of **agoraphobia** suffers multiple fears that center around three main themes: fear of leaving home, of being alone, and of being in a situation where one cannot suddenly leave or obtain help. If agoraphobia progresses, a person may go to almost any lengths to avoid leaving home.

In **social phobia,** which often affects adolescents, a person's central fear is of being humiliated in public. People with this kind of phobia may even balk at eating in a restaurant. They avoid public speaking, parties, and public lavatories; such situations and places may bring blushing, palpitations, sweating, tremors, stuttering, or faintness. As many as 25 percent of professional performers struggle with severe, lifelong performance anxiety—a form of social phobia. A person whose phobia is left untreated may become withdrawn, depressed, and socially incapacitated.

CAUSES

Some **specific phobias** can be explained by early traumatic events, such as the bite of a dog, but the majority have no obvious cause. Most are thought to be produced when an underlying fear or conflict is displaced onto an unrelated object. **Agoraphobia** may develop in response to repeated ***panic attacks.*** Precursors of **social phobia** may be observable early in childhood, but the true cause is unknown.

TREATMENT

The effectiveness of treatment depends partly on the phobia's severity. While some phobias are never completely cured, many people can learn to function effectively, especially after attending phobia clinics and support groups including people who have recovered from phobias.

CONVENTIONAL MEDICINE

For **specific phobias,** treatment by systematic desensitization therapy is highly successful. For example, someone who is afraid of flying may be led through a series of steps, beginning with looking at pictures of airplanes in the relaxed environment of a therapist's office. This is followed by an imaginary trip in an airplane, then a visit to an airport, and finally an actual flight. Each stage should be accompanied by **relaxation** techniques. The support of a trusted person is very important.

Treating **social phobia** usually involves gradual exposure to social situations, along with role playing and rehearsal. Individuals are taught to reduce anxiety and encouraged to be less self-critical and learn appropriate behavior. Medications may also be used. Many musicians, actors, and lecturers reduce their symptoms with ***beta-adrenergic blockers*** (such as ***propranolol***).

The best treatment for **agoraphobia** is to gradually move out into the places and situations that trigger anxiety. Taking small steps each day, in the company of a trusted person, a sufferer eventually learns to cope with situations that once inspired terror. This may be assisted by ***antidepressants*** (such as ***selective serotonin reuptake inhibitors*** or ***tricyclic antidepressants***), which reduce the fear of panic. ***Antianxiety drugs*** may also be used, but with caution because of the risk of dependence. **Relaxation** techniques should be used to facilitate treatment.

ALTERNATIVE CHOICES

Phobias are difficult to treat by yourself. A number of self-help therapies may help to ease the way, but they should be followed only with professional guidance.

AROMATHERAPY

Studies have shown that essential oil of ***lavender*** *(Lavandula officinalis)* can bring relief from anxiety. Carry a small bottle with you; sprinkle on a handkerchief to inhale at stressful moments.

HERBAL THERAPIES

Valerian *(Valeriana officinalis)* tea may ease anxiety. Pour a cup of boiling water over 1 to 2 tsp of the root and steep for 15 minutes.

HYPNOTHERAPY

Hypnosis, in the hands of a skilled professional, may help reduce symptoms, diminish fear, and sometimes uncover the cause of a phobia.

MIND/BODY MEDICINE

Numerous relaxation techniques, including **yoga, meditation,** and **biofeedback** exercises, can help reduce the anxiety that surrounds phobias.

AT-HOME REMEDIES

By taking one small step at a time, most phobic people can reduce their terrors and, in many cases, move beyond them. Work with a trusted friend or therapist. Here are some guidelines:

- Feel free to ask for feedback or a reality check on a feared object or situation: Is it safe? Will it hurt me?
- Practice shifting your thoughts in a positive direction—from "That dog will bite me" to "That dog is tied up and can't hurt me."

P

PREVENTION

- Do regular deep breathing and relaxation exercises, especially when anxiety starts to rise.
- Regular exercise helps burn up adrenaline, which accompanies panic attacks.
- Avoid alcohol, barbiturates, and antianxiety medicine whenever possible; drugs simply mask the symptoms. Also avoid caffeine, which can mimic some of the symptoms of panic attacks. ■

PINCHED NERVE

SYMPTOMS

- tenderness, tingling, or numbness in one part of your body, often a limb.
- prickly, burning, or lacerating pain where a nerve is being irritated, with a dull ache farther along the nerve's length.
- weakness in the affected area; atrophy of muscles because of disuse, so that one arm or leg may look thinner than the other.

See also ***Carpal Tunnel Syndrome, Disk Problems,*** and ***Sciatica.***

CALL YOUR DOCTOR IF:

- the pain persists for several days and does not respond to over-the-counter ***analgesics;*** your doctor may prescribe anti-inflammatory drugs or physical therapy.
- the pain is so great that you are unable to move without severe discomfort; your doctor may want to perform tests in order to rule out other ailments.

Any pressure applied to a nerve by the surrounding tissue will produce irritation and will disrupt the nerve's functioning, with consequences that can range from aches and pains to a loss of feeling or weakening of muscles. The pinching can occur for many reasons—pregnancy, an injury, repetitive motions, or joint disease, to name just a few. It may also occur anywhere in the peripheral nervous system (that is, nerves outside the brain and spine). Nerves passing over a rigid prominence, such as a bone, are particularly vulnerable.

The most typical pinched nerves are the median, ulnar, and radial nerves, which extend down the arms from the shoulders to the hands. Other commonly compressed nerves include the femoral, which extends from the pelvis to the knee; the plantar nerves in your feet; nerves between disks in your spinal column; the peroneal nerve running along the side of your leg; and the sciatic nerve, a large nerve that runs the length of each leg from the base of your spine to your foot *(see **Sciatica**).*

With treatment, a pinched nerve generally heals in a few days to a few weeks. Chronic cases can result from persistent irritation of the affected nerve. In some cases, damage to the nerve can become permanent.

CAUSES

Pressure on a peripheral nerve from the surrounding tissue causes inflammation of the nerve. Such pressure can be the result of injury, disease, and even genetic inheritance. Sometimes the source of the problem is constant repetition of arm or leg movements, common with keyboard operations and assembly-line jobs. *(See **Carpal Tunnel Syndrome.**)*

Another common cause of nerve irritation is a damaged spinal disk—the cushioning between vertebrae. If a disk becomes injured or degenerates, it can tear, allowing the soft jellylike center to bulge out and press on an adjacent nerve. This condition—popularly known as a slipped disk *(see **Disk Problems**)*—tends to occur in the parts of the spine that are the most mobile: the lower

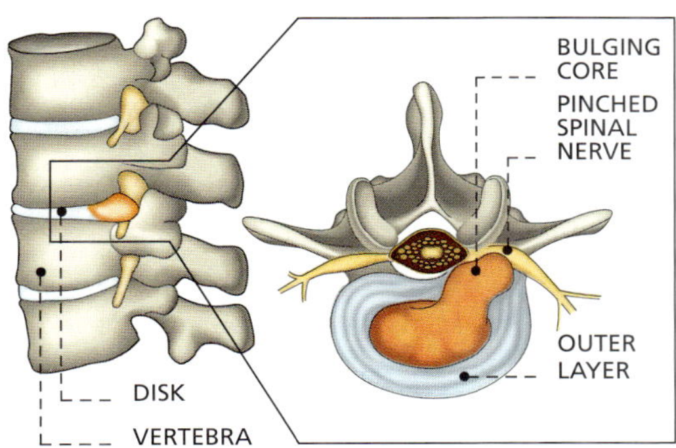

The vertebrae are separated from one another by fibrous pads, or disks *(above)*. The outer layer of the disk is strong and flexible, encasing a soft, jellylike core. When the outer layer is weakened by strain or injury—the condition known as a herniated disk—the inner core can bulge out and press against, or pinch, one of the spinal nerves *(inset)*, resulting in severe pain.

back (lumbar spine) and neck (cervical spine). Heavy lifting, ***obesity,*** and contact sports can contribute to the problem.

DIAGNOSTIC AND TEST PROCEDURES

Your doctor may test your reflexes and look for problems of restricted movement. An EMG test may be performed to determine the motor conduction speed in your arms and legs.

TREATMENT

CONVENTIONAL MEDICINE

Your doctor may advise adjustment or cessation of an activity that is causing pressure on a nerve and may suggest wearing a splint, brace, or some other support. Physical therapy can strengthen surrounding muscles. Anti-inflammatory drugs or a short course of ***corticosteroids*** can promote healing. Small doses of ***amitriptyline*** or another ***tricyclic antidepressant,*** sometimes prescribed for pain, may help if your case is chronic.

ALTERNATIVE CHOICES

In addition to the remedies listed below, **acupuncture** and **yoga** may help relax your muscles and release the pinched nerve.

CHIROPRACTIC

A chiropractor may x-ray your back to measure any abnormalities in your posture. Dislocated vertebrae are manipulated to relieve pressure on nerves and ease pain.

HERBAL THERAPIES

Try a tea combining equal parts of ***St.-John's-wort*** *(Hypericum perforatum),* ***skullcap*** *(Scutellaria lateriflora),* and ***valerian*** *(Valeriana officinalis).*

HOMEOPATHY

For low-back pain that feels better when warmth is applied, try ***Rhus toxicodendron.*** Taking ***Arnica*** when your back pain follows an injury may lessen symptoms. Consult a homeopathic practitioner for proper dosages.

NUTRITION AND DIET

Taking 1,000 mg of lecithin with meals may help regenerate nerves. Nerve impulse conduction may benefit from 2,000 mg daily of ***calcium*** chelate.

AT-HOME REMEDIES

Try the herbal tea discussed above or combine tinctures of all three herbs with the tincture of oats *(Avena sativa);* mix the tinctures together in equal portions and take 1 tsp in a glass of water three times a day.

PREVENTION

Try to avoid tasks that involve repetitive hand, wrist, arm, or shoulder motions. When avoidance is impossible, perform the motions for short periods of time with breaks in between. *(See **Carpal Tunnel Syndrome** for specific guidelines.)* If symptoms begin to appear, consult a physical therapist to learn about possible modifications in the task or the equipment. ■

PLANTAR WARTS

SYMPTOMS

- small, bumpy growths on the soles of the feet, one-quarter inch to two inches in diameter, sometimes with tiny black dots on the surface.
- pinpoint bleeding from warts when they are scratched.
- pain in the soles of the feet when standing or walking.

*(See also the **Visual Diagnostic Guide.**)*

CALL YOUR DOCTOR IF:

- the area becomes red, hot, painful, and tender after treatment; an ***infection*** may have set in.
- you are unsure whether you have a plantar wart or another condition, such as a corn, callus, mole, or skin lesion. Most such growths are harmless, but some can become cancerous.

Plantar warts are tough, horny growths that develop on plantar surfaces—that is, the soles of the feet. Normal standing and walking tends to force them into the skin, and the pressure makes the feet very painful. Like all ***warts,*** they are benign and will eventually go away even without treatment, but in most cases they are too painful to ignore. Plantar warts that grow together in a cluster are known as **mosaic warts.**

CAUSES

Plantar warts are caused by a virus that invades the skin through tiny cuts or abrasions. The warts may not appear for weeks or months after the initial exposure. Like other viral infections, plantar warts are contagious, commonly spread in public swimming pools or communal showers. Virtual epidemics of plantar warts sometimes break out among people who share gym or athletic facilities or who engage in group activities where bare feet are the rule. Because most people build immunity to the virus with age, plantar warts are more common in children than in adults.

TREATMENT

Deciding how to treat your plantar wart may depend on your ability to tolerate the pain that the various treatments can inflict. Folk remedies for treating warts abound, and there is no single treatment that works every time. Conventional treatment focuses on removal, while alternative approaches emphasize gradual remission. Whatever you do, do not try to cut off a plantar wart yourself; let nature or a doctor do the work.

CONVENTIONAL MEDICINE

Your doctor may first try applying salicylic-acid plasters to eliminate the warts. Such treatment may take several weeks to be effective. Burning, freezing with liquid nitrogen dioxide, and surgical removal are more aggressive options for more severe conditions.

ALTERNATIVE CHOICES

In general, alternative treatments emphasize proper nutrition, since a healthy diet will not only enhance your immunity to the virus but help your body combat it. Various substances can be applied directly to the wart as aids to removal.

AROMATHERAPY

Two drops of essential lemon oil in 10 drops of cider vinegar may help remove plantar warts: Apply daily and cover during the day with an adhesive bandage, but leave the wart exposed at night. Or you can put a drop of ***tea tree oil*** (*Melaleuca* spp.) on the center of the wart daily and bandage it. Continue treatment until the wart goes away, which may take several weeks.

You can try strengthening your immune system by massaging your legs with the essential oils of ***rosemary*** *(Rosmarinus officinalis),* geranium *(Pelargonium odoratissimum),* or ***juniper*** *(Juniperus communis)*—or a blend of any two—using long strokes from ankles to thighs.

HERBAL THERAPIES

Various herbal remedies are recommended for removing warts. Whichever herbal remedy you try, first protect the surrounding skin with petroleum jelly and cover the treated wart with a clean bandage. Repeat daily until the warts are gone.

- Apply the juice from ***dandelion*** *(Taraxacum officinale)* stems morning and evening.
- Put a clove of raw ***garlic*** *(Allium sativum) or a* drop or two of garlic oil on the wart twice daily.
- Apply a few drops of yellow cedar *(Thuja occidentalis),* available in either oil or tincture form, to the wart twice daily.

NUTRITION AND DIET

Poor diet can be a factor in persistent or recurring warts. Foods high in ***vitamin A***—eggs, cold-water fish, onions, garlic, and dark green and yellow vegetables such as broccoli, cabbage, Brussels sprouts, squash, and carrots—will help sustain your immune system, as will yogurt and other fermented milk products. You can also consult a nutritional therapist about the potential benefits of supplemental ***vitamins A, B complex, C,*** and ***E;*** L-cysteine; and ***zinc.***

AT-HOME REMEDIES

- Try an over-the-counter topical medication that contains salicylic acid, which is best absorbed by the skin after a bath, a shower, or a soak in warm water. Protect the healthy skin around your warts with petroleum jelly.
- Mix castor oil and baking powder into a paste and apply to the wart nightly. Cover with a bandage until the wart disappears.
- Cut or scrape off some of the white material from the inside of a banana peel—preferably from a green banana, since it is said to have more of the enzymes that help fight the wart-causing virus. Apply a piece of the material to the wart before going to bed, and cover with first-aid tape. Repeat nightly until the condition improves.
- Apply ***vitamin E*** twice daily or ***vitamin A*** nightly; open a capsule of the vitamin, apply the oil to the wart, and cover with a bandage. Continue applications until the wart goes away.
- To ease the pain until the wart is gone, wear a foam pad in your shoe. Cut a hole in the pad at the location of the wart to take pressure off the wart while you are standing or walking.

P

PREVENTION

Protect yourself against exposure to the virus that causes plantar warts by wearing shower shoes, thongs, or rubber swimming shoes whenever you visit a public pool or use a communal shower. Be sure to wash your feet thoroughly with a disinfectant soap after being in an area where the virus can spread. ■

PLEURISY

SYMPTOMS

Pleurisy:

- severe, fleeting, sharp pain in your chest, possibly on one side only, when breathing deeply, coughing, moving, or sneezing.
- severe chest pain that goes away when you hold your breath.

Pleural Effusion:

- shortness of breath.
- a dry cough.

CALL YOUR DOCTOR IF:

- you are experiencing any of the symptoms above, particularly if you have not been diagnosed for the underlying disease; pleurisy and pleural effusion can be symptoms of such serious diseases as ***pneumonia*** and ***lung cancer.***
- the symptoms above are accompanied by fever, no matter how slight. You may have a type of infection called empyema that requires treatment with ***antibiotics.***

Pleurisy, also called pleuritis, is an inflammation of the pleura—the moist, double-layered membrane that surrounds the lungs and lines the rib cage. The condition can make breathing extremely painful and, if not treated promptly, can lead to the development of pleural effusion, in which the area between the membrane's layers, called the pleural space, fills with excess fluid.

Strictly speaking, pleurisy and pleural effusion are not diseases; rather, they are complications of an underlying lung infection or disease, such as ***pneumonia, tuberculosis,*** or systemic ***lupus*** erythematosus. A number of other conditions—most commonly congestive heart failure but including chest injuries, viral infections, rheumatoid ***arthritis,*** and ***cancer***—can also irritate the pleura.

Pleurisy and pleural effusion are generally only as serious as the underlying disease. If you have either of these conditions, you may already be undergoing treatment for the underlying disease; if not, seek medical attention immediately.

CAUSES

The double-layered pleura protects and lubricates the surface of the lungs as they inflate and deflate within the rib cage. Normally, a thin, fluid-filled gap—the pleural space—allows the two layers of the pleural membrane to slide gently past each other. But when these layers become inflamed by an infection in the chest, their roughened surfaces rub painfully together with every breath, sneeze, and cough. This condition is known as pleurisy.

In some cases of pleurisy, excess fluid seeps into the pleural space, resulting in pleural effusion. This fluid buildup usually has a lubricating effect, relieving the pain associated with pleurisy as it reduces friction between the membrane's layers. But at the same time, the added fluid puts tremendous pressure on the lungs, reducing their ability to move freely and causing shortness of breath. In some cases of pleural effusion, this excess liquid becomes infected, causing a condition known as empyema.

DIAGNOSTIC AND TEST PROCEDURES

To diagnose pleurisy, a physician will listen to your chest through a stethoscope as you breathe. If this examination reveals pleural friction rub—the abrasive sound of the pleura's two layers sliding against each other—the diagnosis is clear. Pleural friction rub produces a scraping, raspy sound that occurs at the end of your inhalation and the beginning of your exhalation, and it comes from the area directly over the pleural inflammation. By gently tapping that area on your chest, your doctor might be able to hear a rattling vibration, another indication of pleurisy.

Your doctor may also take x-rays of the area or draw a sample of pleural fluid for analysis. After injecting your back or chest with a local anesthetic, the physician will use a syringe to extract the fluid. The doctor may run tests on the sample to determine, for example, if the underlying cause of the fluid buildup is cancer.

PLEURISY

A lung injury or infection can lead to inflammation of the pleura, a thin, two-ply membrane that encases the lungs and lines the inside of the rib cage. Between the pleural layers is a fluid-filled space that normally cushions the contact between them during respiration. When inflamed, however, the surfaces can become roughened and tender; breathing forces them to rub together, intensifying the pain.

TREATMENT

Conventional medicine usually treats the underlying disease that causes pleurisy or pleural effusion. In some cases of pleural effusion, however, excess fluid must be drained. Alternative treatments may help relieve some of the discomfort associated with these conditions.

CONVENTIONAL MEDICINE

In addition to ***antibiotics*** and other appropriate medications aimed at treating the underlying disease, your physician will probably prescribe anti-inflammatory drugs or ***analgesics,*** such as ***aspirin,*** to remedy the inflammation. Sometimes, a ***codeine***-based cough syrup will be prescribed to control a painful cough.

In the case of pleural effusion, your physician may recommend a ***diuretic*** to help drain excess fluid. As a preventive measure, ***antibiotics*** may also be prescribed to combat empyema. If the amount of pleural fluid is excessive, the doctor may drain it through a tube inserted in your chest, a procedure that requires hospitalization.

ALTERNATIVE CHOICES

The cure for pleurisy and pleural effusion lies with conventional treatment of the underlying disease. Even so, a number of alternative remedies, including **acupuncture,** may alleviate some of the discomfort associated with these conditions.

CHINESE HERBS

The Chinese herb ***ephedra*** *(Ephedra sinica)* is a potent bronchodilator, which can help ease breathing. CAUTION: Large quantities of ephedra have the same effect as large quantities of ***epinephrine;*** do not use the herb if you have ***high blood pressure*** or ***heart disease.*** Prepare an infusion by combining 5 grams ephedra, 4 grams ***cinnamon*** *(Cinnamomum cassia)* sticks, 1.5 grams ***licorice*** *(Glycyrrhiza uralensis),* and 5 grams ***apricot seed*** *(Prunus armeniaca).* Let the mixture steep in cold water for several minutes, then bring it to a boil. Drink it hot. ■

PNEUMONIA

SYMPTOMS

- A combination of low ***fever and chills,*** muscle aches, ***fatigue,*** enlarged lymph nodes in the neck, ***chest pain, sore throat,*** and ***coughing*** are typical symptoms of **viral pneumonia.**
- A combination of high fever, cough with thick yellow-green sputum that may contain blood, shortness of breath, rapid breathing, sharp chest pain that is worse when you breathe deeply, ***abdominal pain,*** and severe fatigue are symptoms of **bacterial pneumonia.**
- Loss of appetite and weight, fever, coughing with sputum, perhaps following a period of unconsciousness, may indicate **aspiration pneumonia**.
- In children, labored and rapid breathing (more than 45 breaths a minute), sudden onset of fever, cough, ***wheezing,*** and bluish skin are general signs of pneumonia.

CALL YOUR DOCTOR IF:

- your symptoms indicate you have any form of pneumonia. You need immediate treatment to recover and avoid complications.
- your sharp chest pain does not respond to prescribed treatment; you have increased shortness of breath; or your fingernails, toenails, or skin becomes dark or develops a bluish tinge after diagnosis. Your lungs are not getting enough oxygen and you need medical assistance.
- you cough up blood; you may need additional treatment for a worsening infection.

P

Pneumonia is the relatively common inflammation caused by various viral, bacterial, and fungal infections, or chemical exposure of the lungs. In response, the lungs become congested with fluids and cells that leak from the affected tissue. If the inflammation is limited to one lobe of one lung, it is classified as **lobar pneumonia;** inflammation spreading from the bronchi to other parts of one or both lungs is **bronchopneumonia.** If both lungs are inflamed, the condition is called **double pneumonia.** Depending on your overall health, pneumonia usually lasts about two weeks, although you may feel exhausted a month or more after it has cleared up.

Viral pneumonia is generally mild; you can usually treat it at home once the doctor has made a diagnosis. **Bacterial pneumonias** are more complex and more serious. Until the development of antibiotics, cases were frequently fatal, and they remain one of the leading causes of death in the U.S. As recently as 1976, **legionnaire's disease** killed 29 people before it was identified and treated as a bacterial pneumonia. Of the many other types of pneumonia, **walking pneumonia** is

EVIDENCE OF INFECTION

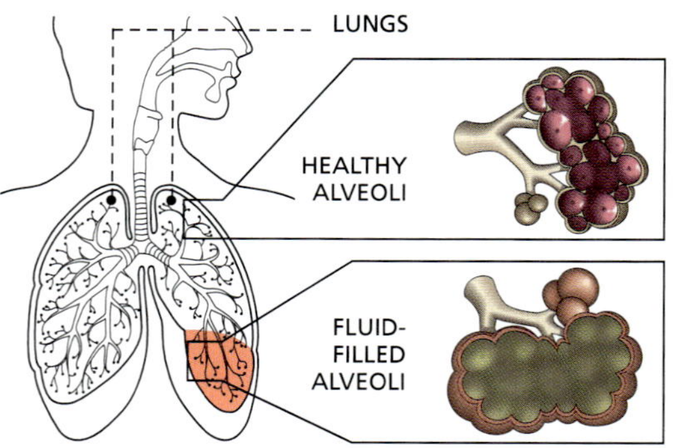

Healthy lungs exchange carbon dioxide in the blood for oxygen through tiny air sacs called alveoli *(inset, top).* A pneumonic infection—whether it is caused by bacterial, viral, or chemical agents—makes tissue in the alveoli swell and fill with fluid *(inset, bottom).* Shallow, labored breathing brought on by an insufficient oxygen supply is often a symptom of pneumonia.

most common in children and in young adults.

Pneumonia is a common complication of many illnesses, and like the ***common cold*** and ***flu,*** any type can be transmitted from one person to another. Patients hospitalized for other ailments may become infected with bacterial pneumonia that is resistant to the usual course of antibiotic treatment. The strains of bacterial pneumonia outside hospitals are usually much less severe and respond readily to antibiotics.

CAUSES

Various common viral organisms are responsible for **viral pneumonia. Bacterial pneumonia** is most commonly caused by *Streptococcus pneumoniae,* sometimes called pneumococcus. The bacterium *Hemophilus influenzae* is often responsible for pneumonia that develops as a complication of ***flu.*** Pneumonia is also on the rise as a result of infection by ***tuberculosis*** bacteria. The Legionella bacterium responsible for **legionnaire's disease** and similar pneumonias can be transmitted through contaminated water from many sources, including hot tubs and air-conditioning units.

Aspiration pneumonia develops when bacteria from the mouth or stomach enter the lungs, generally during sleep, unconsciousness, or a seizure. Such bacteria normally inhabit the digestive tracts of healthy people. A small amount of inhaled mucus won't harm most people, but it can cause lung inflammation in alcoholics or other people with weakened immune systems. Bacteria can also be carried into the lungs by inadvertently inhaling vomit, usually when unconscious.

Pneumocystis pneumonia (PCP) develops when the body's immune defenses are exhausted by ***AIDS,*** Hodgkin's disease, or other diseases that suppress the immune system. It develops as a secondary infection in over half of all AIDS patients, but treatment is readily available.

DIAGNOSTIC AND TEST PROCEDURES

Pneumonia's forms range from a mild condition treatable at home to a potentially fatal infection requiring hospitalization, so you must have a professional diagnosis to guarantee appropriate treatment and a successful recovery. Your doctor will first listen to your chest for crackling noises and tap your chest to check for dull thuds indicating fluid-filled lungs. If necessary, an x-ray can confirm the diagnosis, showing where air sacs in the lungs are filled with fluid and debris. Blood and sputum samples, sometimes obtained by inserting a tube into the lungs, may be tested for microorganisms, but the results are not always conclusive.

ATTENTION!

POSTURAL DRAINAGE

To help clear phlegm out of your lungs, try postural drainage for 5 to 15 minutes three times a day. This technique is physically demanding, so make sure that your doctor approves, and have a support person with you at all times.

Lie on a bed with the top half of your body off the mattress, using your forearms on the floor as support. Cough up phlegm from deep in your lungs and spit it into a container on the floor. At the end of the session, flush the phlegm down the toilet.

If this technique is too strenuous for you, have a friend or family member pound gently with cupped hands on your upper back for several minutes to help loosen chest secretions.

TREATMENT

The goal of treatment for any form of pneumonia is speedy recovery, since complications can set in if the disease is allowed to linger. All treatments include bed rest. Conventional medicine focuses on curing the infection, while alternative treatments may help to ease uncomfortable symptoms.

CONVENTIONAL MEDICINE

For most types of pneumonia, the two essential keys to recovery are bed rest and "productive

P

coughing"—bringing up phlegm and other fluid from your lungs.

If you have a mild case of **viral pneumonia,** you can probably recover at home, taking ***aspirin*** or ***acetaminophen*** to lower your fever and reduce pain, drinking lots of fluids, and eating lightly. If you have **bacterial pneumonia,** your doctor will probably prescribe an ***antibiotic*** such as ***penicillin*** or ***erythromycin.*** You will need to stay in bed until your fever drops and your breathing becomes normal. If your lungs are severely congested, you may need oxygen or to be put on a respirator temporarily, which will require a hospital stay. **Aspiration pneumonia** almost always requires intravenous antibiotics and a lengthy hospital stay. **Pneumocystis pneumonia** is usually treated with bed rest, antibiotics such as pentamidine or ***sulfamethoxazole and trimethoprim,*** and ***decongestants*** to reduce congestion.

A vaccine is available for many identifiable types of bacterial pneumonia, and more are being developed. Vaccination against pneumonia is recommended for everyone over the age of 65, and for people with chronic lung disease, ***sickle cell anemia, heart disease,*** alcoholism, and immune deficiency diseases such as ***AIDS,*** as well as for people whose spleen has been damaged or removed. Vaccines are also available for some forms of influenza and are recommended for older people; a flu shot may protect you from either catching the disease or developing such a serious case that complications like pneumonia set in.

ATTENTION!

BEWARE OF THE BIRDCAGE

Parakeets and lovebirds can transmit psittacosis—a rare form of pneumonia commonly known as parrot fever—to their unsuspecting human owners. Sick birds can spread the infectious microorganism in dust from their feathers, in droppings, or even by biting a finger. Psittacosis symptoms include fever, chills, headaches, muscle aches, loss of appetite, nausea, vomiting, and enlargement of the spleen.

ALTERNATIVE CHOICES

If you are diagnosed as having pneumonia, various alternative therapies may help ease your symptoms and hasten your recovery.

ACUPUNCTURE

Acupuncture on the lung meridian may help your recovery from pneumonia by reducing cough and congestion, making you more comfortable, and improving your energy level. Key points are LU 7 to expel matter from the lungs, LU 5 to stop cough, and LU 1 to relieve chest congestion. Depending on the condition, an acupuncturist may also work on enhancing the immune system. *(See the **Appendix** for information on point locations.)*

AROMATHERAPY

Recovery from pneumonia may be helped if you add the essential oils of ***eucalyptus*** *(Eucalyptus globulus),* ***lavender*** *(Lavandula officinalis),* ***tea tree*** (*Melaleuca* spp.), or pine to a warm bath or a vaporizer for steam inhalation. Do not use steam inhalations if you are asthmatic, because the vapor may irritate your lungs.

BODY WORK

After the fever is gone, **massage** the upper-back muscles to ease chest congestion. Adding a few drops of essential oil of ***eucalyptus*** *(Eucalyptus globulus)* to the massage lotion may help to loosen and release phlegm.

HERBAL THERAPIES

Since clearing the lungs of phlegm is an important part of the healing process, using traditional herbal expectorants to promote coughing can aid recovery. To make your own expectorant, combine 2 oz ***licorice*** *(Glycyrrhiza glabra),* 1 oz wild black cherry *(Prunus serotina)* bark, 1 oz ***coltsfoot*** *(Tussilago farfara),* 1/8 oz ***lobelia*** *(Lobelia inflata),* and 1 oz horehound *(Marrubium vulgare).* Simmer 1 tbsp of the mixture in 1 cup of water for 5 minutes; let the mixture steep for 10 minutes and strain it into a clean container. Adults should

THE ONION OPTION

Try this homemade cough syrup that combines the soothing qualities of honey with the pungent bite of raw onion. Pour honey over slices of raw white onion and let them sit overnight in a covered container. In the morning, strain the mixture into a clean container and discard the onion slices. Take a tablespoonful of the mixture, preferably after warming it slightly, every five or six hours.

drink one cupful every 2 hours. Lobelia can be poisonous, so never use more than the recommended amount. Stop using this mixture if you become nauseated, and never give it to children or pregnant women.

A decoction of pleurisy root *(Asclepias tuberosa)* is recommended to help fight pneumonia. Simmer 1 tbsp of the herb in a cup of water for 10 minutes, steep 5 minutes, and strain; drink four to five times daily.

Eating raw ***garlic*** *(Allium sativum)* or three garlic capsules three times a day is said to help your body fight infection. ***Echinacea*** (*Echinacea* spp.) may help you recover from infection: It can be brewed as tea—1 tsp in a cup of water—taken three times a day. It can also be taken as a tincture, 30 drops four times a day, or in over-the-counter capsules according to label directions.

HOMEOPATHY

Some recommended over-the-counter homeopathic remedies are ***Bryonia, Phosphorus,*** and ***Arsenicum album;*** follow label directions.

NUTRITION AND DIET

- Up to 1,000 mg of ***vitamin C*** an hour may offer substantial benefits in fighting pneumonia if started within two days of onset. Reduce dosage if you develop ***diarrhea.***
- From 25,000 to 50,000 IU of ***vitamin A*** daily, for not more than two weeks, may help support your respiratory and immune systems.
- ***Zinc*** supplements, up to 60 mg daily, may also help your immune system fight infection.
- 600 IU of ***vitamin E*** daily may help support damaged lung tissue.
- If you are taking antibiotics to fight bacterial pneumonia, try *Lactobacillus acidophilus* supplements, either in capsule form or in live yogurt cultures, to help replace your beneficial intestinal bacteria.

AT-HOME REMEDIES

- A heating pad or hot-water bottle on the chest or back for 10-minute periods several times a day can help relieve chest pain. Wrap the pad or bottle in a towel to prevent burning the skin.
- Try a traditional mustard poultice to loosen phlegm. Mix dry mustard with enough warm water to make a thick paste. Spread the paste on thin cotton or cheesecloth, fold, and place on your chest for several minutes, but don't overdo it: Mustard may cause blistering if it is left on bare skin too long.
- Drink plenty of fluids and fresh fruit and vegetable juices to thin lung secretions and make them easier to cough up.

PREVENTION

- Avoid smoking and exposure to tobacco smoke, which significantly damage the hair-like cilia in your respiratory tract that filter irritants from the lungs. Smoking weakens your ability to fight viral and bacterial agents that cause pneumonia.
- Don't drink large amounts of alcohol; alcohol impairs your immune system's ability to fight all sorts of infection, including pneumonia.
- If you are over 60 or suffer from a chronic condition that taxes your immune system, ask your doctor about the advisability of vaccination against pneumonia and seasonal influenza viruses that often lead to pneumonia. ■

POISON IVY

SYMPTOMS

- patches of red, itchy skin, usually followed by small blisters, which fill with a clear fluid and eventually break open.
- Severe cases can develop into swollen, extremely painful areas filled with fluid.
- The rash rarely appears on the soles of the feet or palms of the hand.

CALL YOUR DOCTOR IF:

- your rash stays red and itchy for more than two weeks; you may have another type of contact ***dermatitis, eczema,*** or ***lupus.***
- you have the rash near your eyes or the rash covers a large part of your body. You may need medical intervention.
- you have severe allergic complications, such as generalized swelling, headache, fever, or a secondary ***infection.***
- you have been exposed to or inhale the smoke from burning poison ivy, poison oak, or poison sumac. The toxin is not killed by fire and can cause severe allergic reactions internally as well as externally.

Poison ivy, poison oak, and poison sumac cause a short-lived but extremely irritating allergic form of contact ***dermatitis.*** The rash generally develops within 2 days, peaks after 5 days, and starts to decline after about a week or 10 days. While some people survive exposure without ill effects, complete immunity is unlikely; people who seem immune at one time and place may find themselves vulnerable in other situations.

CAUSES

The leaves, stems, and roots of poison ivy, oak, and sumac plants contain the resin urushiol, minute amounts of which on exposed skin can trigger an inflammatory allergic reaction. Urushiol can be transferred by fingers or animal fur and can remain on clothing, shoes, and tools for a number of months. Scratching the rash does not spread the poison to other parts of the body, but it can prolong the discomfort and cause a secondary infection.

TREATMENT

You can treat most cases of the rash yourself with the application of calamine lotion or over-the-counter topical remedies containing ***antihistamines, benzocaine,*** or ***hydrocortisone.*** A cortisone shot may relieve the itching, particularly within 24 hours of exposure. Oral ***corticosteroids*** or antihistamines may also relieve the symptoms, but both drugs can have unwanted side effects. Don't take oral antihistamines if you are using an antihistamine lotion; the combination may actually make the condition worse. If you have complications from a severe case, you may need to see a doctor. If your case is so severe that general illness develops, your doctor may recommend injections of ***prednisone*** or another corticosteroid drug. *(See **Dermatitis.**)*

ALTERNATIVE CHOICES

Like conventional medicine, various alternative therapies help relieve itching and swelling. In ad-

P

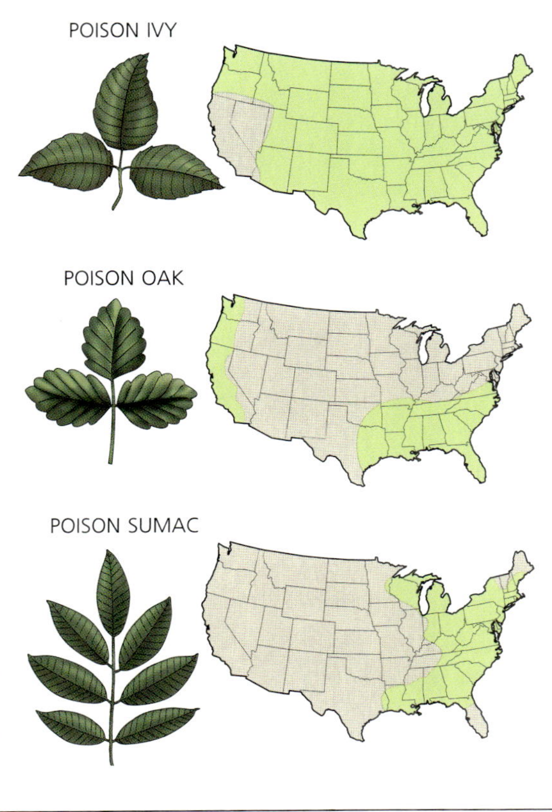

Poison ivy—with its shiny, sometimes reddish-, yellow-, or orange-colored leaves—shares with poison oak a characteristic three-leaf pattern. Poison sumac has paired, pointed leaves, sometimes with greenish white berries. The maps show the distribution of each type.

dition to topical remedies, ***vitamin C*** injections are also said to provide relief.

HERBAL THERAPIES

The leaves of jewelweed *(Impatiens),* which often grows near poison ivy, may neutralize urushiol if wiped over the skin right after contact. For relief from itching, try the following topical remedies:

- a few drops of juice squeezed from the leaves of the common ***plantain*** *(Plantago major).*
- 1 tbsp salt in ½ cup water with enough cosmetic clay to make a paste; add 1 or 2 drops of oil of ***peppermint*** *(Mentha piperita).*
- equal parts ***goldenseal*** *(Hydrastis canadensis)* root powder and green clay, available in health food stores.

HOMEOPATHY

Of all the over-the-counter homeopathic remedies available, ***Rhus toxicodendron***—derived from the poison ivy plant itself—may be the most effective. Follow directions on the label.

AT-HOME REMEDIES

- Wash exposed skin with soap and water within 15 minutes of contact.
- Soothe the itch with calamine lotion or other over-the-counter medication.
- Cover open blisters with sterile gauze to prevent infection.
- Make a paste with water and either cornstarch, oatmeal, baking soda, or Epsom salt, and apply it to the rash. You can also use a paste made with baking soda and a few drops of witch hazel.
- Run hot water over the rash—as hot as you can stand it. The itching will intensify briefly, then abate, giving you several itch-free hours.

PREVENTION

The best way to deal with this poisonous threesome is to learn to recognize the plants, then stay out of reach. If you suspect contact with a poison plant, wash immediately and thoroughly with soap and water—-your skin, clothes, shoes, tools—anything that might have picked up the plant's toxic resin. If you're going into poison-plant country, try one of the barrier lotions available from outdoor suppliers. The old folk tale about eating poison ivy leaves to make yourself immune is just that—a myth: Never eat the leaves or berries of wild plants, many of which can cause dangerous reactions in humans. ■

POSTNASAL DRIP

SYMPTOMS

- a flow of mucus that runs down the back of your throat, ranging in consistency from watery to thick, and often associated with a sore throat, a cough, hoarseness, or the feeling that something is lodged in your throat.
- inadvertent sniffing, snorting, or swallowing of nasal mucus.

CALL YOUR DOCTOR IF:

- you have treated the condition with an over-the-counter decongestant for more than a week without success; or if the condition is accompanied by continued sneezing, wheezing, watery eyes, or persistent shortness of breath. You may be suffering from an ***allergy*** or a form of ***environmental poisoning.***
- the condition is accompanied by a congested nose, fever, pain or abnormal pressure in the nose and face, and thick nasal discharge. You probably have ***sinusitis.***

P

Postnasal drip is an annoying complication of various respiratory ailments and generally disappears after the primary ailment clears up. Mucus is a normal product of the nasal passages, but when too much is produced it finds its way into the throat instead of leaving by way of the nostrils. When the condition becomes chronic—for example, from an ***allergy*** or prolonged ***sinusitis***—mucus can drip into the bronchial tubes, especially at night, inducing coughing and heavy phlegm. Since postnasal drip is most often a symptom of another ailment, the best approach is to identify and treat the underlying condition.

CAUSES

Watery postnasal drip along with itching eyes, nose, palate, and throat (or sneezing, congestion, and watery eyes) is usually **allergic rhinitis** triggered by plant pollen, dust, animal hair, or other allergens. Some people develop postnasal drip when exposed to environmental irritants such as tobacco smoke or airborne contaminants.

If postnasal drip involves thick mucus, a ***sore throat,*** runny and congested nose, ***headache,*** achiness, and reduced sense of taste and smell, you probably have **viral rhinitis**—a ***common cold.*** Intermittent or continual postnasal drip that becomes very pronounced with humidity and temperature changes or periods of emotional ***stress*** may be **vasomotor rhinitis.** This condition can also be a side effect of some prescription drugs.

Thick yellow or greenish mucus can indicate a bacterial or viral respiratory ***infection.*** Whenever thick nasal discharge and postnasal drip are accompanied by fever and congestive pain or pressure in the face, it is probably from ***sinusitis.***

Women who use hormone replacement therapy or estrogen-based birth-control drugs can develop postnasal drip as a side effect, and it can be a minor complication of pregnancy.

DIAGNOSTIC AND TEST PROCEDURES

Laboratory tests of the mucus itself can determine if your postnasal drip is due to an allergy, some form of rhinitis, or another condition. Your

HOMEMADE SALINE

You can buy commercially prepared saline solution, but it's easy to make your own. Mix a teaspoon of table salt and a teaspoon of baking soda in a quart of water. Whenever you need to flush away excess mucus, tilt your head back and spray a small amount of the solution into each nostril. You'll have to buy a small spray bottle—try a well-stocked pharmacy.

doctor will use an illuminating instrument to examine your nasal passages, and if complications from sinus problems are indicated, you may need an x-ray or other imaging procedure.

TREATMENT

Both conventional and alternative treatment will vary depending on whether your symptoms stem from an allergy, a cold, or another condition.

CONVENTIONAL MEDICINE

Over-the-counter ***decongestant*** drops or sprays can help alleviate postnasal drip by opening nasal passages, but prolonged use may make the problem worse. Your system can become temporarily dependent on them and must adjust after you stop their use. If you suffer from ***high blood pressure,*** you should not take oral decongestants without a doctor's approval. Some ***antihistamines*** can make you drowsy; if that happens, look for products with formulas that do not induce sleep.

ALTERNATIVE CHOICES

Alternative treatments to clear postnasal drip rely primarily on ways to thin the offending mucus and allay the underlying causes.

AROMATHERAPY

Inhaling steam can help clear nasal passages. Add essential oils of ***eucalyptus*** *(Eucalyptus globulus),* ***tea tree*** (*Melaleuca* spp.), ***rosemary*** *(Rosmarinus officinalis),* or ***peppermint*** *(Mentha piperita)* to the water in a humidifier during the day, and use the essential oil of ***lavender*** *(Lavandula officinalis)* in the evening for a better night's sleep.

CHINESE HERBS

Chinese medicine relies on mixtures of traditional herbs brewed in water and drunk at prescribed intervals. The Minor Blue Dragon Combination is recommended to reduce nasal drainage; consult an experienced practitioner for the correct amounts of each herb to use for your condition.

HERBAL THERAPIES

Eyebright *(Euphrasia officinalis)* may help dry up postnasal drip; make an infusion or tincture with the leaves and stems, or take two 200 mg capsules of the prepared herb three times daily.

HOMEOPATHY

For postnasal drip with thick yellow-green mucus, try ***Pulsatilla*** (12c) three or four times a day for two days. For postnasal drip associated with symptoms of a ***common cold,*** try ***Nux vomica*** (12c) three or four times a day for two days. For other kinds of postnasal drip, a homeopath will prescribe a remedy for your particular symptoms.

AT-HOME REMEDIES

- Use an over-the-counter cough medicine, or a simple saline solution *(above, left)* as a nasal spray, to help thin postnasal drip mucus.
- Drink lots of water (at least six glasses a day) to help keep the mucus as thin as possible.
- Humidify the air around you, especially in winter. If your heating system does not have a built-in humidifier, you can buy a self-contained unit at most home-supply centers. (Read the directions carefully for cleaning and maintaining a humidifier; improperly cleaned humidifiers can spread germs.) ■

POSTTRAUMATIC STRESS DISORDER

SYMPTOMS

Someone who has experienced severe trauma—war, combat, natural disaster, physical or sexual abuse—or witnessed violence, such as murder or physical abuse, may display one or more of these symptoms:

- repeated flashbacks or recurrent dreams of the event. Children may not remember the event directly but may recall a single image or express their fear by repeatedly playacting an event or action. Their dreams may simply be frightening with no specific content.
- hypervigilance—a preoccupation with possible unknown threats.
- traumatic dreams, sleeping problems.
- outbursts of anger.
- intense distress if exposed to anything resembling the event.
- psychological numbing; inability to relate to others.
- chronic physical symptoms—pain, headaches, irritable bowels.
- in young children, agitated behavior, difficulty concentrating, or developmental regression in such things as toilet training or speech.
- no sense of a future; no expectation of having a family, career, living to old age.

CALL YOUR DOCTOR IF:

- you or your child or other loved one has experienced trauma and shows any of the symptoms.

A few people live through horrible events without experiencing much fear, but most of us react with feelings of horror and helplessness. The degree of a person's reaction—both physical and psychological—to such events determines whether the person will actually develop the condition known as posttraumatic stress disorder (PTSD), whose effects can be long-lasting and disabling. Once known as battle fatigue or shell shock, PTSD is now considered a mental disorder resulting from any sort of deeply shocking experience.

PTSD may begin immediately following the event or may not surface until weeks or months later. Treatment and the passage of time may diminish its duration and its severity. For a few, the symptoms disappear entirely.

Some 31 percent of Vietnam veterans have suffered from it and 15 percent continue to be affected. For battered women, 84 percent reported symptoms soon after the event and 45 percent still suffered a year later. Children are more likely to suffer from PTSD if the trauma is personal—caused by a family member or friend, rather than by a natural disaster. Also, witnessing family violence can be as harsh a trauma for a child as being attacked personally.

As might be expected, people with PTSD also often suffer from various physical ailments, ***depression, drug abuse, phobias,*** or ***panic attacks.***

CAUSES

PTSD is caused by a severely traumatic event that triggers feelings of intense fear, horror, and helplessness. Both its onset and its severity are directly related to the length and severity of exposure; the greater the horror and the longer it lasts, the more likely a person will suffer PTSD and the more severe it is apt to be. This is particularly true of children who experience repeated abuse or witness repetitive family violence.

Some researchers theorize that intense fear may physically damage the part of the brain that processes fear and that this damage may contribute to the symptoms of PTSD—including anger flashes, extreme vigilance, and sleep disturbance.

Risk factors that may contribute to PTSD include a family history of ***anxiety,*** early separation from parents, earlier childhood abuse, or prior exposure to traumas.

DIAGNOSTIC AND TEST PROCEDURES

Diagnosis is based almost exclusively on a report of the patient's full history. This will include recent symptoms; a description of the event; childhood, educational, and work experiences; and relationships with others. Other disorders that often accompany PTSD are ***depression, anxiety,*** and ***drug abuse.***

TREATMENT

The usual treatment for PTSD is a combination of ***antidepressant drugs*** and psychotherapy. Support groups—with or without family members—allow sufferers to work through feelings with others who have had similar experiences.

Alternative treatments include a wide variety of antianxiety techniques, **biofeedback,** and a newly developed therapy called **Eye Movement Desensitization and Reprocessing** *(see **Eye Movement Therapy,** right).*

CONVENTIONAL MEDICINE

To reduce PTSD stress, the antidepressant drug group called ***selective serotonin reuptake inhibitors (SSRIs)*** seems to be the most effective. When psychotherapy is prescribed—whether individual or group—the goal is to encourage the patient to recall all details of the event, express grief, complete the mourning process, and get on with life. For children, this may involve play therapy.

ALTERNATIVE CHOICES

Because PTSD is an anxiety disorder in which the victim is left tense and jittery, the practice of any exercise or relaxation technique is extremely valuable. Choose one or two techniques that you like and practice them daily. (For various options, see ***Anxiety.***)

ACUPUNCTURE

Acupuncture has been shown to ease excessive fear reactions and can reduce traumatic dreams. It works best when combined with psychotherapy. Consult an acupuncturist experienced in treating emotional disorders.

BIOFEEDBACK

In EEG biofeedback (a form of biofeedback also known as neurotherapy), the sufferer retrains his brain's neurological functioning. In controlled studies, some veterans who have suffered for decades have shown great improvement, sometimes total recovery. The patient is attached to an EEG machine and, by listening to the kind and amount of brain waves produced, learns to change them in ways that ultimately affect both behavior and feelings. At least 30 sessions are required to accomplish this, but the technique can result in permanent change.

EYE MOVEMENT THERAPY

A rather astonishing new treatment—known as **Eye Movement Desensitization and Reprocessing (EMDR)**—seems to bring remarkable results. In some clinical studies, EMDR has reportedly brought dramatic improvement in 90 percent of those tested, and it has become standard treatment in some veterans' hospitals.

The technique is relatively simple. The patient visualizes a distressing image from the traumatic event while tracking with his eyes two fingers the therapist moves quickly back and forth across his line of vision. After each set of movements, the client reports any new feelings or forgotten memories he may have. The therapist then repeats the procedure. Each session lasts about 90 minutes and is repeated as often as needed. One Vietnam veteran reported that EMDR accomplished more in one session than conventional counseling had managed in years.

MASSAGE

Massage has proved effective in lowering anxiety and stress for some natural-disaster victims, but it should not be used with anyone who has been physically abused. Massage should be gentle and is best performed by an experienced therapist. ■

PREGNANCY PROBLEMS

SYMPTOMS

Women can expect some or all of these conditions in a normal pregnancy:

- in the first trimester—absence of menstrual flow; minor weight gain; increased urination; enlarged and perhaps sore breasts; **morning sickness** or nausea.
- in the second trimester—significant weight gain (about a pound a week); stretching of the abdominal wall and pelvis; possibly backache, constipation, heartburn, and fetal movement.
- in the third trimester—swollen limbs from fluid retention; leaking breasts; constipation; hemorrhoids; insomnia; discomfort below the rib cage a few weeks before the baby drops at about 36 weeks.

CALL YOUR DOCTOR IF:

- you have severe nausea and vomiting; dehydration; rapid heartbeat; or pale, dry skin. You may have hyperemesis gravidarum, a severe form of **morning sickness.**
- you have vaginal spotting or bleeding. You may be having a **miscarriage** or serious placental complication.
- you have sudden weight gain over a few days, severe headache, and blurred vision. You may have developed **preeclampsia,** a form of ***high blood pressure.***
- you have a fever over 100°F and chills, backache, or blood in your urine. You may have **pyelonephritis,** a ***kidney infection.***
- after the fetus begins to move, you feel decreased movement for more than a day or no movement; you may be experiencing **fetal distress.**

Most pregnancies are medically uneventful and end happily in the successful birth of a healthy baby. But you still have nine months to wonder whether certain physical and emotional discomforts are serious enough for medical intervention or are minor problems that you can deal with on your own.

Your first—and most important—step is signing up for a comprehensive program of prenatal care with a doctor who specializes in pregnancy and childbirth. You and your developing baby will get routine monitoring to make sure everything is going well—and if it isn't, appropriate care for any problems. You and your husband or partner will get confidence-building information about each stage of your pregnancy, including labor, childbirth, and the care and feeding of a newborn.

A pregnant woman is as likely as anyone to get minor illnesses, but when you're pregnant you should always keep your doctor informed so you get proper treatment. Your main responsibility is keeping yourself and your baby well nourished and cared for. That means you need a balanced diet, appropriate exercise, plenty of rest, and a stress-free environment. Above all, don't smoke or use alcohol while you're pregnant, and avoid all drugs except those prescribed by your doctor.

The following text describes what you can do for some of the common health problems you may face during your pregnancy; alternative therapies are included in some cases. Remember, though: You should never hesitate to call your doctor about any discomfort or illness you experience while you're pregnant.

ABDOMINAL PAIN

To relieve sharp pains or cramps from stretched abdominal muscles and ligaments, particularly when sitting or lying down, use a warm heating pad. Regular exercise *(see the box opposite)* will strengthen and tone your abdominal muscles.

BACKACHE

Keep your weight gain under control with proper diet and exercise. Avoid taking ***analgesics;*** instead, use a heating pad to relieve pain. Special exercises to strengthen abdominal muscles can also help reduce backache. *(See **Back Problems.**)* Try a pregnancy girdle or elastic sling to support your abdomen. Wear shoes or shoe inserts designed for pregnant women, and avoid high heels.

Don't stand for long periods and don't stretch to reach high places. Sit straight without slouching, and whenever possible, sit with your legs elevated. Sleep on a firm mattress.

Be careful when lifting heavy loads—especially children. Bend at the knees, keep your back as straight as possible, hold the object or child close to your body, and raise yourself slowly.

Acupressure. Stimulate the Bladder 23 and 47 points, along your lower back, by rubbing vigorously enough with the back of your hand to create heat. Also try pressing the Bladder 48 point. *(See the **Appendix** for information about point locations.)*

Chiropractic. See a licensed chiropractor for treatment of possible spinal misalignment brought about by the stress of the pregnancy.

Massage. Sit backward on a straight chair. Lean over the back with your head resting on your crossed arms. Have the massager use long strokes, working upward and outward from the lower back, avoiding pressure on the spine.

Yoga. Regular yoga practice can help keep your muscles relaxed and toned.

BREAST DISCOMFORT

Wear a bra that gives your enlarged breasts proper support. If your breasts leak small amounts of fluid, use nursing pads in your bra.

BREATHLESSNESS

Keep your weight gain within the recommended limits and maintain good posture, especially when you are sitting. Sleep on your left side, not on your back.

CONSTIPATION

To keep stools soft and bowel movements regular, get plenty of dietary fiber from fresh fruit, vegetables, whole-grain cereals and breads, and dried fruit. Avoid using over-the-counter ***laxatives,*** but try ***psyllium*** *(Plantago psyllium),* an

USEFUL EXERCISES

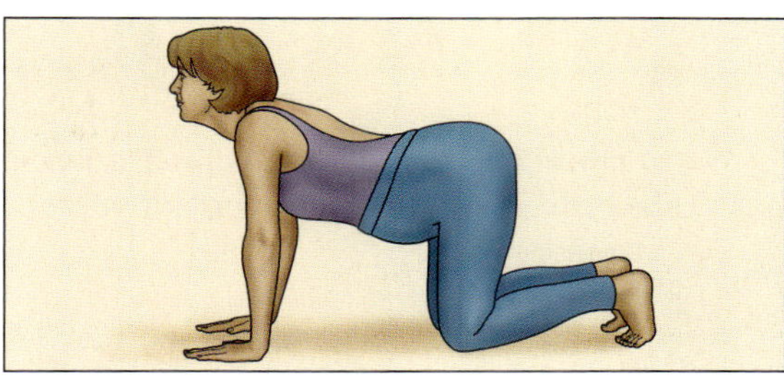

1 To decrease back and abdominal tension and pain, get on your hands and knees, keeping your back flat. Inhale as you arch your back downward, keeping your head and buttocks raised. Hold this position for 5 seconds, then relax and breathe normally.

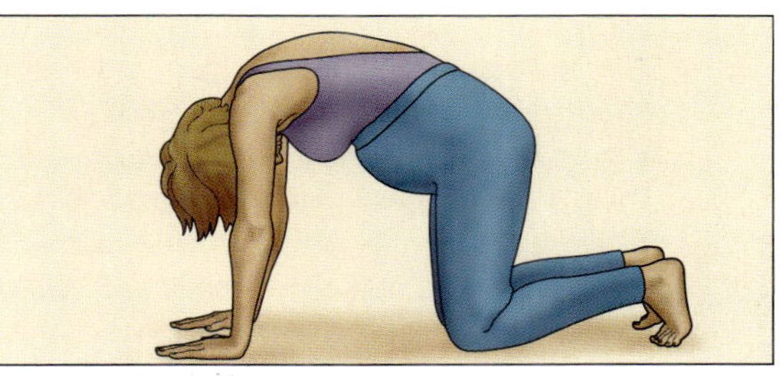

Next, exhale as you arch your back upward, rounding your shoulders and upper spine. Hold this position for 5 seconds, then relax and breathe normally. Slowly repeat this up-and-down sequence 10 times.

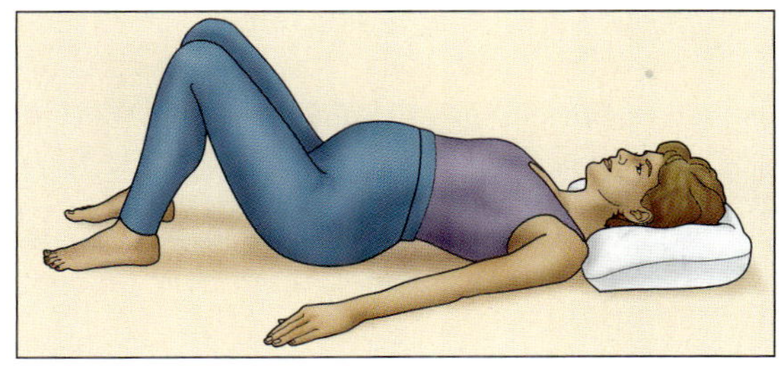

2 Lie on your back with your knees up. Tighten your buttocks and lower abdominal muscles, pressing the small of your back to the floor. Hold the position for 20 seconds, then relax and rest for one minute. Repeat five times.

P

PREGNANCY WARNINGS

- *A growing baby can throw you off balance, so be careful walking and getting out of the shower or tub.*
- *Check with your doctor before you start exercising. Some otherwise normal activities should not be undertaken during pregnancy, and others need to be modified.*
- *Avoid inhalation of or skin contact with chemical household cleaners, paints, and insecticides.*
- *The most dangerous time to take any medication is during the first trimester, when the fetus is developing rapidly and is more vulnerable to injury. Always check with your doctor before taking any over-the-counter or prescription drugs, including those that may have been prescribed before you became pregnant.*
- *Smoking during pregnancy increases the risks of vaginal bleeding, miscarriage, stillbirth, premature birth, low birthweight, and many other potential problems that you and your baby don't need. Smoke-filled rooms, car exhaust, and industrial fumes can also be hazardous to pregnant women: Avoid prolonged exposure to environmental pollutants as best you can.*
- *Several diseases pose special hazards to pregnant women and the unborn child, among them* ***German measles, chickenpox,*** *fifth disease (erythema infectiosum),* ***mumps,*** *cytomegalovirus,* ***chlamydia, gonorrhea, genital herpes, genital warts, syphilis,*** *and* ***AIDS.*** *Check with your doctor immediately if you think you have been exposed to any of them. If possible, get vaccinated against German measles and mumps before pregnancy unless you've had them.*
- *Most couples are able to have sexual intercourse until near the time of birth. Check with your doctor about the advisability of intercourse if you have a history of miscarriages or preterm birth, any* ***infection*** *or bleeding, if the placenta is in an abnormal position (known as placenta previa), or during the last trimester if you are carrying multiple fetuses. Avoid sex after the amniotic sac has broken or fluids leak. If you develop pain or abdominal cramps that continue or worsen more than an hour after having intercourse, call your doctor, your cervix could be dilating.*
- *Avoid having unnecessary x-rays. If you must get an x-ray, be sure to tell the doctor or the technician you are pregnant.*
- *Don't get overheated, avoid exercising in hot and humid weather, and stay out of hot tubs, saunas, and whirlpool baths.*

herbal bulk-forming agent. Drink lots of fluids and exercise regularly.

Acupressure. Pressing the Bladder 48 point may relieve constipation. *(See the* ***Appendix*** *for information on point location.)*

Yoga. Consult a yoga teacher to learn positions that can stimulate the bowel and release constipation.

CONTRACTIONS

Mild, painless uterine contractions usually start sometime after the 20th week of pregnancy. If they cause discomfort, try changing positions. If contractions start coming at regular intervals, notify your doctor.

CYSTITIS

If you develop a ***bladder infection*** or any type of urinary tract infection, ask your doctor about appropriate treatment. A heating pad on your lower abdomen will help relieve the discomfort. *(See also* ***Urinary Problems.****)*

Nutrition and Diet. Several glasses of cranberry juice a day are said to be helpful in preventing urinary tract infections.

DIZZINESS AND FAINTNESS

Slow down when you stand up or get out of bed. Dizziness when you rise too quickly from a sitting or prone position is called **postural hypotension.** If you're in a crowd and start feeling dizzy, step away and get some fresh air; if possible, lie down with your feet elevated or sit with your head between your knees.

EDEMA

Monitor your weight gain throughout your pregnancy. To control swelling in your legs and ankles, wear support hose and avoid standing for long periods. Wear shoes that fit well and give good support, or buy shoe inserts designed especially for pregnant women. Consult a **yoga** teacher to learn positions that can help keep fluid from building up in your legs and ankles.

FATIGUE

Get a full night's sleep and rest with your feet up for at least 15 minutes several times a day.

Acupressure. Stimulate Bladder 23 and 47 points by rubbing your lower back vigorously. Also try pressing the Bladder 10 point. *(See the* ***Appendix*** *for information on point locations.)*

HEADACHES

Make sure you get enough rest, eat regularly, and drink six or more glasses of water daily. Avoid ***aspirin*** or other over-the-counter painkillers except for ***acetaminophen;*** instead, try such stress-reduction techniques as **yoga** or **meditation.** Or try taking a hot bath with a cold pack on your forehead. *(See also* ***Headache.****)*

Acupressure. To relieve a headache, press the Governing Vessel 24.5 point. *(See the* ***Appendix*** *for information on point location.)*

Aromatherapy. Soak a handkerchief or washcloth in cool water with a few drops of ***lavender*** *(Lavandula officinalis)* and place on your forehead.

HEARTBURN

Avoid heavy meals and spicy, greasy, sugary, and acidic foods. Stick to a bland, high-fiber diet, drink lots of fluids, and exercise daily. Don't lie down right after a meal. Raise the head of your bed two to four inches with a stable support such as wooden blocks. *(See also* ***Heartburn.****)*

Acupressure. Pressing Stomach 45 and Spleen 16 may ease the discomfort of heartburn. *(See the* ***Appendix*** *for point locations.)*

Herbal Therapies. After meals, drink tea made from ***chamomile*** *(Matricaria recutita),* ***ginger*** *(Zingiber officinale),* or ***fennel*** *(Foeniculum vulgare).*

HEMORRHOIDS

Hemorrhoids may develop as your pelvis stretches, but they usually disappear after the birth. Eat a high-fiber diet to keep your stool soft, drink lots of fluids, and don't strain during bowel movements. To relieve hemorrhoidal itching or pain, try a warm sitz bath or apply an ice pack or a cloth soaked in witch hazel. Kegel exercises, designed to strengthen the pelvic muscles, can improve circulation in the area. *(See also* ***Hemorrhoids*** *and* ***Incontinence.****)*

Yoga. A yoga teacher can show you floor and inverted positions that can stimulate and improve circulation.

LEG PAINS AND CRAMPS

Wear support hose during the day, and elevate your feet when resting, if possible. Use a heating pad or gentle massage on the back of your thigh to ease ***sciatica.*** When a leg cramp hits, straighten your leg and slowly flex your ankle and toes, massage your calf, or soak your leg in hot water. You may be able to prevent night cramps by wearing socks to bed or by pressing your foot against the bed board. If painful cramps persist, ask your doctor about ***calcium*** or ***magnesium*** supplements.

MORNING SICKNESS

You may feel nauseated at any time of the day, typically in the first trimester. Try eating frequent light meals rather than three full meals. Keep your diet high in protein and complex carbohydrates, and low in sweet and fatty foods. Drink plenty of fluids, and eat fresh fruits and vegetables, which are high in water content. Do not take ***antacids,*** but try 50 mg of ***vitamin*** B_6 three times a day. In general, try to minimize stress in your everyday activities.

Acupressure. Locate the Pericardium 6 point on the inside of your left wrist, breathe deeply, and massage with your right thumb using a deep circular motion for one minute. Repeat on the other wrist. Seasickness straps, available in health stores, press the same point on the wrist. *(See the **Appendix** for information on point locations.)*

Aromatherapy. Add the essential oils of ***lavender*** *(Lavandula officinalis)* and mandarin to your bath, or put 2 drops each of ***peppermint*** *(Mentha piperita)* and sandalwood on a handkerchief and inhale the scent. Massage your abdomen with 2 drops each of peppermint and sandalwood mixed in 2 tsp of a carrier oil such as almond, olive, or sunflower oil.

Herbal Therapies. Try tea made from anise, caraway, ***catnip*** *(Nepeta cataria),* ***fennel*** *(Foeniculum vulgare),* or freshly grated ***ginger*** *(Zingiber officinale).* An infusion of dried ***peppermint*** *(Mentha piperita)* and ***chamomile*** *(Matricaria recutita)* may help your symptoms. Almonds and papaya juice are also said to ease morning sickness.

Homeopathy. Try ***Nux vomica*** (12c) or *Tabacum* (12c) for morning sickness, following label directions.

MOUTH AND GUM DISCOMFORT

Pregnancy can be demanding on your teeth, so see your dentist early in your pregnancy for a checkup and cleaning. Brush your teeth and tongue at least twice a day, and floss regularly. Sugarless gum can be substituted for an after-meal cleaning if it isn't feasible to brush your teeth. Supplemental ***vitamin C, calcium,*** and coenzyme Q10 will strengthen your own teeth and ultimately your baby's. Or try a ***folic acid*** rinse, but do not swallow it.

NASAL CONGESTION OR NOSEBLEEDS

Use a vaporizer to humidify your bedroom at night, and lubricate each nostril with a dab of petroleum jelly during the day to prevent nosebleeds. Avoid nasal sprays, which can constrict blood vessels.

Acupressure. To control nasal congestion, try finger pressure on Bladder 10. *(See the **Appendix** for information on point location.)*

NUMBNESS

Avoid lying on your hands while sleeping. If your hand feels numb when you wake up, shake it over the side of the bed. Soaking the hand in warm water or using a heating pad twice daily may help ease numbness, or try wearing a wrist splint *(see **Carpal Tunnel Syndrome**).* If numbness persists try 50-mg ***vitamin*** B_6 supplements three times a day.

SKIN CHANGES

Rashes from hormone changes during pregnancy generally go away after the baby is born. To prevent freckles or a dark pregnancy mask called **chloasma** on your face, wear a wide-brimmed hat or use sunblock on sunny days. Lubricate dry skin around your abdomen with a moisturizing cream; stretch marks usually fade and decrease after the birth. For heat rash, try to stay as cool as possible and use cornstarch powder under your breasts, on your thighs, or wherever your skin tends to chafe.

TASTE CHANGES

You may find some foods unpalatable and develop a craving for others, especially sweets. Use mouthwash often; chewing gum, mints, or hard candies may also chase away unpleasant tastes. ***Iron*** supplements may leave a bad taste in your mouth; talk to your practitioner if this is a problem.

URINATION PROBLEMS

Kegel exercises *(see **Incontinence**)* can help you to control stress incontinence—losing a small amount of urine when you sneeze, cough, or laugh. You can also use a sanitary napkin. Leaning forward while urinating helps to empty your bladder completely.

VAGINAL DISORDERS

A thin, mild-smelling discharge is normal in pregnancy. Use sanitary napkins, but do not douche without your doctor's approval. Any red or brown discharge is a signal to call your doctor immediately. Vaginal itching and soreness may indicate an ***infection,*** which requires treatment by your doctor. Vaginal ***yeast infections*** may be common in pregnancy and may disappear without treatment after the baby is born. *(See also **Vaginal Problems.**)*

Homeopathy. Check with a homeopath about using ***Sepia*** (9c), or other remedies, to treat mild vaginal disorders.

VARICOSE VEINS

Pregnancy puts extra strain on the blood vessels in your legs. You can get the most benefit from wearing support pantyhose or elastic stockings if you put them on while you are lying down so that body fluids are not gravitating to your legs. Exercise regularly, but don't stand for long periods. Raise your legs above hip level when sitting, if possible. Lie on your side in bed, or put a pillow under your feet. *(See also **Varicose Veins.**)*

Nutrition and Diet. Ask your doctor or a nutritional specialist about taking ***vitamin C*** supplements to strengthen blood vessels.

VISION CHANGES

If your eyes swell from fluid retention and hard contact lenses become uncomfortable, switch to soft lenses or glasses.

C A U T I O N !

BABY ON THE WAY

You can confidently treat many secondary disorders of pregnancy yourself, but only after you discuss the problem and potential treatments with your doctor. Some prescription drugs and over-the-counter medications can be dangerous to unborn babies and pregnant women. This is equally true of herbal preparations, essential oils, or anything you eat or drink. The same cautions apply to acupressure, massage, yoga, and other body work techniques; in fact, most acupuncturists will not treat pregnant women. For your comfort and safety—to say nothing of your baby's—always discuss alternative treatments with trained therapists sensitive to the special aspects of pregnancy. And make sure you have 24-hour access to your doctor to discuss any health questions or concerns. ■

PREMENSTRUAL SYNDROME

SYMPTOMS

The symptoms of premenstrual syndrome recur during the same phase of the menstrual cycle, usually 7 to 10 days before your period begins. They may include any of the following:

- bloating and fluid retention.
- breast swelling and pain.
- acne, cold sores, or susceptibility to herpes outbreaks.
- weight gain of up to five pounds (from retention of fluids).
- headaches, backaches, and joint or muscle aches.
- moodiness, anxiety, depression, or irritability.
- food cravings, especially for sugary or salty foods.
- insomnia.
- drowsiness and fatigue, or conversely, extra energy.
- hot flashes or nausea.
- constipation, diarrhea, or urinary disorders.

A very small number of women with premenstrual syndrome may experience more intense symptoms:

- fits of crying.
- panic attacks.
- suicidal thoughts.
- aggressive or violent behavior.

CALL YOUR DOCTOR IF:

- your symptoms are severe enough to interfere with your normal functions; your doctor may be able to offer treatments that will alleviate your symptoms.

Premenstrual syndrome—commonly known as PMS—is a physical condition characterized by a variety of symptoms that typically recur during a particular phase of the menstrual cycle, usually a week to 10 days before your period begins. Practically every woman experiences at least one PMS symptom sometime in her life, and between 10 and 50 percent of women in the United States suffer from PMS regularly. Specific symptoms vary from woman to woman. Some 5 to 10 percent of women experience symptoms severe enough for them to seek medical help.

PMS is uncommon in adolescents. Although some adolescents do indeed suffer from the syndrome, for most women the symptoms first develop while they are in their twenties.

Women most often affected by premenstrual syndrome are those who have experienced a major hormonal change, as may happen after childbirth, miscarriage, abortion, or tubal ligation. Women who discontinue birth-control pills may also notice an increase in PMS symptoms until their hormone balance returns.

Although PMS has been reported in the medical literature since the 1930s, its validity as a medical condition is a hotly debated subject. Many worry that it will be used to prove women too emotionally and physically unpredictable for certain jobs or responsibilities. Experts point out, however, that the syndrome—although sometimes discomforting—is rarely debilitating.

CAUSES

Numerous theories have been proposed to explain some or all of the symptoms of PMS. Many researchers believe that PMS is the result of a hormonal imbalance, although the precise nature of that imbalance is not certain. An overproduction of the hormone estrogen is sometimes cited; however, most women do not experience PMS at the middle of their menstrual cycle, when estrogen levels are at their peak.

It has also been suggested that a deficiency in a particular hormone—such as estrogen, progesterone, testosterone, or prolactin—may be responsible for PMS, but controlled studies have

P

ruled out these single-hormone theories. Recent research has focused on the monthly fluctuations in brain chemicals known as neurotransmitters, including mood-altering endorphins and monoamines, as a possible cause of the syndrome, but studies have been inconclusive.

Dietary deficiencies, including a lack of ***vitamin B₆*** and essential fatty acids, are also considered a possible cause. One type of PMS, characterized by headache, dizziness, heart pounding, increased appetite, and a craving for chocolate, is thought by some researchers to be the result of a ***magnesium*** deficiency brought on by stress. According to this theory, the craving for chocolate, a food rich in magnesium, helps balance the deficiency; unfortunately, however, the sugar in chocolate also raises blood insulin levels, which can exacerbate the other symptoms.

The fact that identical twins are more likely to share PMS symptoms than are fraternal twins suggests that premenstrual syndrome may have a genetic component.

DIAGNOSTIC AND TEST PROCEDURES

Before making a diagnosis of PMS, your doctor will want to rule out other possible causes of the symptoms by giving you a general physical and pelvic examination. Some doctors take blood samples to check hormone levels in the body, but many PMS experts consider these tests to be of dubious value. Instead, they suggest that the best way of accurately diagnosing PMS is for you to keep a written daily diary of your symptoms for at least two months. Keep a calendar record of when your menstrual period begins and ends, and each evening write down on the calendar any PMS symptoms you had that day. Your doctor can then use this written record not only to confirm a diagnosis but also to help decide on a possible treatment plan.

TREATMENT

You may decide not to treat your PMS symptoms at all. But if they are severe and you seek help, be aware that some treatment approaches are controversial. Remedies for PMS basically fall into two categories: hormonal treatments, prescribed by some conventional doctors, and nutritional and lifestyle changes, prescribed by both conventional and alternative practitioners. Because of the health risks associated with hormonal treatments, many women prefer to try alternative methods first.

CONVENTIONAL MEDICINE

Some doctors prescribe various hormones, most notably estrogen or progesterone, to relieve symptoms. The hormones are given in a variety of forms, including injection and vaginal or rectal suppositories. But hormonal treatments may produce side effects, some of which can be serious, and no controlled studies have definitively shown that these treatments work.

Some doctors prescribe hormone-containing birth-control pills to women with PMS symptoms. Although some women report that the pills alleviate their symptoms, studies have shown that they are not useful for most women with PMS and may in certain cases even worsen symptoms.

Because of the risks associated with hormonal treatments, many conventional doctors prefer approaches that emphasize good nutrition, regular exercise, and other lifestyle changes such as those described below.

ALTERNATIVE CHOICES

A wide variety of alternative treatments may help relieve PMS symptoms. Because PMS is different from one woman to the next, you may have to try several treatments, or a combination of them, before you find the right approach for you.

In addition to the treatments listed below, **acupuncture** treatment or **chiropractic** manipulation may be able to offer relief.

AROMATHERAPY

To relieve anxiety and irritability, try ***lavender*** *(Lavandula officinalis)* or ***chamomile*** *(Matricaria recutita)* oil; ***parsley*** *(Petroselinum crispum)* or ***juniper*** *(Juniperus communis)* oil may also be helpful. Add several drops to a warm bath.

To relieve breast tenderness, try adding 6 to 8 drops of geranium *(Pelargonium odoratissimum)* oil to a warm bath.

CHINESE HERBS

For relief from PMS symptoms, Chinese herbalists sometimes recommend ***dong quai*** *(Angelica sinensis),* which is believed to help balance the body's hormones and have a tonic effect on the uterus and other female organs. Take as a tea or in tincture form (4 to 6 ml) three times a day. Consult a Chinese herbalist for other herb suggestions, tailored to your symptoms.

NUTRITION AND DIET

Dietary changes have been shown to effectively reduce PMS symptoms in some women. Try reducing your intake of caffeine, sugar, salt, dairy products, and white flour, which studies have shown can sometimes aggravate PMS symptoms. Many women also find that eating six or more small meals throughout the day rather than three large ones reduces their symptoms, perhaps by keeping insulin levels more constant.

Some PMS symptoms, such as mood swings, fluid retention, bloatedness, breast tenderness, food cravings, and fatigue, have been linked to a deficiency of ***vitamin*** B_6 or ***magnesium.*** Nutritionists recommend supplements of these nutrients: 50 to 100 mg of vitamin B_6 daily, and 250 mg of magnesium daily, with a gradual increase if necessary. Supplements of ***calcium, zinc, copper, vitamins A*** and ***E,*** as well as various amino acids and enzymes, are also sometimes prescribed. Consult an experienced nutritionist.

Some research has indicated that a dietary deficiency in fatty acids may contribute to PMS. Many women report that taking ***evening primrose oil*** *(Oenothera biennis),* a substance that contains essential fatty acids, is effective. Your healthcare practitioner may recommend that you take one capsule (500 mg) daily throughout the month. If this amount does not bring relief, the dosage may be increased to four capsules a day. Other dosage regimens are also recommended. Consult your healthcare practitioner.

YOGA

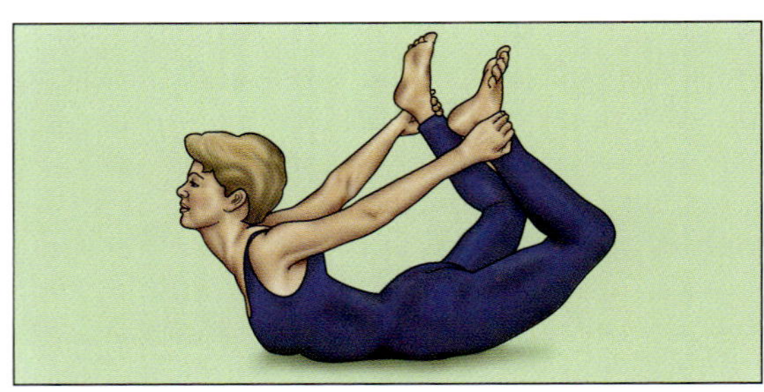

1 To help restore hormonal balance, try the **Bow.** Lie on your stomach, legs bent, and grasp both ankles. While inhaling, squeeze your buttocks and slowly raise your head, chest, and thighs off the floor. Hold for 15 seconds, breathing slowly, and release. Do one time.

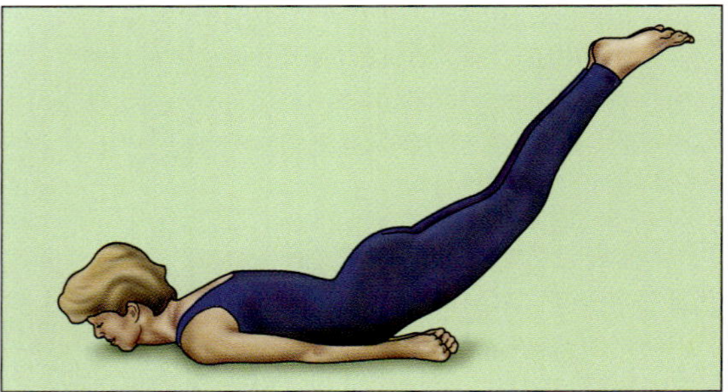

2 The **Locust** tones muscles in the pelvic area. Lie on your stomach, arms at your sides. Squeeze your buttocks as you press down with your arms and fists. Raise your legs, keeping them straight as you press out through the toes and heels. Hold for 15 seconds, then exhale and release. Do once or twice a day.

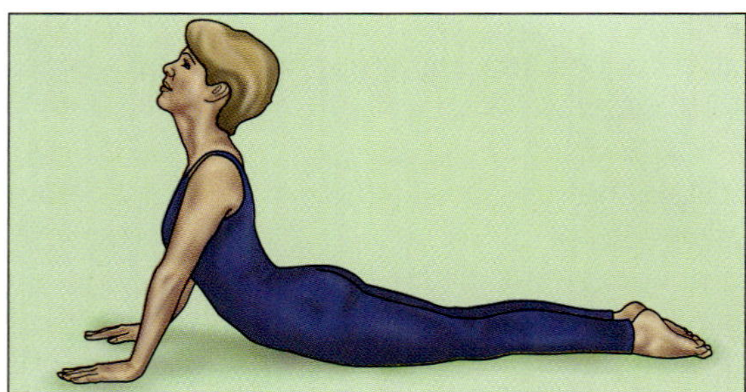

3 You can also try the **Cobra.** Place both hands on the floor, directly under your shoulders, elbows against your body. Inhale and push your chest up while pressing your pelvis and palms against the floor. Hold for 15 seconds, breathing deeply, then slowly relax. Do one or two times.

HERBAL THERAPIES
Herbalists recommend a wide variety of herbs to help alleviate the many symptoms of PMS. ***Chaste tree*** *(Vitex agnus-castus),* for example, is sometimes prescribed because it is believed to help balance the body's hormones and relieve the anxiety and depression associated with PMS. ***Dandelion*** *(Taraxacum officinale),* whose leaves are thought to act as a powerful diuretic, is sometimes used to reduce the bloating and breast swelling caused by premenstrual fluid retention. ***Skullcap*** *(Scutellaria lateriflora),* believed to have a calming effect on the nerves, is also sometimes suggested. For an herbal preparation designed to relieve your particular symptoms, see an experienced practitioner.

HOMEOPATHY
For relief from your specific PMS symptoms, consult an experienced homeopath for individualized remedies and dosages.

LIFESTYLE
Studies have shown that regular exercise lessens PMS symptoms, perhaps by stimulating the release of endorphins and other brain chemicals that help relieve stress and lighten mood. Getting enough sleep is also important for the successful treatment of PMS. Lack of sleep can exacerbate fatigue, irritability, and other emotional symptoms. Experts recommend that people who have trouble getting enough rest stick to a regular sleep schedule. By going to bed and awakening at the same time each day, even on weekends, you may find it easier to get the sleep you need.

MIND/BODY MEDICINE
Various relaxation techniques, such as **yoga** and **meditation,** can be helpful in reducing the anxiety, irritability, and other emotional symptoms that sometimes occur premenstrually. The Cobra and Bow yoga positions *(left)* are particularly recommended for PMS.

ACUPRESSURE

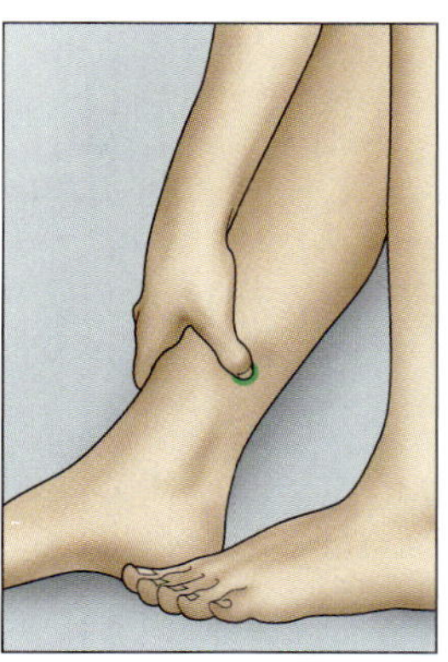

Symptoms of PMS may be relieved by pressing Spleen 6. Place your thumb four finger widths up from your right inside anklebone, near the edge of the shinbone. Press for one minute, then do the same on the other leg. Do two to three times. Do not use SP 6 if you are pregnant.

AT-HOME REMEDIES
- Try to eat a low-fat, high-fiber diet. Avoid salt, sugar, caffeine, and dairy products right before your menstrual period.
- Exercise regularly.
- Try to reduce stress and increase sleep during the week before your period.
- Take recommended vitamin supplements.
- Try to manage your food cravings—particularly for chocolate; giving in to them may actually make your symptoms worse. Reach for fruit instead of sugary treats.
- As your period approaches, take long, warm baths to ease tension and stress.
- Use a hot-water bottle, a heating pad, or castor-oil packs to ease backaches and muscle aches associated with PMS.
- Abstain from alcohol before your period. It can aggravate PMS depression, headaches, and fatigue, and can trigger food cravings.
- Join a PMS support group. Some communities have PMS self-help organizations that meet regularly to provide support and exchange information. Check your phone book or call a local hospital for the name of a group in your area. ■

PROSTATE CANCER

SYMPTOMS

Early prostate cancer rarely causes symptoms. Once a malignant tumor causes the prostate gland to swell significantly, or once cancer spreads beyond the prostate, the following symptoms may be present:

- a frequent need to urinate, especially at night.
- difficulty starting or stopping the urinary stream.
- a weak or interrupted urinary stream.
- a painful or burning sensation during urination or ejaculation.
- blood in urine or semen.

Symptoms of advanced prostate cancer include:

- dull, incessant pain or stiffness in the pelvis, lower back, or upper thighs; arthritic pain in the bones of those areas.
- loss of weight and appetite, fatigue, nausea, or vomiting.

CALL YOUR DOCTOR IF:

- you have difficulty urinating or find that urination is painful or otherwise abnormal. Your doctor will examine your prostate gland to determine whether it is swollen and, if so, whether the problem is caused by a malignant tumor or another kind of ailment.
- you have chronic pain in your lower back, pelvis or upper thighbones, or other bones. Ongoing pain without explanation always merits medical attention. Pain in these areas can have various causes but may be from the spread of advanced prostate cancer.

P

The prostate is a gland in the male reproductive system that helps produce semen, the thick fluid that carries sperm cells. The walnut-sized gland is located beneath a man's bladder and surrounds the upper part of the urethra, the tube that carries urine from the bladder. Prostate function is regulated by testosterone, a male sex hormone produced mainly in the testicles.

Prostate cancer is a major health concern for American men. Although the disease is rare before age 50, experts speculate that most elderly men have at least traces of it. Some 200,000 new cases and 38,000 deaths are attributed to prostate cancer each year in the U.S. For reasons not fully understood, African American men have the greatest incidence of prostate cancer in the world and the highest death rate from the disease. In other parts of the world—notably Asia, Africa, and Latin America—prostate cancer is rare.

Compared with most other cancers, prostate cancer behaves rather strangely. It often lies dormant for years, causing no symptoms and posing no threat to general health. Most men with prostate cancer die of other causes—many without ever realizing that they have the disease. But once prostate cancer "wakes up" and begins to spread, it is dangerous. Although the disease tends to progress slowly, it is generally fatal if it spreads beyond the prostate gland itself.

More than half of diagnosed cases originate in the prostate's posterior section, nearest the rectum. A few rare types originate in the anterior section nearest the urethra. A malignant tumor may grow directly through the prostate gland and spread cancer cells to surrounding tissue, including the rectum and bladder. Cancer cells may also invade the lymphatic system or bloodstream, travel to nearby lymph nodes, and then spread to the bones, liver, lungs, and other organs.

Doctors treating prostate cancer have long been frustrated by not knowing which prostate cancers will remain dormant and which will spread and become life-threatening. Identification of a protein called KAI-1 (named for the gene that controls its production) may make this dilemma obsolete. This protein appears to serve as a "marker" for metastatic, or spreading, prostate cancers. If high levels of KAI-1 are found in can-

DETECTING PROSTATE CANCER

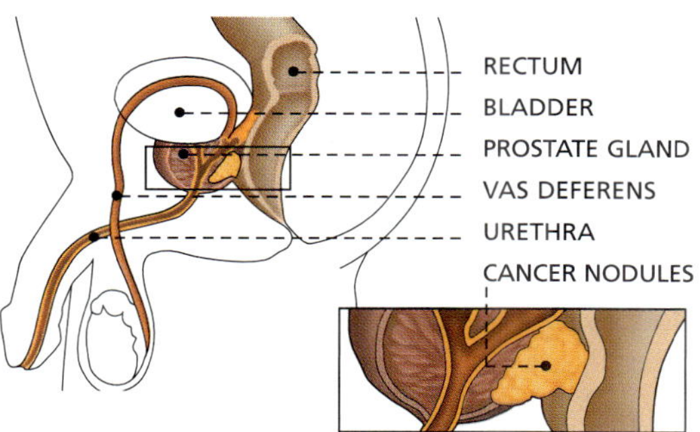

The prostate, a gland about the size of a walnut, encircles a man's urethra just below the bladder *(above, left)*. Prostate cancer typically develops slowly and may be confused with simple enlargement of the gland. A doctor can detect early signs of prostate cancer during a digital rectal exam by inserting a gloved finger into the rectum to feel for telltale nodules *(inset)*.

cerous tissue samples, the prostate cancer is unlikely to spread, or metastasize; if the protein is absent, the cancer is likely to spread.

Cancer that has not spread beyond the prostate gland can be cured. Fortunately, more than half of American men with prostate cancer are diagnosed when the disease is in its early stages. Cancer that has spread beyond the prostate to nearby tissues is rarely curable, but it often can be controlled for years with treatment. Once the cancer becomes widespread, life expectancy ranges from 2 to 3 years. With improved detection and treatment of prostate cancer over the past 30 years, the overall 5-year survival rate has increased from 50 percent to nearly 80 percent.

CAUSES

Prostate cancer affects mainly elderly men. Four out of five cases are diagnosed in men over 65, but less than 1 percent in men under 50. Men with a family history of prostate cancer are three times more likely to die of it than is the general population. On a case-by-case basis, doctors cannot say with certainty what causes prostate cancer, but experts generally agree that diet contributes to the risk. Men who consume great amounts of fat—particularly from red meat and other sources of animal fat—are most likely to develop symptoms of advanced prostate cancer. The disease is much more common in countries where meat and dairy products are dietary staples than in countries where the basic diet consists of rice, soybean products, and vegetables.

The underlying factor linking diet and prostate cancer is probably hormonal. Fats stimulate production of testosterone and other hormones, and testosterone acts to speed the growth of prostate cancer. Theoretically, high testosterone levels spur dormant prostate cancer cells into activity. Some findings suggest that high testosterone levels also influence the initial onset of prostate cancer. Eating meat may be risky for other reasons: Meat cooked at high temperatures produces carcinogens that directly affect the prostate. A few other risk factors have been noted. Welders, battery manufacturers, rubber workers, and workers frequently exposed to the metal cadmium seem to be abnormally vulnerable to prostate cancer.

Researchers know more about what will not cause prostate cancer than what will. No proven link exists between prostate cancer and an active sex life, masturbation, use of alcohol or tobacco, circumcision, infertility, infection of the prostate, or a common noncancerous condition called **benign prostatic hyperplasia (BPH)** that involves an enlarged prostate gland. Most elderly men experience BPH to some degree. The theory that men who have vasectomies are at slightly increased risk for prostate cancer remains unproved.

DIAGNOSTIC AND TEST PROCEDURES

Because most malignant prostate tumors originate in the part of the gland nearest the rectum, many cancers can be detected during routine rectal examinations. Men over 50 should have a rectal exam annually, and most doctors recommend that the exam be supplemented by a prostate-specific antigen (PSA) blood test. PSA is a protein whose concentration tends to increase in the presence of prostate cancer, making it twice as effective as a rectal exam in detecting early prostate cancer; together the two measures offer the best chance of catching prostate cancer while it is localized and most treatable. Prostate cancer may also be discovered incidentally during treatment for ***urinary problems.***

If routine screening arouses suspicion, a doctor will inspect the prostate visually using transrectal ultrasonography. X-rays of the urinary tract, along with blood and urine studies, are performed routinely to aid diagnosis. Performing a biopsy will confirm cancer diagnosis: Guided by ultrasound images, the doctor inserts a needle into the prostate and extracts a small tissue sample from the tumor. A pathologist then studies the sample under a microscope to determine whether cancer cells are present. KAI-1 protein levels and other indicators can determine whether the cancer is likely to spread. If a diagnosed cancer is thought likely to spread, doctors may arrange CT scans, bone scans, chest x-rays, or other imaging tests to determine whether the disease has spread beyond the prostate.

TREATMENT

Now more than ever, doctors have the information necessary to make informed decisions about which early prostate cancers require prompt treatment. Once the decision is made to treat a cancer, other factors, such as a patient's age and general health, affect the type of treatment given. Because decisions about how to treat this cancer are complex, patients should seek a second opinion from a specialist at a major cancer center and should participate in the treatment decision.

CONVENTIONAL MEDICINE

Depending on when the disease is diagnosed, conventional treatment includes some combination of radiation therapy, surgery, and hormone therapy. Localized prostate cancer usually can be cured with conventional surgery, radiation therapy, or cryosurgery—freezing malignant cells with liquid nitrogen. The choice is made on a case-by-case basis and depends on many factors.

The standard operation—a radical prostatectomy—involves the removal of the prostate and nearby lymph nodes. In many cases surgeons can remove the gland without cutting nerves that control penile erection or bladder contraction, making such complications as ***impotence*** or ***incontinence*** less common than in the past. After surgery most men experience some degree of incontinence but eventually regain complete urinary control. Postop patients can manage impotence or incontinence resulting from surgery in a variety of ways. Impotence can be overcome with penile implants or other devices. Incontinence can be managed with special disposable underwear, condom catheters, or penile clamps; in three cases out of four, incontinence can be eliminated altogether with surgically inserted sphincter implants in the urethra.

Radiation therapy may be given as an alternative or follow-up to surgery for cancer that has not spread. If cancer has spread to nearby tissue, radiation is the preferred treatment; it is also used in advanced cases to relieve pain from the spread of cancer to bones. Even advanced cases that cannot be cured may be controlled for years with hormone therapy, sometimes supplemented by other treatments. Hormone therapy slows the cancer's growth by cutting off the testosterone supply, although the treatment's effectiveness may decrease over time. Testosterone can be removed from the bloodstream by surgically removing the testicles or by administering female hormones such as ***estrogen*** or other drugs that block testosterone production. Men generally prefer the testosterone-blocking drug treatment because it is effective, less invasive, and causes fewer side effects than surgery or hormone drugs. If the testicles are removed, the scrotum can be left intact with implants to conceal disfigurement.

If treatment is effective, prostate cancer goes into remission and may never return. All prostate cancer survivors should be examined regularly and have their PSA levels monitored closely. As with other types of cancer, new therapies are being developed for the treatment of advanced prostate cancer. Researchers are using radiation and hormone therapy in innovative ways and are testing the effectiveness of chemotherapy on patients who do not respond to other treatments.

AN ESSENTIAL BLOOD TEST

A tumor marker blood test is designed to measure a specific chemical that often is elevated in the presence of a specific cancer. In this case, the chemical is a protein called prostate-specific antigen (PSA) and the malignancy is prostate cancer. While most tumor marker tests are used to measure the response of various cancers to treatment, the PSA test is considered reliable enough to use in diagnosis.

But as useful as it is, the PSA test is not infallible and therefore cannot be the sole basis for a diagnosis. A man's PSA level tends to rise whenever the prostate becomes enlarged, but the enlargement may or may not be caused by cancer. This means that a higher-than-normal test reading can raise unnecessary alarm—a so-called false-positive reading. A PSA test may also indicate that cancer is not present when in fact it is. Because of its uncertainty, experts recommend that the PSA test be given along with the conventional gloved-finger rectal exam.

The PSA test is easy to give, relatively cheap, and has improved detection of early prostate cancer dramatically. Coupled with rectal exams and the newly developed KAI-1 tumor marker test, the PSA test enables doctors to detect and treat threatening prostate cancers at a very early stage. The American Cancer Society recommends that all men over 50 have an annual PSA test; for information about your local screening site, call 1-800-ACS-2345.

See ***Cancer*** for more information on treatments such as radiation and chemotherapy.

COMPLEMENTARY THERAPIES

Because excess dietary fat appears to promote prostate cancer, reducing fat may help slow the disease's progress. Anyone who has been diagnosed with early prostate cancer should maintain a low-fat, high-fiber, moderately reduced-calorie diet. If dietary fat is shown to play a role in initiating prostate cancer, cutting fat more severely would clearly be an advisable preventive measure for young and middle-aged men, particularly those with a strong family history of the disease.

Studies indicate that men with chronic deficiencies of ***vitamin A*** or ***selenium*** are more likely to develop advanced prostate cancer. Both nutrients can be toxic when taken in excess, so be sure to consult a doctor before taking dietary supplements. Good natural sources of vitamin A include most green and yellow fruits and vegetables, as well as liver, lamb, and turkey.

AT-HOME CARE

Radiation therapy for treating localized prostate cancer is generally well tolerated. Some men, however, may experience ***fatigue, diarrhea,*** uncomfortable urination, dry skin, ***nausea,*** and other unpleasant side effects. Doctors can prescribe medication and suggest other ways to minimize side effects, including those things you can do for yourself. Rest whenever you feel the need, eat light snacks throughout the day rather than having three large meals, and avoid clothes that irritate your skin. For more information, see ***Cancer.***

PREVENTION

To lower your dietary fat, eat more fish, poultry, fresh vegetables, fruits, and low-fat dairy products. In general, eat less red meat; remove skin from poultry before cooking; and cut down on butter, margarine, and oils. To avoid carcinogens created when cooking meats, try poaching or roasting, not frying or barbecuing. ■

PROSTATE PROBLEMS

SYMPTOMS

For an enlarged prostate:
- difficulties in urination, including a weak or intermittent stream, unusual frequency (especially at night), straining, dribbling, or inability to empty the bladder.

For acute prostatitis:
- frequent, difficult urination.
- a burning sensation when urinating.
- sudden fever, chills.
- pain in the lower back and the area behind the scrotum.
- blood in the urine.

For chronic prostatitis:
- frequent, difficult urination.
- pain in the pelvis and genital area.
- painful ejaculation, bloody semen, or sexual dysfunction.

CALL YOUR DOCTOR IF:

- your symptoms lead you to suspect an enlarged or infected prostate. If allowed to progress, prostate problems can lead to bladder stones, generalized infection, or kidney failure.

In addition, an enlarged prostate can be a sign of cancer. *(See **Prostate Cancer.**)*

The prostate is a walnut-sized gland that surrounds the male urethra—the tube that transports urine from the bladder through the penis. Its primary function is to produce an essential portion of the seminal fluid that carries sperm; the prostate also controls the outward flow of urine from the bladder. Because of this dual role, signs of prostate trouble can include both urinary and sexual difficulties.

Prostate problems occur in two principal forms: **enlargement of the prostate,** called BPH (for benign prostatic hyperplasia); and **prostatitis,** a bacterial infection, which may be either sudden and severe **(acute prostatitis)** or milder but persistent or recurrent **(chronic prostatitis).** A chronic infection may follow an acute one.

The signs of **prostate enlargement** generally appear after the age of 45. Typically, the first indication is a need to urinate at night, with the urge gradually increasing over time. Other urination problems may develop: a difficulty or hesitancy in initiating the urine stream; an inability to empty the bladder completely; and dribbling at the end of urination. These signs all have a common origin—the narrowing of the urethra because of growth of the glandular tissue surrounding it. Although the problem varies in severity, few men escape it altogether: Prostate enlargement affects 50 percent of those over 50 and a somewhat astonishing 90 percent of those over 80.

Prostatitis is less common and can occur in younger men or without symptoms of enlargement. While some of the signs resemble those of BPH, others are more typical of infection. **Acute prostatitis** may produce fever, chills, and lower back pain. **Chronic prostatitis** generally brings milder versions of those symptoms and may also cause painful ejaculation, urethral discharge, or sexual dysfunction.

Many men are reluctant to seek treatment for BPH or prostatitis, especially if their discomfort is minor. If either condition progresses toward severe symptoms, the danger can increase sharply. With prostatitis, the infection may reach the testicles and epididymis (a long, coiled tube behind each testicle through which sperm is transported from the testicles). It can also spread to a sexual partner. With BPH, the bladder may eventually

AN ENLARGED PROSTATE

The prostate, a walnut-sized gland in a man's lower abdomen, lies at the base of the bladder and surrounds a section of the urethra, a tube that carries urine and semen out of the body. As indicated below, enlargement of the prostate can put increasing pressure on the urethra, making urination progressively painful and difficult.

be unable to empty itself, and the lingering pools of urine become sites of infection or stone formation. Such urine retention is very painful and should be treated as a medical emergency. If the outflow of urine is blocked, pressure within the bladder may back up to the kidneys, eventually leading to permanent damage.

As the average age of the U.S. population rises, so does the number of men who seek relief from prostate problems. But with BPH, some aspects of the condition, including the chances of its worsening, are still poorly understood. As a result, the field is alive with controversy over when to take medical action and also over the relative merits of standard surgery and newer forms of medical treatment.

CAUSES

Although the molecular mechanisms underlying **prostate enlargement** remain uncertain, the condition seems to stem from age-related changes in hormone balance that begin when a man is in his forties. Testosterone levels in the blood decrease, while other hormone levels rise; the net effect is the increase of a testosterone derivative that stimulates cell growth in the prostate. This results in enlargement and consequent stricture of the urethra within the gland. **Prostatitis** is usually the result of a urinary tract or ***bladder infection*** that has spread into the prostate gland. The infection can be sexually transmitted.

DIAGNOSTIC AND TEST PROCEDURES

If symptoms indicate **prostate enlargement,** a physician will want to determine whether the growth of the gland is benign (BPH) or malignant ***(prostate cancer).*** The physician will insert a gloved finger into the rectum to feel the prostate for hardness or nodules, which can indicate malignancy. A urine sample is taken to detect infection and/or chemical indicators of cancer cells. (In 10 to 20 percent of benign cases, the prostate also harbors such cells.) Ultrasound imaging of the bladder and prostate is usually performed, and the bladder may be examined with a cystoscope. If symptoms suggest **prostatitis,** a urine test will identify the infectious agents. A rectal exam will find the prostate to be very tender and sensitive and will provide a check for coexisting conditions.

TREATMENT

For **prostate enlargement,** be sure that you and your doctor consider the whole range of treat-

SELF-MONITORING

*A primary goal in treating **prostate enlargement** is to reverse the growth of the prostate so the bladder can be emptied and the frequency of urination decreased. In gauging the success of treatment, your physician may suggest that you monitor the rate of urine flow on a regular basis. A reduced flow indicates that prostate growth is further constricting the urethra; an increased flow is evidence that the treatment is working.*

Flow-rate monitoring is a simple chore involving a watch and a container calibrated in cubic centimeters. Calculate the flow rate by measuring the volume of urine voided and the time in seconds it takes to empty your bladder. For example, if the volume voided is 200 cc and the time taken to empty the bladder is 10 seconds, the flow rate is 20 cc per second. A normal flow rate for a man over 50 years of age is at least 15 cc per second.

ment options. Just a few years ago, many physicians felt that surgery was the only solution; today, researchers are proposing an array of new treatment choices, from hormone-blocking drugs to lasers that can remove prostatic tissue without hospitalization.

CONVENTIONAL MEDICINE

Enlarged prostate: When BPH symptoms are mild to moderate, medication may be the appropriate therapy. ***Alpha-1 adrenergic blockers,*** including ***terazosin*** and prazosin, relax the smooth muscles at the bladder neck and urethra, easing urination. Another medication, finasteride, has shown some ability to gradually reduce prostate size and symptoms, though noticeable improvement may take three to six months.

When symptoms are severe or there is evidence of cancer, surgery is usually recommended. About 85 percent of patients experience marked relief of symptoms. In the most common surgery, the patient is placed under anesthesia, but no incision is needed. A small cutting instrument called a resectoscope (*resect* means to remove part of an organ) is passed through the penis and into the prostate by way of the urethra. Using an electrical apparatus at the end of the scope, the surgeon carves away the inner prostate, leaving a hollow shell through which the urine can flow. This procedure is known as TUR, or transurethral resection.

In about 15 percent of cases, TUR can have complications, including possible impotence and urinary incontinence; some patients experience infection or bleeding, and others require a second operation to reopen the urinary tract. For these reasons, and because of the desire of patients to avoid surgery, there is much enthusiasm for nonsurgical resectioning methods. Several kinds of laser resecters, which can be used for outpatients, have shown good results. The instrument is passed through the urethra, as in TUR; the laser is then fired, and the heat quickly coagulates and vaporizes excessive prostate tissue.

Microwave devices, similarly inserted, have been widely employed in Europe and Canada. Recently approved by the FDA, this technique is increasingly available in the U.S. Like laser resections, they can be done in an outpatient setting.

If the prostate is too large for TUR or other methods, the surgeon may recommend open prostatectomy, the removal of the prostate gland via surgical incision.

Prostatitis: A prolonged course of ***antibiotics*** is usually successful in eliminating the infection. Stool softeners, sitz baths, and ***nonsteroidal anti-inflammatory drugs (NSAIDs)*** are prescribed for discomfort. If an infection is neglected too long, antibiotics may not be effective—and it may be difficult to remove the infection even by surgery without causing further complications.

ALTERNATIVE CHOICES

AYURVEDIC MEDICINE

A practitioner may prescribe herbal remedies and exercises to increase circulation and relieve congestion in the prostate.

CHINESE MEDICINE

Prostatitis and urethritis are often considered conditions of damp heat and would be treated accordingly by a practitioner.

HERBAL THERAPIES

An extract of the berries of the ***saw palmetto*** *(Serenoa repens),* a scrubby tree of the American Southeast, is said to shrink an enlarged prostate and relieve symptoms. Other remedies include ***Asian ginseng*** *(Panax ginseng),* flower pollen, ***horsetail*** *(Equisetum arvense),* ***nettle*** *(Urtica dioica),* true unicorn root *(Aletris farinosa),* and the powdered bark of pygeum *(Pygeum africanus),* an evergreen tree.

For **prostatitis,** pipsissewa *(Chimaphila umbellata)* and horsetail are used on a short-term basis to treat infection. Thuja *(Thuja occidentalis)* and pasqueflower *(Anemone pulsatilla)* are also suggested for inflammation of the prostate.

HOMEOPATHY

Numerous medications are available to the homeopathic practitioner for treating prostatic enlargement and prostatitis, among them *Berberis vulgaris* and *Staphysagria.*

NUTRITION AND DIET

Prostate enlargement may respond to nutritional support. In addition, if surgery is elected, good nutrition afterward will speed recovery.

Zinc, which is involved in many aspects of hormonal metabolism, is thought to promote prostate health and reduce inflammation; rich sources of zinc are oysters, wheat bran, whole oatmeal, pumpkinseeds, and sunflower seeds. ***Vitamins C*** and ***E*** may promote prostate health. The amino acids glycine, alanine, and glutamic acid are said to alleviate symptoms. The prostate may also benefit from large amounts of essential fatty acids, as found in flaxseed oil, walnut oil, sunflower oil, soy oil, and ***evening primrose oil.***

YOGA

See the positions illustrated above.

YOGA

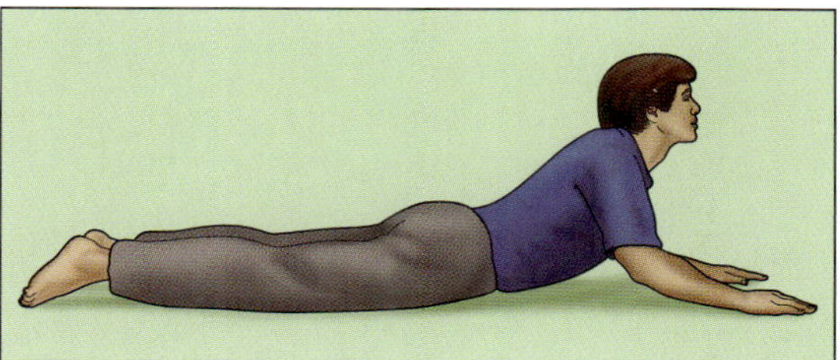

1 Try the modified **Cobra** for an enlarged prostate. Place both forearms on the floor, elbows directly under your shoulders. Inhale and push your chest up while pressing your pelvis against the ground *(above).* Hold for 15 seconds, breathing deeply, then slowly relax.

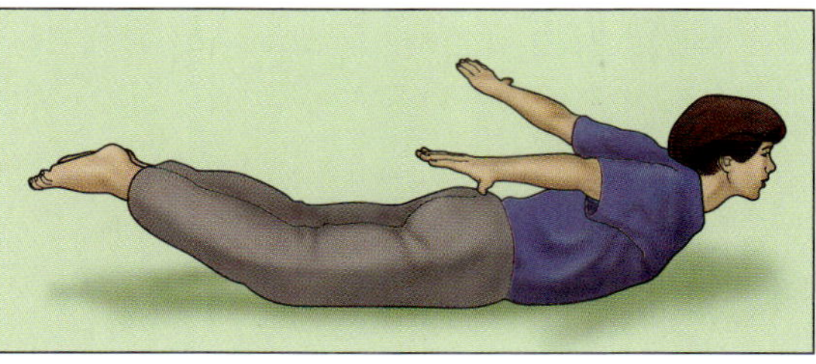

2 Lie on your stomach for the **Boat.** Inhale as you lift your head, chest, arms, and legs off the floor. Stretch your arms behind you and hold the position for 15 or 20 seconds, then exhale as you relax back onto the floor. Do once or twice a day.

PREVENTION

To prevent a recurrence of **chronic prostatitis** and promote prostate health:

- Take warm sitz baths.
- Drink more water; dehydration stresses the prostate.
- Avoid prolonged bicycle riding, horseback riding, or other exercises that irritate the region below the prostate.
- Take supplements of zinc and vitamin C. ■

PSORIASIS

SYMPTOMS

- deep pink, raised patches of skin with white scales, typically on the scalp, knees, elbows, and upper body; mild to severe itchiness.
- pitting, discoloring, and thickening of the fingernails and toenails. If psoriasis develops on the nails, they may separate from underlying skin.
- Red, scaly, cracked skin on the palms of the hands signals **palmar psoriasis;** on the soles of the feet the same condition is **plantar psoriasis.** These forms of psoriasis affect only those areas; the condition can become very inflamed and ooze fluid, making movement very painful.

See also the ***Visual Diagnostic Guide.***

CALL YOUR DOCTOR IF:

- your psoriasis becomes worse after you stop taking heavy doses of ***corticosteroid*** for this or another ailment. You may need a different course of medical treatment.
- your skin inflammation does not respond to any form of treatment; you need to be checked for the possibility of a more serious underlying ailment.

P

Unpredictable, intractable, and unsightly, psoriasis is one of the most baffling and persistent of skin disorders. It is characterized by skin cells that multiply up to 10 times faster than normal, typically on the knees, elbows, and scalp. As underlying cells reach the skin's surface and die, their sheer volume causes raised, white-scaled patches. **Palmar** or **plantar psoriasis,** which affects only the hands or feet, tends to be much more painful and often blisters and oozes.

Though not contagious, psoriasis tends to run in families. Fair-skinned people aged 10 to 40 are particularly susceptible, especially those with a blood relative who suffers from the disorder. Psoriasis is extremely rare among people with dark skin. Outbreaks are triggered by the immune system and can affect other parts of the body, particularly the joints, in which case the condition is called **psoriatic arthritis**. Although psoriasis may be stressful and embarrassing, most outbreaks are relatively benign. With appropriate treatment, symptoms generally subside within weeks.

CAUSES

A variety of factors, ranging from emotional ***stress*** to a streptococcal ***infection,*** can precipitate an episode of psoriasis. As many as 80 percent of patients suffering a flareup report a recent emotional trauma, such as a new job or the death of a loved one. Many doctors believe such external strains serve as triggers for an inherited defect in skin-cell production.

Injured skin, ***obesity,*** and certain drugs—including the painkiller ***ibuprofen*** and the antimalarial medication chloroquine—can aggravate psoriasis. The disease often appears two to three weeks after an infection such as ***strep throat.*** Alcohol consumption clearly makes psoriasis worse, as does a diet high in protein and low in fiber.

TREATMENT

Despite the fact that psoriasis is technically incurable, it responds well to most treatments for ***dermatitis.*** In addition to the conventional therapies below, **light therapy** *(page 708)* is accepted and practiced by conventional doctors.

CONVENTIONAL MEDICINE

A standard treatment recommended by many doctors is to soak in a warm bath for 10 to 15 minutes, then immediately apply a topical ointment such as petroleum jelly, which helps your skin retain moisture. Some doctors recommend salicylic acid ointment, which smooths the skin by promoting the shedding of psoriatic scales. Steroid-based creams are effective; however, because they can have harmful side effects, psoriasis sufferers should be especially careful not to overuse them.

Treatment with capsaicin, a component of ***cayenne*** *(Capsicum frutescens),* may also be effective. Available as an over-the-counter ointment for treating ***shingles,*** it causes the body to block production of an inflammation-causing chemical found in psoriatic skin. It also prevents the body from building blood vessels to the affected area, thereby stemming the abnormal growth of psoriasis. Because capsaicin can burn and severely damage the skin if used incorrectly, try this only under a doctor's supervision.

A topical ointment containing calcitriol, which is related to ***vitamin D,*** has proved as effective as ***hydrocortisone*** creams for treating psoriasis and has fewer side effects. Coal-tar ointments and shampoos can alleviate symptoms, but many psoriasis patients seem vulnerable to the side effects—in particular folliculitis, a pimple-like rash affecting the hair follicles. Some studies also indicate that continued use of such coal-tar products may increase the risk of ***skin cancer.***

Anthralin therapy is generally reserved for severe forms of psoriasis. Anthralin salve is carefully applied to the affected areas and removed after 30 to 60 minutes. All the white scales should be gone, revealing an underlying layer of fresh, normal skin. If not properly applied by a trained therapist, however, anthralin may irritate healthy skin and leave stains that can last several weeks. For persistent, difficult-to-treat cases of psoriasis, many medical doctors also recommend and prescribe **light therapy.**

WHERE PSORIASIS STRIKES

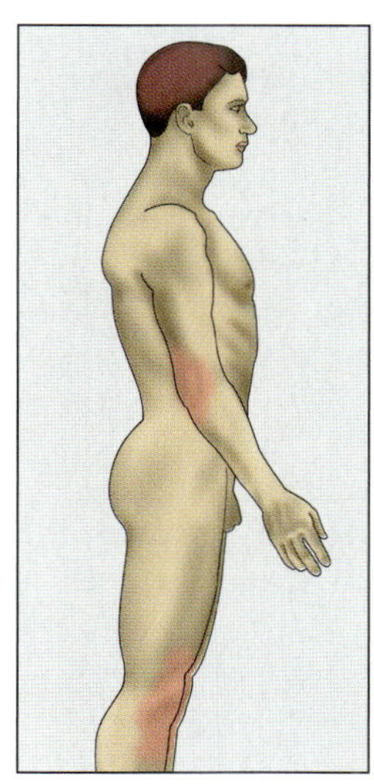

The thick, dry, scaly patches associated with the skin disorder psoriasis can vary greatly in size and appear just about anywhere on the body. The condition most frequently affects the scalp, elbows, and knees, shown in pink at left.

ALTERNATIVE CHOICES

If conventional treatments for psoriasis are not working for you, ask your doctor about the potential benefits of the following alternatives.

AROMATHERAPY

As an alternative to coal-tar shampoos for psoriasis on your scalp, mix together 4 drops of essential oil of cedarwood and 2 drops of ***juniper*** *(Juniperus communis)* or lemon in 1 tbsp almond or olive oil. Apply the mixture to your scalp and leave it on overnight under a shower cap. Shampoo and rinse thoroughly in the morning. Repeat three times a week until the symptoms clear. Since some people are sensitive to essential oils, place a drop on your skin for 30 minutes to be sure you have no adverse reactions.

CLIMATOTHERAPY

Climatotherapy is based on the idea that specific climatic conditions can help or even heal certain diseases. For psoriasis, spending time in the sun can be beneficial. Special facilities at Israel's Dead Sea or other resort locations offer treat-

CAUTION!

Many psoriasis patients choose *corticosteroid* treatments, to avoid the messiness and potential skin-damaging side effects of coal-tar products. Remember that steroid medicines can have serious and far-reaching side effects, too. Excessive or long-term use of steroidal ointments can thin the skin and cause white spots, *acne,* and permanent stretch marks. Used extensively around the eyes, steroidal ointments can, in rare cases, lead to *glaucoma.* Oral corticosteroid treatment may cause psoriasis to flare up again after treatment stops.

People whose psoriasis stubbornly resists conventional treatment should know that the sudden onset of psoriasis may indicate a human immunodeficiency virus (HIV) infection, a precursor to *AIDS.*

ment designed for people suffering from psoriasis and other skin disorders. The combination of sunlight, relaxation, and mineral baths seems to have a therapeutic effect for many people.

HERBAL THERAPIES

Burdock *(Arctium lappa)* root, ***dandelion*** *(Taraxacum officinale)* root, and Oregon grape *(Mahonia aquifolium)* are said to help reduce symptoms of psoriasis. Simmer 1 tbsp of any of these dried herbs in a cup of boiling water for 10 minutes; strain and drink hot, up to three cups a day. You may also take up to 1½ tsp fluidextract of burdock or dandelion root daily.

Evening primrose oil *(Oenothera biennis)* may soothe itching associated with psoriasis. Some doctors believe it's as effective as ***corticosteroids*** with fewer side effects, although people with liver disease or high cholesterol should use it only under medical supervision; pregnant women should not use it, because it can affect their hormone levels. The recommended dose of two 500-mg capsules a day can be costly; flaxseed and borage oils are less expensive alternatives.

Mix tinctures of burdock, ***skullcap*** *(Scutellaria lateriflora),* sourdock *(Rumex crispus),* and cleavers (*Galium* spp.) in equal parts; take 1 or 2 tsp a day. Or steep 1 tbsp of fresh ***nettles*** *(Urtica dioica)* and fresh cleavers in 1 cup boiling water for 10 minutes, strain, and drink two or three cups a day.

A rinse made of dried ***rosemary*** *(Rosmarinus officinalis)* and ***sage*** *(Salvia officinalis)* offers an alternative to tar-based shampoos. Pour a pint of boiling water over 1 oz of each of the herbs and let the mixture steep overnight. Strain and use daily as a hair rinse after each shampoo.

HOMEOPATHY

Don't try to choose homeopathic remedies on your own to treat a chronic, systemic condition such as psoriasis. A homeopath assesses many variables, including the site of the inflammation, as well as the patient's family history and reaction to stress. Remedies homeopaths recommend for psoriasis include ***Sulphur,*** *Graphites,* ***Lycopodium,*** and ***Arsenicum album.***

LIGHT THERAPY

Like other serious or chronic skin disorders, psoriasis may respond to light therapy, or phototherapy. Patients receive timed exposure to ultraviolet radiation, in some cases after taking an oral medication called psoralen. The treatment is repeated several times a week for up to eight sessions per month. Although many doctors and patients report positive results, the treatments can have serious short- and long-term side effects; the drug psoralen is not recommended for pregnant women, because of the potential risk to the developing fetus. While light therapy may not be right for every psoriasis sufferer, it may be worth discussing with your doctor. *(For more on light therapy, see **Dermatitis.**)*

MIND/BODY MEDICINE

The skin, the largest organ in the body, often mirrors turmoil within, so it's no surprise that many psoriasis patients have a history of high ***anxiety,*** low self-esteem, and ***stress***-related problems. Many mind/body techniques help psoriasis patients by addressing the psychological roots and

P

consequences of the disease. In particular, **hypnotherapy, guided imagery,** any of a number of **relaxation** techniques, **biofeedback,** and psychotherapy may be effective.

You can train yourself to relax by trying anything from a brisk half-hour walk every day to self-hypnosis, in which you focus your attention to block out irritating stimuli. If you think internal stress contributes to your condition, make a relaxation technique part of your daily schedule.

NUTRITION AND DIET

Fish oil high in eicosapentaenoic acid (EPA), from such fish as mackerel, herring, and salmon, may help reduce inflammation and itching. Because you would have to eat up to two pounds of fish a day to get enough EPA, try a 1,000-mg fish-oil capsule containing EPA four times a day; or try 1 tbsp cod-liver oil, also high in ***vitamin A,*** once a day.

Vitamin A plays a vital role in the growth and maintenance of skin; when an outbreak of psoriasis occurs, take a megadose of up to 100,000 IU a day for a month under a doctor's supervision, then return to maintenance levels not exceeding 50,000 IU a day. A daily 400 to 1,000 IU of ***vitamin D*** may also help with healing. To avoid the risk of overdose, particularly of these fat-soluble vitamins, ask your doctor to monitor your progress. Always check dosages carefully before giving megasupplements to children.

Vitamin B complex containing ***vitamin*** B_5 and ***vitamin*** B_1 may promote healthy skin; to help fight psoriasis, the suggested dosage is 50 mg three times a day. Rubbing concentrated ***vitamin E*** ointment into your scalp two or three times a week can deter skin damage.

Some research has suggested that eating too much citrus fruit can aggravate psoriasis, and that psoriasis patients, like eczema patients, cannot metabolize fatty acids. To help prevent flare-ups, adopt a diet high in fish and raw vegetables, and low in fatty meats and acidic fruits.

AT-HOME REMEDIES

- For mild forms of psoriasis, try a warm bath followed by an application of topical ointments that help the skin retain water and soothe inflammation. Use ordinary petroleum jelly or vegetable shortening, an over-the-counter ***corticosteroid*** cream, or a salicylic acid ointment. Make sure none of these topical preparations contains additives, preservatives, or perfumes.
- For scalp psoriasis, wash your hair with a coal-tar shampoo or with a mixture of cedarwood and juniper or lemon oils. A rinse with a rosemary-sage solution may also be helpful.
- Sunbathe. Expose areas of inflamed skin, but cover the rest of your body with sunscreen. Avoid overexposure.
- Start a regular exercise or relaxation routine. Allot at least 15 minutes four to five days a week to some activity that relieves stress. ■

PSORIATIC ARTHRITIS

In a trait unique among skin ailments, psoriasis can lead to a complication called psoriatic arthritis, most notably in the joints of the fingers and toes. It afflicts some 5 percent of psoriasis sufferers, with joint inflammation developing shortly before or after the emergence of skin lesions. Symptoms resemble those of rheumatoid ***arthritis,*** *but patients test negative for that disease.*

Doctors frequently treat the skin problem first, because the joint inflammation will usually subside when the skin inflammation is brought under control. Psoriatic arthritis responds well to ***aspirin*** *and* ***nonsteroidal anti-inflammatory drugs (NSAIDs),*** *but patients should avoid the heavy doses of steroids used to treat other forms of arthritis. As with other skin ailments, psoriatic skin lesions can become much worse when steroid dosages are reduced or stopped.*

PUPIL DILATION

Read down this column to find your symptoms. Then read across.

SYMPTOMS	AILMENT/PROBLEM
◆ one pupil is dilated and responds to light less than the other pupil, with no other symptoms.	◆ Holmes-Adie syndrome (a harmless condition in which the pupils respond to light at different rates)
◆ enlarged pupils of equal size that are fixed (do not change in size with changes in light), following a visit to a doctor who put drops in your eyes.	◆ Temporary effect of eye drops specially formulated to temporarily dilate your eyes for an examination
◆ fixed pupils of different sizes, or enlarged pupils of the same size, after taking drugs for any reason.	◆ Side effect of many illegal recreational, over-the-counter, and prescription drugs—especially those containing ***epinephrine,*** such as ***bronchodilators***
◆ one pupil is larger than the other and fixed; the eye may constantly turn outward; double vision; drooping eyelid.	◆ Third nerve palsy—the third cranial nerve is not functioning properly; often a side effect of ***diabetes,*** lead poisoning, ***alcohol abuse,*** or possibly a brain tumor
◆ one pupil is smaller than the other and fixed; eye pain, redness, and/or swelling; tearing; blurred vision.	◆ Uveitis (inflammation of the iris)
◆ over time, one pupil becomes larger than the other and fixed; throbbing eye pain; loss of peripheral vision; seeing halos around lights; possible nausea.	◆ ***Glaucoma***
◆ change in pupil size, or pupil asymmetry, anywhere from a few days to a few weeks after an injury to your head; headache; nausea; drowsiness; dizziness; inability to move arms or legs.	◆ The effects of a head injury, either with or without concussion
◆ pupils of different sizes; fever, vomiting; headache that is worse upon leaning forward; neck stiffness or pain, especially when tilting the chin toward the chest.	◆ ***Meningitis,*** or possibly encephalitis (an ***infection*** of the brain)
◆ pupil dilation accompanied by a sudden, severe headache that may radiate into the neck.	◆ A brain ***aneurysm*** or a migraine ***headache***

WHAT TO DO	OTHER INFO
◆ The first time you experience this, **get emergency medical care;** a single dilated pupil can indicate serious illness, such as ***stroke*** or brain injury.	◆ Holmes-Adie syndrome has no known treatment, but it does not lead to more serious problems.
◆ Pupils should return to normal within a few hours; if they haven't contracted in 24 hours, call your ophthalmologist.	◆ Wear sunglasses or stay in a darkened room if light bothers your eyes.
◆ Ask your doctor about this symptom and your medication regimen; you may need to change.	◆ Your pupils should return to normal as the drug effects wear off.
◆ See your doctor. Treatment depends on the cause of the palsy, and may include ***antibiotics,*** exercises, and possibly surgery.	
◆ See your doctor without delay; without proper treatment (rest, ***corticosteroid*** eye drops, and possibly other medications), uveitis can cause blindness.	◆ Uveitis may occur suddenly, or it may come on gradually over time.
◆ **Get emergency care immediately.** Acute glaucoma can cause blindness in a matter of days; other forms may be managed with surgery and/or medication.	
◆ **Call your doctor now;** you may need emergency treatment for bleeding or blood clotting that is occurring between your skull and brain.	◆ A serious head injury is not always accompanied by unconsciousness. Reduce your risk by using a helmet while riding a bike or motorcycle or while playing contact sports, and by wearing your seat belt in the car.
◆ **Get emergency care immediately.** Without proper treatment, either of these infections can cause death.	◆ One form of meningitis, aseptic meningitis, has identical symptoms but is not serious. A doctor's diagnosis is required.
◆ Call your doctor without delay, unless you have a history of migraines with this symptom; only a physician can tell for sure the difference between migraine and aneurysm.	◆ An aneurysm can be a medical emergency, or it may be treated with medication over the long term.

RABIES

SYMPTOMS

After an incubation period typically of one to three months:

- pain, followed by tingling at the site of the animal bite.
- sensitive skin.

Up to 10 days after the above symptoms appear:

- drooling.
- inability to swallow liquids.
- rage, alternating with periods of calm.
- convulsions.
- paralysis.

CALL YOUR DOCTOR IF:

- you are bitten by a wild or unimmunized animal, or any animal whose immunization status is uncertain. **Call or go to a hospital now;** immediate treatment is vital.
- you are bitten and experience any of the symptoms listed above. **Call or go to a hospital now.**
- you plan to travel to a country where rabies is common; ask your doctor to vaccinate you against rabies.

R

Rabies is a viral brain disease that is almost always fatal if it is allowed to develop and is not prevented with prompt treatment. You may develop it if you are bitten by an infected animal. Carriers of rabies include dogs, cats, bats, skunks, raccoons, and foxes; rodents are not likely to be infected. About 70 percent of rabies cases develop from wild animal bites that break the skin.

The disease is also called hydrophobia (meaning fear of water) because it causes painful muscle spasms in the throat that prevent swallowing. In fact, this is what leads to fatalities in untreated cases: Victims become dehydrated and die.

The incubation period for symptoms can range anywhere from 10 days to two years, but the typical time between the bite and the first appearance of symptoms is one to three months. The first symptoms include a tingling, itching, or cold sensation at the site of the bite, a low fever, and a general sense of illness. This may be followed by chills, difficulty swallowing liquids, restlessness, outbursts of rage, extreme excitability, muscle spasms, and drooling.

A bite from a rabid animal does not guarantee that you will get rabies; only about 50 percent of people who are bitten and do not receive treatment ever develop the disease. But don't take chances. If you are bitten by or have any exposure to an animal that may have rabies, go to the hospital immediately. Treatment virtually ensures that you will not come down with the disease. But any delay could diminish the treatment's effectiveness.

CAUSES

Rabies is caused by a virus that infects the central nervous system—the brain and spinal cord. The virus enters through the skin or mucous membranes, then travels to the brain, where it multiplies and migrates through nerves to other tissues.

DIAGNOSTIC AND TEST PROCEDURES

If you are bitten, your doctor will need to know what kind of animal bit you, and under what circumstances. If the animal is found to be healthy, or if its owner can prove it has been vaccinated

> **CAUTION!**
>
> **See a doctor immediately after you have been bitten by an animal that may have rabies. The longer you wait to get treatment, the greater your risk of developing the disease.**

for rabies, you probably won't need treatment, except to cleanse the wound. But if you're unsure of the animal's health, your doctor should give you the shots that prevent rabies without waiting for any confirmation that the animal was infected.

TREATMENT

As soon as possible after you are bitten, clean the wound thoroughly with soap and water; give it a second scrubbing with an antiseptic, such as hydrogen peroxide. If the wound is superficial and you know the animal has been vaccinated, that's all you'll have to do. Otherwise, call ahead to the nearest hospital and go there immediately.

CONVENTIONAL MEDICINE

Victims of animal bites used to undergo up to 25 painful injections of rabies vaccine in their abdomen. Now treatment consists of a single dose of rabies immunoglobulin and five injections of human diploid cell rabies vaccine given over 28 days. You may also need a shot to prevent ***tetanus*** from setting in.

ALTERNATIVE CHOICES

If you are bitten by an animal that may have rabies, it is imperative that you receive the rabies vaccine. You may try alternative methods in conjunction with conventional medicine to speed healing and reduce discomfort.

AROMATHERAPY

Oil of ***myrrh*** *(Commiphora molmol)* is antiseptic and astringent. Aromatherapists recommend that you apply it directly to a wound to help cleanse it.

CHINESE HERBS

For centuries, doctors of Chinese medicine used ***skullcap*** *(Scutellaria baicalensis)* to treat rabies-related convulsions. Today a qualified practitioner would send you to the emergency room of the nearest hospital. After you received the vaccine, the practitioner might suggest an herbal formula to strengthen your entire system.

HERBAL THERAPY

A compress of ***lavender*** *(Lavandula officinalis)* may help your wound heal faster. ***Echinacea*** (*Echinacea* spp.) is believed to strengthen the immune system to help you recuperate.

HOMEOPATHY

A homeopathic practitioner may give you a remedy to speed wound healing.

AT-HOME CARE

- Cleanse your wound with soap and water, followed by hydrogen peroxide.
- Speed healing by using herbal compresses and aromatic oils.
- Cleanse your system by drinking lots of fruit and vegetable juices.

PREVENTION

- Stay away from strange animals.
- Insist that neighbors obey leash laws.
- If you plan on traveling to an area where rabies is common in domestic animals (India, parts of South America), develop immunity to the virus by getting injections of human diploid cell rabies vaccine. Ask your doctor for details. ■

RASHES

Read down this column to find your symptoms. Then read across.

SYMPTOMS	AILMENT/PROBLEM
For itching skin that is not accompanied by a rash, see ***Itching Skin.*** See also the ***Visual Diagnostic Guide.***	
◆ scaly, itchy, red rash between the toes; may also cause unusual flaking on the soles of the feet; may affect toenails.	◆ ***Athlete's foot***
◆ rash—either localized or diffuse—in an otherwise healthy person.	◆ Contact ***dermatitis; allergies; stress;*** dietary deficiency
◆ rash that progresses rapidly from a simple red flush to small bumps, then a crusted, pimplelike inflammation; extremely itchy.	◆ ***Chickenpox***
◆ red rash in a baby's diaper area.	◆ ***Diaper rash***
◆ tiny pink bumps usually found on the back of the neck and upper back that itch and sting; usually associated with hot, humid weather.	◆ Heat rash
◆ red rash that may resemble a bull's-eye and that fans out several inches from the bite mark; rash is not always obvious; followed by fever, headaches, lethargy, and muscle and joint pain.	◆ ***Lyme disease***
◆ red rash that spreads from face downward and is preceded by fever, cough, and inflamed nasal passages.	◆ ***Measles***
◆ rash that looks similar to the measles rash but is less extensive, lasts for a shorter period of time (usually only three days), and is not accompanied by cough.	◆ ***German measles***
◆ distinctive red, scaly, round or oval patches with normal skin in the center; patches gradually get larger.	◆ Ringworm

WHAT TO DO	OTHER INFO
◆ When you bathe, wash and dry your feet thoroughly, and use an antifungal powder. Keep your feet exposed to the air as much as possible.	◆ ***Tea tree oil*** (*Melaleuca* spp.) ointment may also be effective.
◆ See your doctor to treat severe cases. Consider mind/body techniques, such as guided imagery, to alleviate stress. Consult a nutritionist; a ***zinc*** deficiency may cause a rash.	◆ Stress can play a role as a catalyst for many skin disorders.
◆ Keep a child at home to recuperate and to avoid spreading the disease. Chickenpox is more serious in adults; call your doctor.	◆ The same virus that causes chickenpox causes ***shingles.***
◆ For most cases, use an over-the-counter zinc ointment; consult your pediatrician about more severe or longer-lasting cases.	◆ Diaper rash can be treated with a variety of at-home remedies and alternative therapies. Changing a diaper as soon as it is soiled will help your baby's skin heal.
◆ Cool your body in a cold bath; wear light, loose clothes; avoid excessive heat; avoid activities that cause you to sweat.	◆ Heat rash is caused by blocked sweat glands. Sometimes it affects babies who are overdressed or who have a fever.
◆ Call your doctor if you think you have been bitten by a tick. Get tested for Lyme disease and ***Rocky Mountain spotted fever.*** Treatment involves ***antibiotics.***	◆ If Lyme disease is not treated in its earliest stages with antibiotics, complications of the heart and nervous system may develop.
◆ Call your child's pediatrician. Keep your child at home to recuperate and to avoid spreading the disease.	◆ Serious complications of measles include encephalitis and ***pneumonia.***
◆ Keep your child at home to recuperate and to avoid spreading the disease. If you are pregnant and have been exposed to the virus, call your doctor.	◆ The rubella virus can cause birth defects if transmitted by an infected mother to her unborn child.
◆ Try a topical ***antifungal drug*** such as ***miconazole*** or ***clotrimazole.*** See the ***Visual Diagnostic Guide.***	

R

SYMPTOMS	AILMENT/PROBLEM
◆ pink rash that starts near the wrists and ankles and spreads to the face, torso, palms, and soles of the feet; often accompanied by fever, chills, and severe headaches.	◆ ***Rocky Mountain spotted fever***
◆ light pink, short-lived rash on torso, face, and extremities in children under three years old; occurs three to four days after a fever, lasts less than 48 hours, and does not itch.	◆ Roseola
◆ rash, especially between the fingers and on the wrists, that consists of reddish spots and tiny, grayish lines—the burrows caused by a mother mite digging in with her eggs; extremely itchy.	◆ ***Scabies***
◆ pinpoint lesions on the torso and extremities; raised spots on the tongue; rash peels in five to seven days; sometimes accompanied by fever, headache, vomiting, and chills.	◆ ***Scarlet fever***
◆ painless ulcers on the genitals and sometimes in the mouth, later followed by red, circular, nonitching lesions on the skin, especially on the palms and soles.	◆ ***Syphilis***
◆ bright red rash in a baby's diaper area that does not respond to treatment for standard diaper rash; possibly, white patches in the mouth that leave red sores when wiped away.	◆ Thrush
◆ extremely itchy raised skin lesions with white centers and red rims anywhere on the body; usually part of an allergic reaction to something, such as penicillin or food; extreme heat or cold can also cause an outbreak.	◆ ***Hives***

WHAT TO DO	OTHER INFO
◆ Call your doctor if you suspect you have been bitten by a tick. Get tested for Rocky Mountain spotted fever and ***Lyme disease.*** Spotted fever is life-threatening in adults. ***Antibiotics*** are almost always required.	◆ Despite its name, Rocky Mountain spotted fever is most common in southeast and south-central states.
◆ Allow the rash to run its course without interference from ointments or medication.	◆ Caused by a virus, roseola occurs most often in the spring and fall. The rash usually follows a very high fever (103°F to 105°F). By the time the rash appears, the child is almost fully recovered.
◆ Call your doctor for treatment to kill the mites that cause the disease.	◆ Scabies is highly contagious.
◆ Call your child's pediatrician without delay.	◆ Scarlet fever can cause any of a number of serious complications and can be life-threatening.
◆ Call your doctor. ***Penicillin*** in high doses is usually required. Discontinue all sexual relations until treatment is completed.	◆ Syphilis is usually transmitted through sexual intercourse or oral sex; it can also be transmitted from an infected mother to her unborn baby through the placenta.
◆ See ***Yeast Infections.***	◆ Newborns can contract thrush while passing through the birth canal. In adults, thrush can also be a side effect of several long-term diseases, such as ***diabetes*** and ***leukemia,*** or can appear following an aggressive course of ***antibiotics.***
◆ Oral ***antihistamines*** may provide relief; avoid applying topical ointments since they may obstruct pores.	

R

RAYNAUD'S SYNDROME

SYMPTOMS

- sudden coldness, numbness, or prickly pins-and-needles sensation in the fingers, and possibly toes, when exposed to even a mild drop in temperature—as when walking into an air-conditioned room, for instance. The same symptoms might also be triggered by emotionally stressful situations.
- dramatic color changes in the fingers: When first exposed to cold, fingers turn white, then blue; when rewarmed, they quickly turn red and may throb uncomfortably.

CALL YOUR DOCTOR IF:

- Raynaud's episodes become more intense. Irreversible damage to fingers or toes—a loss of feeling, for example—can occur in serious cases.
- skin ulcers, sores, or discoloration appears on your fingers or toes. These signs suggest that extremities are being severely deprived of blood. In rare cases, gangrene may result.

Raynaud's syndrome, which may afflict up to 1 in 20 Americans, is a circulatory disorder of blood vessels of the extremities. Constriction of those vessels is a normal physiological response to low temperatures, helping the body conserve heat. In Raynaud's syndrome, named for a French physician who first described the condition more than a century ago, nerve receptors in the extremities are overly sensitive to stimulation. Even a slight temperature drop—perhaps the faint chill produced by opening a refrigerator door—will cause a spasmodic closing of the small arteries in the fingers (and sometimes in toes). Typically fingers turn white, then blue, then red, indicating a progression from total blood deprivation to limited blood flow to sudden infusion of oxygenated blood as blood vessels suddenly dilate. Episodes are brief, usually lasting only a few minutes.

The syndrome takes two forms. About 90 percent of cases are of the type called **Raynaud's disease** or **primary Raynaud's**—an isolated condition with no connection to other medical problems. It most often affects women and usually sets in before the age of 40. The remaining 10 percent of cases are termed **Raynaud's phenomenon** or **secondary Raynaud's.** This version, which tends to start later in life, is connected to other medical factors—an underlying disease, for instance, or the long-term use of such vibrating tools as a chain saw or jackhammer.

For most sufferers, Raynaud's syndrome is a mild but maddening condition. Ordinarily, its most serious consequence is a loss of sensitivity in the affected extremity. Very rarely, a severe case results in tissue death and gangrene.

CAUSES

The underlying causes of **Raynaud's disease** are unknown. It afflicts women disproportionately; men account for only about 1 case in 5. It is not thought to be an inherited condition, but it frequently affects more than one family member.

Raynaud's phenomenon has many causes, including such connective-tissue diseases as scleroderma, rheumatoid ***arthritis,*** and ***lupus;*** exposure to certain chemicals and drugs, such as ***beta-adrenergic blockers*** (used to treat ***high blood pressure***) or ergotamine (used to treat migraines); and use of vibrating machinery.

TREATMENT

Relief from Raynaud's is linked to improved circulation. Some exercises may help by forcing blood into the extremities, but relaxation techniques can also work. Of course avoiding triggers—such as cold or nicotine—will decrease the number of attacks.

CONVENTIONAL MEDICINE

For most people, Raynaud's syndrome is not disabling enough to merit prolonged medical care. If attacks are frequent or severe, ***calcium channel blockers*** or other medications—***angiotensin-converting enzyme (ACE) inhibitors,*** for example—may be prescribed, but many people find drugs ineffective. A simple exercise—swinging your arms around like a windmill—will force blood into your extremities and may be as effective as drug therapy.

ALTERNATIVE CHOICES

In addition to trying the treatments discussed below, you might seek professional help from an **acupuncturist, chiropractor, homeopath, osteopath,** or **massage** therapist. Relaxation exercises such as **meditation,** t'ai chi, and **yoga** help relax blood vessels, improving circulation. **Biofeedback** techniques can be used to open blood vessels directly.

CHINESE HERBS

The most common Chinese herbal prescription for Raynaud's syndrome is peony *(Paeonia lactiflora).* **Dong quai** *(Angelica sinensis)* might also be prescribed for cold extremities. Consult a practitioner for dosages.

NUTRITION AND DIET

Simple changes in diet, along with nutritional supplements, can significantly moderate Raynaud's syndrome. Consuming more ***vitamin E, magnesium,*** and fish oils may help reduce blood vessel spasms in the fingers and toes. Fruits, vegetables, seeds, and nuts contain vitamin E. Magnesium is found in seeds, nuts, dark green vegetables, fish, and beans.

AT-HOME REMEDIES

You can train your fingers to resist chills. Starting in a warm room, place your hands in a warm bowl of water for 5 minutes; then move to a cold room or outdoors and again place your hands in warm water, now for 10 minutes. The alternating hot and cold temeratures will improve your circulation and the health of your blood vessels. Repeat the procedure several times a day for as many days as necessary. Eventually, this will produce a conditioned reflex that is the very opposite of the normal one: When exposed to cold, the blood vessels in the fingers will open up rather than close down—without the aid of warm water.

Avoid substances that make you vulnerable to chill. These include nicotine, caffeine, birth-control pills, and most over-the-counter decongestants, cold remedies, or diet pills.

Treat finger or toe infections without delay. When circulation is impaired, even minor infections can become a problem.

PREVENTION

Devise ways to stay warm in your own home or office. Always carry a sweater. Use insulated glasses. Keep fingers and toes dry with talcum powder. Wear socks and mittens to bed. Outdoors, wear loose layers of blended fabrics; shoes made of breathable materials; a hat and, perhaps, earmuffs; and mittens rather than gloves. If you plan to be outside for several hours, try chemical "heaters" in your socks and mittens. Limit your exposure to nicotine; if you smoke, stop. ■

RESPIRATORY PROBLEMS

SYMPTOMS

- wheezing and breathing with effort.
- cough that may bring up phlegm.
- chills and fever.
- fatigue.

Respiratory problems may be accompanied by:

- rapid breathing and rapid heartbeat.
- shortness of breath.
- pain in the chest.
- slight headache.
- overall malaise.
- ***common cold*** symptoms: runny nose, sore throat, and sneezing.

CALL YOUR DOCTOR IF:

- you have a ***common cold*** or ***cough*** that lasts for more than 7 to 10 days and that is not relieved by over-the-counter medications.
- you have a feeling of fullness in your face, pressure behind your eyes, ***postnasal drip,*** and a foul smell in your nose. These are symptoms of ***sinusitis.***
- you have had a cough for a long time, are coughing up colored phlegm, or are short of breath. These may be signs of chronic ***bronchitis, emphysema,*** or ***lung cancer.***
- you have a high fever (101°F or more), chills, pain in your chest, and a cough that brings up bloody phlegm. These may be signs of ***pneumonia*** or other serious illness.
- you have enough trouble breathing to cause you worry or distress; many diseases can make breathing difficult.

Respiratory problems can be divided into three categories: infections of the upper and lower respiratory tracts, such as the ***common cold, sinusitis, pneumonia,*** and ***tuberculosis;*** chronic obstructive lung diseases, such as ***asthma, bronchitis,*** and ***emphysema;*** and occupation-related lung diseases, such as asbestosis and coal miner's disease.

CAUSES

Respiratory infections, which can range from mild to extremely serious, are caused primarily by viruses or bacteria settling in your airways. Your ability to handle these infections depends on such factors as age, the presence or absence of other underlying diseases, and whether or not you smoke.

Chronic obstructive diseases have multiple causes. The chronic inflammation of lung tissue characteristic of ***asthma,*** for example, can be brought on by pollen, irritants, or exercise. The destruction of lung tissue that is the result of ***emphysema*** is caused by excessive smoking or a hereditary enzyme deficiency.

Occupation-related lung diseases can be brought on by an individual's hypersensitivity to work-site substances or by the inhalation of particulate foreign matter, such as asbestos fibers, coal dust, and stone dust (which causes silicosis).

DIAGNOSTIC AND TEST PROCEDURES

Physicians use a variety of diagnostic tests and techniques to evaluate problems in your respiratory tract, including chest x-rays, lung scans, CT scans, analysis of a sputum specimen, and pulmonary function tests.

Invasive tests may be used when specific information is required. An ABG (arterial blood gas) test, for example, measures oxygen and carbon dioxide levels in the blood; a lung biopsy provides tissue samples that can be examined under a microscope.

WHERE PROBLEMS STRIKE

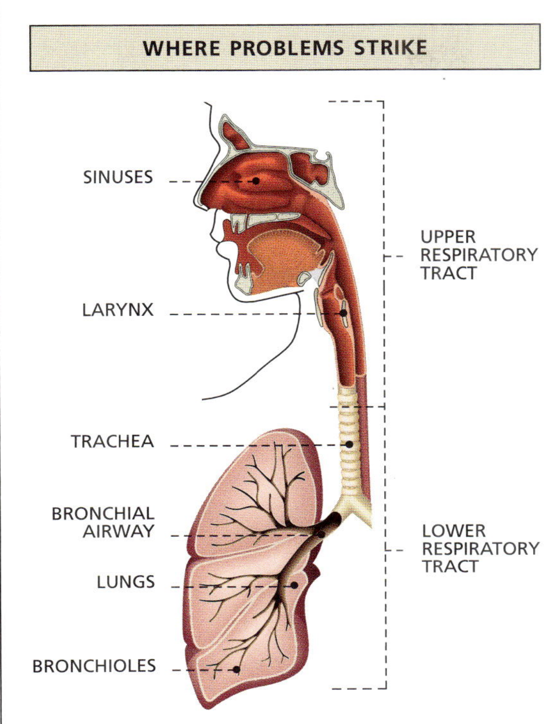

The upper respiratory tract—the sinuses, nose, mouth, and throat—can host ailments such as sinusitis and the common cold. More severe or persistent disorders tend to affect the lower respiratory tract. Asthma and bronchitis involve the trachea and large bronchial airways in the lungs, while pneumonia and emphysema impair the function of microscopic air sacs in the lungs.

TREATMENT

Many respiratory infections usually go away on their own in a week to 10 days. Conventional and alternative therapies offer a range of simple treatments to relieve discomfort.

CONVENTIONAL MEDICINE

If you have a bacterial respiratory infection, your doctor will probably prescribe an appropriate ***antibiotic.*** For the ***common cold, sinusitis,*** and acute ***bronchitis,*** you can make yourself more comfortable with bed rest, plenty of liquids, increased humidity (or steam), and medications for fever or pain. If you smoke, you will be advised to quit. Inhaled medications may help for chronic obstructive diseases such as ***asthma*** and ***emphysema.*** There is no effective treatment for the occupation-related lung diseases asbestosis and silicosis, except to avoid further exposure to respiratory irritants—including secondhand smoke—and if you smoke, to quit.

ALTERNATIVE CHOICES

Alternative therapies may be helpful in relieving symptoms of respiratory problems. Consult an **aromatherapist** or **herbal therapist** for advice on using essential oils and herbs for massages and steam inhalation that may help reduce congestion and soothe inflammation. A practitioner of Chinese medicine might recommend **acupuncture, acupressure,** or various **Chinese herbs. Homeopaths** prescribe a wide range of medications for respiratory problems. Most practitioners agree that your immune system can be strengthened and maintained through good nutrition and healthful dietary practices. Try the recommended daily dosages of ***vitamins A, B complex, C,*** and ***E,*** and the minerals ***zinc*** and ***selenium*** *(see the* ***Appendix****).* The deep breathing exercises of **meditation,** t'ai chi, and **yoga** can help strengthen your lungs.

AT-HOME REMEDIES

During the typical 7- to 10-day course of a respiratory infection, the best remedies for alleviating symptoms are bed rest, plenty of liquids, humidity or steam, and fever or pain medications. ■

R

RESTLESS LEG SYNDROME

SYMPTOMS

- a distinctive tingling or crawling sensation deep in the legs, accompanied by an irresistible urge to move the legs to relieve the sensation.
- occurring most frequently at night, disturbing sleep; during the day, the feeling may prevent you from sitting or standing still for any length of time.
- usually strikes people over the age of 30; becomes more common as people grow older.

CALL YOUR DOCTOR IF:

- you are experiencing any of the above symptoms for the first time; your doctor needs to rule out the possibility of more serious problems, such as ***kidney disease, diabetes, Parkinson's disease,*** deep vein thrombosis *(see* ***Phlebitis****),* ***sciatica,*** or other neurological disorders.

Restless leg syndrome is a neurological disorder that has long baffled doctors and for which a cure remains elusive. People who suffer from the syndrome feel a tingling or crawling sensation deep in their legs and have an overwhelming need to move their legs to relieve the discomfort. Sometimes the arms are also affected. The symptoms often worsen at night, leading some experts to cite this condition as a major cause of ***insomnia*** and other sleep disorders.

Although restless leg syndrome is not health-threatening, it can be uncomfortable and even painful at times. Both drug therapy and simple lifestyle changes offer ways for sufferers to cope. But probably the greatest peace of mind for people with the syndrome comes from knowing that they are not imagining their discomfort.

CAUSES

Restless leg syndrome is believed to be a genetic neurological condition brought on by a chemical imbalance in the brain. Research shows that caffeine can increase the symptoms. The syndrome has also been linked to iron or folic acid deficiencies, especially in people with ***kidney disease.***

TREATMENT

Drug therapy helps many sufferers, so consulting a physician is an important part of treatment.

CONVENTIONAL MEDICINE

Your doctor will want to examine you to rule out other causes for your distress. If you are otherwise in good health, you will probably be started on a course of drug therapy. The principal medicine offering relief is ***clonazepam,*** which acts to stabilize the conduction of nerve impulses. Other drugs that may bring relief include the combination product of carbidopa and ***levodopa,*** a medication used to treat ***Parkinson's disease,*** and the sedatives methadone and ***codeine,*** which are usually prescribed as a last resort because they can be habit-forming. Because all these drugs can produce undesirable side effects and because most people eventually build a tolerance to them, which reduces their effectiveness, your doctor will want to closely monitor your progress while you are receiving drug therapy.

ALTERNATIVE CHOICES

Some sufferers have found that alternative therapies can help lessen or relieve the physical discomfort associated with the condition.

ACUPRESSURE

Applying pressure to Bladder 57 and Stomach 36 in succession may help relieve the tingling sensations of restless leg syndrome. Also try Spleen 6 and Gall Bladder 39. *(See pages 22-23 and the **Appendix** for information on point locations.)*

HERBAL THERAPIES

Herbs with strong sedative qualities may be effective in reducing muscle tension and relieving pain. Such herbs include ***passionflower*** *(Passiflora incarnata)*, ***valerian*** *(Valeriana officinalis)*, and ***black cohosh*** *(Cimicifuga racemosa)*. Cramp bark *(Viburnum opulus)*, an antispasmodic, may also help relax muscles. Seek help from a medical herbalist for appropriate remedies and dosages.

HOMEOPATHY

Homeopathic practitioners frequently treat restless leg syndrome and the insomnia often associated with it with ***Rhus toxicodendron*** and *Cuprum*. Consult an experienced practitioner.

NUTRITION AND DIET

To help correct nutrient deficiencies that may be contributing to your symptoms, take ***vitamin E,*** a multivitamin, or a ***B-complex*** vitamin supplement in standard over-the-counter doses. To offset a folic acid deficiency, a nutritionist might advise you to take ***folic acid*** supplements (400 to 1,000 mcg). Some nutritionists also recommend supplementing the diet with a general food concentrate, such as blue-green algae, which may help correct unidentified nutrient deficiencies. You may also find it helpful to avoid such stimulants as ***caffeine*** and ***decongestants.***

LEG MASSAGE

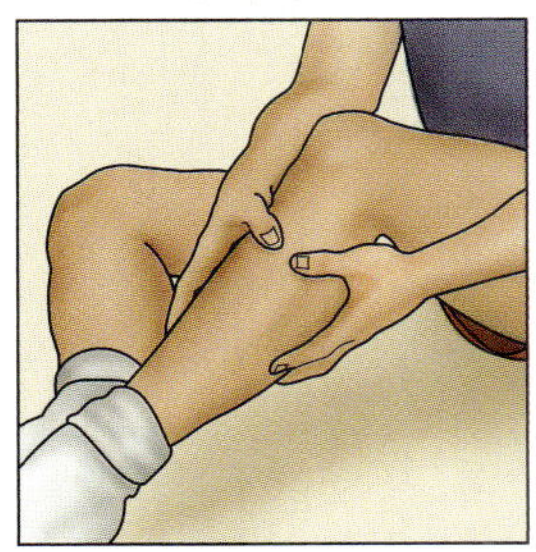

1 Sit on the floor and bend one knee, keeping your foot flat. Grasp your calf in both hands and use your thumbs to find the muscle that runs along the outside of the shinbone below the kneecap. Massage the muscle with your thumbs all the way down to the anklebone.

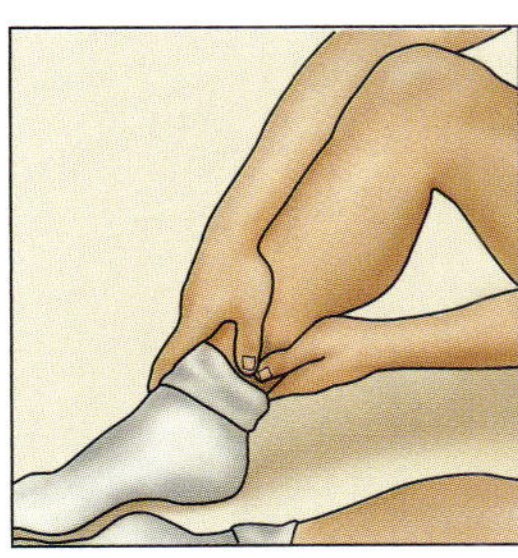

2 Place both thumbs on the inside of your leg near the anklebone. Keeping your hands around your calf for support, massage the inside of the leg vigorously with your thumbs, moving from the ankle up to the knee.

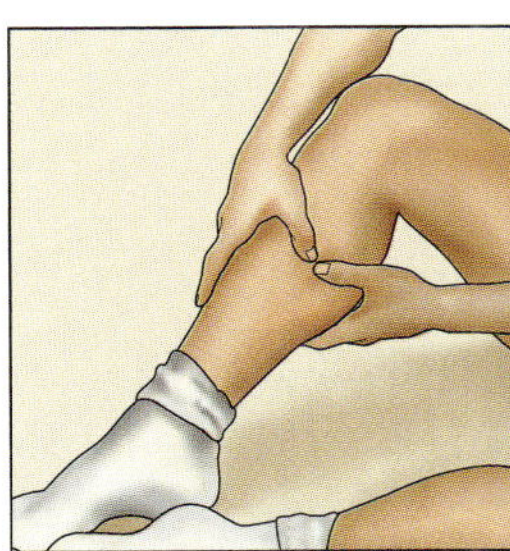

3 Finally, use the thumbs and fingers of both hands to knead the back and sides of your calf muscle. Work from the knee down to the ankle. When you finish massaging one leg, repeat the entire process on the other. Alternately massage both legs several times.

AT-HOME REMEDIES

- Avoid stimulating activities up to three hours before bed; this includes exercising and eating a heavy meal.
- Keep your bedroom quiet and cool; an overly warm room appears to aggravate restless leg syndrome.
- To reduce stress, which can trigger symptoms, practice **relaxation** techniques such as **yoga, biofeedback,** or **meditation.**
- Soak your feet in cool water, which is also said to be effective in bringing relief. Never use ice water, because it can cause nerve damage. ■

R

RHEUMATIC FEVER

SYMPTOMS

- fever.
- a red, raised, latticelike rash, usually on the chest, back, and abdomen.
- swollen, tender, red, and extremely painful joints—particularly the knees or ankles.
- nodules, or small bony protuberances, over the swollen joints.
- sometimes, weakness and shortness of breath.
- sometimes, uncontrolled movements of arms, legs, or facial muscles.

These symptoms often begin one to six weeks after a ***strep throat*** infection has appeared to clear up. Sometimes, however, people with rheumatic fever do not recall having had a sore throat.

CALL YOUR DOCTOR IF:

- you are experiencing the symptoms listed above, particularly if you remember having recently had a sore throat; you may have rheumatic fever and should receive medical attention.
- you have a sore throat without other cold symptoms, accompanied by a fever higher than 101°F; you may have ***strep throat*** and should receive medical attention.
- you experience sudden and unexplained joint pain after recovering from strep throat; the strep infection may have spread and should be medically treated.

A rare but potentially life-threatening disease, rheumatic fever is a complication of untreated ***strep throat,*** caused by streptococcus A bacteria. The main symptoms—fever, muscle aches, swollen and painful joints, and in some cases, a red latticelike rash—typically begin one to six weeks after a bout of strep, although in some cases the infection may have been too mild to have been recognized. Rheumatic fever can also cause a temporary nervous system disorder once known as St. Vitus's dance. Today it is called chorea. People with mild cases of chorea may find it difficult to concentrate or write. More severe cases can cause the muscles of the arms, legs, or face to twitch uncontrollably.

The joints most likely to become swollen from rheumatic fever are the knees, ankles, elbows, and wrists. The pain often migrates from one joint to another. However, the greatest danger from the disease is the damage it can do to the heart. In more than half of all cases, rheumatic fever scars the valves of the heart, forcing this vital organ to work harder to pump blood. Over a period of months or even years—particularly if the disease strikes again—this damage to the heart can lead to a serious condition known as rheumatic heart disease, which can eventually cause the heart to fail. *(See **Heart Disease.**)*

Because of antibiotics, rheumatic fever is now rare in developed countries. In recent years, though, it has begun to make a comeback in the United States, particularly among children living in poor inner-city neighborhoods. The disease tends to strike most often in cool, damp weather during the winter and early spring. In the United States, it is most common in the northern states.

CAUSES

Rheumatic fever results from an inflammatory reaction to certain streptococcus A bacteria. The body produces antibodies to fight the bacteria, but instead the antibodies attack a different target: the body's own tissues. The antibodies begin with the joints and often move on to the heart and surrounding tissues. Because only a small fraction (fewer than 0.3 percent) of people with strep ever contract rheumatic fever, medical experts believe that other factors, such as a weakened immune system, must also be involved in the development of the disease.

DIAGNOSTIC AND TEST PROCEDURES

To determine the presence of streptococcus bacteria, your doctor will do a throat culture. This uncomfortable but painless procedure involves swabbing out a sample of throat mucus for laboratory analysis. It usually takes 24 hours to grow and analyze the culture.

Your doctor will also give you a complete examination, listening to your heart for signs of inflammation and looking for other telltale symptoms, such as arthritis in more than one joint and the small bony protuberances, or nodules, that often appear over the swollen joints.

TREATMENT

Appropriate, often long-term, conventional treatment can greatly lessen the risk of heart disease and other health problems associated with rheumatic fever. Alternative treatments serve as complements to conventional care—helping to ease symptoms of the illness and strengthening the immune system to help avoid recurrent attacks.

CONVENTIONAL MEDICINE

Your doctor will prescribe bed rest and ***penicillin*** to get rid of the streptococcal organisms. To prevent a recurrence of the illness, you may be put on a long-term prescription of ***antibiotics.*** For fever, inflammation, arthritic joint pain, and other symptoms, you may be given ***aspirin*** or an aspirin substitute and perhaps a ***corticosteroid.*** If you have developed rheumatic heart disease, surgery may be necessary to repair damage to the heart.

ALTERNATIVE CHOICES

Your alternative-care practitioner, in consultation with your medical doctor, can provide treatments to supplement the antibiotics prescribed for rheumatic fever. Alternative medicine may also help you boost your immune system and reduce the likelihood of recurrent infections.

HERBAL THERAPIES

To help fight the strep infection behind rheumatic fever, herbalists recommend several herbs with antimicrobial properties. ***Garlic*** *(Allium sativum)* is considered a particularly effective natural antibiotic. Take three cloves a day. If garlic smell becomes a problem, you can try three garlic capsules instead.

Teas made from either ***goldenseal*** *(Hydrastis canadensis)* or ***echinacea*** (*Echinacea* spp.) can also be effective. Drink the brew at least three times a day.

Boneset *(Eupatorium perfoliatum),* sometimes called feverwort, can help relieve the fever and other discomforts of rheumatic fever. Make a tea from the herb; drink it hot and as often as every half-hour.

As a safe heart tonic that helps minimize any long-term damage rheumatic fever may have caused, drink ***hawthorn*** *(Crataegus oxyacantha* or *Crataegus monogyna)* tea daily. Or you can take 30 to 40 drops of hawthorn tincture twice a day.

HOMEOPATHY

After you have recovered from the first attack of rheumatic fever, homeopaths recommend various treatments to avoid further attacks. Remedies include ***Aconite, Mercurius vivus, Bryonia,*** and ***Pulsatilla.*** Consult an experienced homeopath.

R

CAUTION!

Pay attention to sore throats, especially in children. If your child has a severe sore throat without other cold symptoms, accompanied by a fever higher than 101°F, or a milder sore throat that persists for more than two or three days, see a doctor. It may be *strep throat,* which can be treated with antibiotics. ■

ROCKY MOUNTAIN SPOTTED FEVER

SYMPTOMS

- moderate to high fever with chills.
- abrupt and severe headache.
- aching muscles.
- pinkish spots (about one-eighth inch) beginning around wrists or ankles, and spreading to torso, developing on about the fourth day of fever.
- nausea.
- vomiting.
- loss of appetite.
- fatigue.
- abdominal pain.
- hypersensitivity to light.

CALL YOUR DOCTOR IF:

- you develop the symptoms above and you know or suspect that you have been bitten by a tick. Rocky Mountain spotted fever is potentially fatal and must be treated promptly with ***antibiotics.*** Treatment is much less effective if delayed by more than three days.

Although Rocky Mountain spotted fever (RMSF) was named in the West, this tick-borne illness occurs in most states and is most prevalent in southeast and south-central states. While most cases of RMSF are mild and disappear within two weeks, the disease is fatal in up to 20 percent of patients who are not treated; the elderly are especially vulnerable. For those who are diagnosed within a day or two of the appearance of symptoms, antibiotics provide effective treatment.

RMSF is caused by bacteria that are transmitted by the brown dog tick in the East, the Rocky Mountain wood tick in the West, and the lone star tick in the Southwest. Only adult ticks pass this disease to humans. In most tick populations, 1 to 5 percent of ticks harbor the disease.

A tick may spend up to 24 hours on your clothing before biting. It may then feed for several days before dropping off. Because ticks inject an anesthetic similar to lidocaine into the skin, you seldom feel a tick bite.

Symptoms begin 3 to 10 days after the bite. The rash usually begins as very small pinkish spots that turn white when pressed. Later, a tiny red dot that does not whiten when pressed may form at the center of the rash. Initial spots may merge and darken into purplish patches. If the disease is not treated, you may get chills, abdominal pain, nausea, intense headache, mental confusion, and eventually gangrene (tissue death).

When treatment is delayed more than three days after the first symptoms, the death rate is above 6 percent; when started within three days, it is 1.3 percent. Dark-skinned patients have a higher death rate because the rash may be invisible. At greatest risk are campers, dog owners, foresters, children who play outside, and others who spend time outdoors. Almost all cases occur in spring or early summer; some 1,500 cases occur annually. The disease isn't contagious person-to-person.

CAUSES

The organism that causes RMSF, *Rickettsia rickettsii,* is released from a tick's salivary glands 6 to 10 hours after the tick begins feeding. The bacteria then invade human blood-vessel cells and in-

DISEASE-CARRYING TICKS

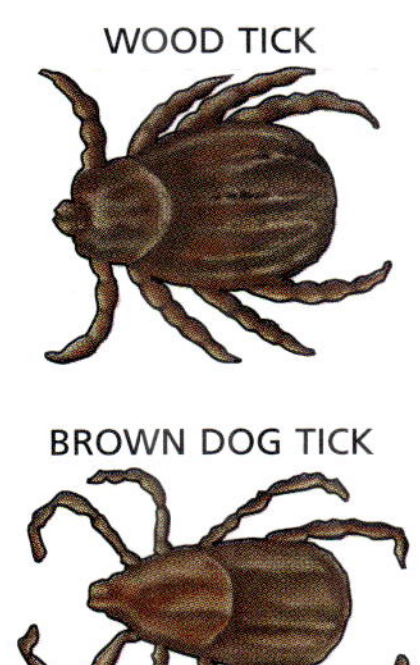

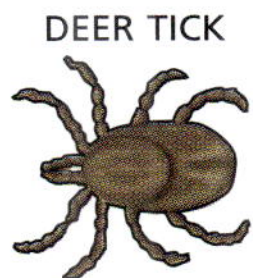

Carriers of Rocky Mountain spotted fever, a potentially fatal disease, include the wood tick *(top)*, found mainly in western states, and the brown dog tick *(middle)*, found mainly in the East. The deer tick *(bottom)*, a carrier of ***Lyme disease,*** is found in many areas and is distinguished by its size: The nymph form that transmits the disease is only slightly larger than the period at the end of this sentence.

terfere with blood clotting throughout the body.

The rash, as well as damage to organs and tissues, is caused by leakage of blood from blood vessels. Vulnerable areas include the lungs, gastrointestinal tract, heart, brain, eyes, and kidneys.

DIAGNOSTIC AND TEST PROCEDURES

In the absence of a known tick bite, RMSF is difficult to diagnose. As many as half of all sufferers do not recall a tick bite. The rash helps distinguish the disease, but it does not appear immediately. Eventually, blood tests that measure antibodies can confirm a diagnosis. But this does not help with early diagnosis, since antibodies are seldom detectable for 10 to 14 days.

During the earliest stage, the rash may be mistaken for measles, but unlike measles, the rash seldom appears on the face.

TREATMENT

Early identification of the disease is critical. The later the diagnosis, the more difficult it is to control the infection.

CONVENTIONAL MEDICINE

Most sufferers can be treated with oral ***tetracycline*** or ***doxycycline.*** Because tetracycline stains developing teeth, pregnant women and patients younger than eight years old may be given oral chloramphenicol, but this treatment may produce ***anemia*** and bone-marrow suppression. Symptoms usually begin to subside within 36 to 48 hours.

PREVENTION

Avoidance, or early removal, of ticks is the best way to prevent RMSF. Take care if you are camping, mowing, gardening, or walking in fields or woods where ticks live. Most ticks live near the ground, so wear shoes and long pants tucked into socks. Spray insect repellent on clothing. Frequent mowing helps suppress tick populations. Inspect ankles, waistline, and hair thoroughly several times a day and at bedtime. Ticks show up best against light-colored clothing, although the color white, heat, and perspiration odor may attract them. Fit your dog or cat with a flea collar.

REMOVING A TICK

If you find a tick on your skin, do not rub or crush it, as this may lead to infection. Some physicians advocate coating the tick first with vegetable or mineral oil, kerosene, or alcohol, which may interfere with its breathing and cause its grip to loosen. Others suggest simply grasping the tick with blunt tweezers (or gloved fingers) as close to the mouthparts as possible and pulling gently upward and outward until it lets go. Do not twist or puncture the tick if possible. After removal, disinfect the attachment site and wash your hands in soap and water. ■

R

SCABIES

SYMPTOMS

- intensely itchy rash with red patches generally located between the fingers, around the wrists, and on the elbows, navel, nipples, lower abdomen, and genitals. The face and scalp are rarely affected.
- pencil-thin lesions that mark where the scabies mites have burrowed into the skin; visible in only about 25 percent of cases.
- itching that is most severe at night.
- scabs that tend to form over scratched areas.

See also the ***Visual Diagnostic Guide.***

CALL YOUR DOCTOR IF:

- you suspect you have scabies; you and anyone else you may come in direct physical contact with need to be treated with a pediculicide (an insecticide that kills mites and lice).
- your lesions appear to ooze or show other signs of infection; the chief complication of scabies is secondary bacterial infections, especially strep and staph.
- you develop an additional rash or have any other adverse reaction after applying the treatment gamma benzene hexachloride (more commonly known as lindane). In rare instances this pediculicide, especially when applied too liberally, has been shown to damage the central nervous system and even cause death.

The contagious skin disease known as scabies can be traced to the insidious action of the mite *Sarcoptes scabiei.* The primary symptom—incredibly itchy, red lesions—results when the female mite burrows into the skin and deposits eggs and feces. Long considered a problem only of the unclean and poor, scabies is actually quite common at all socioeconomic levels. Closed environments such as nursing homes and childcare centers provide ideal breeding grounds for the parasite, which needs a human host to survive. An estimated 300 million new cases spring up each year worldwide. The number of cases in the United States is currently on the rise, probably because more children under the age of five are being cared for in centers.

CAUSES

Scabies mites can survive for only two to three days without a human host, but if they do infest you, it can be very difficult to get rid of them. Transmission almost always occurs through direct person-to-person contact. The telltale red, itchy, pencil-thin lesions usually appear two to three weeks after infestation; the sores are caused by the body's allergic reaction to the mites and their feces.

Since the distinguishing burrow lines show in only about 25 percent of patients, you may have to rely on other signals to determine whether you have been infested. If you find yourself overcome with an overwhelming need to scratch particular areas of your body, especially at night, check with your doctor. People with flaking skin disorders, such as ***eczema*** and ***psoriasis,*** need to be especially vigilant. Because they already tend to have itchy, red skin, they may not notice symptoms until the infestation is widespread.

Contrary to common assumptions, it is highly unlikely that you would contract scabies from your pet; indeed, human skin will not sustain the type of mite often found on dogs, and the pimplelike rash you might get from a canine mite not only is less itchy but may actually clear up on its own.

TREATMENT

To get rid of scabies, those people who are infected and everyone they came in contact with must be treated at the same time. Since the mites can survive for two or three days on almost any surface, including tables and countertops, toys, and linens, all areas must be thoroughly vacuumed and washed. Items that may be difficult to clean, such as stuffed animals, should be bagged and stored for a week.

There has been some controversy about the dangerous side effects of some pediculicides, which kill mites and lice. Several alternatives exist, including herbal remedies, for those who want a more benign (though also potentially less effective) solution.

CONVENTIONAL MEDICINE

A bath with soap and hot water will wash away some of the mites and their debris, but this step alone will not get rid of all the parasites. Most doctors prescribe a pediculicide, which you apply to your skin from the neck down. You may need some assistance with this treatment since you must be certain to cover all areas. Leave the lotion on the skin for 8 to 12 hours and then wash it off. Do not reapply the lotion without your physician's approval.

Gamma benzene hexachloride was at one time the most commonly prescribed pediculicide, but if used improperly, it can attack and permanently damage the central nervous system. Multiple applications, especially in young children, have led to brain damage, paralysis, and seizures. In 1990 the FDA approved the use of permethrin, a cream that works well against scabies without the potent side effects. Permethrin has quickly become the treatment of choice of most dermatologists.

After you rid your skin of mites, you can take an ***antihistamine*** for the itch (which can still rage for days after treatment because of feces left in the burrows) and apply ***corticosteroid*** creams to reduce inflammation.

ALTERNATIVE CHOICES

Like their conventional counterparts, many alternative remedies for eradicating scabies mites are potent and even toxic if taken internally, but many herbs do offer safe relief from itching and inflammation. If mites return after you try an herbal parasiticide, you may want to use the more conventional preparations. The longer the parasites live in your skin, the greater your risk of infection.

HERBAL THERAPIES

Larkspur *(Consolida regalis),* the most effective herbal parasiticide, is poisonous if taken internally. Consult an herbalist for treatment.

HOMEOPATHY

For relief of itching, try taking ***Sulphur*** (6x) every eight hours for up to three days.

AT-HOME REMEDIES

- To relieve itching, add a cup of oatmeal or cornstarch or 1/8 cup of ***chickweed*** to your bath; soak in hot water and scrub with soap, but avoid overscrubbing, which can lead to a skin condition called eczematous scabies.
- Rubbing ***lavender*** *(Lavandula officinalis)* oil into your sores can also help relieve itching.

PREVENTION

The best way to prevent getting scabies is to avoid contact with the mite. For some people, especially those who work in hospitals, day-care centers, and other crowded conditions, that may be difficult. If you contract the parasite, take basic steps to avoid reinfection and infecting others:

- Apply a pediculicide from the neck down and leave it on for at least eight hours; ensure anyone who had physical contact with you also applies it, even if they do not show symptoms.
- Wash all linens, towels, and clothes in hot water; store stuffed animals and other hard-to-wash items in bags for at least a week.
- Wash all tables, chairs, and floors, and vacuum all rugs. ■

S

SCARLET FEVER

SYMPTOMS

Scarlet fever occurs most frequently in children. Its symptoms include:

- bright red or scarlet rash, usually beginning on the neck or chest.
- high fever.
- sore throat.
- tongue coated with red spots.
- swollen glands in neck.
- vomiting.

CALL YOUR DOCTOR IF:

- your child develops symptoms of scarlet fever, especially if the child has recently had ***strep throat.*** Left untreated, scarlet fever may have serious complications affecting the heart, kidneys, and other organs.

Scarlet fever is one of those childhood diseases that have been tamed by ***antibiotics.*** Once a common and dangerous illness, today it is rare and easily managed.

The disease occurs mostly in children between the ages of 2 and 10. After an incubation period of two to five days, it typically starts with a very high fever of up to 104°F. Anywhere from 12 to 48 hours later, a distinctive scarlet rash appears, first on the neck and chest and then all over the body. The rash feels like sandpaper and is most prevalent above the armpits and at the groin. The tongue also becomes swollen and turns bright red. After three days the rash and fever usually disappear, but the tongue may remain swollen for several more days.

Unlike certain other childhood diseases such as ***German measles*** and ***measles,*** scarlet fever cannot be left to run its course; it must be treated or it can lead to ***arthritis, jaundice,*** kidney problems, and ***rheumatic fever.***

CAUSES

Scarlet fever is a contagious infection that is caused by streptococcal bacteria and spread by contact with an infected person or inhalation of the bacteria. Once inside the pharynx or throat, the bacteria multiply and produce a toxin that circulates in the blood and causes the symptoms.

DIAGNOSTIC AND TEST PROCEDURES

Your pediatrician will inspect your child's throat, take a culture, and examine it for the presence of streptococcal bacteria.

TREATMENT

Unless treated with ***antibiotics,*** scarlet fever can have serious complications. Call your pediatrician immediately if you think your child has the disease. Along with taking antibiotics, your child should get plenty of bed rest and drink lots of fruit juice to flush out his system. Cool baths

CAUTION!

Although scarlet fever is easily controlled with antibiotics, it may lead to serious complications if left untreated. Be sure to see your doctor or pediatrician without delay if you think your child may have contracted scarlet fever.

may reduce the fever, and ***acetaminophen*** will help relieve pain. Caution: Don't use ***aspirin,*** which has been associated with Reye's syndrome, a sometimes fatal brain disease whose cause is unknown.

CONVENTIONAL MEDICINE

Your pediatrician will prescribe an antibiotic, such as ***penicillin.*** If your child is allergic to penicillin, he'll be given an alternative, such as ***erythromycin.*** The medicine must be taken for at least 10 days, even if the symptoms disappear sooner. Other family members should also be examined and treated if necessary. Before the advent of ***antibiotics,*** households were quarantined because of scarlet fever, but this is no longer necessary.

ALTERNATIVE CHOICES

A child with scarlet fever must take an antibiotic to kill the infection. Alternative therapies may be used together with antibiotics to accelerate healing and reduce discomfort.

ACUPRESSURE

Ask a qualified practitioner to recommend acupressure massages that will boost your child's immune system and will also help fight the infection more quickly.

AROMATHERAPY

For scarlet fever, aromatherapists recommend inhaling the vapors of ***eucalyptus*** *(Eucalyptus globulus)* oil, which may help antibiotics destroy bacteria. Place a few drops on a handkerchief and inhale through your nose.

CHINESE HERBS

A practitioner of Chinese medicine may prescribe an herbal formula to eliminate toxins and strengthen your child's ability to fight off disease.

HERBAL THERAPIES

Catnip *(Nepeta cataria)* contains chemicals that are thought to reduce fever. Herbalists recommend taking 5 to 10 drops of the extract in a glass of warm water or in peppermint tea three times a day.

Echinacea (*Echinacea* spp.) may help combat the bacteria, ease the rash, and help clear chest congestion. After your child's fever has abated, give him a tea three times a day made with 2 tsp of the powdered root simmered in 1 cup of water for 15 minutes.

HOMEOPATHY

A homeopath may prescribe a remedy to help your child fight off the infection and heal faster. Homeopathic remedies to treat scarlet fever may include ***Ferrum phosphoricum*** (for sore throat and shivering associated with early stages of scarlet fever) and *Kali muriaticum* (for skin rash and white tongue).

NUTRITION AND DIET

Proper nutrition boosts the body's immune system and helps it fight infection. If your child becomes ill, make sure he drinks plenty of fluids to help flush out toxins and prevent dehydration. Citrus juices are a good choice.

PREVENTION

- Stay away and keep your child away from people who have scarlet fever.
- Stay healthy by eating balanced meals and getting plenty of sleep and exercise. ■

SCHIZOPHRENIA

SYMPTOMS

A diagnosis of schizophrenia is considered when a person experiences at least two of the following symptoms:

- delusions.
- hallucinations.
- disorganized speech.
- irrational or catatonic behavior, such as stupor, rigidity, or floppiness of limbs.
- negative symptoms, such as inaction, silence, loss of will.

These symptoms are usually accompanied by a substantial decrease in the ability to interact with others.

CALL YOUR DOCTOR IF:

- you or someone you know experiences the above symptoms. Schizophrenia can be a devastating disorder, and medical care is vital. Be aware that it may not be easy to persuade someone who is becoming mentally ill to acknowledge symptoms or see a physician.

While schizophrenia literally means "split mind," it should not be confused with a "split," or multiple, personality. It is more accurately described as a psychosis—a cluster of severe and prolonged mental disturbances that disrupt normal thought, speech, and behavior.

The onset of schizophrenia is usually characterized by the psychotic symptoms listed at left or by bizarre behavior. But many patients show "negative" symptoms, such as decreased emotional arousal, mental activity, and social drive.

It is seldom useful to talk about subcategories, such as paranoid schizophrenia or catatonic schizophrenia, since individual patients commonly exhibit a variety of symptoms and therapists make different diagnoses. But most schizophrenics do share a range of similar symptoms. For example, they often report a sense of strangeness and confusion about the source of their sensations. They feel great loneliness, anxiety, and an overwhelming sense of being disconnected from others.

A schizophrenic person may think and communicate by private rules, jumping from one idea to another, using vague or repetitive words, or mixing a "word salad" of new words or jumbled phrases. It is common for schizophrenics to be suspicious and resentful. They may sense that their thoughts are stolen, broadcast, or replaced by new information from strangers seeking to control their behavior. They may describe voices that speak directly to them or criticize their behavior.

Schizophrenia normally appears in men when they are in their teens, and in women in their twenties, but the prevalence is about the same. About 1 in 100 people will be treated at some time for schizophrenia. Some patients experience only a single episode and remain symptom free afterward. More commonly, the course of illness fluctuates over several decades, with each recurrence leading to increasing impairment.

CAUSES

Most specialists agree that symptoms are provoked by chemical disturbances of brain function, but no exact mechanism is known. Schizophrenia seems to be a syndrome of multiple causes and types. Genetics seems to play a role, but there is no single "schizophrenia gene." While it is clear that a supportive family can be helpful in preventing relapse, it is also agreed that family strife does not cause schizophrenia.

TREATMENT

The goals of conventional treatment include helping patients toward normal interactions with others, enabling patients to live in the community, and controlling the illness through the smallest effective dosage of medication. A combination of medication and psychotherapy is usually required.

CONVENTIONAL MEDICINE

The modern era of medical treatment for schizophrenia began in 1952 with the use of the tranquilizer chlorpromazine. This drug (and modern relatives like haloperidol) for the first time controlled acute symptoms, reduced hospitalization from years to days, and lowered the rate of relapse by more than 50 percent. However, not everyone responds to these drugs. Long-term control is less successful than short-term alleviation. Also, prolonged medication may bring harmful side effects, especially the neurological muscle disorder known as tardive dyskinesia (TD), which causes involuntary facial movements, such as grimacing and sucking motions.

Clozapine, approved in the U.S. in 1990, has been helping many people unresponsive to other antipsychotic medications without causing TD; it does, however, cause a serious decline in white blood cells in 1 percent of patients, so weekly or biweekly blood tests are required. Risperidone appears to relieve symptoms without this complication. For most patients, lifelong use of ***antianxiety drugs*** is necessary to prevent relapse. Additional drugs, such as ***antidepressants,*** may be used to treat side effects or related symptoms, including stiffness, tremors, and depression.

Psychotherapy by itself is of little value without medication. However, supportive and sympathetic psychotherapy is needed to help the patient diagnosed with schizophrenia understand the disease and reenter society and family life.

ALTERNATIVE CHOICES

Because schizophrenia is such a serious and complex disorder, few therapies are known to be effective. However, research interest in schizophrenia has grown rapidly in recent years.

NUTRITION AND DIET

There is some good evidence that many of the B-complex vitamins, including ***folic acid,*** are helpful as an adjunct to treatment. Also, ***vitamin C*** raises the potency of the antipsychotic haloperidol, and ***vitamin E*** may relieve the symptoms of tardive dyskinesia, especially in its early stages. More controversial is the possibility that ***zinc*** and ***manganese*** are of benefit.

HELP FOR THE SCHIZOPHRENIC

Accepting, nonjudging friends and relatives can help reduce anxiety and the severity of symptoms. Schizophrenics tend to be easily upset by "expressed emotion"; researchers advise family members to reduce criticism and to be as unobtrusive as possible.

Also, sympathetic family members who encourage patients to be active in their own care can help reduce the sense of helplessness. Patients who are in a supportive environment are more likely to accept their medication and to avoid relapses.

Some patients react better to a certain drug, or simply prefer its "feel." It is important to respond to these preferences when possible, and to reinforce efforts toward independence. ■

SCIATICA

SYMPTOMS

- pain radiating through your buttock, down the back of your thigh and leg, often to your foot. The pain can be sharp or dull, shooting or burning, intermittent or continuous. It usually affects just one side of the body. Coughing, sneezing, bending, or lifting may make it worse.
- in some cases, numbness and weakness of the affected area.

CALL YOUR DOCTOR IF:

- the pain is severe and doesn't respond to over-the-counter ***analgesics;*** your physician may prescribe a stronger painkiller and other therapy.
- the pain persists for more than three or four days and is accompanied by leg or foot weakness; this may indicate a more serious neurological problem.

Sciatica, characterized by pain radiating into one or both buttocks and descending the back of the leg, results from compression of the sciatic nerve at the base of the spine. This nerve (one for each side of the lower body) is the longest in the peripheral nervous system, extending through the buttocks and down as far as the foot. The pain can occur along its entire length.

CAUSES

Pressure on a sciatic nerve may be due to poor posture, muscle strain, pregnancy, being overweight, wearing high heels, or sleeping on a too-soft mattress. It can also result from a slipped disk *(see **Pinched Nerve, Back Problems,** and **Disk Problems**)* or inflammation of the sciatic nerve, in some cases caused by osteoarthritis *(see **Arthritis**).*

DIAGNOSTIC AND TEST PROCEDURES

Your doctor may use the so-called straight-leg-raising test—lifting your leg to a 45-degree angle—to help locate the point of pain. Other tests include an x-ray, or an MRI or CT scan.

TREATMENT

CONVENTIONAL MEDICINE

Your physician may prescribe muscle relaxants, ***nonsteroidal anti-inflammatory drugs (NSAIDs),*** systemic painkillers, narcotics, or ***corticosteroids.*** Physical therapy is often recommended, once acute inflammation and pain have subsided. A nutritionist may suggest daily doses of the amino acid DL-phenylalanine taken every other week to help alleviate pain.

ALTERNATIVE CHOICES

BODY WORK

The **Alexander technique,** a system of posture retraining, can teach correct methods of sitting, standing, and moving to prevent future attacks.

CHIROPRACTIC

Soft-tissue and vertebral manipulation may reduce pressure on a sciatic nerve.

HERBAL THERAPIES

Teas made from ***white willow*** *(Salix alba)* bark or meadowsweet *(Filipendula ulmaria)* may relieve joint pain; try ***black cohosh*** *(Cimicifuga racemosa)* for muscle spasms.

HOMEOPATHY

For stiffness that is worse in the morning and at night but improves with heat, try ***Rhus toxicodendron.*** For severe shooting pain extending from your lower back to your ankles that worsens with motion, consider ***Bryonia.*** Consult a practitioner for proper dosages and courses of treatment.

NUTRITION

High doses of ***calcium*** (1,000 mg) and ***magnesium*** (400 mg) at bedtime, along with ***vitamin C*** (500 mg), may be beneficial. Taking 50 mg of ***vitamin*** B_6 three times a day for one week only may also help. Consult a nutritionist for further guidance on taking supplements.

OSTEOPATHY

Slipped disks might benefit from the soft-tissue massage and positioning that osteopaths use to relieve pressure on the sciatic nerve. Consult an osteopath if your sciatica is associated with a strain or muscle injury and improves with exercise but is unrelieved by rest.

AT-HOME REMEDIES

The following remedies might help reduce pain.

- Apply ice to the affected area for 30 to 60 minutes as soon as pain starts. Do this several times a day for two or three days. Thereafter, apply a hot-water bottle at the same intervals.
- Try the following self-massage technique: Lie on your back with your knees bent; relax for several minutes; take a sock containing two soft rubber balls and position them on either side of your spine in the small of your back; allow your body weight to sink into the floor, over the balls. Remove the balls and relax for a few more minutes. Follow the same procedure for your buttocks. If you're having disk problems, check with your doctor before attempting this technique.
- During periods of acute pain, don't pick up anything heavier than 10 pounds, and take the weight of lifted objects in your bent legs and arms, not in your back. Push rather than pull heavy objects.

EXCESS STIMULATION

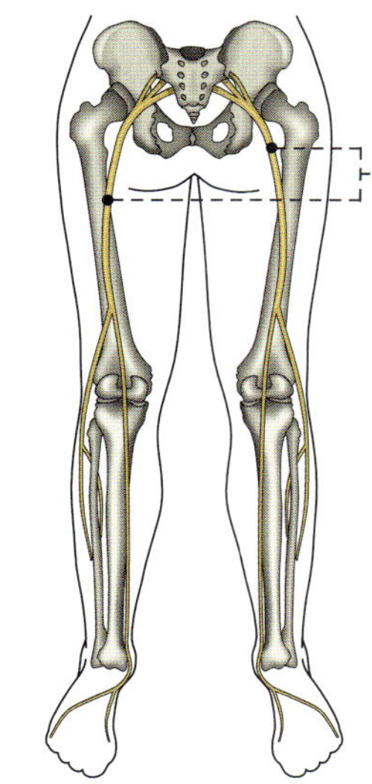

Extending from the tailbone to the toes, the two branches of the sciatic nerve register sensation—including pain—every time the leg is stimulated. Continuous pressure on the nerve, perhaps from a slipped vertebral disk or a fetus in the womb, can send a stream of pain messages along the length of the nerve; the intensity of the pain can range from mild to debilitating.

PREVENTION

- Sleep on a firm mattress on your back or side with your knees bent; avoid sleeping on your stomach. During acute attacks only, sleep with a pillow under or between your knees.
- Adjust the height of your chair so your feet are flat on the floor and your knees are a little higher than your hips; make a habit of sitting with both feet flat on the floor instead of crossing your legs.
- Make sure your chair has firm back support, and sit with your back straight against it. ■

S

SCOLIOSIS

SYMPTOMS

Scoliosis, an abnormal sideways curvature of the spine, may be present if, looking from the rear:

- the entire body seems to tilt to one side.
- the shoulders appear uneven, with one shoulder blade more prominent than the other.
- one leg seems longer than the other.
- the hips appear to be at uneven heights or look as if they have shifted to the right or the left.
- the back looks crooked on bending forward.
- from the front the ribs appear more prominent and spaced more widely apart on one side than the other.

CALL YOUR DOCTOR IF:

- you see any of the symptoms described above. Be especially vigilant if you have a family history of scoliosis. The condition may worsen over time and must be evaluated and treated by a physician in order to arrest its progress.

Scoliosis is a progressive lateral, or sideways, curvature of the spine. People with scoliosis have backs that take on a distinct C- or S-shaped curve that deviates markedly from the normal vertical alignment of the spine *(right).* Scoliosis is sometimes present at birth, although it most often appears between the ages of 10 and 14, becoming increasingly severe as the child grows. The disorder occurs in both boys and girls but tends to be more serious and progress more dramatically in females.

Because scoliosis itself does not generally cause pain, it is sometimes referred to as a "silent" condition. However, if untreated, it may eventually cause painful secondary problems such as ***disk problems, sciatica,*** or ***arthritis.*** In severe cases, the torso may become so twisted and distorted that the heart and lungs are affected, causing chronic fatigue and shortness of breath.

CAUSES

The causes of scoliosis are poorly understood. Doctors suspect that there is a genetic component to scoliosis, although the cause of most cases is unknown. Children who have suffered from diseases of the muscles, bones, or nervous system, such as polio or cerebral palsy, may also develop scoliosis. And in both children and adults, scoliosis may occur following traumatic injuries such as a fractured back, or as a result of conditions that affect the nervous system.

TREATMENT

The standard treatments for scoliosis are exercise, orthopedic bracing, and in severe cases, surgery. For the most part, bracing can only halt the progress of the condition rather than correct any curvature that has already occurred; so it is important to begin early. Scoliosis generally progresses most rapidly during early adolescence, when a youngster's bones are growing at their peak rate. The earlier a child develops scoliosis, the more extensive the curvature will be if it is left untreated.

CURVATURE OF THE SPINE

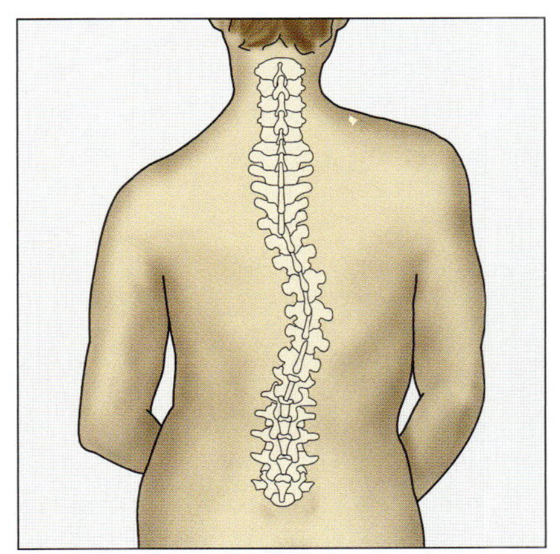

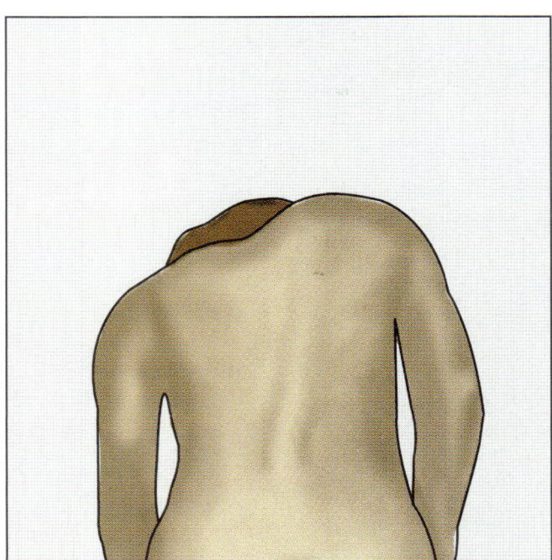

Scoliosis, or sideways curvature of the spine, distorts the carriage of the shoulders and hips by forcing the spine out of its normal alignment *(above, left)*. One shoulder rises higher than normal, while the opposite hip is more prominent. On bending forward *(above, right)*, the back may appear to have a hump on the side of the affected shoulder.

CONVENTIONAL MEDICINE

The treatment a doctor prescribes for scoliosis depends on the patient's degree of spinal curvature. A mild curve of less than 25 degrees can usually be controlled by an exercise program designed to strengthen the torso. Orthopedic body braces, molded to fit the individual's torso and hold it erect, are usually prescribed to manage curves of 25 to 30 degrees or greater. For children and adolescents, the brace is adjusted as the patient grows. It is worn until the skeleton stops growing—at around 16 in most girls and 17 to 18 in most boys.

Curves of 40 degrees or more may call for surgery. Typically, metal rods are implanted alongside the spine, providing an internal splint that corrects the curve. The surgeon also fuses several vertebrae together to straighten and immobilize that section of the spine.

ALTERNATIVE CHOICES

New evidence suggests that the **Alexander technique, chiropractic,** the **Feldenkrais method, massage, osteopathy** and **yoga** may help control the progressive curvature of the spine. **Acupuncture,** or manipulation by a chiropractor or osteopath may also reduce the discomfort of muscular pain or disk problems. Consult a qualified practitioner.

AT-HOME CARE

Consistent long-term care is essential in treating scoliosis. Patients must exercise conscientiously, and those who wear a brace must stick to the prescribed schedule for its use. Typically, a brace is worn 23 hours a day and removed only for bathing and physical therapy—requirements that youngsters find particularly onerous. To help a child cope with a brace, try the following:

- Enlist family, friends, and teachers to provide emotional support.
- Seek the assistance of physicians, orthopedic surgeons, and physical therapists in developing an appropriate exercise program. Encourage your child to engage in activities such as running, fast walking, and dance, all of which can be done while wearing the brace. Exercise won't correct the curvature, but it will improve your child's overall health and muscle tone.
- Watch carefully for signs of chafing and skin breakdown. Have your child wear a snug T-shirt under the brace and use rubbing alcohol to toughen skin that comes in contact with the frame. ■

SEASONAL AFFECTIVE DISORDER

SYMPTOMS

Some or all of these symptoms are present during the fall and winter. Occasionally, seasonal affective disorder (SAD) occurs in summer, but with diminished rather than increased eating or sleeping symptoms.

- ***depression,*** difficulty enjoying life, pessimism about the future.
- loss of energy, inertia, apathy.
- increased sleep, difficulty getting up in the morning.
- impaired functioning: difficulty getting to work on time; tasks that are normally easy seem impossible.
- increased appetite, weight gain.
- carbohydrate cravings.
- desire to avoid people.
- irritability, crying spells.
- decreased sex drive.
- suicidal thoughts or feelings.

For children and adolescents:

- feeling tired and irritable.
- temper tantrums.
- difficulty concentrating.
- vague physical complaints.
- marked cravings for junk food.

CALL YOUR DOCTOR IF:

- you or your child suffers some of these symptoms with the onset of fall and winter and they seem to diminish or dissipate as spring and summer approach.

Seasonal affective disorder (SAD) is an extreme form of the "winter blues," bringing lethargy and curtailing normal functioning. It was only recently recognized as a specific disorder, but since 1982 much has been learned about it and how to treat it. People suffering from SAD undergo extreme differences in mood, as if they were split between a "summer person" and a "winter person."

Although a different kind of SAD can occur in the summer, its most common form begins gradually in late August or early September and continues until March or early April, when the symptoms begin to dissipate. Sufferers have been known to increase their sleep by as many as four hours a night and gain more than 20 pounds as they attempt to "hibernate" the winter away.

Research suggests that SAD may affect 11 million people in the United States each year, and that an additional 25 million suffer a milder form that is indeed called the winter blues. Four times as many women suffer from SAD as men, and it tends to run in families.

As might be expected, geographical location plays the largest role in susceptibility to SAD; the nearer one lives to one of the poles, the greater the incidence. People in Canada or the northern United States are eight times more likely to fall victim to SAD than those living in sunny southern areas like Florida or Mexico.

CAUSES

Researchers are still far from agreement about the precise cause of SAD and suggest it may have more than one cause. Currently, the most likely explanation involves the neurotransmitter serotonin, which during the short days of winter reaches its lowest concentrations in key parts of the brain, causing depression. Whatever the chemical constituents, SAD is triggered by inadequate outdoor light and exacerbated by ***stress.***

For children, the fall onset of SAD comes at the time that school starts, and it is difficult to sort out SAD from other possible reasons for mood changes. Often overlooked by doctors and parents, SAD should be considered a possibility.

DIAGNOSTIC AND TEST PROCEDURES

Because no laboratory test exists for SAD, diagnosis is made on the basis of the patient's history and should be made by a psychiatrist experienced with the disorder. Illnesses with similar symptoms that must be ruled out are underactive thyroid function, chronic viral infections, and ***chronic fatigue syndrome.*** In children, abuse and separation anxiety should also be considered, and in adolescents, substance abuse and ***anxiety*** disorder.

TREATMENT

The most effective treatment for SAD is light therapy, sometimes combined with antidepressant drugs or psychotherapy or both.

CONVENTIONAL MEDICINE

Light therapy can be used in different ways and may employ different types of light boxes, light visors, and lamps. All are designed to bring in extra light to the eyes. Check to be sure a light box filters out harmful ultraviolet light.

In the most common form of light therapy, you sit before a light box of strong fluorescent light (10,000 lux—about 10 to 20 times brighter than ordinary indoor light) for periods varying from 15 minutes to 1½ hours a day. You place the box on a table or desk where you can do paperwork, read, or make phone calls.

Other light sources include larger boxes that stand on the floor, visors with lights attached, and dawn simulators—lights programmed to turn on by your bed on winter mornings before dawn.

Light boxes can be bought for several hundred dollars at special stores. Experts warn against constructing your own light box because of possible damage from ultraviolet light.

Since SAD is a form of ***depression,*** many different types of ***antidepressants*** have been used. The preferred drugs at the present time are the ***selective serotonin reuptake inhibitors (SSRIs),*** because they regulate the brain levels of serotonin and have fewer side effects than many other antidepressants.

ALTERNATIVE CHOICES

Exercise and many other mind/body therapies for ***depression*** can be helpful with SAD. **Massage** may also be a useful adjunct to other therapies. Try three or four massage sessions to see if it works; one session is not enough to judge.

For many centuries, healers believed that certain electrical emissions in the atmosphere—negative ions—improve a person's mood and health. In the last 30 years, scientists have developed small devices that emit negative ions into the atmosphere of a room. The negative ionizer seems particularly helpful for people with SAD (one study showed a 58 percent reduction of depression) and may be a good supplement to light therapy and medications.

NUTRITION AND DIET

People with SAD are apt to overeat in the winter, with special cravings for sweets and starches. One SAD expert recommends that patients avoid snacking on carbohydrate-rich foods and instead recommends balancing carbohydrates with protein or restricting carbohydrate-rich food to a single balanced meal a day.

AT-HOME REMEDIES

- Take a walk at lunchtime when the sun is high. Be outdoors as often as you can.
- Exercise as much as you are able.
- Take winter vacations in places with long days.
- Increase the natural light in your home by trimming low-lying branches near the house and hedges around windows.
- Paint your walls with lighter colors.
- Keep warm and enjoy the fun aspects of winter—such as wood fires, books, music.
- If all else fails and you can manage it, move to a sunnier climate. ■

S

SEXUAL DYSFUNCTION

SYMPTOMS

Sexual dysfunction is broadly defined as the inability to fully enjoy sexual intercourse.

For men, you may have a sexual problem if you:

- ejaculate before you or your partner desires (premature ejaculation).
- do not ejaculate, or ejaculation is delayed (retarded ejaculation).
- are unable to have an erection sufficient for pleasurable intercourse; see ***Impotence.***
- feel pain during intercourse.
- lack or lose sexual desire.

For women, you may have a sexual problem if you:

- lack or lose sexual desire.
- have difficulty achieving orgasm.
- feel anxiety during intercourse.
- feel pain during intercourse.
- feel vaginal or other muscles contract involuntarily before or during sex.
- have inadequate lubrication.

CALL YOUR DOCTOR IF:

you or your partner has

- concerns about your sexual life.
- pain during intercourse. This may indicate infection or illness.
- been exposed to chemicals or ***sexually transmitted diseases.***
- been sexually abused or assaulted.
- a prolonged erection unaccompanied by sexual desire. This condition, called priapism, is serious and requires immediate medical attention.

For couples of any age, sexual dysfunction—the inability of both partners to fully enjoy sexual intercourse—can be an obstacle not only to having children but also to maintaining a positive and loving relationship. Problems of this kind are common, affecting more than half of all couples at some time, according to some studies. While sexual dysfunction rarely threatens physical health, it can take a heavy psychological toll, bringing on ***depression, anxiety,*** and debilitating feelings of inadequacy. Problems may be difficult to resolve without expert help, especially because misinformation is one of the leading causes of sexual dysfunction.

One example of misinformation is that impotence is an unavoidable consequence of aging. In reality, healthy men can enjoy sexual intimacy well into their senior years. Achieving an erection may take 5 to 15 minutes of genital stimulation, however.

Another erroneous belief is that women have no interest in sex after a hysterectomy. Although there may be a decrease in vaginal lubrication if the ovaries are removed along with the uterus, libido (the sex drive) remains intact—and, because any worries about pregnancy are gone, it may even increase.

As people live longer and attitudes change, more older couples desire to prolong the years of healthy sexuality. Sex in old age was at one time thought to be inappropriate and even immoral; now, both physical and emotional intimacy are seen as important to well-being throughout life. Although sexual desire and the frequency of intercourse decline with age, sexual enjoyment and satisfaction do not. For couples in good health, sexual activity, which includes touching and caressing, may continue into the eighties and even nineties.

Sexual dysfunction takes different forms in men and women.

Men: In the male partner of a couple, dysfunction is often associated with anxiety. If a man operates under the misconception that all sexual activity must lead to intercourse and to orgasm by his partner, and if the expectation is not met, he may consider the act a failure. Such an attitude can be a self-fulfilling prophecy.

The most prevalent physical dysfunction in men is premature ejaculation, in which orgasm occurs before or immediately after the penis enters the vagina. This problem, especially common among young men, can lead to performance anxiety, frustration for one's partner, doubts about one's masculinity, and perhaps ***impotence***—itself a common dysfunction.

A more unusual problem is retarded ejaculation, in which orgasm is delayed so long that it satisfies neither partner. A few men experience retrograde ejaculation—in which the semen, rather than emerging from the end of the penis, moves backward into the bladder during orgasm. Rarer still is priapism, a prolonged erection unaccompanied by sexual desire. This condition is potentially dangerous and requires prompt medical attention.

Women: The inability to experience sexual pleasure, known as arousal dysfunction, is one of the most common dysfunctions for a woman. It is difficult to treat and should be discussed with a professional, as well as with her partner.

Some women become aroused but are unable to achieve an orgasm. The fact is that only about one in three women reaches a climax regularly through intercourse alone, without additional stimulation of the clitoris. About 10 percent of women never achieve orgasm. But it is possible and even common to have a pleasurable sex life without orgasm. Lack of orgasm might be considered a dysfunction only if it represents a change or causes anxiety.

Pain during intercourse (dyspareunia) can occur for a variety of reasons, from a simple anatomical problem or vaginal infection to complex and deep-rooted fears, and it can increase at the time of menopause, when there is decreased lubrication of the vagina. If pain persists, it may cause vaginal muscles to contract involuntarily before intercourse, a response known as vaginismus. In some women, this contraction is triggered by the knowledge that sexual activity is about to begin .

Homosexual men and women are also at risk for sexual dysfunction. Knowledge about ***AIDS,*** the difficulties of striving for "safer sex," and the psychological effects of discrimination are just a few of the factors that can give rise to anxieties that depress sexual function.

CAUSES

Many factors, of both physical and psychological natures, can affect sexual response and performance. Injuries, ailments, and drugs are among the physical influences; in addition, there is increasing evidence that chemicals and other environmental pollutants depress sexual function. As for psychological factors, sexual dysfunction may have roots in traumatic events such as rape or incest, guilt feelings, a poor self-image, depression, chronic fatigue, certain religious beliefs, or marital problems.

Men: With premature ejaculation, physical causes are rare—although the problem is sometimes linked to a neurological disorder, prostate infection, or urethritis. Possible psychological causes include anxiety, guilt feelings about sex, and ambivalence toward women.

When men experience painful intercourse, the cause is usually physical—an infection of the prostate, urethra, or testes, or an allergic reaction to spermicide or condoms. Infections can be initiated by sexually transmitted diseases, such as ***chlamydia*** and ***genital herpes.*** Painful erections may be caused by Peyronie's disease, fibrous plaques on the upper side of the penis that often produce a bend during erection. Cancer of the penis or testis and ***arthritis*** of the lower back can also cause pain.

Retrograde ejaculation occurs in men who have had prostate or urethral surgery, take medication that keeps the bladder open, or suffer from ***diabetes***—a disease that can injure the nerves that normally close the bladder during ejaculation.

Women: Dysfunctions of arousal and orgasm may have similar causes. They can be physical (drugs, illness, hormonal deficiencies, gynecologic factors, inadequate stimulation) or psychological (stress, fatigue, depression, performance anxiety, relationship problems). Among the most common are day-to-day discord with one's partner and inadequate stimulation by the partner. Fi-

S

nally, sexual desire can wane as one ages, although this varies greatly from person to person.

Pain during intercourse can occur for any number of reasons, and location is sometimes a clue to the cause. Pain in the vaginal area may be due to infection, such as urethritis; also, vaginal tissues may become thinner and more sensitive during breast-feeding and after menopause. Deeper pain may have a pelvic source, such as ***endometriosis,*** pelvic adhesions, or uterine abnormalities. Pain can also have a psychological cause, such as fear of injury, guilt feelings about sex, fear of pregnancy or injury to the fetus during pregnancy, or recollection of a previous painful experience.

Vaginismus may be provoked by these psychological causes as well. Or it may begin as a response to pain, and continue after the pain is gone. Both partners should understand that the vaginal contraction is an involuntary response, outside the woman's control.

Similarly, insufficient lubrication is involuntary, and may be part of a complex cycle: Low sexual response may lead to inadequate lubrication, which may lead to discomfort and then an even worse response, and so on.

TREATMENT

No matter which partner experiences a sexual dysfunction, it is important for both to understand it. Both may contribute to the problem—and to the solution.

Men: Premature ejaculation is commonly curbed by the "squeeze" technique, a kind of biofeedback. This method has a high success rate, and repeated practice usually leads to better natural control. When you feel that orgasm is imminent, withdraw from the woman's vagina, or signal her to stop stimulation. You (or she) then squeezes gently on the head of the penis with the thumb and forefinger, halting the climax. After 20 or 30 seconds, begin lovemaking again. After several cycles, proceed to ejaculation.

Note that premature ejaculation may signal a more complex disorder whose psychological aspects should be explored in therapy. To rely only on physical control may mask the symptom without resolving the cause.

Retarded ejaculation is often treated by reducing anxiety and learning to control the timing of ejaculation. The sensate focus exercises described in the box at the end of this entry may help; you should withhold penetration until you sense that ejaculation is inevitable.

Retrograde ejaculation may be corrected through surgery that allows the valve at the base of the bladder to close. But it is basically a harmless disorder, causing a problem chiefly if children are desired; in such situations, it may be possible to retrieve sperm from the bladder for artificial insemination *(see **Infertility**).*

When a man lacks sexual desire, the cause may be physical illness, hormonal abnormality, or medications that affect libido. There may also be psychological causes, including depression or interpersonal problems, which a therapist may help identify.

Women: Arousal problems may be difficult to resolve if sexual satisfaction has never been experienced. Therapies are designed to help the patient relax, become aware of feelings about sex, and eliminate guilt and fear of rejection. The sensate focus exercises described at the end of this entry may also help.

In postmenopausal women, scant lubrication can easily be corrected with over-the-counter vaginal lubricants, egg white, or saliva. (Keep in mind that oil-based products can cause infection, however.) Inadequate lubrication in a healthy, premenopausal woman may reflect either a muted sexual response or inadequate arousal by the partner. Explore feelings about sex and seek to eliminate guilt and fear of rejection. Extended foreplay, masturbation, and relaxation techniques may help.

For inability to achieve orgasm, the communication of your desires about sexual foreplay and intercourse to your partner is an essential first step toward satisfaction. Although such treatments as experiential therapy, psychoanalysis, or behavior modification can be beneficial, you must realize that orgasms (let alone simultaneous orgasms) are not necessary to a good sexual relationship.

For pain during intercourse, first make sure there is adequate stimulation and lubrication. A physical exam may reveal a need to medicate for infection, remove scars around the hymen, or gently stretch painful scars at the vaginal opening. ***Endometriosis*** and pelvic adhesions can often be treated by laser to relieve so-called deep pain. Problems related to menopausal change may be relieved with **hormone replacement therapy** *(see **Menopausal Problems**)*. If pain persists, psychotherapy may uncover hidden fears about intercourse. Sensate focus exercises can teach appropriate foreplay and de-emphasize intercourse until both partners are ready. Education can reduce fears of pregnancy or of harm to the fetus.

Vaginismus is difficult to reverse without help. The vaginismus support group, Resolve, recommends psychotherapy or group therapy. If you have a partner, seek therapy together in a safe and supportive environment. To accustom your body to the feeling of penetration, a therapist may recommend inserting a series of vaginal dilators, each slightly larger than the last. You advance at your own pace until you are comfortable inserting a dilator the size of your partner's erection. Contraction and relaxation exercises can teach control of the vaginal muscles and increase sexual responsiveness. Psychotherapy may also increase desire, improve communication skills, and resolve underlying conflicts about sexuality. With therapy and a supportive partner, the improvement rate is good.

ALTERNATIVE CHOICES

Some problems with sexual function are normal. For example, women starting a new or first relationship may feel sore or bruised after intercourse; use an over-the-counter lubricant or egg white. For relaxation, soak in a warm bath; add 5 drops of essential oil of ***lavender*** or clary.

Yoga and **meditation** provide needed mental and physical relaxation for several conditions, such as vaginismus. **Relaxation** facilitates therapy and relieves anxiety about the dysfunction. **Massage** is extremely effective at reducing stress, especially if performed by the partner.

Herbal therapies and **homeopathy** may help improve sexual function; consult a qualified practitioner for specific, individual treatment.

SENSATE FOCUS EXERCISES

The following exercises are valuable not only for dysfunction but also for revitalizing sexual interest and renewing sexuality following a period of inactivity. Remain in each focus area until you are satisfied.

Focus 1. *With the partners taking turns, one is totally receptive for about 15 minutes while the other explores, stimulates, and caresses all parts of the body except genital areas and breasts. The manual stimulation should range from light touch to stroking and rubbing. Lips or other parts of the body may also be used.*

Focus 2. *Continue the various forms of stimulation and expand them to include the genital areas and breasts. The receptive partner should provide feedback on what is most pleasurable. Oral-genital contact is permitted, but hold back from penetration and orgasm.*

Focus 3. *As stimulation continues, proceed to penetration and activities leading to orgasm.* ■

S

SYMPTOMS

Especially if you are a woman, you may experience no symptoms until you have developed serious complications, or you may notice:

- a vaginal, anal, or urethral discharge; the color may be white, yellow, green, or gray, or the discharge may be blood-streaked, and it may have a strong odor.
- genital and/or anal itching or irritation.
- a rash, blisters, sores, lumps, bumps, or warts on or around the genitals.
- burning during urination.
- swollen lymph glands in the groin.
- pain in the groin or lower abdomen.
- vaginal bleeding.
- testicular swelling.
- flulike symptoms.
- painful intercourse.

See also ***AIDS, Chlamydia, Genital Herpes, Genital Warts, Gonorrhea, Hepatitis, Syphilis, Trichomoniasis.***

CALL YOUR DOCTOR IF:

- you have any of the above symptoms. Sexually transmitted diseases are contagious and may result in serious complications or death if left untreated.

Sexually transmitted diseases (STDs), once called venereal diseases, are among the most common contagious diseases. One in four American adults has a sexually transmitted disease, and each year 12 million new cases are reported.

As the name of this group of diseases implies, these infections can be contracted by means of vaginal, anal, or oral sex. You are at high risk if you have more than one sex partner and/or you don't use a condom when having sex.

You are also at high risk for some of these diseases—notably ***AIDS*** and ***hepatitis*** B—if you share needles when injecting intravenous drugs.

Except for AIDS and hepatitis B, sexually transmitted diseases can be cured or managed if they are treated early. But you may not realize you have an STD until it has damaged your reproductive system, vision, heart, or other organs. Also, having an STD weakens the immune system and leaves you more vulnerable to other infections. ***Pelvic inflammatory disease*** is a complication of many STDs that can leave women unable to have children and can even be life-threatening. If you pass an STD to your newborn, the baby may die or suffer blindness and organ damage.

CAUSES

Bacterial STDs include ***chlamydia, gonorrhea,*** and ***syphilis.*** Viral STDs include ***AIDS, genital herpes, genital warts,*** and ***hepatitis*** B. ***Trichomoniasis*** is caused by a parasite. The microbes that cause STDs are found in semen, blood, vaginal secretions, and sometimes saliva. Most of the organisms are spread by vaginal, anal, or oral sex, but some, such as those that cause genital herpes and genital warts, may be spread through skin contact. You can get hepatitis B by sharing personal items, such as razors, with someone who has it.

DIAGNOSTIC AND TEST PROCEDURES

If you are in a high-risk group, ask your doctor to test you for STDs during your annual physical even if you have no symptoms. If you test positive, your sexual partners will require treatment too. STDs may be detected during physical

How to Put On a Condom

Male condom:

- *Always put the condom on before you allow the penis to touch the vagina, mouth, or anus. Always use a latex condom; animal-skin condoms are more porous and may allow microbes to pass. Use water-based lubricants; oil-based lubricants such as petroleum jelly may eat through a condom.*
- *Hold the condom by the tip to squeeze out air. Leave space at the end for semen to accumulate.*
- *Unroll the condom over the erect penis.*
- *Withdraw if the condom breaks or slips off during intercourse; put on a new condom.*
- *After sex, hold the condom at the rim and pull it off slowly, while the penis is still erect.*
- *Use a new condom every time you have sex.*

Female condom, or "pouch":

- *Always insert the polyurethane pouch in the vagina before the penis touches it. Put a water-based lubricant in the pouch.*
- *Squeeze the inner ring of the pouch. Insert the pouch in the vagina as you would a diaphragm.*
- *Using your index finger, push the inner ring as far as it will go; the outer ring stays outside the vagina.*
- *Guide the penis into the pouch. If it slips out of the pouch during sex, guide it back in.*
- *After sex, remove the pouch gently before standing up.*
- *Use a new pouch every time you have sex.*

examination; through Pap smears; and in tests of blood, urine, and genital and anal discharges.

TREATMENT

Don't try to treat an STD yourself. These diseases are contagious and serious. You must see a doctor.

CONVENTIONAL MEDICINE

Bacterial STDs can be cured with ***antibiotics*** if treatment begins early enough. Viral STDs cannot be cured, but you can manage symptoms with medications. There is a vaccine against hepatitis B, but it will not help if you already have the disease.

ALTERNATIVE CHOICES

See entries for specific sexually transmitted diseases for information on alternative therapies.

AT-HOME REMEDIES

- Douche with vinegar, yogurt, or lemon juice solutions to relieve vaginal distress.
- Take ***zinc*** and ***vitamins A, C,*** and ***E*** to boost your immune system and to help treat some skin infections, such as herpes.
- Practice relaxation techniques to ease stress and speed healing.
- Take warm baths and analgesics such as ***aspirin, ibuprofen,*** or ***acetaminophen*** for pain.
- Ask your doctor or pharmacist about other over-the-counter remedies.

PREVENTION

Always avoid sex with anyone who has genital sores, a rash, a discharge, or other disease symptoms. If you are in a high-risk group you should:

- Use latex condoms and water-based lubricants. Remember that condoms are not 100 percent effective at preventing disease.
- Avoid sharing towels or clothing.
- Wash before and after intercourse.
- Get a vaccination for hepatitis B. ■

S

SHINGLES

SYMPTOMS

- slight fever, malaise, chills, upset stomach.
- bruised feeling, usually on one side of your face or body.
- pain (often in the chest) that is followed several days later by tingling, itching, or prickling skin and an inflamed, red skin rash.
- a group or long strip of small, fluid-filled blisters.
- deep burning, searing, aching, or stabbing pain, which may be continuous or intermittent.

*(See also the **Visual Diagnostic Guide**.)*

CALL YOUR DOCTOR IF:

- you suspect an outbreak is beginning; antiviral drugs taken in the early stages may shorten the course of the infection.
- shingles on your face spreads near your eye; get treatment to avoid possible cornea damage.
- the affected area becomes secondarily infected with bacteria (indicated by spreading redness, swelling, a high fever, and pus); ***antibiotics*** can help halt the spread.
- your rash lasts longer than 10 days without improvement; get treatment to avoid potential nerve damage.
- the pain becomes too great to bear; your doctor may prescribe stronger ***analgesics*** or a nerve block.

Shingles is a reactivation of the herpes zoster virus in which painful skin blisters erupt on one side of your face or body. Typical shingles begins with a general feeling of malaise accompanied by a slight fever and a tingling sensation or pain on one side of your body. Within days a rash appears in that same area in a line along the affected nerve, and a group of small, fluid-filled blisters crops up. Typically, this occurs along your chest, abdomen, back, or face, but it may also affect your neck, limbs, or lower back. The area can be excruciatingly painful, itchy, and tender. After one to two weeks the blisters heal and form scabs, although the pain continues.

The deep pain that follows after the infection has run its course is known as postherpetic ***neuralgia.*** It can continue for months or even years, especially in older people. Shingles usually occurs only once, although it has been known to recur in some people.

CAUSES

Shingles arises from the same virus, herpes zoster, that causes ***chickenpox.*** Following a bout of chickenpox, the virus becomes dormant in the spinal nerve cells, but it can be reactivated at a time when the immune system is suppressed—by physical or emotional trauma or a serious illness. Medical science doesn't understand why the virus becomes reactivated in some people and not in others.

TREATMENT

No treatment has yet been discovered to prevent or halt shingles, and although steps can be taken to shorten its duration, frequently the virus must simply run its course. Because the pain following shingles is difficult to manage and can last so long—months or, in rare cases, years—the best approach is early and immediate treatment. Also, early medical attention may prevent or reduce the scarring that shingles can cause.

CONVENTIONAL MEDICINE

Your doctor may suggest medications to reduce inflammation and help you cope with the pain. ***Analgesics*** such as ***aspirin*** or ***acetaminophen*** can alleviate mild pain. Oral, topical, or intravenous use of ***acyclovir,*** an antiviral drug, may help stop progression of the rash. A short course of ***corticosteroids*** either taken orally or applied as a cream can reduce inflammation. Vidarabine monohydrate is another prescription medication that prevents blisters from spreading; it also helps decrease pain and speed healing. Benzoin, available over the counter, may protect irritated skin when applied to unbroken lesions. If the area becomes infected by bacteria, ***antibiotics*** can keep the infection under control. For the pain that lingers after lesions have healed, your doctor may prescribe a ***tricyclic antidepressant,*** which in small doses helps relieve pain.

ALTERNATIVE CHOICES

In addition to the remedies mentioned below, you might want to consult an **acupuncturist** or a **homeopath** for treatments to speed healing or shorten the duration of the disease.

HERBAL THERAPIES

Dabbing or sponging lesions with a solution of lemon balm *(Melissa officinalis)* or **calendula** *(Calendula officinalis)* may reduce inflammation. Make a 50-50 mixture of tincture and boiled, then cooled, water. You can also try three daily applications of a commercially prepared gel made from an extract of ***licorice*** *(Glycyrrhiza glabra),* which appears to interfere with virus growth. An over-the-counter cream made from ***cayenne*** *(Capsicum frutescens)* might decrease the pain of shingles, but it is extremely hot and should be applied only after blisters have healed and never on broken skin.

NUTRITION AND DIET

For relief of postherpetic pain, take 1,200 to 1,600 IU of ***vitamin E*** daily, but for no more than two weeks, only under a doctor's care, and only if you don't have ***high blood pressure.*** To alleviate symptoms once the disease has begun, take 500 mg one to three times a day of the amino acid L-lysine, but only for one week. Studies have shown that this works best if you avoid foods containing the amino acid arginine, such as chocolate, cereal grains, nuts, and seeds.

AT-HOME REMEDIES

- Keep the affected area clean, dry, and exposed to air (without clothes covering it) as much as possible. Don't scratch or burst the blisters. If the pain keeps you from sleeping, snugly bind the area with an elastic sports bandage.
- For the first three or four days, try ice for 10 minutes on, 5 minutes off, every few hours. Later, apply cool, wet compresses soaked in aluminum acetate, available over the counter in the form of astringent solution, powder packets, or effervescent tablets.
- To desensitize nerve endings, crush two ***aspirin,*** mix them with 2 tbsp rubbing alcohol, and apply the paste to lesions three times a day. To cut down on itching, ask your pharmacist to mix 78 percent calamine lotion with 20 percent rubbing alcohol, 1 percent ***phenol,*** and 1 percent ***menthol.*** You can apply this mixture continuously until your blisters scab over. Other remedies for itching include frequent applications of ***vitamin E*** oil, gel from the aloe vera plant, or fresh leeks that have been chopped in a food processor. Dusting colloidal oatmeal powder where clothes rub against your skin can reduce pain.

PREVENTION

Because shingles comes on suddenly, with scarcely any warning, there is little you can do in the way of prevention, but your doctor may be able to avert the pain that follows. Some pain experts have had success using a nerve block during the acute phase of the disease. Administered on an outpatient basis in a hospital to deaden pain and shrink inflammation at the nerve root, a nerve block may act as a preemptive strike against later development of postherpetic neuralgia. ■

SHIN SPLINTS

SYMPTOMS

Shin splints are characterized by pain, aching, and occasionally, swelling anywhere in the lower leg. However, the pain is most often in the locations described below:

- on the front of the leg, toward the inside.
- on the inner side of the leg, toward the back.

CALL YOUR DOCTOR IF:

- you have a hard swelling, numbness, tingling, and severe pain in your lower leg. You may have ruptured a tendon, a condition requiring immediate medical attention.
- you feel pain concentrated in a small area anywhere along the inside part of the lower leg bone. The area is sensitive to the touch and does not seem to "warm up" with sports activity. This could mean that you have a stress fracture, which requires medical evaluation.
- your symptoms persist or worsen after three to seven days. You may have muscle or tendon damage that requires the attention of a doctor.

Shin splints, one of the most common ailments of active people, is a general term referring to pain in the lower leg. Experts differ when explaining what the exact condition is, although most agree that it involves the two muscles that run from the knee to the ankle and the side of the foot, swathing the tibia, or shinbone. These muscles point the foot up and down, and support the arch and the front of the foot to keep it from slapping while walking and running. Injuries that result in small tears in the fibers of these muscles bring on shin splints.

Shin splints may also be related to a condition known as **compartment syndrome,** in which a muscle grows too large for its outer sheath. Stress fractures of the tibia and irritation to the nerves in the shin are also associated with shin splints.

CAUSES

Any unusual or repetitive stress to the lower leg can bring on shin splints. Seasoned athletes and novices alike suffer from the ailment, with runners, cyclists, skiers, and aerobic dancers being especially vulnerable. People who have flat feet, knock-knees, or bowlegs place abnormal stress on their legs and are likely to suffer from shin splints. Poorly cushioned shoes, exercising on unyielding surfaces such as concrete, and poor posture can contribute to the condition.

TREATMENT

Most approaches focus on ensuring adequate rest to allow for healing, followed by a program of strengthening exercises designed to ward off recurrences. It is important to start treatment when the condition first makes itself evident. Ignoring

CAUTION!

If you suffer from *circulatory problems, diabetes,* or *heart disease,* avoid massage and applications of heat or cold until you consult your doctor.

S

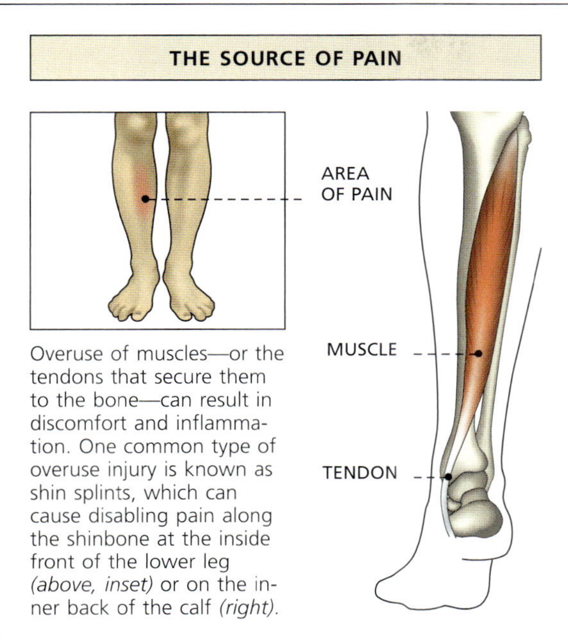

Overuse of muscles—or the tendons that secure them to the bone—can result in discomfort and inflammation. One common type of overuse injury is known as shin splints, which can cause disabling pain along the shinbone at the inside front of the lower leg *(above, inset)* or on the inner back of the calf *(right)*.

the early nagging pain—or attempting to tough it out—will only worsen shin splints.

CONVENTIONAL MEDICINE

Doctors usually recommend the sports medicine therapy RICE (rest, ice, compression, and elevation) as initial treatment for shin splints. *(See box on page 770.)* They often prescribe crutches to keep weight off the injured leg, and ***aspirin*** or ***ibuprofen*** to reduce inflammation and pain. Your doctor may recommend that you see a physical therapist for an exercise program and may suggest ultrasound treatment to relax the muscles, improve circulation, and promote healing.

ALTERNATIVE CHOICES

There are a number of alternative treatments that complement the conventional therapies described above. Many employ massage.

ACUPRESSURE

After gently massaging the affected area, apply gradual, steady pressure to Stomach 36, four finger widths below the kneecap, one finger width outside the shinbone. (The muscle you press is the one that flexes as you move your foot up and down.) The pressure should not cause pain. Try for three minutes, three times a day. *(See the* ***Appendix*** *for more information on locating this point.)*

CHINESE HERBS

A Chinese herbal practitioner might apply a poultice of gardenia *(Gardenia jasminoides),* flour, and wine to reduce swelling and to promote healing. Practitioners also may recommend moxibustion, in which a smoldering piece of ***mugwort leaf*** *(Artemisia argyi)* is held about an inch above the affected area. The process is thought to increase circulation and promote healing. Also perhaps helpful is a massage technique in which the ball of the thumb is used to alternately press hard and rub lightly on the sore area.

AT-HOME REMEDIES

Other than treatments from a physical therapist, you can apply all of the standard conventional and alternative therapies for shin splints at home. Remember RICE. Keep off your feet to rest your legs. Apply ice in alternating intervals, 10 minutes on, 10 minutes off. Wrap your leg in an elastic sports bandage to compress the tissues and counteract swelling. And keep your legs elevated to reduce blood pressure in the inflamed tissues.

PREVENTION

The key to preventing shin splints is finding as many ways as possible to cut down on the stresses that tend to cause the injury. Wear supportive shoes, and check with a podiatrist about inserts to help correct postural difficulties that may contribute to shin splints. Before and after exercising, stretch the muscles in the toes, heel, knee, and lower leg to help condition the muscles and make them more resistant to injury. Be sure to exercise on resilient surfaces such as wood or earth, not on unyielding concrete. ■

SHOULDER PAIN

Read down this column to find your symptoms. Then read across.

SYMPTOMS	AILMENT/PROBLEM
◆ pain in the shoulders and possibly other joints that begins after taking a new medication.	◆ Common reaction to medications such as oral contraceptives, ***penicillin,*** and some ***antianxiety drugs***
◆ pain, stiffness, and swelling in both shoulders; worst upon awakening and dissipates during the day or with rest; may be accompanied by similar symptoms in other joints (especially the fingers); fatigue; possibly, persistent low-grade fever, insomnia, weight loss.	◆ ***Arthritis***
◆ pain at the top, outer part of the shoulder that is worst upon awakening and may subside with normal activity but increases with stretching or exertion; inflammation; redness.	◆ ***Bursitis*** of the shoulder joint
◆ painfully tender and stiff shoulder that hurts more at night and may interrupt sleeping; shoulder may tingle, feel numb, or appear swollen.	◆ ***Tendonitis***
◆ shoulder pain in a specific spot that is worse with movement and follows injury, overexertion, or heavy lifting.	◆ Strained, inflamed, or torn tendon or ligament; torn muscle
◆ moderate to severe shoulder pain and stiffness that has worsened over several weeks; difficulty moving the arm in any direction.	◆ Frozen shoulder (a severe ***inflammation*** of the shoulder joint)
◆ sudden pain in the shoulder joint that accompanies flu or another infection.	◆ Side effect of an ***infection***
◆ sudden, intense shoulder pain; inflammation; shoulder feels hot to the touch, but there is no fever.	◆ Accumulation of crystals in the shoulder joint
◆ a painful, possibly misshapen shoulder that is impossible to move; usually caused by an accident.	◆ Fractured bone or dislocated shoulder joint

WHAT TO DO	OTHER INFO
◆ Ask your doctor about possible alternative medications.	
◆ A ***nonsteroidal anti-inflammatory drug (NSAID)*** or ***aspirin,*** combined with applied heat, can relax muscles and reduce pain and inflammation. Get adequate rest and regular, gentle exercise (such as swimming) to expand your shoulder's range of motion and help suppress symptoms.	◆ Your doctor or chiropractor can suggest many other drugs and procedures that may alleviate pain and inflammation.
◆ Immobilize the shoulder as much as possible. Take ***nonsteroidal anti-inflammatory drugs (NSAIDs), aspirin,*** or the homeopathic remedy ***Bryonia*** (30c) to reduce pain and inflammation.	◆ If bursitis does not heal itself in a few days, call your doctor.
◆ ***Aspirin, ibuprofen,*** or other ***nonsteroidal anti-inflammatory drugs (NSAIDs)*** may relieve pain and swelling. Follow the RICE regimen: rest, ice, compression, and elevation.	◆ Wearing a triangle-shaped sling immobilizes your arm and helps rest your shoulder to promote healing, and is especially helpful when sleeping.
◆ To minimize inflammation and pain, use the RICE regimen: rest, ice, compression, and elevation. *(See **Tendonitis.**)* Call your doctor if pain does not lessen in 24 hours; a torn muscle may require prompt surgery.	◆ Supporting the arm in a sling takes weight off the shoulder and can dramatically reduce pain. The homeopathic remedies ***Arnica*** (30c) and ***Ruta*** (30c) may help speed the healing. See also ***Sprains and Strains.***
◆ Treat as you would ***bursitis.***	◆ Be patient; frozen shoulder can last for six months to several years.
◆ ***Nonsteroidal anti-inflammatory drugs (NSAIDs)*** may lessen the pain.	
◆ See ***Gout.*** Call your doctor. Left untreated, gout can lead to kidney damage.	◆ Gout is caused by uric acid crystals. A related condition, pseudogout, is caused by a type of calcium crystal.
◆ **Seek medical care immediately.** Do not move the arm or shoulder. Whatever its position, stabilize it. *(See **Emergencies/First Aid: Fractures and Dislocations.**)*	◆ Expect to wear a cast or splint for a few weeks to allow healing. The homeopathic remedies ***Arnica*** (30c) and ***Ruta*** (30c) may help speed the healing.

S

SICKLE CELL ANEMIA

SYMPTOMS

- episodes of severe pain, primarily at the joints, in the abdomen, or along the arms and legs.
- fatigue, pallor or ***jaundice,*** and rapid heartbeat, indicating ***anemia.***
- susceptibility to infections.
- in affected children, delayed growth and development, including delayed sexual maturation.
- priapism, a painful, persistent erection; sometimes experienced by affected teenage and adult males.

CALL YOUR DOCTOR IF:

- your infant's hands or feet swell and the baby shows signs of anemia; such symptoms are often the first indication of the disease.
- your affected child has a fever of 101°F or higher, often an indicator of a bacterial infection (which can quickly become fatal); or the child has seizures, becomes irritable, or is lethargic—symptoms of a neurological problem. **Seek emergency medical care immediately.**
- your affected child's abdomen is distended and rigid, and the child shows signs of anemia; this might indicate pooling of blood in the spleen, a life-threatening situation. **Seek emergency medical care immediately.**
- painful episodes persist more than several hours; intramuscular or intravenous pain relievers, or perhaps hospitalization, may be necessary.

Sickle cell anemia is one of the most common forms of an inherited blood disorder called sickle cell disease. People of African descent are at greatest risk. To develop sickle cell anemia, a person must inherit two sickle cell genes. When only one gene is present, a person has another form of sickle cell disease known as sickle cell trait. People with sickle cell trait do not generally experience symptoms except occasionally under low-oxygen conditions, such as when scuba-diving or at high altitudes. They can also pass on the gene, and possibly the disease, to their children.

In addition to having the symptoms of ***anemia,*** people with sickle cell anemia may also experience episodes known as crises, which affect various parts of the body. How often these crises occur varies from person to person. Repeated crises can lead to organ failure and even death.

The vaso-occlusive, or painful, crisis is by far the most common. It causes mild to severe pain in oxygen-deprived tissues, organs, or joints. A painful crisis can be triggered by dehydration, infection, stress, trauma, exposure, lack of oxygen, or strenuous physical activity.

Aplastic and hyperhemolytic crises can lead to severe anemia. In aplastic crises, the bone marrow temporarily stops producing red blood cells. In a hyperhemolytic crisis, the red blood cells break down too rapidly to be replaced adequately. The fourth type of crisis, splenic sequestration, is usually a childhood difficulty that occurs when blood becomes trapped in the spleen, causing the organ to enlarge and possibly leading to death.

Because this disease can be life-threatening, early diagnosis and treatment is vital.

CAUSES

People with sickle cell disease receive a gene for abnormal hemoglobin (the oxygen-carrying protein in red blood cells) from each parent. Red blood cells are normally round and flexible. Cells with abnormal hemoglobin are crescent shaped and less flexible, causing them to break down rapidly, leading to anemia. Viral infections can trigger aplastic and hyperhemolytic crises. Painful crises are caused by the sickled cells becoming trapped in smaller blood vessels and preventing oxygen from reaching surrounding tissues.

DIAGNOSTIC AND TEST PROCEDURES

Sickle cell screening of newborns is required in 30 states. A blood test can identify people with the trait or the disease. Prenatal tests can detect the disease in unborn babies. Genetic testing is available for couples who plan to become parents.

TREATMENT

At present, no cure exists; but with proper management, people with the disease can lead productive lives. If you or your child has sickle cell anemia, be sure to choose a doctor who is very familiar with the disease and its complications.

CONVENTIONAL MEDICINE

It is important to protect an affected child from infections, which can lead to dangerous complications—including death. Because their spleens do not function properly, children with sickle cell anemia are at great risk for such serious infections as ***meningitis, hepatitis,*** peritonitis, osteomyelitis (bone infection), and ***pneumonia.*** In addition to standard immunizations, your child should also receive vaccines for influenza and pneumococcus. Your child's pediatrician will probably also prescribe a preventive course of ***penicillin*** by mouth daily from the age of two months to five years. You will be advised of other preventive steps you can take to avoid crises *(see **Prevention,** below).* In addition, you and your family may be referred to a counselor to deal with the emotional issues of this disease.

During crises, hospitalization will probably be required. Hydroxyurea, a drug used to treat other blood disorders, is being tested in the management of sickle cell anemia in adults; it seems to reduce the severity of painful crises.

ALTERNATIVE CHOICES

Not much is known about the effectiveness of various alternative treatments for sickle cell anemia. **Acupuncture** may be able to help mitigate painful crises. Seek professional advice.

LIFESTYLE

Sickle cell crises can disrupt personal and family life. Parents will want to help an affected child grow up as normally as possible. Let teachers know of your child's illness and teach them how to deal with a crisis; ask them to provide assignments when your child is homebound.

PREVENTION

Avoiding the triggers that can precipitate crises is an important preventive step. Maintaining a good diet, drinking plenty of fluids, taking regular, moderate exercise, and getting enough sleep will help prevent dehydration and fatigue and keep the body strong. To guard against infection, take care of wounds, practice good oral hygiene, and have regular checkups. Children with the disease should be current with all immunizations. ■

ABNORMAL BLOOD CELLS

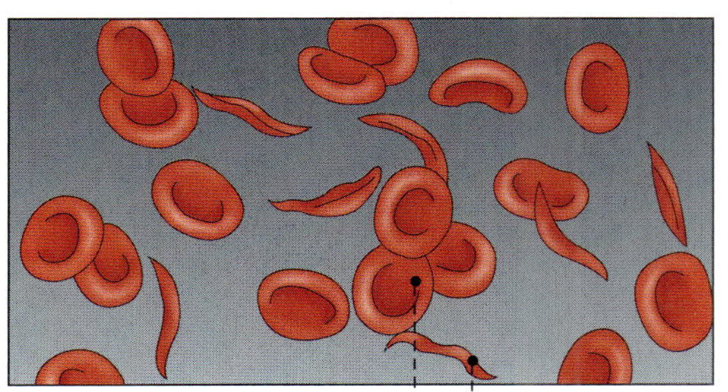

As they deliver oxygen to body tissues, normal, round red blood cells slip easily through tiny capillaries. Cells carrying abnormal hemoglobin—the oxygen-transporting protein in blood—tend to collapse into a crescent, or sickle, shape. Because narrow capillaries cannot accommodate the oddly shaped cells, blood flow is impaired and surrounding tissue is starved of oxygen.

SINUSITIS

SYMPTOMS

- feeling of fullness in the face.
- pressure behind the eyes.
- nasal obstruction, difficulty breathing through the nose.
- ***postnasal drip.***
- foul smell in the nose.
- fever (possibly).
- toothache (possibly).

CALL YOUR DOCTOR IF:

- sinusitis develops into an inflammation around the eye (orbital cellulitis), which could cause damage to the eye and facial nerves.
- the condition does not improve within seven days.
- sinusitis recurs more than three times in a year, and periods between bouts grow shorter; you may have a chronic infection that could become serious.

Sinusitis is an infection or inflammation of the sinuses, the air-filled pockets in the bones of the face. One of the most common healthcare complaints in the United States, sinusitis affects as many as 30 to 50 million Americans a year. Some researchers estimate that as much as 14 percent of the country's population suffers chronic (long-term) sinusitis.

Of all the human body's mysterious components, the sinuses are among the most puzzling. Some scientists believe that the sinuses function mainly as mucus factories for the nose and throat. Others say these hollow chambers help warm the air we breathe, still others that they exist merely to lighten the skull.

All humans have four pairs of sinuses *(below, right),* which connect to the nasal passages through a series of holes and interconnections. Mucus forms on the surfaces of the sinuses, which are also covered with tiny hairs called cilia. When we breathe, the mucus traps dirt brought in by the air; then the cilia push the mucus out through tiny openings that serve as drains. These openings, known as ostia, are very small, in some cases measuring only a few millimeters across. While the frontal, sphenoidal, and ethmoidal sinuses have ostia at the bottom, the maxillary sinuses have their ostia at the top. Consequently, mucus has to drain upward from these cavities, against the pull of gravity. Given that humans walk erect, it's not surprising that sinus problems are common.

CAUSES

Sinusitis occurs when the mucus-producing linings of the sinuses become inflamed, and by far the most frequent cause of this condition is blockage of the ostia. Once these openings are clogged, foreign material can't get out, oxygen levels drop, and bacteria in the nasal cavity slither into the sinuses, causing the sinus walls to swell and fill with pus. If the infection doesn't go away, the body sends in disease-fighting cells to kill the bacteria. Unfortunately, these well-intentioned bodyguards can themselves do considerable damage to the sinus walls. Defender cells can damage the cilia, the hairlike structures that help expel foreign matter. Furthermore, scarring caused by the cells' battles can result in the formation of sores. Large, mushroom-shaped growths called ***nasal polyps*** can also appear inside the nose, interfering with breathing and setting the stage for other problems. Almost invariably, the invading bacteria seek out and colonize adjacent sinuses. More than 40 percent of all sinusitis patients, in fact, are affected in more than one pair of sinuses.

The most common cause of blockage of the ostia is an upper respiratory tract viral infection, such as a ***common cold*** or the ***flu.*** These conditions increase secretions in the nasal passageways, provoke swelling of the sinus walls, and cause the cilia to malfunction. Allergic reactions can have the same effect. ***Hay fever*** often leads to sinusitis, but allergies to dust, animal dander, foods, smoke, and other pollutants can also trigger reactions that result in blocked sinuses.

In some cases, the ostia are blocked by unusual anatomical features—preexisting nasal polyps, a deviated septum, foreign bodies, or tumors, for example. Certain diseases, including ***diabetes*** and HIV infections, can create a predisposition to sinusitis. And people with poorly working mucus and ciliary functions, such as patients with cystic fibrosis, have a better-than-average chance of coming down with the condition. Sinusitis is also common among people with chronic ***tonsillitis*** and ***adenoid problems.***

THE SINUSES

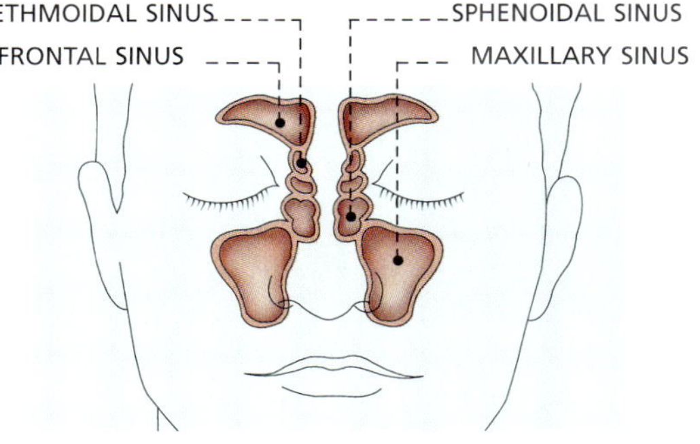

The bones of the face contain air-filled cavities called sinuses. Normally, mucus produced in the sinuses traps debris and drains out through small openings. But if these openings get clogged, foreign material cannot escape. The sinus linings may become inflamed and swollen, causing the pressure, pain, and congestion of sinusitis.

DIAGNOSTIC AND TEST PROCEDURES

In most cases, doctors diagnose sinusitis based on their "clinical impression," or the sum total of your symptoms, medical history, and the results of a physical examination. Some doctors prefer to verify this impression with a test called transillumination. In this procedure, the doctor shines a special flashlight into your nose and examines the roof of your mouth for signs of sinus congestion. Unfortunately, transillumination might not pick up an infection in a deep, distant sinus. Your doctor may also order an x-ray of your sinuses, but even this technique may not be sensitive enough to detect a deep infection.

Doctors often go ahead and assume you have sinusitis and prescribe medications accordingly. If your body doesn't respond after several attempts, they begin other tests. An otolaryngologist (ear, nose, and throat doctor) may insert a tiny tube into your nose and examine the sinuses directly, a technique known as an endoscopy. A CT scan can show swelling in the deep sinuses and reveal any anatomic abnormalities, but even these scans are not always reliable.

TREATMENT

The goal of most treatments is to open up the sinuses and restore proper drainage. If the sinuses are infected with bacteria, it is important to kill the disease organisms before they cause further damage or spread to other sinuses.

CONVENTIONAL MEDICINE

Before you start treating sinusitis, make sure you actually have it; sinusitis can be hard to distinguish from an upper respiratory tract infection, dental disorder, ***asthma,*** or even a ***headache.***

ACUPRESSURE

1 Pressing LI 20 may help relieve the pain, congestion, and swelling of sinusitis. Using the index fingers, gently press the points on either side of your nose. Apply pressure upward, underneath your cheekbones. Breathe deeply and hold for one minute.

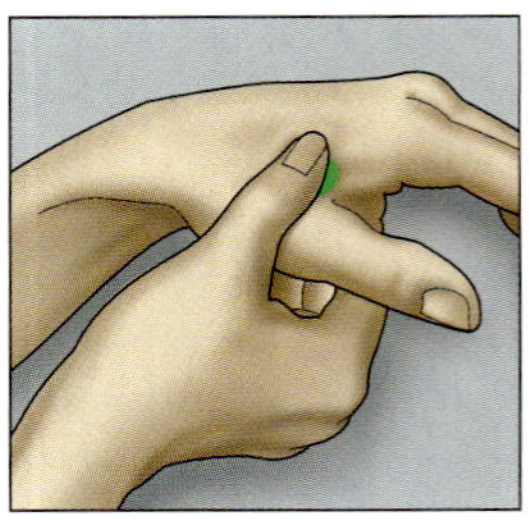

2 To ease headache pain and congestion, try pressing LI 4. With your right thumb, press into the webbing between the thumb and index finger of your left hand. Hold for one minute, then repeat on the other hand. (Do not use if you are pregnant.)

The bugs that most often invade the sinuses are frequent residents of the nose and throat—*Streptococcus pneumoniae* and *Hemophilus influenzae (H. flu).* These pathogens usually respond to such tried-and-true ***antibiotics*** as ampicillin and ***amoxicillin.*** However, because certain strains of *H. flu* have developed resistance to amoxicillin, some doctors prescribe other medications, such as ***sulfamethoxazole and trimethoprim*** and ***cefaclor.*** More-expensive choices are ***loracarbef, amoxicillin and clavulanate, azithromycin,*** and ***clarithromycin.***

Treatment usually lasts 7 to 14 days for acute cases, and from 2 to 3 weeks for chronic or recurrent cases. CAUTION: Stopping the antibiotic treatment prematurely may increase the infection's duration or severity.

Besides antibiotics, many doctors prescribe inhaled steroids such as ***beclomethasone*** or ***triamcinolone*** to reduce inflammation and open the sinuses so they can drain. ***Decongestants*** can also reduce swelling and help unclog the sinuses. Most doctors prefer oral decongestants, including ***pseudoephedrine,*** over nose sprays like ***oxymetazoline*** because sprays can become habit-forming if used for more than three days.

Drugs containing ***guaifenesin*** are used to break up hard, encrusted mucus, but they generally don't work very well. ***Antihistamines*** are not usually prescribed for sinusitis because they tend to make mucus thicker and less able to drain from clogged sinuses. Antihistamines may provide some relief, however, if your condition is caused by ***allergies.***

When sinusitis becomes chronic and other remedies fail, physicians may suggest a sinus washout or surgery. Washout procedures, in which the doctor uses a sterile saline solution to clean out the nasal passages, are rarely performed today. Instead, surgeons prefer surgical techniques such as antrostomy, which involves drilling a hole at the bottom of the frontal sinus to improve drainage. In another procedure, called endoscopic sinus surgery, physicians insert a tiny scope through the nose. Not only does the scope allow doctors to see the insides of the nasal cavities, but it also serves to open clogged passageways and remove dead cells from the sinus wall. Between 80 percent and 90 percent of patients report moderate to complete relief of symptoms with endoscopic surgery. Extremely rare side effects of this procedure include ***meningitis,*** blindness, or double vision *(see* ***Vision Problems****).*

ALTERNATIVE CHOICES

Many alternative therapies are attempts to relieve the pain of sinusitis and open the sinuses for drainage. Others aim to fight infection by boosting the immune system.

ACUPRESSURE

Applying gentle pressure to the face and hands can help ease the pain of sinusitis *(see the illustration above, left).*

ACUPUNCTURE

An acupuncturist will apply medium stimulation to various ear points—adrenal, forehead, internal nose, lung, and near the sinuses—to help drain the sinuses.

AROMATHERAPY

Inhalants of ***eucalyptus,*** pine, or thyme may help break up your clogged sinuses. You may also alleviate the symptoms by holding menthol or eucalyptus packs over your sinuses. Other suggestions: Gently swab your nasal passages with oil of bitter orange, or massage your face with essence of ***lavender*** mixed into vegetable oil.

CHINESE HERBS

The exact makeup of a prescribed mixture depends on whether the sinusitis is "hot" (acute or infectious) or "cold" (chronic or allergic). Either way, the preparation may include the Chinese herb ***ephedra*** *(Ephedra sinica),* a decongestant. (Do not use ephedra if you have hypertension or heart disease.) A number of other Chinese herbs are also helpful in relieving sinusitis symptoms. These include ***honeysuckle*** *(Lonicera japonica),* fritillary bulb *(Fritillaria cirrhosa),* ***tangerine peel*** *(Citrus reticulata),* xanthium fruit *(Xanthium sibiricum),* and ***magnolia flower*** *(Magnolia liliflora).*

HERBAL THERAPIES

Bromelain tablets have been shown in controlled studies to reduce inflammation, nasal discharge, headache, and breathing difficulties. You can give your immune system a boost with ***echinacea*** (*Echinacea* spp.), ***goldenseal*** *(Hydrastis canadensis),* or ***garlic*** *(Allium sativum),* preferably raw. Breathing the steam of clove *(Syzygium aromaticum)* tea or ***ginger*** *(Zingiber officinale)* root tea also provides some relief. To combat excessive mucus production, herbalists suggest elder *(Sambucus nigra)* flower, ***eyebright*** *(Euphrasia officinalis),* ***marsh mallow*** *(Althaea officinalis),* or goldenrod *(Solidago virgaurea).*

HOMEOPATHY

Homeopaths recommend specific remedies for various types of sinusitis discomfort. For acute sinusitis with thick, stringy mucus and pain in the cheeks or the bridge of the nose, use ***Kali bichromicum*** (30c) once or twice a day. For sinusitis with intense facial pain, alternating chills and sweat, and smelly yellow-green discharge from the nose and mouth, use ***Mercurius vivus*** (30c) twice a day. For acute sinusitis with a clear, thin discharge, sneezing, headache, and a stopped-up nose at night, use ***Nux vomica*** (30c) twice a day. For sinusitis with thick, light yellow or green nasal discharge accompanied by low spirits and lack of thirst, use ***Pulsatilla*** (30c) twice a day. If symptoms linger for more than two days, seek the advice of a professional homeopath.

NUTRITION AND DIET

A good healthful diet including fruits and raw green vegetables can help stimulate secretions and break up sinusitis. Nutritionists also suggest the following supplements to the diet: ***vitamin C,*** 500 mg every two hours; bioflavonoids, 1 gram per day; beta carotene *(see* ***vitamin A****),* 25,000 IU per day; and zinc lozenges, 23 mg every two waking hours for up to one week. Stay away from foods that you suspect may trigger an allergic reaction.

AT-HOME REMEDIES

- Inhale steam from a vaporizer, a humidifier, a mixture of hot water and vinegar, or even a cup of tea or coffee. Steam is one of the best and least-expensive remedies for unclogging sinuses.
- Use warm compresses on your nose to help open your sinuses.
- Drink plenty of liquids.
- Practice deep breathing exercises to keep your sinuses open.

PREVENTION

It's difficult to prevent sinusitis, but you can reduce your chances of having your sinuses become infected. First, avoid allergenic substances. Allergens that people don't often think of include the dust in their beds and certain foods, such as dairy products and wheat. Whenever possible, avoid cigarette smoke. Note: People with diabetes, cystic fibrosis, and certain other diseases may be prone to sinusitis. For help in preventing respiratory infections, see ***Common Cold*** and ***Flu.*** ■

SKIN CANCER

SYMPTOMS

The general warning signs of skin cancer include:
- any change in size, color, shape, or texture of a mole or other skin growth.
- an open or inflamed skin wound that won't heal.

Melanoma, the most dangerous type of skin cancer, may appear as:
- a change in an existing mole.
- a small, dark, multicolored spot with irregular borders—either elevated or flat—that may bleed and form a scab.
- a cluster of shiny, firm, dark bumps.

Basal cell carcinoma (BCC) may appear on sun-exposed skin as:
- a pearly or flesh-colored oval bump with a rolled border, which may develop into a bleeding ulcer.
- a smooth red spot indented in the center.
- a reddish, brown, or bluish black patch of skin on the chest or back.

Squamous cell carcinoma (SCC) may appear on sun-exposed skin as:
- a firm, reddish, wartlike bump that grows gradually.
- a flat spot that becomes a bleeding sore that won't heal.

*(See also the **Visual Diagnostic Guide.**)*

S

CALL YOUR DOCTOR IF:

- an existing mole changes size, shape, color, or texture; or you develop a very noticeable new mole as an adult.
- a new skin growth or open sore does not heal or disappear in a few weeks.

All skin cancers originate in the outer layer of skin known as the epidermis. In the normal course of skin rejuvenation, basal cells located at the base of the epidermis move upward to replace dead cells constantly being shed from the skin's surface. Along the way, the round basal cells are transformed into flat squamous cells. Throughout the epidermis are melanocytes, cells that produce a protective pigment called melanin.

Skin cancers fall into two major categories: **melanoma** and **nonmelanoma. Melanoma** is cancer of melanocytes, affecting about 1 in 10 skin cancer patients. It can start in heavily pigmented tissue, such as a mole or birthmark, as well as in normally pigmented skin. Melanoma usually appears first on the torso, although it can arise on the palm of the hand; on the sole of the foot; under a fingernail or toenail; in the mucous linings of the mouth, vagina, or anus; and even in the eye. Melanoma is an extremely virulent, life-threatening cancer. It is readily detectable and always curable if treated early, but it progresses faster than other types of skin cancer and tends to spread beyond the skin. Once this occurs, melanoma becomes very difficult to treat and cure.

The two most common skin cancers, **basal cell carcinoma (BCC)** and **squamous cell carcinoma (SCC),** are **nonmelanomas,** which are rarely life-threatening. They progress slowly, seldom spread beyond the skin, are detected easily, and usually are curable. **BCC,** which accounts for nearly 3 out of 4 skin cancers, is the slowest growing; **SCC** is somewhat more aggressive and more inclined to spread. In addition, there are a few rare nonmelanomas, such as **Kaposi's sarcoma,** a potentially life-threatening disease characterized by purple growths and often associated with ***AIDS.***

Some technically noncancerous skin growths have the potential to become cancerous. The most common are **actinic keratoses**—crusty reddish lesions that may scratch off but grow back on sun-exposed skin. Another precancerous skin growth, **cutaneous horns,** appears as funnel-shaped growths that extend from a red base on the skin.

Every malignant skin tumor in time becomes visible on the skin's surface, making skin cancer the only type of cancer that is almost always detectable in its early, curable stages. Prompt detection and treatment of skin cancer is equivalent to cure.

Skin cancer is by far the most common cancer in the world. Most cases are cured, but the disease is a major health concern because it affects so many people. Over 700,000 cases of nonmelanoma skin cancer are diagnosed annually in the United States alone, and about 32,000 cases of melanoma. Of the 9,000 or so deaths from skin cancer in the U.S. each year, about 7,000 are from melanoma. Skin cancer tends to strike people of light skin color; dark-skinned people are rarely affected, and then only on light areas of the body such as the soles of the feet or under fingernails or toenails. An estimated 40 to 50 percent of fair-skinned people who live to be 65 will develop at least one skin cancer. The incidence of skin cancer is predictably higher in places with intense sunshine, such as Arizona and Hawaii; it is most common in Australia, settled largely by fair-skinned people of Irish and English descent.

TWO SKIN CANCERS

Seen as a pinkish bump on the skin's surface, basal cell carcinoma develops in the bottom, or basal, cell layer of the epidermis, the top layer of the skin *(above, left)*. Melanomas, formed by dark pigment-producing cells called melanocytes, also begin in the epidermis *(above, right)*. Because they often spread through the dermis layer to other parts of the body, melanomas are considered extremely dangerous.

CAUSES

Excessive exposure to sunlight is the main cause of skin cancer. Sunlight contains ultraviolet (UV) rays that can alter the genetic material in skin cells, causing mutations. Sunlamps, tanning booths, and x-rays also generate UV rays that can damage skin and cause malignant cell mutations. **BCC** and **SCC** have been linked to chronic sun exposure, typically in fair-skinned people who work outside. **Melanoma** is associated with infrequent but excessive sunbathing that causes scorching sunburn. One blistering sunburn during childhood appears to double a person's risk for developing melanoma later in life. *(See **Sunburn.**)*

Fair-skinned people are most susceptible because they are born with the least amount of protective melanin. Redheads, blue-eyed blonds, and people with pigment disorders such as albinism bear the greatest risk. But people with many freckles or moles, particularly abnormal-looking ones, may also be vulnerable to melanoma. Workers regularly exposed to coal tar, radium, inorganic arsenic compounds in insecticides, and certain other carcinogens are at slightly higher than normal risk for nonmelanoma skin cancer.

The incidence of skin cancer is rising, even though most cases could be prevented by limiting skin's exposure to ultraviolet radiation. Skin cancer is about three times more common in men than in women, and the risk increases with age. Most people diagnosed with skin cancer are between ages 40 and 60, although all forms of the disease are appearing more often in younger people. If you or any close relatives have had skin cancer, you are more likely to get the disease.

DIAGNOSTIC AND TEST PROCEDURES

If you are in a high-risk group for skin cancer or have ever been treated for some form of the disease, you should familiarize yourself with how skin cancers look *(see the **Visual Diagnostic Guide**)*. Examine your skin from head to toe every few months, using a full-length mirror and hand mirror to check your mouth, nose, scalp, palms, soles, backs of ears, genital area, and between the buttocks. Cover every inch of skin and pay special attention to moles and sites of previous skin cancer. If you find a suspicious growth, have it examined by your doctor or dermatologist.

All potentially cancerous skin growths must be biopsied to confirm a cancer diagnosis. Depending on the suspected type of skin cancer, the biopsy techniques vary slightly but crucially. Any potential **melanoma** requires a surgical biopsy, in which the entire growth is removed with a scalpel. A pathologist then studies the sample under a microscope to determine whether cancer cells are present. If cancer exists and it is melanoma, grains of melanin will be visible in the cancer cells. Skin growths that may be melanoma tumors should never be removed by shaving, burning, or freezing because those techniques do not allow pathologic examination of the growth. Eye melanomas usually are not biopsied because they are virtually unmistakable to an experienced ophthalmologist. If melanoma is diagnosed, other tests may be ordered to assess the degree of cancer spread. Skin growths that are most likely **BCC, SCC,** or other forms of **nonmelanoma** can be biopsied in various ways. Part or all of the growth can be taken with a scalpel, or a thin layer can be shaved off for examination under a microscope.

AND THIS LITTLE PIGGY HAS NONE!

Each of us is defended by an army of immune cells that protect the body from attack. Some immune cells target invaders such as bacteria and viruses; others—including killer T cells—target cancer. T cells easily find and neutralize lone cancer cells that occasionally appear in the body. But if cancer cells begin to multiply faster than T cells can kill them, the T cells appear to surrender, runaway cancer cells continue to multiply, and a tumor develops.

But can T cells be reinforced to counterattack a barrage of malignancy? In the case of melanoma in Sinclair swine, a breed of miniature pigs, the answer seems to be yes. Some 85 percent of Sinclair swine develop melanoma tumors within the first six weeks of life, but over the next month the tumors disappear. Researchers attribute this seemingly miraculous recovery to a special kind of T cell identified in the pigs. By isolating and studying these uniquely endowed killer T cells, researchers hope to develop melanoma treatments that will work in humans.

TREATMENT

Most skin cancers are detected and cured before they spread. Melanoma that has spread to other organs presents the greatest treatment challenge.

CONVENTIONAL MEDICINE

Standard treatments for localized **basal cell** and **squamous cell carcinomas** are safe and effective and cause few side effects. Small tumors can be removed with electric current, frozen with liquid nitrogen, or killed with low-dose radiation. Applying an ointment containing a chemotherapeutic agent called 5-fluorouracil to a superficial tumor for several weeks may also work. Larger localized tumors are removed surgically.

In rare cases where BCC or SCC has begun to spread beyond the skin, tumors are removed surgically and patients are treated with chemotherapy, radiation, or immunotherapy. Some patients with advanced SCC respond well to a combination of retinoic acid (a derivative of ***vitamin A***) and interferon (a type of disease-fighting protein produced in laboratories for cancer immunotherapy). Retinoic acid also seems to inhibit cancer recurrence in patients who have had tumors removed.

Melanoma tumors must be removed surgically, preferably before they spread beyond the skin into other organs or glands. The surgeon excises the tumor fully, along with a safe margin of surrounding tissue and possibly nearby lymph nodes. Neither radiation nor chemotherapy will cure advanced melanoma, but either treatment may slow the disease and relieve symptoms. Chemotherapy, sometimes in combination with immunotherapy—using interferon—is generally preferred. If melanoma spreads to the brain, radiation is used to slow the growth and control symptoms.

Immunotherapy is a relatively new field of cancer treatment that attempts to target and kill cancer cells by manipulating the body's immune system. Some of the most promising developments in the field of immunotherapy have sprung from efforts to cure advanced melanoma. Some researchers are treating advanced cases with vaccines, while others are using drugs such as interferon and interleukin 2 in an effort to stimulate immune cells into attacking melanoma cells more aggressively. Genetic manipulation of melanoma tumors may make them more vulnerable to attack by the immune system. Each of these experimental treatment approaches aims to immunize a patient's body against its own cancer—something the body cannot do naturally. *(See box at left.)*

People who have had skin cancer once are at risk for getting it again. Anyone who has been treated for skin cancer of any kind should have a checkup at least once a year. About 20 percent of skin cancer patients experience recurrence, usually within the first two years after diagnosis.

See ***Cancer*** for more information on treatments such as chemotherapy and radiation.

COMPLEMENTARY THERAPIES

Once skin cancer is diagnosed, the only acceptable treatment is medical care. Alternative approaches may be useful in cancer prevention and in combating nausea, vomiting, fatigue, and headaches from chemotherapy, radiation, or immunotherapy used to treat advanced skin cancer.

NUTRITION AND DIET

Skin experts know that the mineral ***zinc*** and the antioxidant ***vitamins A*** (beta carotene), ***C,*** and ***E*** can help repair damaged body tissue and promote healthy skin. Now researchers are trying to determine whether these and other nutrients might protect skin from the harmful effects of sunlight. To test the theory, selected skin cancer patients are given experimental supplements of these vitamins in the hope of preventing cancer recurrence.

HERBAL THERAPIES

Following the advice of a local herbalist, some light-skinned Zimbabweans have used a crude ointment from the root and bark of the African sausage tree *(Kigelia pinnata)* to treat skin cancer. While initial research indicates that kigelia extract can kill melanoma cells, further study is needed to determine whether or not a kigelia-based drug will effectively treat melanoma in humans.

PREVENTION

If you are susceptible to skin cancer, take the following precautions whenever possible:

- Avoid intense sun exposure by staying out of it from late morning through early afternoon.
- Outside, wear a hat, long sleeves, trousers, and sunglasses that block UV radiation.
- Use a sunscreen with a sun protection factor of 15 or higher whenever you are outside.
- Consider taking a ***B-complex vitamin;*** B vitamins contain a compound called PABA, the active ingredient in many sunscreens.
- Report suspicious skin lesions to a doctor at once, especially if you have abnormal-looking moles or a family history of melanoma.
- Check skin medications with your dermatologist; they may cause increased sun sensitivity.

C A U T I O N !

CHILDREN AND SKIN CANCER

Protect infants from direct sunlight at all times. Start teaching children early about the potential hazards of summer sun and the importance of sun protection. The effects of sun on skin accumulate over a lifetime, and one bad sunburn during childhood significantly increases the risk for melanoma. Women diagnosed with melanoma should not become pregnant until they are completely cured: In rare instances, melanoma cells have spread from a mother to her unborn child. ■

SNEEZING

SYMPTOMS

- A sneeze is usually set off by an irritated nose or a tickling sensation deep in the nasal passages that is relieved by an explosive involuntary expulsion of air.
- Sneezing can itself be a symptom—along with other symptoms such as an itchy, runny, or congested nose or itchy, watery eyes and mouth breathing—of either a head cold *(see **Common Cold**)* or an ***allergy.***

CALL YOUR DOCTOR IF:

- you begin sneezing and experience other allergy symptoms, such as those of ***asthma*** or ***eczema;*** you may have developed a sensitivity to certain irritants that you previously tolerated.

Sneezing is the body's way of eliminating irritants or a foreign object from the nasal passages. People sneeze for four basic reasons. They sneeze when they have a cold, to help clear the nose. They also sneeze when they have allergic rhinitis, or ***hay fever,*** to eliminate allergens from the nasal passages. People with vasomotor rhinitis, a condition characterized by a chronic runny nose, also sneeze occasionally. (The sneezing results from the blood vessels in the nose becoming supersensitive to humidity and temperature, and even to spicy foods.) The fourth common cause of sneezing is nonallergic rhinitis with eosinophilia syndrome, or NARES. People with this condition have the symptoms of chronic rhinitis but do not test positive for allergens. Instead, for some unknown reason, their bodies seem to release histamine, a chemical that produces allergy symptoms such as sneezing.

An occasional sneeze is nothing to worry about. Sneezing that is part of a cold will go away with the cold, usually in about a week. However, persistent sneezing or sneezing accompanied by other allergy symptoms—a runny or congested nose, a sore throat, or itchy, watery eyes—may be worth a trip to the doctor.

CAUSES

Sneezing is caused by an irritant in the nasal passages—anything from ground pepper and tiny foreign objects to pollen, mold, and other allergens.

TREATMENT

Most allergy-related sneezing can be successfully treated with over-the-counter ***antihistamines*** and by home care focused on reducing such allergens as dust, mold, and pet dander. If you have ***hay fever,*** you can also reduce your discomfort by taking appropriate precautions before going outside.

CONVENTIONAL MEDICINE

Your doctor will examine you and discuss your symptoms. You may be referred to an allergist for skin tests. Allergy shots, to desensitize you to a specific allergen, may be recommended. The first line of defense for persistent sneezing is home management and use of over-the-counter or nonsedating prescription ***antihistamines*** to dry the mucous membranes, or ***decongestants*** to shrink swollen blood vessels blocking the nose. Cromolyn sodium, usually prescribed as a nasal spray, helps allergy sufferers by preventing histamine from being released in the body. Cortisone nasal sprays, which reduce inflammation, may also bring relief and are effective for NARES sufferers.

ALTERNATIVE CHOICES

ACUPRESSURE

Steady pressure on the following points may help control sneezing: Triple Warmer 5, Gall Bladder 20, Large Intestine 20, and Large Intestine 4. In addition, pressing your finger across your upper lip, the point of Governing Vessel 26, may help you stop a sneeze. See the illustration above, right, and the ***Appendix*** for more information on point locations.

ACUPUNCTURE

For chronic sneezing, you may wish to consult an acupuncturist, who will examine you and target appropriate points based on the exam.

HERBAL THERAPIES

Hot teas made from either ***red clover*** *(Trifolium pratense)* or ***nettle*** *(Urtica dioica)* are thought to relieve allergy symptoms and make breathing easier by reducing inflammation.

C A U T I O N !

Never stifle a sneeze—you could force mucus into the middle ear or sinuses and cause an infection. In extreme cases, you could burst an eardrum from backed-up air pressure.

ACUPRESSURE

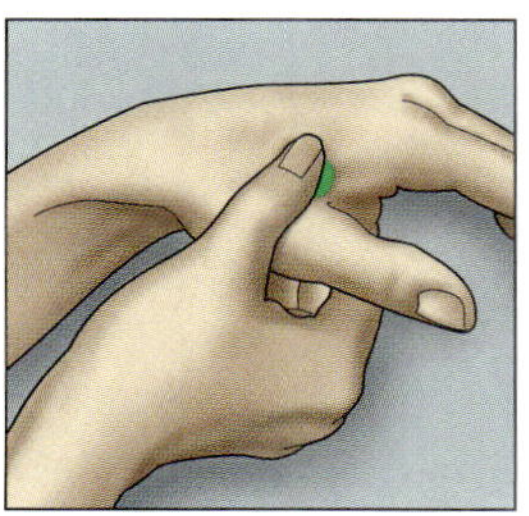

1 To help stop fits of sneezing, press Large Intestine 4, located in the web between the thumb and index finger. Squeeze the web of each hand with the thumb and index finger of the other for one minute. Do not press this point if you are pregnant.

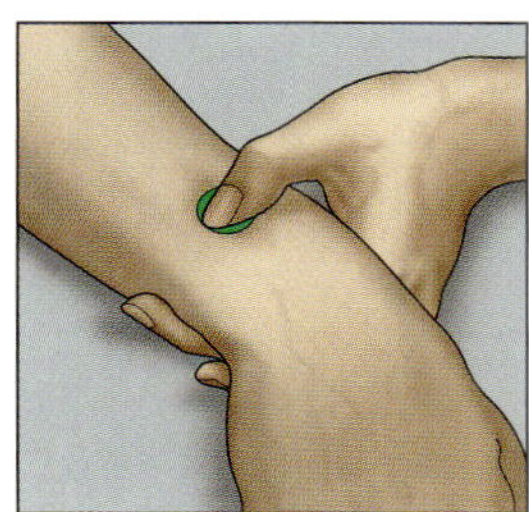

2 Pressing Triple Warmer 5 may help reduce allergic sensitivity. Center your thumb on the top of your forearm, two thumb widths above the wrist joint. Press firmly for one minute, then repeat on the other arm. Do two or three times.

HOMEOPATHY

Depending on your specific symptoms, a homeopathic physician may prescribe one of the following remedies: ***Nux vomica, Pulsatilla,*** or ***Natrum muriaticum.*** Remedies that are derived from pollen or other allergens may also work. For acute sneezing episodes, you may be prescribed ***Arsenicum album,*** *Sabadilla, Euphrasia,* ***Allium cepa,*** or *Dulcamara.*

NUTRITION AND DIET

You will want to seek professional help for allergies. Food allergies may aggravate hay fever. Try eliminating dairy products, food additives, and foods containing chemical residues such as pesticides or steroid hormone residues (often found in meats). Some nutritionists recommend high doses of ***vitamin C*** (3,000 to 6,000 mg, spread evenly throughout the day) as a natural antihistamine.

AT-HOME REMEDIES

Eliminating allergens in the home is one of the surest ways to alleviate chronic sneezing. Follow the suggestions listed for ***hay fever.*** ■

S

SNORING

SYMPTOMS

- rough, hoarse, fluttering noise when breathing during sleep, varying in frequency, pitch, and intensity.

CALL YOUR DOCTOR IF:

- you live with a snorer and note that his or her snoring is very loud or marked by intervals of no breathing at all. The person may have obstructive sleep apnea, a serious respiratory condition.
- you are frequently very sleepy and tired during the day. You could have obstructive sleep apnea, a serious condition that is preventing you from getting enough oxygen during sleep.
- you frequently fall asleep in inappropriate settings, such as at the office or while eating. You could have obstructive sleep apnea or narcolepsy, a disorder that causes sufferers to fall asleep during normal waking hours.

Snoring is usually not a serious problem. Men are 50 percent more likely to snore than women, but most people snore occasionally. Chronic snorers tend to be overweight and middle-aged.

Sometimes, though, snoring can point to a dangerous medical condition. The most serious is obstructive sleep apnea, in which the snorer stops breathing for anywhere from several seconds to two minutes. This results in decreased oxygen in the blood, which leads to fatigue at best and sudden death at worst. If you think you have this disorder, you must seek conventional treatment.

Other potentially troubling problems are also indicated by regular—often loud—snoring that falls into one of two types: moderate (snoring every time a person sleeps, but which may be intermittent or occurs only when the person lies on his back) and heavy (loud snoring throughout sleeping, no matter what position). Fortunately, there are a variety of remedies that can lessen the intensity of snoring, if not eliminate it entirely.

CAUSES

Snoring is caused by vibration of the soft palate (the soft part of the mouth's roof) as the lungs strain to inhale oxygen through obstructed airways. Typically this occurs when the muscles that keep these airways open become too lax; any condition or substance that promotes muscle relaxation—including alcohol; medications such as sleeping pills, cold medicines, or ***antihistamines;*** an overly soft or large pillow; sleeping on one's back; poor muscle tone; or ***obesity***—can have this effect. Obstruction can also be caused by nasal deformities, such as an excessively long soft palate or uvula, or a deviated septum. In children, enlarged adenoids or tonsils often cause snoring. Any ailment that makes bronchial airways constrict, such as ***asthma,*** can lead to obstruction and snoring; smoking, which irritates the passageways, can also make snoring worse.

DIAGNOSTIC AND TEST PROCEDURES

First, your physician will ask about any ***allergies*** you may have, as well as about your eating patterns, what drugs you take, and whether you drink alcohol or smoke. If these are not the culprits, your doctor may examine your throat and nasal passages for any signs of nasal deformities.

If your doctor suspects that you have obstructive sleep apnea, your partner may be asked to keep a diary noting your sleeping patterns, or you may be enrolled in a sleep-monitoring study, which will analyze when and how often you stop breathing during sleep.

TREATMENT

In most cases, snoring requires no medical treatment; going on a diet and cutting out smoking and alcohol usually clear up the problem. Alternative therapies can also help. In more serious cases, however, surgery may be necessary.

CONVENTIONAL MEDICINE

If snoring is light, no treatment may be necessary. If allergies are the cause, your physician will likely prescribe ***antihistamines*** or a nasal ***decongestant.*** Snoring caused by nasal deformities may require corrective surgery to open up the airways. If it is determined that you have obstructive sleep apnea, your doctor will pursue treatment more aggressively, because of the potentially dangerous consequences of the condition.

ALTERNATIVE CHOICES

If your snoring is due to ***allergies, asthma, bronchitis,*** or ***emphysema,*** there are a number of alternative remedies that may help you open up your airways and sleep more peacefully. Refer to the listed ailment entries for treatment advice.

PREVENTION

- Consider losing some weight: Most snorers tend to be overweight, and shedding excess fat has been shown to substantially decrease—if not eliminate—snoring.
- Avoid midnight snacks and alcoholic beverages: Drinking alcohol or eating heavily before going to sleep causes muscles to slacken.
- Avoid sleeping pills or other sedatives: Although they put you to sleep, they relax your neck muscles, making your snoring worse.
- Stop smoking: Smoking causes nasal and bronchial congestion, a major cause of snoring.
- Sleep on your side: While heavy snorers will snore in any position, moderates tend to snore only when sleeping on their backs. One way to avoid this is to sew a pocket onto the back of your nightclothes and insert a tennis ball, which will make it uncomfortable for you to lie on your back and prompt you to turn on your side during sleep.
- Sleep without a pillow: By putting a kink in your neck, pillows can contribute to airway obstruction. ■

OBSTRUCTIVE SLEEP APNEA

Between 1 and 5 percent of adults suffer from a snoring disorder that is no joke: obstructive sleep apnea. The condition, which generally targets men (a reported 9 out of 10 sufferers are men), occurs when breathing stops 30 or more times, for 10 or more seconds in each incident, during a 7-hour sleep period. People with serious cases of the disease may not breathe at all for up to three-quarters of the time that they are asleep. The result is not only oxygen deprivation but also ***high blood pressure;*** *in the very worst cases, the condition can be fatal. If you are a loud, heavy snorer, you may have sleep apnea and should consider enrolling in a sleep-study program, which will monitor your sleep patterns and help develop therapies for your recovery.*

S

SORE THROAT

SYMPTOMS

The classic symptoms of a sore throat include a burning sensation or "scratchiness" in the back of the throat; pain, especially when swallowing; and, perhaps, tenderness along the neck. These symptoms may be accompanied by:

- sneezing and coughing.
- hoarseness.
- runny nose.
- mild fever.
- general fatigue.

CALL YOUR DOCTOR IF:

- you also have a fever higher than 101°F without other cold symptoms; this may indicate a case of ***strep throat*** that needs treatment.
- you also have flulike symptoms that don't get better after a few days; this may indicate infectious ***mononucleosis.***
- any hoarseness lasts longer than two weeks; this could be a sign of ***throat cancer*** or ***oral cancer.***
- your sore throat persists for more than a week and is accompanied by ***postnasal drip;*** this may be a sign of ***allergies*** that require medical attention.
- your sore throat is accompanied by drooling, or you experience difficulty swallowing or breathing; this may indicate an inflamed epiglottis, the structure that overhangs the opening to the larynx, or an abscess in the back of the throat; these two uncommon conditions require medical attention.

Everyone knows what a sore throat feels like. It is one of the most common health complaints, particularly during the colder months of the year, when respiratory diseases are at their peak. Typically the raw, scratchy, burning feeling at the back of your throat is the first sign you'll have of a cold or the flu on the way. But a sore throat can also presage more serious conditions, so you should watch how it develops, and call your doctor if there are any signs that you have more than the run-of-the-mill type.

CAUSES

At least 90 percent of sore throats are caused by inflammation of throat tissue, often triggered by viral infections, including the ***common cold, flu, measles, chickenpox,*** herpes, and infectious ***mononucleosis.*** Bacterial infections, such as ***whooping cough,*** can also lead to a sore throat. The streptococcus bacterium, which produces the illness known as ***strep throat,*** is most commonly at fault, but the bacterium responsible for ***gonorrhea*** can also cause sore throats among people who engage in oral sex.

Living in a dusty or very dry environment can cause a raw and painful throat, as can overuse (or misuse) of the voice, or habitual use of tobacco or alcohol. People who suffer from ***allergies,*** persistent ***coughs,*** or chronic ***sinusitis*** are also prone to sore throats.

In rare cases, a persistent sore throat may be a sign of a potentially cancerous growth in the throat or mouth.

DIAGNOSTIC AND TEST PROCEDURES

If it appears that your sore throat may be the result of a bacterial rather than a viral infection, your doctor may do a throat culture. This painless procedure involves swabbing out a sampling of throat mucus for laboratory analysis. Your doctor's office may be equipped to analyze the culture within a few minutes, or you may have to wait a day or two while the sample is sent to an outside laboratory.

For persistent throat pain, or if other symp-

CURING MORNING SORE THROAT

Some people wake up regularly with a sore throat, which then goes away as the day progresses. This "morning-only" sore throat is often caused by sleeping with your mouth open but can also result from a backup of stomach acids into your throat during the night.

If you think your sore throat may come from sleeping with your mouth open, try a bedroom humidifier or vaporizer (be sure to follow directions for cleaning a humidifier carefully).

If you believe the soreness may be due to a backup of stomach acids, try sleeping on a tilted bed frame. Place bricks or boards under your bed so that the head of the bed is four to six inches higher than the foot. Piling pillows under your head will not help because they will cause your body to bend in a way that will put even more pressure on your esophagus and make the problem worse. Also, avoid eating or drinking anything for an hour or two before going to bed.

toms are present, your doctor may order additional tests to check for other conditions.

TREATMENT

Most sore throats are self-limiting, which means they usually go away on their own without any kind of treatment. In the absence of other symptoms, therefore, you may first want to try alternative treatments for a painful throat. However, if the pain persists or worsens after a few days, you should see your doctor. If left untreated for too long, ***strep throat*** may lead to ***rheumatic fever,*** which can damage the heart, or to acute nephritis, which can damage the kidneys.

CONVENTIONAL MEDICINE

For a bacterial throat infection, such as strep throat, your doctor will probably prescribe ***penicillin***—or, if you are allergic to penicillin, some other ***antibiotic*** such as ***erythromycin***—for 7 to 10 days. To avoid a recurrence, it is very important that you complete the entire course of the antibiotic, even after symptoms have gone away.

Antibiotics are not effective for sore throats caused by viral infections. Your doctor will most likely recommend that you simply rest, drink plenty of liquids, gargle with salt water, and take ***aspirin*** or ***acetaminophen*** if needed for pain relief. Over-the-counter throat lozenges containing a mild anesthetic can also provide relief. CAUTION: Do not give aspirin to a child or young adult with a sore throat, as it may lead to Reye's syndrome, a rare but very serious illness.

ALTERNATIVE CHOICES

See the illustrations on the following page for **acupressure** techniques that may help relieve the pain of a sore throat. In general, alternative therapies are geared toward symptom relief, although in some cases they also address the actual cause of the sore throat.

ACUPUNCTURE

Acupuncture can be very helpful in relieving the pain and reducing the inflammation of a sore throat. A professional acupuncturist will stimulate points along the kidney, large intestine, and stomach meridians. *(See pages 22 and 23 and the **Appendix** for information on point locations.)*

AROMATHERAPY

To increase blood circulation and improve fluid drainage in sore areas, massage your throat and chest with a lotion made with 2 drops each of ***eucalyptus*** *(Eucalyptus globulus)* and ***peppermint*** *(Mentha piperita)* in 2 tsp of a carrier oil such as vegetable or almond oil.

HERBAL THERAPIES

To help fight the infection causing a sore throat, herbalists recommend several herbs with antimicrobial properties. At the first sign of soreness, take three raw cloves of ***garlic*** *(Allium sativum)* a day. (Garlic is a natural antibiotic and antiseptic.) If garlic smell becomes a problem, try four garlic oil capsules instead. Teas made from either ***goldenseal*** *(Hydrastis canadensis)* or ***echinacea*** (*Echinacea* spp.) may also be effective. To make goldenseal tea, pour 1 cup boiling water over 1 tsp powdered herb; let it steep for 10 to 15 minutes, strain, then drink. Repeat three times a day. To make echinacea tea, put 1 to 2 tsp of the root in 1 cup water and bring slowly to a boil; reduce heat and let the tea simmer for 10 to 15 minutes. Cool the tea to a comfortable temperature and drink; repeat three times a day.

Or try a tea made from ***licorice*** *(Glycyrrhiza glabra),* which may help enhance the immune system's defenses against bacteria. Put 1 tbsp of the root in 3 cups water; simmer for 10 to 15 minutes. Drink three times a day. CAUTION: Some forms of licorice affect ***high blood pressure.*** Use licorice for no longer than one week unless under the care of a health practitioner.

To ease the discomfort of a sore throat, drink teas made from ***sage*** *(Salvia officinalis)* or ***chamomile*** *(Matricaria recutita).* A simple lemon tea can also be very soothing. Squeeze the juice of one lemon in 8 oz warm water, add honey to taste, and drink.

A traditional Native American treatment is drinking a tea made from the inner bark of the ***slippery elm*** *(Ulmus fulva).* Put 2 tsp powdered bark in 1 cup water. Bring to a boil and simmer for 10 to 15 minutes.

HOMEOPATHY

Homeopaths prescribe several remedies for sore throats. Consult a homeopathic practitioner or try those listed here.

- If the pain comes on suddenly and is accompanied by great thirst and hoarseness, try ***Aconite*** (6c) three times a day.
- If the pain comes on suddenly and is accompanied by fever, headache, and restlessness, use ***Belladonna*** (6c) three times a day.
- If your sore throat has come on gradually and is accompanied by fatigue, try ***Ferrum phosphoricum*** (6c) three times a day.
- If the back of your throat is red and swollen

ACUPRESSURE

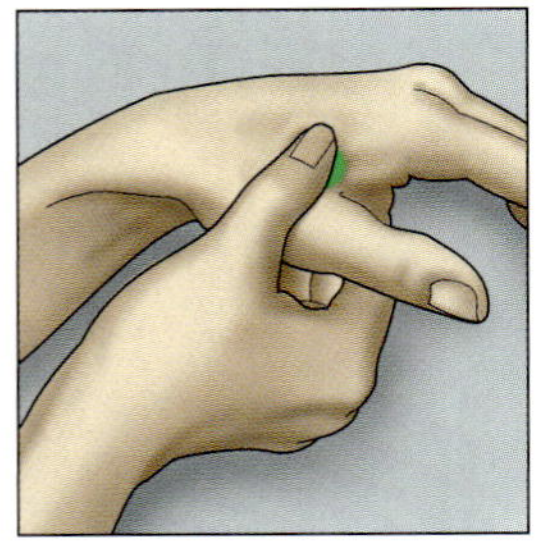

1 For a sore throat from a cold or the flu, try pressing your right thumb into LI 4, between the thumb and index finger of your left hand. Apply firm pressure against the bone above your index finger for one minute, then repeat on the other hand. Do not use during pregnancy.

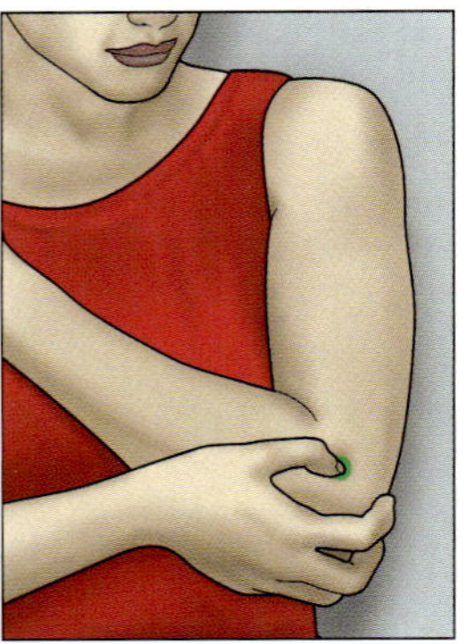

2 Acupressure may help ease the symptoms of a fever due to a cold. Apply pressure with your thumb to LI 11, located at the outer end of the elbow crease on your left arm. Hold for one minute and repeat on the right arm.

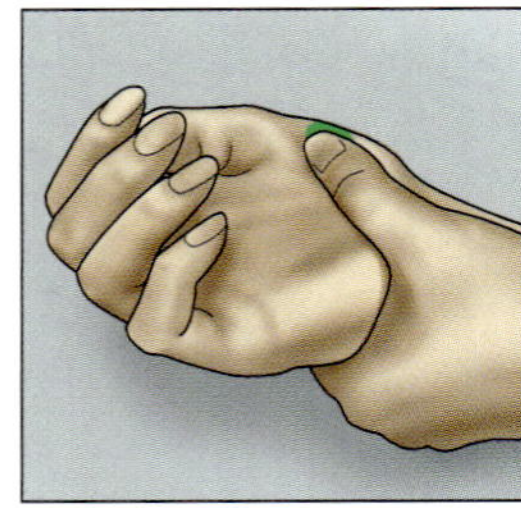

3 To help relieve the discomfort of a sore and swollen throat, try pressure at LU 10. Using your left thumb, apply pressure to the center of the pad at the base of your right thumb. Hold for one minute and repeat on the other hand.

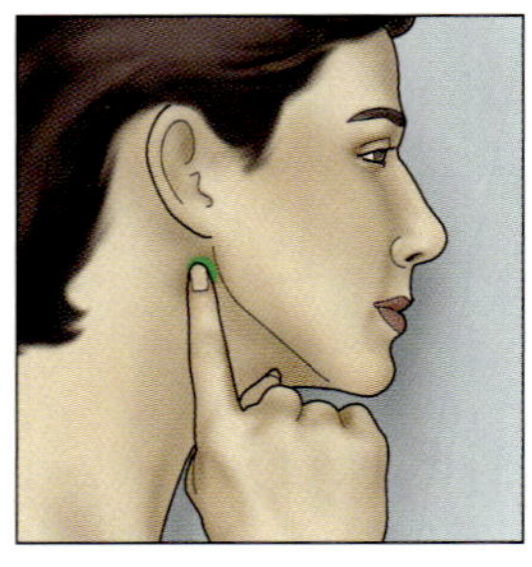

4 To relieve an irritated throat, place your index fingers on SI 17, in the indentations at both corners of your jawbone just below your earlobes. Breathe deeply and press on both sides gently for one minute. These points are very sensitive, so apply pressure slowly and carefully.

and the pain is relieved by cold water or ice, try ***Apis*** (6c) three times a day.

- If your sore throat is accompanied by flulike symptoms, extreme sluggishness, and weakness, use ***Gelsemium*** (6c) three times a day.

NUTRITION AND DIET

At the first sign of soreness, take 500 to 6,000 mg of ***vitamin C*** daily to help fight the cold or other viral infection causing it. CAUTION: Unless your body is accustomed to megadoses of vitamin C, it cannot absorb more than about 1,000 mg every two hours; the excess will be passed off in your urine or, in some cases, result in ***diarrhea.*** Also, if you take a dose at the higher end of this range, drink plenty of fluids to keep the vitamin C from concentrating in your kidneys.

Some practitioners of **naturopathic medicine** attribute repeated sore throats to a ***zinc*** deficiency. Try a daily supplement of 20 to 40 mg.

If you have frequent sore throats, especially ones associated with ear infections, you may have a food allergy. Consult a healthcare practitioner who specializes in food ***allergies.***

AT-HOME REMEDIES

- Get plenty of rest and drink a lot of fluids.
- Take ***aspirin*** or other over-the-counter medication for pain relief.
- Suck on a ***zinc*** lozenge—about 23 mg of zinc—every four hours. Zinc can relieve sore throats and other cold symptoms.
- To help relieve the pain, apply a warm heating pad or compress to your throat. You can also try a warm ***chamomile*** poultice: Mix 1 tbsp dried chamomile flowers into 1 or 2 cups boiling water; steep for five minutes, then strain. Soak a clean cloth or towel in the tea, wring it out, then apply to your throat. Remove the cloth when it becomes cold. Repeat as often as necessary.
- A salt plaster may also help provide relief. Mix 2 cups sea salt with 5 to 6 tbsp lukewarm water; the salt should be damp, but not wet. Place the salt in the center of a dishtowel, then roll the towel along the longer side. Wrap the towel around your neck; cover it with another dry towel. Leave on for as long as you wish.
- Try steam inhalations to ease the pain. Run very hot water in a sink. With a towel draped over your head to trap the steam, lean over the sink while the water is running. Breathe deeply through your mouth and nose for 5 to 10 minutes. Repeat several times a day.

HOMEMADE GARGLES

To wash away mucus and irritants and bring relief from the pain of a sore throat, try any of the following gargles:

- **Salt water:** Mix ½ tsp salt in 8 oz warm water.
- **Sage:** Put 1 to 2 tsp dried leaves in 1 cup boiling water; steep for 10 minutes, then strain and cool until lukewarm.
- **Chamomile:** Steep 1 tsp of the dried herb in 1 cup warm water.
- **Apple cider vinegar:** Mix 2 tsp vinegar in 1 cup warm water.
- **Lemon:** Mix the juice of one lemon in 8 oz warm water.
- **Horseradish:** Mix 1 tbsp pure horseradish, 1 tsp honey, and 1 tsp ground cloves in 8 oz warm water.
- **Raspberry:** Put 1 to 2 tsp raspberry leaf in 1 cup boiling water; steep for 10 minutes, then strain and cool until lukewarm.
- **Cayenne pepper:** Mix the juice of half a lemon, 1 tbsp salt, and ¼ tsp cayenne pepper (or more if you can tolerate it) in ½ cup warm water. The cayenne pepper temporarily reduces the amount of pain-causing chemicals produced by nerve endings in the throat.
- **Aspirin:** Dissolve two tablets crushed aspirin in 1 cup warm water.
- **Hydrogen peroxide:** Make a mixture of half hydrogen peroxide and half warm water.

PREVENTION

If you tend to get recurrent sore throats, replace your toothbrush every month; bacteria can collect on the bristles. Also, be sure to toss an old toothbrush once you've recovered from a sore throat to avoid reinfecting yourself. ■

SPRAINS AND STRAINS

SYMPTOMS

Sprains, which affect joints, and strains, also called muscle pulls, usually occur after a fall or sudden movement that pulls or twists a part of the body violently.

For a sprain:

- pain in the affected joint.
- rapid swelling of a joint, often accompanied by bruising.
- stiffness and difficulty moving a joint.

For a strain:

- sharp pain at the site of an injury, followed by stiffness, tenderness, and in some cases, swelling.

CALL YOUR DOCTOR IF:

- the pain, swelling, or stiffness does not improve in two to three days.
- you feel a popping sensation when you move a sprained joint; this may indicate a serious injury that requires immediate medical treatment.
- you can't move or bear weight on an injured joint. You may have a broken bone.
- the bones in an injured joint don't seem to be aligned properly. The ligaments that hold the joint together may be badly torn, requiring surgical repair.
- an injured muscle does not move at all; it may have torn completely through and may require immediate medical attention.
- you have repeated sprains or strains, indicating a chronic weakness that should be evaluated by a physician.
- you have difficulty moving or walking after straining any back muscle. You may have nerve damage *(see **Back Problems**)*.

Sprains and strains are among the most common injuries, ranging from twisted ankles to aching backs. A **sprain** injures ligaments, the tough, fibrous bands of tissue that connect bones to one another at a joint. A **strain** damages muscle tissue, leaving muscles, or the tendons that attach muscle to bone, stretched or torn.

Given adequate time and rest, most sprained joints or strained muscles will heal themselves. But severe tearing or complete rupture of the affected tissues usually requires surgical repair. And damage caused by a sprain can leave the bones in the affected joint improperly aligned, or the ligaments so stretched and weakened that the joint is particularly vulnerable to future injury. *(See also **Muscle Pain, Tendonitis, Groin Strain, Hamstring Injury.**)*

CAUSES

Anything that places sudden or unaccustomed stress on joints or muscles may cause a sprain or strain. Falls, lifting heavy objects, and the exertion of an unfamiliar sport are common culprits. Being overweight, inactive, or in poor physical condition boosts the likelihood of injury.

THE RICE TREATMENT

Doctors, physical therapists, and athletes all swear by RICE—rest, ice, compression, and elevation—as the standard treatment for the first 48 to 72 hours in muscle, tendon, or ligament injuries. Rest the area immediately to avoid further injury. Apply ice, alternating 10 minutes on, 10 minutes off, to reduce swelling and inflammation. Use elastic bandages to compress the area and reduce swelling. And keep the injured area elevated to promote drainage of fluid.

S

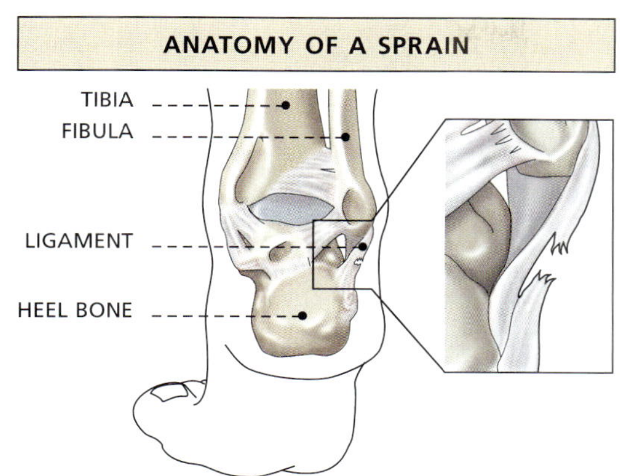

Tough bands of connective tissue called ligaments keep bones in line. In the ankle joint, above, a sudden, quick movement has forced the joint beyond its normal range of motion, causing a sprain. The ligaments are stretched and torn *(inset),* and tissue around the injury has become swollen and the skin discolored. In most cases, a sprained joint will still function but can be painful to use.

DIAGNOSTIC AND TEST PROCEDURES

Your doctor may order x-rays to rule out fracture, or an MRI scan to check for ruptured tissues.

TREATMENT

Treatment of both sprains and strains focuses on control of the initial pain and swelling, followed by adequate rest to allow healing.

CONVENTIONAL MEDICINE

Most sprains and strains heal in two to three weeks. Doctors routinely prescribe rest, ice, compression, and elevation immediately following the injury, along with ***aspirin*** or ***ibuprofen*** to reduce inflammation and pain. Elastic bandages may then be used to support or immobilize the injured area while it heals, and a sprained ankle or knee often calls for crutches to keep weight off the joint. To speed healing, your doctor may also recommend heat or infrared treatments from a physical therapist.

ALTERNATIVE CHOICES

Alternative therapies can help relieve the pain and swelling associated with sprains and strains.

CHINESE HERBS

A practitioner of Chinese medicine may use a poultice of gardenia *(Gardenia jasminoides),* flour, and wine to reduce swelling and promote healing. Massage with the extracted oil of ***safflower flower*** *(Carthamus tinctorius)* is believed to improve circulation, which encourages healing.

HOMEOPATHY

The anti-inflammatory action of homeopathic preparations of ***Arnica*** (6x to 30c), taken orally, may relieve pain.

NUTRITION AND DIET

Research indicates that vitamin supplements may help heal sprains and strains. If your doctor approves, take daily supplements of ***vitamin C*** (1,000 mg), beta carotene *(see **vitamin A**)* (10,000 IU), ***zinc*** (up to 60 mg), ***vitamin E*** (400 IU), and ***selenium*** (50 mcg).

AT-HOME REMEDIES

Once the initial swelling has subsided and you are no longer in acute pain—usually after 48 to 72 hours—you may use a heating pad to relieve soreness and stimulate circulation in the injured area. Massaging the area with an over-the-counter topical cream containing ***aspirin*** or another ***analgesic*** can also alleviate lingering soreness or tenderness.

PREVENTION

The best way to prevent sprains or strains is to keep yourself in good physical shape, so that your muscles, ligaments, and tendons are strong and flexible enough to resist trauma. To prevent recurring injury, ask your doctor for exercises designed to rehabilitate the muscles in the injured area. If you are overweight, ask about an appropriate diet and a general conditioning program. ■

STAPH INFECTIONS

SYMPTOMS

- pain and swelling around a cut or scraped area of skin.
- boils or small, white-headed pimples around hair follicles.
- in infants and young children, blistering and peeling skin.
- swollen lymph nodes in the neck, armpits, or groin.

CALL YOUR DOCTOR IF:

- any pain, swelling, or pus forms around a cut or scraped area of skin; the infection may spread into the bloodstream.
- the lymph nodes in your neck, armpits, or groin become swollen; this can also be a symptom of a variety of other illnesses, including ***mononucleosis, tuberculosis,*** and ***cancer.***
- you have a ***boil*** that is very tender, particularly if it has red lines radiating from it, or if you have fever and chills; the infection may have spread.
- you have a boil or **carbuncle** on or near your lip, nose, cheeks, forehead, or spine; the infection can spread into your brain or spine.
- you have recurrent boils; they may be a sign of ***diabetes.***

S

Staph infections can invade and attack any part of your body, from your skin, eyes, and nails to the inner lining of your heart. Symptoms vary, depending on where the infection develops. Staph infections usually enter the body through an open cut or wound. The infection can spread to adjacent tissue or, through the bloodstream, to distant internal organs, such as the heart or kidneys, where it can become life-threatening. People with a chronic illness, such as diabetes, cancer, or chronic liver or kidney disease, are particularly susceptible to severe staph infections.

Staph infections are known by a variety of names, many of which are also used to describe strep infections. **Folliculitis** is a superficial infection of the hair follicles that produces small, white-headed pustules. Shaving the skin or friction from clothing rubbing against the skin can injure the follicles and cause the infection to erupt. The area where the pustules appear may itch for a day or two beforehand.

Sometimes a staph infection invades the deepest part of the hair follicle, resulting in a large, painful, pus-filled inflammation known as a ***boil.*** Although boils can form anywhere on the body, they are found most frequently on the face, neck, buttocks, and armpits. If one appears on the eyelid, it is known as a ***sty.*** When several separate boils occur simultaneously on the body, the condition is called **furunculosis.**

A **carbuncle** is a cluster of connected boils deep under the skin. Carbuncles are usually found on the upper back or nape of the neck and are more common in men than in women.

Another common staph infection of the skin is ***impetigo,*** characterized by small patches of tiny blisters and pustules that become crusty after breaking open. Less common, but potentially more serious, is **cellulitis,** which occurs in the deeper layers of the skin. It usually begins with a tender swelling and redness around a cut or sore, then gradually spreads into nearby tissue. Red lines may radiate from the infected area to nearby lymph nodes, which may also become infected and swell to two or three times their normal size—a serious condition called **lymphadenitis.**

Infants and young children sometimes develop **scalded skin syndrome,** a staph infection characterized by a blistering, peeling rash. Another staph infection that afflicts mostly children is ***conjunctivitis;*** this causes the eyes to redden and to weep a yellow, watery pus that forms a crust overnight during sleep. **Blepharitis,** a staph infection that involves the edges of the eyelids, can also result in red, crusty eyes. When a staph infection forms around the edges of fingernails, causing swelling and pus-filled blisters, the condition is known as **paronychia.**

A staph infection called **mastitis** can enter the breasts of nursing mothers through cracked, sore nipples, resulting in painful breast abscesses. Menstruating women who use tampons are at risk of developing a potentially life-threatening staph infection, ***toxic shock syndrome.***

Staph infections sometimes spread through the bloodstream to the bones and joints—particularly those of the arms, legs, and spine—where abscesses may then form. The affected joint swells and fills with pus. Left untreated, it may become arthritic and permanently stiff.

If a staph infection spreads to the lungs, staphylococcal ***pneumonia*** can occur; if it spreads to the kidneys, a ***kidney infection*** may develop. Both conditions can be life-threatening. A spreading staph infection can also attack the endocardium, or inner lining of the heart, resulting in bacterial **endocarditis,** a serious condition that can cause permanent damage to the heart. (This condition occurs primarily in intravenous-drug users.) The colon can also become a target of a staph infection, particularly among people who are taking an antibiotic for other ailments. The drug may kill off other kinds of bacteria in the colon, enabling staphylococci to multiply freely.

CAUSES

Staph infections are caused by *Staphylococcus aureus,* a type of bacterium commonly found in the nose, mouth, rectum, or genital area. In fact, at any one time, about 30 to 40 percent of people carry staphylococci in their noses without any symptoms of illness. The bacteria are harmless until they enter the body through a cut, scrape, or other break in the skin. Once they invade the body, the bacteria form pus-containing abscesses. Bacteria that enter the body on contaminated food can cause ***food poisoning.***

DIAGNOSTIC AND TEST PROCEDURES

Your doctor will examine the infection and perhaps take a sample of pus for laboratory analysis to determine if its cause is staphylococci or another kind of bacterium. If your doctor suspects that the infection has spread to other areas of your body, further tests, such as a blood analysis or a lymph node culture, may also be done. If you have recurrent ***boils*** or ***sties,*** your doctor may take a nasal culture to determine whether your nose is harboring staphylococci.

TREATMENT

In mild cases, such as ***boils*** or **folliculitis,** you can clean the infected area yourself with antibacterial soap and apply some of the topical treatments mentioned under **At-Home Remedies.** If the infection persists or worsens, however, you should see your doctor for antibacterial medications to make

STAPH INFECTIONS IN HOSPITALS

Staph infections are easy to pick up in a hospital after a surgical procedure, despite the best efforts of nurses, doctors, and others to keep the hospital a germfree environment. For this reason antibiotics are often prescribed to patients for a full 24 hours following surgery. In cases when the risk is especially high—when the patient is having intestinal surgery, for example—antibiotics are administered before the operation as well as after it.

sure the infection does not lead to serious complications. Alternative treatments to strengthen your immune system can help prevent a recurrence.

CONVENTIONAL MEDICINE

Your doctor will probably give you an oral ***antibiotic,*** such as ***erythromycin*** or dicloxacillin, to clear up the infection. If you have a skin infection, you may be prescribed an antibiotic cream to apply to the infected area. In recurrent cases of ***boils*** or ***sties,*** when a nasal culture has revealed the presence of staphylococci, an antibiotic cream is inserted directly into the nostrils.

Some abscesses must be surgically drained for the infection to heal completely. Your doctor may refer you to a surgeon for this procedure, which can usually be done, using a local anesthetic, right in the surgeon's office. If the infection is severe, you may be hospitalized so that ***antibiotics*** can be administered intravenously.

ALTERNATIVE CHOICES

Your alternative medical practitioner can provide comprehensive treatment for your staph infection. Alternative medicine can also help you to strengthen your immune system so that you can avoid recurrent infections. However, if the infection does not respond to these treatments and worsens or spreads, you should seek conventional treatment with antibiotic medications.

ACUPUNCTURE

In Chinese medicine, any kind of ***boil*** is believed to be caused by excess heat in the body. Treatment therefore consists of stimulating points on the body that can dissipate that heat. Consult a professional acupuncturist.

HERBAL THERAPIES

Several herbs have antibacterial properties that are believed to be helpful in fighting staph infections. They include:

- ***Garlic*** *(Allium sativum):* Take three cloves a day at the first sign of infection; if garlic smell becomes a problem, try three garlic oil capsules instead.

YOGA

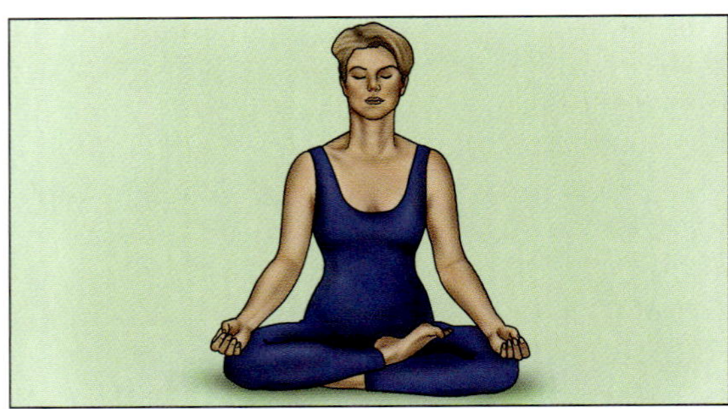

1 To help boost your immune system, try the **Half Lotus:** Bend your left leg and bring the foot close to your body. Bend your right leg and place the foot high on the left thigh. (For **Full Lotus,** place each foot on the opposite thigh.) Hold for five minutes, breathing deeply.

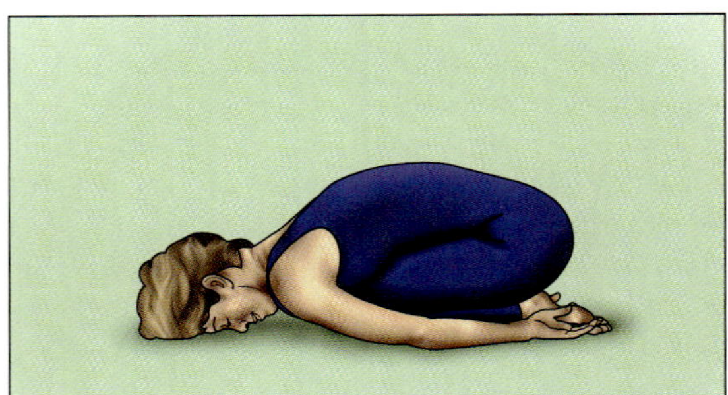

2 The **Child** may help stimulate your immune system by relaxing your body. Sit on your heels, thighs together. Exhale slowly while bending forward from your hips. Move your forehead to the floor. Breathe deeply for 30 seconds, then inhale as you arise. Do once.

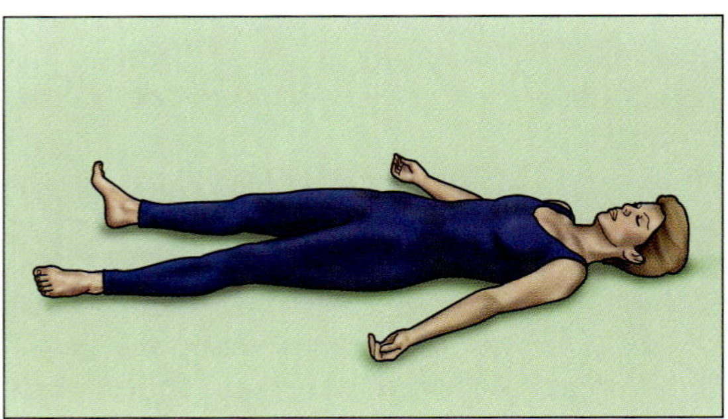

3 Another position that promotes relaxation is the **Corpse.** Lie on your back, with your feet about 18 inches apart and turned out slightly. Place your hands about 6 inches from your hips, palms up. Close your eyes; breathe deeply for 8 to 10 minutes.

- ***Goldenseal*** *(Hydrastis canadensis):* Make a tea from the powdered herb and drink three cups a day.
- ***Echinacea*** (*Echinacea* spp.): Make a tea from the root and drink three cups a day.

To help reduce any swelling of the lymph nodes, use cleavers *(Galium aparine),* an herb believed to be a tonic for the lymphatic system. Make a tea from the dried herb and drink three cups a day; if you prefer, take 2 to 4 ml of a tincture of the herb three times daily.

See also **At-Home Remedies.**

HOMEOPATHY

Staph infections are treated with remedies designed to boost your body's immunity to the infection. Treatments vary according to the type of infection and where it appears on the body. Consult an experienced homeopath.

NUTRITION AND DIET

To help rid your body of the infection and restore your natural immunity, eat plenty of green, orange, and yellow vegetables, which are rich in beta carotene *(see* ***vitamin A****),* and drink 8 to 10 glasses of water each day. To activate your immune system and help your white blood cells fight the infection, take ***zinc*** supplements (30 to 50 mg) daily. In addition, supplements of ***vitamin C*** (1,000 to 5,000 mg spread evenly throughout the day) and bioflavonoids (300 to 2,000 mg daily) may help fight the infection. Recurrent boils or other staph infections can be signs of a poor diet. Consult a nutritionist.

AT-HOME REMEDIES

- To speed healing, place a warm compress such as a warm, wet washcloth on a ***boil*** or ***sty*** for 20 to 30 minutes, three or four times a day. To help prevent scarring, add a few drops of thyme oil, ***lavender,*** or bergamot to the water in which the washcloth is soaked. After the boil or sty has ruptured and the pus has drained, clean the area with warm water and lemon juice or Epsom salt. Keep clean until completely healed. CAUTION: Never squeeze or lance a boil or sty; if you do, you may cause permanent scarring or cause the infection to spread.
- Apply a ***yarrow*** *(Achillea millefolium)* compress to the staph infection. Soak dried or powdered leaves briefly in warm water. Squeeze out most of the water and wrap the leaves or powder in gauze. Place on the infected area of skin.
- Apply a paste made from goldenseal root to the infection. Mix goldenseal root powder with enough water to make a paste. Put it directly onto the infected area of the skin, then cover with a clean, nonporous bandage or cloth. Leave the paste on overnight.
- To prevent a staph infection from spreading while it heals, take showers rather than baths.
- If you have **folliculitis** of the beard, use a new razor blade each day for shaving while the infection is healing.
- If you have a staph infection around the edges of a nail, soak the nail in pure ***tea tree oil*** (*Melaleuca* spp.) for five minutes twice a day until the infection clears. A drop of tea tree oil can also be applied directly to a ***boil.***
- Always wash your hands thoroughly after treating a staph infection.

PREVENTION

- Wash all cuts, scrapes, and wounds with antiseptic soap; keep them clean during healing.
- To keep your staph infection from spreading to other members of your household, do not share towels, washcloths, and bed linens. Change these items daily and launder them in hot water and bleach.
- If you are prone to **folliculitis,** wash your skin with an antibacterial soap before you shave. Soak your razor in rubbing alcohol between shaves, and don't let anyone else use it.
- To avoid ***food poisoning*** caused by staph (as well as other) bacteria, always wash your hands thoroughly before preparing food. If you are recovering from a staph infection, have someone else prepare food so you do not spread the infection to others. ■

STOMACH CANCER

SYMPTOMS

Stomach cancer usually produces no early symptoms other than mild indigestion or loss of weight and appetite, which are symptoms vague enough to be ignored by most people. As the disease advances, the symptoms become more pronounced. Warning signs of stomach cancer may include:

- indigestion, heartburn, abdominal pain, or discomfort aggravated by eating.
- loss of appetite; a bloated or full feeling after eating small amounts of food.
- either diarrhea or constipation; nausea and vomiting after meals.
- general weakness and fatigue.
- dark patches in stool, or blood on stool.
- vomiting blood.

CALL YOUR DOCTOR IF:

- feelings of indigestion or abdominal discomfort persist for more than a few weeks, or if you experience dark stools, an indication of bleeding in the stomach or intestinal tract. You need a thorough medical examination, by either your primary care physician or a gastroenterologist, to find out whether your discomfort is due to a ***stomach ulcer, cancer,*** or some other cause.

Before World War II, stomach cancer—also known as **gastric cancer** or **gastric carcinoma**—was a leading cancer killer in the United States. The disease is now much less prevalent in the U.S., but in Japan, Korea, Latin America, and eastern Europe, it remains one of the most common and lethal cancers.

Almost all stomach cancers start in glandular tissue lining the stomach. A tumor may spread along the stomach wall or may grow directly through the wall and shed cells into the bloodstream or lymphatic system. Once beyond the stomach, cancer can spread to other organs. If treated before it spreads, stomach cancer is curable. A patient whose tumor is removed completely has a good chance of surviving at least five years. Unfortunately, by the time most cases of stomach cancer are diagnosed, the cancer has spread to other organs, making it difficult to treat. Fewer than 1 in 5 patients diagnosed with stomach cancer that has spread to other organs survives five years.

CAUSES

Stomach cancer often originates at the site of an existing ***stomach ulcer,*** although ulcers themselves are not thought to cause the disease. While some stomach ulcers turn cancerous, most do not. For stomach cancer to occur, something has to make normal cells mutate, or reproduce abnormally. Certain dietary agents are linked to stomach cancer: The disease is common among people who frequently eat smoked, pickled, salted, and barbecued foods, all of which contain cancer-promoting nitrites or other nitrogen compounds. Aflatoxins—carcinogenic by-products of a fungus that grows in nuts, seeds, and corn, and in other dried foods stored in humid conditions—also seem to promote stomach cancer. *(See **Food Poisoning, Liver Cancer.**)* Smoking tobacco and drinking alcohol may slightly increase the risk of stomach cancer.

Another suspected promoter of stomach cancer is *Helicobacter pylori,* a bacterium that infects about half of all Americans over the age of 50 and most people in poor regions of Asia and

S

Latin America. Long-term *H. pylori* infection causes chronic stomach irritation and ulcers and may contribute to the development of some stomach cancers. A few other treatable diseases, including ***gastritis,*** gastric polyposis, and pernicious ***anemia,*** are also associated with stomach cancer. Worldwide incidence of stomach cancer is notably higher among coal miners and metal refiners, who inhale certain dust and fumes that contain known carcinogens. In the U.S., stomach cancer occurs twice as often in men as in women, strikes African Americans most frequently, and rarely affects people under 50.

DIAGNOSTIC AND TEST PROCEDURES

When symptoms warrant a thorough examination, a doctor views the stomach with an x-ray or CT scan, or through an orally inserted gastroscope. If a suspicious mass is identified, a biopsy is performed by extracting a tissue sample and studying it under a microscope for cancer cells. If cancer is confirmed, other tests may be run to determine whether the disease has spread.

TUMORS IN THE STOMACH

Aided by strong muscles and gastric juices, the stomach blends and liquefies chewed food for absorption by the small intestine. Cancer typically attacks the stomach's glandular lining *(inset, top)*, often at the site of an ulcer. While cancers can form anywhere in the stomach, they tend to start directly below the junction of the esophagus and the stomach *(inset, bottom)*.

TREATMENT

CONVENTIONAL MEDICINE

If caught early, stomach cancer is treated surgically, sometimes with radiation or chemotherapy beforehand to reduce the tumor's size. Part or all of the stomach is removed, along with surrounding tissue and nearby lymph nodes. Postop patients typically experience ***indigestion*** or ***diarrhea,*** but such side effects can be relieved with medication. Patients whose entire stomachs are removed require regular ***vitamin*** B_{12} injections, because they cannot absorb the nutrient naturally until their systems adjust to digesting food in the intestines.

Most cases of stomach cancer are too advanced at diagnosis to be cured surgically, but radiation, chemotherapy, or limited surgery can relieve symptoms, slow the disease, and possibly prolong life. See ***Cancer*** for more information about treatments.

COMPLEMENTARY THERAPIES

Patients with advanced stomach cancer typically experience significant pain. While medication can offer partial relief, a variety of complementary therapies may also help. Consider **acupuncture** or activities that promote relaxation such as **yoga, massage,** or **meditation.** *(See* ***Cancer.****)*

AT-HOME CARE

Following stomach surgery, people often experience nausea, vomiting, diarrhea, or dizziness after eating. The symptoms usually go away in a few months, but they can be minimized by eating small meals of soft or semiliquid foods, cutting out sweets, and not drinking liquids with meals.

PREVENTION

Studies suggest that drinking green tea and eating plenty of fresh fruits, vegetables, and garlic may help protect against stomach cancer. However, nothing is more preventive than cutting out smoked, pickled, salted, and barbecued foods. ■

STOMACH ULCERS

SYMPTOMS

- burning upper abdominal pain, particularly between meals, early in the morning, or after drinking orange juice, coffee, or alcohol, or taking ***aspirin;*** discomfort is usually relieved after taking ***antacids.***
- tarry, black, or bloody stools.

CALL YOUR DOCTOR IF:

- you have been diagnosed with a stomach ulcer and begin experiencing symptoms of ***anemia,*** such as fatigue and a pallid complexion. Your ulcer may be bleeding.
- you have symptoms of a stomach ulcer and develop severe back pain. Your ulcer may be perforating the stomach wall. **Call your doctor now.**
- you have symptoms of a stomach ulcer and vomit blood or material that looks like coffee grounds, or you pass dark red, bloody, or black stools, or stools that resemble currant jelly. These symptoms indicate internal bleeding; **call 911 or your emergency number now.**
- you have an ulcer and become cold and clammy, and feel faint or actually do faint. These are symptoms of shock, usually resulting from massive blood loss; **get emergency medical treatment.**

There is no clear evidence to suggest that the stress of modern life or a steady diet of fast food causes stomach ulcers, but they are nonetheless common in our society: About 1 out of 10 Americans will suffer from the burning, gnawing abdominal pain of an ulcer sometime in life.

Stomach, or peptic, ulcers are holes or breaks in the protective lining of the stomach, the esophagus, or the duodenum, which is the upper part of the small intestine. The most common type are **duodenal ulcers;** as the name suggests, these affect the duodenum. The second most common are **gastric ulcers,** which develop in the stomach, followed by the comparatively rare **esophageal ulcers,** which form in the esophagus and are typically a result of ***alcohol abuse.***

Duodenal ulcers, whose typical symptoms are recurrent upper abdominal pain and a bloated feeling after eating, are more common in men than women and generally strike between the ages of 40 and 50 years. People between 60 and 70 years old are prime targets for gastric ulcers, whose symptoms are similar to those of duodenal ulcers.

Fortunately, stomach ulcers are relatively easy to treat; in many cases they are cured with ***antibiotics.*** Still, the dangers associated with stomach ulcers—such as ***anemia,*** hemorrhaging, ***pancreatic problems,*** and ***stomach cancer***—are serious, so ulcers should always be monitored by your doctor. There are, however, a variety of self-help and alternative treatments that can aid in relieving pain and in healing ulcers.

CAUSES

Until the mid-1980s the conventional wisdom was that ulcers form as a result of ***stress,*** a genetic predisposition to excessive stomach acid secretion, and poor consumption habits (including overindulging in rich and fatty foods, alcohol, caffeine, and tobacco). It was believed that such influences contribute to a buildup of stomach acids that erode the protective lining of the stomach, duodenum, or esophagus.

While excessive stomach acid secretion certainly plays a role in the development of ulcers, a relatively recent theory holds that bacterial ***infection*** is the primary cause of peptic ulcers. Indeed, research conducted since the mid-1980s has persuasively demonstrated that the bacterium *Helicobacter pylori* is present in 92 percent of duodenal ulcer cases and 73 percent of gastric ulcers.

Other factors also seem to contribute to ulcer formation. Overzealous use of over-the-counter ***analgesics*** (such as ***aspirin, ibuprofen,*** and ***naproxen***), heavy alcohol use, and smoking exacerbate and may promote the development of ulcers. In fact, research indicates that heavy smokers are more prone to developing duodenal ulcers than are nonsmokers, and that people who drink alcohol are more susceptible to esophageal ulcers and those who take aspirin frequently for a long period of time more likely to contract gastric ulcers than those who abstain.

Other studies show that gastric ulcers are more likely to develop in elderly people. This may be because ***arthritis*** is prevalent in the elderly, and alleviating arthritis pain can mean taking daily doses of aspirin or ibuprofen. Another contributing factor may be aging ducts that allow excess bile to seep into the stomach and erode the stomach lining. Also, for no known reason, people with type A blood are more likely to develop cancerous gastric ulcers. Duodenal ulcers tend to appear in people with type O blood, possibly because they do not produce antigens that may protect the stomach lining.

A HOLE IN THE STOMACH

DUODENUM
DUODENAL ULCER
GASTRIC ULCER
STOMACH

A peptic ulcer is a hole or break in the protective lining of the esophagus, the stomach, or the duodenum. Duodenal and gastric ulcers *(inset)* are the two most common forms. They have similar symptoms, most commonly recurring pain in the upper abdomen and a bloated feeling after eating.

DIAGNOSTIC AND TEST PROCEDURES

Noting your symptoms may lead your doctor to suspect that you have a peptic ulcer, but it will not likely help determine the type, because the symptoms of gastric and duodenal ulcers are so similar. To make a specific diagnosis, your doctor may administer several tests.

The most common is a barium x-ray, which allows your doctor to spot the ulcer and determine its type and severity. The test requires you to drink a tracing substance called a "barium milkshake," which in an x-ray will highlight the upper digestive tract. You may be asked to eat only bland, easily digestible foods for two or three days before the test. After drinking the chalky liquid you are strapped to a tilting examining table, which evenly distributes the barium around your upper digestive tract and allows the x-ray to capture images at different angles.

If you do not respond to treatment or if you develop new symptoms, your doctor may perform a gastroscopy, or endoscopic examination, in which a flexible tube is inserted down your throat to give the doctor a direct view of the inside of your esophagus, stomach, and duodenum. This allows the doctor to determine the presence and cause of bleeding, and test for any bacterial infection. During this examination your doctor may also conduct a biopsy to check for cancer.

TREATMENT

Medications are usually used to treat mild to moderate ulcers. If the cause is bacterial, ***antibiotics*** can cure the ulcer. For recurrent, severe cases that do not respond to medication, surgery may be necessary.

Although alternative therapies have been

shown to aid in the relief of symptoms as well as in the healing of ulcers, they should be used only as supplements to conventional treatment.

CONVENTIONAL MEDICINE

The chief goals of treatment are reducing the amount of acid in the stomach and strengthening the protective linings that come in direct contact with gastric acids. This can usually be achieved by taking over-the-counter ***antacids*** containing ***magnesium hydroxide*** and ***aluminum hydroxide*** before meals and at bedtime.

CAN YOU CATCH AN ULCER?

*In 1982, two Australian doctors determined that the bacterium Helicobacter pylori played a significant role in the development of peptic ulcers, and further studies have shown **antibiotics** to be effective in treating ulcers caused by the bacterium. Does this mean that ulcers are contagious?*

The answer is murky. Not everyone infected with the bacterium develops an ulcer, and certainly other factors—such as heredity and excessive use of aspirin, tobacco, and alcohol—increase the chances of getting one. Still, research has shown that infected children are more likely to transmit the bacterium than adults are, a rate that increases in developing countries, where an estimated 80 percent of children are infected.

This does not mean, however, that you should take antibiotics as a preventive measure if you or your child is infected. The best course of action is to consult with your doctor.

Since long-term use of antacids can interfere with the absorption of nutrients, your doctor may prescribe either a proton pump inhibitor or ***histamine H_2 blocker*** as an alternative medication. Histamine blockers reduce stomach acids and heal peptic ulcers 80 percent of the time when taken over a period of four to six weeks. This class of medication includes the generic drugs ***cimetidine, ranitidine,*** and ***famotidine*** among others. Since antacids can reduce the absorption of histamine blockers, your doctor will probably instruct you not to take antacids during this period. Proton pump inhibitors, including the drugs ***omeprazole*** and lansoprazole, help prevent stomach acid production; they are usually taken for four to eight weeks.

If your ulcer is caused by bacterial infection, your doctor may prescribe a combination of ***antibiotics,*** such as ***amoxicillin*** or ***tetracycline*** with metronidazole, along with a bismuth drug and possibly proton pump inhibitors or ***histamine H_2 blockers.***

If these treatments are unsuccessful, or if you have developed serious complications as a result of your ulcer, surgery may be necessary. If your ulcer is hemorrhaging, the surgeon will identify the source of the bleeding (usually a small artery at the base of the ulcer) and repair it. Perforated ulcers—holes in the entire stomach or duodenal wall—must be surgically closed. This is an emergency procedure.

In some cases, a surgical procedure that decreases stomach acid secretion is also warranted. Note, however, that peptic ulcer surgery is done only in emergency situations, because there are many potential complications associated with the procedure, including ulcer recurrence, ***hypoglycemia,*** hematological complications, and dumping syndrome (chronic abdominal pain, diarrhea, vomiting, and/or sweating occurring an hour after eating).

ALTERNATIVE CHOICES

Although you should be monitored by a doctor if you have a peptic ulcer, alternative therapies can help relieve the discomfort of symptoms.

ACUPUNCTURE

Acupuncture targeting the points associated with ***stress, anxiety,*** and stomach/gastrointestinal disorders may help with the treatment of peptic ulcers. Consult a licensed acupuncturist.

HERBAL THERAPIES

Licorice *(Glycyrrhiza glabra),* which stimulates mucus secretion by the stomach, is frequently used in herbal treatments of ulcers. To prepare an infusion, add 1 tsp shredded licorice root to 1 cup water and simmer for 15 minutes. Drink hot, three times a day. Alternatively, try drinking ½ tsp licorice extract mixed with 1 cup water three times a day before meals. (Do not use this treatment for more than a few days at a time.)

MIND/BODY MEDICINE

Biofeedback, meditation, massage therapy, and **yoga** can help you learn how to deal effectively with stress, which increases stomach acid production and irritates ulcers.

NUTRITION AND DIET

Some nutritionists recommend increasing your intake of ***vitamins A*** and ***E*** and ***zinc,*** which increase the production of mucin, a substance your body secretes to protect the stomach lining. Another suggestion may include drinking about a quart of cabbage juice daily; its high content of glutamine is thought to expedite the growth of mucin-producing cells.

AT-HOME REMEDIES

- Cut down on milk. Although it may feel as though milk's coating properties are soothing your ulcer, milk actually stimulates stomach acid secretion, irritating the ulcer.
- Pick appropriate ***antacids.*** Like milk, ***calcium***-containing ***antacids*** can affect stomach acid secretion, so check with your doctor before taking them. Also, don't become dependent on antacids containing a combination of magnesium trisilicate and aluminum hydroxide. These compounds can deplete phosphate levels, causing osteomalacia (bone softening). Experiments suggest that bismuth, an ingredient in some over-the-counter stomach medications, may help destroy the bacterium that causes some peptic ulcers.
- Be cautious when choosing over-the-counter pain relievers. ***Aspirin*** and ***nonsteroidal anti-inflammatory drugs (NSAIDs)*** such as ***ibuprofen*** may not only irritate the ulcer but also prevent a bleeding ulcer from healing. Your best choice may be ***acetaminophen,*** which does not cause or promote stomach ulcers.
- Don't overdose on ***iron*** supplements. Although people with bleeding ulcers can develop ***anemia*** and may need to take iron as a treatment, taking too much can irritate the stomach lining and thus the ulcer. Ask your doctor how much iron you need.
- Learn how to deal with ***stress.*** While there is no evidence that stress causes ulcers, it can exacerbate existing ones. Practicing relaxation techniques—including deep breathing, **guided imagery,** and moderate exercise—can help alleviate stress.

PREVENTION

- Avoid foods that irritate your stomach. Use common sense: If it upsets your stomach when you eat it, avoid it. Everyone is different, but spicy foods and fatty foods are common irritants.
- Eat foods with high fiber content. Fiber has been touted as a cancer-preventing substance, and eating a high-fiber diet can also reduce your chances of developing a duodenal ulcer. Fiber is thought to enhance mucin secretion, which protects the duodenal lining.
- Stop smoking. Heavy smokers are more likely to develop duodenal ulcers than nonsmokers, largely because nicotine is thought to prevent the pancreas from secreting acid-neutralizing enzymes.
- Practice moderation. Heavy consumption of alcohol and aspirin has been shown to contribute to the development of ulcers, so keep your intake to a minimum. ■

STREP THROAT

SYMPTOMS

- ***sore throat*** that comes on rapidly.
- fever, sometimes greater than 102°F.
- back of the throat that is raw and red.
- white pus on tonsils.
- tender, high lymph nodes in neck.
- absence of cough, stuffy nose, or other upper respiratory symptoms.

CALL YOUR DOCTOR IF:

- you quickly develop a fever and sore throat simultaneously; these are the hallmark symptoms of strep throat, which in severe cases can develop into ***rheumatic fever*** if left untreated.

If you're feeling fine one moment, then suddenly your throat is killing you, you're running a high fever, and all your energy has vanished in a haze of illness, you probably have strep throat.

"Strep," in this case, stands for *Streptococcus pyogenes,* a common strain of bacteria that can live in your throat and nose for months without causing any harm. Tests show that about 18 percent of healthy people have the strep bug living uneventfully in their mouths or throats. Once in a while, however, these bugs turn ugly on you. Maybe you've been under too much stress, or your immune system has been overtaxed with fighting a virus such as a ***common cold*** or the ***flu.*** Or perhaps you've picked up a bug from an infected person. Whatever the reason, the normally quiet strep organism can suddenly start spewing out toxins and inflammatory substances to bring on the sore throat and other symptoms.

Although strep throat feels awful, it can be cured easily these days with antibiotics such as ***penicillin*** or ***erythromycin.*** In fact, one of the biggest problems with it is getting people to seek treatment. Because a fever and sore throat are also symptoms of colds and the flu, strep throat is often mistaken for these ailments. But colds and flu normally take several days to develop, and most of the time they are accompanied by a cough, stuffy or runny nose, and headache. A strep throat, by contrast, usually arrives in a hurry and without any other cold or flu symptoms.

Strep throat should never be taken lightly. Untreated, the disease can quickly lead to a more severe illness such as acute nephritis (which can damage your kidneys), ***meningitis,*** or ***rheumatic fever,*** all of which can be fatal.

CAUSES

Although by definition strep throat is caused by the *Streptococcus pyogenes* bug, other bacteria can occasionally invade the throat and cause similar symptoms. Other possible invaders: staphylococcus, neisseria, and *Hemophilus influenzae.*

People usually develop strep throat when their immune systems are not functioning at their peak. ***Stress,*** overwork, exhaustion, and fights with viral infections can weaken the body's defenses and set up attacks of strep throat. And like other throat infections, strep throat also tends to occur during the colder months.

DIAGNOSTIC AND TEST PROCEDURES

In the past, when patients displayed the characteristic red, raw throat, spikes in fever, and white spots on the tongue and tonsils, a careful physician would culture a specimen from the patient's throat and wait 24 to 48 hours for the results. If the test indicated streptococcus, the patient could then start taking antibiotics. To avoid this delay—in which the infection often grew worse—most doctors started patients on antibiotics immediately, not waiting for the results of the culture.

Diagnosis has been made much simpler today as a result of the "quick strep" test. Research indicates that this test, which takes about 20 minutes, is just as accurate as the much slower culture analysis. (If the quick test is not clearly negative and your symptoms strongly suggest strep throat, your doctor may also perform a regular culture.) The beauty of the quick test is that you don't need to take antibiotics without confirmation that the strep organism is the culprit.

TREATMENT

Strep throat is best treated by conventional medicine. For one thing, antibiotics are a quick and surefire cure. Also, the disease can lead to serious complications if left untreated.

CONVENTIONAL MEDICINE

In most cases, a standard dose of ***penicillin,*** taken for 10 days, will eradicate a strep infection without any problems. Most people who are allergic to penicillin can take one of the many kinds of ***cephalosporins.*** For patients who are allergic to both penicillin and cephalosporin, the alternative is usually ***erythromycin.*** Relief from the sore throat should come within 24 to 36 hours after you start taking antibiotics. Doctors recommend throat lozenges and throat sprays to ease the pain for the first few hours.

Frequently, people on ***antibiotics*** notice improvement quickly and stop taking their medications before the course runs out. This practice can have dangerous consequences. Prematurely halting the dosage allows the hardiest strep organisms, those that survived the first doses of antibiotic, to develop resistance to the drug and to bounce back in a more potent form. So even though you may feel better right away, it's important to finish the entire prescription.

ALTERNATIVE CHOICES

Strep throat is one disease in which conventional medicine clearly excels. However, a number of homeopathic remedies may ease the discomfort of a sore throat and related symptoms.

HOMEOPATHY

For a sore throat characterized by a high fever and glassy eyes, use ***Belladonna*** 12x (three times a day). WARNING: Exercise extreme caution when using belladonna, a poisonous member of the nightshade family. For a sore throat that's worse at night, accompanied by a coated tongue and bad breath, use ***Mercurius vivus*** 12x (three times a day). When the sore throat is worse on the left side, particularly at night, and you have swollen glands and difficulty swallowing, use ***Lachesis*** 12x (three times a day). If you feel unusually sensitive to cold and have sharp, sticking pain as well as discharge in the throat, try ***Hepar sulphuris*** 12x (three times a day). If you don't feel better in a day, seek the advice of a professional homeopath.

PREVENTION

The best way to avoid a strep throat is to reduce stress, get plenty of rest, and fortify your body's natural defenses. Nutritional supplements such as ***vitamin C,*** beta carotene *(see **vitamin A**),* and ***zinc,*** along with herbs such as ***echinacea*** (*Echinacea* spp.), ***goldenseal*** *(Hydrastis canadensis),* osha *(Ligusticum porterii),* and ***garlic*** *(Allium sativum),* are all thought to boost the immune system. ■

STRESS

SYMPTOMS

- Physical symptoms may include ***headache, fatigue, insomnia,*** digestive changes, neck pain or ***backache,*** loss of appetite, or overeating.
- Psychological symptoms may include tension or ***anxiety,*** anger, reclusiveness, pessimism, resentment, increased ***irritability,*** feelings of cynicism, and inability to concentrate or perform at usual levels.

CALL YOUR DOCTOR IF:

- you have prolonged or acute symptoms. Excessive stress puts you at risk of other serious disorders, including ***immune problems,*** digestive disorders, ***diabetes, asthma, high blood pressure,*** migraine ***headaches,*** and possibly ***cancer.***
- you have symptoms of stress and any of the following: unusual patterns of sleep, appetite, and moods; physical movement that is unusually agitated or abnormally slow. You may have clinical ***depression.***

Stress is the reaction of our bodies and minds to something that upsets their normal balance. The human response to stressful events is an ancient one, dating back to a time when life was a constant struggle for survival. A good example of stress in action is the way you react when you are frightened or threatened. Your adrenal glands release epinephrine—or adrenaline—a hormone that activates your body's defensive mechanisms: Your heart pounds, your blood pressure rises, your muscles tense, the pupils of your eyes open wide. This cluster of reactions—the fight-or-flight response—concentrates all your body systems on the apparent danger and helps you take the next step, which is either to resist or to retreat.

Of course, not all stressful events are so sudden or so obvious as the threat of bodily harm. Any challenge that overwhelms us—a serious illness, the death of a family member, the loss of a job or a lover—can be stressful to the point of physical and psychological dysfunction. Some of us are especially vulnerable to stressful situations or events, responding in extreme ways to everyday decisions—what to buy at the supermarket, what to wear to the wedding, or how to ask for a raise. But while some people fall to pieces if they are pressed too hard, others are highly productive under pressure. The difference may lie partly in our constitutions, and partly in how we manage our lives.

Continued stress can eventually deplete the body's resources and produce chronic fatigue, loss of appetite or overeating, and other reactions. Coping ability may diminish, causing feelings of insecurity and inadequacy, and possibly leading to ***depression.*** At the same time, the body's immune system becomes disrupted, increasing vulnerability to illness and disease. Unrelieved stress—from real or imagined causes—may bring on hypertension, a recognized factor in ***heart disease*** and some cancers. ***Posttraumatic stress disorder,*** in which symptoms appear immediately or months after a stressful event, can be a protracted and difficult problem.

CAUSES

Stress occurs when there is an imbalance between the demands of life and our ability to cope with them. Certain work is highly stress producing, especially assembly-line jobs or jobs requiring repetitive tasks with dangerous equipment. Events and situations that are difficult to manage typically bring on stress: burnout on the job, financial problems, the loss of or a threat to your security, bereavement, or divorce. A positive experience, such as marriage or a job promotion, can be equally stressful. Other causes are internal: illness, loneliness, pain, or emotional conflict. The effects of such changes, big and little, are cumulative. We can tolerate only so much stress in a given period of time.

DIAGNOSTIC AND TEST PROCEDURES

Diagnosing stress is largely a matter of recognizing and understanding the symptoms—both physical and psychological—in yourself or others. Some researchers have developed more objective diagnostic tools. For example, the Holmes-Rahe questionnaire is helpful in identifying potentially stressful events. The questionnaire scale ranks 43 important life events according to their potential stress value. Not all events are considered "bad," but all involve some kind of change, including a new job, a new home, and the birth of a child.

TREATMENT

You don't have to deal with stress by yourself. A counselor, psychologist, psychiatrist, member of the clergy, or friend can often help you define or resolve a problem that seems unsolvable to you. Developing a stress-abatement routine you trust will help you prepare for an event you know may be stressful.

CONVENTIONAL MEDICINE

If you have symptoms of stress from a specific event, such as a death in the family, your doctor may prescribe an ***antianxiety*** drug, such as ***diazepam.*** While such medications are highly effective if taken for brief periods, they can be addictive if taken for more than a few weeks *(see **Drug Abuse**).*

Your doctor may suggest psychotherapy to pinpoint events or conditions that are stressful to you, and to devise ways of reducing the stress they cause. Group therapy is often valuable for people who share a stressful life situation. Treatment of ***posttraumatic stress disorder*** usually includes counseling and may require antianxiety or ***antidepressant*** medications.

ALTERNATIVE CHOICES

Some treatments once considered alternative are now widely used in the medical community—particularly those designed to promote physical and mental relaxation.

AROMATHERAPY

Essential oil of ***lavender*** *(Lavandula officinalis)* can help reduce stress: Try 5 or 6 drops in a bath, or put 2 or 3 drops on a handkerchief and inhale from time to time.

BODY WORK

By relaxing tense muscles and helping circulation, **massage** helps the mind relax. Between treatments by a trained massage therapist, try self-massaging your temples, neck, shoulders, and face.

HERBAL THERAPIES

A traditional response to stress is to drink a cup of hot tea. Some herbalists suggest ***chamomile*** *(Matricaria recutita),* ***passionflower*** *(Passiflora incarnata),* ***valerian*** *(Valeriana officinalis),* or ***ginseng*** *(Panax quinquefolius)* tea.

LIFESTYLE

Vigorous aerobic exercise can reduce the level of pulse-quickening hormones released during stress and at the same time stimulate a sense of well-being. Even a walk around the block can help reduce anxiety or let off steam. Try to schedule the exercise of your choice—running, swimming, walking—for 30 minutes at least three times a week.

THE "TYPE A" PERSONALITY

Some researchers divide people into two classes: the competitive, hard-charging Type A personalities who thrive on challenge; and the less competitive, calmer Type B. Type A people seem to have a higher risk of heart attack. Some studies show that hostility —not just a fast pace—is the quality most strongly linked with heart disease.

Some experts think Type A people should try to change their behavior, while others think doing so may simply induce more stress or change an essential personality trait. Many if not most Type A people enjoy life in the fast lane. If you think you are a Type A person, work to control hostility and other negative behavior by trying the following strategies:

- *Avoid situations you dislike whenever possible.*
- *Schedule true breaks from work.*
- *Manage your time better.*
- *Penalize Type A actions and reward calm, coping actions.*

Stretching exercises can relax tense upper-body muscles that accompany stress and affect breathing. Rotate your shoulders up, back, and then down. Inhale as the shoulders go back; exhale as they go down. Repeat the exercise four or five times, then inhale deeply and exhale. Repeat the cycle.

MIND/BODY MEDICINE

The **relaxation response** has long been a goal of many Eastern disciplines such as **yoga** and Zen Buddhism. Try this simple routine: Choose a focus word or phrase, for example "peace" or "I'm calm." Sit quietly, relax your body, and breathe slowly and deeply. Say the focus word or phrase each time you exhale. If you lose concentration, simply wait as thoughts pass through your mind, then return to your focus word. Continue for 5 minutes at a time, gradually increasing to 20 minutes. Do the routine at least once a day. Such relaxation exercises, done regularly, can slow your breathing rate, decrease your oxygen consumption, calm your brain-wave rhythms, and lower your blood pressure.

You might also reduce stress through **biofeedback,** identifying the sources of stress and controlling your physical and mental responses. You should learn the proper technique from a professional, then practice at home. Advocates believe that biofeedback can relax specific muscles, alter the brain's electrical activity, reduce heart rate and blood pressure, increase body warmth, and improve gastrointestinal function.

NUTRITION AND DIET

How well you handle stress can be affected by your diet. Because it is easy to neglect nutrition when you are under stress, make an extra effort to eat a balanced diet—plenty of vegetables and fruit, as well as foods high in complex carbohydrates, moderate in protein, and low in fat. Avoid or reduce caffeine consumption: Excessive caffeine has been shown to increase ***anxiety.***

AT-HOME REMEDIES

There are many simple, inexpensive ways to manage stress on your own. For many people, a good way to start is by cutting out artificial stress relievers such as alcohol, which can mask symptoms and may become addictive. Try exercise instead. Take walks. Breathe deeply.

In times of stress, social support is crucial. People with close personal relationships are most likely to recover from serious illness or injury, and stress is no different. The ability to form relationships with people—or pets, for that matter—can be a key to good health.

Start taking a **yoga** class and practice by yourself at home. *(See the illustrations opposite.)* Yoga can relax tense muscles, teach you better breathing, lower your blood pressure, decrease your heart rate, and divert your mind from stress.

Meditation brings relaxation and increased awareness. When you feel stressed, think affirmations such as "I can face this calmly. I feel sure and confident. I control my own life."

Try visualization or **guided imagery** exercises. Visualizing a pleasant situation can bring physical as well as emotional benefits; combine a visualization session with soothing music. Many excellent teachers, books, and tapes are available to help you learn the technique.

Hydrotherapy is easily done at home and highly effective at reducing stress. Soak for 10 to 20 minutes in a tub of very warm water, using half a cup of sea salt and your favorite bath oil.

PREVENTION

While we can't—and perhaps shouldn't try to—change our personality or avoid stressful situations just because they are stressful, we can take common-sense steps to increase our coping ability. Try the following:

- Practice the relaxation and stress-reduction techniques suggested above.
- Cultivate outside interests and plan occasional diversions to break routine habits.
- Set up a regular sleeping schedule and get plenty of rest—without sleeping pills.
- Exercise regularly and vigorously, as appropriate for your age.
- Avoid the learned behaviors of hurry and worry, which can upset your sleeping, eating, and other schedules. Take time to relax and enjoy your life.
- Make a list of things that trouble you. For each one, ask yourself: What's the worst and the best that can happen? Have I done what I can to prepare myself? Is this problem really worth worrying about?
- Laugh more; avoid self-pity; learn to reestablish equilibrium after a stressful event; make an effort to reach out to people.
- When you're facing a stressful situation, remember a bit of folk wisdom: Count to 10 and take a deep breath before saying or doing anything. A deliberate pause can be an instant tranquilizer.

YOGA

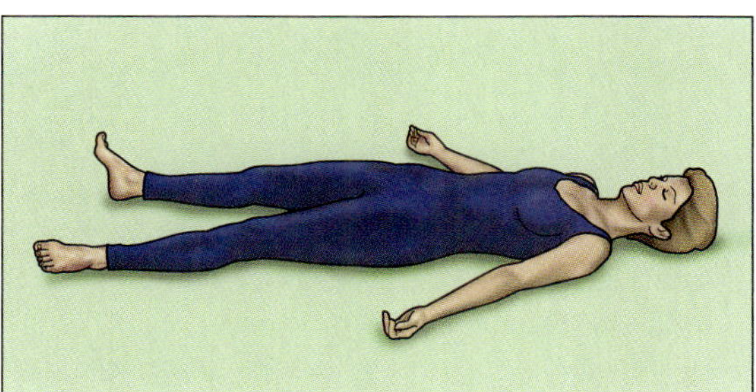

1 Relaxation exercises are good for stress. For the **Corpse,** you should lie on your back, with your feet approximately 18 inches apart and turned out slightly. With palms up, place your hands about 6 inches from your hips. Close your eyes and breathe deeply for 8 to 10 minutes.

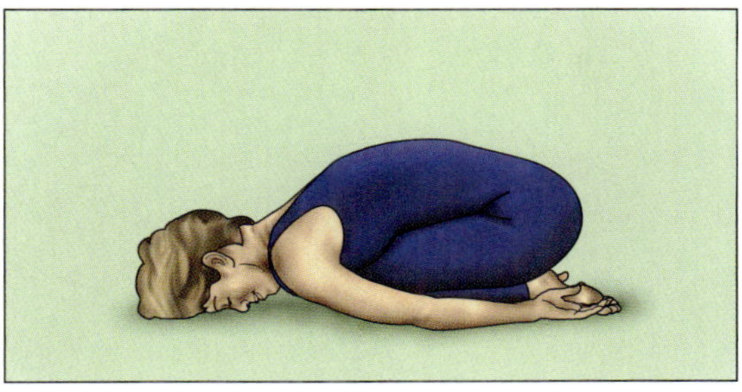

2 The **Child** relaxes the lower back. Sit on your heels keeping your knees together. Exhale and bend from the hips. Extend your upper body over your knees with arms at your sides, palms up, and your forehead to the floor. Breathe slowly, hold for 30 to 60 seconds, then sit up as you inhale.

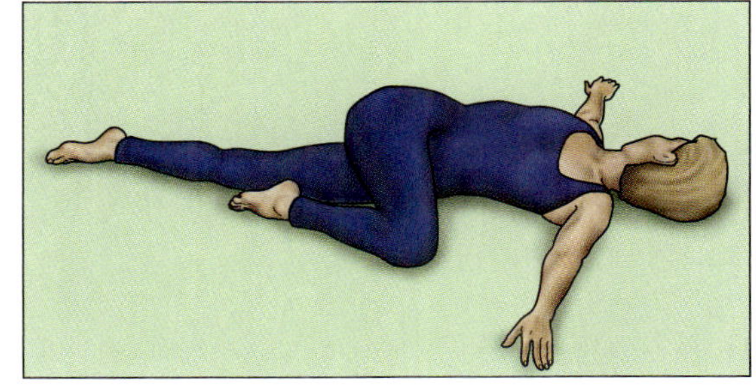

3 The **Knee Down Twist** also relaxes the lower back. Lie on your back with arms out, inhale, and put your right foot on your left knee. Exhale, turn your head to the right, and move your right knee toward the floor to your left. Hold for 15 to 20 seconds. Repeat on the other side. ■

STROKE

SYMPTOMS

- abrupt loss of vision, strength, coordination, sensation, speech, or the ability to understand speech. These symptoms may become more marked over time.
- impairments limited to one side of the body, such as numbness on one side of the face or blindness in one eye.
- sudden loss of balance, possibly accompanied by vomiting, nausea, hiccups, or trouble with swallowing.
- sudden and severe headache followed rapidly by loss of consciousness—indications of a stroke due to bleeding.

CALL YOUR DOCTOR IF:

- you or someone with you manifests any of the signs of stroke. If the symptoms pass quickly, this may indicate a transient ischemic attack (TIA), a brief blockage of blood flow to the brain that is often a forerunner of stroke. Do not ignore this warning sign; medical intervention is essential.

When the blood supply to the brain is disturbed for any reason, the consequences are usually drastic: Control over movement, perception, speech, or other mental or bodily functions is impaired, and consciousness itself may be extinguished. Disruptions of blood circulation to the brain are known as stroke—a disorder that occurs in two basic forms, both potentially life-threatening.

About three-quarters of all strokes are due to blockage of the oxygen-rich blood flowing to the brain. Called **clot strokes,** they are triggered by either a thrombus (a stationary clot that forms in a blood vessel) or an embolus (a clot that travels through the bloodstream and becomes lodged in a vessel). This type of stroke is often preceded by so-called **transient ischemic attacks,** or **TIAs**—episodes of inadequate blood flow that may produce sudden physical weakness, an inability to talk, double vision, or dizziness. With a TIA, circulation and the vital oxygen supply are quickly restored and lasting neurological damage is avoided. With any stroke, however, the interruption of blood flow lasts long enough to kill brain cells, producing irreversible neurological damage.

The second basic type of stroke is **bleeding stroke,** or **cerebral hemorrhage.** It occurs when a brain ***aneurysm*** ruptures or when a weakened or inflamed blood vessel in the brain starts to leak. As blood flows into the brain, the buildup of pressure may either kill the tissue directly or destroy cells by impeding normal circulation to the affected region. This typically produces an excruciating headache, sometimes followed by loss of consciousness. In contrast to clot strokes, which are generally survived, massive bleeding strokes are fatal about 80 percent of the time.

Because of improved treatment and greater public awareness of the dangers of ***high blood pressure,*** the overall death rate from stroke is declining. Nonetheless, stroke remains the third leading cause of death in the United States, behind ***heart disease*** and ***cancer.*** It is also the leading cause of disability and second only to ***Alzheimer's disease*** as a cause of dementia.

Recovery from stroke depends on the extent and location of brain damage. Some stroke victims recover fully; but in the vast majority of cas-

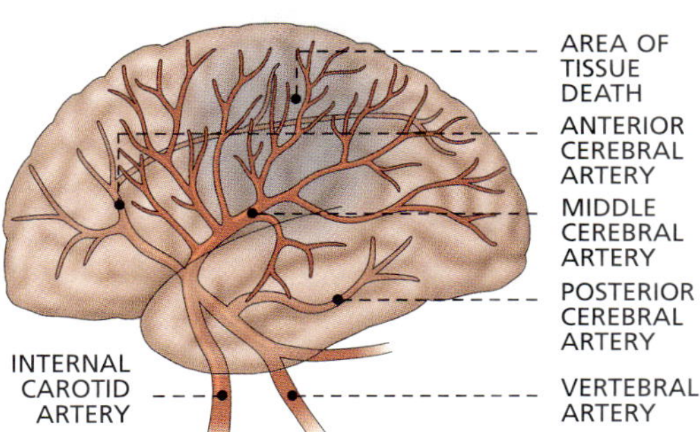

A left-side view of the brain shows the five major vessels responsible for the organ's blood supply. Ruptures or blockages in any of these vessels or their branches can lead to a stroke, in which an insufficient oxygen supply causes tissue death and brain damage. Depending on the part of the brain that is affected, a stroke can result in paralysis, speech dysfunction, loss of vision, or other symptoms.

es, there is lasting physical or mental disability. Weakened stroke victims are also more vulnerable to infectious diseases such as ***pneumonia.*** In addition, ***depression*** often follows a stroke; unless treated, it can significantly hinder recovery.

CAUSES

A **clot stroke** occurs when a blood clot obstructs blood flow to a portion of the brain. The blocked vessel is already narrowed by years' worth of plaque buildup due to ***atherosclerosis.*** The clot that serves as the final plug may be either a stationary blood clot created on the spot, or an embolus composed of blood, plaque, or some other substance that formed elsewhere and traveled to the site. Stroke-triggering blood clots may be produced when blood flow is sluggish. After a ***heart attack,*** for example, clots may form on the damaged heart wall because of slower blood flow there. *(See also* ***Blood Clots.****)*

Bleeding strokes most often stem from weak arteries or aneurysms in the brain that rupture. Arteries are sometimes congenitally weak, but more often they become weak under the strain of ***high blood pressure.*** Bleeding strokes can also result from a leaking **arteriovenous malformation,** a congenital tangle of overgrown blood vessels in the brain.

The vast majority of strokes afflict people over the age of 60. Men are more often affected than women, and African Americans—possibly because of a greater incidence of high blood pressure—more often than Caucasians. A younger person is more apt to have a bleeding stroke, while older people usually suffer clot strokes.

The main controllable risk factors for stroke are high blood pressure, high cholesterol levels (specifically, high LDL cholesterol), a sedentary lifestyle, obesity, the abuse of stimulant drugs such as amphetamines, smoking, use of birth-control pills, and ***stress.***

Incidence of stroke increases in people with a history of TIAs, ***heart disease*** (particularly recent heart attack, atrial fibrillation, or mitral valve disease), excessive blood clotting, or ***diabetes.***

DIAGNOSTIC AND TEST PROCEDURES

When a patient displays strokelike symptoms, a neurologist must not only confirm the symptoms but also identify the type of stroke, its location, and the extent of brain damage. Treatment decisions hinge on all these issues. Testing is typically done quickly, since immediate treatment may limit neurological damage.

The physician first examines the patient and obtains a medical history, if possible. A standard exam includes checking blood vessels in the eyes, listening for unusual noises in the heart and in the prominent carotid arteries of the neck, measuring blood pressure and pulse rate, and testing strength, sensation, and neurological reflexes.

CT or MRI scans are the most critical diagnostic tests for stroke.

TREATMENT

Acute management of stroke should be left to conventional medicine, but many alternative therapies may contribute to stroke prevention and recovery.

CONVENTIONAL MEDICINE

Stroke victims are immediately admitted to the hospital and, in many cases, will be given medication to prevent further brain damage. Normally, **clot strokes** are treated with an ***anticoagulant*** drug called ***heparin.*** Thrombolytic agents, drugs that dissolve blot clots, may reopen blocked blood vessels if they are given shortly after the clot stoke occurs. Emergency surgery might also be required to drain blood that has hemorrhaged into the brain and perhaps to clip a ruptured artery or aneurysm—blocking off the vessel to halt further bleeding.

Once past the critical phase, a stroke patient remains hospitalized until stable. Upon release, patient and doctor carefully review necessary steps for recovery and prevention of future strokes. Advice will likely involve diet and lifestyle changes, ongoing drug treatment, rehabilitative therapy, and possible surgery for critical arterial narrowing.

People at risk of having **bleeding strokes** need to keep their blood pressure low, if possible through diet and lifestyle changes but, when needed, also with medication. These people are also advised not to take ***aspirin*** or ***nonsteroidal anti-inflammatory drugs (NSAIDs),*** including ***ibuprofen.*** If someone has suffered a bleeding stroke because of an aneurysm rupture, other small aneurysms can sometimes be identified and either removed or clipped. Unfortunately, nothing can be done to reverse congenital arterial weakness.

To prevent **clot strokes,** some patients are first advised to take ***aspirin.*** If aspirin proves ineffective, the doctor will probably prescribe ticlopidine, another blood-thinning drug, or ***warfarin*** as a last resort. People at particularly high risk for clot stroke because of an existing heart condition would be treated with ***heparin*** for acute symptoms and warfarin for long-term therapy. In some patients, surgery to prevent future clot strokes might be recommended. The most favored procedure is endarterectomy, to remove plaque from large carotid arteries leading from the neck into the brain. An experimental technique called cerebral angioplasty is used to widen clogged brain arteries.

Another crucial element of stroke treatment, in addition to emergency and follow-up medical care, is rehabilitation. Immediately after a stroke, other parts of the brain can compensate for areas lost to trauma by forming new neurological pathways. Intensive rehabilitative therapy basically aims to enhance the brain's own recovery efforts. A typical program may involve speech, physical, and occupational therapy.

The psychological well-being of victims, families, and caregivers plays a crucial role in rehabilitation. Successful recovery depends on both the quality of care and the positive mind-set of the victim. Several stroke associations offer psychological support via hot lines, discussion groups, and literature.

ALTERNATIVE CHOICES

In addition to the therapies described below, you might want to consult a practitioner of **Chinese medicine** or a **homeopathic** physician for treatment of poststroke complications. **Acupuncture,** for example, is endorsed by the World Health Organization as a viable stroke rehabilitation therapy.

BODY WORK

Several body-work techniques can help restore mobility, promote circulation, and ease muscle tension and stiffness associated with stroke. Among these are **qigong, shiatsu,** and **massage.**

CHIROPRACTIC AND OSTEOPATHY

Chiropractic and osteopathy, two closely related manipulative therapies, can aid post-stroke rehabilitation in numerous ways. By focusing on realignment of the body's skeletal system, they may be able to reduce muscle spasms and stiffness, improve mobility, alleviate nagging pains, and minimize further neurological damage.

HERBAL THERAPIES

A number of scientific studies have shown that ***ginkgo*** *(Ginkgo biloba)* increases cerebral blood flow, so it may be helpful in moderating potential complications of stroke such as memory loss, disturbed thought processes, vertigo, and symptoms of depression. Ginkgo also appears to reduce blood-clot formation. Many other herbs are said to be useful in stroke prevention because of their abilities to improve circulation, reduce clot formation, strengthen and tone blood vessels, and combat atherosclerosis. *(See* ***Aneurysm, Atherosclerosis, Blood Clots, Cholesterol Problems,*** *and* ***High Blood Pressure.****)*

LIFESTYLE

Physical rehabilitation is impossible without regular, gentle aerobic exercise. Swimming in a heated pool is particularly useful for restoring lost motor function and keeping muscles loose.

People at high risk for stroke should not smoke and should eat a low-fat diet. Women at high risk should not take birth-control pills.

MIND/BODY MEDICINE

Techniques that teach the body to relax and the mind to focus on healing can help recovering stroke victims; among other benefits, these techniques can increase tolerance to pain and also alleviate the depression or anger that is common in the wake of a stroke. **Hypnotherapy, meditation,** and **yoga** all can be useful. Some stroke victims working to restore lost muscle control and motor function benefit from **biofeedback.**

NUTRITION AND DIET

Proper diet has much to contribute to stroke prevention, but it can do little to reverse stroke damage. With prevention in mind, your diet should be rich in vitamins, minerals, and other nutrients that combat high blood pressure, excessive clot formation, and atherosclerosis. Particularly noteworthy stroke-deterring nutrients include ***potassium, magnesium, vitamin E,*** and the essential fatty acids contained in fish oils. Some studies suggest that ***selenium*** may also protect against stroke. A low-fat diet, however, is probably the best nutrition-related preventive step you can take for both heart attack and stroke.

A SPIDER-VENOM REMEDY?

Researchers have discovered that compounds in spider venom may be useful in limiting stroke damage. A spider paralyzes its prey by injecting substances that block the action of a chemical called glutamate, which controls muscle movement in insects. Glutamate also exists in the human brain, serving as an important neurotransmitter when it is present in the right quantities. After a stroke, however, damaged neurons release glutamate in such large amounts that it kills surrounding cells. Hence the interest in spider venom: If the venom compounds manufactured by the spider can halt the workings of glutamate in insect prey, perhaps a version of those same compounds can also limit the cascading neuronal death that occurs during stroke in a human.

PREVENTION

Measures that reduce the chances of stroke are the same as those for avoiding ***heart attack:*** Adopt habits that promote cardiovascular health and deter atherosclerosis. The essentials of a healthy lifestyle include eating foods that are low in fat, salt, and cholesterol; exercising regularly; controlling weight; monitoring blood pressure and cholesterol levels; and not smoking.

If your risk of stroke is high because of severe atherosclerosis, high blood pressure, or a history of heart disease, TIAs, or previous strokes, you should see a doctor regularly. When clot stroke is the indicated danger, your doctor may advise an aspirin a day to thin blood. ■

SYMPTOMS

- **sty:** a red, hot, tender, uncomfortable, and sometimes painful swelling near the edge of the eyelid. *(See also the **Visual Diagnostic Guide.**)*
- **chalazion:** a relatively painless, smooth, round bump within a fat gland of the eyelid.

CALL YOUR DOCTOR IF:

- either type of swelling does not subside within a few weeks.
- the swelling interferes with your vision.
- you have pain in the eye.
- you have recurrent sties. A sty can be a symptom of other ailments such as ***diabetes*** and chronic skin problems.

A **sty** is a pimple or abscess on the upper or lower edge of the eyelid that signals an infected eyelid gland. Although sties are usually on the outside of the lid, they can also occur on the underside.

An external sty starts as a pimple next to an eyelash. It turns into a red, painful swelling that usually lasts several days before it bursts and then heals. Most external sties are short-lived.

An internal sty (on the underside of the lid) also causes a red, painful swelling, but its location prevents the pus from appearing on the eyelid. The sty may disappear completely once the infection is past, or it may leave a small fluid-filled cyst or nodule that can persist and may have to be cut open.

A **chalazion** is also a sign of an infected eyelid gland, but unlike a sty, it is a firm, round, smooth, painless bump usually some distance from the edge of the lid.

Sties and **chalazions** are usually harmless and rarely affect your eye or sight. They can occur at any age and tend to recur elsewhere in the lid.

CAUSES

Sties are usually caused by staphylococcal bacteria, which often live in your nostrils. You can transfer the bacteria to your eyelids just by touching your nose and then rubbing your eyes.

A **chalazion** is caused by the blockage of the tiny gland duct that helps lubricate the eyelid. Bacteria may grow within the blocked gland; the resulting inflammation causes the hard bump.

TREATMENT

While painful and unsightly, most **sties** heal within a few days on their own or with simple treatment. **Chalazions,** too, often disappear on their own, but it might take a month or more.

CONVENTIONAL MEDICINE

Typical treatment for a **sty** consists of applying warm compresses to the affected eye for 10 to

15 minutes four times daily for several days. This not only relieves pain and inflammation but also helps the sty ripen faster. Be sure to close your eye while you apply the compresses. When the sty comes to a head, continue applying warm compresses to relieve pressure and promote rupture. Do not squeeze the sty; let it burst on its own.

If sties recur, your doctor may prescribe an ***antibiotic*** ointment or solution. Apply it to the eyelid (with your eye closed) as directed.

Sometimes, if there are staphylococcal infections elsewhere in your body as well, your doctor may prescribe an oral systemic antibiotic such as ***erythromycin.*** If these conservative treatments fail, surgical removal of the sty may be required.

Minor surgery may also be needed to eliminate the cyst that could result from an internal sty. After using a local anesthetic, your ophthalmologist opens the cyst and removes the contents. The eyelid usually heals quickly.

Although a **chalazion** will often disappear on its own, applying warm compresses and perhaps a ***corticosteroid*** ointment will speed the process. The chalazion can also be removed through simple surgery under a local anesthetic. Your doctor then covers the eye for 8 to 24 hours with a pressure patch to control bleeding and swelling.

ALTERNATIVE CHOICES

Although some alternative treatments may be helpful in relieving and preventing eyelid infections, never put any preparations in the eye itself unless specifically directed by a physician. The surface of the eye is easily damaged by some antiseptics and medications. When applying any lotions or compresses to the eyelid, keep your eye closed.

ACUPUNCTURE

In traditional Chinese medicine it is believed that all types of boils, including sties, are caused by heat invasion. To diffuse the heat, a trained acupuncturist may insert needles into BL 54, SP 10, and LI 11 *(see the **Appendix** for point locations).*

HERBAL THERAPIES

To help reduce the pain and inflammation of sties, herbalists recommend professionally prepared eye drops made from ***eyebright*** *(Euphrasia officinalis).* They may also prescribe an oral preparation of ***burdock*** *(Arctium lappa).*

NUTRITION AND DIET

If you have recurrent sties and chalazions, a nutritionist may recommend that you take supplements of ***vitamins A*** and ***C,*** which seem to promote healthy skin. You might also want to try a system-cleansing diet, consuming only raw fruits and vegetables, yogurt, herbal teas, fruit juices, and mineral water for up to a week. Naturopaths believe that this diet, repeated at regular intervals, may keep sties from developing.

AT-HOME REMEDIES

Apply warm compresses four times daily for 10 to 15 minutes for several days for both sties and chalazions. When the sty has come to a head, it will spontaneously rupture. You can also make a compress by wetting a tea bag with warm water and placing it on your eyelid, with your eye closed, for 5 minutes three to four times a day.

PREVENTION

If sties tend to recur, you need to cleanse the outside of your eyelids daily. Put a few drops of very mild baby shampoo into a teacup of warm water and stir. Using a cotton swab, gently brush the mixture over your eyelid once a day, keeping your lids closed. It is very important that you avoid contact of the eyelid with cosmetics, dirty towels, or contaminated hands.

Frequent application of warm compresses at the first sign of an infection will prevent further blockage of the lid glands. To keep the infection from spreading to other members of your household, be sure to use a clean, disposable cloth for compresses and do not share washcloths or towels. ■

S

SUNBURN

SYMPTOMS

- mildly reddish to severely red or purplish skin discoloration; skin feels hot and tender. Sunburn appears 1 to 6 hours after exposure to sunlight and peaks within 24 hours, later fading to tan or brown.
- small, fluid-filled ***blisters*** that may itch and eventually break; flaking or peeling skin that reveals the tender, reddened underlayer.
- red, blistered skin accompanied by chills, fever, nausea, or dehydration. This severe stage of sunburn is considered a second-degree ***burn.***
- pain and irritation of the eye associated with overexposure to ultraviolet rays from sunlight or other sources.

CALL YOUR DOCTOR IF:

- your sunburn blisters and is accompanied by chills, fever, or nausea. Severe sunburn requires professional care to limit the risk of ***infection*** and to prevent dehydration.
- your eyes are extremely painful and feel gritty. You should have your eyes examined by an ophthalmologist to determine whether the corneas are damaged.

Even though light-skinned people have the highest risk of being sunburned, skin of any color can be damaged by the sun's rays. A sunburn is like any other kind of ***burn,*** except that it comes on more slowly. Skin that is reddened and feels hot to the touch can be self-treated and will heal in a matter of days. Sunburned skin that swells or blisters, causing localized pain and overall discomfort, is considered a first-degree burn. A sunburn that results in swelling and extensive ***blisters*** may be accompanied by fever, nausea, and dehydration.

Moderate exposure to sunlight simply darkens light skin, but regular tanning over many years can hasten **photoaging,** characterized by leathery skin, dark spotting, and extensive wrinkling. Long-term exposure, especially in Caucasians over 40, is associated with **actinic keratoses,** a precancerous skin condition. Severe sunburn early in life increases the risk of developing malignant melanoma, a type of ***skin cancer,*** years later.

CAUSES

Of the sun's ultraviolet (UV) radiation that penetrates Earth's atmosphere, UVA radiation generally only tans but may also take part in premature aging and wrinkling. UVB rays cause sunburn and the potential for ***skin cancer.*** Reflected sunlight from sand, water, or snow is as strong as direct sunlight; shade, clouds, clothes, sunglasses, and sunscreens do not offer complete protection. Certain drugs can intensify the harmful effects of UV radiation; if you are concerned about the potential danger, ask your doctor about photosensitivity.

TREATMENT

At-home care will alleviate many of the symptoms of sunburn, but no treatment can undo the damage caused by prolonged exposure to the sun.

CONVENTIONAL MEDICINE

Few cases of sunburn require medical care. If the burn is very painful or widespread, a doctor may prescribe oral ***corticosteroids*** to relieve the discomfort. Treatment for extremely severe cases of sunburn—those involving extensive blistering, dehydration, or fever—usually requires bed rest and possibly hospitalization. *(See **Burns.**)*

ALTERNATIVE CHOICES

HERBAL THERAPIES

Lotions, poultices, and compresses containing ***calendula*** *(Calendula officinalis)* will reduce inflammation. ***Echinacea*** (*Echinacea* spp.) may be used on exposed new skin after peeling or blistering, to help prevent infection. Over-the-counter preparations containing ***aloe*** *(Aloe barbadensis)* are excellent for relieving pain and irritation.

HOMEOPATHY

Cantharis (12x) taken orally every three to four hours for up to two days is recommended for relieving pain and helping to heal blisters.

HYDROTHERAPY

A cool bath laced with several tablespoonfuls of baking soda or cider vinegar can relieve the pain, itching, and inflammation of a moderate sunburn.

AT-HOME REMEDIES

Apply cold compresses or calamine lotion to ease itchiness, take ***aspirin*** to relieve pain, and have a cool bath or shower for overall relief. Drink plenty of water, but avoid alcohol, which dehydrates the skin. Do not break any blisters; doing so will slow the healing process and increase the risk of infection. When your skin peels or the blisters break, gently remove dried fragments and apply an antiseptic ointment or ***hydrocortisone*** cream to the skin beneath. If you feel feverish or nauseated, drink lots of fluids and see a doctor immediately.

PREVENTION

The best way to prevent sunburn is to limit your exposure to direct sunlight, especially between 10:00 a.m. and 3:00 p.m. Take a look at your shadow: If it's shorter than your height, stay under cover.

- If you have to be outside in the midday sun, wear loose-fitting clothes, a broad-brimmed hat, and shoes to protect your feet and ankles.
- Note that radiation exposure is greater at higher altitudes and southern latitudes.
- Any water surface reflects the sun's rays and can double the radiation dose. Protect your skin with a water-resistant sunscreen.
- Protect babies' sensitive skin from strong sunlight, and alert older children to the hazards of overexposure.
- Wear sunglasses that are rated for UV protection. In general, gray, brown, and green lenses block out damaging UV rays in that order from most to least effective. ■

SCREENING THE SUN

Two types of sunscreens are on the market. Physical sunblocks, such as zinc ointment, protect by creating a barrier between your skin and the sun. They're good for small areas, such as the nose and lips, but not for your whole body. Products containing para-aminobenzoic acid (PABA) block virtually all UVB rays but offer only minimal protection against UVA rays.

Sunscreens carry a sun protection factor (SPF); a rating of SPF 15 is recommended for most people, but fair-skinned people who are in the sun all day need more. Apply sunscreen 30 minutes before you go out, and reapply it after a swim. Even if you don't swim, a waterproof sunscreen has more staying power. If PABA gives you a rash, try sunscreens containing cinnamates for UVB protection and avobenzone for UVA protection.

SWALLOWING DIFFICULTY

Read down this column to find your symptoms. Then read across.

SYMPTOMS	AILMENT/PROBLEM
◆ Food you swallow feels like it's not going all the way down; possibly, chest pain when you lie down or bend over; possibly, shortness of breath.	◆ ***Hiatal hernia; heartburn;*** side effect of ***anxiety***
◆ difficulty swallowing, possibly accompanied by a sore throat.	◆ Any of a number of diseases and conditions, including ***tonsillitis;*** respiratory ***allergies; strep throat; laryngitis;*** sores on the vocal cords; diverticula (small hollow pouches of tissue that form in the esophagus wall and may eventually block the esophagus itself); or a throat abscess
◆ While you are eating, food becomes stuck in your throat, perhaps also causing sharp pain.	◆ An object is lodged in your throat
◆ swallowing difficulties that are gradually worsening with time; weight loss of 10 pounds or more in the past six months.	◆ Potentially, ***throat cancer***
◆ sudden, extreme difficulty swallowing; a feeling of drowning or suffocating; quickened pulse; warm and flush skin; possibly, confusion.	◆ ***Allergies;*** possibly, anaphylactic shock (a severe allergic reaction that causes tissues to swell, preventing blood from traveling properly; tissues then become starved for oxygen)

WHAT TO DO	OTHER INFO
◆ See your doctor if you think you have a hiatal hernia. For heartburn, take over-the-counter ***antacids*** and avoid irritants such as fatty and spicy foods, alcohol, tobacco, and caffeine. To alleviate anxiety, find a relaxation technique—such as yoga or meditation—that you're comfortable with and will practice regularly.	◆ For a hiatal hernia, eat four or five small meals a day instead of three larger ones, and eat slowly.
◆ Consult your doctor. Several of the possible causes of your symptoms require professional medical treatment.	◆ If you have a bacterial ***infection, antibiotics*** may clear up the problem. Vocal cord problems include polyps (swellings on the vocal cord membranes) and singer's nodules (calluslike sores), which are usually the result of repeatedly straining the voice. The best treatment is to rest your voice for several weeks.
◆ If you are choking and cannot breathe, use the Heimlich maneuver. *(See **Emergencies/First Aid: Choking.**)* If you can't completely remove the object from your throat or if swallowing is still difficult or pain persists after the object is seemingly removed, **see a doctor immediately.**	◆ If you feel a sharp pain when you try to swallow, do not attempt to "flush" the object down your throat with liquids, because this may damage your esophagus and other tissues.
◆ Call your doctor today. Prompt diagnosis improves the chances of successful treatment.	◆ Throat cancer most often affects those over 40, especially those with a long history of smoking or heavy drinking.
◆ If you suspect anaphylactic shock, **get emergency medical treatment.** *(See **Emergencies/First Aid: Shock.**)* While waiting for emergency care, monitor the patient's breathing and pulse, and give nothing to eat or drink.	◆ The most common cause of anaphylactic shock is sensitivity to the antibiotic ***penicillin.*** If you know you have a strong, specific ***allergy*** (such as an allergy to bee stings), ask your doctor about preparing an emergency kit to help you prevent anaphylactic shock.

SWEATING, EXCESSIVE

Read down this column to find your symptoms. Then read across.

SYMPTOMS	AILMENT/PROBLEM
Normal sweating is the body's way of lowering its temperature. Sometimes, however, the body sweats in excess of what is needed for normal cooling.	
◆ chronic sweating and clamminess, especially of the hands, underarms, and feet.	◆ Hyperhidrosis (chronic sweating)
◆ excessive sweating with chest pain that typically does not recede with rest and lasts a half-hour or more; may be accompanied by nausea, dizziness, or fainting.	◆ ***Heart attack***
◆ nighttime sweats, weight loss, persistent cough, fever, fatigue, and spitting up blood.	◆ Possibilities include lung disease, ***tuberculosis, AIDS,*** or ***cancer***
◆ sweating with high temperature (over 100°F).	◆ Breaking fever (defervescence)
◆ sweating, hot flashes, vaginal dryness, or mood swings.	◆ Menopause
◆ feelings of tension or stress that may cause profuse sweating.	◆ ***Anxiety***
◆ excessive sweating accompanied by two or more of the following: weight loss, increased appetite, anxiety, insomnia; possibly, rapid heartbeat, muscle weakness, hot skin.	◆ Hyperthyroidism (overactive thyroid)
◆ sweating when you are taking a prescription, over-the-counter, or illegal drug; going through withdrawal; or drinking excessively.	◆ Adverse drug reaction; typical effect of drug withdrawal; alcoholism
◆ heat intolerance, increased sweating of the upper body, and decreased or absent sweating of the lower body.	◆ ***Diabetes***

WHAT TO DO	OTHER INFO
◆ See your doctor. In some cases topical aluminum chloride solution is sufficient. For more severe cases, a simple operation severs the nerves that regulate sweating.	◆ Troublesome residual effects of surgery include compensatory sweating elsewhere on the body and continued underarm sweating.
◆ **Call 911 or your doctor now.** See ***Emergencies/First Aid: Heart Attack.***	
◆ See your doctor without delay. ***Lung cancer,*** Hodgkin's disease *(see* ***Lymphoma****),* and ***tuberculosis*** must all be treated promptly. ***AIDS*** patients who seek care early may live for many years.	◆ Sweating may be the only early symptom of Hodgkin's disease or other lymphomas. People with early HIV infection commonly have sweating, as well as a low fever, fatigue, diarrhea, and mild weight loss.
◆ Take plenty of fluids to prevent dehydration. If fever returns, see your doctor.	◆ Profuse sweating is often the body's way of quickly returning its temperature to normal.
◆ See your doctor. Sometimes, an ***antihypertensive drug*** called clonidine can control abnormal temperature in menopause. See ***Menopausal Problems.***	◆ Sweating may also occur when estrogen levels decline after childbirth or at the beginning of the menstrual period.
◆ If your sweating causes embarrassment, see your doctor, who will ask about underlying anxiety and may prescribe medication.	
◆ See your doctor. If you are producing too much thyroid hormone, you may require radiation, surgery, or thyroid-blocking drugs. See ***Thyroid Problems.***	◆ An overactive thyroid causes unpleasant symptoms by speeding up the chemical reactions of your body, both physical and mental.
◆ Discuss these symptoms with your doctor, who may change your prescription medication. See ***Alcohol Abuse*** and ***Drug Abuse.***	◆ Alcohol and large doses of ***aspirin*** or other drugs, such as ***insulin,*** may cause excessive sweating. *(See* ***Diabetes.****)*
◆ See a doctor. This complication of diabetes indicates poor temperature regulation and may lead to hyperthermia and heatstroke.	

SWIMMER'S EAR

SYMPTOMS

Despite its name, you don't have to be a swimmer to get swimmer's ear. The symptoms include:

- itching inside the ear.
- watery discharge from the ear.
- severe pain and tenderness in the ear, especially when moving your head or when gently pulling on your earlobe.
- a foul-smelling, yellowish discharge from the ear.
- temporarily muffled hearing (caused by blockage of the ear canal).

CALL YOUR DOCTOR IF:

- you are experiencing dizziness or ringing in the ears; such symptoms may indicate a more serious problem that needs medical attention.
- you have severe pain; your doctor can provide medications to relieve it.
- you also notice a rash on your scalp or near your ear; you may have seborrheic ***dermatitis,*** for which your doctor can provide treatment.

Known to medical professionals as otitis externa, swimmer's ear is an inflammation of the outer ear canal. Its common name comes from the fact that it often occurs in children and young adults who swim frequently. The inflammation can sometimes lead to an infection that can be very painful.

CAUSES

Swimmer's ear is often caused by excess moisture in the ear from swimming or even routine showering. The moisture causes the skin inside the ear canal to flake—a condition known as ***eczema.*** A break in the skin, which may result from trying to scratch the persistent itch of the eczema, can allow bacteria or (more rarely) a fungus to invade the tissue of the ear canal and cause an infection. Swimming in polluted water, therefore, is a common cause of swimmer's ear; the bacteria in the water find a hospitable home in the moist environment of an inflamed ear canal.

Other skin conditions, such as seborrheic ***dermatitis*** and ***psoriasis,*** can also lead to swimmer's ear. And another common cause is excessive and improper cleaning of wax from the ears. Not only does wax protect the ear canal from excess moisture, but it also harbors friendly bacteria. Removing this protective barrier—particularly with hairpins, fingernails, or other objects that can scratch the skin—makes it easier for an infection to take hold. Hair spray or haircoloring, which can irritate the ear canal, may also lead to an outer ear infection.

TREATMENT

Swimmer's ear is usually not a dangerous condition and often clears up on its own within a few days. With mild infections, therefore, you may want to try alternative treatments first. If the pain worsens or does not improve within 24 hours, you should see your doctor. In rare cases, the infection can spread and damage underlying bones and cartilage.

CONVENTIONAL MEDICINE

Your doctor will probably clean your ear with a cotton-tipped probe or a suction device to relieve irritation and pain. You may be given a prescription ear drop containing a combination of ***hydrocortisone*** to help relieve the itching and an ***antibiotic*** to fight the infection.

If the pain is severe, your doctor may suggest ***aspirin, acetaminophen,*** or some other over-the-counter pain medication. You will also be instructed to keep water out of the infected ear during the healing process. If the infection does not improve within three or four days, your doctor may prescribe an oral antibiotic.

ALTERNATIVE CHOICES

AROMATHERAPY

To improve blood circulation to the area and thus help healing, gently massage the area around the outer ear with an oil made from 3 to 5 drops of either ***eucalyptus*** *(Eucalyptus globulus)* or ***lavender*** *(Lavandula officinalis)* diluted in 1 tsp olive or other vegetable oil. Rub the oil into the temples and neck and on the earlobe.

HERBAL THERAPIES

Mullein *(Verbascum thapsus)* oil, which has anti-inflammatory properties, may help soothe and heal an inflamed ear canal. Put 1 to 3 drops in the infected ear every three hours.

Another useful herb for swimmer's ear is ***garlic*** *(Allium sativum),* which has been shown to act as a natural antibiotic. Combine equal parts garlic juice, glycerin, and a carrier oil, such as olive or sweet almond; put 1 to 3 drops in the infected ear every three hours.

HOMEOPATHY

Homeopaths prescribe a variety of substances to help relieve the pain of swimmer's ear. Consult a homeopathic practitioner for specific remedies, which may include ***Aconite, Apis,*** or *Graphites.*

AT-HOME REMEDIES

- Wash the infected ear canal with an over-the-counter topical antiseptic. Or try a homemade solution made from equal parts white vinegar and isopropyl alcohol. Continue to put a few drops of the solution into the ear every two to three hours. Keep the drops in the ear for at least 30 seconds.
- To relieve pain, place a warm heating pad or compress on the infected ear.
- Take aspirin or another analgesic to ease the pain.
- During the healing process, make sure you keep the infected ear canal dry, even while showering. Use earplugs or a shower cap.

PREVENTION

- Be careful when cleaning your ears. Wipe the outer ear with a clean washcloth. Do not dig into the ear canal, and never use a pointed object.
- Wear earplugs when swimming. Afterward, tilt and shake your head to drain water from your ears.
- Avoid swimming in dirty water.
- Use earplugs or a shower cap to keep your ears dry while showering. Or dry your ears after showering with a hair dryer: Set it on low and hold it about a foot from your ear.
- You can also dry out your ear and help kill germs after swimming or showering by squirting a dropperful of isopropyl alcohol or white vinegar into your ear. Tilt your head so the solution gets to the bottom of the ear canal, then let the liquid drain out.
- To create a protective coating for your ear canal before you go swimming, squirt a dropperful of mineral oil, baby oil, or lanolin into your ear.
- If you wear a hearing aid, take it out as often as possible to give your ear a chance to dry out; a hearing aid can trap moisture in the ear canal. ■

SYPHILIS

SYMPTOMS

There are three stages of syphilis.

- In the first stage, 10 days to 6 weeks after exposure, painless sores appear on the genitals, rectum, or mouth. Lymph nodes near the groin may be swollen as well.
- In the second stage, one week to six months later, a red rash may appear anywhere on the body. You may have flulike symptoms, such as headache, fever, fatigue, loss of appetite, and pain in bones and joints; symptoms may then disappear, and the disease becomes latent, but the bacteria remain in the body.
- In the third stage, which can start anytime from one year to several decades later, joints may be affected, resulting in ***arthritis.*** **Cardiovascular syphilis** develops in approximately 10 percent of patients, causing ***heart disease.*** **Neurosyphilis**, which may cause paralysis, blindness, senility, insanity, or loss of sensation in the legs, develops in about 8 percent of patients.

CALL YOUR DOCTOR IF:

- you experience any of the symptoms above. Syphilis is life-threatening and it's imperative to treat it before it does serious damage to your system.

Syphilis is among the most serious of sexually transmitted diseases. In 1990 some 100,000 cases were reported in the United States—a 40-year high—with the highest incidence occurring in urban populations, among people ages 15 to 39. Epidemiologists attribute the increase to a lack of education about the disease as well as to a rise in the number of prostitutes having unprotected sex. The increase is not reflected among homosexuals or bisexuals, however, presumably because many in that population are using condoms more frequently.

CAUSES

Syphilis is caused by the spirochete bacterium *Treponema pallidum,* which gains entrance to the body through minor cuts or abrasions in the skin or mucous membranes, most often during sexual intercourse. The disease also may be transmitted from mother to child before or during birth.

DIAGNOSTIC AND TEST PROCEDURES

Your doctor will be able to determine whether you have syphilis by examining your blood for antibodies to the disease.

TREATMENT

If caught early, syphilis may be cured with ***antibiotics.*** But if you allow the disease to progress to the third stage, you may suffer irreversible damage to your heart or nervous system. If you have

C A U T I O N !

If you are pregnant, get a syphilis test. The life-threatening disease may be passed to your child before or during delivery. Approximately half of all babies infected with syphilis die before or shortly after birth.

S

syphilis, you'll require follow-up blood tests at regular intervals for at least a year after treatment.

CONVENTIONAL MEDICINE

Penicillin is extremely effective in treating the early stages, and fairly effective in treating the later stages, of syphilis. If you are allergic to penicillin, your physician will give you ***tetracycline*** or ***erythromycin.***

ALTERNATIVE CHOICES

Because syphilis is a serious, potentially life-threatening disease, you must see a doctor as soon as you think you have it. Besides taking penicillin or its derivatives, you can use several alternative therapies to speed healing.

ACUPRESSURE

To treat sexually transmitted diseases, acupressurists work on points that are said to help rid the body of built-up toxins. Several times a day, massage Liver 3, located on top of the foot between the big and second toes, and Liver 8, on the inside of the leg above the knee. Next, press Kidney 3, on the inside of the leg between the anklebone and Achilles tendon. *(See the **Appendix** for more information about point locations.)*

CHINESE HERBS

A doctor of Chinese medicine will give you a unique herbal formula to help clear toxins from the body. Herbs beneficial in the treatment of syphilis include ***Chinese foxglove root*** *(Rehmannia glutinosa)* and ***dong quai*** *(Angelica sinensis).*

HERBAL THERAPIES

Cowboys drank sarsaparilla for a reason: The herb that flavored the popular soft drink was once thought to be the only cure for syphilis, which was rampant in Old West brothels. Sarsaparilla *(Smilax officinalis)* was also used extensively throughout Europe. Trade records from the mid-19th century show that Great Britain alone imported 150,000 pounds a year.

To treat syphilis, some herbalists advocate the following formula: Add 2 tbsp each of sarsaparilla and sourdock *(Rumex crispus)* root to 1 qt boiling water. Simmer for five minutes and add 3½ tsp thyme. Steep covered for one hour. Drink one to three cups per day. Women may use this tea as a douche.

HOMEOPATHY

In addition to prescribing ***antibiotics,*** a homeopathic physician will ask you if any of your ancestors had syphilis or another sexually transmitted disease, on the theory that you could have inherited the tendency to contract syphilis. If so, a homeopath might prescribe a remedy such as *Syphilinum,* to help stimulate your immune system's response to the disease.

NUTRITION AND DIET

One thing you can do yourself to alleviate pain and encourage healing is to watch what you eat. Some nutritionists recommend that you cleanse your body of toxins by fasting for one to three days. Always check with your physician before beginning a fast. To stimulate your kidneys and flush out your system, drink the juices of pomegranate and cranberry or a combination of celery, parsley, and cucumber. Eat a balanced diet and avoid high-fat, salty, processed foods, which may make your system too sluggish to fight off disease.

AT-HOME REMEDIES

- Take a hot bath followed by a cold one to help alleviate the aches and pains associated with syphilis.
- Use acupressure massages, which may help rid your body of toxins.
- Eat a balanced diet to help build up your immune system.

PREVENTION

If you're not in a long-term monogamous relationship, always use a condom when having sex.■

TEETHING PROBLEMS

SYMPTOMS

Although the arrival of your infant's early teeth is a normal development and not an illness, it can be an irritating or painful process for your child and a trying time for you. Indications of teething may include:

- increased fussing, nighttime crying, and clinging from your baby as teeth start pushing out of the gums, usually at about six months.
- drooling and chewing on fingers as more teeth move toward the surface.
- swollen and inflamed gums, especially where a tooth is about to emerge.
- refusal to suck on breast or bottle, because the sucking action hurts inflamed gums.

CALL YOUR DOCTOR IF:

- your teething baby runs a ***fever,*** seems lethargic or irritable, is not responding well to the teething, or has ***diarrhea*** while teething; these symptoms may be signs that your child is ill.
- your teething baby has cold symptoms or a fever and clutches an ear or one side of her face; this may signal ***otitis media.***
- no teeth are present by 12 months of age; this could indicate a harmless inherited tendency to late teething, but it might instead mean some metabolic condition that could cause delayed bone development. Your first call should be to your pediatrician, who later might refer you to a pediatric dentist.

Before birth, a baby's teeth have already developed inside the gums. At around four months, the teeth start moving to the surface. By seven months, your infant probably will be actively teething, with most baby teeth in various stages of eruption—or emergence—from the gums. All 20 baby teeth, appearing in the order indicated below, right, are usually in place before the child is three. Heredity determines the speed at which teeth appear; your children probably will share the same teething pattern. Teething is a good time to start a preventive dental program with regular gum cleaning. Dentists also recommend beginning fluoride treatments at around six months, even if teeth are still under the gum. Fluoride strengthens the teeth by bonding with the calcium and phosphorus in their enamel. Good dental habits learned early will be invaluable when your child begins getting permanent teeth by about seven years of age.

CAUSES

A tooth moving toward the surface of the gum may cause pain and swelling where it will break through. A baby may refuse to suck at this stage because sucking action draws blood to the inflamed area, increasing soreness.

TREATMENT

Because teething is not an illness, the treatment of it is simply a matter of trying to relieve the child's discomfort.

CONVENTIONAL MEDICINE

It is not essential to consult your pediatrician unless your baby has symptoms of illness. If you do seek help for a teething infant with persistent discomfort, the doctor may recommend liquid ***acetaminophen,*** which should be used sparingly (two to four times a day) but usually provides pain relief. Over-the-counter teething medications with a topical anesthetic such as ***benzocaine*** are not recommended, because they can be toxic.

ALTERNATIVE CHOICES

ACUPRESSURE

Practitioners suggest gently pressing Stomach 3 and 4 or massaging Large Intestine 4, found between your child's thumb and index finger on either hand. See the ***Appendix*** for more information on point locations.

HERBAL THERAPIES

Herbalists recommend ***chamomile*** *(Matricara recutita)* tea for inflamed gums; use 3 tsp in your child's food or drink daily, or apply directly to the gums.

HOMEOPATHY

Homeopathic teething remedies are available over the counter. If your child's discomfort is not eased within 24 hours, however, you will want to consult a practitioner for advice. ***Chamomilla*** is considered one of the most effective homeopathic remedies for teething. Other specific remedies that your practitioner might prescribe include ***Aconite, Pulsatilla,*** and ***Belladonna.***

YOUR BABY'S TEETH

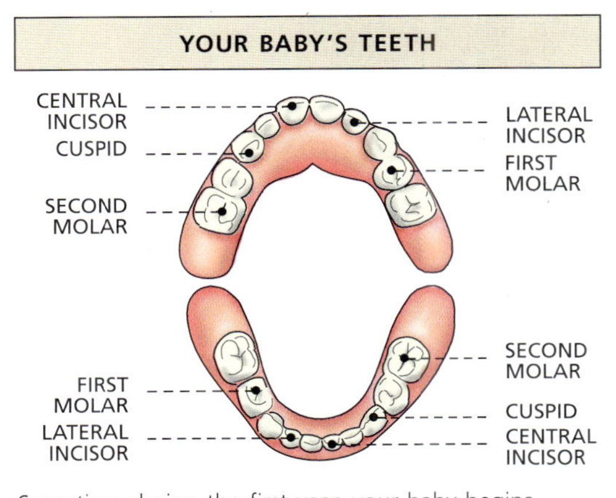

Sometime during the first year, your baby begins teething. The central and lateral incisors appear first. Six to twelve months later the first molars develop, and soon afterward the cuspids. In general, the lower teeth tend to come in before the corresponding upper teeth. By the age of two or a little older the second molars will have appeared, making a full set of 20 primary, or "baby," teeth.

LIFESTYLE

When your child begins teething, you can start cleaning her gums and teeth daily with gauze or a soft toothbrush. When she is two-and-a-half to three, her motor skills will be more developed and you can start teaching her to brush her teeth. At age four, she is ready for her first dental visit.

NUTRITION AND DIET

When weaning your teething child, give her easy-to-digest foods such as baby rice or millet; establish regular feeding times and feed slowly, burping after every feeding. Never let your child teethe on or go to sleep with a bottle of milk or juice; the sugars and starches will encourage tooth decay.

AT-HOME REMEDIES

- A chilled but not frozen teething ring or a chilled wet washcloth can ease soreness and give your child something to chew.
- Wrap an ice cube in a soft cloth and rub it gently on your infant's gums to ease inflammation; keep moving the ice over the gums to avoid damaging tissue.
- Don't let your baby's drooling go unattended; a rash can develop. Put petroleum jelly around your infant's mouth and chin, and use a bib or change the child's clothes if they become saturated from drooling.
- Avoid feeding your child salty or acidic foods, which can aggravate sensitive gums.

CAUTION!

DANGEROUS OLD REMEDY

Never rub alcohol on your teething child's gums! In the past, and occasionally today, liquor has been employed to relieve teething pain. Alcohol may momentarily relieve gum discomfort, but alcohol has a direct toxic effect, and even small quantities can lead to severe hypoglycemia and brain damage. ■

TEMPOROMANDIBULAR JOINT SYNDROME

SYMPTOMS

- pain in front of the ears, especially upon awakening.
- persistent pain in the facial muscles on one or both sides.
- a clicking or popping sensation when opening the mouth or working the jaw.
- difficulty opening the mouth because it feels locked or painful.
- recurring ***headaches.***

CALL YOUR DOCTOR IF:

- you have difficulty opening your mouth following an injury or a blow to the face. You may have dislocated or damaged one or both of your temporomandibular joints.
- you have persistent discomfort in your jaw that does not respond to painkillers, heat, massage, or rest. You may need a specialist's diagnosis and advice about more aggressive treatment to relieve both the symptoms and the cause.

The fact that humans need to speak and eat makes the jawbone one of our busiest moving parts. The twin joints that connect the lower jaw, or mandible, to the temporal bones of the skull are relatively simple hinges with small disks of cartilage to protect the bony surfaces that rub against each other. The jawbreaking term for pain or discomfort in this area is temporomandibular joint (TMJ) syndrome, or myofascial pain dysfunction.

As many as two-thirds of Americans exhibit symptoms of TMJ at some point in their lives, when something as simple as a wide yawn or eating a chewy bagel sets off facial pain or jaw popping. This temporary condition usually resolves itself without treatment or responds quickly to rest and painkillers. In some instances, though, patients feel pain that radiates through the face and around the neck and shoulders, a chronic pattern of TMJ that results from other conditions. Most temporary TMJ discomfort can be helped with inexpensive, at-home remedies; but for a few TMJ sufferers, persistent and sometimes unbearable pain is a serious problem requiring medical treatment. Unfortunately, some health insurers insist on labeling TMJ as a dental rather than a medical problem and object to paying for treatment, a fact that can sometimes discourage sufferers from seeking available help and relief.

CAUSES

Most cases of TMJ are due to excessive strain on the jaw muscles, a displaced disk, or degenerative joint disease—sometimes in combination. The most common cause is strain to the temporalis muscles that open and close the jaw. The strain can stem from unconsciously clenching or grinding the teeth or jutting the jaw forward, as well as from a poor bite caused by misaligned teeth or poorly fitting dentures.

Displacement of one or both of the disks in the jaw's hinges can result from a sudden blow or injury to the head, or simply from hard chewing or a wide yawn. Usually the displaced disk slips back into position without permanently harming the jaw. If such dislocation happens often, however, the jaw may start to pop or click when

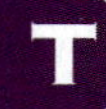

opened, and the joint may become inflamed, stiff, and painful. The effects of degenerative joint disease are similar: Osteoarthritis or rheumatoid ***arthritis*** inflames the joint, causing pain and stiffness. On rare occasions, malnutrition in children can lead to bone deformities that cause TMJ.

THE TEMPOROMANDIBULAR JOINT

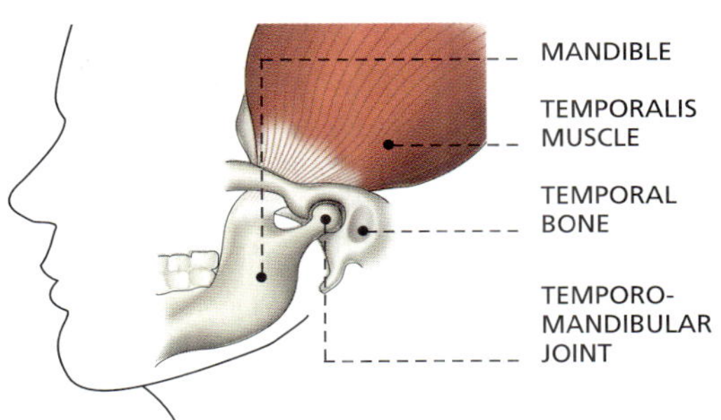

The temporomandibular joint is a hinge that joins the mandible, or jawbone, to the temporal bone of the skull. The large temporalis muscle and other ligaments and muscles keep the joint operating smoothly. If any component is forced out of alignment by such things as muscle tension, arthritis, a head injury, or an uncorrected bite, the joint may not move smoothly and can cause pain.

TREATMENT

Taking a painkiller may ease the inflammation and relieve the pain of TMJ but does not get to the underlying cause of the problem. TMJ sufferers need to assess their entire lifestyle—from potentially avoidable day-to-day stresses to eating foods that strain the jaw. In cases where tooth alignment is at fault, you need to see your dentist.

CONVENTIONAL MEDICINE

Most doctors tell people with mild TMJ to take an over-the-counter ***analgesic,*** massage the area, and limit talking and chewing for a few days—resting the jaw by eating soft or liquid foods. More painful or chronic conditions may require treatment by a dentist, physical therapist, orthodontist, oral surgeon, or behavioral specialist.

Some people unconsciously grind their teeth while sleeping, a condition called bruxism. A dentist can diagnose that problem and fit the patient with a bite guard or splint. A doctor who suspects that TMJ is caused by excessive muscle strain may prescribe a ***muscle relaxant*** such as ***diazepam*** to relieve pain and tension. Since TMJ can be a chronic condition, however, a patient should not rely on such prescription drugs for long-term relief, because of the risk of addiction.

Physical therapy may relieve pain and restore jaw mobility in some cases of TMJ. A physical therapist may recommend massage, moist-heat compresses, ultrasound, or stimulation by interferential electric current to promote circulation and to relieve pain and stiffness. To improve the jaw's range of motion, a therapist may use stretching exercises and may recommend the spray-and-stretch technique, in which the face is sprayed with a numbing coolant and the jaw muscles are stretched. Other physical therapy options include short-wave diathermy and laser treatments. The waves from such treatment reach much deeper than moist-heat applications, and the undulating pressure works like a massage, increasing blood flow to the affected area and reducing inflammation and pain.

Doctors recommend surgery only for extreme cases. The least invasive form, arthroscopy, involves inserting a fiberoptic tube through a small incision and using it to reposition the disk. If arthroscopy fails, open TM joint surgery may be necessary; this entails completely exposing the area and may include a joint replacement. Before making a commitment to surgery, however, a patient should explore all options, potential complications, and side effects and should get a second opinion from another qualified surgeon.

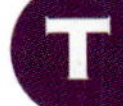

ALTERNATIVE CHOICES

Various alternative therapies can be effective in treating TMJ. A number of herbal remedies may act as sedatives or relax muscles to ease the pain. Many medical doctors acknowledge **biofeedback**'s success rate for controlling stress-related TMJ.

ACUPRESSURE

For patients who feel squeamish about acupuncture needles, acupressure offers a gentle alternative. The acupressure therapist presses points on the stomach meridians, which pass through the area where muscle spasms, stiffness, and pain associated with TMJ are most apt to occur. *(See the illustrations at right.)*

ACUPRESSURE

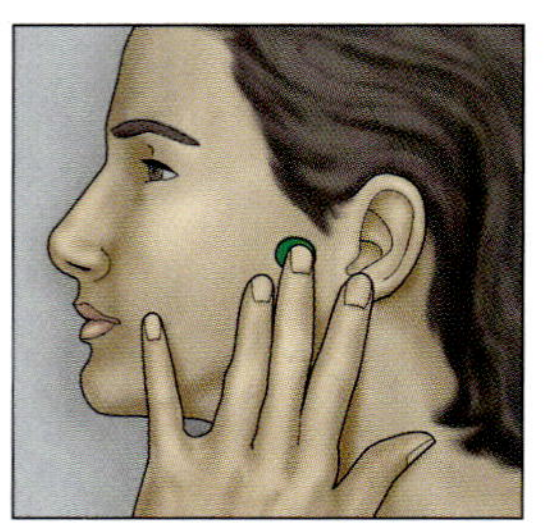

1 Pressing Stomach 7 may ease tension in the jaw. With your middle fingers, feel on either side of your jaw about one thumb width in front of your ears. Find a slight indentation along the upper jaw line, then press steadily for one minute.

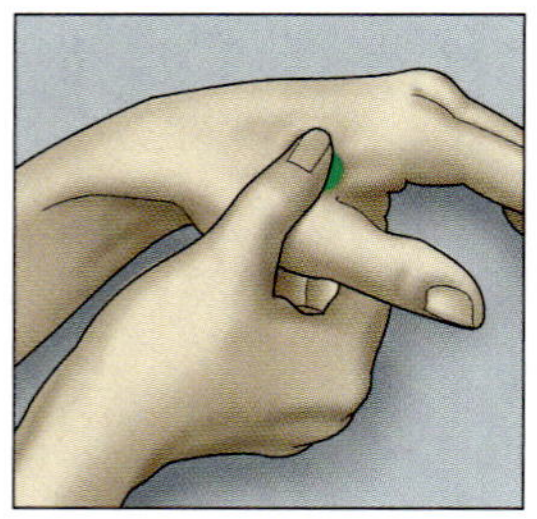

2 To help relieve facial pain caused by TMJ, press Large Intestine 4, located in the web between thumb and index finger. Squeeze the web of each hand with the thumb and index finger of the other for one minute. Do not press this point if you are pregnant.

ACUPUNCTURE

Acupuncture works by relaxing the muscles, which makes it effective for TMJ symptoms that are caused by stress. Like an acupressurist, an acupuncturist will treat points on the stomach meridians for stress-related TMJ, because those meridians pass through the temporomandibular joints.

BODY WORK

When tension is believed to play a role in TMJ, **massage** therapy may provide relief. Two areas can be massaged: One runs from just above and slightly forward of the top of your ear over to your temple; the other is on your jaw about an inch in front of your earlobes. Place a finger on either of these areas, and then open and close your jaw, pressing your teeth together slightly when the jaw is closed. You will feel a muscle pop in and out as it contracts and relaxes. Place your thumb or your index and middle fingers on these areas, and massage lightly in little circles. Doing this for a minute or two at each spot can help relax muscles that cause tension around the joint. For more severe cases of TMJ, consult a professional massage therapist. Techniques that have been reported to help TMJ are deep-tissue **massage,** neuromuscular massage, **Rolfing,** and craniosacral work.

T

CHIROPRACTIC

Chiropractic therapy is recommended for TMJ caused by muscle overuse and strain, rather than by joint damage as in a patient who develops TMJ after whiplash injury in a car accident. A chiropractor not only treats the patient's back and body alignment, but may also use physical therapy, interferential current, ultrasound, or diathermy on the affected joint, any of which can help relax the area and allow the chiropractor to stretch the muscles and manipulate the jaw.

HYDROTHERAPY

A few drops of the essential oils of ***lavender*** *(Lavandula officinalis)* or jasmine *(Jasminum officinale)* in warm bathwater may help you to relax. To reduce inflammation of the TM joints, apply hot and cold compresses. Start with a hot towel for three minutes, then switch to a cold towel for half a minute; repeat two or three times a day for chronic conditions, or more frequently if acute.

MIND/BODY MEDICINE

While **relaxation** techniques, **hypnotherapy,** and **guided imagery** can all alleviate the symptoms of TMJ, **biofeedback** is the most effective mind/body treatment for TMJ. Biofeedback is a drug-free, noninvasive approach to eliminating tension and controlling stress-related pain, and can be self-administered after training by a professional therapist. Using electrical readings from the muscle that moves the jaw, practitioners can train a patient to control the tension in the overall area. Studies have shown that biofeedback works especially well for chronic TMJ sufferers and may help reduce pain and minimize clicking for a longer time than other treatments.

NUTRITION AND DIET

It is important for TMJ sufferers to reduce strain on jaw muscles and joints. Avoid hard foods like raw carrots and apples, and chewy foods like steak and bagels. If the pain in your jaw becomes really unbearable, try fasting or putting yourself on a liquid diet for a day or two; this is especially effective if you also limit talking to when it's absolutely necessary.

From a nutritional standpoint, TMJ patients should consider taking appropriate dosages of bromelain, or the bioflavonoid pyncogenol in combination with ***vitamin C,*** to reduce inflammation; ***calcium/magnesium*** tablets for muscle spasms; or ***B-complex vitamins*** to relieve stress.

OSTEOPATHY

Besides recommending proper dental work, physical therapy, or biofeedback, an osteopathic physician may also use hands-on techniques to help increase the range of motion in the head, neck, shoulders, and upper back. You may be able to find an osteopathic doctor who specializes in TMJ.

AT-HOME REMEDIES

No matter what causes occasional TMJ, you can take ***aspirin*** or a ***nonsteroidal anti-inflammatory drug (NSAID)*** to relieve the pain. If you have an unexplained, persistent headache that's relieved when you put an ice-cream stick between your teeth, you probably have an alignment problem in your jaw area. Stress-related TMJ usually responds well to at-home remedies. But if your pain is caused by poorly aligned teeth or damage to the joint, don't go on a steady painkiller regimen; see a doctor or dentist. Some other suggestions:

- Massage the band of muscles just above and in front of your temples, as well as the larger muscles along your jaw line. Use small circular motions and repeat as needed.
- Mouth guards for football and hockey players might help mild cases of TMJ due to bruxism (teeth grinding). You'll find the guards in sporting-goods stores. Soften the plastic mouthpiece in warm water, then bite down straight and hard to make an imprint of your teeth. Allow the impression to set, then put the guard between your teeth at night when you sleep. If pain or grinding continues for any length of time, see a doctor.

PREVENTION

- To prevent TMJ from unconscious muscle strain or uneven pressure on the jaw, don't sleep with your head tilted or with the entire weight of your head concentrated on your chin—a common practice among people who sleep on their stomachs. Try sleeping on your side, or on your back without a pillow.
- Whenever your jaw hurts, stay away from foods that are hard to chew, and minimize talking.
- If you feel tension in your jaw every morning, you may be unwittingly clenching or grinding your teeth. See a dentist or orthodontist about the advantages of being fitted with a bite guard.

TMJ AND WHIPLASH

For years doctors have found that people who sustain whiplash injuries in car accidents can develop TMJ. Although debate continues about the precise cause, women seem particularly susceptible, possibly because some women's neck muscles are weaker in relation to head size than they are in men, giving the head-snapping momentum greater impact. Studies have shown that whiplash-related TMJ—which occurs without direct impact or pressure on the jaw—may cause clicking, popping, and on occasion some pain, but almost never persists long-term, if treated. ■

T

TENDONITIS

SYMPTOMS

- painful tenderness at or near a joint, especially around a shoulder, wrist, or heel (where it is known as Achilles tendonitis), or on the outside of an elbow (where it is called ***tennis elbow***).
- in some cases, numbness or tingling.
- stiffness that, along with the pain, restricts the movement of the joint involved.
- occasionally, mild swelling at the joint.
- persistence of the soreness, which may last or recur long after the tendon has had time to recover from the original injury.

CALL YOUR DOCTOR IF:

- your pain doesn't ease up in 7 to 10 days. You want to avoid letting chronic tendonitis set in; moreover, you may have another problem such as ***bursitis, carpal tunnel syndrome,*** or ***phlebitis.***
- your pain is extremely severe and accompanied by swelling. You may have a ruptured tendon, which requires immediate medical attention.

Tendonitis is an inflammation in or around a tendon, a band of fibrous tissue that connects a muscle to a bone and transmits the force the muscle exerts. Tendons are designed to withstand bending, stretching, and twisting, but they can become inflamed because of overuse, disease, or injuries that leave them with torn fibers or other damage. The pain can be significant and worsens if damage progresses because of continued use of the joint. Most tendonitis heals in about two weeks, but chronic tendonitis can take more than six weeks, often because the sufferer doesn't give the tendon time to heal. Diseases such as ***diabetes, arthritis,*** and ***gout*** can slow healing.

CAUSES

Tendons can become inflamed when overstressed from any activity. Weekend athletes, who exercise sporadically rather than regularly, are often laid low by sore tendons. But by far the most common cause is repetitive stress—using the same joints for the same stressful movements again and again. This happens not only in sports but also in many types of office work and other situations.

DIAGNOSTIC AND TEST PROCEDURES

Your physician may order x-rays and bone scans in order to rule out bone damage. MRI scans can help determine the severity of damage to a tendon.

TREATMENT

The goals of treatment are to restore movement to the joint without pain and to maintain strength in surrounding muscles while giving the tissues time to heal. Adequate rest is crucial. Returning too soon to the activity that caused the injury can lead to chronic tendonitis or torn tendons.

CONVENTIONAL MEDICINE

As an immediate treatment for tendonitis, doctors and physical therapists recommend what is known as the RICE program: rest, ice, compression, and elevation *(see **At-Home Remedies,** below, right).* They may also suggest ***aspirin*** or ***ibuprofen*** to help reduce inflammation and pain. Ultrasound and whirlpool treatments are employed to relax muscles and tendons, improve circulation, and promote healing. Occasionally, your doctor may prescribe ***corticosteroids.***

Your therapist will probably propose an exercise plan that rests the tendon while strengthening nearby muscle groups and maintaining overall muscle tone. Only gradually will you begin to exercise the tendon itself. Your program may also include "eccentric" exercises, in which you gradually increase use of the injured area, stopping at the first sign of pain. You may work into easy stretching exercises, done several times a day.

TENDONITIS ON THE JOB

If your tendonitis is caused by tasks you perform at work and you cannot rest your injuries while keeping up with your duties, ask your supervisor for help in modifying your work habits. You may want to request a work-site inspection by an ergonomics specialist, who can analyze the situation and suggest changes. Try some stretches before and after work, and plan to take a 5- to 10-minute period each hour to rest the injured area by undertaking tasks that do not involve its use.

ALTERNATIVE CHOICES

CHINESE HERBS

Chinese practitioners might prepare a poultice of gardenia *(Gardenia jasminoides),* flour, and wine, which together with tui na—a type of massage that uses the ball of the thumb to manipulate the affected area—may help to reduce swelling and increase circulation.

HERBAL THERAPIES

For pain, a naturopathic practitioner might suggest ***white willow*** *(Salix alba),* the natural form of aspirin, taken orally. Bromelain, an enzyme found in pineapples, is sometimes taken orally with the aim of reducing inflammation in soft tissues.

HOMEOPATHY

Among the over-the-counter homeopathic remedies suitable for tendonitis symptoms are ***Arnica*** (6x to 30c) as an anti-inflammatory and ***Ruta*** (6x to 12x) as an antispasmodic.

CAUTION!

If you have had a stroke or suffer from circulatory problems, diabetes, or heart disease, avoid massage and applications of heat or cold until you consult your doctor.

NUTRITION AND DIET

Research suggests that vitamin supplements may help heal tendonitis. Ask your doctor about taking daily supplements of ***vitamin C*** (1,000 mg), beta carotene *(see **vitamin A**)* (10,000 IU), ***zinc*** (22.5 mg), ***vitamin E*** (400 IU), and ***selenium*** (50 mcg).

AT-HOME REMEDIES

Remind yourself of RICE. Rest is mainly a matter of remembering not to use the joint, especially not for the same action that injured it. Ice can be in the form of a bag of frozen vegetables if no ice pack is handy. Compression is best provided by a sports bandage wrapping the area snugly, but not painfully tight. For elevation—to reduce blood pressure in the injured area—put your ankle on a footstool or lift your elbow onto a chairside table.

PREVENTION

Include warmups, cooldowns, and stretches in your exercise routine. Vary your exercises. ■

TENNIS ELBOW

SYMPTOMS

- recurring pain on the outside of the upper forearm just below the bend of the elbow; occasionally, pain radiates down the arm toward the wrist.
- pain caused by lifting or bending the arm or grasping even light objects such as a coffee cup.
- difficulty extending the forearm fully (because of inflamed muscles, tendons, and ligaments).
- pain that typically lasts for 6 to 12 weeks; the discomfort can continue for as little as 3 weeks or as long as several years.

CALL YOUR DOCTOR IF:

- the pain persists for more than a few days; chronic inflammation of the tendons can lead to permanent disability.
- the elbow joint begins to swell; tennis elbow rarely causes swelling, so you may have another condition such as ***arthritis, gout, infection,*** or even a tumor.

Doctors first identified tennis elbow (or lateral epicondylitis) more than 100 years ago. Today nearly half of all tennis players will suffer from this disorder at some point, but they account for less than 5 percent of all cases, making the term for this condition something of a misnomer. While people of all ages and races can develop tennis elbow, Caucasian men 30 to 60 years old who work with their hands—carpenters and house painters, for example—are at greatest risk; middle-aged women who do piecework in the garment industry are also highly susceptible.

In recent years cases of tennis elbow have also surfaced in children who play hand-held computer games for extended periods and in office workers who use a computer only rarely but, when they do use one, type intensely for long hours. *(See also **Carpal Tunnel Syndrome.**)*

CAUSES

Tennis players with a lazy, late backhand tend to compensate for their poor footwork and timing by snapping the wrist to come around on the ball. This places a great deal of stress on the relatively delicate common extensor tendon, located on the outside of the elbow, and on the extensor carpi radialis brevis muscle, which helps control the wrist. You can cause the same kind of stress by making aggressive twists with a screwdriver or other implement, or by lifting heavy objects with your elbow locked and your arm extended. Younger people with more supple joints can often get away with straining tissues in this way, but the muscles and tendons of people over 30 are more likely to suffer damage.

The damage consists of tiny tears in a part of the tendon and in muscle coverings. After the initial injury heals, these areas often tear again, which leads to hemorrhaging and the formation of rough, granulated tissue and calcium deposits within the surrounding tissues. Collagen, a protein, leaks out from around the injured areas, causing inflammation. The resulting pressure can cut off the blood flow and pinch the radial nerve, one of the major nerves controlling muscles in the arm and hand.

TENDON INJURY

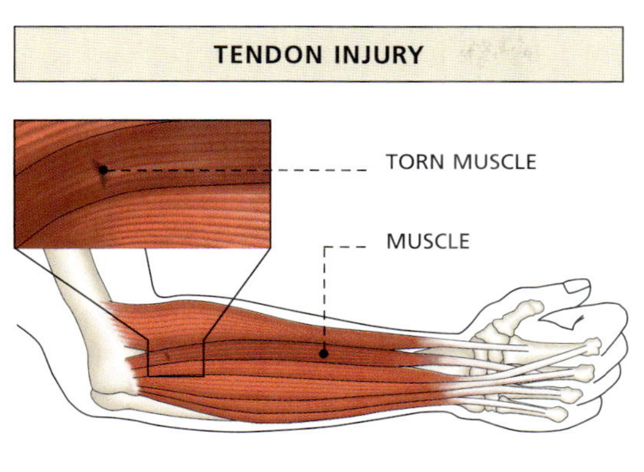

Wrist movement is controlled in part by the extensor carpi radialis brevis muscle. If the extended wrist meets a resisting force, as when hitting a ball with a tennis racket, the excessive pressure and stress can cause the muscle to tear *(above, inset).* Pain and inflammation typically follow the injury.

Tendons, which attach muscles to bones, do not receive the same amount of oxygen and blood that muscles do, so they heal more slowly. In fact, some cases of tennis elbow can last for years, though the inflammation usually subsides in 6 to 12 weeks.

Many medical textbooks treat tennis elbow as a form of ***tendonitis,*** which is often the case, but if the muscles and bones of the elbow joint are also involved, then the condition is called epicondylitis. However, if you feel pain directly on the back of your elbow joint, rather than down the outside of your arm, you may have ***bursitis,*** which is caused when lubricating sacs in the joint become inflamed. If you see swelling, which is almost never a symptom of tennis elbow, you may want to investigate other possible conditions, such as ***arthritis, infection, gout,*** or a tumor.

TREATMENT

The best way to relieve tennis elbow is to stop doing anything that irritates your arm—a simple step for the weekend tennis player, but not as easy for the manual laborer, office worker, or professional athlete.

The most effective conventional and alternative treatments for tennis elbow have the same basic premise: Rest the arm until the pain disappears, then massage to relieve stress and tension in the muscles, and exercise to strengthen the area and prevent reinjury. If you must go back to whatever caused the problem in the first place, be sure to warm up your arm for at least 5 to 10 minutes with gentle stretching and movement before starting any activity. Take frequent breaks.

CONVENTIONAL MEDICINE

Conventional medicine offers an assortment of treatments for tennis elbow, from drug injections to surgery, but the pain will never go away completely unless you stop stressing the joint. Reinjury is inevitable without adequate rest.

For most mild to moderate cases of tennis elbow, ***aspirin*** or ***ibuprofen*** will help address the inflammation and the pain while you are resting the injury, and then you can follow up with exercise and massage to speed healing.

In some patients the body tries to defend the elbow from further damage by contracting the biceps, which then makes it difficult to extend the arm; the entire area can become quite tight. Gentle massage and careful stretching two to four times a week for several weeks will help offset this problem.

For stubborn cases of tennis elbow your doctor may advise ***corticosteroid*** injections, which dramatically reduce inflammation, but they cannot be used long-term because of potentially damaging side effects.

If rest, anti-inflammatory medications, and a stretching routine fail to cure your tennis elbow, you may have to consider surgery, though this form of treatment is rare (fewer than 3 percent of patients). One procedure is for the tendon to be cut loose from the epicondyle, the rounded bump at the end of the bone, which eliminates stress on the tendon but renders the muscle useless. Another surgical technique involves removing so-called granulated tissue in the tendon and repairing tears.

Even after you feel you have overcome a case of tennis elbow, be sure to continue babying your

SHOULD YOU STRAP IT?

Many doctors suggest using a strap or band just below the elbow to support the muscles in the area and take stress off tendons, but research has shown that these devices can reduce circulation and actually impede recovery if used for a prolonged period. Sustained pressure on the inflamed arm may also lead to fibrosis, in which excess connective tissue forms, almost like scar tissue; the resulting trauma can impair circulation and result in a permanent weakening of your arm.

arm. Always warm up your arm for 5 to 10 minutes before starting any activity involving your elbow. And if you develop severe pain after use anyway, pack your arm in ice for 15 to 20 minutes and call your doctor.

ALTERNATIVE CHOICES

Tennis elbow responds well to a variety of alternative therapies. Some you will be able to try on your own, but you should also consider professional help from a **chiropractor, osteopath,** or a practitioner of traditional **Chinese medicine.**

ACUPRESSURE

Deep thumb pressure on Large Intestine 11, located on the inside of the elbow, may help relieve pain. See the ***Appendix*** for more information on locating this point.

ACUPUNCTURE

Acupuncture has an estimated 60 to 70 percent success rate when used on tennis elbow patients—a record that has helped it gain acceptance even in more conservative medical circles. There are a number of acupuncture points that might prove beneficial, so be sure to seek out an acupuncturist who is experienced in treating this or similar types of conditions.

BODY WORK

To prevent recurring bouts of tennis elbow, you need to improve your overall body alignment; proper posture and balance may do more for an ailing joint than drug therapies. Consider seeing a body work specialist or an **osteopath** about techniques such as **Rolfing,** the **Feldenkrais method,** and the **Alexander technique**.

CHIROPRACTIC

Chiropractors, physical therapists, and occupational therapists all commonly use diathermy (a form of electrical stimulation), ultrasound, and **massage** to treat tennis elbow. Electrical and sound currents improve circulation and drainage, which then makes it easier to stretch and massage the affected area. Occasionally, chiropractors and therapists prescribe a splint or band to take stress off the affected tendon or muscle, but be aware that a poor fit or wearing the splint or band for too long can reduce blood flow.

HERBAL THERAPIES

To help relax a tender arm, massage the affected area with oil of ***lavender*** *(Lavandula officinalis)* or ***eucalyptus*** *(Eucalyptus globulus).* ***Cayenne*** *(Capsicum frutescens),* which is available in ointment form in most drugstores, as well as prickly ash *(Zanthoxylum americanum)* oil are believed to increase blood flow and speed healing.

HYDROTHERAPY

If you suffer from recurrent bouts of tennis elbow, consider soaking your arm in warm water for 30 minutes before exercising. Always place the affected joint in ice after a workout.

MIND/BODY MEDICINE

Several studies have demonstrated that **hypnotherapy** may provide effective relief for pain associated with tennis elbow. Consult an experienced practitioner.

OSTEOPATHY

A relatively simple osteopathic treatment known as the counterstrain technique can be done at home. Get someone to rotate your arm in a direction opposite from the one that causes you pain, hold it in that position for 90 seconds, and then release it. Repeat several times a day. This exercise is especially helpful for mild to moderate, but not chronic, forms of tennis elbow. You can also consult an osteopath for more specific guidance on this technique.

AT-HOME REMEDIES

- Take ***ibuprofen*** or ***aspirin,*** or massage eucalyptus or lavender oil into the joint.
- Keep your arm elevated when possible, to reduce inflammation.
- Alternate hot and cold compresses or apply cayenne or prickly ash to the affected area to increase circulation and speed healing.
- For pain relief, apply a warm castor-oil pack to the joint.
- Alternate hot and cold compresses or apply cayenne or prickly ash to the affected area to increase circulation and speed healing.
- Ask a partner to massage the most painful part of your elbow with the convex side of a spoon; be sure that application is aggressive. This treatment hurts tremendously at first but eventually dulls the nerve endings (and thus the pain) and reduces inflammation.

C A U T I O N !

PROPER TENNIS TECHNIQUE

If you have contracted tennis elbow because you play tennis, consider watching the pros. They almost always correct their position relative to the ball by moving their feet rather than altering their arm motion. Most pros have their racket back before the ball clears the net; the weekend hacker usually does not get into the swing until after the ball has bounced after crossing the net. Avoid the temptation to make up for the lost time by twisting your wrist to bring the racket around to meet the ball, especially on your backhand. Otherwise, chances are good that you'll be using an ice pack for the pain and seeing your doctor soon.

PREVENTION

To prevent tennis elbow:

- Lift objects with your palm facing your body.
- Try strengthening exercises with hand weights. With your elbow cocked and your palm down, repeatedly bend your wrist. Stop if you feel any pain.
- Stretch relevant muscles before beginning a possibly stressful activity by grasping the top part of your fingers and gently but firmly pulling them back toward your body. Keep your arm fully extended and your palm facing outward.

To prevent a relapse:

- Discontinue or modify the action that is causing the strain on your elbow joint. If you must continue, be sure to warm up for 10 minutes or more before any activity involving your arm, and apply ice to it afterward. Take more frequent breaks.
- Try strapping a band around your forearm just below your elbow. If the support seems to help you lift objects such as heavy books, then continue with it. Be aware that such bands can cut off circulation and impede healing, so they are best used once tennis elbow has disappeared. ■

TESTICLE PROBLEMS

Read down this column to find your symptoms. Then read across.

SYMPTOMS	AILMENT/PROBLEM
◆ pain that gradually increases, tenderness, and swelling behind the testicle, sometimes with painful urination.	◆ Epididymitis—inflammation of the epididymis, the structure where sperm mature and move from the testicles to the penis
◆ sudden, acute pain and swelling in either testicle; no fever or painful urination, but sometimes nausea and vomiting; often follows strenuous physical exertion, but is usually not related to an injury.	◆ Testicular torsion—twisting of the spermatic cord
◆ swollen vein or veins in the scrotum, almost always on the left side; usually little or no pain; swelling subsides after lying down.	◆ Varicocele—***varicose veins*** in the scrotum
◆ pain, swelling, or discoloration after a fall or a blow to the testicles; sometimes accompanied by nausea and vomiting.	◆ Testicular trauma—a blow or other injury to the testicles
◆ a lump in a testicle that may or may not be painful; when there is pain, it is often worse when lying down.	◆ Possibly a sign of ***testicular cancer***
◆ impotence; absence of sexual desire; infertility; failure to reach puberty by age 15.	◆ Hypogonadism—failure of the testicles to produce adequate amounts of the male hormone testosterone
◆ general pain in the scrotum without an obvious cause.	◆ So-called referred pain from elsewhere in the body

WHAT TO DO	OTHER INFO
◆ See your doctor, who may prescribe bed rest, anti-inflammatory medicine, or—if you have a bacterial infection—***antibiotics.***	◆ May accompany infection of the prostate or urethra, or may follow heavy lifting or prolonged sitting; usually occurs between ages 20 and 40.
◆ **Get medical help immediately.** A twisted spermatic cord reduces blood supply to the testicles and can cause permanent damage.	◆ This is a medical emergency, most common in adolescents, often preceded by less severe but similar painful episodes. The spermatic cord must be untwisted by a physician, and surgery may be required to prevent recurrence.
◆ If you have associated pain, see your doctor for an examination.	◆ Some pain may occur after physical exertion or prolonged standing. About 15 percent of adult men have varicocele, which is a common cause of ***infertility.***
◆ See your doctor. A blood-filled swelling may indicate a ruptured testicle or other injury that should be surgically explored and repaired.	◆ A ruptured testicle can be diagnosed by ultrasound. If there is no rupture, the cause may be a leaking blood vessel. Sitz baths and bed rest with the scrotum elevated may stop internal bleeding.
◆ See ***Testicular Cancer.***	◆ Testicular cancer occurs primarily in men under the age of 35. Some kinds of the disease progress extremely rapidly. Treatment depends on the type of tumor. When treatment is begun promptly, prognosis is usually excellent.
◆ See your doctor for hormone testing and sperm count. Hypogonadism is sometimes treated by hormone replacement.	◆ Infertility may have a genetic cause. Loss of virility after puberty may be caused by drug abuse, damage from radiation therapy or chemical poisoning, or other injury.
◆ See your doctor. Treatment depends on locating the actual source of pain, which may be far from the scrotum. Referred pain is often hard to pinpoint since sensitivity to pain varies from person to person. *(See **Pain, Chronic.**)*	◆ Pain may be transmitted to the scrotum from disorders of the colon, kidneys, or other organs.

TESTICULAR CANCER

SYMPTOMS

The earliest warning signs of testicular cancer usually include:

- a change in size or shape of a testicle.
- swelling or thickening of the testicles.
- a firm, smooth, initially painless, slow-growing lump in a testicle.
- a feeling of testicular heaviness.

Other symptoms of testicular cancer may include:

- ***urinary problems.***
- an abdominal mass or ***abdominal pain.***
- persistent coughing, possibly with blood-tinged sputum.
- shortness of breath.
- loss of weight or appetite; fatigue; lower-***back pain;*** tenderness in the nipples or breast enlargement.
- very rarely, infertility.

CALL YOUR DOCTOR IF:

- you detect any sort of unusual lump or swelling in the scrotum. You should have a thorough physical examination as soon as possible, on the off chance that the abnormality is caused by cancer.

The two testicles, or testes, are glands that produce male hormones and sperm. They hang beneath and behind a man's penis in a pouch called the scrotum. The spermatic cord, composed of the sperm duct, nerves, and blood vessels, connects each testicle to the body. Although testicular cancer is rare, it is the most common type of cancer in men between the ages of 15 and 35. It is much more common in Caucasians than in African Americans and usually is diagnosed when a man is in his mid-thirties.

Almost all testicular cancers are primary—beginning in the testicles themselves. A rare type of testicular cancer arises in the chest or abdomen in traces of embryonic tissue from which the testicles developed in the fetus. Testicular cancer may spread slowly or rapidly, depending on its type, but the path is consistent: Once a malignant tumor penetrates the spermatic cord, cancer cells are free to infiltrate nearby lymph or blood vessels, and they may be carried to abdominal lymph nodes, then to the lungs, then usually to the liver, bones, and possibly the brain.

Thanks to advances in diagnosis and treatment, testicular cancer is among the most curable of cancers, even when advanced, and it is rarely fatal. About 85 percent of patients are diagnosed with localized malignancies that are highly treatable. Improved detection and treatment techniques have raised the overall five-year survival rate above 90 percent. Even if cancer has spread to nearby organs at diagnosis, patients have an excellent chance of surviving at least five years.

CAUSES

What causes testicular cancer is unknown. Ten percent of testicular cancers occur in men born with an undescended testicle, and many cases of father-son incidence have been reported. Men with fertility problems are more likely to develop benign testicular tumors and may be slightly more prone to testicular cancer. Some research suggests that having a vasectomy increases risk, but other studies do not support this conclusion *(see **Testicle Problems**)*. Other suspected but unproven risk factors include a sedentary lifestyle, early puberty, previous ***mumps,*** testicular injury, overexposure to pesticides or radiation, and prenatal conditions related to a mother who was bleeding abnormally, taking ***estrogen,*** or taking diethylstilbestrol (DES) during pregnancy. DES was once given to pregnant women to prevent miscarriage but is no longer marketed in the U.S.

DIAGNOSTIC AND TEST PROCEDURES

Every man should have his doctor explain the steps of testicle self-examination, a simple yet important procedure. He should then physically examine his testicles once a month for signs of abnormality. Any painless lump or swelling in the scrotum may signal cancer. To rule out other possibilities, a doctor may prescribe a course of ***antibiotics*** to see if the mass disappears. If it doesn't, ultrasound imaging and chemical analyses of urine and blood are performed. If cancer is suspected, the testicle is surgically removed and a biopsy is performed to determine the presence and type of testicular cancer. If cancer is diagnosed, other tests will determine whether it has spread. Removal of the second testicle is not standard practice because in most cases it remains cancer free. Removing one testicle usually does not cause infertility, but because further treatment may, patients are advised about sperm banking before treatment proceeds.

WARNING SIGNS

Suspended in a pouch called the scrotum, the male sex glands, or testicles, produce sperm and male hormones. Testicular cancer usually affects only one testicle, typically beginning in the cells that manufacture sperm. Periodic self-examination may detect hard lumps, swelling, or a change in the size or shape of the testicle *(above, right)*—all potential indicators of early testicular cancer.

TREATMENT

CONVENTIONAL MEDICINE

Because it is required for diagnosis, surgical removal of a testicle is unavoidable. If cancer is found, a second operation to remove nearby abdominal lymph nodes usually is performed, and these two operations are often enough to cure limited testicular cancer. In addition to surgery, advanced cases are treated with chemotherapy and sometimes radiation. Nearly all testicular cancer patients achieve remission, but they are urged to have frequent follow-up examinations. If cancer recurs, additional treatment frequently produces another remission. If testicular cancer is not cured by conventional chemotherapy, doctors may advise a bone-marrow transplant to allow higher-dose chemotherapy. *(See **Lymphoma.**)*

See ***Cancer*** for more information on treatments such as chemotherapy and radiation.

COMPLEMENTARY THERAPIES

Although conventional medicine is remarkably successful at curing testicular cancer, simply learning that you have cancer can cause severe emotional distress. Many patients find psychological counseling or support-group therapy helpful in dealing with the emotional consequences.

PREVENTION

Some studies indicate that young men who exercise regularly are less likely to develop testicular cancer. Other research suggests that correcting an undescended testicle surgically before a boy turns 10 minimizes cancer risk. Most important, however, is regular testicle self-examination. ■

TETANUS

SYMPTOMS

You should suspect tetanus if a cut or other wound is followed by one or more of these symptoms:

- stiffness of the neck, jaw, and other muscles, often accompanied by a grotesque, grinning expression.
- irritability.
- uncontrollable spasms of the jaw and neck muscles.
- painful, involuntary contraction of other muscles.

In addition, you may notice restlessness, lack of appetite, and drooling.

CALL YOUR DOCTOR IF:

- you are bitten by an animal or wounded by an object that might be contaminated with dirt, feces, or dust, and you have not been immunized against tetanus or received a booster within the last 10 years. Tetanus infection can be fatal and should be treated as soon as possible.

Tetanus is a dangerous nerve ailment caused by the toxin of a common bacterium, *Clostridium tetani.* Bacterial spores are found in soil—most frequently in cultivated soil, least frequently in virgin soil. They also exist in environments as diverse as animal excrement, house dust, operating rooms, contaminated heroin, and the human colon. If the spores enter a wound that penetrates the skin and extends deeper than oxygen can reach, they germinate and produce a toxin that enters the bloodstream.

This toxin, tetanospasmin, ranks with botulism toxin as the most potent known microbial poison. It is taken up from the blood by the outermost nerves and moves inward toward the spine at a rate of about 10 inches a day. After 7 to 21 days, it begins to short-circuit nerve signals and block the relaxation of muscles. This results in sustained muscle contractions, notably the lockjaw for which tetanus is nicknamed.

Spasms of the jaw or facial muscles may follow, spreading to the hands, arms, legs, and back and blocking the ability to breathe. Spasms are often precipitated by noise or touch. Once tetanus has spread, the mortality rate is approximately 40 percent, even in modern medical facilities.

An estimated one million infants die of tetanus in developing countries each year because of poor hygiene. Since childhood immunization laws were passed in the United States in the 1970s, only about 50 cases a year are reported in this country; about three-quarters are elderly people or people who have never been immunized.

CAUSES

Bacterial spores enter the body by way of animal bites, surgical wounds, needle injection sites, burns, ulcers, and infected umbilical cords—and by the proverbial rusty nail. Be particularly suspicious of any wound caused by a dirty or dusty object that has been outdoors or in contact with soil.

DIAGNOSTIC AND TEST PROCEDURES

Some affected people may experience only pain and tingling at the wound site and some spasms in nearby muscles, but most suffer stiff jaw and neck muscles, irritability, and difficulty swallowing. If muscle spasms develop early, chances of recovery are poor.

It is seldom possible to find either the bacterium or the toxin in a suspected tetanus patient, so diagnosis can be made only on the basis of clinical observations combined with the absence of a history of tetanus immunization.

TREATMENT

If tetanus does develop, seek hospital treatment immediately. This includes a course of ***antibiotics*** and an injection of tetanus antitoxin. You may receive an ***antianxiety drug*** such as chlorpromazine or ***diazepam*** to control muscle spasms, or a short-acting barbiturate for sedation. You may require the aid of an artificial respirator or other life-support measures during the several weeks needed for the disease to run its course.

PREVENTION

Tetanus occurs almost exclusively in people who have not been immunized or whose immunization is not adequate. The fact that you are contaminated with tetanus spores by an animal bite or a wound from a dirty object does not mean, however, that you will necessarily contract a tetanus infection. Much depends on how deep the wound is and how well it is cleaned. The toxin-producing bacteria can thrive only when they are protected from the air by a layer of skin or tissue. Because these bacteria do not flourish in oxygen, it is common practice, when possible, to leave a wound open, without stitches and with only a light gauze dressing, so that the entire area is exposed to air.

Most cases of tetanus develop in people who think their wounds are too small to bother with. *(See **Cuts, Scratches, and Wounds.**)* Even a puncture that barely bleeds can be dangerous; because they are deep, punctures provide a favorable environment for bacteria. Wash the wound thoroughly with soap and a strong stream of water, apply ***antiseptic*** solution, and bandage with a sterile gauze pad. Do not tape the wound closed and do not apply antibiotic ointment, both of which keep air from circulating.

If your wound was caused by an object that may have been in contact with soil, especially if the wound has dead, crushed, or infected tissue, see your doctor quickly—within 24 hours, if possible. He will finish cleaning the wound and cutting away any damaged tissue, a procedure known as debridement.

If you haven't had a tetanus booster shot in the last five years, your doctor will probably give you one. If you've never been immunized, your doctor will quickly give you a shot of human tetanus immunoglobulin, which brings immediate protection that lasts a few weeks. Neither the immunoglobulin shot nor the booster will bring enduring immunity, however, so you will still need the full course of immunization shots if you did not receive them in childhood.

Health officials recommend immunization of infants and children with DPT—diphtheria, pertussis ***(whooping cough),*** and tetanus—vaccine at the ages of 2 months, 4 months, 6 months, 15 months, and about 5 years. After that, most health experts recommend a tetanus booster every 10 years.

If family members have not been immunized against tetanus, encourage them to have it done. Keep a record of tetanus shots, since booster shots given too frequently may cause allergic reactions.

There is evidence that tetanus immunization remains highly effective for much longer than 10 years. Some experts have suggested that a booster in high school and a second booster at the age of 60 provide adequate protection for life.

The most important preventive measure you can take against tetanus, however, is to acquire the initial immunization series. Any adults who have not done so should see their doctor or health department. ■

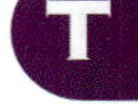

THROAT CANCER

SYMPTOMS

Initially throat cancer causes no symptoms. The earliest warning signs are likely to resemble symptoms of a chest cold. Symptoms caused by a tumor in the upper or lower throat may include:

- nagging cough, hoarseness, or a mild but persistent sore throat.
- difficulty or pain on swallowing.
- traces of blood in sputum.
- ear pain.
- swollen lymph nodes in the neck.

Additional symptoms that may be caused by a tumor in the region directly behind the nose may include:

- partial hearing loss.
- nasal obstruction or nosebleeds.
- ringing in the ears, or ***tinnitus.***
- symptoms of ***otitis media,*** such as pain or pressure in the middle ear.

CALL YOUR DOCTOR IF:

- symptoms resembling those of an upper-respiratory ***infection,*** such as a chest cold, persist for more than two weeks.
- you become suddenly or chronically hoarse for no apparent reason.
- you are a smoker and already have a raspy voice, and you notice another change in your voice.
- lymph nodes in your neck appear swollen.

While any of these symptoms may have other causes, you should have a thorough examination by a nose and throat specialist to get a proper diagnosis.

The throat, or pharynx, is a hollow tube through which food and liquids pass from the mouth to the stomach, and through which air travels to and from the lungs. The throat is divided into three distinct sections: the nasopharynx, located directly behind the nose; the oropharynx, directly behind the mouth and including the tonsils; and the hypopharynx, or lower throat *(illustration, right).*

Most primary throat cancers originate from cells that cover the mucous membrane lining the throat. As the cancer grows, it tends to penetrate through the mucous membrane and muscle layers to surrounding tissues. From there the cancer can spread to lymph nodes in the neck, then to the lungs and other organs. A growing tumor may interfere with hearing, smell, taste, speech, or swallowing. Cancers of the nasopharynx and lower throat often spread early, before they cause obvious symptoms. Cancers of the oropharynx tend to stay localized but eventually will spread unless treated successfully.

Throat cancer is seen about three times more often in men than in women and usually does not occur before age 50. Five-year survival rates range from 50 to 90 percent when throat cancer is diagnosed early, and from 5 to 25 percent for cancer that has spread elsewhere in the body.

CAUSES

Smoking or chewing tobacco and heavy drinking of alcohol cause most cancers of the oropharynx and hypopharynx. Smokers are six times more likely than nonsmokers to develop cancer of these areas, and nearly all people diagnosed with throat cancer are—or once were—smokers. In contrast, the major known risk factor for cancer of the nasopharynx is infection by the Epstein-Barr (E-B) virus.

Inhaling coal or other mineral dust, asbestos, and diesel fumes may increase risk for throat cancer. Poor oral hygiene and regular consumption of salted meats may also contribute. In some cases, throat cancer develops from abnormal tissue growths *(see **Oral Cancer**).*

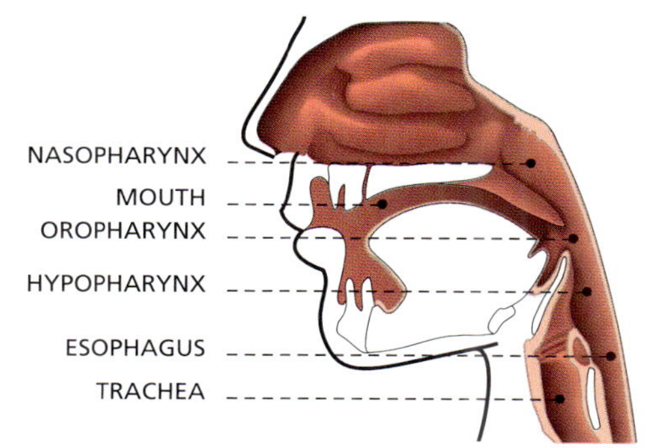

The throat is divided into three sections, any of which can develop cancer. The uppermost section, or nasopharynx, takes in air and mucus from the nasal cavity. Below it lies the oropharynx, a passageway for food and air, and the part of the throat that's visible when you say "aaah." The hypopharynx, or lower throat, delivers food to the esophagus and air to the trachea.

DIAGNOSTIC AND TEST PROCEDURES

You or your physician may be able to see abnormal growths in your oropharynx but not in the nasopharynx or the hypopharynx, which must be examined with mirrors or a fiberoptic scope. Any suspicious lesion, tumor, or swollen lymph node should be biopsied, or a test for the E-B virus should be made. If cancer is detected, imaging scans can help establish how widespread the disease has become.

TREATMENT

Provided throat cancer has not spread beyond lymph nodes by the time of diagnosis, treatment removes all traces of the disease, remission is obtained, and in at least half of all cases, the cancer is cured. But treatment for throat cancer is typically risky and complex; depending on a tumor's location and stage of development, doctors must consider the impact of treatment on the patient's speech and other essential functions.

CONVENTIONAL MEDICINE

Specific treatment for throat cancer depends first on the tumor's location. Patients with cancer of the nasopharynx typically receive high-dose radiation to the head and neck, perhaps following chemotherapy to shrink tumors. This treatment cures more than 80 percent of early cancers and more than half of moderately advanced cases.

Small tumors of the oropharynx usually are treated with radiation in order to avoid disfigurement and other complications. If the cancer does not respond adequately or is too advanced, surgery is indicated, sometimes preceded by chemotherapy or followed by radiation.

Although small tumors of the hypopharynx may be treated with radiation alone, most localized hypopharyngeal cancers require surgery, possibly preceded by chemotherapy or followed by radiation. The cancerous portion of the throat is removed, followed by reconstructive surgery. After throat surgery, many patients need physical therapy to help regain the ability to speak, swallow, and chew. Radiation may be used to relieve symptoms and slow the progress of advanced cancers that cannot be treated surgically.

AT-HOME CARE

If radiation treatment to the head and neck causes mouth discomfort and a sore and scratchy throat, try the following:

- Ask your oncologist about appropriate medications and advice on how to ease side effects.
- Eat soft or semiliquid foods and drink liquids throughout the day to keep your mouth and throat moist.
- Ask your dentist about proper mouth care during and after treatment. *(See **Oral Cancer.**)*

PREVENTION

If you smoke or chew tobacco, stop. If you have a tendency to abuse alcohol, get counseling or medical help to bring the problem under control. ■

T

THYROID PROBLEMS

SYMPTOMS

Hyperthyroidism:
- weight loss despite increased appetite.
- increased heart rate, higher blood pressure, and increased nervousness, with excessive perspiration.
- more frequent bowel movements, sometimes with diarrhea.
- muscle weakness, trembling hands.
- development of a ***goiter.***

Hypothyroidism:
- lethargy, slower mental processes.
- reduced heart rate.
- increased sensitivity to cold.
- tingling or numbness in the hands.
- development of a ***goiter.***

Subacute thyroiditis:
- mild to severe pain in the thyroid gland.
- the thyroid feels tender to the touch.
- pain when swallowing or turning your head.
- appearance of these symptoms shortly after a viral infection, such as the flu, mumps, or measles.

CALL YOUR DOCTOR IF:

- you are feverish, agitated, or delirious, and have a rapid pulse; you could be having a thyrotoxic crisis, a sudden and dangerous complication of **hyperthyroidism.**
- you feel intensely cold, drowsy, and lethargic; you could be experiencing a myxedema coma, a sudden and dangerous complication of **hypothyroidism** that can cause unconsciousness and possibly death.

Through the hormones it produces, the thyroid gland influences almost all of the metabolic processes in your body. Thyroid disorders can range from a small, harmless ***goiter*** that needs no treatment to life-threatening ***cancer.*** The most common thyroid problems involve irregular production of thyroid hormones. Too much of these vital body chemicals results in a condition known as **hyperthyroidism.** Insufficient hormone production leads to **hypothyroidism.**

The four parathyroid glands, located at the four corners of the thyroid gland, function independent of the larger gland and are responsible for regulating blood levels of calcium, necessary for the growth and maintenance of bones and teeth. Imbalances in their hormone secretion can result in hyperparathyroidism or hypoparathyroidism, which in turn can adversely affect bone development. Although the effects can be unpleasant or uncomfortable, most thyroid problems are not serious if properly diagnosed and treated.

CAUSES

All types of **hyperthyroidism** are due to an overproduction of thyroid hormones, and the condition can occur in several ways: In ***Graves' disease,*** the release of excess hormones is triggered by an autoimmune disorder *(see **Immune Problems**)*. At other times, nodules called toxic adenomas develop in the thyroid gland and begin to secrete thyroid hormones, altering the normal flow and upsetting the body's chemical balance; certain ***goiters*** may contain several of these nodules. In **subacute thyroiditis,** inflammation of the thyroid causes the gland to "leak" excess hormones, resulting in temporary hyperthyroidism. Although rare, hyperthyroidism can also develop from pituitary gland malfunctions or from cancerous growths in the thyroid gland.

Hypothyroidism, by contrast, stems from an underproduction of thyroid hormones. Since your body's energy production requires certain amounts of thyroid hormones, a drop in hormone production leads to lower energy production. A common cause of hypothyroidism is Hashimoto's thyroiditis, an autoimmune disorder in which white blood cells gradually replace thyroid tissue, which then comes under attack by immune-system proteins called antibodies. Hypothyroidism can also result when the thyroid gland has been surgically removed or chemically destroyed as treatment for hyperthyroidism. And if you are exposed to excessive amounts of iodide—perhaps from a hidden source such as cold and sinus medicines, or from certain medical tests—you may be at greater risk for developing hypothyroidism, especially if you have had thyroid problems in the past. Untreated for long periods of time, hypothyroidism can bring on a myxedema coma, a rare but potentially fatal condition that requires immediate hormone injections.

Hypothyroidism poses a special danger to newborns and infants, as a lack of thyroid hormones in the system at an early age can lead to the development of cretinism (mental retardation) and dwarfism (stunted growth). Most infants now have their thyroid levels checked routinely soon after birth; if they are hypothyroid, treatment begins immediately. In infants, as in adults, hypothyroidism can be due to a pituitary disorder, a defective thyroid, or lack of the gland entirely. A hypothyroid infant is unusually inactive and quiet, has a poor appetite, and sleeps for excessively long periods of time.

Although cancer of the thyroid gland is the most common endocrine malignancy other than ovarian cancer, it is still quite rare. You might have one or more thyroid nodules for several years before they are determined to be cancerous. People who have received radiation treatment to the head and neck earlier in life, possibly as a remedy for acne, tend to have a higher-than-normal susceptibility to thyroid cancer.

DIAGNOSTIC AND TEST PROCEDURES

A doctor can diagnose **hyperthyroidism** and **hypothyroidism** by looking at the levels of certain hormones in your blood. Doctors usually take readings of hormones secreted by the thyroid itself, and also of thyroid-stimulating hormone (TSH), a chemical released by the pituitary gland to trigger hormone production in the thyroid.

When you are **hypothyroid,** higher quantities of TSH are circulating in your blood as your body attempts to foster increased production of thyroid hormones; the reverse is true with hyperthyroidism, in which TSH levels are below normal and circulating thyroid-hormone levels are high.

To determine the cause of **hyperthyroidism,** doctors often use radioactive iodide uptake tests, which track the amount of iodide absorbed by the thyroid gland during a set time period. Iodide is a key ingredient in the manufacture of thyroid hormone, so the amount of iodide the thyroid absorbs is a reliable indicator of how much hormone the gland is producing. For this test, you must swallow a small amount of radioactive iodide in liquid or capsule form. After a predetermined wait, the doctor places an instrument over your neck to measure how much of the radioactive iodide has gathered in your thyroid.

If the results of this test suggest that the gland is collecting excessive amounts of iodide, the doctor may then conduct a radioactive iodide uptake scan. In this test, the physician uses a special film to create a picture that shows the exact location of the radioactive iodide in your thyroid gland. The scan will reveal, for example, if the iodide is collecting in adenomas, indicating that the nodules are responsible for the excess hormone. If the scan shows that the iodide is spread equally throughout the tissue, the whole thyroid is involved in the excess production.

Some practitioners believe that blood tests may not be sensitive enough to detect milder forms of **hypothyroidism.** Instead, they advocate monitoring your body's basal (resting) temperature. To track your basal temperature accurately, you must closely follow certain guidelines: Shake the thermometer below 95°F at night and place it where you can reach it without getting out of bed. The following morning, before you get out of bed, take your temperature via your armpit for 10 minutes while staying as still as possible. Keep records of your temperature for at least three days. (Women should do this during the first two weeks of the menstrual cycle, as their basal temperature may rise during the latter half.) Normal body basal temperatures fall between 97.4°F and 97.8°F. If your basal temperature is consistently low, you could be mildly hypothyroid.

T

If you have one or more adenomas, your practitioner will want to keep careful records of when they were first found and how they develop, since not all adenomas produce excess thyroid hormone. In fact, most of these nodules are not malignant, especially if they remain the same size over long intervals. (Cancerous tissue, by contrast, will undergo noticeable growth.) Nodules that appear suddenly are typically fluid-filled cysts and are often benign. If blood tests indicate that the nodules are producing excess thyroid hormone, and if you have other symptoms, your practitioner will treat you for **hyperthyroidism.**

In any case, you should receive periodic checkups if you have a nodule on your thyroid gland, since you may become hyperthyroid in the future. If your blood tests show elevated hormone levels, your doctor may recommend other tests, including radioactive iodide uptake tests and scans that indicate whether the nodules are "hot" or "cold." Hot nodules, or those that are actively trapping iodide, are rarely cancerous. But cold nodules—those showing low iodide concentrations—indicate a possible malignancy and need to be investigated further.

One type of thyroid cancer can be diagnosed through a simple blood test that measures levels of a hormone involved in bone formation. In most cases, however, doctors check for thyroid cancer by performing a biopsy, which involves drawing cells from the suspect nodule with a fine needle to determine if the tissue is malignant.

TREATMENT

For thyroid disorders stemming from the over- or underproduction of thyroid hormones, both conventional and alternative treatments offer varied methods to restore hormone levels to their proper balance. Conventional treatments rely mainly on drug therapy and surgery. Alternative treatments attempt to relieve some of the discomfort associated with thyroid conditions, or to improve the function of the thyroid gland through a variety of approaches ranging from diet supplements and herbal remedies to lifestyle changes and special exercises. You should always receive a professional evaluation for any thyroid disorder; most of these conditions require a course of treatment beyond the scope of home care alone.

CONVENTIONAL MEDICINE

Treating **hyperthyroidism** requires suppressing the manufacture of thyroid hormone, while **hypothyroidism** demands hormone replacement. Conventional medicine offers extremely effective techniques for lowering, eliminating, or supplementing hormone production. Before deciding which therapy is best for you, your doctor will make an evaluation based on your particular thyroid condition as well as your age, general health, and medical history.

Thyroid hormone production can be suppressed or halted completely with a radioactive iodide treatment, antithyroid medication, or surgery. If your doctor decides that radioactive treatment is best, you will be asked to swallow a tablet or liquid containing radioactive iodide in amounts large enough to damage the cells of your thyroid gland and limit or destroy their ability to produce hormones. Occasionally more than one treatment is needed to restore normal hormone production, and many patients actually develop hypothyroidism as a result of this procedure.

If you start using antithyroid medications such as propylthiouracil or methimazole, which are usually administered in tablet form, your hyperthyroid symptoms should begin to disappear in about six to eight weeks, as hormones already in your system run out and the medication starts to impair the thyroid's hormone production. However, you will need to continue taking the medication for about a year. After that time, you will also need to receive periodic medical exams to make sure that the condition has not returned.

Surgery is often recommended for people under 45 when their hyperthyroidism is due to toxic adenomas, since these nodules tend to be resistant to radioactive iodide. Once the tissue is removed surgically, hormone levels typically return to normal within a few weeks.

Although **subacute thyroiditis** can bring on temporary hyperthyroidism, this condition usually does not require medical treatment, and any pain associated with the inflamed thyroid can generally be alleviated with ***acetaminophen*** or ***aspirin.*** If over-the-counter drugs don't help, a physician may prescribe ***prednisone*** or dexamethasone for a short period of time. Since both of these drugs may encourage the development of stomach ulcers and the loss of bone mass, however, ask your doctor if you should also be taking ***calcium*** supplements.

Hypothyroidism calls for a lifelong regimen of hormone replacement therapy. No surgical techniques or conventional drugs can increase the thyroid's hormone production once it slows down. Although hormones from animal extracts are available, doctors generally prescribe synthetic forms of thyroid hormone, such as ***levothyroxine.*** Side effects are rare, but some patients experience nervousness or chest pain while taking these drugs; usually, adjusting the levels of medication will alleviate any unpleasant effects. However, if you are also taking ***tricyclic antidepressants, anticoagulant*** drugs, or ***digitalis,*** or if you have ***diabetes,*** make sure that you and your practitioner discuss any possible interactions or other complications.

Thyroid cancer is usually treated by surgically removing either the cancerous tissue or the whole thyroid gland, a procedure known as a thyroidectomy. If the cancer has spread beyond the thyroid, any other affected tissue, such as the lymph glands in the neck, will also be removed.

ALTERNATIVE CHOICES

Though the alternative choices available to you for thyroid problems will not completely suppress or replace thyroid hormones, they are often used to strengthen the thyroid itself or to alleviate some of the unpleasant symptoms.

CHINESE HERBS

Several herbal mixtures may help relieve symptoms in cases of **hyperthyroidism:** baked ***licorice*** *(Glycyrrhiza uralensis)* combination, ***bupleurum*** *(Bupleurum chinense)* and dragon bone combination, or bupleurum and peony combination. See a practitioner for guidance and supplies.

HERBAL THERAPIES

For relief from the symptoms of **hyperthyroidism,** try 4 parts bugleweed (*Lycopus* spp.), 2 parts motherwort *(Leonurus cardiaca),* 2 parts ***skullcap*** (*Scutellaria* spp.), and 1 part ***hawthorn*** (*Crataegus* spp.) in a tincture three times a day.

For insomnia due to **hyperthyroidism,** combine equal parts of ***valerian*** *(Valeriana officinalis)* and ***passionflower*** *(Passiflora incarnata)* in a tincture and take half an hour before bedtime.

In the case of **hypothyroidism,** you can prepare a tea made from bladder wrack *(Fucus vesiculosus)* to improve thyroid function. Three times daily, pour 1 cup boiling water on 2 tsp bladder wrack and steep for 10 minutes before drinking. Bladder wrack can also be taken in capsule form three times daily.

LIFESTYLE

Aerobic exercise for 15 to 20 minutes a day is excellent for maintaining good thyroid function. Regular physical activity is especially important if you are hypothyroid. (Check with your doctor before starting an exercise program.)

NUTRITION AND DIET

For **hypothyroidism,** avoid cabbage, peaches, rutabagas, soybeans, spinach, peanuts, and radishes, as these foods can interfere with the manufacture of thyroid hormones. Supplements of ***vitamin C, vitamin E,*** riboflavin ***(vitamin B_2),*** ***zinc, niacin*** (vitamin B_3), pyridoxine ***(vitamin B_6),*** and tyrosine might help boost thyroid production. However, if you have **hyperthyroidism,** eating the foods listed above might help lower your body's production of thyroid hormone.

YOGA

For many people, the Shoulder Stand position, at least once daily for 1 to 2 minutes, can help improve overall thyroid function. CAUTION: Do not do this position if you have high blood pressure or glaucoma. Lie on your back and lift your legs up so your hips are off the floor. Supporting your hips with your hands, extend your legs vertically. Make sure your body weight is supported by your shoulders, not your head and neck. Release slowly, while exhaling. ■

TICS AND TWITCHES

SYMPTOMS

- a brief, flicking sensation confined to a small part of the body, such as the eyelid; usually indicative of a harmless involuntary muscle contraction.
- a repetitive, uncontrollable, purposeless contraction of an individual muscle or group of muscles, typically in the face, arms, or shoulders; may be a sign that you have a tic related to a minor psychological disorder, a condition related to a brain disorder, or trigeminal ***neuralgia.***
- intense, longer-lasting trembling or shaking of a body part or of the entire body; could be symptomatic of caffeine poisoning, alcohol withdrawal, an overactive thyroid gland *(see **Thyroid Problems**)*, or ***Parkinson's disease.***

CALL YOUR DOCTOR IF:

- your condition consists of unexpected trembling movements that occur only when the affected body part is at rest; you need to be checked for the possibility of ***Parkinson's disease.***
- your tic or twitch is persistent or recurs often; you may be having minor seizures, or you may have a neurological disorder or other condition of a serious nature.

Tics and twitches are defined as involuntary contractions of a muscle or group of muscles. They come in many forms and have a variety of causes—some trivial and some serious.

CAUSES

Movements such as shoulder shrugging, mouth twitching, and erratic blinking may be signs of a minor psychological disturbance. They most often develop in children ages 7 to 14 as a result of anxiety, and usually stop within a year; some cases may persist into adulthood. The disorder occurs in up to 25 percent of children, and boys

TOURETTE'S SYNDROME

Tourette's syndrome is perhaps the best-known involuntary movement disorder. Named after Georges Gilles de la Tourette, the French neurologist who first described the condition in 1885, it usually starts in childhood and persists throughout life. It is a neurological abnormality of unknown cause and is up to four times more common in men.

Tourette's can be mild, with only minor involuntary twitches, or more severe and progressive. Symptoms may include continual grimacing, and violent jerking of the head and neck, as well as the arms and legs. As Tourette's progresses, involuntary noises such as grunts, coughing, and barking may occur; in 50 percent of cases, patients occasionally shout out expletives.

There is no cure for Tourette's, but some forms can be successfully managed. Antipsychotic drugs such as haloperidol may provide temporary relief from jerking and vocal outbursts.

exhibit symptoms three times as often as girls.

Caffeine poisoning (which can result from drinking five or more cups of coffee within 12 hours) and alcohol withdrawal may also manifest themselves in involuntary movements, including trembling or shaking. *(See **Alcohol Abuse.**)*

Tics or twitches are sometimes caused by neurological disorders, in which case they are referred to as dyskinesia. *(See **Parkinson's Disease.**)* This condition may result from brain damage at birth, head trauma, or use of the antiemetic (vomit suppressant) drug metoclopramide, or drugs to treat psychiatric ailments. Dyskinesia includes muscle spasms, repetitive fidgets, jerking or writhing movements, or a combination of these symptoms.

Other medications, such as phenothiazines and central nervous system stimulants, can also cause temporary twitching, as can fatigue and stress. The condition can also be hereditary.

ACUPRESSURE

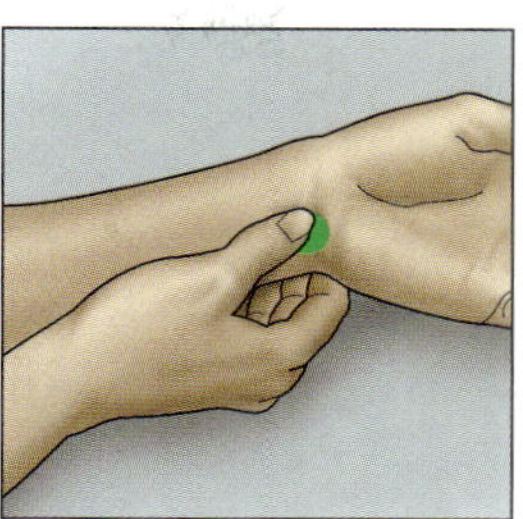

1 Anxiety-induced sleeping problems may be improved by pressing Heart 7, located along the crease on the inside of the wrist, directly in line with the little finger. Squeeze firmly between thumb and index finger for one minute, then repeat on the other hand.

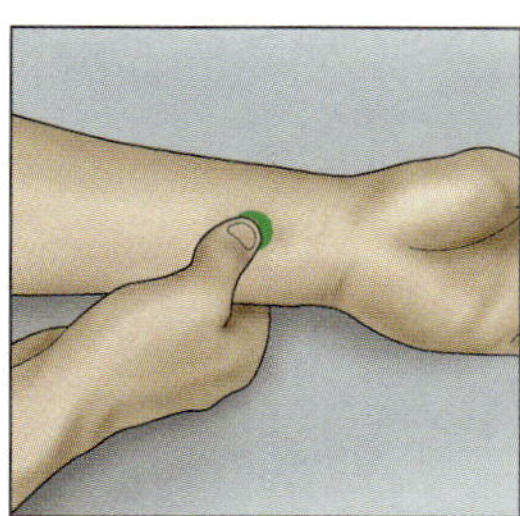

2 To help calm nerves, press Pericardium 6. Place your thumb in the center of your inner wrist, two finger widths from the wrist crease and between the two bones of the forearm. Press firmly for one minute, three to five times, then repeat on the other arm.

TREATMENT

CONVENTIONAL MEDICINE

Tension-related tics or twitches usually disappear on their own, especially if you take steps to reduce ***stress.*** Dyskinesia caused by a particular drug may be treated by simply stopping use of the drug. When it is caused by other factors, effective treatment is harder to determine. Your physician will probably have to prescribe a series of drugs before an effective one is found.

If tics are severe and persistent and there is no clear physical cause, your doctor may prescribe antianxiety ***benzodiazepine*** drugs or antipsychotic drugs. You can tell whether caffeine may be responsible for your twitching or trembling by not drinking caffeinated beverages for several hours to see if your symptoms disappear. You may need to cut down on your caffeine intake.

ALTERNATIVE CHOICES

Alternative remedies for various forms of tics and twitches may relieve discomfort as you wait out the symptoms of your disorder, or they may serve as a complement to your physician's prescribed treatment. In addition to the treatments listed below, **acupuncture, acupressure** *(above),* **yoga,** and **massage** may also relieve symptoms.

HERBAL THERAPIES

Taking a 1-ml dose of ***hops*** *(Humulus lupulus)* in tincture form three times a day may relieve symptoms of facial tics and twitches.

NUTRITION AND DIET

If alcohol abuse has been a problem, it is important to maintain a healthful diet after you stop drinking; a high-dose multivitamin and mineral supplement may also be helpful in easing symptoms of alcohol withdrawal.

AT-HOME REMEDIES

Avoid fatigue, stress, and caffeine: They can aggravate minor tics and twitches. If your eyelid is twitching, gently massage the area. If caffeine poisoning is a regular concern, replace caffeinated beverages with fruit juices. In addition, herb teas, coffees made from roasted cereal grains and dandelion roots, and carob to replace chocolate in drinks and sweets are viable substitutes. ■

TINNITUS

SYMPTOMS

- a noise in the ears, such as ringing, roaring, buzzing, hissing, or whistling; the noise may be intermittent or continuous.
- sometimes, hearing loss.

CALL YOUR DOCTOR IF:

- you have tinnitus; it could be a symptom of an underlying health problem, such as ***high blood pressure*** or an underactive thyroid *(see **Thyroid Problems**)*, that can be treated.
- the noise is accompanied by pain or pus in the ear; these may be signs of an ear infection.
- the noise is accompanied by dizziness; this may be a sign of ***Ménière's disease*** or a neurological problem. **Seek medical care immediately.**

Tinnitus, or ringing in the ears, is the sensation of hearing ringing, buzzing, hissing, chirping, whistling, or other sounds. The noise can be intermittent or continuous, and can vary in loudness. It is often worse when background noise is low, so you may be most aware of it at night when you're trying to fall asleep in a quiet room. In rare cases, the sound beats in sync with your heart.

Tinnitus is very common, affecting an estimated 50 million adults in the United States. For most people the condition is merely an annoyance. In severe cases, however, tinnitus can cause people to have difficulty concentrating and sleeping. It may eventually interfere with work and personal relationships, resulting in psychological distress. About 12 million people seek medical help for severe tinnitus every year.

Although tinnitus is often associated with hearing loss, it does not cause the loss; nor does a hearing loss cause tinnitus. In fact, some people with tinnitus experience no difficulty hearing, and in a few cases they even become so acutely sensitive to sound that they must take steps to muffle or mask external noises.

Some instances of tinnitus are caused by infections or blockages in the ear, and the tinnitus often disappears once the underlying cause is treated. Frequently, however, tinnitus continues after the underlying condition is treated. In such a case, other therapies—both conventional and alternative—may bring significant relief by either decreasing or covering up the unwanted sound.

CAUSES

A wide variety of conditions and illnesses can lead to tinnitus. Blockages of the ear due to a buildup of wax, an infection *(see **Otitis Media**)*, or rarely, a tumor of the auditory nerve can cause the unwanted sounds, as can a perforated eardrum. But perhaps the most common source of chronic tinnitus is prolonged exposure to loud sounds. The noise causes permanent damage to the sound-sensitive cells of the cochlea, a spiral-shaped organ in the inner ear. Carpenters, pilots, rock musicians, and street-repair workers are among those whose jobs put them at risk, as are people who work with chain saws, guns, or other loud devices or who repeatedly listen to loud music. A single exposure to a sudden extremely loud noise can also cause tinnitus.

Certain drugs—most notably ***aspirin,*** several types of ***antibiotics,*** and quinine medications—can contribute to the condition as well. In fact, tinnitus is cited as a potential side effect for about 200 prescription and nonprescription drugs.

The natural process of aging can result in a deterioration of the cochlea or other parts of the ear and lead to tinnitus. Tinnitus is also associated with ***Ménière's disease,*** a disorder of the inner ear, and otosclerosis, a degenerative disease of the small bones in the middle ear. Other medical conditions that can cause ringing in the ears include ***high blood pressure, allergies, anemia,*** and an underactive thyroid *(see **Thyroid Problems**).* Tinnitus can also be a symptom of a disorder of the neck or jaw, such as ***temporomandibular joint syndrome*** (TMJ).

For reasons not yet entirely clear to researchers, ***stress*** seems to worsen tinnitus.

DIAGNOSTIC AND TEST PROCEDURES

To determine whether the underlying cause of your tinnitus is a medical condition for which treatment can be prescribed, your doctor will give you a general physical exam, including a careful examination of your ears. Be sure to inform your doctor of all medications you are taking. If the source of the problem remains unclear, you may be sent to an otologist or an otolaryngologist (both ear specialists) or an audiologist (a hearing specialist) for hearing and neurological tests. As part of your examination by these specialists, you may be given a balance test called an electronystagmography. An imaging technique, such as an MRI or a CT scan—which might reveal a structural problem—may also be recommended.

TREATMENT

Because tinnitus may be a symptom of an underlying medical condition, the first step is to treat that condition. But if the tinnitus remains after treatment or if it results from exposure to loud noise, health professionals recommend various nonmedical options that may help reduce or mask the unwanted noise. Sometimes, tinnitus goes away spontaneously, without any intervention at all.

If you are having difficulty coping with your tinnitus, you may find counseling and support groups helpful *(see the **Appendix**).* Ask your doctor for a referral.

CONVENTIONAL MEDICINE

If the cause of your tinnitus is excessive earwax, your physician will clean out your ears with a cotton-tipped probe or a suction device. If you have an ear infection, you may be given a prescription ear drop containing ***hydrocortisone*** to help relieve the itching and an ***antibiotic*** to fight the infection.

In cases where otosclerosis or a tumor is diagnosed, surgery may be necessary. If your tinnitus is the result of ***temporomandibular joint syndrome,*** your doctor will probably refer you to an orthodontist or other dental specialist for appropriate treatment.

For people with chronic tinnitus, drug treatments can offer some success. Lidocaine, a medication used for the treatment of certain types of abnormal heart rhythms, has been shown to relieve tinnitus for some people, but it must be given intravenously and its effect does not last long.

If your tinnitus is accompanied by some hearing loss, a hearing aid may be helpful. Many people have also benefited from tinnitus maskers, devices resembling hearing aids that play a sound more pleasant than the internal noise produced by the tinnitus. A newer device is a tinnitus instrument, which is a combination of hearing aid and masker. Another therapeutic technique, known as auditory habituation, uses a device that generates a certain type of white noise that is quieter than the tinnitus sound; the brain learns to habituate to, or ignore, the tinnitus noise. You must be tested and fitted for any of these devices so that their sounds will cover the particular frequency of noise you hear.

ACUPRESSURE

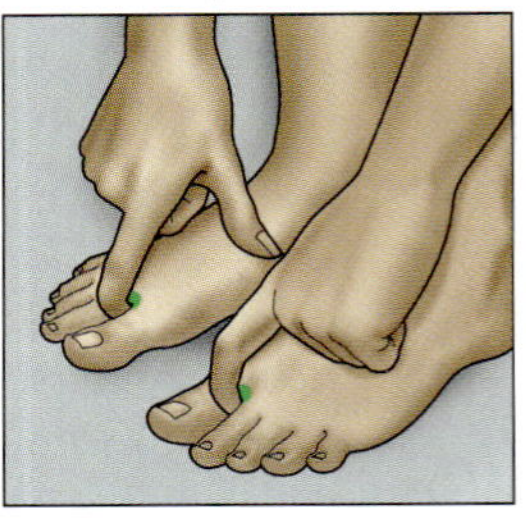

1 Pressure on Liver 2 may relieve stress brought on by a balance disorder. Press into the web between the big and second toes of both feet, angling the pressure toward the base of your big toe. Press firmly and hold for one minute.

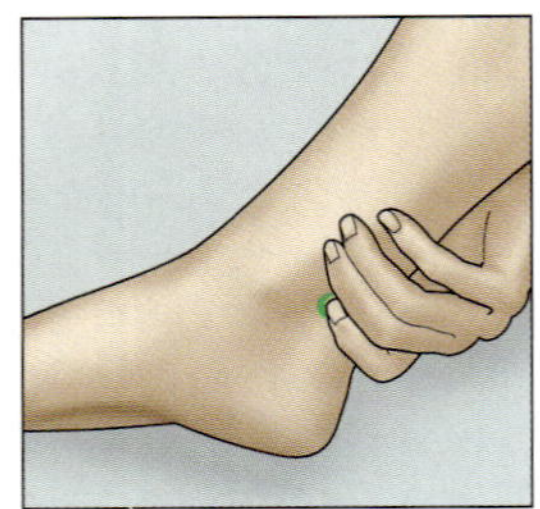

2 If you have ringing in your ears or earache pain, press the Kidney 3 point, between your Achilles tendon and the inside of your anklebone. Use your index finger to apply firm pressure toward the back of the ankle. Hold for one minute and repeat on the other foot.

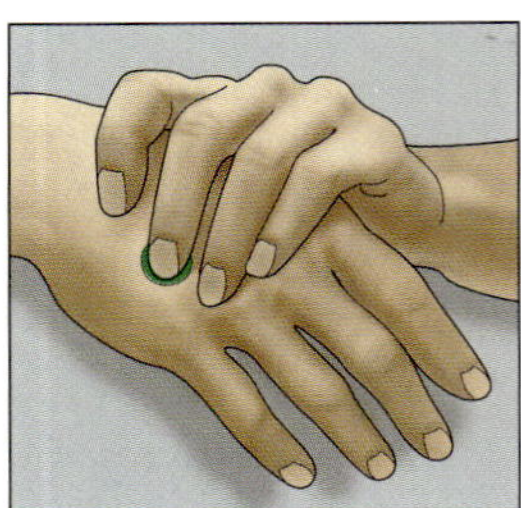

3 Applying pressure to Triple Warmer 3, in the groove on the back of the hand directly between and behind the fourth and fifth knuckles, may help relieve earache pain. Press gently and hold for one minute, and repeat on the other hand.

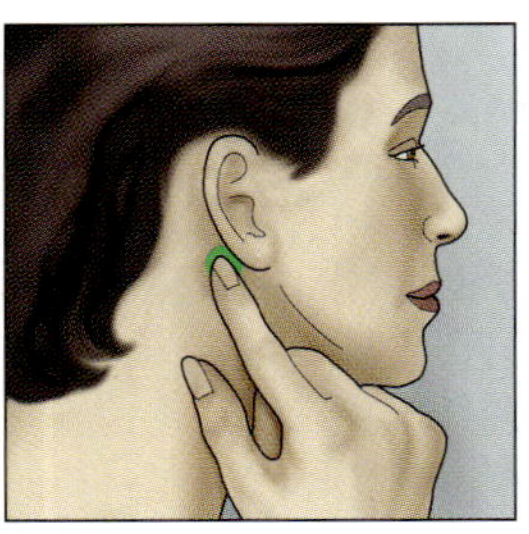

4 To help relieve ear pain, press your index fingers into Triple Warmer 17, the indentation behind your earlobes. These points may be tender, so press gently. Breathe deeply and hold for two minutes.

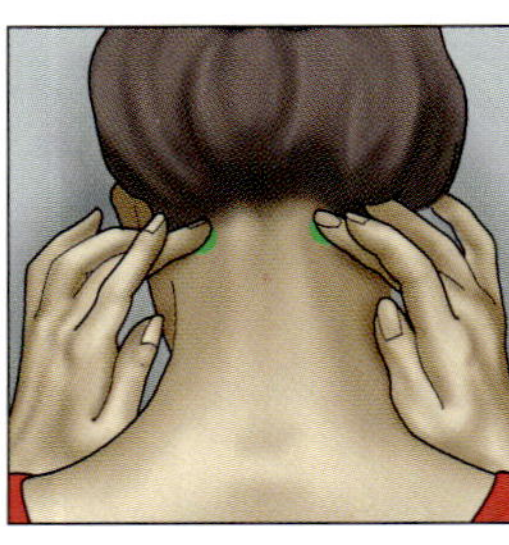

5 If ringing is worse when your neck is tense, place middle fingers one to two inches apart on Gall Bladder 20, the hollow areas on the sides of the neck at the base of the skull. With eyes closed, breathe deeply and tilt your head back; press up for one to two minutes.

ALTERNATIVE CHOICES

In addition to the therapies mentioned below, **Chinese herbs** may relieve tinnitus; consult a Chinese herbalist for the appropriate treatment. See the illustrations at left for **acupressure** and at right for **yoga** techniques that may help with your tinnitus.

ACUPUNCTURE

Acupuncture may help decrease the level of the tinnitus sounds you hear. The condition is believed to result from a disturbance in the flow of energy, or chi, to the liver or kidney. Consult a professional acupuncturist for treatment.

BIOFEEDBACK

Studies have shown that biofeedback can help people cope with their tinnitus, apparently by relieving stress. Patients are trained to relax the forehead muscles, which tighten during times of stress, and to warm their hands and feet. Ask your physician for a referral to a qualified biofeedback practitioner.

BODY WORK

Practitioners of the **Alexander technique** sometimes use postural training of the neck to help people with tinnitus, particularly in cases accompanied by vertigo. The technique is believed to improve the flow of blood to the ear.

CHIROPRACTIC

Manipulation that loosens the neck and improves blood supply to the ears may be beneficial in some cases. An **osteopath** can provide similar treatment.

HERBAL THERAPIES

Ginkgo *(Ginkgo biloba)* has been found useful in minimizing the distress of tinnitus. Take 80 to 120 mg of the dried herb or ½ to 1 tsp of the liquid extract daily. Don't expect immediate results from ginkgo; you may need to take the remedy for several weeks before experiencing any relief.

YOGA

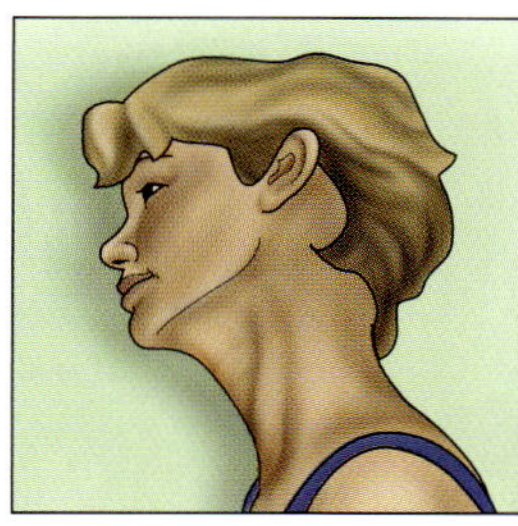

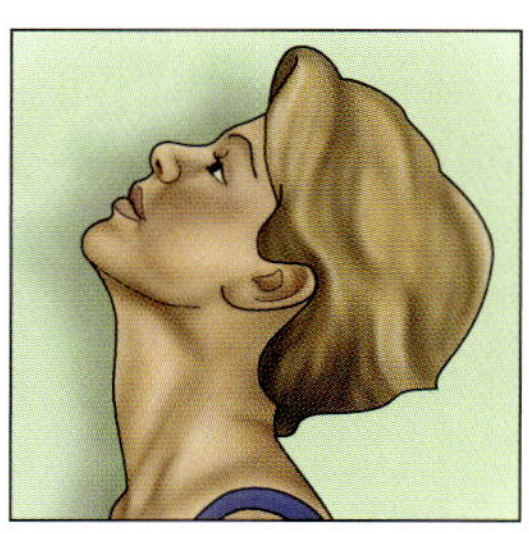

Head movements may help release tension in the shoulder and neck areas. This will expand the neck muscles and increase circulation. Exhale and slowly move your right ear toward your right shoulder and hold for 10 seconds *(top);* inhale and bring your head up, then repeat on the left side. Exhale as you slowly place your chin to your chest and hold for 10 seconds. Lift your head as you inhale, then exhale as you ease your head backward with your chin up *(bottom);* hold for 10 seconds. Inhale as you slowly bring your head back to the starting position. Do twice daily.

HOMEOPATHY

Several homeopathic remedies are prescribed for tinnitus. A homeopathic practitioner may prescribe one of the following:

- ◆ If the noise is a buzzing or hissing sound, *Chininum sulphuricum.*
- ◆ If the noise is a ringing sound with no other symptoms, *Kali iodatum.*
- ◆ If the noise is a roaring sound and is accompanied by some hearing loss, *Salicylicum acidum.*
- ◆ If roaring sounds are accompanied by a tingling sensation and by the feeling that the ears are blocked, *Carboneum sulphuratum.*

LIFESTYLE

Regular exercise that increases blood circulation to the head may help bring some relief from tinnitus. Try running, fast walking, swimming, biking, or some other aerobic activity. Be aware that after beginning an exercise program you may experience a slight worsening of your tinnitus before you notice an improvement.

MIND/BODY MEDICINE

Some people report that through self-hypnosis they can successfully "turn off" the unwanted sound created by their tinnitus for hours or even days at a time. A trained hypnotherapist may be able to teach you to adjust the volume of your tinnitus using an imaginary dial or other device. This form of **hypnotherapy** works only for people who are able to go into a moderately deep trance.

NUTRITION AND DIET

To improve blood circulation to your ears, reduce the saturated fat and cholesterol in your diet. ***Niacin*** supplements—100 to 6,000 mg a day—can also help lower cholesterol. WARNING: Do not take higher doses of niacin without being monitored by a professional because it can have side effects, such as liver toxicity.

Research has shown that a high percentage of people with tinnitus are deficient in ***vitamin B_{12}.*** Nutritionists recommend that you get 6 mcg of the vitamin daily. In addition, some evidence indicates that ***vitamin A*** supplements (5,000 to 10,000 IU a day) may be at least partially effective against tinnitus.

AT-HOME REMEDIES

- ◆ Avoid alcohol, smoking, and caffeine; they can make tinnitus worse.
- ◆ Cut down on salt in your diet. Salt can cause fluid to build up in your ears, worsening tinnitus.
- ◆ Avoid loud noises, which can aggravate a case of tinnitus you already have.
- ◆ If you have trouble sleeping because of the noise in your ears, try turning on a radio, which can mask the unwanted sound with soothing music. Or record a "white noise" tape, such as of running water, and play it whenever you need relief.
- ◆ Avoid too much ***aspirin,*** which can make tinnitus worse. ■

TONSILLITIS

SYMPTOMS

For tonsillitis:
- a very sore throat with red, swollen tonsils; there may be a white discharge or spots on the tonsils.
- swollen and tender lymph nodes in the neck under the jaw.
- a low-grade fever and headache accompanying the other symptoms.

For tonsillar abscess:
- in addition to inflamed tonsils, severe pain and tenderness around the area of the soft palate, at the roof of the mouth, and difficulty swallowing.
- distinctively muffled speech, as if the child is speaking with a mouthful of mashed potatoes, caused by swelling from the abscess.

CALL YOUR DOCTOR IF:

- your child has symptoms of tonsillitis.
- your child has tonsillitis and starts drooling or having difficulty breathing, which may indicate a **tonsillar abscess**.
- your child has trouble breathing at night or experiences noisy breathing or episodes of sleep apnea, in which the child stops breathing for brief periods while asleep; these symptoms may indicate ***adenoid problems*** or overgrown tonsils.
- your child has recurrent bouts of tonsillitis; surgery may be indicated.
- your child is not responding to ***antibiotics*** and has fever or pain, as well as white spots or a discharge on the tonsils; this may indicate ***mononucleosis*** or another infection.

The tonsils are masses of lymphatic tissue located at the back of the throat. They produce antibodies designed to help your child fight respiratory infections. When these tissues themselves become infected, the resulting condition is called tonsillitis.

Tonsillitis most commonly affects children between the ages of three and seven, when tonsils may play their most active infection-fighting role. But as the child grows, the tonsils shrink, and infections become less common. Tonsillitis is usually not serious, unless a **tonsillar abscess** develops. When this happens, the swelling can be severe enough to block your child's breathing. Secondary ear infections ***(otitis media)*** and ***adenoid problems*** are other complications.

CAUSES

Most tonsil infections and tonsillar abscesses in elementary school-age children are caused by the streptococcal bacterium, the same organism that causes ***strep throat.*** Cold or influenza viruses sometimes also cause tonsillitis.

TREATMENT

To check your child's tonsils, place the handle of a spoon on her tongue and ask the child to say "aaahhh" while you direct a light on the back of her throat. If the tonsils look bright red and swollen, call your pediatrician.

CONVENTIONAL MEDICINE

Your pediatrician will examine your child's tonsils and take a throat culture to check for strep throat. To check for a **tonsillar abscess,** the doctor will examine the tonsils and soft palate. If he discovers an abscess, he may drain it. For either a strep infection or an abscess, the doctor will prescribe an ***antibiotic*** such as ***penicillin*** or ***erythromycin.*** Be sure to give your child the full course; if unchecked, strep bacteria can cause serious autoimmune disorders such as nephritis or ***rheumatic fever.*** To ease pain, the doctor may

T

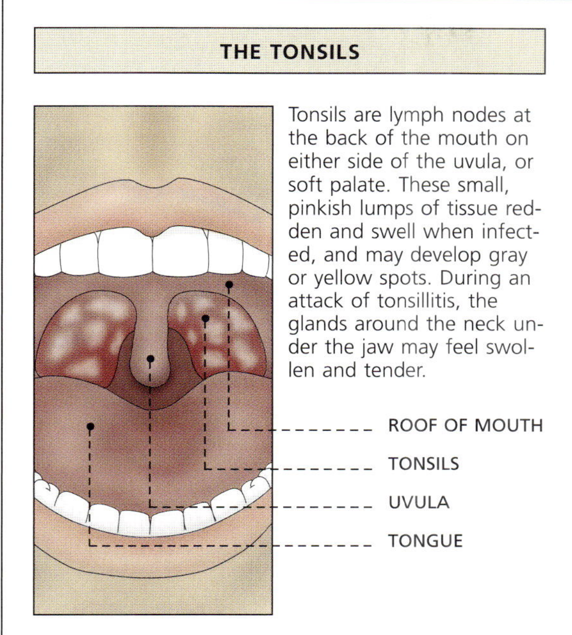

Tonsils are lymph nodes at the back of the mouth on either side of the uvula, or soft palate. These small, pinkish lumps of tissue redden and swell when infected, and may develop gray or yellow spots. During an attack of tonsillitis, the glands around the neck under the jaw may feel swollen and tender.

also recommend ***acetaminophen.*** (Do not give your child ***aspirin,*** which has been linked to Reye's syndrome.) Severe cases may warrant a tonsillectomy *(see **Prevention,** below).*

ALTERNATIVE CHOICES

Some alternative therapies are effective in relieving the symptoms of tonsillitis. But be sure to first get a throat culture to rule out strep throat, which must be treated with antibiotics. A **tonsillar abscess** should be treated by a medical doctor before you start any alternative method.

CHINESE MEDICINE

A practitioner of Chinese medicine may advise acupressure to relieve a sore throat, or acupuncture to combat chronic tonsillitis. Herbalists may recommend the over-the-counter remedy Honeysuckle and Forsythia Powder, thought to help soothe a sore throat in the early stages of tonsillitis.

HERBAL THERAPIES

To reduce inflammation, medical herbalists suggest drinking a tea made from cleavers (*Galium* spp.): Add 1 tsp dried herb to 1 cup boiling water. A gargle made from ***sage*** *(Salvia officinalis)* is thought to help fight infection: Add 2 tsp to boiling water and steep for 10 minutes. Let your child gargle with the tea (as warm as she can tolerate it) for 5 minutes several times a day.

HOMEOPATHY

After determining if your child is suffering from acute or chronic tonsillitis, a homeopath may recommend one of the following remedies: for inflamed tonsils, ***Belladonna, Hepar sulphuris,*** or ***Mercurius vivus;*** for chronic enlarged tonsils, *Baryta carbonica* or ***Calcarea carbonica.***

OSTEOPATHY

Osteopaths treat tonsillitis and tonsillar abscesses with the same surgical and drug therapies offered by conventional medical doctors but may also try gentle soft-tissue manipulation techniques to encourage lymphatic drainage.

AT-HOME REMEDIES

- A saltwater gargle can relieve soreness. Dissolve ½ tsp salt in a glass of warm water and let the child gargle as needed to ease pain.
- Ice cream or frozen yogurt, especially after a tonsillectomy, will relieve soreness and soothe your child.
- A cool-mist humidifier will increase moisture in the room and soothe a child's sore throat. Aim the mist away from your child so that it does not spray directly at her face, and change her clothes if they become damp.

PREVENTION

Tonsillectomy, the surgical removal of the tonsils, is performed much less frequently today than in years past. Doctors now generally recommend the operation only in serious cases, such as when tonsillar abscess is a recurring problem. If surgery is performed, your child may need to be hospitalized for a day or two and her throat will be sore for four or five days. ■

TOOTHACHE

SYMPTOMS

- aching or sharp pain in tooth when biting or chewing.
- soreness in teeth, gums, or jaw.

CALL YOUR DENTIST IF:

- your gums are painful, red, and swollen; you may have an impacted tooth or a gum disease. *(See **Gum Problems.**)*
- you experience continuous bouts of throbbing pain in a tooth, or the tooth is extremely sensitive to heat or cold; you may have tooth decay (a cavity) that requires a new or replacement filling. If the decay is advanced, you may need root canal work. You may also have a tooth abscess, a serious infection requiring emergency treatment.
- you have a sharp pain in your tooth, your tooth feels long or loose, and you have a fever. See your dentist immediately; you may have a tooth abscess.

A toothache can be caused by something as simple as a piece of food wedged between your gum and tooth—in which case relief involves no more than rinsing or flossing away whatever is causing the pain. But if the pain is not so easily eliminated, you probably have a dental disorder that can cause serious problems if you don't visit your dentist.

Tooth decay cannot be cured, but its progress can be halted through conventional dental care. Other causes of dental pain include impacted teeth—teeth that grow at odd angles—and gum disease, which inflames the area around a tooth so much that you cannot tell if the pain is coming from the tooth or from the tissue around the tooth. *(See **Gum Problems.**)*

Prevention of tooth decay is the best way to avoid toothaches. Alternative remedies may help alleviate the discomfort of symptoms, but conventional treatment is absolutely necessary to stop decay or infection from spreading.

CAUSES

The major cause of **tooth decay** is dental plaque—a substance composed of the bacteria, acids, and sugars in your mouth—which corrodes the protective enamel on your teeth. Initially, you may have no symptoms; but as decay develops, you may feel stabbing pain whenever you eat something hot, cold, sweet, or sour.

If decay goes untreated, bacteria infect the underlying dentin and eventually the pulp, or fleshy core, of the tooth. To fight ***infection,*** pus floods the pulp, causing a painful abscess. If left untreated, abscesses can damage the jawbone or sinus and lead to generalized ***blood poisoning.***

Impacted teeth are common in people in their late teens and early twenties, who are getting in their third molars, or wisdom teeth. Wisdom teeth are often too big for the jaw and thus do not fully emerge from the gum or grow in at odd angles; they press against neighboring teeth or trap food particles, causing pain and infection.

Toothaches may also be caused by pressure from sinus congestion, by tooth grinding, or by a blow to the face.

TOOTH DECAY

GUM
ENAMEL
DENTIN
PULP
DECAY

Plaque buildup can erode a tooth's protective enamel, causing decay and infection of the underlying dentin. If left untreated, the infection can spread to the pulp, or fleshy core, of the tooth. As the body attempts to fight the infection, a painful, pus-filled abscess may form at the root of the tooth, possibly causing damage to the gum, jawbone, or even the sinuses.

JAWBONE
ROOT
ABSCESS

TREATMENT

CONVENTIONAL MEDICINE

For most tooth decay, your dentist will remove the decayed portion and fill the cavity with a durable material. If the decay is serious, you may need a root canal, which involves removing the pulp, sealing the opening, and then capping the tooth with a crown. For abscesses, a dentist will likely first prescribe an ***antibiotic.*** If damage is so severe that a root canal is impossible, or if a tooth is impacted, extraction is the usual treatment.

ALTERNATIVE CHOICES

You must see a dentist for aches that you suspect may be related to tooth decay, but alternative treatments may ease the pain in the meantime.

ACUPRESSURE

Apply deep pressure to the webbing between index finger and thumb (LI 4) to relieve dental pain; massaging this area with an ice cube may also help. Do not press this point if you are pregnant.

HERBAL THERAPY

Rubbing clove oil *(Syzygium aromaticum)* or ***myrrh*** *(Commiphora molmol)* on the gum around a painful tooth helps numb it.

AT-HOME REMEDIES

Try the following remedies to relieve your pain.

- Rinse with salt water; if rinsing doesn't work, floss gently to pry out any trapped particles.
- Numb your gums: Sucking on ice for a minute numbs the gum surrounding a painful tooth.
- Keep cool: Though a hot compress may ease pain, if your toothache is caused by an infection, heat will cause the disease to spread.

PREVENTION

- Brush and floss after eating; use a nonabrasive, fluoride-based toothpaste. Beware so-called whitening agents; they often contain abrasives that can wear down enamel.
- Cut down on sweets and carbohydrates.
- Get your teeth cleaned professionally every six months, and make sure a dentist examines your teeth annually.

HYPERSENSITIVE TEETH

If a tooth reacts just to heat or cold, you could have dentinal hypersensitivity. More than 40 million Americans feel pain caused by the wearing away of enamel and exposure of dentin. It's brought on by age, receding gums, dental surgery, or excessive brushing with whitening toothpastes or hard-bristled brushes. You can help relieve hypersensitivity by using a toothpaste made for sensitive teeth and a toothbrush with soft bristles. ■

T

TOXIC SHOCK SYNDROME

SYMPTOMS

In a woman who is menstruating or has just completed a menstrual period; or in a new mother or any recent surgery or burn patient:

- high fever—over 102°F.
- vomiting and/or diarrhea.
- a rash resembling a sunburn with peeling skin, especially on fingers and toes.
- dizziness or mental confusion.
- pale and clammy skin, signaling a rapid drop in blood pressure; if toxic shock is left untreated at this stage, it will quickly lead to loss of consciousness, cardiac and respiratory failure, and death.

CALL YOUR DOCTOR IF:

- you have the symptoms above, which can develop suddenly. Toxic shock can dangerously lower blood pressure, resulting in life-threatening shock *(see also* ***Emergencies/First Aid****).* **Seek treatment immediately.**

Toxic shock syndrome is a sudden, potentially fatal condition brought on by the release of toxins from an overgrowth of a bacterium *(Staphylococcus aureus)* commonly found in many women. It is widely known to affect menstruating women, especially those who use superabsorbent tampons. The body responds with the classic symptom of shock: a precipitous drop in blood pressure, which deprives vital organs of oxygen and can lead to death.

This disease reached the headlines in the 1970s after the deaths of several young women who were using a certain brand of superabsorbent tampon; that brand was later removed from the market. Toxic shock syndrome is still primarily a disease of menstruating women who use tampons—especially superabsorbent tampons; however, it has also been linked to the use of menstrual sponges, diaphragms, and cervical caps. A woman who has recently given birth is also at increased risk for developing toxic shock. But the condition is not limited to these factors alone: Its victims also include both men and women who have been exposed to *Staphylococcus aureus* bacteria while recovering from surgery, a burn, or an open wound.

More than a third of all cases of toxic shock involve women under 19 years of age, and up to 30 percent of women who have had the disease will suffer a recurrence. The reason for this is unclear; however, it means that if you have ever suffered toxic shock, you must be especially alert to the symptoms of its onset so that you can get immediate medical care.

People who die from toxic shock are killed by the body's acute response to toxins released by *Staphylococcus aureus* bacteria. Victims suffer what is known technically as **hypotensive shock,** in which the heart and lungs are overburdened to the point that they stop working.

If you are menstruating and have a high fever with vomiting, especially if you have been wearing tampons, you must get medical help right away. If you are wearing a tampon, menstrual sponge, diaphragm, or cervical cap when you are taken sick, remove it immediately, even before calling your doctor.

CAUSES

The primary cause of toxic shock syndrome is a toxin produced by the bacterium *Staphylococcus aureus*. This organism is one of several related staph bacteria that often cause skin infections in burn victims and hospital patients weakened by surgery. These bacteria are not rare; in fact, *Staphylococcus aureus* is normally—and harmlessly—present in the vagina.

Exactly why and how *Staphylococcus aureus* causes toxic shock syndrome is not completely understood; what is known is that two conditions are necessary. First, the bacteria need an environment in which they can grow rapidly and release toxins. Then the toxins must have a way of getting into the bloodstream, where they trigger serious, life-threatening symptoms.

One theory holds that a tampon saturated with blood can serve as a medium conducive to rapid bacterial growth. What the tampon is made of seems to matter: Polyester foam apparently provides a better growth medium than either cotton or rayon fibers.

In cases that involve the use of menstrual sponges, diaphragms, and cervical caps, either the device had been in the vagina for an exceptionally long time—more than 30 hours—or, in the case of the sponge, pieces of the sponge had been retained in the vagina. (Either situation may provide a favorable environment for growth.)

The way in which bacterial toxins enter the bloodstream may also be related to tampon use. According to researchers, sliding a tampon into place in the vagina may make microscopic tears in its walls, rupturing tiny blood vessels. A superabsorbent tampon—especially if left in overlong, or if used when the menstrual flow is light—can also dry out the vagina, making such tearing even more likely.

Researchers investigating the causes of toxic shock syndrome have ruled out certain factors. Feminine deodorant sprays and douches, underwear, and other clothing do not play a role, and the condition is also unrelated to the victim's menstrual history, drug or alcohol use, cigarette smoking, swimming or bathing, or sexual activity.

TREATMENT

Toxic shock syndrome requires immediate emergency care in a hospital setting. If you suspect you are suffering an attack, get medical help as soon as possible. If your doctor is not available, call 911 or get to a hospital emergency room right away; have someone take you because you may quickly become too shaky to drive yourself.

CONVENTIONAL MEDICINE

Treatment for this life-threatening condition must be aggressive. Your doctor or emergency-care specialist should start by giving you ***antibiotics*** specific to a ***staph infection,*** to kill the bacteria and limit further release of toxins. Other urgent steps—necessary to control your body's response to the toxins and to support vital functions—include blood transfusion and intravenous administration of fluids and electrolytes to stabilize your blood pressure. Some cases call for a ventilator, which will temporarily breathe for you. Caregivers will monitor your vital signs constantly during the acute phase of this disease.

PREVENTION

Using regular tampons increases your risk of developing toxic shock syndrome far less than using superabsorbent ones. Nevertheless, the most conservative preventive approach would involve switching to sanitary napkins. You may also decrease risk somewhat by taking the following steps:

- Minimize your use of tampons. You might alternate tampons with sanitary napkins during the day, and use napkins at night.
- Use the least absorbent tampon that will control your menstrual flow; change tampons at least every eight hours. Be sure to remove the last tampon when your period is over.
- If you use a menstrual sponge, diaphragm, or cervical cap, remember to remove it when it is not needed. Under no circumstances should you leave any such device in for more than 24 hours. Wash your diaphragm or cervical cap in warm, soapy water after each use. ■

T

TRENDING

Read down this column to find your symptoms. Then read across.

SYMPTOMS	AILMENT/PROBLEM
◆ shaky hands; you regularly drink coffee, colas, or tea.	◆ Effects of caffeine
◆ trembling (shaking that you cannot control) after taking a new medication.	◆ Side effects of a medication
◆ trembling; feelings of anxiety, fear, or anger.	◆ An inherited tendency to tremble in response to ***stress*** or other strong emotional states
◆ trembling; hunger; weakness; excessive perspiration; nervousness and confusion; lightheadedness; possibly, headache or irregular heartbeat.	◆ ***Hypoglycemia*** (abnormally low levels of blood sugar)
◆ weight loss despite increased appetite; nervousness; trembling; excessive perspiration; irregular heartbeat; fatigue; protruding eyes; enlarged thyroid gland that you may be able to feel with your fingers.	◆ ***Graves' disease***
◆ weakness and fatigue; trembling; weight loss; irregular heartbeat; possibly, lack of appetite.	◆ One of many forms of hyperthyroidism
◆ tremor in your hand, fingers, head, or voice that increases with fatigue or strong emotion, and gradually worsens with time.	◆ Essential tremor, a harmless but annoying shaking
◆ trembling between bouts of heavy drinking; broken facial capillaries; flushed face; chronic diarrhea.	◆ Effects of chronic overconsumption of alcohol
◆ trembling accompanied by slow, jerky movements; unsteady balance; indistinct speech; trouble swallowing; age over 50.	◆ ***Parkinson's disease***
◆ trembling with numbness, tingling; double or blurred vision; weakness; muscle spasms or paralysis; mood swings; incontinence.	◆ ***Multiple sclerosis***

WHAT TO DO	OTHER INFO
◆ Reduce your caffeine consumption; talk to your healthcare practitioner if you experience headaches, nausea, irritability, or other withdrawal symptoms.	◆ Some practitioners believe it is possible to develop a physical addiction to coffee even if you drink only two cups a day.
◆ Many medications, either alone or in combination with others, can cause trembling or other side effects. Check with your doctor or pharmacist about possibly changing your medication.	◆ Make sure that your doctor and pharmacist have a complete list of all the medications you are taking.
◆ See your doctor soon for an accurate diagnosis. See ***Anxiety, Panic Attack, Phobias, Stress.***	◆ Try breathing exercises, yoga, and/or aerobic exercise to help you relax and keep emotions from becoming overwhelming.
◆ Eat something sweet; this may boost your blood sugar level in 5 to 20 minutes.	◆ Eating frequent, small meals that are high in complex carbohydrates and protein yet low in sugar will often keep hypoglycemia attacks at bay.
◆ See your doctor for an accurate diagnosis and treatment.	◆ Graves' disease is most likely to occur between the ages of 30 and 40.
◆ See your doctor for an accurate diagnosis and treatment. See ***Thyroid Problems.***	◆ With treatment, most people with hyperthyroidism lead a normal life.
◆ See your doctor about treatment.	◆ The most common movement disorder in the United States; essential tremor does not lead to more serious problems.
◆ Reduce your alcohol consumption; see ***Alcohol Abuse.***	
◆ See your doctor for an accurate diagnosis and treatment.	◆ Medication can significantly slow the progress of Parkinson's disease. Acupuncture and homeopathy may also be heplful.
◆ See your doctor for diagnosis; the form of the disease will determine treatment.	◆ Multiple sclerosis can affect every part of the body. Be open to a variety of alternative treatments to see which works best for you.

T

TRICHOMONIASIS

SYMPTOMS

If you're a woman, you may have no symptoms at all, or you may experience:
- a greenish yellow, frothy vaginal discharge with a pronounced odor.
- vaginal itching or irritation.
- painful intercourse.
- pain in the lower abdomen.
- vaginal bleeding.

If you're a man, you'll probably have no symptoms, or you may experience some discomfort when urinating.

CALL YOUR DOCTOR IF:

- you experience any of the above symptoms. Trichomoniasis is contagious and can lead to complications. Women shouldn't assume that the problem is simple vaginitis *(see **Vaginal Problems**)*.

Trichomoniasis—a parasitic infection spread primarily through sexual intercourse—is not serious, but it is contagious. In 70 percent of cases, it produces no symptoms, which makes it notoriously difficult to diagnose. In women who do have symptoms, discomfort may persist for a week to several months and may be more pronounced right after menstruation or during pregnancy. Left untreated, the parasite may infect tissues throughout the urinary tract and reproductive system. In women, vulnerable sites for infection include the vagina, urethra, cervix, bladder, and various glands. In men the infection may spread to the urethra, prostate gland, seminal vesicles, and epididymis.

The parasite that causes trichomoniasis likes an alkaline environment. Women have a greater chance of getting the disease if they use oral contraceptives, are pregnant, or frequently use commercial douches, all of which can increase alkaline levels in the body.

CAUSES

The culprit behind trichomoniasis is a protozoan parasite called *Trichomonas vaginalis*. Usually transmitted through intercourse, the parasite may also be acquired from toilet seats, locker room benches, damp towels, and bathing suits.

DIAGNOSTIC AND TEST PROCEDURES

Your doctor may want to examine your vaginal or urethral discharge under a microscope or test your urine. Trichomoniasis occasionally shows up on Pap smears in women with no symptoms. Your best bet is to get tested during your annual physical if you think you may have been exposed to the organism.

TREATMENT

Nine out of ten people with trichomoniasis are cured with a single course of ***antibiotics.*** Stubborn cases require larger doses administered over longer periods of time.

CONVENTIONAL MEDICINE

The drug most commonly used to fight trichomoniasis is metronidazole, which comes in tablet form; few other drugs are as effective. Metronidazole is viewed with caution by some physicians because of test results showing it to cause birth defects and cancer in animals. But no studies have proved it harmful to humans. If you take metronidazole, you may experience side effects such as nausea, vomiting, or a metallic aftertaste. You can minimize discomfort by taking the drug during or immediately after a meal. Also, don't drink alcohol within 24 hours of taking the medicine; if you do, you may experience severe abdominal pain and vomiting.

ALTERNATIVE CHOICES

Besides taking antibiotics, you can try alternative treatments to help speed healing.

ACUPRESSURE

A doctor of Chinese medicine may recommend that you flush out toxins by massaging acupressure points Liver 3, between the big and second toes, and Liver 8, on the inside of the leg above the knee. Also try kneading Kidney 3, on the inside of the leg between the anklebone and the Achilles tendon. Use any of these techniques at home several times a day. *(See the **Appendix** for more information about point locations.)*

AROMATHERAPY

Aromatherapists believe that oil of bergamot *(Citrus bergamia)* may help dry up irritating discharges. Douche with it or add it to your bath.

CHINESE HERBS

A practitioner of Chinese medicine may prepare a prescription for you with herbs such as ***gentiana*** *(Gentiana scabra),* ***Chinese foxglove root*** *(Rehmannia glutinosa),* and ***angelica root*** *(Angelica pubescens).*

HERBAL THERAPIES

Herbalists say that you can reduce inflammation and discharges by douching with teas of ***calendula*** *(Calendula officinalis),* ***myrrh*** *(Commiphora molmol),* and thuja *(Thuja occidentalis).*

HOMEOPATHY

A homeopathic physician may prescribe a remedy to strengthen your entire system. A complete consultation is necessary to determine which remedy is right for you.

NUTRITION AND DIET

Antibiotics destroy beneficial as well as disease-causing organisms in your body. Replace the beneficial ones by eating live-culture yogurt or by taking a *Lactobacillus acidophilus* supplement and *Bifidobacterium* in a glass of water twice a day, away from food.

To promote healing and boost immunity, nutritionists recommend that you supplement a balanced diet with ***zinc*** and ***vitamins A, C,*** and ***E.***

AT-HOME REMEDIES

Women who douche frequently with commercial chemical products may raise their risk of developing trichomoniasis. But if you have the infection, use one of the following natural douches once a day, while lying in a warm bath:

- vinegar douche: 1 tsp vinegar to 1 qt warm water.
- live-culture yogurt or a solution of *Lactobacillus acidophilus* (½ tsp to 1 cup of water).

To increase parasite-killing acidity, you may add to either douche the juice of one lemon. CAUTION: Do not douche if you are pregnant.

PREVENTION

- Use a condom when having sex.
- Don't share towels or swimsuits.
- Shower immediately after swimming in a public pool.
- Wash before and after intercourse. ■

T

TUBERCULOSIS

SYMPTOMS

- at first, only a mild cough or, often, no symptoms.
- fatigue.
- weight loss.
- cough, with occasional bloody sputum.
- slight fever, night sweats.
- pain in the chest, back, or kidneys, and perhaps all three.

CALL YOUR DOCTOR IF:

- you exhibit any of the above symptoms, especially if you live in crowded conditions, are malnourished, or have the virus that causes ***AIDS.*** (Note: Virtually all of the symptoms of tuberculosis can be confused with those of other diseases; bloody sputum, for example, is also a symptom of ***pneumonia.***)
- you have been exposed to someone with active tuberculosis.

Tuberculosis, commonly referred to as TB, is a chronic bacterial infection that can spread through the lymph nodes and bloodstream to any organ in your body but is usually found in the lungs. In their active state, TB bacteria in essence eat away at the tissue of infected organs, possibly resulting in death. But the organisms usually remain inactive after entering the body; thus, most infected people will never develop the active form of the disease if they receive proper care.

Because the bacteria that cause tuberculosis are transmitted through the air, the disease can be quite contagious. However, it is nearly impossible to catch TB simply by passing an infected person on the street. To be at risk, you must be exposed to the organisms constantly, by living or working in close quarters with someone who has the active disease. Even then, because the bacteria generally stay dormant after they invade the body, only 10 percent of people infected with TB will ever come down with the active disease. The remaining 90 percent will show no signs of infection, nor will they be able to spread the disease to others. Dormant infections can eventually become active, though, so even people without symptoms should receive medical treatment.

Once widespread, TB became relatively rare with the help of antibiotic therapies developed in the 1950s. Today, however, a new and highly resistant form has emerged, creating a public-health hazard in many large cities worldwide. If you have TB—in its active or dormant state— you must seek conventional medical treatment.

CAUSES

Tuberculosis is generally caused by exposure to microscopic airborne droplets containing the bacterium *Mycobacterium tuberculosis,* also called the tubercle bacillus. The disease is almost never transmitted through clothes, bedding, or other personal items. Because most people with TB exhale only a few of these germs with each breath, you can contract the disease only if you are exposed to an infected person for a long time. If you spend 8 hours a day for six months, or 24 hours a day for two months, with someone with

A RESISTANT MENACE

Two decades ago, the United States surgeon general announced that tuberculosis was a disease of the past. He spoke too soon: The disease has since resurfaced in a potent new form that has once again turned TB into a public-health hazard. This new form, called multidrug-resistant TB (MDR-TB), is caused by strains of the bacterium M. tuberculosis that, through mutation, have developed the ability to resist two or more antibiotic drugs. Even with treatment, roughly half of all MDR-TB patients die. This mortality rate matches that of patients with regular TB who received no medical care at all.

an active case of TB, you have a 50 percent chance of acquiring the disease.

People who are malnourished or who live in close quarters stand the greatest chance of contracting tuberculosis. Therefore, the conditions that accompany poverty, although not a cause of tuberculosis, certainly contribute to its ability to spread. Healthcare workers, long-term hospital patients, and prison workers or inmates also face a greater-than-normal risk of becoming infected with TB.

DIAGNOSTIC AND TEST PROCEDURES

You will generally have no symptoms if you are infected with TB. In fact, you may not even be aware that you have the disease until it is revealed through a skin test, perhaps during a routine checkup. The Mantoux skin test is the most reliable detector of TB. A medical practitioner injects a small amount of liquid material between the top two layers of skin on your arm. If a red welt develops at that site over the next day or so, you are probably infected with TB, though not necessarily in its active form. X-rays of your lungs will usually reveal if the disease has spread.

TREATMENT

Anyone with tuberculosis must be monitored by a doctor. If you have the infection—but not the active disease—your doctor will probably prescribe an ***antibiotic*** drug called isoniazid (INH) as a preventive measure. If you have the active disease, your physician will most likely prescribe broad-spectrum antibiotics.

CONVENTIONAL MEDICINE

For patients who are infected with tuberculosis organisms but do not have the active disease, doctors usually administer preventive therapy. This usually involves a daily dose of isoniazid and periodic checkups. If you have the active disease, regularly monitored treatment by a doctor is crucial. You will probably be given a combination of several ***antibiotics,*** which may include INH, rifampin, pyrazinamide, or ethambutol.

ALTERNATIVE CHOICES

If you have TB, you must be supervised by a conventional doctor. Alternative therapies may help alleviate some symptoms of the disease, but they cannot replace medical treatment.

HERBAL THERAPIES

An herbalist might recommend three cups per day of an infusion from elecampane *(Inula helenium),* or 20 to 40 drops from a tincture of this herb three times a day. The plants are thought to have antibacterial properties that guard against further infection.

NUTRITION AND DIET

Because malnutrition contributes to the activation of TB bacteria, a balanced diet is essential for people with tuberculosis. Many nutritionists also recommend ***vitamins A, C,*** and ***E,*** along with the mineral ***zinc,*** as these are believed to help keep mucous membranes healthy. ■

URINARY PROBLEMS

Read down this column to find your symptoms. Then read across.

SYMPTOMS	AILMENT/PROBLEM
◆ pink or red (bloody) urine.	◆ Any of a variety of diseases and conditions, including ***prostate problems, kidney stones, kidney cancer,*** or ***kidney disease;*** a reaction to a medication or food
◆ painful urination.	◆ Any of a variety of diseases and conditions, including ***bladder infection, kidney stones,*** urinary blockage, or ***bladder*** or ***prostate cancer***
◆ desire to urinate more frequently or with greater urgency than usual.	◆ Any of a variety of diseases and conditions, including ***gonorrhea,*** urethritis (inflammation of the urethra), cystitis (a ***bladder infection***), prostatitis (a ***prostate problem***), ***kidney stones,*** or ***bladder cancer***
◆ dwindling amounts of urine or no urine production at all.	◆ Dehydration; ***kidney disease***
◆ excessive thirst and passing abnormal amounts of urine (more than three quarts a day).	◆ Any of a variety of diseases and conditions, including a chemical imbalance, ***diabetes,*** or psychological problems; a side effect of long-term lithium therapy for ***manic-depression***
◆ cloudy (pus-containing) urine, possibly with a foul odor.	◆ Cystitis (a ***bladder infection***)
◆ urinary leakage, dripping, or uncontrollable urges to urinate.	◆ ***Incontinence***
◆ inability or only partial ability to empty the bladder.	◆ Any of a variety of conditions, including a narrow urethra, an enlarged prostate gland (a ***prostate problem***), bladder or urethral stones, psychological problems, or in children, an impaired urethral valve.

WHAT TO DO	OTHER INFO
◆ See your doctor without delay. Although blood in the urine is not always a cause for concern, it may indicate a serious underlying disorder. For more information about treatment, see the various entries listed at left.	◆ Urine that turns pink or red soon after a sore throat or upper respiratory infection may be a sign of a serious kidney problem.
◆ See your doctor. For more information about treatment, see the various entries listed at left.	◆ A nonburning pain when urinating may indicate an abnormal blockage within the bladder or urethra, while a burning pain usually indicates a urinary tract infection.
◆ See your doctor. For more information about treatment, see the various entries listed at left.	◆ How often you need to pass urine each day depends on several factors, including personal habit, the amount of fluid you take in, and the strength of your bladder muscles.
◆ Drink fluids to replenish your body, but avoid drinks containing alcohol or caffeine. If you are not dehydrated but the amount of urine you are passing seems insufficient, your kidneys may be failing. This can be a medical emergency; **call your doctor now.**	◆ To avoid dehydration, drink plenty of fluids during hot weather, even if you do not feel thirsty.
◆ See your doctor. Depending on its cause, the condition may resolve itself or it may require drug therapy.	◆ Some types of drugs, particularly ***diuretics,*** can cause an increase in urine production.
◆ See your doctor. Cystitis, a bacterial bladder infection, is usually treated with ***antibiotics.***	◆ Pus is caused by large numbers of white blood cells, an indication of an ***infection.***
◆ See your doctor, who will suggest a remedy. Incontinence is neither a normal nor an inevitable part of aging, and can often be treated successfully.	◆ Urinary incontinence has several causes, including infection, medications, depression, restricted mobility, and hormone deficiency. Most problems can be corrected by medication or counseling; surgery is sometimes required.
◆ **Call your doctor now.** The inability to urinate even when you feel the urge is a medical emergency.	

UTERINE CANCER

SYMPTOMS

Uterine cancer causes no symptoms at onset. Symptoms usually appear as the malignancy begins to grow, but 5 percent of women with uterine cancer experience no symptoms until the disease spreads to other organs. The most likely symptoms are:

- abnormal vaginal bleeding. Before menopause, this means unusually heavy menstrual periods or bleeding between periods. After a woman enters menopause, this means any vaginal bleeding, unless she is on hormone replacement therapy (HRT). Postmenopausal women on HRT may have monthly bleeding that resembles menstruation and that may mask symptoms of uterine cancer; any unusual or heavy bleeding should be reported to the doctor.
- vaginal discharge that may range from pink and watery to thick, brown, and foul smelling.
- an enlarged uterus, detectable upon pelvic examination.
- unexpected weight loss; weakness and pain in the lower abdomen, back, or legs. This occurs once the cancer has metastasized, or spread to other organs.

CALL YOUR DOCTOR IF:

- you experience abnormal vaginal bleeding or discharge. Abnormal bleeding is not a symptom of menopause and should not be construed as such. It should be brought to your doctor's attention immediately. Uterine cancer usually doesn't occur before menopause, but it can appear around the time menopause begins.

In women of childbearing age, the uterine lining—the endometrium—thickens each month and prepares to receive a fertilized egg. If no egg is fertilized, the extra layers of tissue and blood are shed and expelled through menstruation. Various conditions—benign and malignant—can affect the uterus. Fibroid tumors on the uterine wall are benign, not precancerous, and women who have them are not at increased risk for uterine cancer. Endometrial hyperplasia is the most serious benign uterine condition, and in some women it evolves into uterine cancer. *(See **Endometriosis.**)*

Most uterine cancers arise in the endometrium and are called **endometrial cancer** or **endometrial carcinoma.** The more aggressive **uterine sarcoma** arises in the muscular wall of the uterus and accounts for less than 5 percent of all cases. (Only endometrial cancer is addressed here.) If left untreated, endometrial cancer can penetrate the uterine wall and invade the bladder or rectum, or it can spread to the vagina, fallopian tubes, ovaries, and more distant organs. Fortunately, endometrial cancer grows slowly and usually is detected before spreading very far. Of the 32,000 American women diagnosed annually with this cancer, more than 80 percent will be cured.

CAUSES

High-risk candidates for uterine cancer include postmenopausal women who began menstruating early; went through menopause late; suffer from ***obesity, diabetes,*** or ***high blood pressure;*** have few or no children; or have a history of ***infertility,*** irregular menstrual periods, or endometrial hyperplasia. Women taking the drug ***tamoxifen*** to treat ***breast cancer*** are at very slightly increased risk, but women who have taken birth-control pills are only half as likely to develop the disease after menopause as those who have not.

Susceptibility to endometrial cancer is linked to how much the endometrium has been exposed to estrogen "unopposed" by progesterone. The reason is simple: With a high level of cell division, the chance of cancerous cell mutation increases, and while estrogen stimulates cell division, progesterone suppresses it. Modern hormone replacement therapy (HRT) for postmenopausal women utilizes low-dose formulations of ***estrogen*** combined with progesterone, which pose minimal risk for endometrial cancer. Nonetheless, women on HRT should be examined regularly for signs of uterine cancer.

DIAGNOSTIC AND TEST PROCEDURES

Pap smears, which screen for ***cervical cancer,*** detect a small number of uterine cancers before symptoms develop. Otherwise, uterine cancer is usually diagnosed by the appearance of symptoms. If a tissue biopsy confirms the diagnosis, imaging tests, blood studies, and ultimately surgery can determine the stage of the disease.

TREATMENT

Conventional medicine successfully cures most women of uterine cancer. Deciding which treatment to use depends on the stage of the cancer as well as on the patient's age and general health.

WHERE CANCER DEVELOPS

Each month during childbearing years, the lining of a woman's uterus, known as the endometrium, prepares a layer of dense tissue to receive a fertilized egg. If no egg is fertilized, this extra tissue is shed during menstruation. After menopause the endometrial cells are at risk of becoming cancerous *(above, inset)*. Fortunately, most uterine cancers are slow growing and have a high cure rate.

CONVENTIONAL MEDICINE

Surgery is standard treatment for uterine cancer that has not begun to metastasize, or spread. The preferred treatment for early endometrial cancer is total hysterectomy, in which the uterus, cervix, ovaries, and fallopian tubes are removed. This extensive surgery may be enough to cure early cancer and is most likely to deter recurrence. If the disease has begun to spread beyond the uterus, the patient is given radiation therapy after surgery, in the hope of wiping out the remaining cancer cells. Some doctors also recommend radiation when the cancer has not spread but is already large.

Patients with widespread (metastatic) uterine cancer usually receive hormone therapy to slow the cancer's growth. Chemotherapy or radiation might also be given to reduce the size and number of metastatic tumors. Such treatment is rarely curative but can prolong life and relieve symptoms. If it successfully destroys distant tumors, and the cancer is confined to the urogenital organs, surgery may then be performed.

Patients in remission need checkups every few months for several years. If cancer recurs, it usually happens within three years. Caught early, recurrent cancer may be cured with aggressive radiation therapy or further surgery. *(See **Cancer** for more information on treatments.)*

COMPLEMENTARY THERAPIES

To help cope with the emotional difficulties of having uterine cancer, patients might consider joining a support group. Counseling is especially beneficial for premenopausal women who become depressed after a hysterectomy, knowing that they can no longer bear children.

PREVENTION

Have a Pap smear and pelvic exam annually. If you are of childbearing age, discuss the pros and cons of taking birth-control pills with your doctor. At any age, it pays to control your weight and fitness through exercise and a low-fat diet. ■

U

UTERINE PROBLEMS

SYMPTOMS

- heavy, prolonged, or irregular bleeding, with pain in the lower abdomen or back, which may indicate **fibroids** (benign uterine tumors).
- difficulty urinating and moving bowels, urine leaks when you laugh or cough, backaches; you may have a **prolapsed uterus.**
- bleeding between periods or bleeding after menopause, which may sometimes indicate ***uterine cancer.***
- chronic, abnormal premenopausal bleeding, known as **dysfunctional uterine bleeding.**

CALL YOUR DOCTOR IF:

- you feel a sharp or chronic pain low in the abdomen. You may have **fibroids** or another serious pelvic disorder such as acute ***pelvic inflammatory disease*** or ***endometriosis.*** **Call your doctor now.**
- your periods are excessively heavy. This may lead to ***anemia*** and may also be symptomatic of **fibroids, dysfunctional uterine bleeding,** ***uterine cancer,*** or other uterine problems.

The uterus is a muscular, hollow, pear-shaped organ located in the pelvic cavity behind the bladder and in front of the rectum. The lower portion narrows into the cervical opening, which leads to the vagina. The fallopian tubes are attached on either side of the upper portion of the uterus. The uterus is lined with a mucous membrane called the endometrium, whose state changes with the phases of the menstrual cycle. During normal reproduction a fertilized egg implants itself in the wall of the uterus. It is here that the embryo develops into the fetus, which grows and is nourished until birth.

Normally, the uterus is tipped forward somewhat, but in 20 percent of women it is retroverted (inclined backward). Usually this normal variation in the position of the uterus is present at birth, but changes may be caused by tumors, ***pelvic inflammatory disease,*** or ***endometriosis.*** A retroverted uterus is usually harmless.

Abnormal endometrial bleeding is referred to as **dysfunctional uterine bleeding.** Such bleeding, which occurs as menorrhagia (heavy menstruation or bleeding longer than 8 days), metrorrhagia (bleeding between periods), or chronic polymenorrhea (a cycle that is less than 18 days), may cause iron deficiency ***anemia.***

A **prolapsed uterus** occurs when the uterus descends from its normal position in the lower abdomen. In severe cases the uterus is visible through the vulva. The disorder is most common in middle-aged women who have had children weighing more than eight pounds at birth, but it may also occur in childless women. In recent years incidents of uterine prolapse have become rarer because women are having fewer children.

Occurring specifically in or on the uterus, **fibroids** are benign tumors, or growths of the muscles and fibrous tissue. Fibroids vary in size, usually grow slowly, and may occur inside the uterus, within the uterine wall, or on the outside surface of the uterus. They occur in more than 20 percent of women over 35 years old. For unknown reasons fibroids are more common in African American women.

Although they are usually not problematic, fibroids may cause enlargement and distortion of the uterus and make it difficult to become preg-

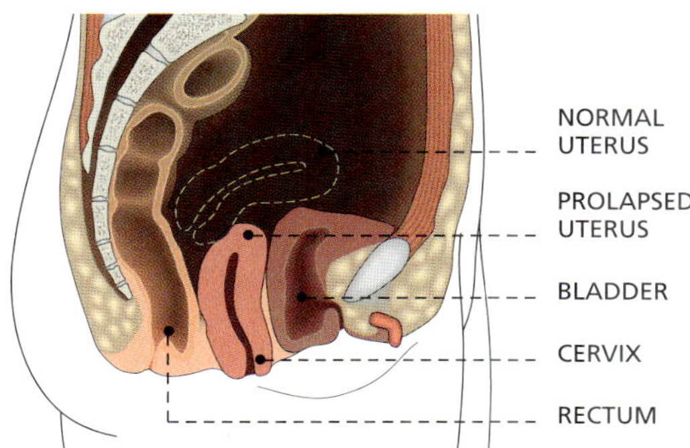

Aging, obesity, or repeated childbirth can weaken the muscles and ligaments in a woman's pelvis, allowing the uterus to prolapse, or slip out of place. A third-degree prolapse brings the head of the cervix flush with the opening of the vagina. In the severe case of prolapse above, the uterus—along with the bladder—protrudes outside the vagina.

nant. Sometimes a fibroid attached to the uterine wall may become twisted or may outgrow its blood supply, causing it to be starved for blood and oxygen. When this happens, you may suddenly feel a sharp pain in your abdomen. See your physician without delay to have this fibroid tumor removed.

Fibroids may cause bladder or bowel pressure or make intercourse painful for you. If they cause your period to become excessively heavy, you could develop ***anemia.*** Often, however, there are no symptoms at all. Because fibroids are affected by hormones, they have a tendency to enlarge during pregnancy and, if you are not undergoing estrogen replacement therapy, shrink after menopause.

CAUSES

Although the cause of **fibroids** is not known, their growth is related to hormones. Because of this, oral contraceptives, estrogen replacement therapy, and pregnancy may cause fibroids to grow and expand.

Dysfunctional uterine bleeding occurs when unchecked estrogen stimulation occurs in the endometrium. Several disorders that are characterized by high estrogen levels, including ovarian tumors, ***obesity,*** and anovulation (suppressed ovulation) in women in their late thirties and forties, may cause dysfunctional uterine bleeding.

The most common cause of a **prolapsed uterus** is the stretching of the support ligaments that hold it in place. Such stretching often occurs in childbirth. Being overweight may also contribute to and possibly exacerbate the condition.

For more information on the causes and treatment of uterine cancer, see ***Uterine Cancer.***

DIAGNOSTIC AND TEST PROCEDURES

Often, **fibroids** are brought to your attention only when your physician feels them during a routine pelvic examination. To verify their presence, an ultrasound scan may be performed.

An endometrial biopsy (or, in cases of extremely heavy bleeding, a dilation and curettage) may be performed, which, along with your history, will confirm a diagnosis of **dysfunctional uterine bleeding.**

A **prolapsed uterus** is usually easily identifiable on examination by a physician. A swollen vaginal wall is a telltale sign. During a pelvic exam, when the speculum is inserted, you may be asked to cough, allowing your physician to see the uterus prolapse.

TREATMENT

Formerly, a physician's all-purpose treatment for uterine disorders was to perform a hysterectomy, but with advances in medicine and growing interest in women's health issues, many other treatment options, both conventional and alternative, are now available.

CONVENTIONAL MEDICINE

Treatment for **fibroids** varies and should be approached according to your specific medical situation. This is very important because a hysterectomy—removal of the uterus—is commonly recommended to women with fibroids but may not be necessary. If your fibroids are not causing you any problems, you may want to consider doing nothing. Not all fibroids grow. Even large fibroids may not cause any symptoms, and most fibroids shrink after menopause. But you should monitor their growth by having an examination every six months.

To help prevent further fibroid growth, your physician may recommend that you stop taking oral contraceptives or abandon any hormone replacement therapy programs, both of which supply the body with synthetic estrogen. Gonadotropin releasing hormone (GnRH) agonists may be prescribed to shrink fibroids as presurgical treatment, but these drugs are expensive and should not be taken for more than six months to avoid the risk of developing ***osteoporosis.*** Also, GnRH agonists may cause early symptoms of menopause, and once use of the drug is stopped, the fibroids are likely to return.

Fibroids may be removed surgically in a procedure known as a myomectomy. Unless your growths are causing severe abdominal pain or you want to have more children, this major surgical procedure is usually not recommended. In 10 to 30 percent of cases the fibroids have been shown to return within five years after a myomectomy is performed.

In most women who suffer from **dysfunctional uterine bleeding,** birth-control pills, which contain hormones, may be prescribed to regulate the menstrual cycle. This treatment does not cure the physical disorder, but it is a comfortable way of eliminating your symptoms and at your physician's discretion may be used up until menopause. Progestins or gonadotropin releasing hormones (GnRH) may also be prescribed to control bleeding, but they take more than 30 days to show any effect and have many side effects.

A hysterectomy may be offered as treatment for severe uterine problems, including uncontrollable heavy bleeding and constant pain or frequent urination caused by fibroids pushing against your bladder.

A procedure known as an endometrial ablation controls bleeding by destroying the endometrium with lasers. Endometrial ablation is a viable alternative to a hysterectomy because it is less invasive.

A vaginal hysterectomy, in which the uterus is removed through the vagina, may be necessary if your **prolapsed uterus** is so displaced that it projects beyond the vulva.

If you prefer not to have surgery, your physician may insert into the vagina a plastic device known as a pessary, which sits in the vagina like a diaphragm to hold the uterus in place. Although a pessary will help support the uterus, it must be replaced every three to six months and is thus not a long-term solution.

ALTERNATIVE CHOICES

Many of these alternative therapies will ease the symptoms of your uterine disorder, but use them only as a complement to conventional treatment. In addition to the treatments listed below, **Chinese herbs** and **guided imagery** may help shrink fibroids; **yoga** may alleviate dysfunctional uterine bleeding.

ACUPRESSURE

Cramps that sometimes accompany the menstrual flow and **fibroids** may be treated with a kind of "first aid" acupressure that focuses on specific pressure points for temporary relief of pain. Beneficial points include Spleen 6, Spleen 8, Liver 3, and Conception Vessel 4. See the ***Appendix*** for point locations.

BODY WORK

Massage and **t'ai chi** may increase energy flow to the pelvis, which may help shrink fibroids.

HERBAL THERAPIES

Combine equal amounts of the tinctures of blue cohosh *(Caulophyllum thalictroides),* ***black cohosh*** *(Cimicifuga racemosa),* and ***chaste tree*** *(Vitex agnus-castus).* Take ½ tsp of this mixture three times a day as a tonic thought to improve the vitality of your uterus. For cramping, add 1 part ***wild yam*** *(Dioscorea villosa)* to the mixture.

ALTERNATIVES TO HYSTERECTOMY

A hysterectomy has traditionally been the indicated treatment for uterine problems, but this procedure is usually necessary only in extreme conditions. The following are alternative choices you should discuss with your physician.

For fibroids:

- *gonadotropin releasing hormone (GnRH) agonist therapy, which shrinks fibroids.*
- *myomectomy, a surgical procedure to remove fibroids; will control bleeding and symptoms of pressure.*

For prolapsed uterus:

- *pelvic floor exercises to strengthen the muscles that support the uterus.*
- *a pessary, a plastic device inserted in the vagina to hold the uterus in place.*

For dysfunctional uterine bleeding:

- *GnRH therapy and progestins, which may control bleeding.*
- *endometrial ablation, a procedure in which lasers are used to destroy the endometrium to control bleeding.*

HOMEOPATHY

Seek treatment from a professional homeopath. ***Pulsatilla, Belladonna,*** *Sabina,* and ***Sepia*** are among the remedies that may be prescribed for your uterine disorder.

LIFESTYLE

If heavy bleeding is symptomatic of your **fibroids,** you should try to lighten your daily routine and get more rest during your period.

NUTRITION AND DIET

Increasing fiber intake and reducing fat intake will lessen your estrogen production and restore hormone balance, which may effectively combat fibroid growth. Incorporating more ***vitamin C,*** bioflavonoids—found in citrus fruits, red onions, and leafy vegetables—and ***vitamins A*** and ***E*** may also be effective against fibroid growth. A high-fiber diet in the case of a **prolapsed uterus** or **fibroids** will ease difficulty with moving your bowels.

Multivitamin and mineral supplements, along with a high-fiber, low-fat diet that includes vegetables and whole-grain products, may help balance hormone levels that may contribute to uterine problems.

AT-HOME REMEDIES

When **fibroids** occur on the outside of the uterus (subserous fibroids), you may become aware of a mass on your abdomen. Lying down and placing a hot pack or hot-water bottle on the lower abdomen lessens pain. The hot packs should be applied three times a week for at least 60 minutes each time. Pelvic floor exercises (also known as Kegel exercises) to strengthen the uterine-support ligaments and to control urination are frequently recommended by physicians to help hold your **prolapsed uterus** in place. You can learn to exercise these muscles by stopping and starting your urine flow. Once you are familiar with the targeted muscles, practice tightening and relaxing them. Initially, 5 sets of the exercises are recommended, 10 times a day. At your own pace you may graduate to 10 sets, 10 times a day.

PREVENTION

Generally, uterine disorders are not caused by anything in particular that can be avoided. They are, however, closely related to estrogen levels and the phases, or malfunctions, of the menstrual cycle. While maintaining a low-fat, high-fiber diet, getting plenty of rest, and avoiding stress will not render you completely immune to uterine disorders, they are a step in the right direction.■

VAGINAL PROBLEMS

SYMPTOMS

- your vulva is inflamed and itches; you may have **vulvitis.**
- the skin of the vulva is thick and has developed white patches; this may indicate a condition called lichen sclerosis or ***cancer*** of the vulva. See your doctor for diagnosis.
- increased vaginal discharge with an offensive odor and burning, itching, and pain; you may have **vaginitis.**
- you have been sexually or psychologically abused and experience muscle constriction and pain at any attempt to penetrate the vagina; you may have **vaginismus.**
- an abnormal discharge, bleeding, and/or a firm lesion on any part of the vagina; you may have **vaginal cancer.** *(See **Cancer, Cervical Cancer,** or **Uterine Cancer.**)*

CALL YOUR DOCTOR IF:

- your bleeding is not caused by menstruation. If you are taking oral contraceptives, it may only be breakthrough bleeding. Otherwise, you may have dysfunctional uterine bleeding. *(See **Uterine Problems.**)* If you are pregnant, there may be a complication in the pregnancy. Postmenopausal bleeding sometimes indicates ***uterine cancer.***
- you have lower-abdominal pain along with fever, menstrual disturbances, abnormal discharge, and/or painful sex. You may have a pelvic ***infection.***
- you use tampons, a diaphragm, or a contraceptive sponge and you develop a high fever or rash. You may have ***toxic shock syndrome.***

The vagina is the part of the female reproductive system that connects the cervix (the entrance to the uterus) with the vulva, the skin folds that enclose the urethral and vaginal openings. This passage, composed of elastic, muscular walls, is lubricated by its own secretions and by mucus-producing glands in the cervix.

The vagina is self-cleaning. As the secretions, or discharge, flow downward, dead cells and other substances are flushed out. The amount and nature of your vaginal discharge will vary at different stages of your menstrual cycle, but some discharge is almost always present. A normal vaginal discharge is clear or white.

Vaginitis is an umbrella term meaning inflammation of the vagina. Yeast causes vaginal ***yeast infections,*** which are the most common form of the disorder. Other vaginal infections include **bacterial vaginosis** and sexually transmitted diseases such as ***gonorrhea, trichomoniasis,*** and ***chlamydia.*** Itching, irritation, an abnormal discharge, and inflammation may accompany these disorders. Vaginal infections are very common and treatable.

Bacterial vaginosis commonly occurs in the reproductive years. For unknown reasons there may be a change in the balance of naturally occurring bacteria in the vagina that allows disease-causing bacteria to dominate. The predominant sign of this condition is a fishy-smelling discharge, but many women with this infection exhibit no symptoms, which is also true for ***chlamydia*** and ***gonorrhea.*** To safeguard yourself, you should be routinely tested during your regular gynecological exam.

Overgrowth of fungal yeast cells may also upset your vagina's chemical balance. The result is a vaginal yeast infection, which is generally characterized by itching and soreness and may also produce a white, cottage-cheese-like discharge. Yeast infections are more likely to develop in women who are diabetic, on birth-control pills or antibiotics, or pregnant, but an estimated 75 percent of all women will have a yeast infection at least once in their lifetime. Many will suffer from recurring yeast infections, which are most frequent between the ages of 16 and 35. Vaginal yeast infections may cause pain during

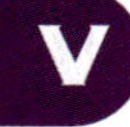

THE FEMALE REPRODUCTIVE SYSTEM

UTERUS
CERVIX
VAGINA
OVARY
FALLOPIAN TUBE

The female reproductive system consists of the ovaries, fallopian tubes, uterus (or womb), cervix, and vagina. The muscular, elastic walls of the vagina form a passageway between the internal sexual organs and the external genitalia. The vagina is subject to several kinds of infections, few of which are serious. Some vaginal infections, however, can lead to complications that deserve medical attention.

urination or during sexual intercourse or both.

Vaginal infections are generally not serious; but, while vaginal yeast infections primarily cause discomfort and annoyance, sexually transmitted infections such as ***gonorrhea*** and ***chlamydia*** have been found to be associated with an increased risk for ***pelvic inflammatory disease*** or other complications. Because of the vulva's proximity to the vagina, **vulvitis** often accompanies vaginitis and the inflammation is usually caused by the same organisms.

Vaginal cancer, accounting for only 2 percent of all gynecological cancers, occurs primarily in women over the age of 50. The severity of vaginal cancer depends on its type and exact location. Varieties include squamous cell carcinoma and clear cell adenocarcinoma. Once cancer appears on the vagina, it may spread to surrounding tissues, including the bladder, rectum, vulva, and pubic bone.

The involuntary constriction of the lower-vaginal muscles is called **vaginismus.** Vaginismus is a sexually related psychological disorder. The spasming of the muscles may be painful, and it interferes with penile penetration or the insertion of other objects such as a speculum or tampon. Sufferers of this disorder usually fear sexual intercourse and associate it with pain.

CAUSES

Bacterial vaginosis is primarily caused by *Gardnerella vaginalis* or *Mobiluncus* dominating the vaginal flora, but several other bacteria may also cause the disease. ***Stress*** or a new sexual partner may cause a change in the vaginal flora, which makes this infection more likely.

Vaginal ***yeast infections*** are caused by one of four varieties of the *Candida* fungus. Nearly 80 percent of vaginal yeast infections are caused by overgrowth of *Candida albicans.* This unchecked growth may be caused by a significant change in your diet or the use of ***corticosteroids*** or ***antibiotics*** prescribed to treat another disorder.

Vulvitis may be caused by chemical irritation or an allergic reaction to products such as soaps or douches. A viral, bacterial, or fungal infection, decreasing estrogen levels in menopausal women, or cancer may also lead to the disorder.

Vaginismus has psychological origins. It occurs most often after sexual trauma such as incest or rape. Negative conditioning with regard to sexuality may also cause the disorder.

Between the 1940s and 1970s, diethylstilbestrol (DES), a synthetic estrogen, was prescribed for women at high risk of miscarriage. (The drug was later found to be ineffective in preventing miscarriage.) Young women whose mothers took DES during pregnancy have an increased incidence of clear cell adenocarcinoma.

DIAGNOSTIC AND TEST PROCEDURES

A variety of tests may be ordered to diagnose **vulvitis**. Most cases may be identified with a pelvic exam, but a blood test or tests for sexually transmitted disease, if suspected, may also be administered. If your vulvitis persists, a biopsy to test for malignancy may be a necessary precaution.

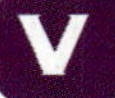

If **vaginismus** is suspected, your physician will discuss your sexual history with you, paying special attention to psychological factors. A pelvic exam will rule out the possibility of physical disorders and confirm the involuntary constriction of the muscles surrounding the vagina.

Diagnosis of the form of **vaginitis** you may have is made by identifying which organism has caused your infection. This is determined by taking a sample of discharge and viewing it under a microscope. Once you have been diagnosed with a vaginal yeast infection, you can usually recognize the symptoms if it recurs.

The diagnosis of vaginal cancer is usually based on thorough examination with a colposcope and biopsy of any suspicious-looking areas.

TREATMENT

Whether conventional or alternative, treatment for most vaginal disorders is aimed at maintaining proper bacterial balance and soothing your irritation and discomfort.

CONVENTIONAL MEDICINE

For postmenopausal cases of **vulvitis** or **bacterial vaginosis** your physician may prescribe ***antibiotics*** or estrogen suppositories or topical cream to thicken and lubricate vaginal tissues. For other cases of bacterial vaginosis your physician will prescribe an antibiotic cream such as metronidazole or clindamycin or oral metronidazole. Because an infection commonly passes back and forth between sexual partners, your partner may also need to be treated.

Once your physician diagnoses your vaginal irritation as a vaginal yeast infection, an ***antifungal drug,*** such as nystatin, ***miconazole,*** or ***clotrimazole*** will be prescribed either in a vaginal suppository or as a topical cream. If you suffer from recurring vaginal yeast infections, many over-the-counter treatments are available. These products, which come in vaginal inserts, creams, and suppositories, are, like those prescribed by your physician, either clotrimazole or miconazole.

Because **vaginismus** is of a psychological nature, professional individual and couples' sexual therapy is the best approach.

Cancer can be a life-threatening disease. Your physician's familiarity with your specific case of vaginal cancer will lead to a combination of treatments appropriate for you. In the early stages topical chemotherapy and laser surgery are usually recommended. These treatments are aimed at preserving and maintaining a functional vagina. This is possible, however, only if the condition is caught early. Surgery is primarily recommended when the tumor is extensive. Advanced forms of vaginal cancer are usually treated with radiation therapy. Most cases of vaginal cancer are treated by gynecologists with specialized training in cancer diagnosis and treatment. *(See **Cancer** for more information on forms of treatment.)*

ALTERNATIVE CHOICES

The following are supplemental therapies that, along with your physician's prescribed treatment, may ease your recovery. **Chinese herbs** are an additional supplemental therapy that may effectively treat vaginal problems.

HERBAL THERAPIES

Incorporate fresh ***garlic*** *(Allium sativum)* into your diet; it has antibacterial, antifungal, and antiviral properties and may be effective in treating **vagini-**

ATTENTION!

PRODUCTS THAT CAN IRRITATE

Many women may not be aware that their itching and burning may be caused by irritation from products such as soaps, bath oils and crystals, spermicides, swimming pool chlorine, feminine-hygiene sprays, perfumed douches or lubricants, scented or colored toilet paper, or perfumed pads and tampons. If your physician cannot detect an infection as the cause of your irritation, then an allergy or sensitivity to these commercial products is the likely culprit. Stop using suspect items. Try cool soaks in a tub and add Epsom salt if desired.

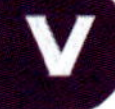

tis, including vaginal yeast infections. A fresh, peeled garlic clove wrapped in gauze may be inserted in the vagina to help treat **bacterial vaginosis.** This insert should be changed twice daily.

If itching or minor irritation is a symptom of your vaginitis, bathe with an infusion of fresh ***chickweed*** *(Stellaria media)* for relief. (Pour 1 cup of boiling water on 1 to 2 tsp of the herb, steep for 5 minutes, and let cool.) To reduce inflammation associated with **vulvitis** and infectious discharge of bacterial vaginosis, an herbal douche may bring relief. To make, pour 1 cup of boiling water over 1 to 2 tsp of ***calendula*** *(Calendula officinalis)* and steep for 10 to 15 minutes; let cool before using the tea as a douche.

HOMEOPATHY

The following remedies taken three or four times a day for one or two days may be used for minor vaginal problems. A smelly, yellow discharge with severe burning, swelling, and soreness may be treated with *Kreosotum* (12c); for itching and a white or yellow discharge, ***Sepia*** (12c) is recommended; ***Pulsatilla*** (12c) may aid in treating a thick, creamy yellow-green discharge. See a professional homeopath if your condition does not clear up.

Many over-the-counter homeopathic mixtures to treat vaginal yeast infections are available under brand names at your local drugstore.

LIFESTYLE

If you have recurrent vaginal infections, discontinue use of tampons for six months. In addition, avoid sexual intercourse while your symptoms of vaginal yeast infection or bacterial vaginosis are still apparent.

Wearing cotton panties and avoiding pantyhose and tight clothing will aid in keeping the vagina cool and dry, which may help prevent vulvitis and forms of vaginitis.

NUTRITION AND DIET

Monitor your sugar level if you have a vaginal yeast infection. If you are susceptible to these infections, eating yogurt containing active cultures may help to maintain the natural bacterial flora of the vagina.

AT-HOME REMEDIES

Incorporating *Lactobacillus acidophilus* into your diet may be helpful for treating vaginal yeast infections. A paste can be made from refrigerated capsules, available at health food and nutrition stores. Pour the *Lactobacillus acidophilus* powder into the palm of your hand and add water to create a pasty substance that may be introduced into the vagina using a vaginal applicator or your finger.

Regular sexual intercourse in postmenopausal women may help prevent dryness and thinning of the vaginal walls, although it could increase the likelihood of **vaginitis.** The activity stimulates blood flow in the area, which keeps vaginal tissue supple.

Discussing inhibitions with a trained sex therapist may be therapeutic for **vaginismus** sufferers.

Always wipe from front to back to avoid infection from any organisms that may be present in fecal matter.

PREVENTION

A well-balanced diet always aids in the maintenance of good health. Many women seem to be prone to vaginal infection, while others are rarely affected. Maintaining good hygiene and always using condoms are the best defenses against vaginitis. If you suspect a vaginal infection, do not douche for 24 hours before seeing your physician, as this may wash away secretions that aid in the diagnosis of your disorder.

A true case of **vaginismus** is caused by fear rather than physical abnormality. The best prevention for this disorder is a healthy home environment where sexuality is not made to seem dirty but rather, when appropriate, is discussed in an open, honest, factual manner. If you have suffered sexual abuse or trauma, you should seek professional help. ■

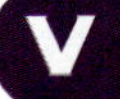

VARICOSE VEINS

SYMPTOMS

- prominent dark blue blood vessels, especially in the legs and feet.
- aching, tender, heavy, or sore legs; often accompanied by swelling in the ankles or feet after standing for any length of time.
- Bulging, ropelike, bluish veins indicate **superficial varicose veins.**
- Aching and heaviness in a limb, sometimes with swelling, but without any prominent or visible blue vein, may signal a **deep varicose vein.**
- Discolored, peeling skin; skin ulcers; and constant rather than intermittent pain are signs of **severe varicose veins.**

CALL YOUR DOCTOR IF:

- swelling becomes incapacitating, or if the skin over your varicose veins becomes flaky, ulcerous, discolored, or prone to bleeding. You may want to have the veins removed to avoid further discomfort and prevent potentially more serious circulatory problems.
- you have red varicose veins. This may be a sign of ***phlebitis,*** a serious circulatory condition.
- you cut a varicose vein. Control the resulting burst of blood *(see page 48 in **Emergencies: First Aid**)* and have the vein treated to prevent complications.

Varicose veins usually announce themselves as bulging, bluish cords running just beneath the surface of your skin. They can appear anywhere in the body but most often affect legs and feet. Visible swollen and twisted veins—sometimes surrounded by patches of flooded capillaries known as spider-burst veins—are considered **superficial varicose veins.** Although they can be painful and disfiguring, they are usually harmless. When inflamed, they become tender to the touch and can hinder circulation to the point of causing swollen ankles, itchy skin, and aching in the affected limb. *(See also **Hemorrhoids.**)*

Besides a surface network of veins, your legs have an interior, or deep, venous network. On rare occasions, an interior leg vein becomes varicose. Such **deep varicose veins** are usually not visible, but they can cause swelling or aching throughout the leg. Deep varicose veins may be sites where ***blood clots*** can form. Deep vein inflammation, or thrombophlebitis, in the thighs and pelvis may lead to a pulmonary embolism, a potentially fatal condition.

Varicose veins are a relatively common condition, and for many people they are a family trait. Women are at least twice as likely as men to develop them. In the United States alone, nearly 10 percent of all adult men and 20 percent of adult women are affected by them to some degree, bringing the total affected to more than 20 million people.

CAUSES

To circulate oxygen-rich blood from the lungs to all parts of the body, your arteries have thick layers of muscle or elastic tissue. To push blood back to your heart, your veins rely mainly on surrounding muscles and a network of one-way valves. As blood flows through a vein, the cuplike valves alternately open to allow blood through, then close to prevent backflow.

Varicosity results from a chronic increase in blood pressure, which dilates the vein. When the vein walls are pushed apart, the valves no longer seal properly, making it difficult for the muscles to push the blood "uphill." Instead of flowing

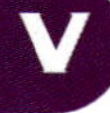

from one valve to the next, the blood begins to pool in the vein, increasing venous pressure and the likelihood of congestion while causing the vein to bulge and twist. Because superficial veins have less muscular support than deep veins, they are more likely to become varicose.

Any condition that puts excessive pressure on the legs or abdomen can lead to varicosity. The most common pressure inducers are pregnancy, ***obesity,*** and standing for long periods. Chronic ***constipation*** and—in rare cases—tumors also can cause varicose veins. Being sedentary likewise may contribute to varicosity, because muscles that are out of condition offer poor blood-pumping action. The likelihood of varicosity also increases as veins weaken with age. Contrary to popular belief, sitting with crossed legs will not cause varicose veins, although it can aggravate an existing condition.

VALVES IN VEINS

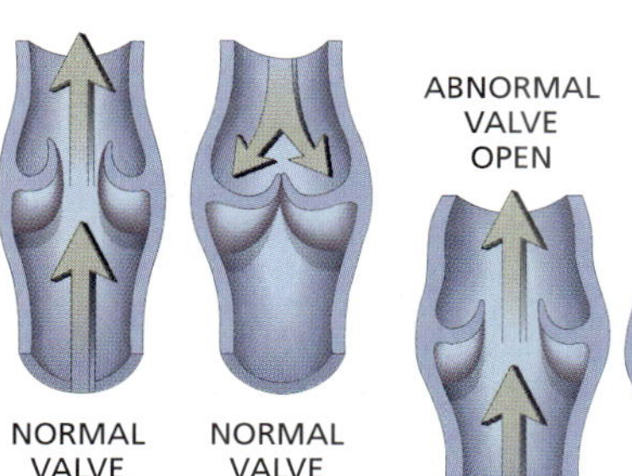

A normal valve in a vein opens to let blood flow toward the heart and seals tightly to prevent backflow. When a vein is weakened or stretched by excessive pressure, the valve cannot close properly. Blood backs up in the vein, causing it to swell and twist. Varicose veins, characteristically bluish purple in color, are most often seen close to the skin, but they can occur in deep tissue.

TREATMENT

A mild case of varicose veins does not usually require a doctor's care. You can find relief from the discomfort of varicose veins with basic at-home treatment and various alternative remedies.

CONVENTIONAL MEDICINE

Superficial varicose veins normally do not require medical attention, but they should not be ignored. To relieve the discomfort, your doctor may recommend elastic support stockings, which you can buy in most pharmacies and medical supply stores. Support stockings help your leg muscles push blood upward by concentrating pressure near the ankles. Put them on before you get out of bed in the morning. Raise your legs in the air and pull the stockings on evenly; they should not feel tight in the calf or groin. You should wear them all day.

To alleviate occasional swelling and pain, your doctor will probably suggest an over-the-counter anti-inflammatory drug such as ***aspirin*** or ***ibuprofen.*** If you notice skin around a varicose vein becoming ulcerous or discolored, or if you have continuing pain with no obvious outward signs, contact a doctor at once about the possibility of **deep varicose veins.**

Varicose veins can be eliminated by one of several methods. Spider veins can be removed quite simply through laser treatment. A mild case of **superficial varicose veins** can be treated by sclerotherapy: A chemical known as a sclerosing agent is injected into the vein to collapse its walls so it can no longer transport blood. More severe cases may merit surgical removal, or stripping. Unfortunately, no treatment can prevent new veins from becoming varicose. Before pursuing a particular treatment, discuss all options with a dermatologist or vascular surgeon.

ALTERNATIVE CHOICES

To cope with varicose veins, try a two-pronged strategy of natural remedies to ease the discomfort and preventive maintenance to keep your body fit and strong.

AROMATHERAPY

With numerous oils to choose from, you can tailor aromatherapy to your particular needs. Oil

V

of ***rosemary*** *(Rosmarinus officinalis)* massaged gently into an affected area may help stimulate circulation by causing capillaries to dilate. Oils of cypress and ***chamomile*** *(Matricaria recutita)* may soothe swelling and inflammation and help relieve pain.

BODY WORK

Regular **massage** can significantly alleviate discomfort associated with varicose veins. A trained massage therapist starts at the feet and massages your legs up to the hips and along the lymphatic system, to mobilize congested body tissues. Other techniques, such as **reflexology** and **acupressure,** may also prove helpful in alleviating symptoms of varicose veins.

HERBAL THERAPIES

Many herbs have long histories of folk use in the treatment of varicose veins, and some have undergone extensive scientific study. ***Ginkgo*** *(Ginkgo biloba),* ***hawthorn*** *(Crataegus laevigata),* and ***bilberry*** *(Vaccinium myrtillus)* are all reported to strengthen blood vessels and improve peripheral circulation. Tinctures or topical ointments of horse chestnut *(Aesculus hippocastanum)* and ***butcher's-broom*** *(Ruscus aculeatus)* are also recommended for toning veins while reducing inflammation; butcher's-broom can also be prepared as tea.

For skin irritation associated with varicose veins, try a lotion made of distilled witch hazel *(Hamamelis virginiana).* To disperse buildup of a protein called fibrin that makes skin near varicose veins hard and lumpy, try eating more ***cayenne*** *(Capsicum frutescens),* ***garlic*** *(Allium sativum),* onion, ***ginger*** *(Zingiber officinale),* and pineapple, which contains bromelain, an enzyme that promotes breakup of fibrin.

HOMEOPATHY

For long-term treatment of varicose veins, a homeopath may prescribe a constitutional remedy in the potency and dosage best suited to your symptoms. ***Pulsatilla*** is one remedy that is commonly prescribed.

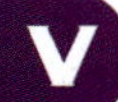

For immediate relief from specific symptoms, you can try over-the-counter homeopathic remedies: *Hamamelis,* or witch hazel, cream in a 6x to 15c solution applied to an area that is bluish and perhaps bruised may relieve soreness. *Hamamelis* 6x to 15c can also be taken internally as directed on the label for general relief. ***Belladonna,*** 12x or 12c potency four times a day, is recommended for red, hot, swollen, and tender varicose veins.

HYDROTHERAPY

Sponging or spraying legs with cold water can relieve aches and pain from **superficial varicose veins.** Hot and cold baths may slow the progression of varicose veins on the feet and ankles: Dip your feet in warm water for 1 to 2 minutes, then cold water for half a minute, and alternate for 15 minutes. You might even add an aromatherapy oil to the water.

LIFESTYLE

Maintaining your overall fitness—both nutritionally and physically—is most essential to preventing varicose veins from developing. Aerobic exercise totaling 30 minutes a day several times a week will help you keep your weight down while toning and strengthening veins. You might start your morning with a brisk walk, for example, or finish your day with a swim or bike ride.

If you already have varicose veins, you can help control them with a program of specially designed exercises, preferably under the direction of a trained exercise therapist attuned to the condition's particular needs.

MIND/BODY MEDICINE

Yoga's stretching and relaxation techniques can be particularly beneficial for varicose veins. Certain positions, such as the Plow, Half Shoulder Stand, and Shoulder Stand *(see the **Appendix**),* promote circulation and the drainage of blood from the legs. The deep-breathing exercises you learn to practice in yoga may further alleviate discomfort by getting more oxygen into the bloodstream.

NUTRITION AND DIET

Diet plays a critical role in any varicose vein treatment program. Your goals are to promote better circulation and keep weight in check. Ex-

SWITCH YOUR BED

Varicose vein sufferers are told to elevate their feet when resting or sleeping. But before you rush to the bedroom armed with pillows and bricks—or start building a makeshift ramp at the end of your bed—consider changing the bed itself. By switching to a hospital-style adjustable bed, you can keep your feet raised all through the night, and you'll have the added benefit of low back pain relief. Another option—perhaps more attractive to the home decorator—is a well-designed waterbed. Waterbeds adapt their contour to fit your body, minimizing the discomfort to tender veins where they come in contact with the mattress.

tra body fat increases water retention and puts pressure on the legs and abdomen, aggravating varicosity. To decrease body fat, eat foods that are low in fat, sugar, and salt, and high in fiber. To promote a healthy flow of nutrients and waste through the body, make fruits, vegetables, and whole grains the mainstays of your diet, and drink plenty of fluids, especially water.

Certain vitamins and bioflavonoids—natural substances found in many fruits and vegetables—may improve varicose veins; try 500 mg of ***vitamin C*** and 400 IU of ***vitamin E*** daily. Bioflavonoids are beneficial because they promote the absorption of vitamin E. Among bioflavonoids, rutin is used routinely to treat varicose veins. It is present in many foods, including citrus fruits, apricots, blueberries, blackberries, cherries, rose hips, and buckwheat. A lesser-known bioflavonoid, quercetin, suggests promise in treating varicose veins. You can now buy bioflavonoids as nutritional supplements.

AT-HOME REMEDIES

You can minimize the discomfort of varicose veins in your legs. To ease painful swelling and inflammation, rest frequently, wear support stockings, and take one or two ***aspirin*** or ***ibuprofen*** tablets daily until the condition clears. If you like to sit with your legs crossed, cross them at the ankles rather than the knees for better circulation. Better yet, take a break and put your feet up; periods of rest with your feet a few inches above your heart level let gravity work in your favor, helping pooled blood drain from your legs. To further improve circulation, women should avoid high heels in favor of flat shoes and should wear loose clothing.

PREVENTION

- Exercise regularly! Staying fit is the best way to keep your leg muscles toned, your blood flowing, and your weight under control.
- Eat foods low in fat, sugar, and salt. Drink plenty of water. Take supplements of ***vitamins C*** and ***E,*** both critical to blood-vessel health.
- If your daily routine requires you to be on your feet constantly, stretch and exercise your legs as often as possible to increase circulation and reduce pressure buildup.
- If you smoke, quit. Studies show that smoking may contribute to elevated blood pressure, which in turn can aggravate varicosity.
- If you're pregnant, be sure to sleep on your left side rather than on your back to minimize pressure from the uterus on the veins in your pelvic area. This position will also improve blood flow to the fetus. ■

SYMPTOMS

- Blurred vision when you are looking at distant objects indicates that you are **nearsighted,** or myopic.
- Blurred vision when you are looking at objects nearby indicates that you are **farsighted,** or hyperopic.
- Vertical or horizontal lines that appear blurry or irregular indicate **astigmatism.**
- Flashing-light sensations, tiny objects floating in your eyes, or a sudden loss of central or peripheral vision may indicate **retinal detachment.**
- Difficulty distinguishing between red and green in dim light is a sign that you are **color-blind.**
- Difficulty distinguishing objects in dim light is a sign of **night blindness.**

For symptoms of other vision ailments, see ***Cataracts, Eye Problems, Glaucoma,*** and ***Macular Degeneration.***

CALL YOUR DOCTOR IF:

- you experience symptoms of **retinal detachment;** you need immediate medical treatment to prevent potential blindness.
- you become unusually sensitive to bright light; you may have an inflamed iris.
- you have a foreign object in your eye that will not flush out with water; you risk scarring or infecting the eye.
- your contact lenses become uncomfortable; you may have an infection, abrasion, or foreign body in the eye.
- a cut or blow to your eye affects your vision; you may have internal bleeding or a fracture of the bone around your eye.

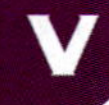

Your eyes are your body's most highly developed sensory organs. In fact, a far larger part of your brain is dedicated to the functions of eyesight than to those of hearing, taste, touch, or smell. We tend to take eyesight for granted, yet when vision problems develop, most of us will do everything in our power to restore our eyesight to normal.

The most common forms of vision impairment are errors of refraction—the way light rays are bent inside the eye so images can be transmitted to the brain. **Nearsightedness, farsightedness,** and **astigmatism** are examples of refraction disorders. **Retinal detachment, color blindness,** and **night blindness** are systemic disorders of the eye that lead to distorted or inaccurate vision. ***Cataracts, conjunctivitis, glaucoma,*** and ***macular degeneration*** are other diseases of the eye that respond in varying degrees to medical treatment.

CAUSES

Nearsightedness and **farsightedness** have to do with the way the eye brings images into focus on the back of the eyeball, where 10 layers of light-sensitive nerve tissue make up the retina. **Nearsightedness,** or myopia, which affects about 20 percent of the population, is the result of images being focused in front of the retina rather than on it *(right),* so distant objects appear blurred. A nearsighted person holds a book close to the eyes when reading and has to sit in the front of the classroom or movie theater to see clearly. The condition runs in families and affects men and women equally, usually appearing in childhood and stabilizing in the twenties.

Farsightedness, or hyperopia, is the opposite of nearsightedness: The lens of the eye focuses images slightly behind the retina, making nearby objects appear blurry. Children often overcome mild farsightedness through a natural process called accommodation: As the eye grows, the eye muscles contract, bringing the focal point forward onto the retina. With age, the eye's natural ability to accommodate tends to diminish.

Astigmatism, often associated with near- or farsightedness, occurs when the eye lacks a sin-

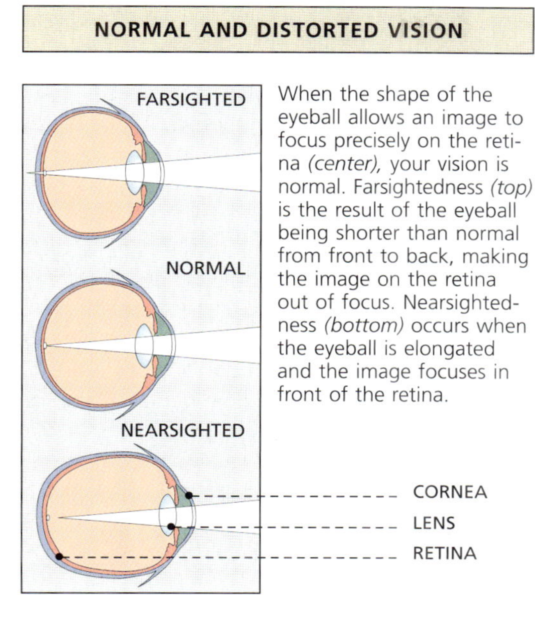

When the shape of the eyeball allows an image to focus precisely on the retina *(center),* your vision is normal. Farsightedness *(top)* is the result of the eyeball being shorter than normal from front to back, making the image on the retina out of focus. Nearsightedness *(bottom)* occurs when the eyeball is elongated and the image focuses in front of the retina.

gle point of focus. The condition is a result of an uneven curvature of the cornea or, in some cases, an abnormality in the lens. People with astigmatism have a random, inconsistent vision pattern, in which some objects appear clear and others blurry. Astigmatism is usually present from birth and neither improves nor worsens over time.

Presbyopia is blurred vision at normal reading distance. It typically starts at about age 40 and is the reason many older people use glasses.

Retinal detachment occurs when a part of a retinal layer is pulled out of place, or when a hole or tear occurs. Although a detached retina is not painful, it is definitely a medical emergency. If the retina is not reattached to its source of nutrients promptly, the cells die and blindness can result. Risk factors for the condition include nearsightedness, previous eye surgery or injury, and congenital thinness of retinal tissue.

Color blindness is a disorder of the retina's light-sensitive cone cells, which respond to colors. Most people with color blindness see colors normally in bright light but have difficulty distinguishing reds and greens in dim light. Color blindness occurs mostly in men, afflicting 8 percent of the male population. It is extremely rare for someone to be totally color-blind—that is, able to see only shades of gray.

Night blindness—difficulty seeing in dim light—occurs when the retina's rod cells, which distinguish light from dark, begin to deteriorate. The precise cause is unclear, but it may be linked to a liver disorder, a vitamin-A deficiency, or a disease of the retina, such as retinitis pigmentosa, an inherited disorder.

Eyestrain does not affect your vision, but it accompanies some vision disorders and may bring on a ***headache.*** It is often the result of eye muscles becoming strained from holding the same focus too long. If you wear prescriptive lenses, eyestrain may be an indication that you need new glasses or a different prescription. Eye exercises or resting the eyes every 30 minutes helps relieve eyestrain, especially if you work with computers.

DIAGNOSTIC AND TEST PROCEDURES

Annual eye examinations by your ophthalmologist are essential to monitor the health of your eyes and diagnose suspected disorders. Checking the external and internal portions of your eye and your eye's movement will reveal crossed eyes or other forms of strabismus *(see **Eye Problems**).*

A Snellen test employs letters of decreasing size to determine the sharpness of your vision and to detect nearsightedness, farsightedness, and astigmatism. An ophthalmologist will examine the cornea using a slitlamp microscope to detect signs of clouding in the lens of the eye, known as a ***cataract.*** Examinations with an ophthalmoscope can reveal abnormalities of the retina, macula, and optic nerve.

TREATMENT

If routine testing indicates that your vision is impaired, conventional treatment calls for wearing corrective glasses or contact lenses, practicing sensible eye care, and, in some cases, having corrective surgery. Almost 60 percent of the population wears corrective lenses, and that number in-

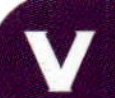

creases dramatically after the age of 65. A far smaller percentage ever need surgery for vision disorders, but those who do benefit from sophisticated, highly successful procedures.

CONVENTIONAL TREATMENT

Conventional treatment for disorders such as **nearsightedness, farsightedness,** and **astigmatism** depends primarily on corrective prescription lenses. Disorders such as ***cataracts, macular degeneration,*** and **retinal detachment** require surgical treatment.

To treat **nearsightedness** your ophthalmologist will usually prescribe lenses to focus visual images correctly on the retina. Normally you have a choice between wearing conventional eyeglasses and contact lenses. As an alternative to corrective lenses, or in severe cases, surgical techniques are used to treat nearsightedness. Radial keratotomy is a surgical procedure in which tiny, spokelike incisions are made in the cornea, flattening the center and focusing images correctly on the retina. Each eye is examined and operated on individually, and success is relatively good. More than three-quarters of those who have had the surgery report corrected or partially corrected vision. The procedure has potential complications, however: Vision may be erratic, the cornea may become infected, and there is some risk of the cornea's rupturing.

Excimer laser treatment may offer results similar to those of radial keratotomy. The laser beam removes microscopic amounts of tissue from the center of the cornea. This effectively flattens the cornea so that light rays focus correctly on the retina.

If **farsightedness** has not accommodated naturally and the disorder persists into adulthood, glasses or contact lenses can be prescribed, but they usually are not necessary until age 40 or older. People typically seek treatment for farsightedness when they begin to complain of eyestrain, especially at the end of the day.

For **astigmatism,** the accepted prescription is a lens that will correct or neutralize the effect of the uneven cornea. You will normally have a choice between glasses and contact lenses.

Some cases of **retinal detachment** can be corrected with laser surgery, which has a high rate of success. If the peeling or tearing of the retina is extensive, additional corrective surgery may be necessary.

ALTERNATIVE CHOICES

Alternative remedies rely on correcting mineral and vitamin deficiencies that may contribute to vision problems and on relieving the strain of overworked eyes. They can complement medical remedies prescribed by an ophthalmologist to treat your particular vision disorder.

ACUPRESSURE

Traditional Chinese relaxation therapy calls on the natural healing powers of your body to soothe overworked eyes, to ease headaches, and to relieve eyestrain from reading or working at a computer for extended periods.

If you are **nearsighted** or **farsighted,** or suffer from **astigmatism,** try the exercises Chinese children use to start the school day:

- Place both thumbs against the upper eye socket next to the bridge of your nose and knead vigorously.
- Pinch the bridge of your nose with your thumb and forefinger, then squeeze repeatedly.
- Using both forefingers, press and knead the bone under your eyes next to your nose.
- Place your forefingers on your temples at the side of your head behind your eyes and knead.

HERBAL THERAPIES

A daily 200-mg dose of ***bilberry*** *(Vaccinium myrtillus)* is reported to be useful for improving microcirculation, the flow of blood in the vessels of the eye, particularly for people with **night blindness** and **nearsightedness.**

HOMEOPATHY

If you develop **eyestrain** and your eyes are sore after a period of close work, the recommended over-the-counter remedy is ***Ruta*** in 12x potency, three or four times a day for two days.

NUTRITION AND DIET

To help strengthen the retina, people with **night blindness** can take up to 25,000 IU of ***vitamin A*** in fish liver oil daily. ***Zinc,*** which is found in high concentrations in oysters, may be helpful for night blindness. It is said to aid in adaptation to darkness and to strengthen the retina. ***Selenium, magnesium,*** and ***vitamin C*** supplements are antioxidants reported to prevent deterioration of the retina, especially in diabetics.

AT-HOME REMEDIES

When your eyes feel tired or overworked, take time to rest and reinvigorate them. Lie down in a dark room or sit quietly with your eyes covered. To soothe sore eyes and refresh puffy, red eyelids, try this old-fashioned remedy: Put a thick slice of fresh cucumber over each closed eyelid and relax for 15 to 30 minutes.

For itchy or irritated eyes, try a refreshing herbal eyewash. Steep 2 or 3 tsp of ***chamomile*** *(Matricaria recutita)* flowers or 2 tsp of dried ***eyebright*** *(Euphrasia officinalis)* in a pint of boiling water. Allow the brew to cool and strain out the residue. Put ½ tsp in an eyecup and rinse each eye several times a day.

PREVENTION

Resting your eyes when they are overworked is the first line of defense against vision problems. Eye exercises and a well-balanced, nutritious diet will help your eyes remain healthy and your vision acute.

Maintenance of your healthy eyesight depends on getting sufficient ***vitamin A,*** which plays a key role in the eye's ability to adjust to different degrees of light. To help prevent or postpone vision disorders, you should cut your consumption of refined sugar. If you smoke, stop. Do everything possible to stay away from tobacco smoke, exhaust fumes, and other kinds of polluted air. Finally, do not let yourself get overtired. When your body is rested, your circulation improves and your eyes get the supply of oxygenated blood they need.

COMMON MYTHS ABOUT YOUR EYES

Contrary to popular belief, the following activities may temporarily strain your eyes, but they will not impair your vision:

- *reading in poor light.*
- *reading without your glasses.*
- *wearing the wrong glasses.*
- *working at a computer for long periods of time.*
- *sitting close to a television screen or computer monitor.*

EYE EXERCISES TO RELIEVE EYESTRAIN

- When using a computer or doing concentrated activity such as sewing or reading, rest your eyes for 5 minutes at 30-minute intervals. Look away from your work; close your eyes and then gently massage them with your fingers.
- Blink regularly. This action helps prevent evaporation of the tear film that protects the cornea. Blinking also breaks the continuous focus when you have been reading or looking at a computer screen, increasing the amount of concentrated activity you can perform.
- If you are driving for long stretches, alternately focus on the dashboard and a faraway object. Changing the focus periodically will relax your eye muscles and prevent eyestrain.
- Palm your eyes. Sit comfortably, breathe deeply, and cover your eyes with the palms of your hands for 2 minutes.
- Breathe deeply for several minutes. Roll your head around with a circular motion while stretching your neck and shoulders, then turn your head from side to side and up and down, repeating several times.
- While yawning, stretch and maneuver the muscles of your face to relieve tension. ■

VITILIGO

SYMPTOMS

- White patches of skin are often located symmetrically on both sides of the body; borders of the irregularly shaped spots may be raised.
- Patches can appear at any time, though their appearance is often stress related.
- Patches are most common in exposed areas such as the face, neck, and hands but can emerge anywhere.
- Hair may gray and the whites of the eyes may change color.

CALL YOUR DOCTOR IF:

- the depigmentation is severe enough to affect your self-esteem and social activities; there are many treatments available that can offset the effects of vitiligo.

As many as two million people in the United States have this disease, which results in white patches on the skin. Sometimes the patches appear symmetrically; for example, you may have almost identical patterns on your right and left index fingers.

The first signs of pigment loss often appear before you reach age 20, and there may be cycles of rapid loss of color followed by little or no change. The dormancy period can last for years.

The progression of the disease varies. One patient might develop a few spots at first and then nothing more happens for years, while another might lose all skin pigmentation in six months. Emotional or physical stress can be contributing factors.

Vitiligo itself does not endanger your health, but it is sometimes associated with ***thyroid problems,*** pernicious ***anemia,*** Addison's disease (decreased adrenal gland function), and alopecia areata (patches of ***hair loss***). For most patients, however, the greatest risk is loss of self-esteem.

CAUSES

Doctors don't know what causes vitiligo, though the disease does tend to run in families; up to a third of all patients have a relative who also suffers from the condition. Chemical agents such as phenol (often used as a disinfectant) and catechol (used in dyeing and tanning), as well as emotional and physical stress, may precipitate the onset of vitiligo.

The underlying problem is that cells called melanocytes cease producing melanin, which gives skin its color. There are three prominent theories on why this happens in vitiligo patients: Abnormal nerve cells might injure nearby pigment cells; the body might be destroying its own tissue (an autoimmune response) because it perceives the pigment cells as foreign; or pigment-producing cells might self-destruct (autotoxic response), leaving a toxic residue that destroys new pigment cells. Whatever the cause, the problem is never life-threatening and rarely even a health risk.

TREATMENT

Most treatments for vitiligo involve drawing more pigmented cells to the skin's surface. A therapy known as psoralen ultraviolet A (PUVA), which combines an oral drug and ultraviolet light, has proved particularly effective, especially for patients in advanced stages of the disease.

Alternative medicine has little to offer for vitiligo patients, since the only way to influence the progression of the disease is to alter the body's production of melanin or to transplant healthier cells to the affected areas. Certain relaxation techniques, however, may prove helpful if you find that stress triggers episodes of depigmentation.

CONVENTIONAL MEDICINE

There are two basic approaches to treating vitiligo: trying to restore normal pigment, or depigmenting the rest of the skin—which makes the skin very pale but uniform in color. For mild forms of the disease doctors usually start with topical ***corticosteroids,*** which have a good record of restoring small patches. In instances where vitiligo has affected more than 20 percent of the body's surface, PUVA treatments are commonly prescribed. At least half of all vitiligo patients regain pigment in most areas with these treatments.

Researchers continue to hunt for alternatives to PUVA therapy because of its many side effects, including liver damage, ***cataracts*** and other ***eye problems,*** a phototoxic reaction that causes skin blistering, and ***nausea.*** Khellin, derived from the roots of the *Ammi visnaga* plant, has proved to be an effective substitute. It does not induce phototoxicity, though at high doses it can cause nausea, ***dizziness, insomnia,*** and an increase in liver enzyme levels.

If vitiligo has created patches on more than half of your skin, you might consider having the remaining color removed—a process known as depigmentation. Before you take this step, however, consider that it can take months to years to complete and is irreversible. The drug of choice, a combination of monobenzone and hydroquinone, destroys melanocytes. Potential side effects include contact ***dermatitis,*** severe itching, abnormally dry skin, pigment deposits in the cornea, and graying hair.

RECOGNIZING VITILIGO

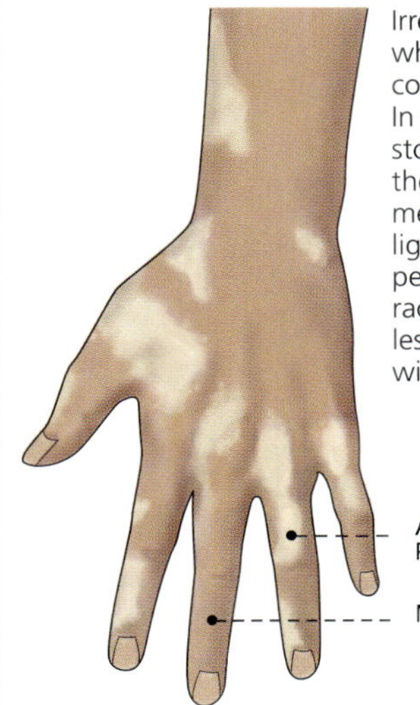

Irregular patches of stark white skin against normal coloration signals vitiligo. In this disorder, the body stops producing melanin, the substance that pigments the skin of both light- and dark-skinned people. Vitiligo has no racial preferences, but it is less noticeable in people with light skin.

ALTERNATIVE CHOICES

Homeopathic therapy is probably the best alternative for vitiligo patients who want to avoid potent conventional medicines. Consult a professional about a homeopathic treatment plan.

To reduce the stress that can aggravate vitiligo, try **mind/body** relaxation techniques such as **guided imagery, yoga,** or **hypnotherapy.**

AT-HOME REMEDIES

To properly treat vitiligo you must see a doctor. One step you can take at home that might help is to expose patches of affected skin to the sun (while protecting healthy skin with a sunscreen). The ultraviolet radiation from the sun may promote repigmentation. ■

VOMITING

Read down this column to find your symptoms. Then read across.

SYMPTOMS	AILMENT/PROBLEM
For other conditions that may involve vomiting, see also ***Nausea.***	
◆ vomiting that appears to be brought on by a specific situation, such as a long car trip or a stressful encounter.	◆ ***Motion sickness; anxiety***
◆ small amounts of vomiting; burning chest pain (heartburn); difficulty swallowing; shortness of breath.	◆ ***Hiatal hernia***
◆ vomiting, headache, nausea; symptoms may be worse with exposure to bright light.	◆ Migraine ***headache;*** possibly ***meningitis***
◆ vomiting preceded by intense dizziness, to the extent that everything around you appears to spin; possibly, ringing in your ears.	◆ Inner ear disorder; possibly ***Ménière's disease***
◆ diarrhea, vomiting, nausea, and fever lasting 48 hours or less, sometimes after you eat rich, spicy, or possibly spoiled foods, drink an excessive amount of alcohol, or ingest a drug you have never taken before.	◆ ***Gastroenteritis*** (also called stomach flu or intestinal flu)
◆ vomiting accompanied by fever, lower abdominal pain, and frequent, malodorous, and/or painful urination.	◆ ***Kidney infection***
◆ recurrent vomiting accompanied by yellowish skin and/or whites of eyes.	◆ ***Jaundice***

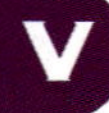

WHAT TO DO	OTHER INFO
◆ For motion sickness, ask your doctor about preventive treatment such as ***antinausea drugs*** that you can take before you travel. For anxiety, find a relaxation technique—such as yoga—that you're comfortable with and will practice regularly. See also ***Stress.***	◆ ***Ginger*** *(Zingiber officinale)* capsules may alleviate motion sickness, as may acupressure.
◆ See your doctor for an accurate diagnosis. Over-the-counter ***antacids*** are often the first line of defense against ***heartburn;*** avoiding stomach irritants such as alcohol, tobacco, and caffeine can also help.	◆ A maneuver known as the stomach pull, performed by naturopathic physicians and osteopaths, may treat hiatal hernias.
◆ If you suspect meningitis, **call 911 or your emergency number now.** Migraines may respond to various ***analgesics*** (over-the-counter and prescription varieties).	◆ While meningitis requires emergency medical treatment, symptoms of migraine headache may be relieved by a variety of alternative choices. Herbalists often recommend taking a daily 125-mg capsule of ***feverfew*** *(Chrysanthemum parthenium)* to prevent migraines.
◆ See your doctor. You may need ***antibiotics*** to clear up an ear infection.	
◆ Rest, drink plenty of fluids, and eat bland foods. You may need an ***antibiotic*** if your stomach bug is the result of a bacterial infection.	◆ Take care not to let vomiting persist, or your body will lose important fluids and become dehydrated. To prevent dehydration, drink room-temperature beverages such as water, fruit juice, or soda that has been allowed to go flat.
◆ Call your doctor today. You may need prescription ***antibiotics*** to treat the infection.	◆ If you are prone to kidney infections, drinking cranberry juice daily may keep them at bay. Cranberry capsules are also available.
◆ Call your doctor. There are many possible causes of jaundice, and some are serious.	◆ If your skin is yellow but the whites of your eyes are still white, you likely have carotenemia, not jaundice. Carotenemia is a harmless effect of high levels of the pigment carotene in the body and can be brought on by a diet rich in leafy green vegetables, carrots, and oranges.

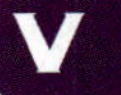

SYMPTOMS	AILMENT/PROBLEM
◆ vomiting accompanied by severe pain in or around one eye.	◆ ***Glaucoma***
◆ vomiting, fever, headache, nausea; unusual sleepiness and/or confusion; possibly, staggered walk.	◆ ***Meningitis;*** encephalitis (inflammation of the brain, usually caused by a virus transmitted by mosquitoes); Reye's syndrome (a neurological disorder typically seen in children, which may occur after ***aspirin*** has been given for an infection or ***chickenpox***)
◆ nausea and vomiting; whitish bowel movements; dark urine.	◆ ***Hepatitis***
◆ intense, recurrent abdominal pain that is not relieved by vomiting; loss of appetite.	◆ ***Appendicitis; stomach ulcer;*** possibly ***stomach cancer***
◆ vomit that smells like feces, accompanied by constipation.	◆ Intestinal obstruction (the intestines are blocked); possibly, ***colorectal cancer***
◆ headache, vomiting, drowsiness, confusion and/or aberrant behavior.	◆ Possibly, ***brain cancer*** or an ***aneurysm***
◆ severe headache that occurs several hours or days after a head injury; nausea and possibly vomiting; drowsiness, confusion; dilation of one or both pupils.	◆ Concussion (neurological problems caused by head trauma); severe cases may also include bleeding within the skull
◆ vomit containing blood or material that looks like coffee grounds.	◆ Internal bleeding, possibly from a ***stomach ulcer, stomach cancer,*** or ***throat cancer***
◆ You are—or may be—in the first three months of pregnancy, and have vomited on several days of the past week or more.	◆ Normal effects (sometimes called morning sickness, though it can occur any time of day) often felt during the first three months of pregnancy

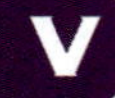

WHAT TO DO	OTHER INFO
◆ Call your doctor today. Depending on the type of glaucoma, you may need ***beta-adrenergic blockers*** to reduce eye pressure or surgery to help the eye drain fluid.	◆ Blindness may occur in as little as three to five days with some types of glaucoma. Early, fast treatment is essential.
◆ **Call 911 or your emergency number now.** Each of these illnesses is serious; Reye's syndrome in particular escalates quickly and can be fatal.	◆ To avoid Reye's syndrome, never give ***aspirin*** to a child with fever; use ***acetaminophen*** instead.
◆ **Call 911 or your emergency number now.** You may need emergency care.	◆ Improved nutrition and a specific diet may help in recovery.
◆ **Call your doctor now.** An accurate diagnosis is essential. Appendicitis requires immediate surgery.	◆ In the United States, 1 in 15 people gets appendicitis. It is most common between ages 10 and 30.
◆ **Call 911 or your emergency number now.** Intestinal obstruction can be fatal within hours if left untreated. Successful treatment of colorectal cancer depends on an early and accurate diagnosis.	◆ Scar tissue from a previous surgery is the most frequent cause of intestinal obstruction.
◆ **Call 911 or your emergency number now;** these are serious conditions that may require immediate surgery.	
◆ **Call 911 or your emergency number now.** Although a mild concussion may not require medical treatment, there is no way to tell if bleeding is occurring. Bleeding within the skull is a medical emergency.	◆ Prevent head trauma whenever you can by using seat belts in vehicles and wearing helmets for sports such as bicycling, in-line skating, and ice skating.
◆ **Call 911 or your emergency number now.** Internal bleeding calls for prompt intervention, as well as a follow-up evaluation to determine its cause.	
◆ Try not to let your stomach become empty, which seems to make morning sickness worse. Eat soda crackers or other breads frequently to prevent nausea or to calm existing nausea. See ***Pregnancy Problems.***	◆ ***Vitamin*** $\boldsymbol{B_6}$ may help combat morning sickness, but consult with your doctor before trying any supplements, medications, or therapies.

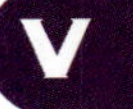

WARTS

SYMPTOMS

- Common warts are small, hard, rough lumps that are round and elevated; they usually appear on hands and fingers and may be flesh-colored, white, pink, or granulated.
- Digitate warts are horny and fingerlike, with pea-shaped bases; they appear on the scalp or near the hairline.
- Filiform warts are thin and threadlike; they commonly appear on the face and neck.
- Flat warts appear in groups of up to several hundred, usually on the face, neck, chest, knees, hands, wrists, or forearms; they are slightly raised and have smooth, flat, or rounded tops.
- Periungual warts are rough, irregular, and elevated; they appear at the edges of fingernails and toenails and may extend under the nails, causing pain.

See also ***Genital Warts*** and ***Plantar Warts*** and the ***Visual Diagnostic Guide.***

CALL YOUR DOCTOR IF:

- over-the-counter remedies don't work.
- you are a woman and develop ***genital warts,*** which in rare cases may indicate ***cervical cancer.***
- you are older than 45 and discover what looks like a wart; it may instead be a symptom of a more serious skin condition, such as ***skin cancer.***
- warts multiply and spread, causing embarrassment or discomfort.
- you notice a change in a wart's color or size; this could indicate ***skin cancer.***

After acne, warts are the most common dermatological complaint. Three out of four people will develop a wart (verruca vulgaris) at some time in their lives. Warts are slightly contagious, and you can spread them to other parts of your body by touching them or shaving around infected areas. Children and young adults are more prone to getting warts because their defense mechanisms may not be fully developed, but it is possible to get a wart at any age.

CAUSES

Warts are caused by the human papilloma virus (HPV), which enters the skin through a cut or scratch and causes cells to multiply rapidly. Usually, warts spread through direct contact, but it is possible to pick up the virus in moist environments, such as showers and locker rooms.

DIAGNOSTIC AND TEST PROCEDURES

In most cases you don't need to undergo tests for other conditions if you develop a wart. But if you're over 45, your doctor may want to examine the growth, possibly after removing it, to ensure that it is benign.

TREATMENT

Nearly every doctor says that the best treatment for warts is no treatment at all. Most people develop an immune response that causes warts to go away by themselves. One-fifth of all warts disappear within six months, and two-thirds are gone within two years. However, if your wart doesn't disappear, or if it's unsightly or uncomfortable, you can try self-treatment or seek help from your doctor.

CONVENTIONAL MEDICINE

If you decide to treat your own wart, your first-choice remedy should be an over-the-counter medication in liquid, gel, pad, or ointment form. Most of these contain salicylic acid, the main constituent of ***aspirin,*** which softens abnormal skin cells and dissolves them.

First, soak the wart in warm water for five minutes to help the medication penetrate the skin. Then gently rub off dead skin cells with a washcloth or pumice stone. Before applying the medicine, coat the area around the wart with petroleum jelly to keep the medicine away from healthy or sensitive skin.

If over-the-counter treatment fails, your doctor can remove a wart by:

- freezing it with liquid nitrogen.
- burning it off with electricity or a laser.
- excising it (a minor surgical procedure).
- dissolving it by wrapping it in a plaster patch impregnated with salicylic acid.

Any of these treatments can cause scarring, so instead you may want to ask your doctor about a prescription patch that clears up warts by delivering a continuous dose of medication.

ALTERNATIVE CHOICES

CHINESE HERBS

A doctor of Chinese medicine may place a slice of ***ginger*** *(Zingiber officinale)* root on top of the wart and cover it with smoldering ***mugwort*** *(Artemisia).* The burning herb enables the ginger to release its antiviral constituents. This process is called indirect moxibustion.

HERBAL THERAPIES

Several herbs contain chemicals thought to fight viruses and help treat skin conditions. Herbalists recommend applying the sticky juices of ***dandelion*** *(Taraxacum officinale),* milkweed *(Asclepias syriaca),* and celandine *(Chelidonium majus).* An ointment of thuja *(Thuja occidentalis)* applied four or five times a day may also help.

HOMEOPATHY

Homeopathic medicines for warts include *Causticum, Nitric acid,* and *Antimonium crudum.*

NUTRITION AND DIET

To strengthen your immune system, eat dark green and yellow vegetables, which contain ***vitamin A,*** as well as onions, ***garlic,*** Brussels sprouts, cabbage, and broccoli, which contain ***sulfur.*** Supplements to help fight off warts include beta carotene, L-cysteine, ***zinc,*** and ***vitamins B complex, C,*** and ***E.***

AT-HOME REMEDIES

There are countless folk cures for warts. One that may have some validity is rubbing the wart with a slice of raw potato or the inner side of a banana skin; both contain chemicals that may dissolve the wart. You might also try any of the following applications:

- ***vitamins A*** and ***E,*** which are generally good for skin conditions.
- a paste of crushed ***vitamin C*** tablets and water.
- over-the-counter medicines or a paste of crushed ***aspirin;*** both contain wart-dissolving salicylic acid.
- ***aloe*** *(Aloe barbadensis),* ***dandelion,*** or milkweed juices.
- cotton soaked in fresh pineapple juice, which contains a dissolving enzyme.

PREVENTION

Practice good hygiene, and eat balanced meals high in vitamins A, C, and E to boost your immune system. Avoid stress, which can compromise your immunity, and learn to relax.

CAUTION!

Be sure your growth is a wart. It could be any of several benign skin growths, such as a mole or a *corn or callus,* but there is also a chance it could be a form of *skin cancer.* Warts are usually pale, skin-colored growths with a rough surface. If your growth doesn't look like this, play it safe and see a doctor. Also check with your doctor if a wart's appearance changes. ■

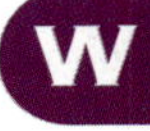

WHEEZING

SYMPTOMS

- a whistling sound and labored breathing, particularly when exhaling; sometimes accompanied by a mild feeling of tightening in the chest.

CALL YOUR DOCTOR IF:

- wheezing is accompanied by a fever of 101°F or above. You may have an upper-respiratory infection such as acute ***bronchitis.***
- breathing is so difficult that you feel that you are suffocating. This is either a sign of a severe ***asthma*** episode or an allergic reaction *(see **Allergies**)*; **get emergency medical help immediately.**
- you wheeze most days and cough up greenish or gray phlegm. You may have chronic ***bronchitis*** or ***emphysema.***
- you begin wheezing suddenly and cough up frothy pink or white phlegm. This may be a sign of ***heart disease;* get emergency medical help immediately.**

Many people with respiratory ***allergies*** know that bouts of wheezing almost always come with the arrival of ***hay fever*** season. Mild wheezing may also accompany respiratory infections such as acute ***bronchitis*** or ***emphysema.*** But the characteristic whistling sound of wheezing is the primary symptom of the chronic respiratory disease ***asthma.***

A variety of conventional and alternative remedies can alleviate wheezing. However, you should be regularly monitored by a conventional doctor if you have asthma, severe allergies, chronic bronchitis, or emphysema.

CAUSES

The whistling sound that characterizes wheezing occurs when you attempt to breathe deeply through bronchial passages that are constricted or excreting excess mucus due to allergy, infection, or other irritation. With your lungs' airways partially blocked, your bronchial muscles may tighten because of increasing anxiety. This makes the wheezing worse, because it is more difficult for you to exhale completely.

In some people, wheezing is the result of asthma or allergic reactions to pollen, chemicals, pet dander, dust, foods, or insect stings. People with acute bronchitis also produce excess mucus in the respiratory tract, which can cause the lungs' passageways to become blocked. People with these respiratory diseases may also be more vulnerable to developing allergies. Wheezing may also be caused by cystic fibrosis or obstruction from a foreign body.

DIAGNOSTIC AND TEST PROCEDURES

To determine the cause of your wheezing, your physician will ask you questions to determine if you have allergies. For example, if you have no history of lung disease and you always wheeze after eating a certain food or at a certain time of year, your doctor may suspect that you have a

YOGA

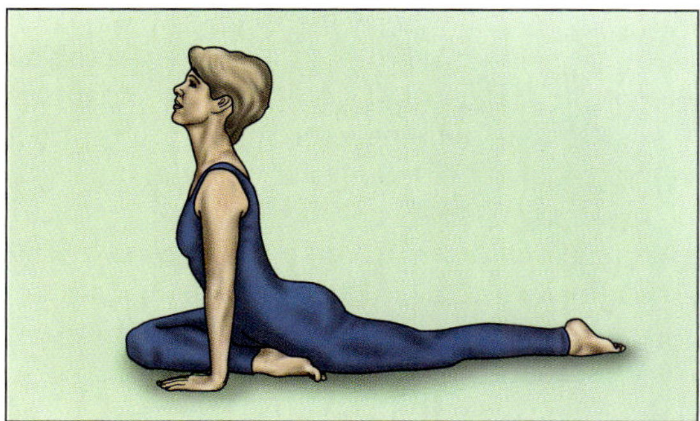

The **Pigeon** may enhance breathing. From a kneeling position, slide your left leg straight behind you. Take a deep breath and stretch up through your torso while arching your back slightly. Hold the position for 20 or 30 seconds, breathing deeply. Exhale and relax. Repeat with the other leg.

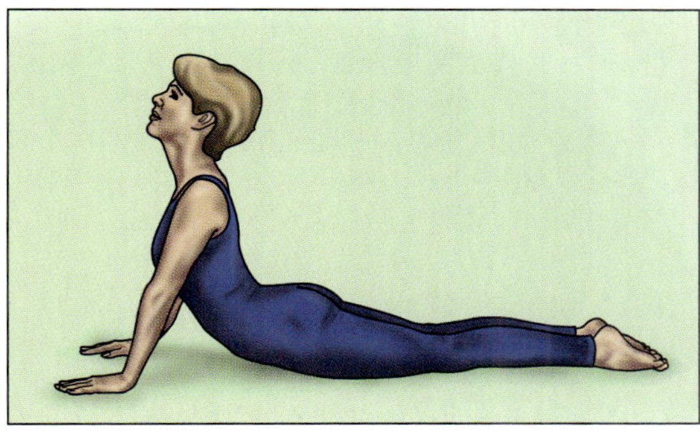

To ease wheezing spasms, try the **Cobra.** Place both hands on the floor, directly under your shoulders, elbows against your body. Inhale and push your chest upward, straightening your arms while pressing your pelvis against the ground *(above).* Hold for 20 seconds, breathing deeply, then slowly relax.

food or respiratory allergy. There are a variety of tests your doctor may use to determine the exact nature of your allergy, including skin tests and blood tests. Your doctor may also administer a pulmonary function test to evaluate the volume of air moving through your bronchial passages. If your wheezing appears related to chronic bronchitis or emphysema, your doctor may also want to take x-rays.

TREATMENT

You must see a conventional medical doctor to determine the cause of your wheezing and receive treatment for it. Alternative therapies, however, can help ease discomfort.

CONVENTIONAL MEDICINE

If your wheezing is caused by ***asthma,*** your doctor will probably prescribe ***bronchodilators,*** drugs that help dilate the constricted airways. If you have ***allergies,*** your doctor will almost certainly prescribe ***antihistamines,*** drugs that counteract the allergy-producing chemicals in your body. If you have acute ***bronchitis,*** your doctor will probably prescribe an ***antibiotic*** to clear up your respiratory infection; generally, any mild wheezing that accompanies acute bronchitis disappears when the infection does. In cases of chronic bronchitis or ***emphysema,*** your doctor may prescribe an ***expectorant,*** to clear excess mucus, or a ***bronchodilator.*** In emergencies, when wheezing is so severe that it is difficult or impossible for you to breathe, a medical team may administer a shot of ***epinephrine*** to open clogged respiratory passages.

ALTERNATIVE CHOICES

Many alternative therapies for asthma may be effective for wheezing. See ***Asthma*** for specific suggestions, including **Chinese medicine, reflexology,** and **herbal therapies.** But remember: If you have asthma, serious allergies, chronic bronchitis, or emphysema, you need to be monitored regularly by a conventional physician.

YOGA

Several postures may help relieve wheezing by teaching you how to control your breathing and release stress. Particularly effective positions include the Pigeon, Cobra, Sphinx, and Bridge. See the illustrations at left. *(See also the **Appendix** for more information on yoga positions.)* ■

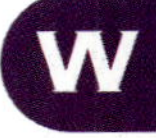

WHOOPING COUGH

SYMPTOMS

- in the early stage, a runny nose, a persistent cough, and sometimes a low-grade fever.
- after 7 to 14 days, severe spasms of coughing, in which each cough is followed by a high-pitched whooping sound as the person forces air over a swollen larynx (voice box). Young babies are often too weak to make the whooping sound.
- sometimes, vomiting after coughing episodes.
- particularly in infants under two months, interrupted breathing (apnea), during which the infant's lips may turn blue from lack of oxygen.

CALL YOUR DOCTOR IF:

- your child has not been vaccinated against whooping cough and has recently been exposed to the illness.
- you suspect your child has whooping cough, especially if the child has a cold and cough that have lasted a week or more.
- your child's lips turn blue and your child experiences periods of breathing poorly, an indication of severe respiratory distress. **Seek emergency medical care immediately.**
- your child still seems unwell with a persistent cough and fever after the whooping cough spells have cleared up; the child may have developed a secondary respiratory infection, such as ***pneumonia*** or ***bronchitis.***

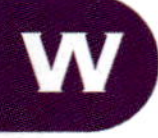

Whooping cough, a highly contagious respiratory infection, is considered one of the most serious of traditional childhood diseases. Most states require children to be vaccinated against it. If untreated, it can cause lung damage and recurrent bronchial infections; in infants, it can lead to brain damage and even death. It is most often associated with very young children, but teenagers and adults can also become infected, though usually much less seriously. Fortunately, it has become uncommon in the U.S. because of the widespread immunization of children.

The first symptoms—usually a runny nose, dry cough, and mild fever—begin about 7 to 10 days after exposure. After another week, the characteristic cough may develop: violent spasms of coughing followed by a high-pitched whooping sound, though in babies this sound is often muted. The person may cough up copious amounts of thick saliva, and vomiting is common. This coughing phase usually lasts up to 6 weeks; during this time patients are susceptible to secondary infections that can be quite serious. The last phase is a recovery period of up to a month, during which the patient regains strength.

CAUSES

Whooping cough is caused by the *Bordetella pertussis* bacterium. It is spread by airborne droplets from a cough or sneeze or through contact with contaminated sheets or clothing.

TREATMENT

Whooping cough requires prompt medical treatment; delay can lead to serious complications, particularly in children.

CONVENTIONAL MEDICINE

A pediatrician will probably prescribe ***erythromycin,*** an ***antibiotic*** that can be effective in reducing the length and severity of the infection, especially if started in the first 10 days of illness. ***Codeine*** may be prescribed to relieve coughing.

In severe cases or if your child is under a year old, hospitalization may be required to prevent dehydration and to permit quick administration of oxygen should the patient have difficulty breathing.

ALTERNATIVE CHOICES

Alternative therapies, which are primarily aimed at relieving the cough, should be used only in conjunction with conventional medicine.

ACUPRESSURE

To relieve a severe cough, try pressing Bladder points 43, 12, or 13. See pages 22-23 and the ***Appendix*** for information on point locations.

HERBAL THERAPIES

For cough relief, try wild black cherry *(Prunus serotina)* bark syrup, a favorite remedy with children. Other herbs that might help relieve the cough include sundew *(Drosera rotundifolia),* thyme *(Thymus vulgaris), and* ***mullein*** *(Verbascum thapsus).* Consult a medical herbalist for dosages.

HOMEOPATHY

Homeopathic remedies can help supplement conventional care. See a trained practitioner, whose remedies may include *Carbo vegetabilis, Drosera,* or *Coccus cacti.*

OSTEOPATHY

Manipulation of the spinal segments of the chest and ribs may encourage lymphatic drainage and reduce the severity of the cough.

AT-HOME CARE

- To help ease coughing spasms, have your child sit up and lean forward. Keep a bowl nearby to catch any phlegm that may be coughed up.
- If your child is vomiting, try feeding him immediately afterward, when it may be easier to keep food down.
- Increase liquids to offset dehydration and to thin mucus.
- To aid your child's breathing, use a cool-mist humidifier. Direct the mist away from your child and change any clothes or bedding that becomes damp. Use a humidifier with a humidistat, which keeps the air from becoming too humid, and make sure both the water and the humidifier stay clean to prevent mold and other germs from growing.
- Keep your child away from cigarette smoke, which can aggravate respiratory distress.

C A U T I O N !

If your child is producing a lot of mucus, don't give him cough suppressants. Such medications will prevent him from effectively expelling mucus from a blocked airway.

PREVENTION

The DPT (diphtheria, pertussis, and tetanus) vaccine is given in five doses between the ages of two months and six years. The vaccine has been shown to be 90 percent effective when the child receives all five doses; however, it does not provide permanent immunity. Five years after the final dose, a previously immunized child is no longer protected. Reimmunization is not recommended, however, because the vaccine can trigger severe side effects in older children and adults. Because some family members may no longer be immune to the illness, doctors often recommend that others in the family take a 10-day preventive course of ***erythromycin*** when a child comes down with whooping cough.

Minor reactions to the DPT vaccine—mild fever, fretfulness, and drowsiness—are common. But if your child develops a very high fever, persistent crying, or convulsions, he may be having a severe reaction to the vaccine. **Seek emergency medical care immediately.** Fortunately, such reactions are very rare. Most medical experts believe that the risks of whooping cough far exceed the risks of the vaccine. ■

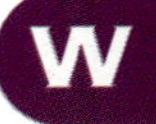

SYMPTOMS

- Severe anal itching especially at night, restlessness, and difficulty sleeping may indicate **pinworms.**
- Itching on the soles of your feet suggests **hookworms;** in some cases this may be accompanied by a rash, coughing bloody sputum, and fever, followed by loss of appetite, diarrhea, palpitations, anemia, and fatigue.
- Nausea, diarrhea, abdominal pain, dizziness, changes in appetite, and fatigue indicate a **large tapeworm**—probably originating in beef, pork, or fish.
- Loss of appetite and weight, irritability, diarrhea, abdominal pain, and vomiting are symptoms of **small tapeworms**—originating in a rodent or dog.
- Diarrhea and cramping that last up to a week, followed by fever, muscle pain, conjunctivitis, and facial swelling around the eyes are signs of **trichinosis.**
- Wheezing, coughing, or other breathing difficulties, followed by vomiting, stomach pain, and bloating, suggest **ascariasis.**
- Small red lesions that may itch—followed by coughing, wheezing, or bronchitis; diarrhea; abdominal pain; and flatulence—are signs of **threadworms.**

CALL YOUR DOCTOR IF:

- you experience any combination of the listed symptoms; you need a medical diagnosis for the possibility of worms.

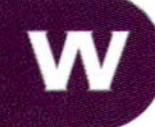

Parasitic **roundworms** and **tapeworms** that infest humans come from unsanitary living conditions and poor food preparation. They range in size from half-inch pinworms to tapeworms more than 30 feet long. Of the roundworms, **pinworms** and **ascarids** (the worms that cause **ascariasis**) are the most common parasites affecting children in the United States. **Trichinosis** is a disease caused by a microscopic roundworm; if not treated, the worm larvae can cause muscle damage and cardiac or neurological complications. **Hookworms** are roundworms that live on blood, glucose, and oxygen they suck from the intestinal wall, often causing ***anemia.*** Like **hookworms, threadworms** can spread to the lungs and cause chronic coughing; both types often infest people sharing living quarters, as in prisons or mental institutions.

The several types of **tapeworms** that infest humans are generally not harmful unless they penetrate the intestinal wall and move to another part of the body. Any worm infestation can lead to respiratory or cardiovascular complications, but most are easily treated and cause no lasting harm.

CAUSES

Most **roundworms** share a similar life cycle inside the body, but their methods of infestation differ. **Pinworms** live in people's lower intestinal tracts. The female worm leaves the anus to deposit eggs in the anal area at night. This produces an irritating itch that—when scratched—transfers the eggs to the host's fingers; the eggs can thus spread by touch through an entire household. If inadvertently eaten, the eggs hatch in the intestines and the cycle continues. The roundworm that causes **ascariasis** can enter the body in unwashed or raw food contaminated with the worm's eggs; it may also be picked up from soil that contains the eggs. **Hookworms** and **threadworms** enter the body in contaminated drinking water or through bare feet. The larvae migrate to the small intestine, where they may live for several years, taking nutrients from the intestinal walls. Their eggs are excreted in feces; if the infested feces contaminate soil, the cycle is repeated. You can contract the roundworm that causes **trichinosis** by eating raw or undercooked pork or game, which may contain living worm larvae encased in cysts. After digestive juices dissolve the cysts, the larvae circulate through the blood and the lymphatic system before digging into muscle and forming a cyst with new larvae.

Tapeworms also enter the body in raw or undercooked beef, fish, or pork. In rare cases, children may swallow tapeworm-infested fleas or lice that live on vermin or household pets.

DIAGNOSTIC AND TEST PROCEDURES

A physician may diagnose **pinworms** by using a piece of sticky tape to pick up any eggs that may be around the anal area; the tape is then checked under a microscope. The worm itself is sometimes visible in stool samples or around the anus. **Roundworms, hookworms, threadworms,** and **tapeworms** can be diagnosed from stool samples as well, and sometimes tapeworm segments are found in bedding or clothes. To diagnose **trichinosis,** a physician will test samples of blood or muscle tissue.

TREATMENT

CONVENTIONAL MEDICINE

Most worms respond to medicines specific to the type of worm. **Hookworms** and **threadworms** are treated with pyrantel or mebendazole. Doctors usually treat **pinworms** with three oral doses of mebendazole, two weeks apart. Since the eggs can spread, everyone in the household must be treated. Washing all bed linens and clothing is essential to eradicate all pinworm eggs. You can relieve itching in the anal area with petroleum jelly.

Most cases of **trichinosis** are mild and do not need medication; if symptoms are severe, the medicine of choice is mebendazole. Trichinosis that spreads to the respiratory, cardiovascular, or central nervous system is rare and is treated with ***corticosteroids*** to fight inflammation.

After you have completed a course of treatment, have your doctor repeat the diagnostic tests to make sure the worms are gone. If not, another course of treatment may be necessary. **Tapeworms** may not clear your system for up to five months.

ALTERNATIVE CHOICES

Once you have seen a doctor for an accurate diagnosis, alternative treatments can be used to flush worms from your system.

HERBAL THERAPIES

Check with a licensed herbalist about using these herbs, since they can be toxic:

- For **pinworms** and **roundworms**, steep 1 or 2 tsp wormwood *(Artemisia absinthium)* in a cup of boiling water for 10 to 15 minutes; drink three times daily. Over-the-counter tinctures of wormwood and ***black walnut*** *(Juglans nigra)* are also recommended; follow dosages on the labels.
- For **roundworms** and **threadworms,** steep 1 tsp dried tansy *(Tanacetum vulgare)* or 2 tsp dried balmony *(Chelone glabra)* in a cup of boiling water for 10 to 15 minutes; drink three times daily. Avoid tansy if you are pregnant.

NUTRITION AND DIET

Pineapple, papaya juice, and pumpkin seeds are all said to be tough on worms. Try over-the-counter grapefruit-seed extract to flush worms out of your intestines; follow dosage directions on the label.

PREVENTION

- Make sure children always wash their hands after going to the bathroom and before eating.
- Keep fingernails short to reduce the chances of picking up **pinworm** eggs underneath them.
- Have all your four-legged pets checked and treated for worms in the spring and fall.
- Avoid **trichinosis** by thoroughly cooking pork.
- Wash thoroughly in hot, soapy water tools and utensils that come in contact with raw meat.
- Always wear shoes in areas where **hookworms** and **threadworms** may live in the soil, particularly in the southeastern U.S. ■

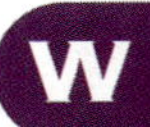

YEAST INFECTIONS

SYMPTOMS

- painless white patches in your mouth or throat that may come off when you eat or brush your teeth; this indicates **oral thrush,** most common in infants, the elderly, and ***AIDS*** patients.
- white patches in the mouth and throat, sometimes associated with painful swallowing; these are symptomatic of **esophageal thrush,** a potential complication of ***AIDS.***
- peeling skin on the hands, especially between the fingers, and swollen nail folds above the cuticle; possibly painful, red, and containing pus.
- itchy or burning shiny, pink rash with a scaly or blistered edge in the folds of the skin. This indicates **intertrigo.**
- in women, vaginal itching and irritation; redness and swelling of the vulva; unusually thick, white discharge; and pain during intercourse. These are signs of a **vaginal yeast infection,** also known as **moniliasis.**
- in men, red patches and blisters at the end of the penis and around the foreskin, possibly accompanied by severe itching and pain. These are symptoms of **balanitis.**

CALL YOUR DOCTOR IF:

- you have any of the symptoms for the first time; you need a professional evaluation before beginning treatment.
- the infection does not respond to treatment or recurs; you may have a more serious disorder such as ***diabetes*** or an HIV infection.

Yeast, or fungal, infection—sometimes called **candidiasis**—takes many forms. Yeast infections often develop where a moist environment encourages fungal growth, especially on the webs of fingers and toes, nails, genitals, and folds of skin. *(See **Athlete's Foot.**)* **Oral thrush** is a painless, often recurrent infection of the mouth and throat; it is common in babies, young children, and the elderly, but can affect all ages. **Moniliasis** is a painful vaginal yeast infection experienced by many women, most commonly during pregnancy or treatment with ***antibiotics.*** *(See **Vaginal Problems.**)* **Balanitis** is a less common but equally irritating infection of the penis. *(See **Penile Pain.**)* **Systemic yeast infections** can occur in cases of ***diabetes, AIDS,*** and other ailments or drug treatments that suppress the immune system.

CAUSES

Candida albicans is a fungal organism, or yeast, that thrives in your mouth, gastrointestinal tract, and skin; your body produces bacterial flora that keeps it in check. When fungal growth exceeds the body's ability to control it, yeast infection develops. This can happen when you are weakened by illness or upset by ***stress.*** Modern ***antibiotics*** that treat many ailments can actually kill the bacteria that otherwise control fungal outbreaks.

Yeast infections are common among dishwashers and people whose hands are often in water, in children who suck their thumbs or fingers, and in people whose clothing retains body moisture. The ***diaper rash*** called **candidal dermatitis** is caused by yeast growth in the folds of a baby's skin. Diabetics are especially prone to yeast infections because they have high levels of sugar in their blood and urine and a low resistance to infection—conditions that encourage yeast growth. In rare cases the candida fungus may invade the bloodstream through an intravenous (IV) tube or urinary catheter. If the infection travels to the kidneys, lungs, brain, or other organs, it can cause serious systemic complications, but these develop only in people who are seriously ill or who have other health problems that weaken the immune system, such as drug addiction or ***diabetes.***

DIAGNOSTIC AND TEST PROCEDURES

To diagnose **oral thrush,** a doctor will examine the white patches and may take a sample for testing. To check for **vaginal yeast infection,** a doctor may take a vaginal wet smear. If your physician thinks you have a **systemic yeast infection,** a blood, stool, or tissue sample will be tested for the fungus.

TREATMENT

Treatment will depend on your specific condition but will focus on counteracting the growth of the yeast organism that causes the infection.

CONVENTIONAL MEDICINE

Your doctor will probably treat **oral thrush** with an ***antifungal*** medication such as ***clotrimazole*** or ***ketoconazole.*** Babies with oral thrush are typically given nystatin with a dropper. Infections of the skin or nails can be treated with topical applications of clotrimazole. For **vaginal yeast infection,** an over-the-counter intravaginal cream containing ***miconazole*** or clotrimazole is typically suggested. If over-the-counter medications are not effective, your doctor may prescribe a cream with ***terconazole*** or an oral antifungal drug containing fluconazole. If your doctor determines that you have a **systemic yeast infection,** you may get intravenous doses of amphotericin or flucytosine.

ALTERNATIVE CHOICES

Alternative remedies can strengthen the immune system to resist yeast infections, and can treat specific yeast infections and prevent recurrence.

HERBAL THERAPIES

For healing yeast infections on your skin, apply full-strength ***tea tree oil*** (*Melaleuca* spp.) two to three times daily; a slight burning sensation is normal, but discontinue if the treatment is painful. An over-the-counter salve containing ***usnea*** (*Usnea* spp.) and ***yarrow*** *(Achillea millefolium)* is good for rashes in children over two years of age.

CHRONIC YEAST INFECTION

Although the diagnosis is not universally accepted, some doctors recognize a condition called chronic candidiasis, or chronic yeast infection, that may affect the gastrointestinal, nervous, endocrine, and immune systems. Treatment focuses on eliminating predisposing factors, such as prescription or over-the-counter drugs, foods with high refined-sugar or yeast content, high-carbohydrate vegetables, and milk products. Your doctor may also test you for underlying conditions, such as ***diabetes*** *or* ***thyroid problems.***

An herbal remedy for chronic yeast infection is tea brewed from 1 to 2 grams of dried root of ***barberry*** *(Berberis vulgaris) or* ***goldenseal*** *(Hydrastis canadensis) in a cup of boiling water, taken three times a day. With your doctor's approval, you may want to try taking daily supplements of 45 mg* ***iron,*** *45 mg* ***zinc,*** *and 200 mcg* ***selenium*** *(avoid higher doses of selenium).*

HOMEOPATHY

Numerous homeopathic remedies are used to treat yeast infections; ask a licensed homeopath about which one best suits your symptoms.

PREVENTION

- If work keeps your hands in water for long periods, wear rubber gloves. When you're done, wash your hands and apply a mild prescription or over-the-counter antifungal cream.
- Wear cotton or silk underclothes, which, unlike nylon and other synthetics, allow excess moisture to evaporate. Wash and dry your underclothes thoroughly; change them often. ■

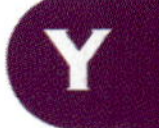

INDEX OF CONVENTIONAL AND NATURAL MEDICINES

More than 350 drugs, herbs, and homeopathic remedies are described in this index of medicines. Included are the most frequently prescribed and most widely used medicines in each of five categories: prescription drugs, over-the-counter drugs, Western herbs, Chinese herbs, and homeopathic remedies. The category to which each entry belongs is identified by an icon beside its name. A key to the icons appears below and at the bottom of each right-hand page of this index.

You can learn about a prescription or over-the-counter drug by looking up its class, such as analgesics—a designation based on the drug's effects on the body. Each drug is also listed by its generic name, such as acetaminophen, which indicates its active ingredient. You can also look up brand names in the general index, beginning on page 1118, which will tell you the generic name under which the medication is listed here. If your brand is not listed in the index, check your drug's package label for the generic name and look that up. If you consult the class entry, which summarizes the characteristics of the generic drugs in that class, you may find a more extensive explanation of side effects, interactions, and the way a given set of drugs acts on the body. Cross references from a generic drug to its class and from a class to its component generics will help guide you.

Natural medicines include herbs and homeopathic remedies. Western herbs are listed by their common names; Chinese herbs are listed by their common English, rather than Chinese, names; and homeopathic remedies are listed by their Latin names. See "About Herbal Preparations" and "About Homeopathic Remedies" *(pages 1025-1027)* for more information.

Whenever you are prescribed a medication, there are several important questions that you should consider asking your doctor or your pharmacist:

- What are the alternatives to medication?
- Is the generic version of the drug as effective as the brand-name variety?
- How should the drug be stored?
- What should I do about missed or delayed doses?
- How long before the drug starts to work?
- When can I expect to see an improvement?

It is important to tell your doctor—or doctors, if you are being treated by more than one—about all the prescription and over-the-counter drugs, vitamins, herbs, and homeopathic remedies you currently use, especially if your doctor plans to give you a new prescription. Medicines that heal when taken alone may provoke serious side effects when combined with other drugs or herbs. Older patients frequently need to take several medications at the same time and should be especially cautious about possible adverse interactions.

Most doctors recommend that you avoid using medicines during pregnancy, unless they are clearly needed, as they might be if, for example, you have epilepsy or a serious infection. With careful monitoring by a physician, women who use medicines for such illnesses can have safe deliveries and healthy babies.

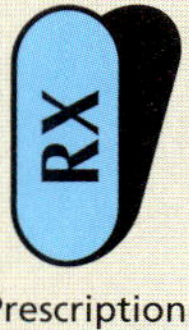

Prescription Drug (Rx)

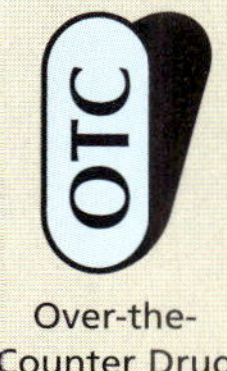

Over-the-Counter Drug

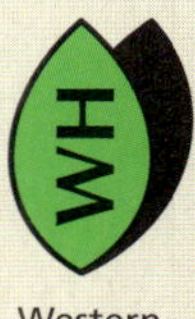

Western Herb

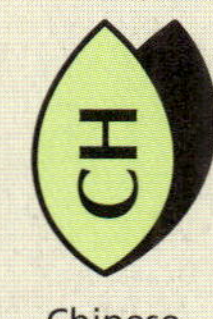

Chinese Herb

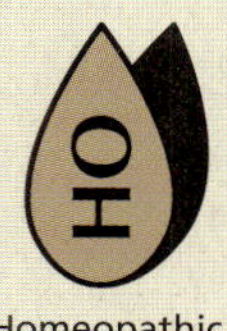

Homeopathic Remedy

A

ACETAMINOPHEN

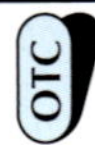

DRUG CLASS
Analgesics

BRAND NAMES
Acetaminophen-only brands: Tylenol, Tylenol Extra Strength

Acetaminophen-containing combinations for colds: Chlor-Trimeton Allergy-Sinus Headache Caplets, Comtrex, Contac, Drixoral, TheraFlu, Triaminic Sore Throat Formula, Tylenol in various forms, Vicks DayQuil or NyQuil in Liquid or LiquiCaps

Combinations for pain: Excedrin Extra-Strength, Tylenol in various forms

Combinations for sleep: Excedrin PM, Tylenol PM

GENERAL DESCRIPTION
A pain reliever as well as a fever reducer, acetaminophen is a good alternative to aspirin, particularly for people who are allergic to aspirin or who are taking warfarin. One drawback is that acetaminophen does not reduce inflammation, so it is not effective for such conditions as swelling, redness, or menstrual cramps. If you seek relief from inflammation, try aspirin or a nonsteroidal anti-inflammatory drug.

TARGET AILMENTS
- fever.
- headaches, muscle aches, pain, or injuries.

SIDE EFFECTS
Serious (rare, if taken in recommended doses):
Hypersensitivity reaction (rash, hives, itching); kidney damage (lower-back pain, sudden reduction in urine output); liver damage (pain or swelling in the upper abdominal area) or hepatitis (jaundice); blood disorder (unusual sore throat or fever); anemia (unusual tiredness); platelet disorder (unusual bruising or bleeding; black, tarry stools; bloody or cloudy urine). If you notice any of these symptoms, discontinue use and call your doctor immediately.

SPECIAL INFORMATION
- Acetaminophen can cause or exacerbate liver problems, so you should avoid alcoholic beverages when taking this drug. If you are too sick to eat, even moderate overdoses of acetaminophen can cause serious liver damage, possibly leading to convulsions, coma, and death. If you already have liver disease, use acetaminophen with caution, preferably under a doctor's supervision.
- Don't take more than the recommended dose. Persistent pain or high fever may indicate serious illness. If pain persists for more than 10 days or fever lasts for 3 days, contact your physician.
- If an overdose occurs, seek emergency help. Possible symptoms of overdose include nausea, vomiting, increased sweating, loss of appetite, and abdominal pain, although in some cases there are no symptoms. Treatment must start within 24 hours to prevent severe liver (and possible kidney) damage.
- To avoid involuntary overdose, be careful when combining this drug with other medications that contain acetaminophen. Read labels carefully.

POSSIBLE INTERACTIONS
Alcohol: risk of liver damage.

Anticoagulants (oral): if acetaminophen is taken regularly and in high doses, this combination can lead to an increased anticoagulant effect.

Aspartame: possibly hazardous for phenylketonuria patients.

Aspirin: risk of increased side effects of both drugs when combination is taken over a long period.

Barbiturates (except butalbital): reduced acetaminophen effect. Taking too much acetaminophen in combination with barbiturates also increases the risk of liver damage.

Isoniazid: risk of liver damage.

Nonsteroidal anti-inflammatory drugs (NSAIDs): risk of increased side effects of either drug when combination is taken over a long period.

Zidovudine (AZT): increased blood levels of zidovudine and risk of serious side effects.

ACONITE

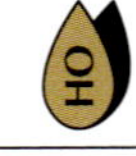

LATIN NAME
Aconitum napellus

GENERAL DESCRIPTION
Aconite grows throughout the mountainous regions of Europe, Russia, and central Asia, producing clusters of bluish violet flowers that hang from the stem like monks' cowls, giving the plant its common name, monkshood. Highly toxic, aconite was the preferred poison of the ancient Greeks. Administered in very small doses, it produces mental and physical restlessness and tissue inflammation. For this reason, homeopathic physicians prescribe *Aconite* for patients who seem distressed or fearful and complain of thirst and unbearable aches and pains that accompany their illnesses.

For homeopathic use, the whole plant—except the root, which is the most poisonous part—is gathered while in full bloom and pounded to a pulp. Juice is pressed from the pulp and mixed with alcohol, then diluted to nontoxic levels.

For more information on homeopathic medicine, see page 1027.

TARGET AILMENTS
- angina, arrhythmia, anxiety induced by sudden shock, arthritis, asthma, bronchitis, colds and flu, croup, fevers with rapid onset and chills that may be accompanied by restlessness or thirst, eye inflammations with burning pain and sensitivity to light, laryngitis, sore throat, middle ear infections, toothaches with a sensitivity to cold water.

PREPARATIONS
Aconite is available over the counter in various potencies, in both tablet and liquid form, at selected stores and pharmacies. Consult your practitioner for more precise information.

SIDE EFFECTS
None expected.

ACYCLOVIR

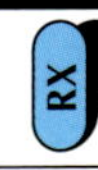

DRUG CLASS
Antiviral Drugs

BRAND NAME
Zovirax

GENERAL DESCRIPTION
Introduced in 1979, acyclovir is an antiviral drug that has been used to treat various types of herpes, shingles, and chickenpox infections. It is also used to fight other viral diseases, including mononucleosis and the Epstein-Barr virus.

Acyclovir hinders viral reproduction by inhibiting the expression of genetic material (DNA) in the virus and in infected cells, thus slowing or stopping the organism's spread. Acyclovir may be used in tablet, liquid suspension, or topical form, depending on the ailment and the patient's condition. For herpes and chickenpox, for example, it may be used topically. Otherwise, it is taken orally. The FDA is currently reviewing acyclovir for approval to over-the-counter status.

TARGET AILMENTS

- genital herpes: herpes simplex.
- herpes simplex in patients with compromised immune systems (people with cancer or HIV, for example).
- chickenpox in patients with compromised immune systems.
- shingles in patients with compromised immune systems.
- herpes simplex encephalitis (brain infection).

SIDE EFFECTS

Not serious:
Gastrointestinal upsets (such as nausea), lightheadedness, headache; with topical preparation: mild burning, stinging, itching, or skin rash. Call your doctor if these symptoms persist or become bothersome.

Serious:
None expected for short-term treatment outside a hospital setting.

SPECIAL INFORMATION

- Use caution when taking acyclovir if you are pregnant or breast-feeding. Although no adverse effects are known to have resulted from its use in such cases, the drug can cross the placenta and affect the fetus, and it can pass to nursing infants through breast milk.

POSSIBLE INTERACTIONS

Zidovudine (AZT): increased toxicity; profound drowsiness and lethargy.

AGASTACHE

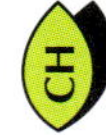

LATIN NAME

Agastache rugosa

GENERAL DESCRIPTION

The leaves, stems, and flowers of agastache are most often used to treat disorders that affect the digestive tract. This plant is also known as patchouli or pogostemon. An aromatic herb grown throughout China, agastache is classified in Chinese herbal medicine as acrid and slightly warm. Harvested in June and July, the best-quality agastache has many soft, thick, and fragrant leaves.

TARGET AILMENTS

- nausea and vomiting, diarrhea and dysentery, morning sickness, swelling of the abdomen, reduced appetite, and colds without fever. (Take internally.)

PREPARATIONS

Agastache is available in Chinese pharmacies, Asian markets, and Western health food stores, where it is in the form of dried leaves or powder.

Combinations: The herb, appearing in several preparations with other Chinese herbs, should not be cooked for more than 15 minutes or it will lose its fragrant quality. In combination with pinellia and atractylodes (black), it may be prescribed for nausea and vomiting, bloating of the chest and abdomen, reduced appetite, and diarrhea. A mixture of agastache with coptis and bamboo shavings is used by Chinese herbalists for certain types of vomiting. Practitioners of Chinese medicine also recommend agastache together with grains-of-paradise fruit for morning sickness. Consult a Chinese medicine practitioner for information on dosages and additional herbal combinations.

SIDE EFFECTS

None expected.

SPECIAL INFORMATION

- Do not use agastache when there are what Chinese medicine calls heat signs. These include symptoms such as fever, thirst, and sweating.

AIDS TREATMENT

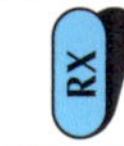

GENERIC NAMES

Reverse transcriptase inhibitors: abacavir, adefovir, delavirdine, didanosine, efavirenz, lamivudine, nevirapine, stavudine, zalcitabine, zidovudine, zidovudine plus lamivudine

Protease inhibitors: amprenavir, indinavir, nelfinavir, ritonavir, saquinavir

GENERAL DESCRIPTION

These powerful antiviral drugs are used in combination to treat people who are infected with the human immunodeficiency virus (HIV), which causes acquired immunodeficiency syndrome (AIDS). None of these drugs will cure AIDS or rid the body of HIV, but they may help stave off the worst symptoms of disease for several years in some people.

Antiviral drugs work to slow down the virus by inhibiting its ability to propagate itself. Reverse transcriptase inhibitors act by restricting the ability of the virus to make copies of itself; protease inhibitors interfere with the proper production of proteins required for the infection of new cells.

A problem with this group of drugs is that the virus often becomes resistant to them within a few years. Also, they can cause serious side effects. Combining drugs is the most helpful form of treatment. Two or three reverse transcriptase inhibitors are often combined, with the addition of a protease inhibitor. The drugs may later be given in different combinations, with substitution of one or more, as resistance develops. Protease inhibitors are often active against strains of HIV that become resistant to reverse transcriptase inhibitors.

The best tolerated of the reverse transcriptase inhibitors is lamivudine; the best tolerated protease inhibitors are nelfinavir and saquinavir.

TARGET AILMENTS

- HIV infection (with or without symptoms).
- AIDS.
- HIV prevention in individuals with occupational exposure to HIV (such as healthcare personnel).
- HIV prevention in the unborn children of pregnant women with AIDS or HIV.

SIDE EFFECTS

Consult your doctor and pharmacist about the reactions you might expect and about any symptoms you find troublesome.

SPECIAL INFORMATION

- WARNING: An overdose of these drugs can be dangerous, causing seizures, loss of coordination, severe nausea and vomiting, or extreme weakness. Contact a poison control center or seek emergency treatment if you have taken more than the prescribed amount.
- Using any of these drugs does not lower the risk of transmitting HIV to other people through blood contamination or sexual contact. Appropriate precaution must be taken to avoid spreading HIV.
- If you are pregnant and HIV positive, consult your doctor about possible benefits and risks of these drugs.

Zidovudine (AZT) reduces the risk of HIV transference from mother to baby.

POSSIBLE INTERACTIONS

There are many potential interactions between drugs in this group and other medications, both prescription and over the counter. The interactions between them also vary. Consult your doctor before taking any other drug while you are undergoing therapy with these antivirals.

ALBUTEROL

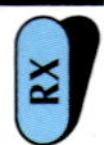

DRUG CLASS
Bronchodilators

BRAND NAMES
Proventil (inhalation aerosol, inhalation solution, tablets), Ventolin (inhalation aerosol, inhalation solution), Volmax (tablets)

GENERAL DESCRIPTION
Albuterol, an antiasthmatic drug that acts by relaxing the muscles in the bronchial tubes, is commonly prescribed for symptoms of acute bronchial asthma. The drug is also used to reduce the frequency and severity of recurrent asthma attacks and exercise-induced bronchospasms. Albuterol is available in inhaler and tablet form. See ***Bronchodilators*** for information on side effects and possible drug interactions.

SPECIAL INFORMATION
- Do not take more than the recommended dosage, especially in inhalant form. Overuse of this drug can cause heart-rhythm irregularities.

ALFALFA

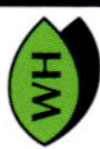

LATIN NAME
Medicago sativa

GENERAL DESCRIPTION
The alfalfa plant, bearing blue and purple blossoms, is considered a nutritional supplement and a general tonic. Its leaves, growing in groups of three, are thought to nourish the body by stimulating the appetite, acting as a phytoestrogen and diuretic, and providing such nutrients as fiber, protein, calcium, trace minerals, and vitamins E, K, and carotene.

TARGET AILMENTS
- inflammation of the bladder, bloating or water retention, menopause, indigestion, constipation, halitosis. (Take internally.)

PREPARATIONS
Over the counter:
Alfalfa is available as tincture, prepared tea, capsules, dried leaves, concentrated powder extract, or sprouts.

At home:
Tea: Steep 1 to 2 tsp dried leaves per cup of water for 5 to 10 minutes. Drink 3 cups a day.

Nutrition: Add sprouts or powdered alfalfa to soups, salads, or sandwiches.

SIDE EFFECTS

Not serious:
Alfalfa may cause stomach upset and diarrhea. If it does, stop using the herb and inform your physician.

SPECIAL INFORMATION
- WARNING: Avoid eating alfalfa seeds, because they contain relatively high levels of the toxic amino acid canavanine. Ingesting large quantities of alfalfa seeds over a long period of time may lead to pancytopenia, a blood disorder that causes the deterioration of both platelets, responsible for blood clotting, and white blood cells, which fight infections.
- Alfalfa contains saponins, chemicals thought to destroy red blood cells. Consequently, anyone suffering from anemia should use alfalfa only under the direction of an herbalist or a licensed healthcare professional.
- If you are pregnant, check with a practitioner before ingesting this herb. Alfalfa seeds contain stachydrine and homostachydrine, which promote menstruation and in some cases can lead to miscarriage.
- If you have a predisposition to systemic lupus erythematosus, do not use this herb. The canavanine in alfalfa is believed to reactivate this disease in some people who are in remission.
- Although scientists have found no direct evidence, some herbalists believe, on the basis of animal studies, that alfalfa can help the body to ward off heart disease and strokes by delaying the absorption of cholesterol and dissolving plaque deposits on the arterial walls.

ALISMA

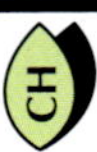

LATIN NAME
Alisma plantago-aquatica

GENERAL DESCRIPTION
The rhizome of the alisma plant, also known as water plantain, is prescribed by herbalists to treat malfunctions of the kidney and bladder. Alisma is often prescribed as a diuretic (a substance that releases body fluids), and this effect may stem from a high concentration of potassium, a mineral that helps to flush out urine. Since its action is mild and it does not dry out the body excessively, alisma can be taken by weak, elderly patients, for whom other such medications are too strong. The herb is classified as cold, bland, and sweet in traditional Chinese medicine. Literally translated as "marsh drain," alisma grows in the swamps of China's Fujian, Jianxi, and Sichuan provinces. The best quality of fresh herb is a lustrous, powdery, white plant.

TARGET AILMENTS
- difficulty in urination, edema (swelling caused by retention of fluids), diarrhea, dysentery, and symptoms that Chinese herbalists associate with kidney deficiencies, including a burning sensation in the urinary tract, tinnitus (ringing in the ears), or dizziness. (Take internally.)

PREPARATIONS
Alisma is available in bulk form at Chinese pharmacies, Asian food markets, and Western health food stores. It can be purchased by the ounce.

Combinations: In a mixture with grains-of-paradise fruit, alisma may be prescribed for patients with distended stomachs and abdomens who also have low production of urine. Consult a Chinese herbalist for information on specific dosages and additional herbal combinations.

SIDE EFFECTS

Serious:
Although alisma may be safe when taken in moderation, it can irritate the intestinal tract, and prolonged use can lead to gastroenteritis.

SPECIAL INFORMATION
- Do not use alisma when there is a clear, thin vaginal discharge.
- Healthy subjects taking alisma often increase their output of urine and excrete more sodium and urea than usual.

ALLIUM CEPA

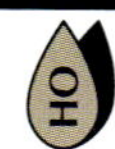

LATIN NAME
Allium cepa

GENERAL DESCRIPTION
Cultivated worldwide, *Allium cepa,* otherwise known as red onion, has been used in folk medicine for centuries. This common garden vegetable has been applied to the skin in poultices for acne, arthritis, and congestion, and used internally to clear the intestines of worms. Modern-day herbalists find onion useful for treating conditions as varied as earaches, hemorrhoids, and high blood pressure. Homeopathic practitioners consider *Allium cepa* a remedy for conditions that are accompanied by the same symptoms as those brought on by exposure to red onions—watering eyes and a burning, runny nose.

For the homeopathic preparation, red onions are harvested in midsummer. The bulbs are pounded to a pulp and then mixed with water and alcohol through several stages of extreme dilution.

Like most homeopathic prescriptions, *Allium cepa* was developed as a remedy by observation of the reactions of healthy individuals to a series of undilute doses. The mental, emotional, and physical changes induced by *Allium cepa* were then cataloged. When a homeopathic practitioner encounters a patient with a set of symptoms that matches the cataloged symptoms brought on by *Allium cepa,* the practitioner then prescribes it in an extremely dilute form. It is presumed that in this highly dilute dosage, *Allium cepa* can counter the symptoms that it induces when it is at full strength. For more information on homeopathic medicine, see page 1027.

TARGET AILMENTS
- colds with sinus congestion that shifts from side to side in the head; coughs that cause a ripping, tearing pain in the throat; watery and inflamed eyes, hay fever; neuralgic pains; earaches. (Take internally.)

PREPARATIONS
Allium cepa is available over the counter in various potencies, in liquid or tablet form, at selected stores and pharmacies. Consult your homeopathic practitioner for more precise information.

SIDE EFFECTS
None expected.

ALOE

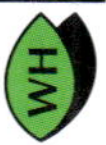

LATIN NAME
Aloe barbadensis

GENERAL DESCRIPTION
This tropical herb, with long, light-green leaves and sagging purple-and-yellow blooms, yields two therapeutic substances. The first, a translucent gel obtained from the inner leaves, works externally to relieve minor burns, skin irritations, and infections; taken internally, aloe gel provides relief from stomach disorders. It is thought to function by inhibiting bradykinin, a pain-producing agent. In addition it is believed to contain magnesium lactate, an effective antihistamine. Among its ingredients are several that reduce inflammation. Aloe gel is used as a beauty aid and moisturizer because it contains polysaccharides, which act as emollients to soothe, soften, and protect the skin.

The second remedy contained in the aloe plant is a bitter, yellow juice known as latex, found just beneath the surface of the leaves. Latex acts as a powerful laxative.

TARGET AILMENTS
- digestive disorders, gastritis, stomach ulcers. (Use aloe gel internally.)
- constipation. (Use aloe latex internally.)
- minor burns, infection in wounds, insect bites, skin irritations, bruising, chickenpox, sunburn, poison ivy, acne. (Use aloe gel externally.)
- irritated eyes. (Use aloe gel externally.)

PREPARATIONS
Over the counter:
Aloe is available as powder, fluidextract, powdered capsules, bottled gel, or latex tablets.

At home:
Eyewash: Dissolve ½ tsp powdered aloe gel in 1 cup water. Add 1 tsp boric acid to accelerate the healing process. Pour the solution through a coffee filter before applying to the eyes.

Bath: Add 1 to 2 cups aloe gel to a warm bath to relieve sunburn or skin lesions.

Combinations: Use aloe gel with wheat-germ oil and safflower flower to reduce bruising.

SIDE EFFECTS
Not serious:
The use of aloe may result in allergic dermatitis, intestinal cramps, or diarrhea. Try a lower dosage or stop using the product.

SPECIAL INFORMATION
- WARNING: Do not exceed the recommended dose of aloe latex. If taken in excess, its powerful laxative chemicals can cause intestinal cramps leading to ulcers or irritated bowels.
- If you are pregnant or have a gastrointestinal illness, take aloe internally only in consultation with an herbalist or a licensed healthcare professional.

A

ALPHA$_1$-ADRENERGIC BLOCKERS

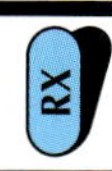

GENERIC NAMES
doxazosin, terazosin

GENERAL DESCRIPTION
Members of a general category of medicines known as antihypertensives, alpha$_1$-adrenergic blockers are used primarily to treat high blood pressure (hypertension). They work by selectively blocking nerve endings called alpha receptors; the blockage allows the blood vessels to relax and expand, which enables blood to pass through more easily and lowers blood pressure.

Alpha$_1$-adrenergic blockers can be used alone or in conjunction with other drugs, such as beta-adrenergic blockers or diuretics. These drugs do not cure high blood pressure, but they do help control it.

Doxazosin and terazosin are also used to relax the muscles in the prostate gland and increase urine flow. They will not, however, shrink an enlarged prostate. For more information, see entries for generic drugs listed above. For information on other drugs used to treat high blood pressure, see ***Antihypertensive Drugs.***

TARGET AILMENTS
- high blood pressure.
- benign prostatic hyperplasia (benign enlargement of the prostate).

SIDE EFFECTS
Not serious:
Nasal congestion, headache, fatigue, nausea, indigestion, nervousness, weakness, irritability, skin rash, blurred vision, drowsiness. These effects should subside as you adjust to the drug. Check with your doctor if these or other symptoms persist or are bothersome: You may need a dosage adjustment.

Serious:
First-dose effect: Alpha$_1$-adrenergic blockers can cause marked low blood

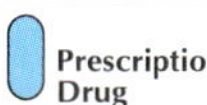
Prescription Drug
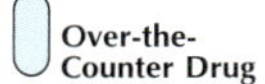
Over-the-Counter Drug
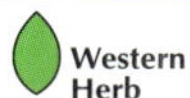
Western Herb
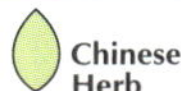
Chinese Herb
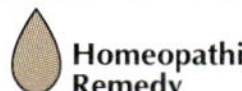
Homeopathic Remedy

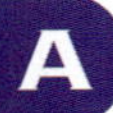

pressure. Common symptoms include lightheadedness, dizziness, vertigo, palpitations, and fainting. You are most likely to experience these symptoms if, when you first start taking the drug, you rise too quickly from a sitting or prone position, drink alcohol, exercise strenuously, or stand for long periods of time, especially in hot weather. Check with your doctor immediately.

SPECIAL INFORMATION

- Avoid driving and hazardous tasks for 24 hours after the first dose, after a dosage increase, or after resumption of treatment.
- The effects of these drugs on pregnant women, nursing mothers, and children under 12 years of age are not yet known. Use only if directed by your physician.
- Before taking these drugs, tell your doctor if you have previously experienced an unusual or allergic reaction to any of the alpha blockers or have encountered dizziness, faintness, or lightheadedness with other drugs. Inform your doctor if you have a history of mental depression, stroke, or impaired circulation to the brain; coronary artery disease; impaired liver function or active liver disease; impaired kidney function; or any plans to undergo surgery in the near future.
- To minimize dizziness, take the first dose at bedtime. Dosages must be adjusted on an individual basis.
- $Alpha_1$-adrenergic blockers may affect some laboratory tests. Effects may include a mild decrease in white blood cell counts, certain cholesterol ratios, and blood sugar levels.
- The symptoms of prostate cancer are similar to those of benign prostate enlargement. Ask your doctor to test for prostate cancer before starting $alpha_1$-adrenergic treatment.

POSSIBLE INTERACTIONS

Alcohol: can intensify the blood pressure-lowering actions of this medicine and increase the chances of fainting or dizziness.

Drugs that lower blood pressure, such as beta-adrenergic blockers and diuretics: may increase the effects of the $alpha_1$-adrenergic blockers, possibly affecting the duration and severity of the first-dose (low-blood pressure) symptoms.

Estrogens and indomethacin: may reduce the blood pressure-lowering effect.

ALPRAZOLAM

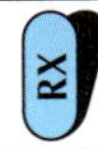

DRUG CLASS
Antianxiety Drugs [Benzodiazepines]

BRAND NAME
Xanax

GENERAL DESCRIPTION
Alprazolam is used for short-term management of anxiety disorders and anxiety associated with depression. It is also used to treat panic disorder. Since this drug can become habit forming, alprazolam is not used to treat the anxiety and stress of everyday living. See ***Benzodiazepines*** for further information on side effects and possible drug interactions.

SPECIAL INFORMATION
- Be careful not to confuse the brand names Xanax and Zantac. Zantac is the brand name for ranitidine, a drug used to treat ulcers.
- The following effects on sexual and reproductive function have been noted with alprazolam: increased or decreased libido, sexual dysfunction, menstrual disorders.

ALUMINUM HYDROXIDE

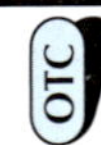

DRUG CLASS
Antacids

BRAND NAMES
Some types of Maalox and Mylanta

GENERAL DESCRIPTION
Aluminum hydroxide is an aluminum-containing antacid used to relieve upset and sour stomach, heartburn, acid indigestion, and some types of ulcers. The most common adverse effect is constipation. See ***Antacids*** for more information, including facts about side effects and possible drug interactions.

SPECIAL INFORMATION
- Do not take an aluminum-containing antacid if you have or are at risk for Alzheimer's disease; some evidence suggests that excess aluminum may be a contributing factor in the disease.
- Avoid aluminum-containing antacids if you are on kidney dialysis; aluminum toxicity could result.

AMILORIDE

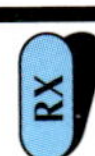

DRUG CLASS
Diuretics

BRAND NAME
Midamor

GENERAL DESCRIPTION
Like other diuretics, amiloride is used to remove excess fluid from the body by increasing urine production, thereby lowering blood pressure. Amiloride is among the group of medicines called potassium-sparing diuretics; it prevents the excess loss of potassium, a frequent consequence of the excretion of body fluids. This drug is usually used in combination with nonpotassium-sparing diuretics. See ***Diuretics*** for more information, including side effects and drug interactions.

SPECIAL INFORMATION
- Because amiloride inhibits potassium excretion, you should not take potassium supplements (including salt substitutes, which often contain potassium) or eat large quantities of potassium-rich foods (such as bananas) while on this medication. Excess potassium can lead to heart-rhythm problems.

AMITRIPTYLINE

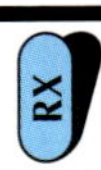

DRUG CLASS
Antidepressants [Tricyclic Antidepressants (TCAs)]

BRAND NAME
Elavil

GENERAL DESCRIPTION
Since 1961, the tricyclic antidepressant amitriptyline has been used in the treatment of depression. The drug acts on the nervous system by restoring levels of the vital brain chemicals serotonin and norepinephrine. Amitriptyline may also be used to treat peptic ulcers and, when combined with other medications, to alleviate chronic pain. See ***Antidepressants*** for information about side effects and possible drug interactions.

AMLODIPINE

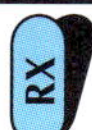

DRUG CLASS
Calcium Channel Blockers

BRAND NAME
Norvasc

GENERAL DESCRIPTION
Amlodipine, introduced in 1986, is a calcium channel blocker used to treat hypertension and angina. Like other drugs in its class, amlodipine inhibits the passage of calcium into body cells, thus slowing the contraction of the heart and arteries, dilating the arteries, and lowering blood pressure. These actions also reduce the rate and pumping force of the heart and may block spasms of the coronary arteries, thus lessening angina. See ***Calcium Channel Blockers*** for information on side effects and possible drug interactions.

AMOXICILLIN

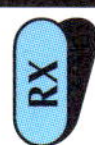

DRUG CLASS
Antibiotics [Penicillins]

BRAND NAMES
Amoxil, Polymox, Trimox, Wymox

GENERAL DESCRIPTION
Introduced in 1969, amoxicillin is a penicillin antibiotic commonly used to treat genitourinary tract infections, gonorrhea, otitis media, sinusitis, pharyngitis, and other bacterial infections caused by certain strains of staph, strep, and *E. coli.* For more information on side effects and interactions, see ***Penicillins.***

AMOXICILLIN AND CLAVULANATE

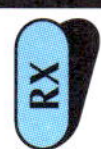

DRUG CLASS
Antibiotics [Penicillins]

BRAND NAME
Augmentin

GENERAL DESCRIPTION
Introduced in 1982, amoxicillin and clavulanate is a combination antibiotic drug. Clavulanate reinforces amoxicillin's ability to destroy bacteria. This combination and the single drug amoxicillin are used to treat some of the same bacterial infections, including otitis media, sinusitis, and other infections of the respiratory tract, and infections of the skin and urinary tract. For more information, see ***Penicillins.***

▼POSSIBLE INTERACTIONS

Disulfiram: do not take this drug with amoxicillin and clavulanate.

ANALGESICS

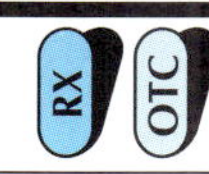

GENERIC NAMES
Acetaminophen, aspirin

Caffeine [Adjunct Therapy]

Methyl Salicylate [Topical Analgesic]

Cox-2 Inhibitors: celecoxib, rofecoxib

Nonsteroidal Anti-Inflammatory Drugs (NSAIDs): diclofenac, etodolac, flurbiprofen, ibuprofen, ketorolac, nabumetone, naproxen, oxaprozin

Opioid Analgesics: codeine, hydrocodone, oxycodone, propoxyphene

GENERAL DESCRIPTION
Analgesics are drugs that relieve pain. Many have been used for centuries for their ability to reduce suffering. Some offer relief by affecting the brain and nervous system; these are called narcotic pain relievers. Nonnarcotic pain relievers act at the site of the pain, usually by relieving inflammation.

Sometimes two or more analgesics are combined to increase the effectiveness or the range of their action. Analgesics have side effects that depend on their mode of action and also on individual response. Some can cause drowsiness or a severe allergic reaction, while others may affect the digestive system or blood vessels. For more information about a specific analgesic, see the entries for the generic drugs and their subclasses listed on page 888.

ANEMARRHENA

LATIN NAME
Anemarrhena asphodeloides

GENERAL DESCRIPTION
The rhizome of the anemarrhena plant is used to treat fever and other ailments that Chinese medicine practitioners associate with yin deficiency, a disorder distinguished by what Chinese medicine regards as heat signs; these include symptoms such as fever, chills, headache, thirst, sweating, and a rapid pulse. Anemarrhena is classified in traditional Chinese medical practice as bitter and cold. It grows in China's Hebei province, where it is harvested in autumn. A high-quality specimen of this herb appears large, thick, and hard, and has a white cross section.

TARGET AILMENTS
Take internally for:
- high fever and thirst accompanied by a rapid pulse.
- coughing that brings up thick, yellow phlegm.
- night sweats, low-grade fever, afternoon fever.
- certain types of dizziness and vertigo.
- ulcers in the mouth, bleeding gums.
- abnormally high sex drive and nocturnal emissions.

PREPARATIONS
Anemarrhena is available in bulk at Chinese pharmacies, Asian markets, and Western health food stores. Practitioners sometimes recommend a preparation of the herb cooked in salt water to treat the kidneys.

Combinations: In a mixture with phellodendron, anemarrhena is used to treat night sweating, dizziness, and vertigo. The herb is also combined with fritillaria to treat coughing and bringing up phlegm. Chinese herbalists mix anemarrhena with scrophularia and Chinese foxglove root for ulcers in the mouth.

Check with a Chinese medicine practitioner for information on appropriate dosages and other herbal combinations.

▼SIDE EFFECTS

None expected.

SPECIAL INFORMATION
- Anemarrhena has demonstrated possible antibiotic effects in laboratory tests. It is used in Chinese medicine to deal with infection.

ANESTHETICS

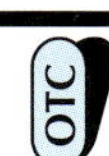

GENERAL DESCRIPTION
Over-the-counter anesthetics are topical

medications frequently used to block pain and discomfort by deadening nerve endings. They are used on all body surfaces and in easily accessible areas inside the body, such as the mouth and esophagus.

Although the most commonly used over-the-counter anesthetics are for mouth pain, the drugs are also found in preparations used to treat minor burns, sunburn, and rectal pain (from hemorrhoids), and to aid in medical examinations and minor surgical procedures. These medications have relatively few side effects except when used excessively, which results in their absorption into the bloodstream, or when they trigger an allergic or hypersensitivity reaction, which may appear as local irritation and reddening of the application site. For information about a specific anesthetic drug, see ***Benzocaine.***

ANGELICA ROOT

LATIN NAME
Angelica pubescens

GENERAL DESCRIPTION
Chinese medicine practitioners prescribe *Angelica pubescens* as a pain reliever. They believe the root of this plant alleviates the pain and numbness in joints and muscles—especially of the lower body—attributed in Chinese medicine to cold, damp weather conditions. This aromatic herb with its thick, glistening roots is classified as acrid, bitter, and warm according to the tenets of traditional Chinese medicine.

TARGET AILMENTS
Take internally for:
- acute and chronic pain in the lower back and legs that is sensitive to cold, damp weather.
- mild headache and toothache that respond to changes in the weather.

PREPARATIONS
The herb is available in bulk at Chinese pharmacies, Asian food markets, and Western health food stores.

Combinations: A mixture with Chinese wild ginger and gentiana macrophylla root is prescribed for pain and numbness in the neck, back, and legs. When combined with ephedra stem, it is used for body aches with colds and flu, if the patient is not perspiring. This herb is also mixed with a root known as siler in a remedy for numbness in the legs.

Angelica root is related to notopterygium root, which is regarded as a better treatment for pain in the upper back and shoulders. Chinese herbalists often use these two herbs together. For example, a headache remedy is created when angelica root is combined with notopterygium, another root called cnidium *(Ligusticum chuanxiong),* and a fruit known as vitex.

Consult a Chinese medicine practitioner for information on specific dosages as well as additional herbal combinations.

SIDE EFFECTS
None expected.

SPECIAL INFORMATION
- WARNING: Do not use angelica root when there are what Chinese medicine calls heat signs. These include symptoms such as fever, thirst, sweating, and a rapid pulse.
- In laboratory experiments, angelica root apparently has relieved pain in mice.
- This herb has slowed the growth of bacteria in a test tube study.

ANGIOTENSIN-CONVERTING ENZYME (ACE) INHIBITORS

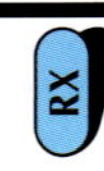

GENERIC NAMES
benazepril, captopril, enalapril, lisinopril, quinapril, ramipril

GENERAL DESCRIPTION
Angiotensin-converting enzyme (ACE) inhibitors block an enzyme in the body that is essential for the production of a substance that causes blood vessels to constrict. As a result, these drugs relax blood vessels, thereby lowering blood pressure and putting less stress on the heart. Some ACE inhibitors also increase the heart's ability to pump blood. For more information, see the entries for the generic drugs listed above.

TARGET AILMENTS
- high blood pressure.
- sometimes congestive heart failure (when used in conjunction with digitalis preparations and diuretics).

SIDE EFFECTS
Not serious:
Dry, persistent cough; headache, fatigue, nausea, diarrhea, loss of sense of taste, temporary skin rash, low blood pressure or dizziness on suddenly rising or changing position. Call your doctor if these effects become bothersome.

Serious:
Fainting, persistent skin rash, joint pain, drowsiness, numbness and tingling, abdominal pain, vomiting, diarrhea, excessive perspiration, fever, chills, chest pain, heart palpitation, jaundice (yellowing of skin or eyes). Call your doctor right away. Get medical attention immediately if you notice swelling of your face, tongue, or vocal cords or have difficulty swallowing or breathing; this reaction can be life-threatening.

SPECIAL INFORMATION
- WARNING: These drugs should not be taken during pregnancy because they have been associated with death of the fetus and newborn baby.
- ACE inhibitors cause an increase in blood levels of potassium. Do not use salt substitutes (which contain potassium) or other potassium-rich products, including low-salt milk, without first consulting your doctor. Such products could increase the potassium in your blood to dangerous levels, leading to heart-rhythm problems.
- Because your first dose of an ACE inhibitor may cause a sudden drop in blood pressure, your doctor may recommend that you take the first dose at bedtime.
- Do not abruptly stop taking these drugs. Your doctor may tell you to reduce the dosage gradually.
- Some of these drugs, especially captopril, cause photosensitivity, an increased sensitivity to the sun that may result in serious, unexpected sunburn.
- Use caution during hot weather or while exercising; ACE inhibitors may cause increased perspiration, leading to dehydration and reduced blood pressure.
- Let your doctor know if you have arthritis or kidney disease, or if you are on a strict low-sodium diet or taking diuretics.

POSSIBLE INTERACTIONS

Alcohol: increased ACE inhibitor effects, leading to much lower blood pressure.

Central nervous system stimulants (including pseudoephedrine, an over-the-counter decongestant): reduced ACE inhibitor effect.

Estrogens: fluid retention, possibly raising blood pressure.

Indomethacin, NSAIDs, salicylates (such as aspirin): may decrease the effects of ACE inhibitors (especially captopril) and prevent the drugs from lowering blood pressure.

Lithium: lithium toxicity, which can lead to stupor, coma, and seizures.

Other medications that lower blood pressure, such as beta-adrenergic blockers, calcium channel blockers, diuretics, levodopa, nitrates, and opioid analgesics: increased hypotensive (blood pressure-lowering) effect of both combined medications.

Potassium products and diuretics that do not eliminate potassium from the body (such as amiloride, spironolactone, and triamterene): increased potassium blood levels, leading to heart-rhythm problems.

ANTACIDS

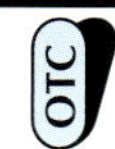

GENERIC NAMES
aluminum hydroxide, calcium carbonate, magnesium hydroxide, sodium bicarbonate and citric acid.

GENERAL DESCRIPTION
Antacids relieve the occasional unpleasant symptoms that accompany heartburn, acid indigestion, and sour stomach. The drugs work to neutralize excess gastric acid in the stomach, and as a result they help to heal and reduce the pain of ulcers. Many popular antacid preparations are combinations of different generic drugs.

Taken regularly over a long period of time, some calcium-containing antacids may help prevent osteoporosis and other conditions associated with calcium deficiency. For more information, see entries for the generic drugs listed above.

TARGET AILMENTS
- upset stomach, heartburn, acid indigestion, sour stomach.
- ulcers.
- calcium deficiency (calcium carbonate).

SIDE EFFECTS

Not serious:
Mild constipation; laxative effect or diarrhea; chalky taste in the mouth; stomach cramps, nausea, or vomiting; belching; flatulence; white specks in the stool. Call your doctor if these problems persist.

Serious:
Contact your doctor immediately if you notice any of the following symptoms: swelling of the wrist, foot, or lower leg; bone pain; severe constipation; dizziness; mood changes; muscle pain, weakness, or twitching; nervousness or restlessness; slow breathing; irregular heartbeat; fatigue; pain upon urinating or frequent need to urinate; change in appetite.

SPECIAL INFORMATION
- Except under special circumstances determined by your doctor, antacids should not be used if you have impaired renal function or if you have high levels of calcium in your blood, a condition known as hypercalcemia.
- If you have any of the following conditions, you and your doctor will have to weigh the benefits and risks of taking the different types of antacids: symptoms of appendicitis, gastrointestinal or rectal bleeding of undiagnosed cause, intestinal obstruction, or sensitivity to aluminum, calcium, magnesium, simethicone, or sodium bicarbonate medications.
- Before taking antacids, check with your doctor if you have had a colostomy or ileostomy, or if you have any of the following: cirrhosis, congestive heart failure, edema, colitis, diverticulitis, diarrhea, constipation or fecal impaction, hemorrhoids, sarcoidosis (a rare disease manifested by lesions in the skin, eyes, lungs, and lymph nodes), or hypophosphatemia (abnormally low concentrations of phosphates in the blood).
- Children under the age of six should not take antacids without a doctor's approval.
- Notify your doctor if you develop symptoms such as black, tarry stools or vomit the consistency of coffee grounds. These are indications of bleeding in the stomach or intestines.
- Although antacids are considered safe if taken in low doses and for short periods (under two weeks), pregnant and nursing women should consult a doctor first; antacids containing sodium may increase fluid retention.
- Any long-term antacid therapy—such as the treatment of ulcers—should be administered by a doctor.
- Combination antacids, such as aluminum and magnesium or calcium and magnesium, have the advantage of offsetting either constipation or diarrhea.
- Antacids are most effective when taken on an empty stomach.
- Because they can affect the rate of absorption of other drugs, antacids should not be taken within one to two hours of many other oral medications. Ask your doctor or pharmacist for guidance.
- If taken for any length of time, antacids can have a rebound effect that worsens your symptoms when you stop taking the medication.
- Calcium carbonate and sodium bicarbonate antacids can cause milk-alkali syndrome, which is characterized by headaches, nausea, irritability, and weakness. In time, milk-alkali syndrome can lead to kidney disease or failure.

POSSIBLE INTERACTIONS
Staggering medication times is one way to avoid undesirable drug interactions.

Anticholinergics, digoxin, phenothiazines, quinidine, warfarin: antacids are known to interfere with the effectiveness of these drugs.

Aspirin and other salicylates: antacids may increase excretion of these drugs, lessening their effectiveness. Do not take aspirin or other salicylates within three to four hours of antacids.

Cellulose sodium phosphate: the ability of this drug to reduce hypercalciuria (excretion of abnormally large amounts of calcium in the urine) may be lessened when it is taken with calcium antacids.

Enteric-coated medications: antacids may cause the enteric coating to dissolve too rapidly, resulting in gastric irritation. Do not take these medications within one to two hours of antacids.

Iron: decreased iron absorption. Space doses of iron and antacids as far apart as possible (12 hours).

Isoniazid (oral): absorption of this antitubercular drug may be delayed and decreased when taken with antacids.

Ketoconazole (antifungal drug): absorption of ketoconazole may be reduced when taken within three hours of antacids.

Mecamylamine: antacids may prolong the effects of this high blood pressure drug. Do not take mecamylamine with antacids.

Methenamine: this drug, used to treat urinary tract infections, may be less effective when taken with antacids.

Phenytoin should not be taken within two to three hours of antacids, since antacids may decrease absorption of this seizure-control drug.

Quinolones: reduced effectiveness of quinolones and fluoroquinolones.

Sodium polystyrene sulfonate (a cholesterol-reducing drug): risk of kidney failure and alkalosis.

Tetracycline (antibiotic): decreased absorption of tetracycline; do not take this drug within three to four hours of antacids.

Vitamin D: if taken concurrently with antacids containing either magnesium or calcium, vitamin D can result in abnormally large amounts of either mineral in the blood.

ANTIACNE DRUGS

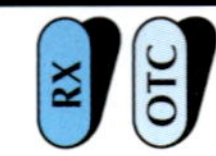

GENERAL DESCRIPTION

The antiacne drug class includes a number of over-the-counter and prescription medicines commonly advertised to treat acne and oily skin. These drugs, applied to the skin as creams, gels, lotions, or solutions, may work in several ways. Some affect the skin itself, acting as drying agents to reduce oiliness, or as agents that promote cell growth and sloughing or peeling of the skin. Others may have antiseptic or antibacterial action, or a combination of actions.

Most of these drugs cause local irritation and reddening of the skin, which may lessen with time. You should not use them if your skin is inflamed by sunburn, windburn, cuts, or abrasions. More serious side effects may include blistering or changes in skin color.

Absorption of antiacne drugs through the skin into the bloodstream is generally negligible, but these medications may produce side effects if absorbed in sufficient amounts. These include dizziness, headache, nausea, diarrhea, and ringing in the ears. For further information on a specific generic antiacne drug, see ***Tretinoin.***

ANTIANXIETY DRUGS

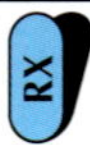

GENERIC NAMES

alprazolam, buspirone, diazepam, lorazepam

GENERAL DESCRIPTION

Drugs in this class are prescribed to manage anxiety disorders and relieve symptoms of anxiety. They may also be used to treat panic disorder. These drugs should not be used for the anxiety and stress associated with everyday living. Certain antianxiety drugs are potentially habit forming (addictive). Antianxiety drugs also vary in the amount of time they take to start working and in their duration of action: For example, the effects of alprazolam and other benzodiazepines start after the first dose, while those of buspirone (a nonbenzodiazepine) can take as long as two weeks. For information about side effects and possible drug interactions, see the entries for the generic drugs listed above.

ANTIBIOTICS

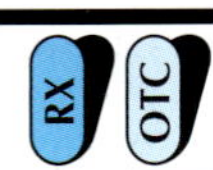

GENERIC NAMES

nitrofurantoin

Carbacephems: loracarbef

Cephalosporins: cefaclor, cefadroxil, cefixime, cefprozil, cefuroxime, cephalexin

Erythromycins: azithromycin, clarithromycin, erythromycin

Fluoroquinolones: ciprofloxacin, ofloxacin

Ophthalmic Antibiotics: erythromycin, tobramycin

Penicillins: amoxicillin, amoxicillin and clavulanate, penicillin V

Sulfonamides in Combination: sulfamethoxazole and trimethoprim.

Tetracyclines: doxycycline, tetracycline

Topical Antibiotics: bacitracin, chlorhexidine, mupirocin, neomycin, polymyxin B

GENERAL DESCRIPTION

Antibiotics are a large class of drugs used against bacterial infections, such as strep throat, otitis media, and other infections of the respiratory tract, eyes, or skin. Bactericidal antibiotics kill bacteria by attacking bacterial cell walls. Bacteriostatic antibiotics prevent bacteria from reproducing, thus enabling the body's defenses to overcome the infection. Antibiotics are not effective against fungal infections or against viruses, such as those that cause colds.

Because antibiotics target bacteria and not fungi, the drugs can disturb the body's normal balance of fungi and bacteria. This imbalance may be manifested as a fungal superinfection, such as a yeast infection, or in symptoms of diarrhea or gastrointestinal disturbances. To help restore your body's normal bacteria, some doctors recommend eating yogurt that contains *Lactobacillus acidophilus* culture or taking acidophilus tablets during antibiotic therapy and for a week afterward. For more information about a specific antibiotic, see the entries for the generic drugs and their subclasses listed (in bold) on page 891.

SPECIAL INFORMATION

- To prevent reinfection, take the full course of your prescription, even if you feel better before you've taken all the medicine.

ANTICANCER DRUGS

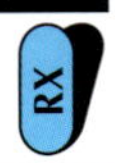

GENERAL DESCRIPTION

Medications in the anticancer drug class are used against the various forms of cancer, such as leukemia, lymphoma, and cancers of the prostate, colon, ovaries, and breasts. The drugs, used in treatment regimens known as chemotherapy, generally work by preventing the growth of abnormal, tumor-forming cells. Some drugs in this class are thought to block the effects of hormones that may stimulate cancer cell growth.

Side effects of anticancer drugs include loss of appetite, nausea and vomiting, diarrhea, temporary hair loss, skin rash, itching, darkening of the skin and fingernails, and unusual fatigue. For information about a specific drug used to treat breast cancer, see ***Tamoxifen.***

ANTICOAGULANT AND ANTIPLATELET DRUGS

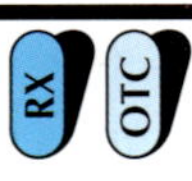

GENERIC NAMES

Rx: dipyridamole, heparin, warfarin

OTC: aspirin

GENERAL DESCRIPTION

Anticoagulants and antiplatelets decrease the blood's clotting ability. They are generally used as a secondary form of prevention for diseases in which the formation of harmful blood clots may cause serious problems. Although sometimes called blood thinners, these drugs do not really thin the blood or dissolve existing blood clots. They stop clots from growing larger and prevent new clots from forming in the blood vessels.

Antiplatelets (aspirin, dipyridamole) and anticoagulants (heparin, warfarin) can be used alone or in combination. The drugs and dosages must be carefully balanced for each patient. See also entries for generic drugs listed above.

TARGET AILMENTS

These drugs are prescribed as prophylaxis, to reduce the risk of:

- blood-clot formation in the veins (phlebitis).
- blood-clot formation in the lungs (pulmonary thromboembolism).
- blood-clot formation in the brain (cerebral thrombosis).
- heart attack, stroke, and atrial fibrillation.
- blood-clotting complications during or after surgery.

SIDE EFFECTS

Not serious:
See individual generic entries.

Serious:
The most serious effects of these drugs, whether used alone or in combination, are too much bleeding (excess anticoagulation, or overdose) and internal bleeding. Call your doctor immediately if you experience any of the following:

Early signs of excess anticoagulation (or overdose): unexplained bruising or purplish areas on the skin, bleeding from gums, heavy bleeding from cuts or wounds, unusually heavy nosebleeds or menstrual periods.

Signs of internal bleeding: backache or back pain; abdominal swelling or pain; blood in urine; tarry or bloody stools; constipation; coughing up or vomiting blood; joint stiffness, pain, or swelling.

SPECIAL INFORMATION

- Pregnant and nursing women should check with a physician before taking dipyridamole or heparin. If you are pregnant or nursing, you should not take aspirin. Warfarin may cause birth defects.
- These medications must be taken as directed by your physician.
- Do not use a given drug if you have had an allergic reaction to it in the past.
- Do not use these drugs without telling your physician if you have had a heart attack, uncontrolled high blood pressure, ulcers, or a stroke.
- Tell your doctor if you have or have had low blood pressure, an impaired kidney or liver, a bleeding disease or disorder, chest pains, allergies, asthma, colitis, diabetes, active tuberculosis, a recent childbirth, medical or dental surgery, spinal anesthesia, x-rays, a bad fall, heavy bleeding or menstrual periods, diarrhea, or any other medical problem. Also, tell your doctor if you are using an intrauterine device (IUD) for birth control or a catheter.
- Antiplatelets and anticoagulants may affect some lab tests. Before undergoing a lab test, be sure to advise the practitioner administering the test that you are taking the drug.
- Tell your pharmacist, dentist, and physician that you are taking the medicine. You may be advised to carry a medication identification card.
- Avoid dangerous activities that might cause injuries. Be sure to report all falls and blows to your doctor. Internal bleeding may occur without symptoms.
- Avoid eating foods rich in vitamin K, such as green leafy vegetables. Vitamin K decreases the anticoagulant effect of these drugs

POSSIBLE INTERACTIONS

Anticoagulant drugs seem to be involved in more drug interactions than any other class of drug. Be sure to let your healthcare professional know if you are taking any other medicine (prescription or over the counter) including aspirin, vitamins, laxatives, and antacids.

ANTICONVULSANT DRUGS

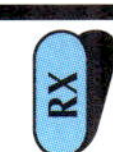

GENERIC NAMES

carbamazepine, phenytoin, valproic acid

GENERAL DESCRIPTION

The anticonvulsant drug class contains a number of medications used in the treatment of epilepsy. Although the exact mechanisms by which these drugs work are unknown, anticonvulsants appear to inhibit the sudden spread of excessive or abnormal electrical impulses in the brain, thereby limiting or preventing epileptic convulsions.

Anticonvulsants are not curatives, but they can reduce the possibility of seizure-related brain damage. They are usually prescribed, either alone or in combination, to control specific types of epileptic seizures. Since every case of epilepsy is unique and all anticonvulsants have toxic effects when taken in large dosages, a period of trial and error is usually needed to determine the appropriate drug and dosage. For more information, see entries for the generic drugs listed on page 892. See also ***Benzodiazepines,*** specifically ***Clonazepam*** and ***Diazepam.***

SPECIAL INFORMATION

- Possible side effects include skin rashes, headache, nausea, dizziness, confusion, and unsteadiness. Driving and hazardous activities should be avoided. You may be advised to wear a bracelet or carry an identification card stating which anticonvulsant drug you are taking.

ANTIDEPRESSANTS

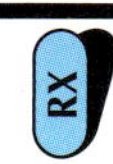

GENERIC NAMES

bupropion

Selective Serotonin Reuptake Inhibitors (SSRIs): fluoxetine, paroxetine, sertraline

Tricyclic Antidepressants: amitriptyline, doxepin, nortriptyline

GENERAL DESCRIPTION

Antidepressants are a class of nonnarcotic drugs that restore the normal levels of neurotransmitters such as serotonin and norepinephrine in the brain. Subclasses of antidepressants include tricyclic antidepressants (amitriptyline, doxepin, and nortriptyline) and selective serotonin reuptake inhibitors such as fluoxetine. Although the drugs in each subclass are somewhat distinct in structure and mode of action, they have similar uses and side effects. A few appear to be effective for nondepressive diseases such as phobias. For more information, see entries for the individual generic drugs listed above; also see ***Monoamine Oxidase (MAO) Inhibitors*** for other antidepressant medications.

TARGET AILMENTS

- major depressive disorders.
- obsessive-compulsive disorders.
- phobias.
- alcohol dependence (fluoxetine).
- eating disorders.
- chronic severe pain, especially in migraine headaches, cancer, and severe arthritis (nortriptyline).

SIDE EFFECTS

Not serious:
Dizziness on changing position; drowsiness; mild tiredness or weakness; dry mouth; headache; increased appetite or cravings; weight gain; nausea or, less frequently, diarrhea; increased sweating or insomnia; photosensitivity. Let your doctor know if these symptoms persist or become troublesome.

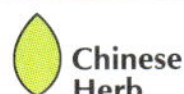

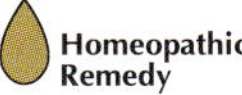

Serious:
Blurred vision, confusion, delirium, hallucinations; paralytic ileus (blockage of intestines, possibly indicated by abdominal pain or swelling, difficulty in breathing, and severe constipation), difficulty in urination, eye pain from aggravated glaucoma, tremors, changes in heartbeat, nervousness, restlessness, Parkinson's-like symptoms (shuffling walk, stiffness in the extremities). Rarely: allergic reactions, skin rash or spots, bruising or bleeding, jaundice, sore throat, fever, ringing in the ears. Call your doctor immediately if you notice these symptoms. You may be reacting to the drug or taking too much.

SPECIAL INFORMATION

- Antidepressants may cause drowsiness. When taking these drugs, use care while driving, operating machinery, or performing tasks that require mental alertness.
- These drugs, especially fluoxetine, can trigger manic attacks in individuals with manic-depression. Be sure to tell your doctor if you have manic-depression.
- Antidepressants can affect blood sugar (glucose tolerance) tests by causing fluctuation in blood sugar levels.
- Fluoxetine may exacerbate suicidal tendencies in some individuals. Be sure to tell your healthcare provider if you have experienced thoughts of suicide or believe you may be susceptible to such thoughts. The doctor may want to prescribe a different drug.
- The full effects of an antidepressant drug may not occur for several weeks.
- If you are pregnant, nursing, or planning a pregnancy, check with your doctor before taking antidepressants.

POSSIBLE INTERACTIONS

Alcohol and other drugs that depress the central nervous system: increased antidepressant effects, leading to problems such as respiratory depression or very low blood pressure.

Anticoagulant drugs (such as warfarin): Tricyclic antidepressants may increase the anticlotting activity.

Anticonvulsants: decreased effectiveness of anticonvulsants, making seizures more likely.

Antihistamines: increased antihistamine action, including any side effects; antihistamines may also increase the action of antidepressants, including any side effects.

Barbiturates: decreased effectiveness of tricyclic antidepressants.

Digitalis preparations: using fluoxetine or sertraline with heart medications may increase blood levels of both the antidepressant and the heart drugs, increasing the risk of side effects.

Lithium: taking fluoxetine or sertraline with lithium could increase blood levels of lithium, leading to toxicity.

MAO inhibitors: severe, possibly fatal reactions such as seizures, tremor, and coma because of additive effects of the drugs.

Other antidepressants: combining antidepressants will likely increase the action of one or both drugs, leading to increased side effects.

Thyroid medications: combining tricyclic antidepressants with thyroid drugs may increase the effects, including side effects, of both medications.

ANTIDIABETIC DRUGS

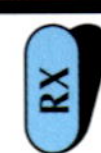

GENERIC NAMES
acarbose, insulin, metformin

Oral Hypoglycemics: glipizide, glyburide

GENERAL DESCRIPTION
The specific medication used to treat diabetes depends on which type of the disease you have. Oral hypoglycemics and other drugs are prescribed for non-insulin-dependent diabetes, commonly known as Type 2 diabetes. Insulin-dependent diabetes (Type 1) can be controlled only through injections of insulin, a hormone normally produced by the pancreas. A program of diet and exercise, used in conjunction with antidiabetic drugs, is vital to controlling both types of the disease.

Oral hypoglycemic drugs stimulate the release of existing insulin in people whose bodies are capable of producing insulin. These drugs do not lower blood sugar on their own but work with a prescribed regimen of diet and exercise to perform effectively. Other drugs, such as acarbose and metformin, may be prescribed to help decrease blood sugar levels.

Injected insulin provides necessary amounts of insulin in people whose bodies are not capable of producing the chemical. Insulin does lower blood sugar by itself, although it works most effectively in combination with a prescribed program of diet and exercise. For more information, including facts about side effects and possible interactions with other medications, see ***Glipizide, Glyburide, Insulin,*** and ***Oral Hypoglycemics.***

ANTIDIARRHEAL DRUGS

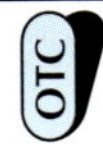

GENERIC NAMES
attapulgite, bismuth subsalicylate, loperamide

GENERAL DESCRIPTION
Over-the-counter antidiarrheal drugs are used for the short-term control and symptomatic relief of diarrhea. Diarrhea can vary in intensity from mild (3 to 4 loose, watery stools a day) to severe (10 or more per day), and may be accompanied by weakness, flatulence, pain, fever, or vomiting.

Antidiarrheal drugs work in different ways. Attapulgite, a claylike substance, binds and inactivates the intestinal irritants that are causing the problem. Bismuth subsalicylate and loperamide seem to stop diarrhea and cramps by slowing down the movements and contractions of the intestinal tract. For more information, see entries for the generic drugs listed above.

TARGET AILMENTS

- acute diarrhea: the sudden onset of loose stools in an otherwise healthy person. The cause may be infectious, toxic, dietary, drug induced, or the result of various ailments. Infectious diarrhea, especially in children in the United States, is usually viral in origin.
- traveler's diarrhea: a form of acute infectious diarrhea afflicting tourists in foreign lands. It is usually caused by various bacteria found in contaminated food or water.
- chronic diarrhea: persistent or recurrent bouts of diarrhea associated with inflammatory bowel disease.

SIDE EFFECTS

When used at the recommended dosage for no more than two days, these drugs rarely cause side effects.

Not serious:
You may experience mild constipation. Bismuth subsalicylate sometimes causes a harmless grayish black stool and a darkened tongue. Check with your doctor if the diarrhea does not decrease after one or two days, or if you develop a fever.

Serious:
Bismuth subsalicylate can be toxic if taken in very large doses. See overdose symptoms below. Although very rare, the following side effects of loperamide might indicate a more dangerous bowel problem: constipation, bloating, loss of appetite, and stomach pain with vomiting and nausea. Call your doctor promptly if you develop any of these, or a skin rash.

SPECIAL INFORMATION

- It is possible to take too much over-the-counter medication. Symptoms of bismuth subsalicylate overdose include anxiety, confusion, depression, fast or deep breathing, headache, sweating, muscle spasms or weakness, nausea, vomiting, stomach pain, ringing in the ears, and trembling. Check with your doctor immediately.
- Diarrhea can cause excessive fluid loss. Call your doctor as soon as possible if you have any signs of dehydration, including decreased urination, lightheadedness and dizziness, wrinkled skin, dryness of mouth, or increased thirst.
- When you use antidiarrheal drugs, it is vitally important that you replace lost fluids by drinking large quantities of water and other clear liquids (such as decaffeinated colas and tea, ginger ale, and broth). Eat only gelatin for the first 24 hours. The next day you may eat bland foods, such as bread, crackers, cooked cereals, and applesauce. Other beverages and foods may make the condition worse.
- Antidiarrheals are not recommended for children under three years of age or for geriatric patients. If used, follow your doctor's instructions.
- Do not use antidiarrheals if you have a fever or your stool contains blood or mucus: These are symptoms of dysentery, an infection of the lower intestinal tract. Contact your doctor.
- Antidiarrheal drugs have different functions. Some combat the symptoms of diarrhea; some are directed against the cause; and others try to counter some of the effects of the ailment. A number of antidiarrheal drugs are available only by prescription. If over-the-counter medications do not solve the problem, see your doctor.

POSSIBLE INTERACTIONS

Alcohol, sleeping pills, and tranquilizers: may increase depressant and sedative effects.

Antibiotics and narcotic pain medicine: may cause severe constipation if taken with antidiarrheals.

ANTIFUNGAL DRUGS

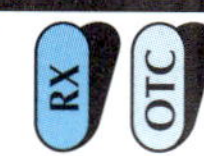

GENERIC NAMES

Rx: clotrimazole, ketoconazole, miconazole, terconazole

OTC: clotrimazole, ketoconazole, miconazole, tolnaftate

GENERAL DESCRIPTION

Antifungal drugs are used to treat a wide variety of conditions, including fungal infections of the skin, lungs, mouth, groin, hands, feet, and nails. Ringworm infections, including athlete's foot and jock itch, are among the best-known groups of skin disorders for which these drugs are used. Some antifungal medications are also used to treat yeast infections of the mouth (oral thrush); skin folds and hands; urethra, penis and foreskin (balanitis); and vagina.

Antifungal drugs work in different ways to interfere with the growth and reproduction of fungal cells or, in strong concentrations, to destroy fungal cells. These medications can be topical, vaginal, or systemic (acting throughout the body), and are available as creams, suppositories, lotions, powders, sprays, shampoos, lozenges, and oral tablets. For more information, see entries for the generic drugs listed above. Also see ***Vaginal Antifungal Drugs*** for information about a subclass of medications commonly used to treat vaginal yeast infections.

TARGET AILMENTS

- yeast infections (candidiasis) of the vulva and vagina, mouth, skin, hands, and internal organs.
- ringworm (tinea) of the body, scalp, nails, hands, feet (athlete's foot), and groin (jock itch); also, tinea versicolor, a ringworm infection that produces white-brown patches on the skin.
- fungal diseases of the lungs.
- fungal skin infections (tropical).
- seborrheic dermatitis; dandruff.

SIDE EFFECTS

Not serious:
Mild skin irritation in the infected area; headache, drowsiness, dizziness, nausea or vomiting, stomach pain, constipation or diarrhea. Call your doctor if these side effects persist or become bothersome.

Serious:
Topical preparations may cause an allergic skin reaction, such as a rash or hives. Vaginal preparations may cause redness, stinging, burning, or itching of the genitals; abdominal cramps or menstrual irregularities; or itching and burning of a sexual partner's penis. Call your doctor if you experience any of these side effects.

SPECIAL INFORMATION

- Do not use any topical antifungal medications if you have had an allergic reaction to another drug of this type. Check first with your physician or pharmacist.
- Although ringworm medications are available in over-the-counter form, be sure your condition has been correctly diagnosed before treating it yourself.
- Vaginal antifungal creams and suppositories are inserted directly into the vagina, usually at bedtime, for a period of one to seven days.
- Systemic antifungal medications (ketoconazole) are available in oral suspension and tablet form. They are used to treat a variety of disorders, including pneumonia and urinary tract infections.
- Topical lotions, creams, powders, and sprays are applied directly to the skin to treat fungal skin infections.
- Because they are massaged into the skin, creams and ointments are more effective than sprays and powders for the treatment of skin infections. Be sure to wash and thoroughly dry the infected area before use.
- Spray and powder forms of antifungal medications are effective in preventing fungal skin infections.
- It is very important to medicate the entire area when treating an active fungal infection. If you have athlete's foot, for example, you need to apply the medication between all toes, to the skin around each toenail, and to the sole of the foot. Both feet should be treated with the same thorough care.
- Pregnant and nursing women should avoid antifungal medications, unless administered under a doctor's care.
- Because fungi thrive in moist conditions, avoid tight-fitting shoes and underwear made with synthetic fibers during treatment; wear cotton underwear instead.

POSSIBLE INTERACTIONS

No interactions are expected with most topical and vaginal forms of antifungal drugs. See ***Ketoconazole*** for a list of drugs and other substances you should avoid while taking systemic antifungal medications.

A

ANTIGASTROESOPHAGEAL REFLUX DRUGS

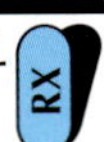

GENERAL DESCRIPTION

Drugs in this class target gastroesophageal reflux disease, a digestive disorder affecting the lower esophageal sphincter, the muscle that connects the esophagus to the stomach. The condition results when stomach contents back up into the esophagus, causing the unpleasant sensations known as heartburn and acid indigestion. The problem, which often occurs during pregnancy and is more common in middle age, can usually be corrected through alterations in your diet and meal schedule. Eating shortly before bedtime, for example, is more likely to produce the disorder than eating several hours earlier.

Antigastroesophageal reflux drugs act by strengthening the lower esophageal sphincter to inhibit backflow, and by speeding up the emptying of stomach contents into the intestines. Medications known as histamine H_2 blockers, a subclass of antiulcer drugs, are also used to treat chronic gastroesophageal reflux. For information about these drugs, see ***Histamine H_2 Blockers,*** as well as individual entries for ***Cimetidine, Famotidine, Nizatidine,*** and ***Ranitidine.***

ANTIHISTAMINES

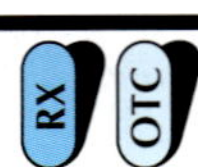

GENERIC NAMES

Rx: diphenhydramine, loratadine, promethazine

OTC: brompheniramine, chlorpheniramine, clemastine, dexbrompheniramine, diphenhydramine, doxylamine, triprolidine

GENERAL DESCRIPTION

Antihistamines block the action of histamine, a natural substance the body releases when fighting infection and in allergic reactions; histamine causes the runny nose, watery eyes, congestion, and hives or itching associated with allergies. Antihistamines are used primarily to relieve the symptoms of allergies and colds, although they cannot cure the underlying conditions. Since a common side effect of these drugs is drowsiness, some antihistamines are used as sleeping aids. See entries for generic drugs listed above for additional information.

TARGET AILMENTS

- nasal and respiratory allergies (seasonal and nonseasonal), including hay fever.
- the common cold (although antihistamines alone are not effective for most cold symptoms).
- allergic skin reactions (to poison ivy, insect bites, or drugs, for example).
- insomnia (though not astemizole, loratadine, and terfenadine).
- motion sickness (diphenhydramine and promethazine).

SIDE EFFECTS

Not serious:
Drowsiness in varying degrees—avoid driving or operating machinery until you know how the antihistamine you are taking affects you; dizziness, weakness, and slower movement and reaction time; dryness of the mouth, nose, or throat; nervousness, restlessness, and insomnia, especially in children; upset stomach, nausea, and change in bowel habits.

Serious:
In rare cases, cetirizine and loratadine may cause fainting or irregular heart rhythms that can be life-threatening. Call your doctor immediately if you notice any change in your heartbeat.

Skin reactions (itchiness, rash, inflammation) are an uncommon side effect of topical antihistamines. If you think antihistamines are causing these symptoms, discontinue use and tell your doctor.

SPECIAL INFORMATION

- Antihistamines are considered unsafe for women who are pregnant or nursing.
- Many antihistamines are considered unsafe for children under the age of 12. Some are appropriate if the child's dosage is determined by a physician or, in the case of OTC drugs, printed on the label. Children may be more susceptible to side effects than adults.
- To avoid drowsiness, take less of the drug or try another antihistamine. Some antihistamines, such as cetirizine and loratadine, do not cause drowsiness, and over time you may develop a partial tolerance to the drugs that do.
- Some antihistamines, especially loratadine, may cause palpitations, fainting, cardiac arrest, or other serious heart disorders if taken in dosages that are even slightly higher than those recommended. Follow the dosage instructions carefully.
- If antihistamines give you an upset stomach, nausea, diarrhea, or other gastrointestinal problems, take the pills with meals or with milk.
- Check with your doctor before using antihistamines if you have asthma, glaucoma, an enlarged prostate, a stomach ulcer, a bladder obstruction, or liver disease; the drugs may exacerbate these conditions.

POSSIBLE INTERACTIONS

Alcohol: likely to increase the sedative effects of certain antihistamines; do not drink when you take these drugs.

Antianxiety drugs; barbiturates or other sedatives: do not take with antihistamines, as the combination may result in excessive sedation.

Clarithromycin, erythromycin, itraconazole, and ketoconazole: may interfere with the body's metabolism of loratadine and cause life-threatening cardiac problems. WARNING: Do not combine these drugs with loratadine.

MAO inhibitors: can cause hypotension and dryness of the respiratory passages when taken with antihistamines. Do not combine these with antihistamines.

ANTIHYPERTENSIVE DRUGS

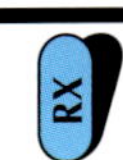

GENERAL DESCRIPTION

Antihypertensives are drugs used to control high blood pressure (hypertension) in the 40 million Americans who have this disorder. The particular antihypertensive drug that is used depends, in part, on the severity of the condition.

Antihypertensive medications include diuretics; calcium channel blockers; angiotensin-converting enzyme (ACE) inhibitors; and sympathetic nerve inhibitors, which act either centrally (in the brain) or peripherally (in the blood vessels) to block signals from the brain that tell the arteries to constrict.

For information on specific generic drugs used to treat high blood pressure, see ***Guanfacine*** and ***Valsartan.*** Also see ***Alpha$_1$-Adrenergic Blockers, Angiotensin-Converting Enzyme (ACE) Inhibitors, Beta-Adrenergic Blockers, Calcium Channel Blockers,*** and ***Diuretics.***

ANTI-INSOMNIA DRUGS

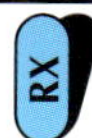

GENERAL DESCRIPTION

The anti-insomnia drug class (sometimes called the sedative-hypnotic class) includes a large number of drugs used in the treatment of sleeping problems. Since insomnia is often related to psychological or physical disorders, the choice of medication will depend on the underlying condition. Certain benzodiazepines, a subclass of antianxiety drugs, are often prescribed for people in acute distress, although diphenhydramine, an antihistamine, may be an acceptable milder alternative. Antipsychotic and antidepressant drugs with sedative effects are also used if warranted. For information on a nonbenzodiazepine sleeping pill prescribed for the short-term relief of insomnia in adults, see ***Zolpidem***.

ANTI-ITCH DRUGS

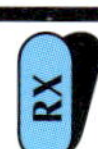

GENERAL DESCRIPTION

Anti-itch drugs include antihistamines that have antipruritic, or anti-itch, properties. These medications are used to relieve itching due to allergies or anxiety-induced skin irritations. For more information on a specific generic drug used to treat itching, see ***Hydroxyzine.***

ANTIMIGRAINE DRUGS

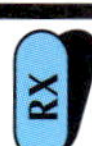

GENERAL DESCRIPTION

Antimigraine drugs are used to treat classic migraine headaches (those preceded by the warning sensation known as an aura) as well as common migraines (those without an aura). If you suffer from more than three migraine headaches per month, your doctor may suggest that you regularly take drugs that help prevent migraine attacks, such as beta-adrenergic blockers, calcium channel blockers, anti-inflammatory drugs, or antidepressants. If you have only one or two mild-to-moderate migraines per month, your doctor may recommend that you take vasoconstrictive drugs, anti-inflammatory medications, or opioid analgesics at the first sign of a headache.

The most effective drugs for the relief of migraine pain are the vasoconstrictors, which work by narrowing dilated blood vessels and thereby reducing the amount of blood flowing through them. Swollen cranial blood vessels are believed to be a major cause of migraine headaches. For more information on a specific generic drug used to treat migraines, see ***Sumatriptan***.

ANTINAUSEA DRUGS

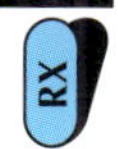

GENERAL DESCRIPTION

The antinausea drug class (sometimes called the antiemetic class) includes a large number of drugs used in the control of nausea and vomiting. These uncomfortable symptoms may be caused by or associated with a number of factors, ranging from motion sickness to psychosis. Appropriate treatment is determined by the cause of the nausea and by the needs and condition of the individual. See ***Prochlorperazine*** for information on a specific drug that is sometimes prescribed for short bouts of flulike nausea but is usually used to control severe nausea induced by surgery, radiation therapy, chemotherapy, and other drugs.

ANTI-PARKINSONISM DRUGS

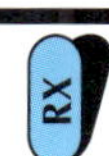

GENERAL DESCRIPTION

Anti-Parkinsonism drugs are used to control the trembling, stiffness, and other symptoms that characterize Parkinson's disease, a neurological disorder that causes a gradual degeneration of nerve cells in the portion of the midbrain that controls body movements. The disease can be brought on by viral infections or exposure to environmental poisons such as carbon monoxide and manganese, but in most cases the cause is unknown.

Anti-Parkinsonism drugs work by supplying the brain with dopamine, a necessary chemical that Parkinson's patients have in deficient amounts. Dopamine is critical for proper transmission of the nerve impulses that control muscle movement. For more information on a specific generic drug used to treat Parkinson's disease, see ***Levodopa.***

ANTISEPTICS

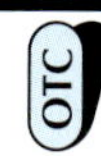

GENERAL DESCRIPTION

Antiseptics are generally used to inhibit the growth of bacteria and reduce the likelihood of infection. These drugs are most often used topically to cleanse minor cuts, scrapes, and burns and rid them of germs. Antiseptics are usually combined with one another or with other ingredients, such as alcohol, iodine, hydrogen peroxide, thymol, benzocaine, eucalyptol, menthol, methyl salicylate, or camphor. Depending on the other chemicals in the combination, antiseptic preparations may also have analgesic or local anesthetic properties, temporarily reducing pain and itching where applied on the skin. Such preparations are sometimes used to relieve the discomfort associated with poison ivy rashes, insect bites, toothaches, teething, fever blisters, and other soreness of the gums and mouth.

When used according to package labels, side effects are extremely rare, although antiseptics should never be swallowed, used near the eyes, or used to treat diaper rash. For more information on a specific generic antiseptic drug, see ***Phenol.***

ANTISPASMODIC DRUGS

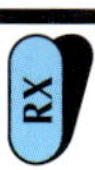

GENERAL DESCRIPTION

Antispasmodic drugs reduce muscle spasms in the gastrointestinal tract, airways, bladder, and urethra. They are used to treat many disorders, including asthma, urinary incontinence, motion sickness, irritable bowel syndrome, infant colic, and peptic ulcers. The drugs work by preventing involuntary muscle contractions and inhibiting glandular secretions (such as saliva, bronchial mucus, and stomach acids). For information about a drug used to reduce muscle spasms in the gastrointestinal tract, see ***Dicyclomine.***

ANTIULCER DRUGS

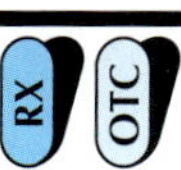

GENERIC NAMES

omeprazole, sucralfate

A

Histamine H_2 Blockers: cimetidine, famotidine, nizatidine, ranitidine

GENERAL DESCRIPTION

Antiulcer drugs are used to treat disorders associated with the overproduction of stomach acid, such as gastritis, gastroesophageal reflux, multiple endocrine neoplasia, Zollinger-Ellison syndrome, and, most commonly, ulcers of the stomach and duodenum (first portion of the small intestine). In general, antiulcer drugs work by inhibiting the production of the stomach's digestive juices, most notably hydrochloric acid and the digestive enzyme pepsin. Individual drugs achieve this effect in different ways.

Medications among the subclass of antiulcer drugs known as histamine H_2 blockers (including cimetidine, famotidine, nizatidine, and ranitidine) block the stomach's response to the chemical compound histamine, thereby reducing the secretion of hydrochloric acid. The drug omeprazole reduces the production of hydrochloric acid by inhibiting the action of enzymes in the acid-producing cells of the stomach lining. The exact mechanism of sucralfate is not completely understood, but the drug is believed to inhibit the digestive action of pepsin. It may also form a coating over stomach and duodenal ulcers, protecting them from the erosive effect of hydrochloric acid.

TARGET AILMENTS

- duodenal ulcer; gastric ulcer.
- upper gastrointestinal bleeding associated with gastric ulcer or duodenal ulcer, or with gastritis.
- Zollinger-Ellison syndrome, multiple endocrine neoplasia, and other conditions characterized by an overproduction of stomach acid.
- gastroesophageal reflux.
- gastrointestinal symptoms associated with the use of nonsteroidal anti-inflammatory drugs (NSAIDs) and aspirin.

SIDE EFFECTS

The side effects of the various antiulcer medications differ from drug to drug, and may include the following.

Not serious:
Rare or infrequent: dizziness, lightheadedness, constipation, mild drowsiness, headache, mild diarrhea, skin rash, itching or other skin problems, muscle or joint pain, hair loss, temporary impotence and decreased libido, breast enlargement and tenderness (in women or men), abdominal pain, heartburn, indigestion, nausea, gas, appetite loss, dry mouth or skin, insomnia, depression or anxiety.

Serious:
Unusual bruising or bleeding, unusual fatigue, rapid or irregular heartbeat, delirium or hallucinations, shortness of breath, bronchospasm (tightness in the chest), confusion, vomiting, numbness or tingling in the fingers or toes, jaundice, mouth ulcers, inflammation of the pancreas (severe abdominal pain accompanied by vomiting or fever), black, tarry stools (sign of internal bleeding), vomit the consistency of coffee grounds, combined weakness, fever, and sore throat (signs of bone marrow depression). If any of these effects occur, contact your doctor immediately.

SPECIAL INFORMATION

- Do not take these medications if you have had any unusual or allergic reaction to an antiulcer drug in the past.
- Avoid antiulcer drugs if you are pregnant or nursing.
- Be sure to inform your doctor if you have any other medical problems, especially kidney or liver disease or any disease that causes obstruction of the gastrointestinal tract.
- Antiulcer drugs can interfere with the accuracy of some laboratory tests. Be sure to tell the person giving you a lab test that you are taking one of these drugs.
- Remember that some medications—such as aspirin and nonsteroidal anti-inflammatory drugs (NSAIDs)—and certain foods and drinks, including citrus products and beverages that are carbonated, alcoholic, or caffeinated, may irritate your stomach and make your problem worse.
- Check with your doctor before using antacids concurrently with an antiulcer drug.

POSSIBLE INTERACTIONS

Antiulcer drugs interact with many prescription and over-the-counter medications, some of which are listed below. Be sure to inform your doctor of any other drugs you may be taking.

Alcohol, caffeine, carbonated drinks, citrus foods, tobacco: may stimulate secretion of stomach acid and slow ulcer recovery rate; drinking alcoholic beverages while taking a histamine H_2 blocker may also increase blood levels of alcohol.

Alprazolam, carbamazepine, diazepam, digitalis preparations, glipizide, metoprolol, oral anticoagulants (including aspirin, dipyridamole, heparin): histamine H_2 blockers may increase the effects and possibly the toxicity of these drugs.

Antacids: reduced effects of antiulcer drugs. Sometimes switching to another type of antacid or taking the antacid and the antiulcer drug at different times of the day can eliminate this problem. Consult your doctor. Avoid aluminum-containing antacids while taking sucralfate; the combination may lead to weakening of the bones and other symptoms of aluminum toxicity.

Aspirin: stomach irritation.

Cimetidine, ciprofloxacin, digoxin, ofloxacin, phenytoin, ranitidine, tetracycline, theophylline, warfarin: sucralfate may decrease the effectiveness of these drugs; omeprazole may increase the effects of phenytoin and warfarin.

Iron: absorption of iron into the body may be inhibited by omeprazole.

Ketoconazole: omeprazole and histamine H_2 blockers may inhibit the absorption of ketoconazole into the body.

ANTIVIRAL DRUGS

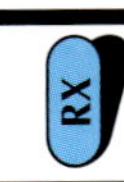

GENERAL DESCRIPTION

Antivirals, a class of drugs introduced in recent decades, are used to treat viral infections ranging from the flu to herpes and AIDS. Each antiviral medication is usually effective against only one virus, although in some cases a single antiviral drug is useful against several organisms in a viral class. (Because viruses differ greatly from bacteria, antibiotics do not work against viral diseases.) For more information, see ***AIDS Treatment*** and ***Acyclovir***.

APIS

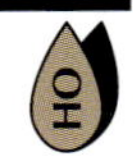

LATIN NAME

Apis mellifica

GENERAL DESCRIPTION

The medicinal value of *Apis,* the scientific name for the honeybee, may date to ancient Egypt, where bees were a symbol of power, wealth, and health. Egyptian doctors revered honey over all other healing substances, and extensive methods of beekeeping were already in practice in 4000 B.C. It is not the honey but the bee itself, however, that is used in homeopathic medicine.

This remedy is made from the body

of the honeybee; it is used to treat those patients whose ailments are accompanied by symptoms similar to the results of a bee sting, for example redness and swelling, and also patients who express behavior considered beelike, such as restlessness or irritability. To prepare this remedy, the entire live honeybee is crushed and highly diluted by mixing it into a water-alcohol base.

For more information on homeopathic medicine, see page 1027.

TARGET AILMENTS

- bites and stings, especially those that swell and burn or itch; conjunctivitis; edema (accumulation of fluids in body tissues) and conditions of general swelling such as hives and food allergies; headaches that include sudden, stabbing pains; red, swollen joints; mumps. (Take internally.)

PREPARATIONS

Apis is available over the counter in various potencies, in both liquid and tablet form, at selected stores and pharmacies or from your homeopathic practitioner. Consult your practitioner for more precise dosage information.

SIDE EFFECTS

None expected.

APRICOT SEED

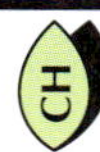

LATIN NAME

Prunus armeniaca

GENERAL DESCRIPTION

Practitioners of Chinese medicine frequently use the inner kernel of apricots to relieve bronchial ailments. These seeds, also known as bitter almonds, are believed to serve as an expectorant, expelling mucus from the lungs, and also as an agent to stop coughing. In addition apricot seeds are prescribed as a laxative. In traditional Chinese medicine, apricot seeds are classified as bitter and slightly warm.

TARGET AILMENTS

- coughing and wheezing, bronchitis, asthma, emphysema, constipation. (Take internally.)

PREPARATIONS

Apricot seeds or decoctions such as cough syrups are available at Chinese pharmacies, Asian markets, and Western health food stores.

Combinations: Chinese medicine practitioners recommend treating dry coughs with apricot seed and either white mulberry leaf or a tuber known as ophiopogon. The choice, depending on the nature of the cough, should be made in consultation with an herbalist, who can give you information on specific dosages and other herbal combinations.

SIDE EFFECTS

Serious:

Excessive doses can lead to dizziness, nausea, vomiting, and headache, and this, in turn, can progress to spasms, dilated pupils, erratic heartbeat, coma, and death.

SPECIAL INFORMATION

- WARNING: Patients should take care with this herb, since it includes a poisonous substance. In the human body, the components of apricot seed break down into several products, including prussic acid, which is highly toxic. Chinese herbalists have reported that a dose of 50 to 60 kernels of apricot seed can kill adults, while just 10 kernels can be fatal in children. Activated charcoal and syrup of ipecac are recommended as antidotes to overdoses.
- Use caution in using apricot seed to treat children or patients with diarrhea.
- In a clinical experiment, a paste of apricot seed and sugar seemed to benefit patients with chronic bronchitis. Some users, however, suffered bouts of headache and nausea.

POSSIBLE INTERACTIONS

Some Chinese medicine practitioners believe that apricot seeds should not be taken in combination with astragalus, skullcap, or kudzu root.

ARNICA

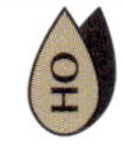

LATIN NAME

Arnica montana

GENERAL DESCRIPTION

Arnica, sometimes called mountain daisy, grows wild across the higher elevations of Europe, northern Asia, and parts of the United States. Mountain climbers in the Alps have traditionally chewed arnica after a long day's hike to relieve muscle aches. Homeopathic practitioners prescribe *Arnica* for bruises, sprains, strains, and other types of accidents that are sudden and may induce shock. The flowers, leaves, stem, and root of arnica are crushed to a pulp and soaked in alcohol; they then undergo the homeopathic dilution process, which renders the substance nontoxic.

For more information on homeopathic medicine, see page 1027.

TARGET AILMENTS

Take internally for:

- blood blisters caused by a blow to the affected area; broken bones, sprains, strains, and other sudden injuries with swelling, tenderness, and pain, where posttrauma shock is a threat.
- bruises, especially if *Arnica* is given before the skin begins to turn black and blue; sore and swollen joints, as in rheumatism; head pain; pain and swelling after surgery; toothache and pain from dental work.
- groin strain.

PREPARATIONS

Arnica is available over the counter in various potencies, in both tablet and liquid form, at selected stores and pharmacies. Consult your practitioner for more precise information.

SIDE EFFECTS

None expected.

ARSENICUM ALBUM

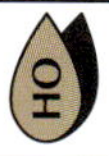

LATIN NAME

Arsenicum album

GENERAL DESCRIPTION

This remedy, also called *Ars alb* by homeopathic practitioners, is an extremely dilute form of arsenic, a metallic poison derived from the chemical element of the same name. Weak preparations of arsenic have had a history of medicinal use; but slow accumulation of the element in body tissues can cause chronic poisoning, leading to gastrointestinal disorders, nausea, dehydration, and even paralysis and death. In step with the homeopathic theory that like cures like, *Ars alb* is preferred by practitioners to treat patients with various digestive complaints that are accompanied by signs of dehydration and burning pains, the same symptoms that are induced by *Ars alb.*

In its homeopathic form, arsenic is separated from other metals like iron, cobalt, and nickel by baking at high temperatures. The extracted powder is

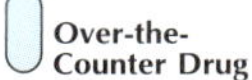

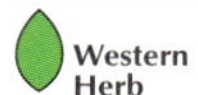

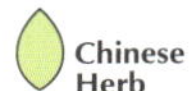

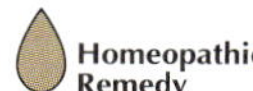

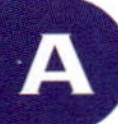

then finely ground and weakened by mixing successively greater amounts of milk sugar with the poison.

For more information on homeopathic medicine, see page 1027.

TARGET AILMENTS

- angina; anxiety disorders and panic attacks; asthma; hay fever; burns that form blisters; chronic skin problems; high fevers accompanied by chills; recurrent headaches; dry, hacking coughs; colds accompanied by excessive, watery nasal discharge and frequent sneezing; colitis, indigestion, food poisoning; Crohn's disease, influenza, insomnia, and exhaustion brought on by an illness and coupled with restlessness. (Take internally.)

PREPARATIONS

Ars alb is available over the counter in various potencies, in both liquid and tablet form, at selected stores and pharmacies. Consult your practitioner for more precise information.

SIDE EFFECTS

None expected.

ASHWAGANDA

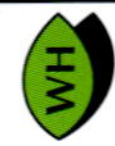

LATIN NAME

Withania somnifera

GENERAL DESCRIPTION

Identified by clusters of tiny green-and-yellow flowers, this small shrub from India is believed to strengthen the body and to serve as a source of energy. Sought after for its roots, leaves, and berries, ashwaganda is thought to aid in restoring muscles, body tissues, and bone marrow. It is commonly prescribed as a medicinal supplement for people recovering from an illness or suffering from excessive fatigue. Ashwaganda also has a reputation as an aphrodisiac, and according to tradition, it is believed to help prevent male sterility and other sexual ailments.

TARGET AILMENTS

- loss of muscular strength, multiple sclerosis, rheumatism, fatigue, infertility, sexual debility, indigestion, heart disease, male sterility, hay fever. (Take internally.)
- carbuncles, inflammations, swelling, sores. (Apply medicated oil externally.)
- ringworm. (Apply a compress to the affected area.)

PREPARATIONS

Over the counter:
Available as tincture, dried roots and leaves, powder.

At home:
Tea: Boil 1 oz ashwaganda root in 1 cup water for 15 to 20 minutes. Drink up to 2 cups a day.

Milk decoction: Combine 1 oz ashwaganda root, 1 cup milk, and 4 cups water. Heat over low flame for 30 minutes to two hours, until water evaporates. Drink 2 cups daily. Add honey, raw sugar, or syrup to sweeten.

Medicated oil: Combine 2 oz crushed ashwaganda leaves, 1 cup castor oil, and 4 cups water. Heat over low flame for four to eight hours, until water is evaporated.

Compress: Soak a clean cloth in the tea and apply directly to the affected area.

SPECIAL INFORMATION

- Do not eat ashwaganda berries. They may cause severe gastrointestinal pain.
- Do not use ashwaganda if you are pregnant.

ASPIRIN

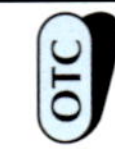

DRUG CLASSES

Analgesics; Anticoagulant and Antiplatelet Drugs

BRAND NAMES

Alka-Seltzer Plus Cold Medicine, Anacin Caplets, Bayer (various forms), Bufferin (various forms), Ecotrin, Excedrin Extra-Strength

GENERAL DESCRIPTION

Since its introduction in 1899, aspirin has become one of the most popular over-the-counter pain relievers, used for headache, arthritis, muscle aches, and minor injuries. Aspirin also suppresses fever, and as an anti-inflammatory medication it reduces inflammation associated with menstrual cramps, arthritis, bursitis, and other conditions.

As an antiplatelet drug, aspirin is used once a day in very low dosages to reduce the risk of heart attack, stroke, and postsurgical problems that can develop when a blood vessel is obstructed by blood clots. It may be used alone or in combination with dipyridamole or one of the anticoagulant drugs. Aspirin works by preventing the production of thromboxane, a powerful stimulator of blood platelet activation. For more information, see ***Anticoagulant and Antiplatelet Drugs*** and ***Analgesics.***

SIDE EFFECTS

Not serious:
Aspirin can sometimes cause stomach irritation, but for four out of five people this side effect is minimal if the drug is used as prescribed.

Serious:
Gastric ulceration (black or bloody stools, stomach pain, vomiting of blood). In large doses, aspirin can cause ringing in the ears, hearing loss, headache, dizziness, and nausea. Discontinue use and call your doctor.

SPECIAL INFORMATION

- Aspirin may increase the chance of excessive bleeding in some people. Do not take aspirin to prevent stroke, heart attack, or blood clots unless it has been prescribed by your doctor.
- Do not give aspirin to children or teenagers with fevers. Aspirin can provoke a potentially fatal liver inflammation called Reye's syndrome in young people if the drug is used to treat a fever or viral infection such as chickenpox or influenza.
- Pregnant and nursing women should not use aspirin.
- Before any type of surgery, let your doctor or dentist know if you use aspirin regularly for its antiplatelet action. Your doctor may tell you to discontinue aspirin during the week or two before surgery.

ASTHMA THERAPY

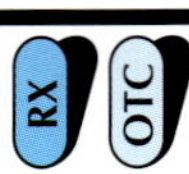

GENERAL DESCRIPTION

Asthma therapy involves the use of several classes of prescription and over-the-counter drugs to relieve the symptoms associated with asthma. While none of these drugs represents a cure, each can be effective in alleviating symptoms that interfere with normal breathing. Some of these drugs are used for acute asthma attacks, while others are taken for long-term therapy. For information on a specific asthma drug, see ***Cromolyn.*** Also see ***Bronchodilators*** and ***Corticosteroids,*** as well as the individual entries for the corticosteroid drugs ***Beclomethasone, Prednisone,*** and ***Triamcinolone.***

ASTRAGALUS

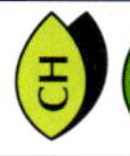

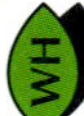

LATIN NAME
Astragalus membranaceus

GENERAL DESCRIPTION
The perennial plant astragalus, or milk-vetch root, has sprawling stems and pale-yellow blooms. Western herbalists believe that substances known as polysaccharides in this herb stimulate the immune system and generally strengthen the body, speeding metabolism, promoting tissue regeneration, and increasing energy. In traditional Chinese medicine astragalus is regarded as sweet and slightly warm.

TARGET AILMENTS
Chinese:
- chronic colds, general weakness and fatigue, loss of appetite, spontaneous perspiration, diarrhea, blood abnormalities or deficiencies resulting from excessive bleeding. (Take internally.)

Western:
- chronic colds and flu, AIDS, cancer, and chronic fatigue. (Take internally in conjunction with conventional medical treatment.)

PREPARATIONS
Over the counter:
Astragalus is available as prepared tea, fluidextract, capsules, dried root.

At home:
Chinese: Combine 1 part honey, 4 parts dried root, and a small amount of water in a wok. Allow mixture to simmer until the water evaporates and the herbs are slightly brown.

Combinations: For spontaneous perspiration, astragalus is mixed with Asian ginseng. As an immune system stimulant, the herb is combined with siler. Blood abnormalities are treated with a mix of astragalus and dong quai. Herbalists combine astragalus and atractylodes (white) for diarrhea. Astragalus with rhubarb root and bupleurum is aimed at uterine disorders.

Western:
Tea: Boil 1 oz astragalus root in 1 cup of water for 15 to 20 minutes.

SIDE EFFECTS
None expected.

SPECIAL INFORMATION:
- Pregnant women should check with their practitioners before using.
- Astragalus has been used for centuries in *fu-zheng* therapy, the treatment of ailments by strengthening the body's natural defense mechanisms. The concept of fu-zheng therapy was recently acknowledged by Western medical researchers who examined astragalus's effect on the immune system of cancer patients undergoing chemotherapy and radiation. Although not conclusive, the results of these studies suggest that astragalus had a positive effect on these cancer patients. Check with your doctor before using astragalus in this capacity.

ATENOLOL

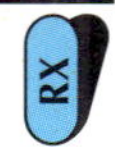

DRUG CLASS
Beta-Adrenergic Blockers

BRAND NAME
Tenormin

GENERAL DESCRIPTION
Introduced in 1973, atenolol is a beta blocking drug prescribed to help manage angina, high blood pressure (hypertension), and heart attack (myocardial infarction). By blocking the action of major body chemicals in the heart, blood vessels, and certain muscles, the drug reduces the oxygen requirement of the heart and relaxes blood vessels. These actions result in lower blood pressure and decreased angina.

Atenolol is a cardioselective beta blocker, meaning it primarily affects the muscles in the heart; at higher doses it also affects the bronchial and vascular muscles. See ***Beta-Adrenergic Blockers*** for warnings and information on side effects and possible drug interactions.

ATORVASTATIN

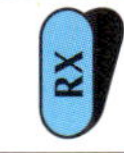

DRUG CLASS
Cholesterol-Reducing Drugs

BRAND NAME
Lipitor

GENERAL DESCRIPTION
Atorvastatin is an HMG-CoA reductase inhibitor, a type of drug that lowers the levels of cholesterol and other blood fats. It works by blocking a liver enzyme needed for the production of cholesterol. Atorvastatin is useful for lowering cholesterol in patients who may be at risk for heart disease and in patients with coronary atherosclerosis. For more information, see ***Cholesterol-Reducing Drugs***.

SPECIAL INFORMATION
- If you become pregnant while taking this drug, stop using it immediately and inform your doctor. Nursing women should take this medication only under a doctor's supervision.

POSSIBLE INTERACTIONS

Erythromycin, immunosuppressants, and niacin: severe muscle pain or kidney failure.

Gemfibrozil: may affect the absorption and excretion of atorvastatin; do not take concurrently.

ATRACTYLODES (WHITE)

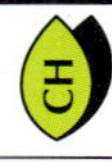

LATIN NAME
Atractylodes macrocephala

GENERAL DESCRIPTION
The aromatic rhizome of the herb known as atractylodes (white) is primarily a tonic. Classified in traditional Chinese medicine as bitter, sweet, and warm, it is believed to improve digestion and counter fatigue. A good specimen is large, firm, and fragrant, with a yellowish white cross section.

TARGET AILMENTS
Take internally for:
- diarrhea, fatigue, lack of appetite, vomiting, chronic gastroenteritis; spontaneous sweating; abdominal pain and bleeding during pregnancy; edema (the accumulation of fluid in the body) and reduced urination.

PREPARATIONS
Over the counter:
The herb is available fresh and in dried form from Chinese pharmacies, Asian markets, and some Western health food stores.

At home:
Dried atractylodes is used to treat edema and bloating. To stop diarrhea, the dried herb is stir-fried before it is decocted.

Combinations: A mixture with unripened bitter oranges is prescribed for loss of appetite. Vaginal discharges are treated with a preparation containing both white and gray atractylodes. Poria,

A

cinnamon twig, and atractylodes make a preparation for chest congestion. Combined with astragalus and wheat chaff, the herb is believed to provide relief from spontaneous sweating. Consult a Chinese herbalist for information on specific dosages and other herbal combinations.

SIDE EFFECTS

None expected.

SPECIAL INFORMATION

- In several experiments on animals, the herb has indicated a strong diuretic effect, while tests on humans have shown mixed results.
- Animal experiments have also shown a lowering of blood glucose as a result of taking atractylodes.

ATTAPULGITE

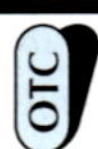

DRUG CLASS

Antidiarrheal Drugs

BRAND NAME

Kaopectate

GENERAL DESCRIPTION

Attapulgite is taken after each loose bowel movement to treat mild-to-moderate acute diarrhea. For chronic diarrhea, attapulgite should be used only for temporary relief of symptoms until the cause can be determined. See ***Antidiarrheal Drugs*** for more information.

POSSIBLE INTERACTIONS

The presence of attapulgite in your body might prevent the absorption of other medications. Avoid taking other medications within two to three hours of taking attapulgite.

AUCKLANDIA

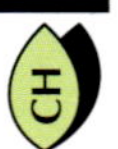

LATIN NAME

Aucklandia lappa

GENERAL DESCRIPTION

Aucklandia root is used for several abdominal disorders. Its Chinese name literally means "wood fragrance"; in English it is sometimes known as costus root or saussurea. Classified by Chinese medicine practitioners as acrid, bitter, and warm, it is grown mainly in China's Yunnan province, although it also appears in Sichuan and Tibet.

TARGET AILMENTS

- diarrhea, lack of appetite, abdominal pain or distention, nausea, and vomiting. (Take internally.)

PREPARATIONS

Over the counter:
Aucklandia is available in bulk at Chinese pharmacies, Asian food markets, and some Western health food stores.

At home:
For treatment of diarrhea, it should be toasted for greater effectiveness and is usually added to a mixture of herbs during the last five minutes of cooking.

Combinations: When mixed with green tangerine peel, aucklandia is given to patients suffering from indigestion or pain and swelling in the abdomen. Chinese herbalists recommend a preparation of aucklandia and coptis to treat the type of diarrhea that feels burning and explosive. Another mixture, with grains-of-paradise fruit, is prescribed for abdominal pain, loss of appetite, nausea, vomiting, morning sickness, and diarrhea. In combination with rhubarb root and betel nut, aucklandia is used to treat swelling of the abdomen accompanied by diarrhea.

Consult a Chinese herbalist for information on specific dosages and additional herbal combinations.

SIDE EFFECTS

Aucklandia is not recommended for use alone when patients suffer either from a loss of body fluids or from what Chinese medicine practitioners call heat signs, such as fever or thirst.

SPECIAL INFORMATION

- In laboratory studies using guinea pigs, extracts of the herb have shown some ability to clear out the bronchial tubes and reduce blood pressure.

AZITHROMYCIN

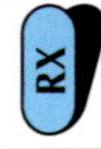

DRUG CLASS

Antibiotics [Erythromycins]

BRAND NAME

Zithromax

GENERAL DESCRIPTION

Azithromycin, an antibiotic introduced in 1991, is a long-acting derivative of erythromycin. The drug's action varies with the type of bacteria it is being used to fight. Azithromycin kills some bacteria outright and stops the growth and reproduction of others.

TARGET AILMENTS

- respiratory tract infections (including pharyngitis and sinusitis caused by strep), bronchitis, some types of pneumonia; skin and soft-tissue infections; chlamydial infections.

SIDE EFFECTS

Not serious:
Yeast infections; abdominal pain, mild diarrhea, nausea; dizziness, headache, fatigue. Consult your doctor if these effects persist.

Serious:
Inflammation of the colon (diarrhea, cramps, vomiting, and fever). Kidney inflammation (fever, joint pain, rash). Anaphylactic reaction (severe itching, rash, or difficulty breathing). Angioedema (swelling of the face, mouth, neck, hands, and feet). Discontinue use and contact your doctor immediately.

SPECIAL INFORMATION

- Tell your doctor if you are allergic to erythromycin, clarithromycin, or troleandomycin; you might also be allergic to azithromycin.
- Let your doctor know if you have impaired kidneys, an impaired liver, or a history of drug-induced colitis.
- Don't use azithromycin during pregnancy unless your doctor prescribes it. Avoid this drug if you are nursing.

POSSIBLE INTERACTIONS

Antacids containing aluminum, calcium, or magnesium: decreased azithromycin effect. Take azithromycin one hour before or two hours after taking antacids.

Anticoagulants: increased anticoagulant effect, risk of bleeding.

Carbamazepine: increased carbamazepine effect, possible toxicity.

Cyclosporine: increased cyclosporine effect, possible toxicity.

Digoxin: increased digoxin effect, possible toxicity.

Ergotamine: possible ergotamine toxicity.

Phenytoin: increased phenytoin effect, possible toxicity.

Theophylline: increased theophylline effect, possible toxicity.

Triazolam: increased triazolam effect, possible toxicity.

BACITRACIN

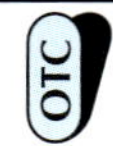

DRUG CLASS
Antibiotics [Topical Antibiotics]

BRAND NAME
Neosporin

GENERAL DESCRIPTION
Bacitracin is available by itself and in combination with neomycin and polymyxin B as an over-the-counter topical antibiotic. This combination is used to prevent infections in minor cuts, scrapes, and burns. For side effects and other information, see ***Topical Antibiotics.***

BARBERRY

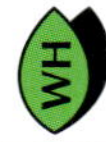

LATIN NAME
Berberis vulgaris

GENERAL DESCRIPTION
The root bark of barberry, an eight-foot-high shrub identified by its yellow root and dainty yellow blooms, is prescribed for several liver ailments. Herbalists also use the herb to reduce blood pressure, aid digestion, and fight infection. These effects on the body are attributed to the herb's active ingredients called isoquinoline alkaloids, which include berberine, berbamine, and oxyacanthine.

TARGET AILMENTS
Take internally for:
- jaundice, hepatitis, anemia, indigestion, constipation, diarrhea, heartburn, swollen spleen, gallstones, hangover.

Gargle with barberry tea for:
- sore throat.

Use as a compress for:
- inflamed eyelids, conjunctivitis (pinkeye), skin infection.

PREPARATIONS
Over the counter:
Barberry is available as root, fluidextract, and powder.

At home:
Tea: Boil 1 oz barberry root in 1 cup water for 15 to 20 minutes. Let it cool. Drink up to 3 cups a day as needed for up to 7 days. Add honey to sweeten.

Compress: Soak a clean cloth in barberry tea and apply it directly to the infected area.

Combinations: To cleanse the liver, combine 1 part barberry root, 1 part wild yam, 1 part dandelion, ½ part licorice root. Simmer 1 oz in 1 pt water for 10 minutes. Strain through a coffee filter. Drink 2 oz three or four times daily.

SIDE EFFECTS
Not serious:
You may experience upset stomach, diarrhea, nausea, vomiting, dizziness, or faintness. If these symptoms persist, check with a practitioner.

Serious:
In large doses, barberry may cause convulsions or drastic lowering of blood pressure, heart rate, or respiration. If any of these occur, stop using the herb immediately and inform your practitioner.

SPECIAL INFORMATION
- WARNING: Do not take barberry if you are pregnant, because of its stimulant effect on the uterus.
- Use only in consultation with an herbalist or licensed healthcare professional if you have heart disease or chronic respiratory problems.

BAYBERRY

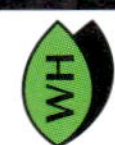

LATIN NAME
Myrica spp.

GENERAL DESCRIPTION
Early North American settlers valued bayberry for the wax from its berries, which they used to make candles. The grayish bark of the bayberry tree, a native American evergreen that can grow 35 feet tall, contains myricitrin, an antibiotic that in addition promotes sweating, which in turn can reduce fever; it also stimulates the flow of bile. The herb is therefore prescribed today to alleviate fever and diarrhea. Myricitrin is also an expectorant, helping to remove mucus from the lungs. And some herbalists regard bayberry as a stimulant for the circulatory system.

Bayberry, however, is less popular today than it was in the 19th century, when it was heavily publicized as a treatment for colds, influenza, fever, and diarrhea. Two commonly used species of bayberry are *Myrica cerifera* and *Myrica pensylvanicum.*

TARGET AILMENTS
Take internally for:
- dysentery, diarrhea, sore throat, canker sores.

Apply externally for:
- poor circulation, varicose veins, hemorrhoids.

PREPARATIONS
Over the counter:
Bayberry is available as tinctures, fluidextract, capsules, powder, dried root, bark, and berries.

At home:
Decoction: In 1 pt water, boil 1 tsp powdered root bark for 10 to 15 minutes. Add a little milk and drink it cool, up to 2 cups a day.

Gargle: The same preparation can be used as a gargle or mouthwash.

Fomentation: Soak a cotton towel in a hot herbal tea or decoction and apply to the affected area. To retain the heat, place a layer of plastic over the hot towel, then cover with a heating pad or a cloth soaked in hot water.

SIDE EFFECTS
Not serious:
Large doses may cause nausea and vomiting. If these persist, call your doctor.

SPECIAL INFORMATION
- WARNING: The herb affects the body's electrolyte balance, retaining sodium but depleting potassium in the body. This in turn can lead to high blood pressure and edema (water retention). Consult your practitioner for advice. Individuals with high blood pressure, edema, kidney disease, congestive heart failure, gastrointestinal conditions, or any type of imbalance between sodium and potassium should consult with a doctor before using bayberry.
- Do not use this herb if you have a history of cancer. Bayberry contains a high proportion of tannins, chemicals that in laboratory studies seemed to promote cancer.
- Do not use bayberry if you are pregnant.

BECLOMETHASONE

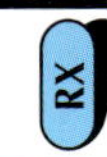

DRUG CLASS
Corticosteroids

BRAND NAMES
Beconase AQ, Vancenase AQ, Vanceril

GENERAL DESCRIPTION
Beclomethasone is a potent adrenal corticosteroid, available in nasal spray

B

and oral inhalant forms. Introduced in 1976, this drug is normally prescribed when a person does not respond to other treatments. Oral inhalant forms are used to treat bronchial asthma. They are intended to prevent, not relieve, acute asthma attacks. Concurrent use of bronchodilators in tablet, nasal spray, or oral inhalant form may increase the effects of beclomethasone.

As a nasal spray, beclomethasone is used to treat severe seasonal or perennial hay fever (allergic rhinitis) when decongestants are inadequate (although clearing your nasal passages with a decongestant spray before using beclomethasone may improve the drug's effect). Some systemic absorption may occur with long-term use of beclomethasone. See ***Corticosteroids*** for more information.

SIDE EFFECTS

Not serious:
White patches in the mouth, throat, or nose; throat irritation; stuffy or runny nose, and burning or dryness inside the nose. See your doctor if these symptoms persist or if there is no improvement in your condition in three weeks.

Serious:
None expected with low-dose, short-term use.

BELLADONNA

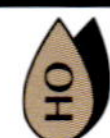

LATIN NAME
Belladonna

GENERAL DESCRIPTION
Belladonna, a highly toxic plant also known as deadly nightshade, grows wild across Europe, producing yellow flowers in July and dark-red berries in late summer. Its name, meaning "beautiful woman" in Italian, dates from the Renaissance, when ladies of Italy dilated their pupils with belladonna eye drops for a doe-eyed appearance. Belladonna poisoning brings on a range of symptoms, including a dry mouth and hot, flushed skin, nausea, convulsive movements, and delirium. Homeopathic practitioners prescribe *Belladonna* for illnesses that are accompanied by these same symptoms. All parts of the belladonna plant are gathered for use in the homeopathic remedy. The plant is crushed and pressed, and the extracted juice is mixed with alcohol in an extremely dilute preparation.

Like most homeopathic prescriptions, *Belladonna* was developed as a remedy by observation of the reactions of healthy individuals to a series of undilute doses. The mental, emotional, and physical changes induced by *Belladonna* were then cataloged. When a homeopathic practitioner encounters a patient with a set of symptoms that matches the cataloged symptoms brought on by *Belladonna,* the practitioner then prescribes it in an extremely dilute form. It is presumed that in this highly dilute dosage, *Belladonna* can counter the symptoms that it induces when it is at full strength.

For more information on homeopathic medicine, see page 1027.

TARGET AILMENTS
- common cold, flu, sore throat, earache with excruciating pain, high fever accompanied by chills but with no signs of thirst, acute inflammatory arthritis, acute bursitis, gallstones, colic, measles, mumps, acute diverticulitis (a colon disorder), neuralgia (pain along a nerve), sunstroke, acutely inflamed varicose veins, painful toothache, painful menstrual periods, teething pains in infants, breast-feeding complications, especially when the breasts are engorged and inflamed. (Take internally.)

PREPARATIONS
Belladonna is available over the counter in various potencies, in both liquid and tablet form. Consult your practitioner for more precise dosage information.

SIDE EFFECTS

None expected.

BENAZEPRIL

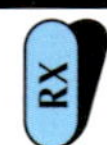

DRUG CLASS
Angiotensin-Converting Enzyme (ACE) Inhibitors

BRAND NAME
Lotensin

GENERAL DESCRIPTION
Introduced in 1991, the ACE inhibitor benazepril is prescribed for control of high blood pressure (hypertension). The drug works by blocking a body enzyme that is essential for the production of a substance that causes blood vessels to constrict. This action relaxes arterial walls, lowering blood pressure. Benazepril is also used to treat congestive heart failure.

TARGET AILMENTS
- high blood pressure.
- sometimes congestive heart failure (when used in conjunction with digitalis preparations and diuretics).

SIDE EFFECTS

Not serious:
Dry, persistent cough; headache, fatigue, nausea, diarrhea, loss of sense of taste, temporary skin rash, low blood pressure or dizziness on suddenly rising or changing position. Call your doctor if these effects become bothersome.

Serious:
Fainting, persistent skin rash, joint pain, drowsiness, numbness and tingling, abdominal pain, vomiting, diarrhea, excessive perspiration, fever, chills, chest pain, heart palpitation, jaundice (yellowing of skin or eyes). Call your doctor right away. Get medical attention immediately if you notice swelling of your face, tongue, or vocal cords or have difficulty swallowing or breathing; this reaction can be life-threatening.

SPECIAL INFORMATION
- WARNING: These drugs should not be taken during pregnancy because they have been associated with death of the fetus and newborn baby.
- ACE inhibitors cause an increase in blood levels of potassium. Do not use salt substitutes (which contain potassium) or other potassium-rich products, including low-salt milk, without first consulting your doctor. Such products could increase the potassium in your blood to dangerous levels, leading to heart-rhythm problems.
- Because your first dose of an ACE inhibitor may cause a sudden drop in blood pressure, your doctor may recommend that you take the first dose at bedtime.
- Do not abruptly stop taking these drugs. Your doctor may tell you to reduce the dosage gradually.
- Use caution during hot weather or while exercising; ACE inhibitors may cause increased perspiration, leading to dehydration and reduced blood pressure.
- Let your doctor know if you have arthritis or kidney disease, or if you are on a strict low-sodium diet or taking diuretics.

POSSIBLE INTERACTIONS

Alcohol: increased ACE inhibitor effects, leading to much lower blood pressure.

Central nervous system stimulants (including pseudoephedrine, an over-the-counter decongestant): reduced ACE inhibitor effect.

Estrogens: fluid retention, possibly raising blood pressure.

Indomethacin, NSAIDs, salicylates (such as aspirin): may decrease the effects of ACE inhibitors (especially captopril) and prevent the drugs from lowering blood pressure.

Lithium: lithium toxicity, which can lead to stupor, coma, and seizures.

Other medications that lower blood pressure, such as beta-adrenergic blockers, calcium channel blockers, diuretics, levodopa, nitrates, and opioid analgesics: increased hypotensive (blood pressure-lowering) effect of both combined medications.

Potassium products and diuretics that do not eliminate potassium from the body (such as amiloride, spironolactone, and triamterene): increased potassium blood levels, leading to heart-rhythm problems.

BENZOCAINE

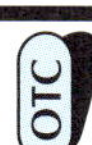

DRUG CLASS
Anesthetics

BRAND NAMES
Anbesol, Orajel

GENERAL DESCRIPTION
Benzocaine is an over-the-counter local anesthetic (derived from the same source as the sunscreen preparation PABA) that is frequently used to relieve pain and discomfort in the mouth and on the skin or mucous membranes. The drug works by deadening nerve endings so that they do not transmit pain messages to the brain. Most side effects associated with local anesthetics are caused by excessive applications or individual sensitivity to the anesthetic. Benzocaine is more likely to cause sensitivity reactions than most other anesthetics.

TARGET AILMENTS
- pain associated with minor skin and mouth problems, such as toothache and canker sores.

SIDE EFFECTS

Not serious:
None expected.

Serious:
Rarely, allergic reactions such as skin rash, hives, redness, and itching at the site of application; large hivelike swellings on the skin or in the mouth or throat; burning, stinging, and swelling not present before application. Call your doctor to determine whether you used too much medication or are sensitive to benzocaine.

Overdose symptoms include dizziness, headache, tiredness, blurred vision, irregular heartbeat, or ringing in the ears. Call your doctor immediately.

SPECIAL INFORMATION
- Benzocaine should not be used on areas where irritation, infection, or bleeding is present unless your doctor directs you to do so. Benzocaine can cause excess irritation or become absorbed into the bloodstream, leading to overdose symptoms.
- Do not use benzocaine if you are sensitive or allergic to PABA, since the two are chemically similar.

BENZODIAZEPINES

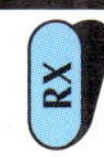

GENERIC NAMES
alprazolam, clonazepam, diazepam, lorazepam, temazepam, triazolam

GENERAL DESCRIPTION
Benzodiazepines are used to treat anxiety, insomnia, muscle spasms, and convulsions. They work by enhancing the action of a natural chemical in the brain that acts to depress certain areas of the central nervous system.

Some benzodiazepines can be used to treat any of the conditions listed below, but most have one or two primary uses. For example, alprazolam is used mainly for anxiety, clonazepam for convulsions, temazepam and triazolam for insomnia. Though benzodiazepines can cause physical and psychological dependence, they are considered particularly useful because they have fewer toxicity problems, fewer side effects, and less abuse potential than other drugs used for the same purposes. For more information, see the entries for the generic drugs listed above.

TARGET AILMENTS
- anxiety and panic disorders (alprazolam, diazepam, lorazepam).
- insomnia (lorazepam, temazepam, triazolam).
- convulsions or seizures (clonazepam, diazepam as an adjunct).
- skeletal muscle pain and spasticity (diazepam as an adjunct).
- alcohol withdrawal (diazepam).
- presurgery anxiety (diazepam, lorazepam). Used as an adjunct to anesthesia.

SIDE EFFECTS

Not serious:
Clumsiness or unsteadiness, lethargy, dry mouth, nausea, change in bowel habits. Tell your doctor if these symptoms persist or become bothersome.

Temporary amnesia (especially "travelers' amnesia" when taken to treat insomnia associated with jet lag). Contact your doctor if you are having difficulty with your memory.

Serious:
Drowsiness, dizziness, blurred vision, persistent or severe headache; allergic reaction (rash or itching), although rare; confusion; depression; changes in behavior (outburst of anger, difficulty concentrating); hallucinations; uncontrolled movement of body or eyes; muscle weakness; chills, fever, or sore throat. Rarely: jaundice, low blood pressure, anemia, or low platelet count (unusual bruising or bleeding). Tell your doctor about these symptoms right away.

SPECIAL INFORMATION
- Benzodiazepines can impair your alertness, judgment, and coordination. Avoid driving and performing hazardous activities until you experience how the drug affects you.
- Let your doctor know if you have narrow-angle glaucoma, a liver or kidney impairment, chronic respiratory disease, myasthenia gravis, depression, sleep apnea, or a history of drug abuse or addiction. Benzodiazepines may exacerbate these conditions.
- Benzodiazepines can cause sleep apnea in people with chronic respiratory disease, such as emphysema.
- Benzodiazepines can cause physical and psychological dependence, sometimes after only one or two weeks, but usually after prolonged use.
- People with a history of drug or alcohol abuse are at a greater risk of psychological dependence on benzodiazepines.
- Never combine alcohol with benzodiazepines; the combination can cause dangerous central nervous system and respiratory depression.

- Do not abruptly stop taking these drugs. Sudden cessation can provoke withdrawal symptoms, including seizures; irritability; insomnia; confusion; mental depression; hypersensitivity to pain, noise, or light; and feelings of suspicion and distrust. Slowly reduce the dosage under your doctor's guidance.
- Tolerance may increase with prolonged use; as your body adjusts to the benzodiazepine, the drug becomes less effective. Never increase the dose without consulting your doctor, because the risk of benzodiazepine dependence increases with higher doses.
- Do not take benzodiazepines if you are pregnant or breast-feeding.

POSSIBLE INTERACTIONS

Alcohol, anticonvulsants, antihistamines that cause drowsiness (clemastine, diphenhydramine), barbiturates, MAO inhibitors, opioids, tricyclic antidepressants: increased sedative effects, such as excessive mental (central nervous system) depression, sleepiness, and slow or shallow breathing. It is very important that you avoid taking benzodiazepines in combination with any of these drugs.

Antacids: may slow the absorption of benzodiazepines. Separate from benzodiazepine dose by an hour.

Beta blockers, cimetidine, disulfiram, erythromycin, ketoconazole, omeprazole, oral contraceptives, probenecid: may prolong the amount of time benzodiazepines remain in your body, leading to increased benzodiazepine effects and possible toxicity.

Cigarette smoking: decreased benzodiazepine effects.

Clozapine: risk of profound hypotension (low blood pressure), slow or shallow breathing, cessation of breathing, and cardiac arrest leading to death.

Isoniazid: increased effect and possible toxicity of diazepam and triazolam. This interaction also may occur with other benzodiazepines.

Levodopa: decreased levodopa effect.

Rifampin: decreased effect of diazepam and possibly of other benzodiazepines.

Valproic acid: increased benzodiazepine effects, including mental depression; risk of certain types of seizures if taken with clonazepam.

Zidovudine: risk of zidovudine toxicity.

BETA-ADRENERGIC BLOCKERS

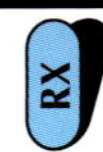

GENERIC NAMES

atenolol, metoprolol, nadolol, propranolol, timolol (oral and ophthalmic)

GENERAL DESCRIPTION

Also known as beta blockers, these drugs interfere with the action of certain parts of the nervous system, thereby slowing the heart rate and nerve impulses to the heart and other organs. This in turn results in lowered blood pressure and decreased angina. The first of the beta-blocking drugs to be developed (including nadolol, propranolol, and timolol) are called nonselective agents because they work in the whole body and can be used to treat a variety of medical conditions.

The newer beta blockers, among them atenolol and metoprolol, are called cardioselective because they target beta receptors in the muscles of the heart and blood vessels. These drugs are particularly useful for treating heart disorders such as angina and arrhythmia. For more information, see the individual entries for the generic drugs listed above.

TARGET AILMENTS

- heart disease, especially angina (pain), heart attack (myocardial infarction), and abnormal heart rhythms.
- high blood pressure (hypertension).
- migraine headaches (propranolol, timolol).
- tremors (propranolol).
- schizophrenic and anxiety disorders (propranolol and timolol).
- alcohol withdrawal (atenolol and propranolol).
- glaucoma (timolol).

SIDE EFFECTS

Not serious:
Decreased sexual ability, drowsiness, weakness, trouble sleeping, upset stomach, nervousness, change in bowel habits. Consult your doctor if these effects continue or are bothersome.

Serious:
Bronchospasm (trouble in breathing), congestive heart failure (swelling of feet or lower legs, shortness of breath), dizziness, mental depression, prolonged reduced circulation (cold hands and feet), fast or irregular heartbeat, chest pain, sudden shortness of breath, sweating, trembling and weakness. Call your doctor immediately.

See ***Timolol*** for side effects of an ophthalmic (eye drop) form of a beta-adrenergic blocker.

SPECIAL INFORMATION

- Beta-adrenergic blockers can make you drowsy, dizzy, and lightheaded. Avoid activities that require alertness, such as driving, until you know how you react to these drugs.
- Tell your doctor if you are planning surgery or have any of the following conditions, which beta-adrenergic blockers may complicate: allergies, bronchial asthma, or emphysema; congestive heart failure; diabetes mellitus; hyperthyroidism; impaired liver or kidneys; mental depression; myasthenia gravis; poor circulation or circulatory disease.
- Do not use beta blockers if you have a bronchospastic disease, bronchial asthma, or a severe chronic obstructive pulmonary disease.
- Beta blockers can both mask the symptoms of low blood sugar and cause a severe rise in blood sugar in patients with diabetes mellitus.
- Beta-adrenergic blockers can increase the severity of allergic reactions to drugs, food, or insect stings. Contact your doctor immediately if a severe allergic reaction occurs.
- Suddenly stopping these drugs may cause or increase heart problems. Dosage must be reduced gradually under your doctor's supervision.
- Before taking these drugs, let your doctor know if you are pregnant or nursing.

POSSIBLE INTERACTIONS

Beta blockers may interact with many over-the-counter and prescription medications, including the following:

Aminophylline, theophylline: decreased clearance of these drugs and possible toxicity.

Antacids (aluminum hydroxide or magnesium): decreased beta-blocker absorption. Take antacid four hours before or two hours after beta blocker.

Antidiabetic drugs, insulin: increased risk of high blood sugar and impaired recovery from hypoglycemia.

Antihypertensive drugs (including calcium channel blockers, clonidine, and guanabenz): increased antihypertensive effect.

Antipsychotic drugs (thioridazine, chlorpromazine): increased effects of both combined drugs, producing excessively low blood pressure, slowed heart rate, and difficulty breathing.

Cimetidine: increased beta-blocker effect.

Ephedrine, epinephrine, and isoproterenol: decreased effects of these drugs; risk of increased blood pressure.

Estrogens: decreased antihypertensive effect of beta blockers.

MAO inhibitors: combination can cause hypertension. Do not take beta blockers until 14 days after discontinuing MAO inhibitors.

Nonsteroidal anti-inflammatory drugs (NSAIDs), such as ibuprofen: reduced beta-blocker effect.

Phenothiazines: increased effects of both combined drugs.

BETAMETHASONE

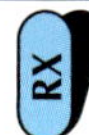

DRUG CLASS
Corticosteroids

BRAND NAME
Lotrisone (with clotrimazole)

GENERAL DESCRIPTION
Lotrisone, a combination of the corticosteroid drug betamethasone and the antifungal medication clotrimazole, is used to destroy fungi and relieve any accompanying skin inflammation. See ***Antifungal Drugs, Clotrimazole,*** and ***Corticosteroids*** for more information.

BILBERRY

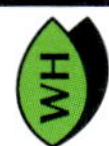

LATIN NAME
Vaccinium myrtillus

GENERAL DESCRIPTION
Herbalists have long valued the berries and leaves of the bilberry, a wild shrub that grows in Europe and North America. British pilots in World War II ate bilberry jam before flying night missions, to enhance their night vision. Small laboratory studies since then have indicated that the berries help other eye problems, such as glaucoma, cataracts, and macular degeneration (a common cause of blindness in adults). Bilberry's healing effects probably stem from chemicals known as anthocyanosides in the berries.

Some European herbalists claim that bilberry anthocyanosides may protect the arteries by reducing deposits that can lead to heart attacks, strokes, and high blood pressure. Dried berries work directly on the small intestine and are used to treat diarrhea. Herbalists have also prescribed bilberry leaves to lower blood sugar in diabetics.

TARGET AILMENTS
Take internally for:
- eyestrain, cataracts, glaucoma, macular degeneration, nearsightedness, night blindness, constipation, vomiting, diarrhea, dysentery, stomach cramps.

Apply externally for:
- spider veins, varicose veins, hemorrhoids, burns, skin problems.

PREPARATIONS
Over the counter:
Bilberry is available as tinctures, fluidextract, dried leaves, and berries.

At home:
Eat fresh or dried berries alone or mixed with apple powder to treat diarrhea.

Tea: Boil 2 to 3 tsp leaves in 1 cup water. Drink 1 cup per day for vomiting and stomach cramps. Use externally as a wash for skin problems and burns.

Decoction: Use 1 cup water with 1 tsp dried berries and simmer for 10 to 15 minutes. Drink 1 to 2 cups a day, cold.

SIDE EFFECTS
Not serious:
The use of fresh bilberries can cause diarrhea in some individuals.

SPECIAL INFORMATION
- WARNING: If the leaves are consumed over a long period of time, they can be poisonous. Do not exceed the recommended dose.

BIOTA

LATIN NAME
Biota orientalis

GENERAL DESCRIPTION
Biota comes from the leafy twig of the arborvitae shrub. Among its various uses, this herb is prescribed to control bleeding and to heal burns. And in laboratory experiments with animals, preparations of biota seem effective as expectorants. According to the principles of traditional Chinese medicine, this herb is astringent, bitter, and slightly cold.

TARGET AILMENTS
Take internally for:
- bleeding disorders such as vomiting and coughing up blood, dry coughing that fails to bring up phlegm, bleeding gums, blood in the stool or urine, and uterine bleeding.

Apply powdered form externally for:
- burns.

PREPARATIONS
Biota leaves are available in bulk, and they can be purchased in dried form in Chinese pharmacies, Asian markets, and some Western health food stores. A powdered form is available for treatment of burns. It should be applied as soon as possible after the burn.

Combinations: Two mixtures that contain biota may be prescribed to prevent bleeding. In one, the fresh herb is combined with the leaves of fresh lotus and fresh mugwort; in the other, biota is mixed with mugwort leaf and dried ginger. A blend of biota and cattail pollen is recommended for excessive bleeding from the uterus. And a preparation containing biota and jujube dates is used for patients with chronic dry coughs. Chinese herbalists can provide information on dosages and additional herbal combinations.

SIDE EFFECTS
Large doses or prolonged use of the herb may lead to dizziness, nausea, and vomiting.

SPECIAL INFORMATION
- Low concentrations of the herb in alcohol extractions appeared to inhibit the growth of tuberculosis and streptococcus bacteria in a test-tube trial.
- In human tests, oral preparations containing the herb slightly reduced the time it took to stop bleeding from gastric and duodenal ulcers, compared with a control group using standard therapy.

BISMUTH SUBSALICYLATE

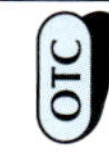

DRUG CLASS
Antidiarrheal Drugs

BRAND NAME
Pepto-Bismol

GENERAL DESCRIPTION
Bismuth subsalicylate is used to treat diarrhea. Because it appears to inhibit intestinal secretions, it is also effective in preventing symptoms of traveler's diarrhea and can be taken regularly during the first two weeks of travel. This

drug is also used to treat symptoms of gastric distress or upset stomach, including heartburn, acid indigestion, and nausea. See ***Antidiarrheal Drugs.***

SPECIAL INFORMATION
- Advise your healthcare professional if you have had allergic reactions to other salicylates, including aspirin.
- If taken in higher doses and for longer periods to prevent traveler's diarrhea, this drug may intensify some of the symptoms of dysentery, gout, kidney disease, stomach ulcers, and hemophilia and other bleeding problems. If you have any of these conditions, consult your doctor first before taking the drug.
- Bismuth subsalicylate may have an effect on some laboratory tests. Be sure to tell the healthcare practitioner performing the test that you are taking the medication.

POSSIBLE INTERACTIONS

Antidiabetic drugs (oral): may reduce blood sugar levels.

BLACK COHOSH

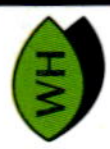

LATIN NAME
Cimicifuga racemosa

GENERAL DESCRIPTION
The knotty black rhizome and root of black cohosh contain substances that act like the female hormone estrogen. A leafy perennial, it is prescribed for several menstrual and menopausal conditions. In Germany, black cohosh is a key ingredient in the three drugs used most often to treat menopausal disorders. Black cohosh also acts as a sedative and is believed to promote urination, dry up discharges of fluid, aid in expelling mucus from the lungs, and relieve spasmodic conditions such as the coughs that accompany whooping cough and tuberculosis. Laboratory tests on animals suggest that one of the components of black cohosh, actein, may help in the treatment of high blood pressure.

TARGET AILMENTS
Take internally for:
- menstrual discomfort, menopausal disorders, premenstrual stress, headache, diarrhea, bleeding gums, spasmodic coughs, high blood pressure.

Apply externally for:
- sciatica, neuralgia, muscle spasms, rheumatism.

PREPARATIONS
Over the counter:
Black cohosh is available as tinctures, syrup, capsules, fluidextract, and also as dried root and rhizome.

At home:
Decoction: Boil ½ tsp powdered rootstock per cup of water for 30 minutes and let cool. Take as much as a cup per day, 2 tbsp at a time. To take away the bitter taste, add lemon and honey.

Combination: Mix the dried herb with skullcap, wood betony, passionflower, and valerian to make a mild tranquilizer.

SIDE EFFECTS

Not serious:
Prolonged use may irritate the uterus.

Serious:
Overdoses or use for long periods can cause dizziness, diarrhea, nausea, vomiting, abdominal pain, headaches, joint pains, lowered heart rate, hypertension, flushing. If any of these symptoms develop, stop using black cohosh and call your doctor immediately.

SPECIAL INFORMATION
- WARNING: Because it can potentially cause serious side effects, use black cohosh only under medical supervision.
- WARNING: Individuals suffering from congestive heart failure or any other type of heart disease should not use black cohosh.
- Do not use if you are pregnant, because it can cause premature labor.
- Do not take the herb if you have been advised not to take contraceptive pills.

BLACK WALNUT

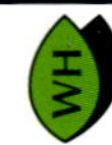

LATIN NAME
Juglans nigra

GENERAL DESCRIPTION
Native Americans used the bark of the black walnut, a tree that grows in the eastern U.S., to treat skin problems such as ringworm. They drank a tea made from the bark as a laxative, and they chewed on the bark to relieve headache pain. Today black walnut's bark, leaves, fruit rind, and liquid extracts are prescribed by herbalists for constipation, fungal and parasitic infections, and mouth sores. Black walnut is rich in tannins and contains a large amount of iodine, which makes it a good antiseptic. Also, the herb is believed to relieve toxic blood conditions. And some evidence indicates that, if used internally over a long period, the herb will help eliminate warts caused by viruses.

TARGET AILMENTS
Take internally for:
- constipation, intestinal worms and parasites, warts, mouth sores.

Apply externally for:
- ringworm, scabies, eczema, herpes, psoriasis, sores, pimples, athlete's foot, jock itch, cold sores.

PREPARATIONS
Over the counter:
Black walnut is available as tinctures, extract, dried bark, leaves, and fruit rind.

At home:
Decoction: Simmer the green husk in boiling water for 10 to 15 minutes. Take 1 tbsp three or four times a day.

Gargle: Use the decoction as a mouthwash or gargle to treat mouth sores.

Extract: Rub on the affected area twice a day.

Poultice: Make a poultice from the green rind of black walnut and apply to the sites of ringworm.

SIDE EFFECTS

None expected.

SPECIAL INFORMATION
- Do not use if you are pregnant.
- Fresh green husks may irritate your skin.

BLESSED THISTLE

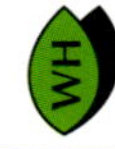

LATIN NAME
Cnicus benedictus

GENERAL DESCRIPTION
During the Middle Ages, blessed thistle was used to treat bubonic plague. Modern herbalists consider the aboveground parts of this annual plant a remedy for a range of problems. A component of blessed thistle is the chemical cnicin, an anti-inflammatory agent that also stops bleeding. In addition extracts from the plant contain more than a dozen antibacterial compounds. Blessed thistle is also used to induce vomiting in individuals who have taken poisons, and to regu-

late menstrual cycles. This bitter herb, sometimes known as St. Benedict's thistle, is used in the liqueur Benedictine.

TARGET AILMENTS

Take internally for:

- poor digestion, fever, headache, colic, gas, diarrhea.

Apply externally for:

- cuts and wounds, fever, shingles.

PREPARATIONS

Over the counter:

Blessed thistle is available as a tincture, extract, and dried herb.

At home:

Tea: Steep 1 tsp dried herb in ½ cup boiling water. Drink 1 cup to 1½ cups a day, unsweetened, for problems with digestion.

Poultice: Mash leaves and other parts, and apply to chilblains, wounds, and sores.

Combinations: Used with cramp bark, blue cohosh root, and ginger to treat menstrual difficulties.

SIDE EFFECTS

Not serious:

Overdoses can cause vomiting.

SPECIAL INFORMATION

- WARNING: Use recommended amounts and only under a doctor's supervision. Blessed thistle is a strong emetic and induces vomiting very effectively.
- During pregnancy, avoid blessed thistle and any compounds that include the herb.
- Avoid using blessed thistle if you have an ulcer, because blessed thistle stimulates gastric activity.

BLOODROOT

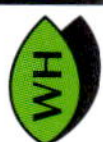

LATIN NAME

Sanguinaria canadensis

GENERAL DESCRIPTION

Named for the crimson extract made from its root, bloodroot not only looks forbidding but is potentially toxic and can cause severe side effects if ingested in excess. For this reason, herbalists prescribe the root of this perennial plant primarily as an external remedy to relieve eczema, venereal blisters, rashes, and other skin disorders. Only rarely is the bitter herb taken internally, and that is when herbalists recommend it for respiratory disorders such as bronchitis. Bloodroot is a major ingredient in many mouthwashes and toothpastes because of its ability to kill the bacteria that can lead to gingivitis (gum disease) and the buildup of plaque. Its key components are the antibacterial isoquinoline alkaloids.

TARGET AILMENTS

- gingivitis. (Use as toothpaste and mouthwash.)
- congestion of the lungs, bronchitis, asthma, headaches, head colds. (Take bloodroot internally.)
- fungus, athlete's foot, venereal blisters, rashes, eczema, ringworm, warts. (Apply bloodroot externally.)

PREPARATIONS

Over the counter:

Bloodroot is available as tincture and dried root; it is also an ingredient in several commercial dental products.

At home:

Tea: Prepare by boiling 1 oz bloodroot in 1 cup water for 15 to 20 minutes. Drink three times daily.

Combinations: Bloodroot can be blended with horehound and elecampane to relieve congestion. It can be mixed with red sage and a pinch of cayenne to treat pharyngitis (irritation of the throat).

SIDE EFFECTS

Serious:

High doses can cause burning in the stomach, vomiting, nausea, slowing of the heart rate, impaired vision, intense thirst, and dizziness. Stop using immediately if these symptoms develop, and consult your practitioner.

SPECIAL INFORMATION

- WARNING: Bloodroot is potentially toxic. Take it internally only under the supervision of an herbalist or licensed healthcare professional.
- Avoid using bloodroot internally during pregnancy.
- Bloodroot has a long folk history in the treatment of cancer, and it is currently the subject of studies and experiments. It contains sanguinarine, a constituent that is thought to impede the formation of tumors.

BLOOD VISCOSITY-REDUCING AGENTS

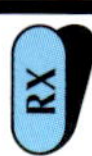

GENERIC NAME

pentoxifylline

GENERAL DESCRIPTION

Blood viscosity-reducing agents are used to improve the flow of blood through small blood vessels, thereby decreasing pain—particularly in the legs—caused by poor blood circulation. Unlike anticoagulants and antiplatelets, these drugs are true "blood thinners": They reduce the viscosity (thickness, stickiness) of red blood cells and improve their flexibility, thus easing the flow of blood throughout the body. See ***Pentoxifylline*** for more information about a blood viscosity-reducing agent used to bring relief from leg cramps and other symptoms associated with peripheral vascular disease, a chronic blood-vessel disorder in which the inflexibility of red blood cells causes poor blood circulation in the arms or legs.

BONESET

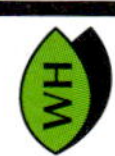

LATIN NAME

Eupatorium perfoliatum

GENERAL DESCRIPTION

A tall, hardy plant, boneset has nothing to do with setting bones; it is used to treat fever. Native Americans took boneset for fever-producing illnesses such as cholera, dengue fever, and typhoid. It then became one of the most popular herbs among the colonists, who kept it on hand for colds and other ailments that give rise to fever. Today herbalists still recommend boneset, also called feverwort and sweat plant, for the aches and pains that accompany fever, especially during bouts of influenza. Boneset also helps clear mucus from the respiratory tract. It is also often used for arthritis and rheumatism. Herbalists use the leaves and flower tops, which are harvested as soon as the plant blooms in late summer.

TARGET AILMENTS

Take internally for:

- fever, colds, flu, coughs, congestion in the upper respiratory tract, arthritis, and rheumatism.

B

PREPARATIONS
Over the counter:
Available in health food stores as dried leaves and flowers, and as tinctures.

At home:
Infusion: Pour 1 cup boiling water onto 2 to 3 tsp dried herb and let steep for 10 to 15 minutes. Drink as hot as possible. For fever or flu, drink a cup every half hour up to 4 cups in 6 hours, and only 6 cups in a 24-hour period. To mask the very bitter taste of boneset, mix it with an herbal tea or add honey and lemon.

SIDE EFFECTS

Large doses of boneset can cause nausea, vomiting, or diarrhea. Do not exceed the recommended dosage; call your doctor if you experience adverse reactions.

SPECIAL INFORMATION
- WARNING: Do not use fresh boneset. It contains a toxic chemical, called tremerol, that can cause vomiting, rapid breathing, and at high doses, possibly coma and death. Drying boneset removes the tremerol.
- If you have a history of alcoholism, liver disease, or liver cancer, consult your herbalist before taking boneset; it contains pyrrolizidine alkaloids, which are toxic to the liver.
- Because of its toxic effects, you should not take boneset for more than two weeks at a time.

BROMPHENIRAMINE

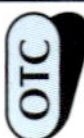

DRUG CLASS
Antihistamines

BRAND NAMES
Dimetapp in various forms

GENERAL DESCRIPTION
Brompheniramine is an antihistamine drug with mild sedating effects. See ***Antihistamines.***

BRONCHODILATORS

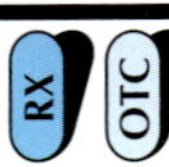

GENERIC NAMES
Rx: albuterol, epinephrine, ipratropium, salmeterol, terbutaline, theophylline

OTC: ephedrine, epinephrine, theophylline

GENERAL DESCRIPTION
Bronchodilators relax the muscles in the bronchial tubes and the blood vessels of the lungs by inhibiting certain body chemicals. Some of these drugs also act as central respiratory stimulants to make breathing easier. This relieves spasms and improves lung capacity, thereby alleviating the symptoms of bronchial asthma and bronchitis.

Theophylline (found naturally in commercial tea and related to the caffeine found in coffee) acts mainly on the muscles of the respiratory tract. Other bronchodilators act on the sinuses and upper respiratory tract. All of these drugs may act on the heart, arteries, and veins, especially if taken in large doses. For this reason bronchodilators can affect blood pressure and heart function.

TARGET AILMENTS
- anaphylactic shock from severe allergic reactions.
- acute bronchial asthma.
- chronic, recurrent bronchial asthma.
- bronchitis.
- emphysema.
- hay fever and cold symptoms (ephedrine).
- other chronic obstructive pulmonary diseases.
- heart-rhythm problems and cardiac arrest (epinephrine).
- exercise-induced bronchospasms.

SIDE EFFECTS

Not serious:
Mild nausea, weakness, insomnia, nervousness or restlessness. Call your doctor if these effects become bothersome.

Serious:
Change in blood pressure, change in heartbeat (irregular or pounding, for example), trembling, breathing problems, weakness, anxiety, nervousness, dizziness, lightheadedness, muscle cramps, or nausea or vomiting. Rarely, chest pain or discomfort. Let your doctor know right away if you experience these side effects.

SPECIAL INFORMATION
- These drugs (especially ephedrine and epinephrine) can cause adverse effects in individuals with high blood pressure, diabetes, heart disease, seizures, peptic ulcers, or thyroid or prostate problems. If you have any of these conditions do not use bronchodilators—even in their over-the-counter forms—without your doctor's permission.
- WARNING: Your body can build up tolerance to bronchodilators used as inhalants, causing them to become less effective. If this happens, discontinue the drug and tell your doctor. Do not increase the dose. Increasing the dose can lead to serious, perhaps fatal bronchial constriction.
- Women who are pregnant or breast-feeding should consult a doctor before using these drugs.

POSSIBLE INTERACTIONS

Alcohol: increased stomach problems because these drugs have common gastrointestinal effects.

Alpha and beta blockers: these drugs decrease the action of bronchodilators, especially ephedrine and epinephrine.

Blood pressure medicines, including diuretics: bronchodilators may decrease the actions of these medicines.

Caffeine and other central nervous system stimulants: increased nervousness and insomnia.

Diabetes medications, including insulin: decreased effectiveness of diabetes medications.

Heart medications (such as digoxin): heart-rhythm problems.

Levodopa: increased heart-rhythm problems. Your doctor may need to adjust your dosage.

Lithium: theophylline may decrease the effectiveness of lithium.

MAO inhibitors: possible effects on the heart or blood vessels.

Nitrates: decreased effectiveness of nitrates in relieving angina.

Other antiasthmatic drugs: do not combine these drugs unless your doctor directs you to do so or unless your prescription contains a combination. Using two bronchodilators may increase the side effects, especially on the heart.

Phenytoin: serious cardiovascular effects, such as heart-rhythm problems or very low blood pressure.

Thyroid medications: increased bronchodilator effect.

Tricyclic antidepressants and maprotiline: increased effects of bronchodilators on the heart and cardiovascular system.

BRYONIA

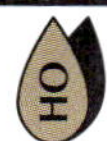

LATIN NAME
Bryonia alba

GENERAL DESCRIPTION
Bryonia, or wild hops, is a creeping vine commonly found along hedgerows and in forests across southern Europe. Its medicinal value was known to the Greeks, who used the root as a purgative and may have given the plant its name, derived from *bryo,* meaning "to thrust or sprout," a reference to how quickly the vine grows. Accidental ingestion of the root can cause tissue inflammation, severe vomiting, and diarrhea violent enough to cause death. Homeopathic physicians prescribe their dilute solutions of *Bryonia* for illnesses that are accompanied by similar symptoms. The homeopathic remedy is prepared from the root, which is harvested in early spring. An extract pressed from the root pulp is mixed with alcohol into an extremely dilute solution.

Like most homeopathic prescriptions, *Bryonia* was developed as a remedy by observation of the reactions of healthy individuals to a series of undilute doses. The mental, emotional, and physical changes induced by *Bryonia* were then cataloged. When a homeopathic practitioner encounters a patient with a set of symptoms that matches the cataloged symptoms brought on by *Bryonia,* the practitioner then prescribes it in an extremely dilute form. It is presumed that in this highly dilute dosage, *Bryonia* can counter the symptoms that it induces when it is at full strength.

TARGET AILMENTS
Take internally for:
- arthritis with sharp, sticking pains; backaches centered in the small of the back; bursitis.
- colds accompanied by chest congestion; painful coughs; sore throat, with pain upon swallowing; influenza; severe headaches that are worsened by light, sound, or any motion; dizziness.
- nausea, vomiting, constipation, gastritis (stomach inflammation), acute diverticulitis (a colon disorder), stomach flu, migraine headaches.
- inflammation during breast-feeding.

PREPARATIONS
Bryonia is available over the counter in various potencies, in both liquid and tablet form. Consult your practitioner for more precise information.

SIDE EFFECTS
None expected.

BUCHU

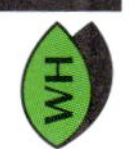

LATIN NAME
Agathosma spp.

GENERAL DESCRIPTION
The leaves of this southern African shrub contain an oil that increases the production of urine. African people used it for urinary problems long before they had contact with Europeans. In the 17th century Dutch settlers in South Africa used it to treat urinary tract infections and kidney stones. In 1847, buchu was introduced in the U.S. and hailed as a cure-all. Today Western herbalists continue the tradition, prescribing buchu for urinary tract infections and as a diuretic, and also for treating premenstrual syndrome and high blood pressure.

TARGET AILMENTS
Take internally for:
- urinary tract disorders, acute bladder inflammation and infections, irritable bladder, kidney stones, painful urination.

PREPARATIONS
Over the counter:
You can obtain buchu dried and as a tincture at health food stores. The herb is also found in Fluidex and Odrinil, two commercial diuretics used to treat premenstrual syndrome.

At home:
Infusion: Add 1 to 2 tsp dried, crumbled leaves to 1 cup boiling water and let steep for 10 minutes. Drink up to three times a day.

Combinations: Mix buchu with uva ursi, yarrow, or couch grass to treat cystitis (bladder inflammation). Combine buchu with corn silk or marsh mallow for dysuria (painful or difficult urination).

SIDE EFFECTS
Not serious:
Too large a dose of buchu can cause stomach upset or diarrhea.

SPECIAL INFORMATION
- WARNING: Diuretics such as buchu may deplete the body's potassium levels, so be sure to eat more potassium-rich foods, such as bananas and fresh vegetables, while taking buchu.
- If you are pregnant, consult your doctor before taking buchu or any other diuretic.
- If you plan to treat high blood pressure with buchu, do so only under a doctor's care as part of a larger treatment plan.
- Avoid buchu if you have a history of kidney disease; its oil content may be too irritating.

BUCKTHORN

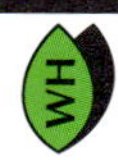

LATIN NAME
Rhamnus purshiana

GENERAL DESCRIPTION
The bark and the black, pea-sized berries of the buckthorn tree act as a laxative so strong that Western herbalists advise using it only as a last resort, after other laxatives have failed. Its effectiveness stems from chemicals known as anthraquinones; these substances exert an extremely powerful purgative effect. You should use the herb only in consultation with your doctor.

TARGET AILMENT
- constipation. (Take internally, with care.)

PREPARATIONS
Over the counter:
Buckthorn is available as a tincture and in dried form. It is a component of the commercial laxative Movicol.

At home:
Decoction: Boil 1 tsp dried buckthorn in 3 cups water and steep 30 minutes. Drink cool, 1 tbsp at a time, before bed.

Tincture: Take ½ tsp before bed.

Combination: Mix ½ tsp each of dried buckthorn bark, chamomile, and fennel seed, and steep in 1 cup boiling water for 10 minutes. Drink at bedtime.

SIDE EFFECTS
Serious:
Fresh buckthorn can cause vomiting, violent diarrhea, and stomach cramps. Consult a doctor immediately.

SPECIAL INFORMATION
- WARNING: Do not take fresh buckthorn. Dry both the berries and the bark for a year or two before using. For faster drying, put the berries or bark in an oven at 250°F for several hours.
- WARNING: Do not use buckthorn for

more than two weeks at a time. It can cause lazy bowel syndrome, in which the stool cannot be moved without chemical stimulation. If this occurs, consult a doctor.

- WARNING: Do not use buckthorn if you are pregnant or nursing, or if you have chronic gastrointestinal problems like hemorrhoids, ulcers, and colitis.
- Do not use buckthorn with any other laxatives.

BUMETANIDE

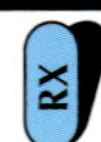

DRUG CLASS
Diuretics

BRAND NAME
Bumex

GENERAL DESCRIPTION
Bumetanide, a fast-acting and powerful diuretic, is prescribed to eliminate excess body fluid and to treat high blood pressure (hypertension). Introduced in 1983, the drug acts by increasing urine production, thereby removing water from the body and helping to reduce swelling and blood volume. However, because this medication belongs to a group known as nonpotassium-sparing diuretics, salts containing minerals such as sodium, potassium, and calcium are also eliminated; this can sometimes lead to muscle cramps and serious cardiovascular side effects. For information on additional side effects and possible drug interactions, see ***Diuretics.***

SIDE EFFECTS
Not serious:
Although uncommon, chest and muscle pain and problems with sexual performance may occur with use of this drug. Let your doctor know if you are troubled by these effects.

BUPLEURUM

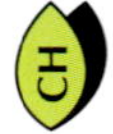

LATIN NAME
Bupleurum chinense

GENERAL DESCRIPTION
The long, coarse root known as bupleurum is often used to reduce certain types of fever and to treat irritability and feelings of frustration. Sometimes called hare's ear or thorowax root, it is characterized in traditional Chinese medicine as bitter, acrid, and cool.

TARGET AILMENTS
Take internally for:
- low-grade fevers.
- malaria and malaria-like disorders.
- alternating chills and fever, typically accompanied by a bitter taste in the mouth, pain in the side, irritability, vomiting, or difficulty in breathing.
- prolapse of the uterus (fallen uterus).
- dizziness and vertigo combined with pain in the chest, and tenderness in the side or breast, often accompanied by emotional irritability.
- menstrual problems, such as premenstrual syndrome, irregular menstruation, and cramps.
- pressure in the chest, bloated abdomen, nausea, and indigestion.

PREPARATIONS
The root is available in bulk in Chinese pharmacies, Asian markets, and some Western health food stores. Chinese pharmacies also offer mixtures containing the root.

Combinations: White peony root mixed with bupleurum is prescribed for vertigo, dizziness, chest pain, and painful menstrual periods. Irregular menstruation, premenstrual syndrome, and certain kinds of depression may be treated with a blend of bupleurum and field mint. Bupleurum is often combined with bitter orange fruit to alleviate pressure in the chest, abdominal pain, poor appetite, and irregular bowel movements. Chinese herbalists sometimes mix small amounts of licorice with bupleurum to treat hepatitis. For information on specific dosages and additional herbal combinations, consult your Chinese medicine practitioner.

SIDE EFFECTS
Too large a dose of the herb can cause nausea or vomiting.

SPECIAL INFORMATION
- Clinical experiments have indicated that the herb may be able to reduce fever resulting from infections of the upper respiratory tract.
- In test-tube studies, preparations of bupleurum seem to have inhibited the growth of tuberculosis bacteria, as well as influenza and polio viruses.

BUPROPION

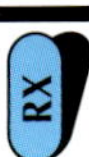

DRUG CLASS
Antidepressants; Smoking Cessation Drugs

BRAND NAMES
antidepressant: Wellbutrin

smoking cessation drug: Zyban

GENERAL DESCRIPTION
Bupropion is prescribed to treat depression or as an aid to quit smoking. This medication appears to alleviate depression by blocking certain chemicals necessary for nerve transmission in the brain and to boost dopamine and norepinephrine levels in the brain, reducing symptoms of nicotine withdrawal. See ***Antidepressants*** and ***Smoking Cessation Drugs*** for additional information.

SPECIAL INFORMATION
- Warning: Do not take bupropion if you have a seizure disorder. The drug may cause you to have more frequent seizures.
- Bupropion has not been tested as a long-term treatment for depression. Your doctor should monitor your condition if you take the antidepressant for longer than 8 weeks.
- Unlike other antidepressants, bupropion does not adversely affect sexual function.
- Other drugs may alter the metabolism of bupropion. Inform your doctor of all other medications you are taking, including over-the-counter drugs.

BURDOCK

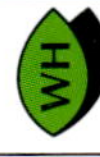

LATIN NAME
Arctium lappa

GENERAL DESCRIPTION
For several centuries, herbalists have prescribed burdock root to cure a wide range of illnesses. Today, some practitioners use burdock to treat urinary tract infections, arthritic conditions, external wounds, and skin ulcers. This herb works best in conjunction with professional medical treatment. The root has brown bark and a white, spongy interior that hardens when dried. Burdock got its name from its tenacious burrs and from *dock,* the Old English word for "plant."

TARGET AILMENTS

Take internally for:

- fungal and bacterial infections; skin disorders such as eczema and psoriasis, which cause dry, scaly skin; urinary tract infections; rheumatism; arthritis.

Apply externally for:

- wounds and skin conditions.

PREPARATIONS

Over the counter:

Burdock is available as dried powder, slices of root, and tinctures. You can find the fresh root in the vegetable sections of health food stores.

At home:

Decoction: Add 1 tsp burdock root to 3 cups water and boil for 30 minutes. Drink up to 3 cups a day to treat genital and urinary tract irritations.

Compress: Soak a clean cloth in burdock tea and place it on the skin to speed healing of wounds and skin ulcers.

Combinations: Burdock can be mixed with yellow dock, red clover, or cleavers and taken orally for skin disorders. Consult an herbalist for more information.

SIDE EFFECTS

Burdock may cause stomach discomfort if too much is taken. Do not exceed recommended dosages.

SPECIAL INFORMATION

- WARNING: Do not use burdock if you are pregnant; it stimulates the uterus.
- Laboratory trials on animals indicate that burdock has possible antitumor activity.
- Do not give burdock to children younger than 2 years of age. Older children and people over 65 should start with lower-strength doses, increasing them if needed.

BUSPIRONE

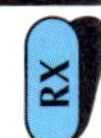

DRUG CLASS

Antianxiety Drugs

BRAND NAME

BuSpar

GENERAL DESCRIPTION

Buspirone is a nonbenzodiazepine antianxiety drug whose actions on the body appear to be complex and are not clearly understood. Compared with other antianxiety drugs, buspirone may be slow to take action; its effects generally begin after two weeks, and the total treatment time may be three to four weeks. Among its advantages, buspirone produces milder side effects, as well as less sedation. Since it is not addicting, buspirone can be used in patients who may be prone to addiction, such as alcoholics. See ***Antianxiety Drugs*** for an overview of this class.

TARGET AILMENTS

- anxiety disorders or short-term treatment of anxiety symptoms.

SIDE EFFECTS

Not serious:

Nausea, sore throat, nasal congestion. Call your doctor if symptoms continue or are bothersome.

Serious:

Dizziness, drowsiness, nervousness, lightheadedness, excitement, blurred vision, persistent or severe headache, ringing in the ears, chest pain, shortness of breath, fainting, confusion, muscle weakness, uncontrolled movements of the body, numbness or tingling in the hands or feet. Contact your doctor immediately.

SPECIAL INFORMATION

- Buspirone has milder sedative effects than other antianxiety drugs and no withdrawal symptoms. However, you should not use buspirone unless it is clearly needed. Prolonged periods of use may increase the likelihood of serious side effects.
- Avoid driving and working near heavy machinery until you learn how this drug affects you.
- Do not use this drug if your liver or kidneys are impaired.
- Do not use buspirone if you are pregnant or breast-feeding.

POSSIBLE INTERACTIONS

Alcohol, anticonvulsants, antihistamines, barbiturates, benzodiazepines, muscle relaxants, opioid analgesics, sedatives, tricyclic antidepressants:
Taking buspirone in combination with any of these drugs may cause excessive sedation.

Digoxin: possible increased digoxin effect.

Haloperidol: possible increased haloperidol effect.

MAO inhibitors: significantly increased blood pressure. Do not combine these drugs with buspirone.

BUTCHER'S-BROOM

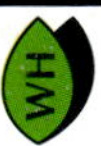

LATIN NAME

Ruscus aculeatus

GENERAL DESCRIPTION

Butcher's-broom acquired its name because ancient Mediterranean butchers used the scrubby stems and leaves of the tough plant to sweep meat scraps off their cutting boards. Its medicinal use dates to classical Greece, when physicians applied its roots and rhizomes to swellings and prescribed it as a laxative and diuretic. Today herbalists believe its rhizomes have anti-inflammatory properties, and they use it to treat disorders of the veins. Butcher's-broom is an astringent that puckers up the insides of veins. Among its active ingredients are two steroidal components called ruscogenin and neuroscogenin, which appear to narrow blood vessels.

TARGET AILMENTS

- circulation disorders of the legs such as varicose veins; hemorrhoids and other rectal inflammation and bleeding. (Use internally or externally.)

PREPARATIONS

Over the counter:

Butcher's-broom is available in dry bulk, capsules, ointment, and tincture.

At home:

Tea: Put 2 tsp powdered root in 1½ pt boiling water. Simmer slowly in a covered container for about 30 minutes. Drink cold, 2 to 3 tbsp, six times a day.

Compress: Soak a clean cloth in tea, and apply.

Ointment: Apply small amounts to hemorrhoids until inflammation is cleared.

SPECIAL INFORMATION

- Consult your doctor for a diagnosis of circulatory problems before using any remedy.

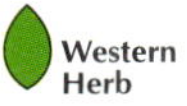

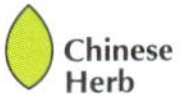

C

CAFFEINE

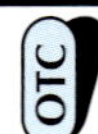

DRUG CLASS
Analgesics [Adjunct Therapy]

BRAND NAMES
Anacin, Excedrin Extra-Strength, Vivarin

GENERAL DESCRIPTION
Caffeine, obtained from both natural and synthetic sources, has been used for centuries as a mild central nervous system stimulant. It works by stimulating all parts of the central nervous system, affecting the heart, lungs, other organs, and muscles. Caffeine also affects the blood vessels by temporarily increasing the heart's rate, contraction force, and output. While these effects usually produce no change in blood pressure for healthy individuals, you should avoid caffeine if you have high blood pressure.

Caffeine increases the production of stomach acids. Other effects include a slight diuretic action, a decrease in uterine contractions, and a temporary increase in blood sugar. Some people develop a tolerance to caffeine. When caffeine is used for a long period, abrupt discontinuation can produce withdrawal symptoms such as headache, irritability, dizziness, and unusual tiredness.

TARGET AILMENTS
- fatigue.
- pain. Caffeine is used as an adjunctive (additive) treatment in combination with analgesics, such as aspirin, to enhance relief.
- migraine and other vascular headaches; used with ergot preparations.

SIDE EFFECTS

Not serious:
Mild stimulation of the central nervous system (jitters), mild digestive upset, mild nausea, insomnia. Call your doctor if these symptoms become bothersome.

Serious:
Excessive stimulation such as dizziness, increased heart rate, nervousness, tremors; digestive upsets such as nausea, vomiting, diarrhea. Let your doctor know if you have these effects. You may have taken too much caffeine. Overdose symptoms include those above plus headache, vision disturbances such as seeing flashes or lights, delirium, fever, increased sensitivity to pain, ringing in ears.

SPECIAL INFORMATION
- There has been some controversy regarding the use of caffeine by pregnant or nursing women. Although no proof of birth defects has been found, caffeine does cross the placenta and small amounts also pass into breast milk. Caffeine can cause hyperactivity and insomnia in infants. For this reason, pregnant and nursing women should use caution and limit their intake of caffeine.
- Caffeine's effects on children have not been studied.

POSSIBLE INTERACTIONS

Barbiturates: combining these drugs may decrease the action of both.

Beta blockers: combining these drugs may decrease the action of both.

Bronchodilators: taking caffeine with these may increase stimulation and other side effects.

Cimetidine (ulcer medicine), antacids and supplements that contain calcium: may decrease the elimination of caffeine, possibly increasing its effects.

Disulfiram (for alcohol dependency): may decrease the elimination of caffeine, thus intensifying its effects.

Erythromycin and troleandomycin: may decrease the elimination of caffeine, possibly increasing its effects.

Iron supplements: decreased iron absorption.

Lithium: may increase lithium elimination, decreasing lithium's effectiveness.

MAO inhibitors: combining with large amounts of caffeine may produce heart arrhythmias or severe hypertension.

Oral contraceptives: decreased action of caffeine.

Other central nervous system stimulants (amphetamines, pseudoephedrine): may add to stimulation and other adverse effects.

Other sources of caffeine or theobromines (related to caffeine) such as tea, coffee, chocolate: may produce an additive effect making side effects more likely.

CALCAREA CARBONICA

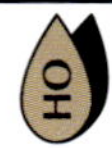

LATIN NAME
Calcarea carbonica

GENERAL DESCRIPTION
Calcarea carbonica, or calcium carbonate, is a source of calcium, one of the most abundant natural elements in the human body. Essential to cell structure and bone strength, calcium comes from many materials, including chalk, coral, and limestone. Perhaps as a reflection of its body-building properties, *Calcarea carbonica,* also called *Calc carb,* is used by homeopathic physicians for conditions that are accompanied by symptoms of exhaustion, depression, and anxiety. Calcium carbonate prepared for homeopathic use is ground from oyster shells and used at full strength.

TARGET AILMENTS
- lower-back pain, broken bones that are slow to heal, sprains from overexertion, muscle cramps, constipation, chronic ear infections, eye inflammations, headaches, insomnia brought on by anxiety, eczema, allergies, teething problems, gastritis, gallstones, childhood diarrhea, menstrual problems, asthma, palpitations, arthritis. (Take internally.)

PREPARATIONS
Calcarea carbonica is available over the counter in various potencies, in both liquid and tablet form, at selected stores and pharmacies. Consult your practitioner for more precise instructions.

SIDE EFFECTS

None expected.

CALCIUM CARBONATE

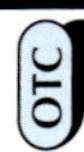

DRUG CLASS
Antacids

BRAND NAMES
Rolaids, Tums

GENERAL DESCRIPTION
Calcium carbonate is a calcium-containing antacid drug that relieves the symptoms of upset and sour stomach, heartburn, acid indigestion, and ulcers. This medication is also used to help prevent calcium-deficiency diseases such as osteoporosis. See ***Antacids*** for more information, including facts about side effects and possible drug interactions.

CALCIUM CHANNEL BLOCKERS

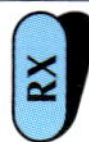

GENERIC NAMES
amlodipine, diltiazem, isradipine, nifedipine, verapamil

GENERAL DESCRIPTION
Calcium channel blockers block the passage of calcium into body cells. This action helps slow the contraction of the heart and arteries, thereby dilating the arteries, lowering blood pressure, and preventing some heart spasms. These drugs are used alone or in carefully selected combinations with other heart and blood pressure medications. For more information, see entries for the generic drugs listed above.

TARGET AILMENTS
- angina.
- heart-rhythm problems (especially diltiazem or verapamil).
- high blood pressure.
- Raynaud's syndrome (nifedipine).
- prevention of migraine headaches.

SIDE EFFECTS

Not serious:
Gastrointestinal upset (nausea, diarrhea, constipation), weight gain, increased appetite, drowsiness, tiredness, lightheadedness, headache, flushing. Call your doctor if these effects become troublesome.

Serious:
Heart problems, such as congestive heart failure, heart-rhythm irregularities, or increased angina (heart pain); low blood pressure; swelling of the lower extremities; allergic reactions, such as skin rash; bleeding or tender gums (rare). Contact your doctor immediately.

SPECIAL INFORMATION
- Recent findings have prompted warnings from some healthcare professionals about the safety of calcium channel blockers, particularly large doses of the short-acting form of nifedipine. Before using any of these drugs, be sure to discuss this matter thoroughly with your doctor. If you are already taking a calcium channel blocker, do not stop the medication without first consulting your doctor.
- Pregnant and nursing women should use calcium channel blockers only if clearly needed.
- Let your doctor know if you are suffering from low blood pressure (hypotension), heart or kidney disease, or pulmonary congestion.

POSSIBLE INTERACTIONS

All heart drugs, including digoxin, nitroglycerin, beta blockers, and angiotensin-converting enzyme (ACE) inhibitors: calcium channel blockers taken in combination with a heart medication may increase the effect of any of the drugs. However, it is not uncommon for these drugs to be prescribed together. If you are taking more than one of these medications, your doctor will want to monitor your reactions closely.

Alcohol: increased effect of calcium channel blockers, leading to dangerously low blood pressure; do not drink alcohol while being treated with these drugs.

Anti-inflammatory drugs, including nonsteroidal anti-inflammatory drugs (NSAIDs): decreased effect of calcium channel blockers.

Blood pressure drugs: can interact with calcium channel blockers, increasing the effect of any of the combined drugs and leading to excessive lowering of blood pressure.

Calcium supplements: may decrease the action of calcium channel blockers.

Carbamazepine, theophylline: increased blood levels of these medications.

Cimetidine: may increase the effects of some calcium channel blockers by interfering with stomach action.

Cyclosporine: taking calcium channel blockers with cyclosporine may cause toxic levels of cyclosporine to accumulate in the blood.

Drugs that reduce blood pressure either directly or indirectly, such as monoamine oxidase (MAO) inhibitors or opioid analgesics: calcium channel blockers may increase the hypotensive action of these drugs, possibly leading to dangerously low blood pressure. Your doctor may have to adjust your dosage of all medicines.

Estrogens: may elevate blood pressure and thus increase the need for calcium channel blockers.

Lithium: nausea, vomiting, diarrhea, or tremors.

Rifampin: reduced effect of calcium channel blockers.

CALCIUM POLYCARBOPHIL

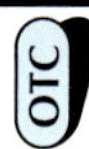

DRUG CLASS
Laxatives

BRAND NAME
FiberCon

GENERAL DESCRIPTION
Calcium polycarbophil is a bulk-forming laxative drug used to relieve both constipation and diarrhea. This type of laxative should be considered the first choice in treating constipation. It may also be especially beneficial to people on low-fiber diets and to those with irritable bowel syndrome (spastic colon), diverticulitis, or hemorrhoids. See ***Laxatives*** for information about side effects and possible drug interactions.

SPECIAL INFORMATION
- When taking this laxative, be sure to drink plenty of water or other fluid to avoid obstruction of the throat and esophagus. Taking this medication without enough liquid may cause choking.
- This laxative is slow acting; you may not experience its effects for 12 to 72 hours after taking it.

CALENDULA

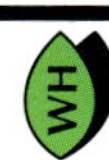

LATIN NAME
Calendula officinalis

GENERAL DESCRIPTION
The therapeutic use of calendula originated in ancient Egypt and spread to Europe. Many varieties of the plant exist, one of which is the common marigold. Calendula's medically active parts are its flowers. A natural antiseptic and anti-inflammatory agent, calendula is one of the best herbs for treating wounds, skin abrasions, and infections. Taken internally, it also helps alleviate the symptoms of indigestion and other gastrointestinal disorders. Calendula's healing power appears to come from components known as terpenes. One of these, calenduloside B, is known as a sedative and for its healing effect on ulcers.

TARGET AILMENTS
Take internally for:
- indigestion, gastric and duodenal ulcers, gallbladder problems.

Use as a gargle for:
- sore throat, cold sores.

Apply externally for:
- cuts, wounds, sores, burns; skin rashes from measles, chickenpox, and other eruptive skin diseases; diaper rash; athlete's foot and other fungal infections.

PREPARATIONS

Over the counter:
Calendula is available in several forms for both internal and external use. You can find lotions, ointments, oils, tinctures, and fresh or dried leaves and florets.

At home:
Rub lotions, ointments, and oils on injuries, rashes, and infections, as needed.

Poultice: Mash up the leaves, then apply directly to minor burns or scalds.

Infusion: Steep 1 oz dried herb in 1 pt boiling water. For acute internal symptoms, drink two to four times a day until symptoms lessen.

Combinations: A mixture of marsh mallow root, American cranesbill, and calendula may help digestive problems. Calendula is often combined with slippery elm and applied to soothe skin inflammations and wounds. A mixture of goldenseal, calendula, and myrrh makes an antiseptic lotion.

SPECIAL INFORMATION
- Calendula flowers can be made into an oil for external use and to ease earaches and other infections.

CAMPHOR

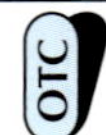

BRAND NAME
Vicks VapoRub

GENERAL DESCRIPTION
A resin from a type of cinnamon tree, camphor has been used for centuries as an insect repellent and as a medication for minor skin irritations. By itself or in combination with menthol, phenol, or methyl salicylate, camphor is found in many over-the-counter products, ranging from pain-relieving liniments to decongestants and cough suppressants.

Camphor is absorbed rapidly through the skin and by inhalation. Exposure to high concentrations of the substance can result in serious, even toxic side effects. Because deaths have occurred from camphor poisonings, the FDA has banned all products with a camphor concentration greater than 11 percent, including camphorated oil.

TARGET AILMENTS
- cough.
- nasal congestion.
- pain from arthritis and minor skin irritations.
- minor cuts and scrapes (as an antiseptic).

▼SIDE EFFECTS

Not serious:
Minor irritation when applied to skin. Call your doctor if the irritation is troublesome.

Serious:
Headache, dizziness, delirium, hallucinations, restlessness, confusion, tremors, jerky motions, convulsions, drowsiness, shallow breathing, coma. These symptoms indicate overdose or poisoning. In rare cases, death can result from respiratory failure or extreme convulsions. If any of these symptoms occur, call your doctor or poison control center immediately.

SPECIAL INFORMATION
- Because it can affect the developing fetus or pass to an infant through breast milk, camphor is not considered safe for pregnant or nursing women.
- Do not apply camphor to deep or serious wounds, since this may allow the drug to enter the bloodstream.

CANTHARIS

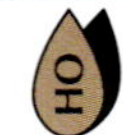

LATIN NAME
Cantharis

GENERAL DESCRIPTION
Popularly known as Spanish fly, cantharis is actually a beetle found in southern France and Spain. It produces an irritant so caustic that the skin will blister if exposed to it.

Cantharis has had a long career in medicine, used for all manner of disorders from baldness to rheumatism, even as an aphrodisiac. In high concentrations, the irritant can be toxic, prompting abdominal cramps and burning pains in the throat and stomach, vomiting of blood, diarrhea, kidney damage, convulsions, coma, and death. Homeopaths prescribe *Cantharis* for patients whose ailments are coupled with symptoms like those of cantharis poisoning.

According to homeopathic tradition, the beetles are collected at daybreak, when they are still sluggish from the cool of the night, and heated in the steam of boiling vinegar until dead. The beetles are then crushed and mixed with successively greater amounts of milk sugar, a pharmaceutical process called trituration. The resulting powder is highly dilute.

Like most homeopathic prescriptions, *Cantharis* was developed as a remedy by observation of the reactions of healthy individuals to a series of undilute doses. The mental, emotional, and physical changes induced by *Cantharis* were then cataloged. When a homeopathic practitioner encounters a patient with a set of symptoms that matches the cataloged symptoms brought on by *Cantharis,* the practitioner then prescribes it in an extremely dilute form. It is presumed that in this highly dilute dosage, *Cantharis* can counter the symptoms that it induces when it is at full strength.

TARGET AILMENTS
- bladder infections or cystitis, with a constant desire to urinate accompanied by blood and pain during urination; sunburns, scalds, and blistering second-degree burns. (Take internally.)
- stings or bites with intense burning.

PREPARATIONS
Cantharis is available over the counter in various potencies, in liquid and tablet form, at selected stores and pharmacies. Consult your homeopathic practitioner for more precise information.

▼SIDE EFFECTS
None expected.

CAPTOPRIL

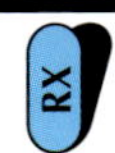

DRUG CLASS
Angiotensin-Converting Enzyme (ACE) Inhibitors

BRAND NAME
Capoten

GENERAL DESCRIPTION
Introduced in 1979, the ACE inhibitor captopril is prescribed for the control of high blood pressure (hypertension) and congestive heart failure. The drug works by blocking a body enzyme essential for

the production of a substance that causes blood vessels to constrict. This action relaxes arterial walls, lowering blood pressure and decreasing the work load of the heart. For increased effectiveness in lowering blood pressure, captopril is sometimes combined with hydrochlorothiazide. See ***Angiotensin-Converting Enzyme (ACE) Inhibitors*** for information on side effects and possible drug interactions.

CARBACEPHEMS

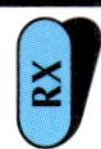

GENERIC NAME
loracarbef

GENERAL DESCRIPTION
Carbacephem drugs, a subclass of antibiotics, work in much the same way as penicillins and cephalosporins to kill growing bacteria. Loracarbef is the only carbacephem antibiotic on the market. See ***Loracarbef*** for information about side effects and possible interactions.

CARBAMAZEPINE

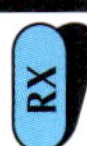

DRUG CLASS
Anticonvulsant Drugs

BRAND NAME
Tegretol

GENERAL DESCRIPTION
When first introduced in 1962, carbamazepine was approved as a pain reliever for rare forms of neuralgia. It is now used primarily in the control of several types of epileptic seizures, including tonic-clonic (grand mal) seizures, partial seizures, and mixed seizure patterns. Carbamazepine is considered a first-choice anticonvulsant drug due to its low toxicity and the rarity of serious adverse effects. For more information, see ***Anticonvulsant Drugs.***

TARGET AILMENTS
- certain types of epileptic seizures.
- relief of pain in trigeminal (tic douloureux) and glossopharyngeal neuralgia. However, carbamazepine should never be used to relieve ordinary aches and pains.

SIDE EFFECTS

Not serious:
Constipation; impaired urination; dry throat and mouth; water retention; mild nausea and vomiting; loss of appetite; drowsiness; fatigue; increased sensitivity to sunlight (sunburn, rash, itching, redness); headache; dizziness; unsteadiness; and confusion. Consult your doctor if these or other effects persist or are bothersome.

Serious:
Blurred or double vision; severe dermatitis; bone marrow depression (weakness, fever, abnormal bleeding or bruising); liver damage (jaundice); behavioral changes (agitation, hostility); and mental depression. Call your doctor at once.

SPECIAL INFORMATION
- Do not use carbamazepine if you: have had an allergic reaction to it or to any tricyclic antidepressant drug in the past; are nursing or in the first three months of pregnancy; have a blood cell disorder, a bone-marrow disorder, or an active liver disease.
- Tell your doctor if you: are taking any other drugs (prescription or over the counter); consume more than two alcoholic drinks a day; have a history of kidney or liver disease, thrombophlebitis, or a severe mental depression or disorder; are planning any medical or dental surgery requiring a general anesthesia.
- If you are over the age of 60, this drug may aggravate glaucoma, angina, and prostate problems.
- Carbamazepine should be taken with food to lessen stomach upset and improve absorbency.
- Routine testing for early indications of bone-marrow or blood cell toxicity is essential.
- Carbamazepine may affect blood cell counts, liver function tests, urine pregnancy tests, and various blood tests.
- Do not abruptly discontinue the drug or switch to another anticonvulsant drug unless advised to do so by your physician.
- Sudden withdrawal can cause a series of uninterrupted seizures.

POSSIBLE INTERACTIONS

Anticoagulants, doxycycline, oral contraceptives with estrogen, and valproic acid: carbamazepine can decrease the effect of these drugs.

Monoamine oxidase (MAO) inhibitors and lithium: may cause severe toxic reactions when taken with carbamazepine.

Tranquilizers, narcotics, alcohol, sedatives, and hypnotics: increased sedative effects.

CARISOPRODOL

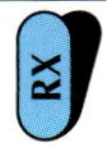

DRUG CLASS
Muscle Relaxants

BRAND NAME
Soma

GENERAL DESCRIPTION
Carisoprodol is used to rapidly relieve acute pain associated with muscle strains and spasms. Although its exact mechanisms are unknown, the drug has a sedative effect and it appears to block chemical pain messages from traveling to the brain. Carisoprodol is most effective if used in conjunction with rest, physical therapy, and other medications, such as analgesics.

TARGET AILMENTS
- acute, painful muscle strains and spasms

SIDE EFFECTS

Not serious:
Dizziness, drowsiness, flushed face, hiccups, lightheadedness, nausea, vertigo. Infrequently: headache, irritability, insomnia. Call your doctor if these side effects persist or become bothersome.

Serious:
Allergic reactions such as itching, welts on skin, skin rash, difficulty breathing, weakness. Uncommonly: agitation, confusion, depression, enlarged pupils, fainting, rapid heart rate, speech problems, temporary paralysis of arms and legs, tremors, vision problems, vomiting. Discontinue use and call your doctor immediately.

SPECIAL INFORMATION
- Women who are pregnant or nursing should take this medication only under a doctor's supervision.
- This medication may cause drowsiness. Use caution while taking carisoprodol if you must drive or perform other tasks requiring alertness.
- Carisoprodol should be used with caution by patients who have kidney or liver problems.

POSSIBLE INTERACTIONS

Alcohol: Increased effects of alcohol.

Antidepressants, sedatives, tranquilizers: Altered effects of these drugs. Consult your doctor before combining carisoprodol with any of these drugs.

CATNIP

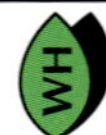

LATIN NAME
Nepeta cataria

GENERAL DESCRIPTION
Herbalists have used the flowers and leaves of catnip, an aromatic member of the mint family, for more than 2,000 years. Today it is prescribed for easing digestion, calming nerves, and relieving muscle spasms, including menstrual cramps. Cats are strongly attracted to catnip and may become intoxicated by eating it; but the herb has no such effect on humans.

TARGET AILMENTS
Take internally for:
- indigestion, gas, tension, difficulty in sleeping, colds, flu, bronchial congestion, fever, colic in infants, menstrual cramps.

Apply externally for:
- cuts and scrapes.

PREPARATIONS
Over the counter:
Catnip is available in dried bulk flowers and leaves, tincture, and tea bags.

At home:
To treat minor cuts and scrapes, press crushed catnip leaves into them before washing and bandaging them.

Infusion: Pour 1 cup boiling water onto 2 tsp dried leaves and steep for 10 to 15 minutes. Drink three times a day.

Combinations: Mix with boneset, elder, yarrow, or cayenne for colds.

SIDE EFFECTS

Not serious:
Catnip can produce an upset stomach. If this occurs, discontinue use and call your doctor.

SPECIAL INFORMATION
- Avoid catnip during pregnancy.
- You can give weak, cool infusions to infants with colic. For other children and people over 65, start with weak preparations and increase the strength as necessary.

CAYENNE

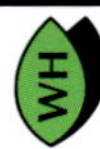

LATIN NAME
Capsicum frutescens

GENERAL DESCRIPTION
Herbalists regard cayenne as a powerful tonic. The seed-sized fruit stimulates the heart and promotes blood circulation, improves digestion, and boosts energy. Like other species of hot garden pepper, such as chili or tabasco, cayenne contains the natural stimulant known as capsaicin. Cayenne was widely grown in Central and South America in pre-Columbian times; it was carried to Spain and Europe after the early voyages of discovery.

TARGET AILMENTS
Take internally for:
- poor circulation, indigestion, gas, physical or mental exhaustion, and lowered energy or vitality, particularly in the elderly.

Apply externally for:
- pain, including that of arthritis and diabetes, strains, sore muscles and joints, the need to stimulate blood flow or to stop external bleeding.

PREPARATIONS
Over the counter:
Cayenne is available as powder, capsules, tincture, or oil.

At home:
Rub the oil on sprains, swelling, sore muscles, and joints to ease pain.

Infusion: Pour 1 cup boiling water onto ½ to 1 tsp cayenne powder and steep for 10 minutes. Mix 1 tbsp of the infusion with hot water and drink as needed.

Gargle: Combine cayenne with myrrh to treat laryngitis and as an antiseptic wash.

SIDE EFFECTS

Not serious:
In large doses, cayenne can produce vomiting, stomach pain, and a type of intoxication. Do not exceed prescribed dosages.

SPECIAL INFORMATION
- Because it is hot and spicy as an infusion or tincture, cayenne can cause mild nausea when first taken. It's best to start with a small amount and increase gradually to the recommended dosage.
- Do not use cayenne on open cuts, sores, or broken skin.
- If you have an ulcer, use cayenne only with the consent of your physician.

CEFACLOR

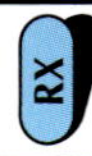

DRUG CLASS
Antibiotics [Cephalosporins]

BRAND NAME
Ceclor

GENERAL DESCRIPTION
Introduced in 1979, cefaclor is a cephalosporin antibiotic used to treat certain types of pneumonia and otitis media, as well as strep throat and infections of the skin, skin-structure, and urinary tract. For more information see ***Cephalosporins.***

CEFADROXIL

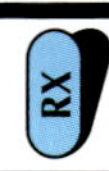

DRUG CLASS
Antibiotics [Cephalosporins]

BRAND NAME
Duricef

GENERAL DESCRIPTION
A cephalosporin antibiotic introduced in 1977, cefadroxil is used to treat infections of the urinary tract, upper respiratory tract, and skin. For information about side effects and interactions, see ***Cephalosporins.***

CEFIXIME

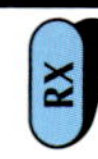

DRUG CLASS
Antibiotics [Cephalosporins]

BRAND NAME
Suprax

GENERAL DESCRIPTION
Introduced in 1986, cefixime is a cephalosporin antibiotic used to treat respiratory tract infections such as pharyngitis and otitis media, as well as uncomplicated gonorrhea and urinary

tract infections. For more information, see ***Cephalosporins.***

CEFPROZIL

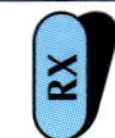

DRUG CLASS
Antibiotics [Cephalosporins]

BRAND NAME
Cefzil

GENERAL DESCRIPTION
Introduced in 1991, cefprozil is a cephalosporin antibiotic used to treat skin infections and respiratory tract infections such as pharyngitis, otitis media, and bronchitis. For more information see ***Cephalosporins.***

SPECIAL INFORMATION
- People with the congenital disorder phenylketonuria should avoid cefprozil in oral suspension, which contains phenylalanine.

CEFUROXIME

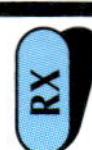

DRUG CLASS
Antibiotics [Cephalosporins]

BRAND NAME
Ceftin

GENERAL DESCRIPTION
A cephalosporin antibiotic introduced in 1976, cefuroxime is used to treat respiratory tract infections, such as otitis media, as well as gonorrhea and infections of the urinary tract and skin. This drug is often taken with food to mask its strong, bitter taste. See ***Cephalosporins*** for more information.

CELECOXIB

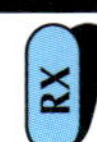

DRUG CLASS
Nonsteroidal Anti-Inflammatory Drugs (NSAIDs) [COX-2 Inhibitors]

BRAND NAME
Celebrex

GENERAL DESCRIPTION
Celecoxib is used to treat two types of arthritis: osteoarthritis and rheumatoid arthritis. Like other COX-2 inhibitors, this drug is less likely to cause ulcers and stomach bleeding than other NSAIDs and it does not decrease blood clotting time. Celecoxib has been approved as a cancer prevention drug in people at high risk for colon cancer due to the genetic disorder familial adenomatous polyposis. It is in clinical trials to determine if it can prevent colon, skin, esophageal, and bladder cancers in the general population. For additional information about this drug, see ***COX-2 Inhibitors.***

CENTRAL NERVOUS SYSTEM STIMULANTS

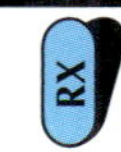

GENERAL DESCRIPTION
The central nervous system (CNS) stimulant class includes a number of drugs that are used to treat various organic, psychological, and behavioral disorders, such as attention deficit disorders, narcolepsy, depression, and obesity. Amphetamines and cocaine are major drugs in this class. Minor drugs include appetite suppressants, bronchodilators, caffeine, and the sympathomimetics.

Abuse or chronic use of CNS stimulants can result in drug dependence or addiction. For this reason, dosages must be prescribed on an individual basis, and physician supervision is essential. For information on a specific generic drug used primarily in the treatment of attention deficit disorders in children and in the control of narcolepsy, see ***Methylphenidate.***

CEPHALEXIN

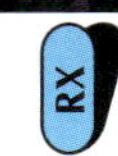

DRUG CLASS
Antibiotics [Cephalosporins]

GENERAL DESCRIPTION
Introduced in 1969, cephalexin is a cephalosporin antibiotic used to treat respiratory tract infections, such as otitis media, as well as bacterial infections of the skin, bones and joints, and genitourinary tract. For more information, see ***Cephalosporins.***

CEPHALOSPORINS

GENERIC NAMES
cefaclor, cefadroxil, cefixime, cefprozil, cefuroxime, cephalexin

GENERAL DESCRIPTION
Cephalosporins, a subclass of antibiotics related to penicillins, act by destroying growing bacteria. They do not kill fungi or viruses, such as those responsible for colds and the flu. Your doctor may prescribe these drugs if you have an infection caused by bacteria resistant to penicillins. Cephalosporins are available in forms that can be taken orally or injected.

TARGET AILMENTS
- otitis media.
- infections of the respiratory tract, genitourinary tract, skin, or soft tissue.
- serious infections of the blood, bones, joints, abdomen, lungs, or heart.

SIDE EFFECTS

Not serious:
Mild nausea, mild diarrhea, yeast infections of the mouth (sore mouth or tongue) or of the vagina (vaginal itching or discharge). Tell your doctor when convenient.

Serious:
Dizziness, serum sickness (fever accompanied by joint pains and rash), severe diarrhea, a severe allergic reaction, unusual bruising or bleeding, or severe stomach cramps. Call your doctor immediately.

SPECIAL INFORMATION
- Let your doctor know if you have ever had an allergic reaction to a cephalosporin drug or to penicillins, penicillamine, or a penicillin derivative. Your doctor may decide to prescribe a different drug. About 10 percent of people with allergies to penicillin are also allergic to cephalosporins. Reactions range from mild rashes and fever to life-threatening anaphylaxis.
- Tell your doctor if you have kidney or liver impairment, phenylketonuria, or a history of bleeding disorders or gastrointestinal disease; cephalosporins can exacerbate these conditions.
- Take the full course of your prescription, even if you feel better before finishing the medication; otherwise, the infection may return.
- These drugs may cause false-positive results for the Clinitest urine glucose test. (They do not affect results of

Clinistix or Tes-Tape.) Cefuroxime causes false-negative results in some blood glucose tests.
- Cephalosporins may be taken on a full or on an empty stomach. While most of these drugs are absorbed more quickly on an empty stomach, cefuroxime is better absorbed when taken with food.
- If possible, avoid taking these drugs if you are pregnant or breast-feeding.
- Cephalosporins also kill "good" intestinal bacteria that keep harmful fungi and intestinal bacteria in check. Eating yogurt containing *Lactobacillus acidophilus* culture or taking acidophilus tablets may help restore the body's normal bacteria.
- Prolonged use of any antibiotic drug can lead to fungal infections, including candidiasis, or to bacterial infections such as pseudomembranous colitis.

POSSIBLE INTERACTIONS

Aminoglycosides (amikacin, gentamicin, kanamycin, neomycin, netilmicin, streptomycin, tobramycin): risk of kidney failure.

Bacteriostatic drugs (tetracycline, erythromycin, chloramphenicol, sulfonamides): may impair cephalosporins' bacteria-killing action.

Loop diuretics: risk of kidney failure.

Nephrotoxic drugs (vancomycin, colistin, polymyxin B): risk of kidney failure.

Probenecid: decreases the kidneys' ability to excrete cephalosporins. Possible cephalosporin toxicity. However, this combination is sometimes prescribed to treat serious infections that require high, prolonged serum levels of cephalosporins.

CHAMOMILE

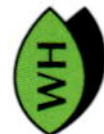

LATIN NAME
Matricaria recutita

GENERAL DESCRIPTION
Of the three types of chamomile plant, the most popular and thoroughly studied is German chamomile, used medicinally around the world for thousands of years. Modern herbalists have identified elements in the oil of the chamomile flower that appear to calm the central nervous system, relax the digestive tract, and speed the healing process.

TARGET AILMENTS
Take internally for:
- stomach cramps, gas and nervous stomach, indigestion, ulcers, menstrual cramps, insomnia, colic, bladder problems.

Apply externally for:
- swelling and pain in the joints, skin inflammation and sunburn, cuts and scrapes, teething pain, varicose veins, hemorrhoids, sore or inflamed eyes.

Use as a gargle for:
- gingivitis and sore throat.

PREPARATIONS
Over the counter:
Available as prepared tea, tincture, essential oil, and dried or fresh flowers.

At home:
Tea: Pour 8 oz boiling water over 2 tsp chamomile flowers and steep for 10 minutes. Drink 1 cup three or four times daily, or dilute and use as an eye compress *(see below).*

Compress: Strain the tea through a coffee filter and dilute with an equal amount of water. Always use fresh tea (less than 24 hours old) and refrigerate unused portions. (Bring the dilute tea to room temperature before using it.) To make the compress, pour the liquid on a cloth and apply to the closed eye. Discontinue if your eye becomes irritated.

Fomentation: Apply three or four times daily to sore muscles; sore, swollen joints; varicose veins; and burns and skin wounds.

Herbal bath: Run bathwater over 2 or 3 oz chamomile flowers tied in cloth, or add no more than 2 drops essential oil of chamomile to bathwater.

SIDE EFFECTS
None expected.

SPECIAL INFORMATION
- Allergies to chamomile are rare. However, anyone allergic to other plants in the daisy family (chrysanthemums, ragweed, and asters, for example) should be alert to possible allergic reactions to chamomile, ranging from contact dermatitis to anaphylaxis (itching, rash, and difficulty breathing).

CHAMOMILLA

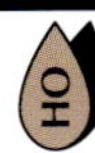

LATIN NAME
Chamomilla

GENERAL DESCRIPTION
Chamomilla is made from the flowering German chamomile plant common in Europe. The whole plant is crushed, and its juices are mixed with equal parts of alcohol, then succussed. In homeopathy, *Chamomilla* is considered to work best for people who are extremely sensitive to pain, irritable, impatient, and implacable. *Chamomilla* patients sweat easily and are sensitive to wind and chills. *Chamomilla* is most often given to children who work themselves into violent temper tantrums.

Like most homeopathic prescriptions, *Chamomilla* was developed as a remedy by observation of the reactions of healthy individuals to a series of undilute doses. The mental, emotional, and physical changes induced by *Chamomilla* were then cataloged. When a homeopathic practitioner encounters a patient with a set of symptoms that matches the cataloged symptoms brought on by *Chamomilla,* the practitioner then prescribes it in an extremely dilute form. It is presumed that in this highly dilute dosage, *Chamomilla* can counter the symptoms that it induces when it is at full strength.

TARGET AILMENTS
- irritability; toothaches aggravated by cold air and warm food; painful menstrual periods with severe cramping and a feeling of anger or restlessness; extremely painful earaches; teething pain, especially if the child is irritable; difficulty getting to sleep; painful diarrhea, especially in children.

PREPARATIONS
Chamomilla is available over the counter or from your homeopathic practitioner. Consult your practitioner for dosage information.

SIDE EFFECTS
None expected.

CHASTE TREE

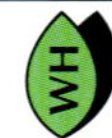

LATIN NAME
Vitex agnus-castus

GENERAL DESCRIPTION
Since ancient times, herbalists have used the berries of the chaste tree, sometimes known as chasteberries, to manipulate the functioning of the female reproductive system. Chaste tree's natural compounds seem to aid in regulating the menstrual cycle by bringing into balance the female sex hormones, estrogen and progesterone. Besides treating menstrual irregularities, chaste tree is prescribed for relieving premenstrual syndrome and to counter symptoms of menopause. It also aids in readjusting the body after withdrawal from long-term use of birth-control pills, preventing miscarriage in the first three months of pregnancy, and promoting lactation. In past eras, the herb was used to dampen the sexual longings of Roman women whose husbands were abroad on military expeditions and to curb the sex drives of medieval monks. Paradoxically, chaste tree has also had a reputation as an aphrodisiac.

TARGET AILMENTS
- premenstrual syndrome, menstrual irregularities, symptoms of menopause, prevention of miscarriage, promotion of lactation, hormone-related constipation, endometriosis (disorder of the uterine lining), fibroid cysts that occur in smooth muscle tissue, acne in both male and female teenagers. (Take internally.)

PREPARATIONS
Over the counter:
Chaste tree is available as berries, powder, dried herb, capsules, and tincture.

At home:
Tea: Pour 1 cup boiling water onto 1 tsp ripe berries and let them infuse for 10 to 15 minutes. Drink three times a day.

SPECIAL INFORMATION
- Chaste tree seems to regulate hormonal imbalances within 10 days, and relief from premenstrual syndrome may be noticeable by the second menstrual cycle. For optimal benefit, however, the herb should be taken for six months or longer.
- Discontinue the herb after the third month of pregnancy, since it may cause premature production of milk.

CHICKWEED

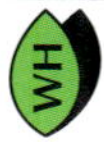

LATIN NAME
Stellaria media

GENERAL DESCRIPTION
Rubbed on the body, this common weed is one of the best herbs for relieving the discomfort of insect bites and other itchy skin conditions. The components of chickweed known as saponin glycosides exert a soothing effect on the skin. Taken internally, chickweed has a similar soothing and moistening effect on the lungs and stomach.

TARGET AILMENTS
Take internally for:
- sore throat, congestion in the lungs, stomach and duodenal ulcers, rheumatism.

Apply externally for:
- cuts; wounds; bites from mosquitoes and other insects; eczema, psoriasis, and other itching skin irritations; boils, abscesses, skin ulcers; scalp conditions.

PREPARATIONS
Over the counter:
Chickweed is available in dried bulk, oil, ointment, and tincture.

At home:
Tea: Pour 1 cup boiling water onto 2 tsp dried herb and steep for five minutes. Drink a cup three times a day to reduce itching.

Bath: Pour either a strong infusion or fresh herbs into the bathwater to relieve itching.

Cool drink: Combine a handful of fresh herbs with pineapple juice, process in the blender, and strain. This drink may relieve skin irritation and rheumatism.

Ointment: Add marsh mallow root to the fresh herbs and juice, and blend.

Poultice: Grind up fresh leaves and apply to leg ulcers.

SPECIAL INFORMATION
- You can eat as much fresh chickweed as you want, for its therapeutic effects. Chickweed is high in vitamin C, and the fresh herb can be eaten raw in a salad or as a cooked green.
- Juice squeezed from the leaves with a mortar and pestle is particularly effective in healing scalp problems.
- Because it contains vitamin C, chickweed has been used as a remedy for scurvy.

CHICORY

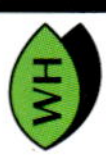

LATIN NAME
Cichorium intybus

GENERAL DESCRIPTION
A somewhat scraggly plant with blue flowers, chicory flourishes both in gardens and in the wild, and has been known to doctors at least as far back as the first century AD. Although it has many medicinal uses, chicory is often used as a food additive. The plant's leaves, like other leafy green vegetables, can be added to a salad or served by themselves, and the roasted and ground chicory root is a common addition to coffee in Europe as well as in the United States. Chicory added to coffee complements the popular drink, for experiments have shown that lactucin and lactucopicrin (two of the substances in chicory that make it taste somewhat bitter) may counteract the effects of caffeine by their sedative action on the central nervous system.

Chicory is believed to be a laxative and is also said to increase the flow of bile. It may in addition be suitable for treating gout and rheumatism, because it acts as a mild diuretic, increasing the elimination of fluid from the body. Chicory leaves have also been used in compresses to treat skin inflammations and swellings.

TARGET AILMENTS
Take internally for:
- caffeine-induced rapid heartbeat; jaundice, spleen problems, gallstones; gastritis and other digestive difficulties; rheumatism; gout.

Apply externally for:
- skin inflammations.

PREPARATIONS
Over the counter:
Chicory is available in bulk as green leaves and dried roots.

At home:
Tea: Simmer 1 tsp rootstock or dried herb with ½ cup water and strain; drink 8 to 12 oz per day for jaundice, spleen problems, gallstones, or gastritis.

Nutrition and diet: Squeeze 1 tbsp juice from the chicory stem with your hands and take it in milk or water three times daily. Use the fresh greens in a salad, or sauté them as a side dish.

SIDE EFFECTS

Not serious:
If your skin becomes red, swollen, or irritated after you handle chicory, cover

C

your hands with gloves and treat the irritated area as needed.

CHINESE FOXGLOVE ROOT

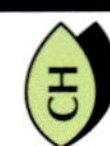

LATIN NAME
Rehmannia glutinosa

GENERAL DESCRIPTION
The thick, reddish yellow Chinese foxglove root is cooked in wine and used as a tonic. The cooked form of the root is often used in treating disorders associated with aging. It is classified as sweet and warm in traditional Chinese medicine.

TARGET AILMENTS
Take internally for:
- lightheadedness, palpitations, blurred vision, or floaters in vision.
- insomnia or the inability to be still and restful.
- chronic low-grade fever and night sweats.
- constipation with dry, hard stools.
- irregular menstruation or uterine bleeding, especially after childbirth.
- low-back pain and weak knees; weak, stiff joints.
- hearing loss and tinnitus (ringing in the ears).
- premature graying of hair.

PREPARATIONS
The prepared root and the raw version are available from Chinese pharmacies, Asian markets, and some Western health food stores. When you order, specify that you want the cooked version, which is made by soaking the root in rice wine with spices such as cardamom.

Combinations: A mixture with gelatin is prescribed for coughing and vomiting blood, nosebleeds, and bleeding from the uterus. Practitioners also use combinations of the cooked root with cornus and Chinese yam, or with freshwater turtle shell, to treat lightheadedness, insomnia, forgetfulness, and related symptoms. See a Chinese medicine practitioner for information on dosages and further herbal combinations.

SIDE EFFECTS
- Grains-of-paradise fruit is often added to preparations of Chinese foxglove root to prevent side effects such as diarrhea, nausea, and abdominal pain.

SPECIAL INFORMATION
- WARNING: Individuals who have digestive problems or a tendency to gas and abdominal bloating are advised to use this herb carefully; the cooked herb can distend the abdomen and cause loose stools.
- In a trial with a small number of patients, raw Chinese foxglove root was used to treat rheumatoid arthritis. Some improvement in rheumatic symptoms was shown over a period of about six months.

CHINESE MOTHERWORT

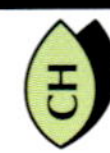

LATIN NAME
Leonurus heterophyllus

GENERAL DESCRIPTION
In a literal translation of its Chinese name, *yì mu cao,* motherwort means "benefit mother herb," and indeed the leaves are popular among Chinese women as a treatment for menstrual difficulties. When seeking the best variety, look for thin stems and pure green coloring. In traditional Chinese medicine, motherwort is classified as acrid, bitter, and slightly cold.

TARGET AILMENTS
Take internally for:
- irregular menstruation or light menstrual flow, premenstrual abdominal pain, uterine fibroids, postpartum abdominal pain, infertility.
- difficulty in urinating and edema (swelling caused by retention of fluids), particularly when accompanied by blood in the urine.

PREPARATIONS
Chinese motherwort is available as leaves or powder in Chinese pharmacies, Asian food markets, and some Western health food stores.

Combinations: The herb is often mixed with red peony root, dong quai, and aucklandia to regulate the appropriate timing of the menstrual cycle and alleviate the pain and discomfort of menstruation. Herbalists prescribe a combination with imperata to treat edema associated with the kidney disease nephritis. And a mixture containing Chinese motherwort, polygonati, pyrrosia leaves, and musk mallow seeds is used to treat kidney stones and bloody urine. Check with a Chinese medicine practitioner for information on dosages and additional combinations.

SIDE EFFECTS
None expected.

SPECIAL INFORMATION
- WARNING: Do not use this herb if you are pregnant. In laboratory trials it has caused rabbits to miscarry.
- In a clinical test, the herb seemed effective in causing the uterus to contract after childbirth.
- The seeds of this plant also are thought to have medicinal properties. They are used for certain types of uterine bleeding.

CHINESE YAM

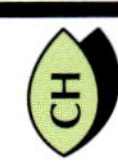

LATIN NAME
Dioscorea opposita

GENERAL DESCRIPTION
Chinese yam, a thick, firm root with a white cross section, is used as a tonic. Classified as neutral and sweet in traditional Chinese medicine, the herb is harvested in the winter in the mountains of Hunan and many other Chinese provinces.

TARGET AILMENTS
- weak digestion with diarrhea and fatigue, reduced appetite, frequent urination, excessive vaginal discharge, chronic coughing and wheezing, symptoms that accompany diabetes. (Take internally.)

PREPARATIONS
Chinese yam is available as a fresh or dried vegetable in Chinese pharmacies, Asian food markets, and some Western health food stores. For symptoms of diabetes, slices of the fresh root are steeped in hot water to make a tea.

Combinations: A mixture of Chinese yam, poria, and atractylodes (white) may be prescribed for loose, watery stools. Chinese yam and codonopsis root make up a preparation used to treat fatigue, general weakness, and reduced appetite. Consult a Chinese medicine practitioner for information on dosages and other herbal combinations.

SIDE EFFECTS
None expected.

SPECIAL INFORMATION
- If symptoms include abdominal swelling and pain, do not use Chinese yam.

POSSIBLE INTERACTIONS

Do not take Chinese yam with kan-sui root.

CHLORHEXIDINE

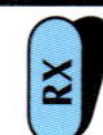

DRUG CLASS
Antibiotics [Topical Antibiotics]

BRAND NAME
Peridex

GENERAL DESCRIPTION
Chlorhexidine is used as an oral rinse in the treatment of gingivitis. By reducing the amount of bacteria in the mouth, the drug helps reduce inflammation (redness and swelling) and bleeding in the gums. For side effects and other information, see ***Topical Antibiotics.***

CHLORPHENIRAMINE

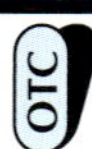

DRUG CLASS
Antihistamines

BRAND NAMES
Alka-Seltzer Plus Cold Medicine, Chlor-Trimeton, Comtrex Multi-Symptom Cold Reliever, TheraFlu, Triaminic Nite Light, Triaminic Syrup, Triaminicol Multi-Symptom Relief, some types of Tylenol Cold for adults and for children

GENERAL DESCRIPTION
Chlorpheniramine is an antihistamine with mild sedating effects. See ***Antihistamines.***

CHOLESTEROL-REDUCING DRUGS

GENERIC NAMES
atorvastatin, cholestyramine, colestipol, gemfibro-zil, lovastatin, pravastatin, simvastatin

GENERAL DESCRIPTION
As their name suggests, cholesterol-reducing drugs are used to alter levels of cholesterol and other fats in the blood. These fats combine with proteins to form lipoproteins. It has been shown that high levels of low-density lipoprotein (LDL) cholesterol increase the risk of heart disease, whereas high levels of high-density lipoprotein (HDL) seem to protect against it. These drugs help both to reduce the "bad" LDL cholesterol and to raise the "good" HDL cholesterol.

Cholesterol-reducing drugs are usually prescribed only after diet modification has failed to lower blood cholesterol levels. The medicines serve as a supplement to a proper diet and exercise program. They will not cure cholesterol disorders, but they do help to control them. No one drug is appropriate for treating all cholesterol disorders.

There are four major groups of cholesterol-reducing drugs: antihyperlipidemic (gemfibrozil); HMG-CoA reductase inhibitors (atorvastatin lovastatin, pravastatin, simvastatin); bile acid-binding resins (cholestyramine, colestipol); and niacin. The drugs work alone or in carefully prescribed combinations to normalize blood lipid levels. Some work by inhibiting the synthesis of cholesterol and lipoproteins. Others accelerate the clearance of lipoproteins in the bloodstream or hasten their breakdown and elimination. For more information, see entries for the generic drugs listed above.

TARGET AILMENTS

- the major types of cholesterol disorders, particularly those in which high levels of blood fats (cholesterol and triglycerides) have been linked to an increased risk of heart disease.

SIDE EFFECTS

Not serious:
Mild stomach pain; diarrhea; heartburn; nausea and vomiting; dizziness; headache.

Serious:
Severe stomach pain with nausea and vomiting; unusual tiredness or weakness.

SPECIAL INFORMATION

- If you are pregnant or nursing, check with your doctor before using any of these drugs. Atorvastatin, lovastatin, pravastatin, and simvastatin are not recommended if you are nursing, pregnant, or planning to become pregnant.
- Do not use any of these drugs if you have had an allergic reaction to them in the past.
- Do not use these drugs without telling your physician if you have or have had impaired liver or kidney function, gallstones or gallbladder disease, peptic ulcers, bleeding disorders, allergies, alcohol abuse, convulsions, organ transplants, cataracts or visual problems, chronic muscular disorder, gout or diabetes, low blood pressure, constipation, major surgery (or plan surgery soon), or any other medical problem.
- Carefully follow the special diet your doctor has recommended: This is essential if the medication is to work effectively.
- See your doctor regularly to have your progress measured and monitored.
- Do not stop taking the medication without first checking with your doctor; your blood cholesterol levels may increase again.
- Cholesterol-reducing drugs may affect the results of laboratory tests. Be sure to inform the healthcare practitioner performing the test if you are taking any of these drugs.
- Before undergoing emergency treatment or medical or dental surgery, be sure to tell your healthcare practitioner if you are taking any of these drugs.

POSSIBLE INTERACTIONS

Anticoagulants (such as warfarin): increased or decreased blood-thinning effects.

Oral medications: cholestyramine and colestipol interfere with the absorption of nearly every other drug, as well as with vitamins A, D, E, and K. Be sure to take your other medications at different times of the day.

CHOLESTYRAMINE

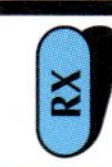

DRUG CLASS
Cholesterol-Reducing Drugs

BRAND NAME
Questran

GENERAL DESCRIPTION
Introduced in 1959, cholestyramine is in the group of medicines known as bile acid-binding resins. These drugs lower blood levels of cholesterol by binding to the bile acids from which cholesterol is made and removing them from the body. See also ***Cholesterol-Reducing Drugs.***

SIDE EFFECTS

Not serious:
Belching, bloating.

Serious:
Constipation; weight loss; black, tarry stool.

SPECIAL INFORMATION

- Never take this drug in dry form, as it may cause you to choke. Mix powder as directed with water or fruit juice.
- Cholestyramine may interfere with your body's ability to absorb certain nutrients. While on this medication, you may need to take supplements of vitamins A, D, E, and K; folic acid; and calcium. Consult your doctor.

POSSIBLE INTERACTIONS

Other medications should be taken two hours before or four to six hours after taking cholestyramine.

CHRYSANTHEMUM FLOWER

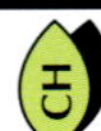

LATIN NAME

Chrysanthemum indicum

GENERAL DESCRIPTION

The wild chrysanthemum, growing throughout China, is valued for its anti-inflammatory effects. The best flowers for medicinal purposes are yellow and fragrant, with an acrid, bitter taste. In traditional Chinese medicine the herb is characterized as acrid, bitter, and slightly cold. It is harvested in the fall, when the flowers bloom.

TARGET AILMENTS

Take internally for:

- headaches, dizziness, and hearing problems.
- hypertension (high blood pressure).

Apply externally as a compress or wash:

- eye problems, such as conjunctivitis, red or dry eyes, blurred vision, and spots in front of the eyes.

PREPARATIONS

Fresh or dried flowers are available in bulk at Chinese pharmacies, Asian food markets, and some Western health food stores. They make a cooling drink.

Combinations: A mixture of chrysanthemum flowers with honeysuckle flowers and other herbs is a formula for colds and flu. A combination of the flowers with prunella and white mulberry leaf is prescribed for painful, red, swollen eyes. Chrysanthemum flowers mixed with honeysuckle are taken for toxic sores. Modern practitioners use a blend containing chrysanthemum, honeysuckle, and dandelion *(Taraxacum mongolicum)* to treat hypertension (high blood pressure). Check with a Chinese medicine practitioner for details of dosages and additional herbal combinations.

SIDE EFFECTS

None expected.

SPECIAL INFORMATION

- Use cautiously if there is diarrhea.
- The herb has a strong antibiotic effect.

CICADA

LATIN NAME

Cryptotympana atrata

GENERAL DESCRIPTION

A winged insect with a large head, the cicada is recognized by its characteristic chirping sound. The molted skin of the creature is used as a treatment for skin rashes, sore throats, and other ailments. In traditional Chinese medicine cicada is characterized as sweet and slightly cold.

TARGET AILMENTS

Take internally for:

- swollen, sore throat with loss of voice.
- skin rashes, particularly during the early stage of measles or chickenpox.
- red, painful, swollen eyes and blurred vision.
- high fever in childhood illnesses such as measles, which can cause convulsions, spasms, delirium, and terrifying nightmares in children.

PREPARATIONS

Dried cicada can be obtained at Chinese pharmacies. Look for yellow, lightweight skins.

Combinations: A blend with field mint is prescribed to ease itchy, red eyes and also to bring the rash out in the early stage of measles, to help shorten the duration of the illness. Herbalists may add chrysanthemum flowers *(Chrysanthemum morifolium)* and white mulberry leaves to strengthen the mixture's fever-reducing qualities. Another treatment for the early stage of measles is a blend of cicada skins with kudzu root and great burdock fruit. A preparation containing cicada skins and sterculia seeds may be prescribed for hoarseness. Check with a Chinese medicine practitioner for details of dosages and other herbal combinations.

SPECIAL INFORMATION

- WARNING: Be careful about using cicada if you are pregnant, because it might prompt a miscarriage. Check with a Chinese herbalist.

CIMETIDINE

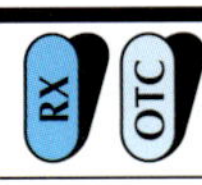

DRUG CLASS

Antiulcer Drugs [Histamine H_2 Blockers]

BRAND NAMES

Rx: Tagamet

OTC: Tagamet HB

GENERAL DESCRIPTION

Cimetidine is used both to treat and to prevent ulcers of the stomach and duodenum (upper intestine). It is also prescribed for other conditions characterized by an overproduction of stomach acid, such as Zollinger-Ellison syndrome and gastroesophageal reflux (in which stomach acid flows backward into the esophagus). In some cases, cimetidine is used to help stop upper gastrointestinal bleeding. Cimetidine has also been used experimentally to treat kidney cancer.

In the over-the-counter form, cimetidine is used not for ulcers but to relieve acid indigestion and heartburn. Although the OTC version is a lower dose of cimetidine than the prescription form, essentially the same interactions apply, though the side effects are milder.

Belonging to the subclass of antiulcer drugs known as histamine H_2 blockers, cimetidine works by blocking the stomach's response to the chemical compound histamine, thereby reducing the secretion of the digestive juice hydrochloric acid. For more information on side effects and possible drug interactions, see ***Antiulcer Drugs.***

SIDE EFFECTS

Not serious:
Mild diarrhea, skin rash, hives, dizziness, headache, blurred vision, fatigue, muscle and joint pain. Contact your doctor if these symptoms continue or become bothersome.

Serious:
Confusion, nervousness, delirium and hallucinations, slowed or irregular heartbeat, abnormal bleeding or bruis-

ing, combined weakness, fever, and sore throat (signs of bone-marrow depression), hair loss, enlarged or painful breasts (in women or men), male impotence, jaundice. Call your doctor immediately.

SPECIAL INFORMATION

- Inform your doctor if you have a history of arthritis, kidney or liver disease, organic brain syndrome, asthma, or low sperm count.
- Avoid this drug if you are pregnant or nursing.
- Cimetidine may affect the results of some medical tests, including blood cholesterol levels, liver function tests, and sperm counts. Inform the person giving you the test that you are taking this medication.
- This drug may inhibit your body's ability to absorb vitamin B_{12}. Talk to your doctor about B_{12} supplements.

POSSIBLE INTERACTIONS

This drug interacts with many prescription and over-the-counter medications, some of which are listed here. Make sure you inform your doctor of any other drugs you may be taking.

Alcohol: cimetidine may interfere with the elimination of alcohol from the body, prolonging alcohol's intoxicating effects.

Antacids: blocked absorption of cimetidine; space dosages of cimetidine and antacids at least an hour apart.

Anticancer drugs: increased risk of blood disorders.

Anticoagulants (such as warfarin), oral antidiabetic drugs, benzodiazepines, calcium channel blockers (such as amlodipine and diltiazem), carbamazepine, metoprolol, pentoxifylline, phenytoin, propranolol, theophylline, triamterene, tricyclic antidepressants: increased effects of these drugs, possibly leading to toxicity.

Digoxin: decreased digoxin effect.

Enteric-coated tablets: changes in stomach acidity may cause these drugs to dissolve prematurely in the stomach; avoid taking enteric-coated medications with cimetidine.

Iron, ketoconazole, tetracycline: decreased absorption of these drugs into the body.

Tobacco: smoking may block the beneficial effects of cimetidine.

CIMICIFUGA

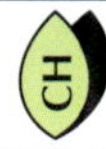

LATIN NAME

Cimicifuga foetida (or *Cimicifuga dahurica*)

GENERAL DESCRIPTION

Otherwise known as bugbane, cimicifuga has medicinal properties in the root, which should have a black skin without rootlets. The Chinese name of this herb literally translated means "ascending hemp," an allusion to its alleged ability to lift the patient's energy level. Depending on the species of cimicifuga, the cross section of the root is white, light green, or gray. Chinese herbalists, following traditional medical practice, characterize cimicifuga as acrid, sweet, and cool.

TARGET AILMENTS

Take internally for:

- skin rashes, including those of measles; headache accompanying measles.
- sore teeth and gums, canker sores, and sore throats.
- prolapse (dropping) of the uterus, rectum, or bladder.

PREPARATIONS

Cimicifuga is available in dried form at Chinese pharmacies, Asian food markets, and some Western health food stores.

Combinations: When it is combined with great burdock fruit and indigo, the blend brings out skin rashes, such as those that accompany measles. This action helps the disease run its course faster. A mixture with coptis is prescribed for swollen gums, toothache, and ulcers of the mouth and tongue. It is taken internally and also rubbed on the affected areas. Together with bupleurum it is used to treat prolapses of internal organs, and also diarrhea. A Chinese medicine practitioner can provide details of dosages and additional herbal combinations.

SIDE EFFECTS

Beware of taking too much cimicifuga: It may cause headaches, vomiting, tremors, and gastroenteritis.

SPECIAL INFORMATION

- WARNING: Although cimicifuga effectively brings out the skin rash caused by measles in its early stage, the herb should not be used when the disease has fully developed.
- WARNING: This herb should not be taken by patients with breathing difficulties.

CINNAMON BARK

LATIN NAME

Cinnamomum cassia

GENERAL DESCRIPTION

A popular stimulant in Chinese medicine, cinnamon is harvested from trees usually after they have reached seven years of age. Its outer bark is the common spice; the inner bark contains more oil and has stronger medicinal effects. Cinnamon bark is used to treat abdominal disorders, menstrual pain, infertility, and some forms of asthma. Characterized as hot, acrid, and sweet according to traditional Chinese medicine, the best quality has a thick skin and is oily and fragrant.

TARGET AILMENTS

- poor digestion, lack of appetite, diarrhea with undigested food, abdominal spasms.
- excessive urination, impotence, and lack of sexual desire.
- menstrual pain alleviated by applying cold packs, lack of menstruation, infertility.
- wheezing from asthma caused by exposure to cold.

PREPARATIONS

Cinnamon bark is available fresh or dried at Chinese pharmacies, Asian food markets, and some Western health food stores. It is normally taken in the form of powder, pill, or tincture, in which the crushed bark is mixed with alcohol.

Combinations: Chinese herbalists prescribe cinnamon bark together with the roots of Asian ginseng and of Chinese foxglove cooked in wine to treat palpitations of the heart and shortness of breath. A Chinese medicine practitioner can advise you on dosages and additional herbal combinations.

SIDE EFFECTS

Serious:

Large doses can cause changes in breathing, dilation of blood vessels, and convulsions.

SPECIAL INFORMATION

- WARNING: Use this herb cautiously if you are pregnant.
- WARNING: Do not use the herb

C

when there is fever, inflammation, or hemorrhaging.
- In a clinical trial, an alcohol-based preparation of the bark, injected at an acupuncture point associated with the lung, seemed to have a beneficial effect on bronchial asthma.
- Cinnamaldehyde, a major constituent of cinnamon bark, has shown tranquilizing and pain-relieving effects in mice.

CINNAMON TWIG

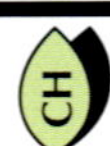

LATIN NAME
Cinnamomum cassia

GENERAL DESCRIPTION
Cinnamon twigs, sometimes called cassia twigs, are prescribed for colds, influenza, arthritis, and minor gynecological problems. Those of good quality can be discerned by their strong fragrance and brownish red color. While cinnamon twigs have many properties in common with cinnamon bark, Chinese herbalists use each part of the plant to treat a different set of ailments. Cinnamon twigs are characterized in traditional Chinese medicine as warm, acrid, and sweet.

TARGET AILMENTS
Take internally for:
- colds, influenza, and low-grade fever accompanied by chills.
- arthritis and rheumatism.
- gynecological problems such as painful menstruation or uterine fibroids.

PREPARATIONS
Cinnamon twigs can be purchased in Chinese pharmacies, Asian markets, and some Western health food stores.

Combinations: A preparation containing cinnamon twigs and licorice that has been fried with honey is recommended by Chinese herbalists for palpitations and shortness of breath. When mixed with evodia fruit, the herb is prescribed for abdominal pain and menstrual disorders. Consult a Chinese medicine practitioner about dosages and additional herbal combinations.

SIDE EFFECTS
Be careful about using cinnamon twigs if you are pregnant or if you menstruate heavily, because they may cause more bleeding or difficulties with the pregnancy.

SPECIAL INFORMATION
- Do not use the herb to treat cases of influenza with high fever.
- Preparations of cinnamon twig have shown a possible antibiotic effect against organisms such as staphylococcus and salmonella.
- The herb is considered a diuretic.

CIPROFLOXACIN

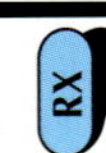

DRUG CLASS
Antibiotics [Fluoroquinolones]

BRAND NAME
Cipro

GENERAL DESCRIPTION
Introduced in 1984, ciprofloxacin is a synthetic fluoroquinolone that is used to treat a number of infections, including bone and joint infections, bacterial gastroenteritis, and chancroid infections (genital ulcers) caused by *Hemophilus ducreyi*. For more information, see ***Fluoroquinolones.***

SPECIAL INFORMATION
- Ciprofloxacin may be taken with meals (to prevent stomach upset); food does not affect overall absorption of the drug.
- Take ciprofloxacin at least two hours before or six hours after antacids and similar drugs. (See ***Fluoroquinolones*** for further instructions.)

POSSIBLE INTERACTIONS

Alkalizers (urinary), such as sodium bicarbonate, and citrates: these drugs reduce the solubility of ciprofloxacin in urine and can, in rare instances, lead to crystalluria (crystals in urine) or kidney toxicity.

Cyclosporine (immunosuppressant): increased blood levels of cyclosporine. Your doctor may have to adjust your dose of cyclosporine.

Phenytoin (anticonvulsant): reduced phenytoin levels and effectiveness.

Theophyllines (asthma drugs): ciprofloxacin may inhibit metabolism of these drugs, increasing the risk of adverse effects and theophylline toxicity.

CLARITHROMYCIN

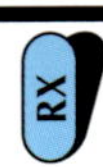

DRUG CLASS
Antibiotics [Erythromycin]

BRAND NAME
Biaxin

GENERAL DESCRIPTION
Clarithromycin, an antibiotic introduced in 1991, is a type of erythromycin but has fewer side effects than other drugs in that class. Clarithromycin's action varies with the type of bacteria it is used to fight. It kills some and stops the growth and reproduction of others.

TARGET AILMENTS
- respiratory tract infections, including sinusitis, pharyngitis due to strep, tonsillitis, bronchitis, and some types of pneumonia.
- infections of the skin and soft tissue.
- AIDS-related infections due to *Mycobacterium avium* or *Mycobacterium intracellulare.*

SIDE EFFECTS

Not serious:
An unusual taste in the mouth, abdominal pain, mild diarrhea, nausea, headache, yeast infections. Consult your doctor if symptoms are prolonged or bothersome.

Serious:
Unusual bleeding or bruising, possibly signaling a blood disorder; inflammation of the colon (diarrhea that lasts more than 24 hours, cramps, fever). Discontinue use and call your doctor immediately.

SPECIAL INFORMATION
- Some infections may require 14 days of treatment. Take the full course to prevent bacteria from becoming resistant to the medicine.
- Tell your doctor if your kidneys or liver is impaired. You may need to have your dose adjusted.
- Let your doctor know if you are allergic to erythromycin, azithromycin, or troleandomycin, because you may also be allergic to this drug.
- Do not use clarithromycin during pregnancy unless clearly needed. Avoid using this drug while nursing.

POSSIBLE INTERACTIONS

Rifabutin: decreased clarithromycin effect.

Zidovudine: decreased zidovudine effect.

(See ***Erythromycin*** for other possible interactions.)

CLEMASTINE

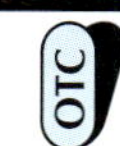

DRUG CLASS
Antihistamines

BRAND NAME
Tavist, Tavist-D

GENERAL DESCRIPTION
Clemastine is an antihistamine with mildly sedative effects. See ***Antihistamines.***

CLONAZEPAM

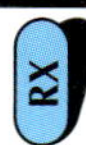

DRUG CLASS
Antianxiety Drugs [Benzodiazepines]

BRAND NAME
Klonopin

GENERAL DESCRIPTION
Introduced in 1977, clonazepam is a benzodiazepine that is prescribed alone or in combination with other drugs to control epileptic absence (petit mal) seizures as well as myoclonic and akinetic seizures. See ***Benzodiazepines*** for information on side effects and possible drug interactions.

SPECIAL INFORMATION
- Do not confuse the brand name Klonopin with the generic name Clonidine. Clonidine is used to treat high blood pressure.

CLOTRIMAZOLE

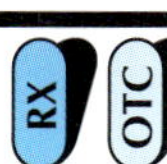

DRUG CLASS
Antifungal Drugs

BRAND NAMES
Rx: Lotrisone

OTC: Lotrimin AF

GENERAL DESCRIPTION
Clotrimazole, available in topical or vaginal preparations, is used to treat a great variety of yeast and ringworm infections of the mouth, throat, skin, and vaginal tract. For information on side effects and possible drug interactions, see ***Antifungal Drugs.*** Also see ***Vaginal Antifungal Drugs*** for information about medications commonly used to treat vaginal yeast infections.

SPECIAL INFORMATION
- Lotrisone, a combination of clotrimazole and betamethasone, is an antifungal-corticosteroid medication. Its purpose is to destroy fungi and relieve any accompanying skin inflammation. See ***Betamethasone.***

CNIDIUM SEEDS

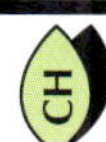

LATIN NAME
Cnidium monnieri

GENERAL DESCRIPTION
Cnidium seeds grow throughout China and are prescribed typically for skin complaints. A good specimen is round, dusky yellow, and fragrant. Chinese medicine practitioners, following the tenets of their traditional medicine, categorize the seeds as acrid, bitter, and warm.

TARGET AILMENTS
- itching skin, eczema, scabies, ringworm; or itchy, weeping skin lesions, especially in the genital area. (Apply externally.)
- vaginal discharge. (Use as a douche.)
- male impotence, female infertility. (Take internally.)

PREPARATIONS
Over the counter:
Cnidium seeds are available in bulk at Chinese pharmacies, Asian markets, and some Western health food stores. They can occasionally be found in pill and powder form in combinations.

At home:
For eczema and other skin disorders, soak the skin with a cnidium seeds solution, or use as a douche for vaginal problems.

Combinations: A mixture with the roots of the sophora and stemona herbs is prescribed for itchy, weeping skin lesions. Another preparation, containing cnidium seeds and calomel, is often applied to skin lesions associated with acute flareups of eczema, genital eczema, and scabies. Chinese herbalists also recommend an oral preparation of cnidium seeds mixed with cuscuta and schisandra for impotence or infertility. Consult a Chinese medicine practitioner for advice about dosages and other herbal combinations.

SIDE EFFECTS
None expected with recommended dosage.

SPECIAL INFORMATION
- Do not use cnidium seeds for hot, sore skin that is excessively dry.

POSSIBLE INTERACTIONS
Chinese herbalists caution against prescribing cnidium seeds at the same time as bark of the tree peony root, croton seed, or fritillaria.

CODEINE

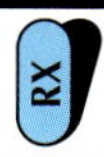

DRUG CLASS
Analgesics [Opioid Analgesics]

BRAND NAME
Tylenol with Codeine

GENERAL DESCRIPTION
The narcotic codeine, frequently combined with other analgesics such as acetaminophen and aspirin, has been prescribed for decades for moderate pain relief. Codeine has a calming effect on the brain and nervous system and also helps control coughing by suppressing the cough reflex. Although the drug is less habit-forming than most other opiates, it should be used with caution. See ***Opioid Analgesics*** for information about side effects and possible drug interactions.

CODONOPSIS ROOT

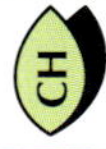

LATIN NAME
Codonopsis pilosula

GENERAL DESCRIPTION
The codonopsis root is the basis of a tonic for patients suffering from lethargy and related symptoms. Classified as sweet and neutral in traditional Chinese medicine, the root should be thick,

C

moist, and tight-skinned. Herbalists consider it milder and safer than Asian ginseng, and often use it as a substitute for the stronger herb. Codonopsis grows throughout northeastern China.

TARGET AILMENTS
Take internally for:
- diabetes.
- chronic cough and shortness of breath.
- prolapsed (fallen) uterus, stomach, or rectum.
- lack of appetite, fatigue, and tired limbs.
- diarrhea and vomiting.
- excessive thirst.

PREPARATIONS
Codonopsis is available in bulk form at Chinese pharmacies, Asian markets, and some Western health food stores. It is included in several preparations designed as tonics.

Combinations: Codonopsis mixed with atractylodes (white) is prescribed for reduced appetite, diarrhea, and vomiting, while a combination with astragalus is recommended in cases where shortness of breath is added to these symptoms. A preparation containing the roots of codonopsis and dong quai in addition to Chinese foxglove root cooked in wine is given to patients suffering dizziness, weakness, and lassitude. See a Chinese medicine practitioner for information on dosages and appropriate herbal combinations.

SIDE EFFECTS
None expected.

SPECIAL INFORMATION
- In laboratory tests, oral and intravenous doses of codonopsis increased the red blood cell counts and hemoglobin levels in rabbits.
- Codonopsis has improved the endurance of mice in a laboratory trial.

POSSIBLE INTERACTIONS
Some Chinese herbalists believe that codonopsis is incompatible with veratrum.

COIX

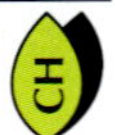

LATIN NAME
Coix lachryma jobi

GENERAL DESCRIPTION
The seeds are the functional parts of the coix plant, which is also known as Job's-tears, a kind of barley. The full, round, white fruit is used as a food, and its seeds can be ingested over a long period of time without producing side effects other than a feeling of dryness. In traditional Chinese medicine the seeds are categorized as sweet, bland, and slightly cold. The fruit is grown throughout China and harvested at the end of fall when the seeds have ripened.

TARGET AILMENTS
Take internally for:
- urinary difficulty, marked by edema (retention of body fluids).
- carbuncles.
- lung or intestinal abscesses.
- diarrhea.
- coated tongue (symptomatic of digestive problems).
- arthritic pains from weather changes.
- fever accompanied by inadequate urination.
- plantar warts.

PREPARATIONS
Coix seeds are available in bulk at Chinese pharmacies, Asian food markets, and some Western health food stores. The herb can also be obtained in tablet form from some Chinese pharmacies.

Combinations: A preparation of coix mixed with poria mushrooms, kudzu root, and atractylodes (white) is often prescribed for traveler's diarrhea, weak digestion, nausea, vomiting, diarrhea, constipation, morning sickness, bloating, and cramps. When combined with winter melon seed, aduki beans, and akebia caulis, coix is given for inadequate urination. Other combinations are prescribed for diarrhea and internal abscesses. Consult a Chinese medicine practitioner for information on herbal preparations and dosages.

SIDE EFFECTS
None expected, except a feeling of dryness.

SPECIAL INFORMATION
- Practitioners urge pregnant women to use the seeds with caution, because of the herb's drying effect on body tissues.
- Laboratory studies show that oil made from the seeds seems to reduce or eliminate muscle spasms in frogs.
- Clinical trials have indicated an effect of the oil from coix seeds on breathing: Low doses of the oil appear to stimulate breathing, while high doses seem to inhibit it. The oil also may cause dilation of the bronchial tubes.

COLESTIPOL

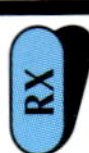

DRUG CLASS
Cholesterol-Reducing Drugs

BRAND NAME
Colestid

GENERAL DESCRIPTION
Introduced in 1974, colestipol is in the group of medicines known as bile acid-binding resins. These drugs lower blood levels of cholesterol by binding to the bile acids from which cholesterol is made and removing them from the body. For more information, see ***Cholesterol-Reducing Drugs.***

SIDE EFFECTS

Not serious:
Belching, bloating.

Serious:
Constipation; loss of weight; black, tarry stool.

SPECIAL INFORMATION
- Never take this drug in dry form, as it may cause you to choke. Mix powder as directed with water or fruit juice.
- Colestipol may interfere with your body's ability to absorb certain nutrients. While on this medication, you may need to take supplements of vitamins A, D, E, and K; folic acid; and calcium. Consult your doctor.

POSSIBLE INTERACTIONS
Other medications should be taken two hours before or four to six hours after colestipol.

COLTSFOOT

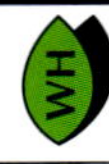

LATIN NAME
Tussilago farfara

GENERAL DESCRIPTION
As far back as 2,000 years ago, Asians and Europeans were using coltsfoot as a cough suppressant for respiratory ailments, and both the dried flowers and the leaves are still used as a gentle expectorant and cough suppressant. They contain a substance called mucilage, which may be responsible for soothing the respiratory tract. Another ingredient of coltsfoot leaves is zinc, which may help heal injured skin tissue. Today

coltsfoot is banned in Canada, but in the United States the Food and Drug Administration classifies it as an herb with "undefined safety." Coltsfoot contains an alkaloid that can seriously damage the liver; and a Japanese study concluded that the flower buds may be carcinogenic. Many practitioners in Europe and the United States, however, still use coltsfoot routinely on a short-term basis to treat coughs and other respiratory ailments.

TARGET AILMENTS

- coughs, asthma, bronchitis, whooping cough, and emphysema. (Take internally.)
- burns, swellings, skin ulcers, inflammations, and insect bites. (Apply externally.)

PREPARATIONS

Over the counter:
Available in tincture, capsules, and in bulk.

At home:
Tea: Pour 1 cup boiling water onto 1 to 3 tsp dried flowers or leaves and steep for 10 minutes. Drink three times a day, as hot as possible.

Compress: Soak a pad in a coltsfoot infusion for several minutes, wring out, then apply to the affected area.

Combinations: For coughs, coltsfoot is often combined with white horehound and mullein; for bronchitis, coltsfoot is mixed with garlic or echinacea.

SIDE EFFECTS

Serious:
Fever, nausea, vomiting, loss of appetite, diarrhea, jaundice, or pain in the upper-right abdomen may result from using coltsfoot. Stop taking the herb and call your doctor immediately.

SPECIAL INFORMATION

- WARNING: Do not give coltsfoot to children under two years old, pregnant or nursing women, alcoholics, or anyone with liver disease.
- WARNING: If you decide to use coltsfoot, take only medicinal amounts under a practitioner's supervision for short periods of time.

COMFREY

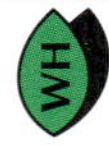

LATIN NAME
Symphytum officinale

GENERAL DESCRIPTION
Praised for centuries by herbalists throughout the world, who still use it to treat disorders ranging from cuts to cancer, comfrey nevertheless is rejected by many practitioners in the United States as too dangerous for any type of internal use. Comfrey contains pyrrolizidine alkaloids, which can cause liver damage when consumed in large amounts. The active agent in comfrey is allantoin, which fosters the growth of new cells. Although the dried roots and leaves are used for medicinal purposes, the comfrey root contains up to twice as much allantoin as the other parts. While its internal use remains questionable, comfrey can be used safely on external injuries such as cuts and other wounds.

TARGET AILMENTS

- wounds, cuts, insect bites, bruises, ulcers, and inflammations. (Apply externally.)

PREPARATIONS

Over the counter:
Comfrey is available in dry bulk.

At home:
Poultice: Sprinkle a powder made from dry comfrey over cuts, bruises, insect bites, or wounds, and cover with a clean cloth.

SPECIAL INFORMATION

- WARNING: The American Herb Products Association has placed comfrey on its restricted list and suggests that this herb be used for external ailments only.

CONJUGATED ESTROGENS

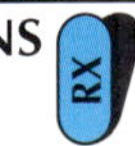

DRUG CLASS
Estrogens and Progestins

BRAND NAME
Premarin, Premphase, Prempro

GENERAL DESCRIPTION
Like other estrogens, conjugated estrogens may be prescribed to replace a woman's estrogen at natural menopause or after removal of the ovaries or uterus, thereby lessening any resulting symptoms such as hot flashes. The drugs are also thought to be effective in preventing osteoporosis and cardiovascular disease. For more information, see ***Estrogens and Progestins.***

COPTIS

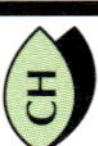

LATIN NAME
Coptis chinensis (or *Coptis deltoidea*)

GENERAL DESCRIPTION
The rhizome of the coptis plant, sometimes called Chinese goldthread, is an antibiotic and fever-reducing herb frequently prescribed by Chinese medicine practitioners. It contains the antimicrobial substance berberine, which seems to inhibit many of the bacteria that cause dysentery. Look for a reddish yellow cross section in *Coptis chinensis,* the form most often available commercially, or for a pure yellow cross section in *Coptis deltoidea.* Chinese herbalists characterize the herb as cold and bitter.

TARGET AILMENTS

Take internally for:

- high fever with irritability, disorientation, or delirium.
- dysentery with hot, burning diarrhea.
- nosebleeds.
- bright-red blood in the urine, stool, or vomit.
- bad breath or belching with bad odor.

Apply externally for:

- toothache, swollen gums, ulcers of the tongue and mouth; red, painful eyes.

PREPARATIONS

You can obtain coptis in bulk at Chinese pharmacies, Asian food stores, and some Western health food stores. It is also possible to buy the medication in tablet form. Look for a powder or ointment for external use to treat eye problems.

Combinations: With skullcap and gardenia, coptis forms a preparation to treat conditions marked by high fever, irritability, dry mouth and throat, and dark urine. Combined with Chinese foxglove root, coptis is prescribed for insomnia and delirium, and also for serious illnesses with high fever. Coptis and aucklandia are mixed to treat dysentery. And a combination of coptis and Chinese wild ginger, usually with gypsum, is used for toothaches, swollen gums, and ulcers of the tongue and mouth. Consult a Chinese medicine practitioner for advice about dosages and other herbal combinations.

SIDE EFFECTS

Serious:
This herb can injure the spleen and stomach if used over long periods.

C

SPECIAL INFORMATION
- In clinical trials, coptis seemed to have some effect in treating scarlet fever, typhoid fever, and diphtheria.
- Local administration of coptis preparations has improved cases of inflammatory bowel disease, anal fissures, and infections of the vagina caused by protozoa.

POSSIBLE INTERACTIONS

Some herbalists believe that coptis should not be taken with pork. They also advise patients to avoid the herb in combination with chrysanthemum flowers *(Chrysanthemum morifolium),* scrophularia, dictamnus root bark, and silkworm. Coptis is also believed to counteract the beneficial effects of coltsfoot flower and achyranthes root.

CORNUS

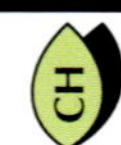

LATIN NAME
Cornus officinalis

GENERAL DESCRIPTION
Chinese practitioners use cornus berries in several medicinal tonics. Known also as Asiatic cornelian cherry fruit and Asiatic dogwood, it is prescribed for kidney and bladder disorders and for menstrual irregularity. Grown in several parts of China, it is harvested in October and November, when the fruit becomes purplish red. The best variety is fat, thick, soft, and seedless. Traditional Chinese medicine attributes sour and slightly warm characteristics to cornus.

TARGET AILMENTS
Take internally for:
- excessive urination, incontinence, impotence, and other symptoms related to kidney and bladder problems.
- excessive sweating.
- lightheadedness with weakness of the back and knees.
- excessive menstrual bleeding or prolonged menstruation.

PREPARATIONS
The berries are available at Chinese pharmacies, Asian food markets, and some Western health food stores.

Combinations: A preparation designed to overcome urinary frequency, tinnitus (ringing in the ears), and low-back pain contains cornus berries as well as Chinese foxglove root, Chinese yam, and other minor ingredients. A blend of cornus and Cherokee rose hip is prescribed for urinary incontinence. Check with a Chinese herbalist for recommended doses and additional combinations.

SIDE EFFECTS

None expected.

SPECIAL INFORMATION
- While cornus is believed to have low toxicity, herbalists warn against prescribing it for some forms of painful, difficult urination involving infection or cystitis.
- Laboratory tests indicate that cornus may have an antibiotic effect on staphylococcus bacteria.
- In tests with animals, cornus increased urination and reduced blood pressure.

POSSIBLE INTERACTIONS

Some Chinese herbalists advise against using cornus in combination with the herbs platycodon, siler, and stephania.

CORTICOSTEROIDS

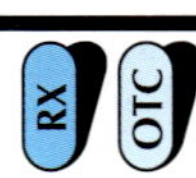

GENERIC NAMES
Rx: beclomethasone, betamethasone, mometasone furoate, prednisone, triamcinolone

OTC: hydrocortisone

GENERAL DESCRIPTION
The term corticosteroids refers both to natural hormones produced by the adrenal glands and to synthetic versions of these hormones. Corticosteroids are powerful drugs, prescribed for a variety of conditions ranging in severity from skin rash to multiple sclerosis. Because they affect almost all parts of the body, these drugs must be used with caution.

Corticosteroid medications are available in topical creams, nasal inhalers and sprays, lung inhalers and sprays, and oral forms (tablets, syrup, and solutions). For more information, see individual entries for each of the generic drugs listed above.

TARGET AILMENTS
- skin disorders, for symptomatic relief of rash, inflammation, itching; treatment of psoriasis, eczema, sunburn, and other skin diseases. (Hydrocortisone, mometasone furoate, and triamcinolone.)
- nasal inflammations (seasonal and chronic), including hay fever (allergic rhinitis), and nonallergic inflammation of the nasal passages. (Beclomethasone and triamcinolone.)
- respiratory ailments such as severe asthma. (Beclomethasone and triamcinolone.)
- rheumatic disorders (arthritis, bursitis, tendonitis), ulcerative colitis, Crohn's disease. (Prednisone.)
- itchiness and inflammation associated with fungal infections such as athlete's foot, jock itch, and yeast infections. (Betamethasone, in combination with the antifungal drug clotrimazole.)

SIDE EFFECTS

Not serious:
Topical corticosteroids: mild and transient skin rash, burning, irritation, dryness, redness, itchiness or scaling. Other corticosteroids: stomach upset, increased or decreased appetite, restlessness, dizziness, sleeplessness, change in skin color, unusual hair growth on face or body.

Serious:
Eye pain, loss of or blurred vision; stomach pain or burning; black, tarry stools; severe and lasting skin rash, hives, or burning, itching, or painful skin; blisters, acne, or other skin problems; nausea or vomiting; high blood pressure; foot or leg swelling; rapid weight gain; fluid retention (edema); unusual bruising; menstrual irregularities; prolonged sore throat, fever, cold, or other sign of infection. Contact your doctor immediately.

SPECIAL INFORMATION
- Topical corticosteroids should be used with caution if you are allergic to other corticosteroids; if you have an infection or thin skin at the treatment site; if you have or have had cataracts, glaucoma, diabetes, or tuberculosis.
- Corticosteroid topical creams, as well as nasal and oral sprays or inhalers, may be absorbed into your system after prolonged use. Tell your doctor if you are taking any other medication, and watch for any significant side effects or possible drug interactions.
- Ask your doctor about the risks and benefits of corticosteroid treatment if you have or have had any of the following conditions: HIV infection or AIDS, heart disease, hypertension, ulcerative colitis, diabetes, diverticulitis, gastritis or peptic ulcers, recent chickenpox or measles, candidiasis or other fungal infections, glaucoma, herpes simplex, liver or kidney disease, myasthenia gravis, osteoporosis, anastomoses, lupus, tuberculosis, recent intestinal problems, or any infection, such as a cold or flu.
- One of the actions of corticosteroids

is to suppress your immune system, thereby making you more susceptible to opportunistic infections. Corticosteroids can also mask symptoms of infection that occur while you are taking the drugs; because the symptoms will not appear, an infection may worsen without your being aware of it.
- Prolonged use of corticosteroids can cause birth defects. Pregnant and nursing women should avoid these drugs.
- Prolonged use of corticosteroids increases the risk of osteoporosis, cataracts, glaucoma, Cushing's syndrome (moon face), and diabetes. It can also reactivate tuberculosis.
- Check with your doctor before you stop using these drugs. It may be necessary to reduce the dosage gradually to avoid serious consequences.

POSSIBLE INTERACTIONS

See ***Prednisone.***

CORYDALIS

LATIN NAME
Corydalis yanhusuo

GENERAL DESCRIPTION
Grown in China's Zhejiang, Hubei, Hunan, and Jiangsu provinces, the corydalis root is considered among the most effective painkillers in traditional Chinese medicine. Herbalists use it alone or in combination to treat almost any kind of pain. It does not seem to cause addiction or to have toxic side effects. The best roots are large, hard, and bright yellow on the inside. According to the tenets of traditional Chinese medicine, corydalis is an acrid, bitter, and warm herb.

TARGET AILMENTS
- pain of many varieties, including abdominal and chest pain, and pain resulting from traumatic injuries, menstruation, rheumatism, and arthritis. (Take internally.)

PREPARATIONS
Corydalis is available in Chinese pharmacies, Asian markets, and some Western health food stores. Toasting or frying in vinegar enhances its effects in cases of menstrual pain and pain caused by trauma. The powdered form of the root is an extremely strong painkiller.

Combinations: Mixed with cnidium root *(Ligusticum chuanxiong),* it is prescribed for body aches and headaches. In combination with fennel, it is used for abdominal pain and hernial disorders. Herbalists prescribe a preparation containing corydalis and cinnamon bark for painful menstruation. Consult a Chinese medicine practitioner for information on appropriate dosages and additional combinations.

SIDE EFFECTS

None expected.

SPECIAL INFORMATION
- WARNING: Pregnant women should not use corydalis.
- In clinical tests, the root has shown a slight hypnotic effect on many animal species, causing a lack of alertness.

COUGH SUPPRESSANTS

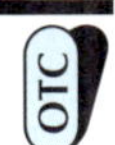

GENERAL DESCRIPTION
Cough suppressants (antitussives) are used to reduce the intensity and frequency of the dry, nonproductive, temporary type of cough associated with allergies, colds, and the flu. Cough suppressants should not be used with a productive (phlegm- or mucus-producing) cough unless the cough is extremely bothersome or disrupts sleep.

Some cough suppressants work in the brain to suppress the cough reflex; others act on the throat and bronchial passages to soothe irritation and relax the muscles. For more information on a potent, nonnarcotic drug found in many over-the-counter products, see ***Dextromethorphan.*** For information about other drugs that help suppress the cough reflex, see ***Codeine, Hydrocodone,*** and ***Opioid Analgesics.***

COX-2 INHIBITORS

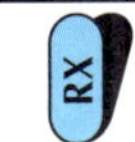

GENERIC NAMES
celecoxib, rofecoxib

GENERAL DESCRIPTION
The COX-2 Inhibitors relieve pain and inflammation by blocking the effects of the COX-2 enzyme active at sites of inflammation without inhibiting the effects of the COX-1 enzyme, which acts to protect the stomach and helps form blood clots. Because of this selectivity for the COX-2 enzyme, these drugs are less likely to cause ulcers and stomach bleeding than other, nonselective nonsteroidal anti-inflammatory drugs (NSAIDs), although these side effects may rarely occur. Unlike other NSAIDs, these drugs do not interfere with blood clot formation and so do not increase bleeding time. For more information, see ***Celecoxib*** and ***Rofecoxib.***

TARGET AILMENTS
- osteoarthritis, rheumatoid arthritis (celecoxib).
- osteoarthritis, acute pain, painful menstrual cycles (rofecoxib).

SIDE EFFECTS

Not serious:
headache, indigestion, nausea, diarrhea, sinus inflammation, edema. Call your doctor if these symptoms persist or become bothersome.

Serious:
Gnawing or burning stomach pain, black or tarry stools, vomiting. Rarely, stomach pains, ulcers. Discontinue use and call your doctor immediately.

SPECIAL INFORMATION
- Do not take COX-2 inhibitors if you have ulcers or stomach bleeding, allergies to aspirin or other NSAIDs, or severe kidney or liver problems.
- Do not take these drugs if you are pregnant or nursing.
- Do not take celecoxib if you are allergic to sulfa drugs, aspirin, or other nonsteroidal anti-inflammatory drugs (NSAIDs).

POSSIBLE INTERACTIONS

Angiotensin-converting enzyme (ACE) inhibitors: decreased ACE inhibitor effect.

Antacids: Decreased absorption of rofecoxib.

Warfarin: Bleeding problems. Warfarin dosages may need to be adjusted.

CROMOLYN

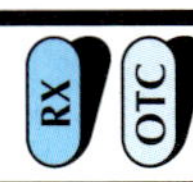

DRUG CLASS
Asthma Therapy

BRAND NAME
Rx: Intal

OTC: Nasalcrom

C

GENERAL DESCRIPTION

Cromolyn is an antiasthmatic and antiallergenic drug used to prevent bronchial asthma episodes and bronchospasm caused by allergens, dry air, airborne pollutants, or other triggering factors. The drug, available as a pill, powder, oral inhalant, and nasal spray, can also be used immediately before exercise to control exercise-induced bronchial problems. Because cromolyn is not fast acting, it should not be used for relief during acute asthma attacks.

Cromolyn is also used to treat congestion and other nasal symptoms of allergy. In some cases, it is combined with other medications for additive therapeutic effects. See ***Asthma Therapy, Bronchodilators,*** and ***Corticosteroids*** for more information on asthma medications.

TARGET AILMENTS

- bronchial asthma attacks.
- bronchospasm from all sources (including environmental irritants and exercise).
- respiratory allergies.
- allergic rhinitis (nasal spray).

SPECIAL INFORMATION

- Pregnant and nursing women should use caution when taking this drug; however, no adverse fetal effects have been linked to oral inhalation of cromolyn. It is not known whether cromolyn shows up in breast milk, but small amounts of the drug do occur in the body following oral inhalation. Check with your doctor.
- If you have a history of heart arrhythmias or coronary artery disease, let your doctor know; cromolyn inhalants may affect your condition.

SIDE EFFECTS

Not serious:
Cough and hoarseness; less frequently, dryness of the mouth or throat, sneezing, nasal congestion, watery eyes, throat irritation. Call your doctor if these effects become troublesome. If you experience an unpleasant taste, there is no need to call your doctor.

Serious:
Uncommonly, swelling of the face, lips, eyelids, hands, feet, inside of mouth; increased bronchospasm (more wheezing, chest tightness, trouble breathing); difficult, painful, or frequent urination; joint pain or swelling; severe or continuous headache; nausea; vomiting; skin rash, hives, or itching. Rarely, difficulty swallowing; pneumonia (chest pain, chills, severe breathing difficulty, sweating, wheezing). Call your doctor immediately if you experience these effects.

POSSIBLE INTERACTIONS

Cortisone drugs: increased cortisone effect. Your doctor may decrease your cortisone dosage.

Ipratropium (asthma inhalant): increased cromolyn effect.

CUSCUTA

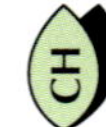

LATIN NAME

Cuscuta chinensis

GENERAL DESCRIPTION

A common parasitic growth on plants, cuscuta yields grayish yellow seeds, also known as Chinese dodder seeds, that have medicinal effects. Among other uses, they are prescribed to prevent miscarriages. The seeds are considered to have sweet, acrid, and neutral characteristics in traditional Chinese medicine.

TARGET AILMENTS

Take internally for:

- impotence, nocturnal emissions, premature ejaculation, prostate problems.
- frequent urination, incontinence, loose stools or diarrhea with lack of appetite.
- habitual or threatened miscarriages.
- backache from muscular weakness.
- dizziness, tinnitus (ringing in the ears), blurred vision.

PREPARATIONS

Cuscuta seeds are available in bulk from Chinese pharmacies, Asian markets, and some Western health food stores.

Combinations: Practitioners recommend a mix of cuscuta seeds, psoralea fruit, and eucommia bark for premature ejaculation. A preparation of cuscuta and astragalus seeds *(Astragalus complanatus)* may help blurred vision, dizziness, and tinnitus. And a mixture of cuscuta, Japanese teasel root, mulberry mistletoe stems, and eucommia bark is often prescribed to prevent threatened miscarriages. Check with a Chinese medicine practitioner for further combinations and doses.

SIDE EFFECTS

None expected.

SPECIAL INFORMATION

- The herb is not recommended for use by patients with constipation and scanty, dark urine.

CYCLOBENZAPRINE

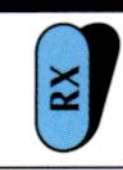

DRUG CLASS

Muscle Relaxants

BRAND NAME

Flexeril

GENERAL DESCRIPTION

Cyclobenzaprine is used along with other medications to relieve acute pain associated with muscle spasms. Although not actually a sedative, the drug acts to reduce muscle hyperactivity, thereby producing a sedative effect. By reducing pain and tightness in muscles, cyclobenzaprine helps restore motion in affected areas of the body and can allow patients to sleep more restfully. Chemically related to tricyclic antidepressants, cyclobenzaprine may cause such side effects as sedation in some individuals.

TARGET AILMENTS

- acute, painful muscle spasms.

SIDE EFFECTS

Not serious:
Dryness of the mouth, blurred vision; dizziness or lightheadedness; drowsiness. Rarely: headache, confusion, nervousness, general run-down feeling, tiredness; numbness, tingling, pain, or weakness in hands or feet; muscle twitching, trembling, or weakness, insomnia; gastrointestinal problems (such as stomach cramps, diarrhea); pounding heartbeat, changes in the sense of taste. Call your doctor if these symptoms become troublesome.

Serious:
Allergic reactions, including swelling of the face, lips, or tongue; skin rash, hives, or itching; mania, unusual dreaming, clumsiness, fainting, severe disorientation, depression, ringing in the ears; yellow skin; heart-rhythm problems, low blood pressure, breathing difficulties. Call your doctor if you experience these effects; you may be having an adverse reaction to cyclobenzaprine, or you may have taken too much.

SPECIAL INFORMATION

- Women who are pregnant or nursing

should take this medication only under a doctor's supervision.

- Since cyclobenzaprine may reduce saliva production, you should maintain good dental hygiene to avoid problems such as caries and periodontal disease.
- This medication may cause drowsiness. Use caution while taking cyclobenzaprine if you must drive or perform other tasks requiring alertness.
- Before taking this drug, tell your doctor if you have glaucoma, urinary retention, congestive heart failure, hypertension, or arrhythmia.

POSSIBLE INTERACTIONS

Since cyclobenzaprine is closely related to tricyclic antidepressants, drug interactions specific to those drugs may also apply to cyclobenzaprine. See ***Tricyclic Antidepressants*** for more interaction information.

Any central nervous system depressant (including sedatives, antihistamines, MAO inhibitors, and alcohol): may boost effects of the combined drugs while also increasing risks associated with side effects.

CYPERUS

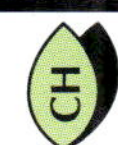

LATIN NAME

Cyperus rotundus

GENERAL DESCRIPTION

The root of a plant found in marshy areas and river bottoms throughout China, cyperus is considered one of the best menstrual regulators known to traditional Chinese medicine. Practitioners also prescribe it for digestive problems. Sometimes called nut-grass rhizome, this fragrant root at its best is large, solid, and reddish brown. In traditional Chinese medicine cyperus is classified as acrid, slightly bitter, and neutral.

TARGET AILMENTS

- irregular menstruation, menstrual cramps, digestive problems such as gas and bloating, depression, moodiness, and instability. (Take internally.)

PREPARATIONS

The cyperus root is available in bulk from Chinese pharmacies, Asian markets, and some Western health food stores. To increase its pain-reducing effects, practitioners suggest frying the root in vinegar; and to speed its action, they recommend cooking it in wine.

Combinations: A preparation of cyperus, bupleurum, and white peony root is prescribed for pain and bloating in the chest, sides, and breasts. Combined with aucklandia and finger citron fruit, it makes a treatment for pain in the upper abdomen, indigestion, vomiting, and diarrhea. A preparation of cyperus, dong quai, and cnidium root *(Ligusticum chuanxiong)* is often prescribed for irregular menstruation, while a mixture of cyperus, bupleurum, and trichosanthes fruit is recommended for breast swelling during menstruation. For information on specific dosages and other herbal combinations, consult a Chinese medicine practitioner.

SIDE EFFECTS

None expected.

SPECIAL INFORMATION

- In laboratory experiments, injections of the herb under the skin have increased the pain thresholds of mice.

D

DAMIANA

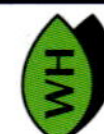

LATIN NAME
Turnera diffusa

GENERAL DESCRIPTION
Since 1874, when damiana became commercially available in the United States, its effectiveness as an aphrodisiac has been touted by some even as it was being dismissed by herbalists and the public. It has been used as a food additive in sweets, baked goods, and liqueurs, and a few of its believers have smoked the leaves and reported a high lasting about 90 minutes. Although some contemporary herbalists think damiana has no medicinal value, others recommend it to support the nervous and endocrine systems. How damiana renders this support has not been proved, but anecdotal evidence suggests that the herb is useful in testosterone production and may stimulate the central nervous system, aiding in the alleviation of depression. It is prescribed to reduce anxiety, depression, or mood disorders of a sexual origin.

Damiana may promote digestion and serve as a laxative; it is believed that the minute quantities of volatile oil in the leaf can stimulate the genitourinary tract. The leaves also contain an antimicrobial agent that may be effective in the urinary tract.

TARGET AILMENTS
Take internally for:
- hormone-based disorders such as impotence, hormone imbalance.
- prostate problems and ailments of the urinary tract.
- depression, anxiety, listlessness.
- poor libido.

PREPARATIONS
Over the counter:
Damiana is available in dry bulk, tinctures, and capsules.

At home:
Tea: Steep 1 to 2 tsp dried leaves in 1 cup boiling water for 10 to 15 minutes, and drink three times daily.

Combinations: For nervous anxiety or depression, damiana can be combined with any or all of the following: oats, skullcap, or kola.

SIDE EFFECTS

Not serious:
Too much damiana can cause insomnia and headaches. Discontinue use.

DANDELION

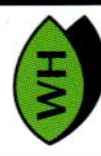

LATIN NAME
Taraxacum officinale

GENERAL DESCRIPTION
Long before the European colonists introduced dandelion to the native population of North America, the herb had an established niche in the Chinese and Ayurvedic medical traditions of Asia, the Middle East, and Europe. Dandelion acts as a natural diuretic while also supplying potassium, a nutrient often lost through diuretic use. The plant is rich in vitamins A and C—antioxidants that are believed to help prevent cancer. The young leaves can be eaten fresh or used in herbal preparations.

TARGET AILMENTS
- poor digestion, gallbladder problems, inflammation of the liver, and disorders such as congestive heart failure and high blood pressure that require diuretic treatment.
- As a supplemental diuretic, dandelion may help relieve symptoms associated with high blood pressure, congestive heart failure, premenstrual syndrome, menstrual pain, and general joint pain.

PREPARATIONS
Over the counter:
Available in tinctures, prepared tea, capsules, and dried or fresh leaves or roots.

At home:
Tea: Prepare by steeping 1 tbsp dried or 2 tsp fresh leaves per cup of boiling water for 10 minutes. Drink as many as 4 cups a day.

Decoction: Simmer 1 tbsp fresh or dried root per cup of water for 15 minutes. Drink as many as 4 cups a day.

Nutrition and diet: Add fresh leaves to a salad, or blend in a juicer with other green vegetables. Use with barberry for liver and gallbladder problems. Use with yarrow for water retention.

SIDE EFFECTS

Not serious:
Allergic dermatitis, stomach upset, diarrhea, flulike symptoms, liver pain. Discontinue use and call your doctor when convenient.

SPECIAL INFORMATION
- If any of the following conditions apply, use dandelion only in consultation with a professional herbalist or naturopath: pregnancy, heart condition, inflamed stomach or colon, liver or gallbladder disease. Consult an herbalist if you plan to use the herb longer than two or three months.
- Use low-strength preparations for adults over 65 and children between the ages of 2 and 12. Do not give to children younger than 2.
- See also ***Diuretics.***

DANDELION

LATIN NAME
Taraxacum mongolicum

GENERAL DESCRIPTION
While the Chinese dandelion differs slightly from the Western variety, both have roots with similar medicinal properties. Chinese medical practitioners use dandelion frequently for hepatitis, stomach disorders, and fluid retention. Dandelion root, according to traditional Chinese medicine, is characterized as bitter, sweet, and cold.

TARGET AILMENTS
Take internally for:
- hepatitis, jaundice, and other liver conditions.
- poor lactation in nursing mothers.
- painful and difficult urination.
- red, painful, swollen eyes.

Use both internally and topically for:
- abscesses, boils, carbuncles, and sores, particularly on the breast.

PREPARATIONS
Dandelion is available in bulk form from Chinese pharmacies, Asian markets, and some Western health food stores. It is also possible to obtain it in tablet form.

Combinations: Mixed with trichosanthes fruit, fritillaria, and myrrh, dandelion root is applied to breast abscesses, carbuncles, and furuncles. Dandelion blended with chrysanthemum flower *(Chrysanthemum morifolium)* and skullcap is used to treat red, swollen eyes. A preparation that contains dandelion and honeysuckle flower is prescribed for painful, deep-rooted boils. Adding forsythia fruit and chrysanthemum flower strengthens the effect. Consult your herbalist for information on additional combinations and doses.

SIDE EFFECTS

Overdoses of the herb can cause mild diarrhea; some preparations using Chinese dandelion root may cause heartburn.

SPECIAL INFORMATION
- Test-tube studies suggest that the herb may kill staphylococcus and other bacteria that resist other antimicrobial treatments.

DECONGESTANTS

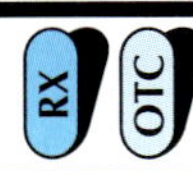

GENERIC NAMES
Rx: phenylpropanolamine
OTC: oxymetazoline, phenylpropanolamine, pseudoephedrine

GENERAL DESCRIPTION
Available as sprays or pills in over-the-counter and prescription form, decongestants relieve nasal and sinus congestion and headaches by constricting blood vessels in the nose and other parts of the respiratory system. Because the drugs affect certain receptors in the nervous system, high doses (above recommended amounts) may produce central nervous system side effects. Some of those used orally are chemically related to amphetamines and are banned for athletic use.

Decongestants come in both pill and spray forms, depending on the desired effect. Nasal sprays give the fastest results and are used for short-term treatment of nasal congestion. Use of these sprays for extended periods of time or at higher-than-recommended doses may result in nasal irritation or rebound congestion (nasal stuffiness, swelling, and redness without underlying illness).

In pill form, decongestants are used alone or in combination with other drugs to relieve the symptoms of colds, allergies, and other respiratory problems. Usually, decongestant pills do not produce rebound congestion and therefore are useful for long-term treatment of nasal congestion. Decongestant pills can also be used to treat problems caused by pressure changes during air travel. For more information, see individual entries for the generic drugs listed above.

TARGET AILMENTS
- congestion of the nose and sinuses caused by allergy or upper-respiratory infection.
- congestion of Eustachian tubes, which join the ear with the nose and throat (pseudoephedrine).
- bronchial asthma (phenylpropanolamine).
- obesity (phenylpropanolamine, used as an appetite suppressant).
- urinary incontinence (phenylpropanolamine).

SIDE EFFECTS

Not serious:
Mild nervousness, restlessness, insomnia, dizziness, lightheadedness, nausea, dryness of mouth or nose, rebound congestion.

For spray and topical forms: sneezing; burning, stinging, or dryness of nose. Call your doctor if these symptoms continue or become troublesome.

Serious:
Severe headache, nervousness, restlessness, insomnia, pounding or irregular heartbeat, high blood pressure. Contact your doctor immediately.

SPECIAL INFORMATION
- In rare cases, phenylpropanolamine has been associated with serious cardiovascular side effects, including severe high blood pressure and heart-rhythm problems, as well as psychotic problems, such as hallucinations and seizures. These effects are associated with high doses of phenylpropanolamine and may be more likely in individuals with similar preexisting problems, such as high blood pressure or neurologic or psychiatric disease.
- Check with your doctor before taking any decongestants if you have cardiovascular disease (including angina, coronary artery disease, and hypertension), hyperthyroidism (overactive thyroid), diabetes, or glaucoma. Decongestants may exacerbate these conditions.

POSSIBLE INTERACTIONS

Anticoagulant (blood-thinning) drugs: decreased anticoagulant effect.

Beta blockers: oral decongestants can lessen the effectiveness of beta blockers, causing hypertension.

Digitalis preparations: taking these drugs with oral decongestants may result in heart-rhythm problems.

High blood pressure drugs containing rauwolfia: decreased effectiveness of oral decongestants.

MAO inhibitors: increased stimulant action of oral decongestants, causing effects such as hypertension and heart-rhythm problems.

Stimulants (such as other decongestants, amphetamines, caffeine): increased stimulant effects, leading to excessive nervousness, insomnia, irregular heart rhythm, or seizures.

Tricyclic antidepressants (such as amitriptyline): increased action of oxymetazoline and phenylpropanolamine, making serious central nervous system side effects more likely.

DESOGESTREL

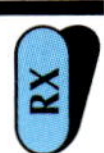

DRUG CLASS
Estrogens and Progestins

BRAND NAMES
Desogen, Ortho-Cept

GENERAL DESCRIPTION
Desogestrel is a progestin that is used in combination with estrogens as a contraceptive. See ***Estrogens and Progestins*** for information about side effects and possible drug interactions.

DEVIL'S CLAW

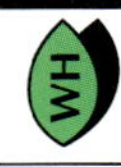

LATIN NAME
Harpagophytum procumbens

GENERAL DESCRIPTION
An extremely bitter herb, devil's claw grows in arid regions in southern and eastern Africa, where the root is collected at the end of the rainy season. Traditionally, the dried root was made into a tea used to treat indigestion, fevers, and blood disorders, while the fresh root was used for an ointment to put on boils and skin lesions.

Since the herb's active ingredient, harpagoside, is believed to reduce pain and inflammation, devil's claw is sometimes recommended for arthritis; this usage, however, was not validated when the herb was clinically tested. Herbalists do recommend trying devil's claw for arthritis on a case-by-case basis, especially if the arthritis is accompanied by severe pain and swelling.

Some herbalists believe that devil's claw is helpful in the treatment of liver and lymphatic disorders, and it also may lower blood sugar levels. It is also used to stimulate the appetite and aid digestion. Since it must be imported from Africa, devil's claw is very expensive.

TARGET AILMENTS
Take internally for:
- arthritis, gout.
- liver dysfunctions, chronic gallbladder disorders, digestive problems.
- diabetes

Apply externally for:
- skin lesions and boils.

D

PREPARATIONS

Over the counter:
Devil's claw is available in bulk and in tinctures and capsules.

At home:
To make a decoction: Put ½ to 1 tsp devil's claw ground to a powder in 1 cup boiling water; simmer for 15 minutes and strain; drink three times a day for at least one month.

Compress: Soak a pad in an infusion of devil's claw for several minutes; wring out and apply to the affected area.

Combinations: Devil's claw can be used with bogbean, celery seed, and meadowsweet for arthritis.

SPECIAL INFORMATION

- Check with your practitioner before using devil's claw if you are pregnant.
- Do not use devil's claw if you have an acute gallbladder attack or an ulcer.

DEXBROMPHENIRAMINE

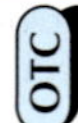

DRUG CLASS
Antihistamines

BRAND NAMES
Drixoral Cold and Flu, Drixoral Cold and Allergy

GENERAL DESCRIPTION
Dexbrompheniramine is an antihistamine with mild sedating effects. It is usually sold in combination products with decongestants. See ***Antihistamines***.

DEXTROMETHORPHAN

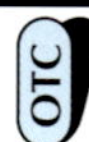

DRUG CLASS
Cough Suppressants

BRAND NAMES
Some types of Comtrex, Contac, and TheraFlu; Vicks DayQuil Liquid or LiquiCaps, Dimetapp DM Elixir, NyQuil, Robitussin-CF, Robitussin-DM, Triaminic Nite Light, Triaminic Sore Throat Formula, Triaminic DM Syrup, Triaminicol Multi-Symptom Relief, Tylenol Cold (adult and children)

GENERAL DESCRIPTION
Dextromethorphan is the main ingredient in a large number of widely available over-the-counter cough suppressants (antitussives) and common cold medications. The drug is used for the temporary relief of dry coughs caused by the common cold or flu. It should not be used for chronic coughs or for coughs that produce secretions.

Like codeine, from which it is derived, dextromethorphan inhibits the cough reflex by acting directly on the cough center, located in the medulla of the brain. Unlike codeine, however, dextromethorphan is not a narcotic. When taken at the recommended dosages, it lacks analgesic and addictive properties and does not depress respiration. For more information, see ***Codeine, Cough Suppressants,*** and ***Opioid Analgesics***.

TARGET AILMENTS
- dry, nonproductive, and temporary coughing.

SIDE EFFECTS

Not serious:
Mild drowsiness, mild dizziness, stomach pain, nausea or vomiting. Call your doctor if these symptoms persist or are bothersome.

Serious:
Adverse effects at the recommended nonprescription dosages are mild and rare; for overdose symptoms, see **Special Information** below.

SPECIAL INFORMATION
- Overdose symptoms include confusion, hyperactivity, feeling of intoxication, lack of coordination, hallucinations, irritability, and severe nausea and vomiting. Seek immediate medical help.
- Do not take dextromethorphan if you have had an allergic reaction to any medications containing this drug.
- Before taking dextromethorphan, consult your doctor if you have asthma or impaired liver function, or if your cough is producing mucus or phlegm.
- Use dextromethorphan medication only as instructed by your doctor or the label directions. Take it only as long as needed; some reports suggest that this drug may be habit-forming if you use too much for too long.
- Check with your doctor if your cough persists for more than 7 to 10 days or if it is accompanied by a skin rash, high fever, or continuing headache. These symptoms may indicate the presence of other medical problems.

POSSIBLE INTERACTIONS

Central nervous system depressants (anesthetics, antidepressants, antihistamines, anti-insomnia drugs, barbiturates, benzodiazepines, muscle relaxants, narcotics or prescription pain medicines, tranquilizers): increased sedative and depressant effects.

MAO inhibitors: disorientation, psychotic behavior, coma.

DIAZEPAM

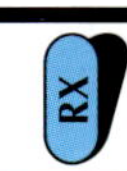

DRUG CLASS
Antianxiety Drugs [Benzodiazepines]

BRAND NAME
Valium

GENERAL DESCRIPTION
Since 1963, diazepam has been used to reduce anxiety and nervous tension. Despite its history of being overprescribed, particularly in the years immediately following its introduction, diazepam is effective in up to eighty percent of anxiety patients and is now considered one of the drugs of choice for treating mild to moderate anxiety. However, diazepam should not be used for the stress and anxiety of everyday living. Like other benzodiazepines, the drug is potentially habit-forming, especially when used for extended periods of time or at high dosages. Diazepam may also be used to treat acute alcohol withdrawal and presurgery anxiety, and as an adjunct treatment for skeletal muscle spasms and seizure disorders. See ***Benzodiazepines*** for more information on side effects and other possible drug interactions.

POSSIBLE INTERACTIONS

Isoniazid: increased diazepam effect and possible toxicity.

Phenytoin: possible phenytoin toxicity.

Rifampin: decreased diazepam effect.

DICLOFENAC

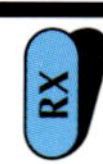

DRUG CLASS
Analgesics [Nonsteroidal Anti-Inflammatory Drugs (NSAIDs)]

BRAND NAME
Voltaren

GENERAL DESCRIPTION
Diclofenac is an NSAID available in timed-release form for treating symptoms of rheumatoid arthritis, osteoarthritis, and arthritis of the spine. This drug is also used for general pain relief and for alleviating menstrual discomfort. See ***Nonsteroidal Anti-Inflammatory Drugs (NSAIDs)*** for side effects and additional drug interaction information.

POSSIBLE INTERACTIONS

Antidiabetic drugs and insulin: diclofenac may either increase or decrease the hypoglycemic effect of antidiabetic drugs.

DICYCLOMINE

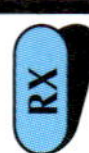

DRUG CLASS
Antispasmodic Drugs

GENERAL DESCRIPTION
Introduced in 1954, dicyclomine is an antispasmodic drug used to reduce muscle spasms in the gastrointestinal tract. The drug works in two ways: It acts directly on the smooth muscles of the gastrointestinal tract. Dicyclomine also has an anticholinergic effect, meaning that it inhibits the action of a body chemical called acetylcholine. This prevents muscles in the GI tract from contracting, thereby eliminating spasms.

TARGET AILMENTS
- irritable bowel syndrome (spastic colon).
- infant colic.

SIDE EFFECTS

Not serious:
Altered sense of taste; decreased perspiration; nasal congestion; insomnia; dizziness; drowsiness; constipation; dry mouth, ears, and throat. Call your doctor if these effects become bothersome.

Serious:
Hives or skin rash, intense itching, headaches, difficulty urinating, nausea and vomiting, confusion or delirium, agitation, heart palpitations, blurred vision, dilated pupils, eye pain, difficulty swallowing and breathing, muscle weakness, lightheadedness, feeling of faintness. Discontinue use and contact your doctor immediately.

SPECIAL INFORMATION
- Do not give this drug to infants under the age of six months.
- Do not use dicyclomine if you have ulcerative colitis, paralytic ileus (obstruction of the bowel), urinary retention, myasthenia gravis (muscle weakness), gastroesophageal reflux, esophagitis, or an allergic reaction to anticholinergic drugs.
- Before taking this medication, inform your doctor if you have glaucoma, hypertension, angina, coronary artery disease, congestive heart failure, tachycardia, asthma or bronchitis, an enlarged prostate, ulcerative colitis or a peptic ulcer, or if you have kidney, liver, or thyroid disease. You should also tell your doctor if you plan to have surgery within two months that will require anesthesia.
- If you are pregnant, consult your doctor and weigh the benefit-to-risk ratio of taking this drug.
- Dicyclomine passes into breast milk and lessens the flow; avoid the drug if you are nursing.
- Take this medication 30 minutes before meals and at bedtime.
- Prolonged use of dicyclomine can result in chronic constipation and possible fecal impaction.
- Dicyclomine may cause drowsiness or blurred vision; use caution when driving or operating machinery.

POSSIBLE INTERACTIONS

Antacids and some antidiarrheal drugs: decreased dicyclomine effect.

Ketoconazole: decreased ketoconazole effect.

Other anticholinergics, amantadine, antihistamines, certain antiviral drugs, benzodiazepines, buclizine, MAO inhibitors, meperidine, methylphenidate, orphenadrine, phenothiazines, quinidine, tricyclic antidepressants: increased dicyclomine effect.

Potassium chloride: risk of intestinal ulcers.

DIGITALIS PREPARATIONS

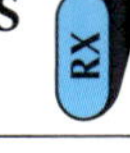

GENERAL DESCRIPTION
In use for decades, digitalis preparations have been the drugs of choice in treating various heart ailments, including congestive heart failure and some heart arrhythmias. Originally obtained from plants of the foxglove genus, most digitalis preparations are now produced synthetically because the potency of plant parts is highly variable.

Digitalis preparations are effective, but toxicity is a major concern with their use, since the effective dose is often only slightly smaller than a toxic dose. For information about a specific digitalis preparation, including side effects and possible interactions with other drugs, see ***Digoxin.***

D

DIGOXIN

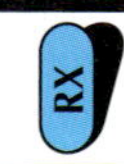

DRUG CLASS
Digitalis Preparations

BRAND NAME
Lanoxin

GENERAL DESCRIPTION
Digoxin is a digitalis preparation that has been used since 1934 to strengthen the heart and to treat heart arrhythmias. Digoxin interacts with many over-the-counter and prescription drugs.

TARGET AILMENTS
- congestive heart failure (all degrees).
- prevention and treatment of heart arrhythmias (atrial fibrillation and flutter; atrioventricular tachycardia; and paroxysmal nodal tachycardia).

SIDE EFFECTS

Not serious:
None expected; all side effects are potentially serious.

Serious:
Slow or irregular heartbeat; in children, fast heartbeat; visual disturbances, such as blurred vision or halos around objects; drowsiness, confusion, or depression; headache; fainting; digestive problems, such as pain in the lower stomach, diarrhea, nausea, vomiting, or loss of appetite; unusual tiredness or weakness; allergic reactions (rare), such as skin rash or hives. Call your doctor immediately if you experience any of these effects.

SPECIAL INFORMATION
- Do not discontinue this medication without your doctor's knowledge; to do so might cause heart problems.
- Check your pulse if directed by your doctor; be sure to report any low pulse rate (less than 60 beats per minute) to your doctor immediately.
- Digoxin can cross the placenta and affect the fetus, and it can pass to infants through breast milk. Pregnant and nursing women should therefore

use caution when taking this medication. The dosage often must be reduced for women who have given birth recently (within six weeks).
- Avoid all over-the-counter antacids as well as cough, cold, allergy, and diet drugs, except when advised otherwise by your doctor.

POSSIBLE INTERACTIONS

Following is a partial list of the drugs and other substances that can interact with digoxin. To compensate for these interactions, your doctor may have to adjust the dosages of digoxin and any other drugs you may be taking.

Amiodarone (an antiarrhythmia drug): increased amounts of digoxin circulating in the blood, which can lead to heart-rhythm problems.

Antacids, antidiarrheal drugs (such as kaolin and pectin), antiulcer drugs (including sulfasalazine), dietary fiber, laxatives: inhibited absorption of digoxin, reducing its effectiveness.

Calcium channel blockers: increased amounts of digoxin circulating in the blood, possibly leading to heart-rhythm problems.

Diuretics: may increase or decrease the effects of digoxin.

Erythromycin: increased absorption of digoxin into the body, thereby increasing its actions and side effects.

Fluoxetine: increased digoxin effects.

Indomethacin, a nonsteroidal anti-inflammatory drug (NSAID): increased amounts of digoxin circulating in the blood.

Other antiarrhythmia drugs, calcium supplements, rauwolfia (an antihypertensive drug): increased heart arrhythmias.

Potassium supplements (salts): increased risk of excess potassium, possibly leading to heart-rhythm problems; do not take potassium supplements with digoxin.

Quinidine or quinine: increased blood concentration of digoxin.

Stimulant drugs, such as amphetamines or over-the-counter decongestants: increased risk of heart-rhythm problems.

DILTIAZEM

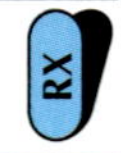

DRUG CLASS
Calcium Channel Blockers

BRAND NAMES
Cardizem, Dilacor XR

GENERAL DESCRIPTION
The calcium channel blocker diltiazem has been used since 1977 to treat heart-rhythm problems, hypertension, and angina. Like other drugs in its class, diltiazem works to inhibit the passage of calcium into body cells. This dilates the arteries and slows the contraction of the heart and arteries, thereby decreasing the work load on the heart and lowering blood pressure. See ***Calcium Channel Blockers*** for information on side effects and possible drug interactions.

DIPHENHYDRAMINE

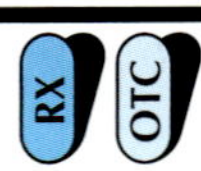

DRUG CLASS
Antihistamines

BRAND NAMES
Rx: Benadryl

OTC: Benadryl, Excedrin PM, Tylenol Cold Night Time Medication Liquid, Tylenol PM

GENERAL DESCRIPTION
Introduced in 1946, diphenhydramine was one of the first antihistamines. Its sedating and drying effects are more pronounced than those of the newer antihistamines. Diphenhydramine is used to treat symptoms of allergies, insomnia, chronic cough, vertigo, and mild Parkinson's disease. One form of diphenhydramine, a drug called dimenhydrinate, is used to treat motion sickness. See ***Antihistamines***.

DIPYRIDAMOLE

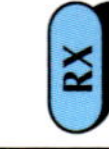

DRUG CLASS
Anticoagulant and Antiplatelet Drugs

GENERAL DESCRIPTION
Introduced in 1959, dipyridamole is used to prevent the formation and migration of blood clots (thromboembolism) following heart valve surgery and in other heart and blood conditions. It may be used alone or in combination with aspirin or one of the anticoagulants. Dipyridamole seems to inhibit the action of certain enzymes, thus preventing the aggregation of blood platelets (the smallest type of blood cell) and reducing the chance of blood clot formation. For more information, see ***Anticoagulant and Antiplatelet Drugs.***

SIDE EFFECTS

Not serious:
Dizziness, lightheadedness, flushing, weakness, stomach irritation.

Serious:
Chest pains, severe headaches, low blood pressure, rash, breathing problems, wheezing, runny nose, chest tightness.

POSSIBLE INTERACTIONS

Aspirin: taken concurrently, aspirin may make it possible to reduce the dosage of dipyridamole; it may also lessen the drug's side effects. Do not take aspirin for this purpose without first consulting your doctor.

DIURETICS

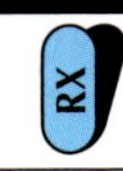

GENERIC NAMES
amiloride, bumetanide, furosemide, hydrochlorothiazide, indapamide, potassium chloride (adjunct therapy), triamterene

GENERAL DESCRIPTION
Diuretics, sometimes referred to as water pills, work by increasing the elimination of fluids from the body through urination. This action lowers blood volume (and blood pressure), helps reduce swelling, and decreases excess fluid in body tissues. During the excretion of fluid, minerals such as sodium, potassium, magnesium, and calcium are also eliminated, a side effect that can cause problems with the heart, muscles, and other organs.

The heart, in particular, can be affected by either too much or too little potassium. For this reason, doctors often prescribe newer, so-called potassium-sparing diuretics (such as amiloride or triamterene), which are designed to lessen the excretion of potassium. In some cases, supplements of potassium chloride are prescribed to restore supplies of that mineral lost through the use of diuretics. For more information, see entries for each of the generic drugs listed above.

TARGET AILMENTS
- general edema (swelling caused by water retention), especially of the ankles and feet.

- edema associated with various medical conditions, including congestive heart failure and cirrhosis of the liver.
- high blood pressure (hypertension).

SIDE EFFECTS

Not serious:
Headache, blurred vision, diarrhea, dizziness or lightheadedness when getting up (orthostatic hypotension), increased risk of sunburn. Let your doctor know if these symptoms continue or become troublesome.

Serious:
Diuretics can cause dehydration or an electrolyte imbalance, which can result in the following symptoms: nausea or vomiting, fatigue or weakness, irregular or weak pulse, increased thirst, dry mouth, muscle pain or cramps, mood changes, mental confusion. In rare cases, diuretics may cause bleeding in urine or stools, unusual bruising, or a skin rash. Tell your doctor immediately if you experience any of these symptoms. You may be advised to lower your dosage and increase your intake of fluids and minerals.

SPECIAL INFORMATION

- Taking diuretics in hot weather or while engaged in heavy exertion can cause a dangerous loss of fluids or minerals. Watch for signs of dehydration (fatigue, dizziness, headache, nausea).
- Your doctor will closely monitor your potassium levels to prevent heart-rhythm problems. If you are not taking a potassium-sparing diuretic, you may be given a potassium supplement (such as potassium chloride). If you are currently taking a potassium-sparing diuretic, you should avoid potassium supplements, salt substitutes (which are high in potassium), and potassium-rich foods such as bananas.
- When potassium-sparing diuretics are suddenly discontinued after prolonged use, a rebound effect may occur, causing a rapid and potentially dangerous buildup of potassium in the body. Gradual discontinuation of these diuretics is important to prevent potassium toxicity.
- Because diuretics have both known and suspected effects on glucose (blood sugar) levels, people with diabetes or who have been diagnosed with borderline diabetes should have their blood sugar levels monitored closely.

POSSIBLE INTERACTIONS

Alcohol: increased action of diuretics.

Amiodarone: low calcium blood levels and subsequent heart arrhythmias.

Anticoagulants (such as coumarin derivatives or heparin): thiazide diuretics and furosemide may decrease the action of these drugs.

Antigout medications (including probenecid): thiazide diuretics may increase blood uric acid levels. Your doctor may need to adjust your dosage of the antigout medicine.

Digitalis and other heart drugs: though thiazide diuretics and furosemide are sometimes taken with heart medications, such combinations can increase the risk of potassium loss and additional heart-rhythm problems. Your doctor will closely monitor your progress.

Foods high in potassium (such as bananas and low-salt milk), salt substitutes, potassium supplements: may lead to potassium toxicity if ingested in sufficient amounts while taking a potassium-sparing diuretic.

Lithium: thiazide diuretics and furosemide may increase the risk of lithium toxicity.

Nonsteroidal anti-inflammatory drugs (NSAIDs), especially indomethacin: reduced effectiveness of diuretics.

Oral antidiabetic drugs, insulin: in rare cases, diuretics may interfere with these medicines or raise blood glucose levels.

Other blood pressure drugs, including angiotensin-converting enzyme (ACE) inhibitors: although diuretics are frequently taken with medications to lower blood pressure, caution should be exercised to ensure that blood pressure does not go too low.

DOCUSATE

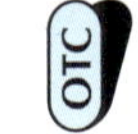

DRUG CLASS
Laxatives

BRAND NAMES
Colace, Correctol, some types of Ex-Lax

GENERAL DESCRIPTION
Docusate, a stool-softening type of laxative, is used to relieve constipation. Stool softeners are often taken as a prophylactic to prevent straining during bowel movements after heart attacks, childbirth, or rectal surgery, or when hemorrhoids are present. See ***Laxatives*** for information about side effects and possible drug interactions.

SPECIAL INFORMATION

- This type of laxative should never be taken with mineral oil; stool softeners increase the toxicity of mineral oil.
- Docusate is often used in combination with the laxative phenolphthalein, which in rare cases can cause side effects ranging from skin rashes and kidney problems to breathing difficulty and cardiac arrest.

DONG QUAI

LATIN NAME
Angelica sinensis

GENERAL DESCRIPTION
Also known as Chinese angelica root, dong quai is used by Chinese herbalists as a treatment for several gynecological complaints. Look for a long, moist, oily plant as the source of the root, which has brown bark and a white cross section. The fragrant herb is characterized as sweet, acrid, bitter, and warm, according to traditional Chinese medicine.

TARGET AILMENTS
Take internally for:

- menstrual irregularity, lack of menstruation, painful or insubstantial menstruation.
- stabbing pain, pain caused by traumatic injury.
- poor blood circulation, pale complexion, possible anemia.
- carbuncles that, according to traditional Chinese medicine, arise from stagnant blood; abscesses; sores.
- lightheadedness, blurred vision, heart palpitations.

PREPARATIONS
This root is widely available in bulk and in tablet form at Chinese pharmacies, Asian markets, and Western health food stores. You should avoid the herb if it is dry or has a greenish brown cross section. Frying the herb in vinegar or wine improves its tonic effect on blood circulation. Toasting it to ash increases its ability to stop bleeding.

Combinations: Mixed with astragalus, dong quai provides a tonic for treating fatigue and other symptoms associated with loss of blood. A blend of dong quai, white peony root, Chinese foxglove root cooked in wine, and cnidium root *(Ligusticum chuanxiong)* is prescribed for menstrual irregularity and similar conditions. Dong quai is also combined with honeysuckle flowers and red peony root to form a preparation that reduces the swelling and alleviates the pain of abscesses and sores. Consult a Chinese medicine practitioner for further information on mixtures and doses.

D

SIDE EFFECTS

None expected if used as directed.

SPECIAL INFORMATION

- You should not take dong quai during the early stages of pregnancy.
- Check on the use of this herb with your Chinese medicine practitioner if you have diarrhea or abdominal bloating; it is not recommended in some cases.

DOXAZOSIN

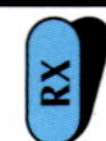

DRUG CLASS

Alpha$_1$-Adrenergic Blockers

BRAND NAME

Cardura

GENERAL DESCRIPTION

Introduced in 1986, doxazosin is one of several alpha-adrenergic blocking agents used in the treatment of high blood pressure. It can be used alone or in combination with other drugs, depending on the degree of hypertension. For more information, see ***Alpha$_1$-Adrenergic Blockers.***

SPECIAL INFORMATION

- You should not take doxazosin if you have ever had an allergic or unusual reaction to it, or to terazosin or prazosin.

DOXEPIN

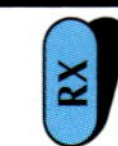

DRUG CLASS

Antidepressants [Tricyclic Antidepressants (TCAs)]

GENERAL DESCRIPTION

Introduced in 1969, doxepin is among the group of drugs called tricyclic antidepressants, commonly prescribed in the treatment of depressive illnesses. Like other antidepressants, this drug works to restore serotonin and other brain chemicals to their normal levels. Doxepin is also used to treat some kinds of chronic pain, peptic ulcers, and urticaria (hives, skin ulcers). See ***Antidepressants*** for information about side effects and possible drug interactions.

DOXYCYCLINE

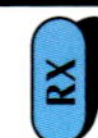

DRUG CLASS

Antibiotics [Tetracyclines]

GENERAL DESCRIPTION

Introduced in 1967, doxycycline is a semisynthetic tetracycline antibiotic, used for the same ailments as other tetracyclines and for certain additional conditions. These include use by short-term travelers for the prevention of malaria in areas where the disease is resistant to other preventives. Doxycycline is also used to prevent and treat traveler's diarrhea in high-risk patients. For more information, see ***Tetracyclines.***

SPECIAL INFORMATION

- Unlike most other tetracyclines, doxycycline may be taken with food, milk and other dairy products, or carbonated beverages with no expected decrease in action.

POSSIBLE INTERACTIONS

Barbiturates and anticonvulsants (such as carbamazepine or phenytoin): decreased doxycycline effect, possibly requiring increased dosage of doxycycline or use of another tetracycline.

DOXYLAMINE

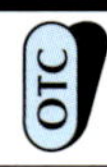

DRUG CLASS

Antihistamines

BRAND NAME

NyQuil

GENERAL DESCRIPTION

Doxylamine is used to treat symptoms such as a runny nose and congestion. Because it causes drowsiness, it is also used as a mild sedative-hypnotic to induce sleep. See ***Antihistamines.***

ECHINACEA

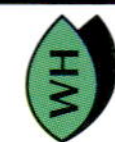

LATIN NAME
Echinacea spp.

GENERAL DESCRIPTION
Echinacea was among the herbs frequently used by Native Americans of the southwest plains in poultices, mouthwashes, and teas. Now a popular garden perennial, the plant displays purple blossoms and grows as high as five feet. Herbalists value the dried root of echinacea for its broad-based action against many types of viral and bacterial illnesses such as colds, bronchitis, ear infections, influenza, and cystitis. Laboratory testing shows that it contains echinacoside, an ingredient that may have antibiotic effects. Another ingredient, echinacein, is believed to block some mechanisms that enable infectious viruses or bacteria to invade body tissue.

In the laboratory, echinacea seems to bolster the immune system's white blood cells in their battle against foreign microorganisms; it may increase the production of T cells, which join other white blood cells in the fight against infectious agents.

Echinacea can also be effective as a topical medicine for eczema and other skin problems.

TARGET AILMENTS
Take internally for:
- colds, influenza, and other respiratory illnesses, mononucleosis, ear infections, septicemia (blood poisoning), and bladder infections.

Apply externally for:
- boils, cuts, burns, abscesses, wounds, stings, hives, insect bites, eczema, and herpes.

PREPARATIONS
Over the counter:
Available in dried form in bulk, and in teas, capsules, and tinctures.

At home:
Tea: Boil 2 tsp dried root in 1 cup water, and simmer for 15 minutes. Drink three times daily.

Combinations: Use echinacea with yarrow or uva ursi to treat cystitis.

SIDE EFFECTS
None expected.

SPECIAL INFORMATION
- Do not use echinacea continuously for more than a few weeks.
- Do not give echinacea to children younger than two years old; start with minimal doses for older children and older adults.
- Check with your doctor before using echinacea if you are pregnant or nursing.

ENALAPRIL

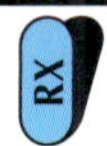

DRUG CLASS
Angiotensin-Converting Enzyme (ACE) Inhibitors

BRAND NAME
Vasotec

GENERAL DESCRIPTION
Like other ACE inhibitors, enalapril relaxes arterial walls, thereby lowering blood pressure and reducing the work load of the heart. For these reasons the drug, introduced in 1985, is used to manage high blood pressure (hypertension) and congestive heart failure. Enalapril is sometimes combined with hydrochlorothiazide for increased blood pressure-lowering action. See ***Angiotensin-Converting Enzyme (ACE) Inhibitors*** for information on side effects and possible drug interactions.

EPHEDRA

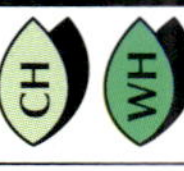

LATIN NAME
Ephedra sinica

GENERAL DESCRIPTION
With its jointed, barkless branches that bear few leaves, the ephedra plant has been used by traditional Chinese healers for thousands of years. The roots and aboveground parts of this herb have been adopted by Western practitioners as a bronchial decongestant and remedy for asthma, hay fever, and the common cold. Its active ingredients are ephedrine, pseudoephedrine, and norpseudoephedrine, all central nervous system stimulants. Ephedrine affects the body by opening bronchial passages; this activates the heart, increasing blood pressure and speeding up metabolism. For this reason, herbalists warn that excessive use of ephedra can lead to nervousness, insomnia, and high blood pressure. In the United States, several states have set restrictions on the strength of over-the-counter products containing ephedra.

Known as *ma huang* in China, ephedra grows abundantly throughout the northern provinces of this country. It is described in traditional Chinese medicine as acrid, bitter, and warm.

TARGET AILMENTS
Chinese:
- fever and chills, coughing, wheezing, nasal and chest congestion, indigestion, stomachache. (Take internally.)
- joint swelling (in combinations).

Western:
- colds, asthma, hay fever, nasal and chest congestion, influenza, obesity. (Take internally.)

PREPARATIONS
Over the counter:
Available as fluid extract, tablets, dried bulk herb.

At home:
Chinese: Prepare by combining dried herbs and water in a wok. Simmer over low heat for 15 minutes.

Combinations: For fever and chills, ephedra is mixed with cinnamon twig. A combination of ephedra and apricot seed is used for coughing and wheezing. For indigestion and stomachaches ephedra is mixed with licorice. Congestion is treated by ephedra combined with dried ginger.

Western: A tea is prepared by boiling 1 tsp ephedra with 1 cup water for 15 to 20 minutes. Drink up to 2 cups a day.

SIDE EFFECTS
Not serious:
Insomnia, dry mouth, nervousness, irritability, headache, dizziness.

Serious:
Increased blood pressure, increased heart rate, heart palpitations. If any of these symptoms develop, stop using ephedra immediately and consult your physician.

SPECIAL INFORMATION
- WARNING: Do not take ephedra if you are pregnant or have heart disease, diabetes, glaucoma, or an overactive thyroid gland (hyperthyroidism).
- WARNING: Ephedra is an ingredient in several weight-loss aids. Its effectiveness in this regard, however, derives from its accelerating effect on the metabolism, considered an unwanted side effect; consequently, many healthcare professionals warn against using it to aid in losing weight.
- If you are taking any medication, consult your physician before using this herb.

- Do not take ephedra for more than 4 weeks.
- Use low-strength preparations for children or adults over 65. Do not administer to children under age 2.
- WARNING: Because ephedra can cause a number of side effects—and in rare cases, death—consult a practitioner before using it.

EPHEDRINE

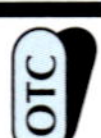

DRUG CLASS
Bronchodilators

BRAND NAMES
Primatene Dual Action Formula, Primatene Tablets

GENERAL DESCRIPTION
Ephedrine, a synthetically produced drug chemically similar to the herb ephedra, is a decongestant that also works as a bronchodilator. It is used to reduce the frequency and severity of recurrent asthma attacks. Ephedrine is available in liquid and tablet form, sometimes in combination with aspirin or acetaminophen. See ***Bronchodilators*** for further information about side effects and possible drug interactions.

SIDE EFFECTS
Not serious:
Dryness of nose and throat, rebound congestion.

EPINEPHRINE

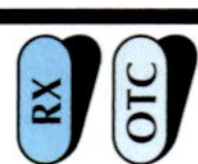

DRUG CLASS
Bronchodilators

BRAND NAMES
Rx: Adrenalin Chloride Solution, Ana-Kit, EpiPen, Sus-Phrine

OTC: Primatene Mist, Primatene Mist Suspension

GENERAL DESCRIPTION
Since 1900, epinephrine has been used to relieve the symptoms of bronchial asthma and allergic nasal congestion. In the form of eye drops, the drug is used to manage glaucoma. Other uses include the emergency treatment of heart problems and anaphylactic shock.

See ***Bronchodilators*** for information about side effects and possible drug interactions.

ERYTHROMYCIN

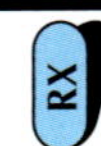

DRUG CLASS
Antibiotics [Ophthalmic Antibiotics; Erythromycins (systemic)]

BRAND NAMES
Ophthalmic: Ilotycin

Systemic: E.E.S., E-Mycin, Ery-Tab, Erythromycin Base Filmtab, Erythrocin, PCE

GENERAL DESCRIPTION
Erythromycin, which was introduced in 1952, and other drugs in its class, are used to treat many of the same infections for which penicillins are prescribed. Depending on its target and its concentration, erythromycin may kill bacteria outright (bactericidal action) or stop the growth and spread of bacteria (bacteriostatic action) by keeping the organisms from manufacturing protein. Once their growth has been halted, the bacteria can be eliminated by the body's defenses. Erythromycin is particularly useful for people who are allergic to penicillin or tetracycline.

When it is used for the eyes in the form of a solution or ointment, erythromycin has fewer side effects than it does when taken orally or by injection for systemic problems. The various systemic forms of this drug include erythromycin estolate, erythromycin stearate, erythromycin ethylsuccinate, and erythromycin base.

TARGET AILMENTS
Ophthalmic:
- eye infections due to strains of strep, staph, *Hemophilus influenzae*, and other bacteria. (Erythromycin is also used to prevent conjunctivitis in newborns who have been exposed to chlamydia or gonorrhea.)

Systemic:
- respiratory tract infections, including pharyngitis and sinusitis caused by strep; otitis media; some types of pneumonia; whooping cough; and legionnaire's disease.
- amoebic dysentery.
- infections of the skin and soft tissue.
- nonspecific urethritis.
- gonorrhea and syphilis.
- chlamydial infections.
- rheumatic, congenital, or valvular heart disease; used in short-term therapy before dental or upper-respiratory surgery to prevent endocarditis, or in continuous therapy to prevent strep infections.

SIDE EFFECTS
Not serious:
Systemic: mild nausea, oral candidiasis (sore mouth or tongue), vaginal candidiasis, unusual fatigue. Call your doctor when convenient.

Serious:
Ophthalmic: eye irritation that develops and persists after you begin using this drug; also itching, redness, or swelling. These symptoms may indicate an allergy or superinfection. Discontinue use and call your doctor right away.

Systemic: diarrhea, abdominal cramps, vomiting, and fever. Call your doctor if these symptoms are severe or prolonged.

Hearing loss; jaundice (pale stools, dark urine, yellow eyes or skin); anaphylactic reaction (rash, redness, itching, and hives). Discontinue use and call your doctor right away.

SPECIAL INFORMATION
- With long-term use, antibiotics can interfere with the actions of "good" bacteria and fungi that normally populate the intestines, mouth, and vagina; this may cause diarrhea and fungal infections, such as candidiasis. If you get a fungal infection while taking an antibiotic, continue the medication but call your doctor to find out how to treat these problems. Eating yogurt containing *Lactobacillus acidophilus* culture, or taking acidophilus tablets, can help restore the "good" bacteria that help keep the fungi in check.
- Before starting erythromycin therapy, let your doctor know if you have ever had an allergic reaction to this drug or if you have ever used erythromycin estolate.
- Tell your doctor if you have hearing loss, cardiac arrhythmias, an impaired liver, or if you are susceptible to allergies (asthma, eczema, or hives). The systemic forms of this drug may exacerbate these conditions.
- If you are pregnant, avoid erythromycin estolate, which can cause liver toxicity during pregnancy. A number of health professionals consider other forms of erythromycin to be safe for pregnant women. However, if you're pregnant or nursing, be sure to tell your doctor before taking any form (systemic or ophthalmic) of this drug.

POSSIBLE INTERACTIONS

Ophthalmic:
None expected. While the body's absorption of erythromycin through the eyes is negligible, you should tell your doctor about any other medicine you are using to avoid possible interactions.

Systemic:

Acidic fruits or juices: decreased effect of erythromycin; do not consume within an hour of taking erythromycin.

Alcohol: possible liver damage.

Alfentanil: increased alfentanil effect.

Aminophylline: possible aminophylline toxicity.

Anticoagulants: increased anticoagulant effect, risk of bleeding.

Bactericidal antibiotics (penicillins, cephalosporins): erythromycins decrease the effectiveness of these drugs.

Carbamazepine: possible toxicity of both drugs.

Chloramphenicol: increased chloramphenicol effect.

Cyclosporine: possible toxicity of both drugs, risk of kidney damage.

Digoxin: possible digoxin toxicity.

Ergotamine: possible ergotamine toxicity; impaired circulation, tingling, and burning pain in hands and feet.

Lincomycin: decreased lincomycin effect.

Lovastatin: risk of rhabdomyolysis, a severe muscle disease.

Midazolam: increased midazolam effect.

Phenytoin: possible toxicity of both drugs.

Theophylline: possible theophylline toxicity.

Triazolam: increased triazolam effect.

ERYTHROMYCINS

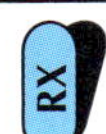

GENERIC NAMES
azithromycin, clarithromycin, erythromycin

GENERAL DESCRIPTION
Introduced in 1952, erythromycins are a subclass of antibiotics used to treat many of the same bacterial infections for which penicillins are prescribed. See the entries for the generic drugs listed above for information about side effects and possible interactions.

ESTRADIOL

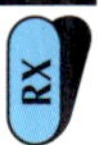

DRUG CLASS
Estrogens and Progestins

BRAND NAMES
Alora, Climara, Estrace, Estraderm, Fempatch, Vivelle

GENERAL DESCRIPTION
Used in estrogen replacement therapy to restore natural estrogen, estradiol is used to treat symptoms of menopause and to prevent osteoporosis and atherosclerosis after surgical removal of the uterus or ovaries. Estradiol is available in pill form and as a skin patch. See ***Estrogens and Progestins*** for information about side effects and possible drug interactions.

ESTROGENS AND PROGESTINS

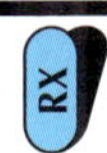

Estrogens: conjugated estrogens, estradiol, estropipate, ethinyl estradiol, mestranol

Progestins: desogestrel, ethynodiol diacetate, levonorgestrel, medroxyprogesterone, norethindrone, norethindrone acetate, norgestimate,norgestrel

GENERAL DESCRIPTION
Estrogens and progestins are natural and synthetic hormones or hormonelike substances that have strong effects on the reproductive organs of animals. The drugs, used for birth control and to treat a range of hormone-related medical conditions, also affect the heart, circulatory system, bones, and other organs. Your doctor will select an oral contraceptive based on the relative strength and proportion of each ingredient to best fit your menstrual cycle.

TARGET AILMENTS
- estrogen- and progestin-deficiency conditions, such as hot flashes, vaginal dryness, and other symptoms occurring at natural menopause or after surgical removal of the ovaries; the drugs can also be prescribed for women who have little or no ovarian function for other reasons.
- birth control (oral contraceptives, implants, injections).
- possible use in prevention of osteoporosis and heart disease in postmenopausal women.
- palliative treatment of advanced inoperable cancers: breast cancer in women and, occasionally, prostate cancer in men.
- abnormal uterine bleeding (medroxyprogesterone).

SIDE EFFECTS

Not serious:
Acne; mild nausea; diarrhea; vomiting; headache; migraine headache; abdominal pain; decrease or increase in appetite; weight gain or loss; fluid retention or swelling of ankles, feet, breasts; breast tenderness; changes in sexual desire; sodium retention. Less frequent: blotchy spots on skin, increased body hair, loss of hair on scalp, photosensitivity, intolerance to contact lenses, mild dizziness, local skin irritation (with skin patch). Let your doctor know if these symptoms persist or become bothersome.

Serious:
Lumps in the breasts, enlargement of the breasts, changes in menstrual bleeding, spotting, painful or frequent urination, fainting, jaundice, pain or swelling of the upper abdomen, pain in the stomach or right side of the abdomen, increased blood pressure, skin rash not associated with skin patch, dark-colored or new mole, cataracts, vaginitis (itching, irritation, or thick whitish discharge). Let your doctor know if you experience these symptoms.

Get medical attention immediately if you experience any of the following: severe pain in leg, chest, or abdomen; sudden headaches; changes in speech, vision, or breathing; weakness or numbness in extremities. (These symptoms may indicate blood clots.)

SPECIAL INFORMATION
- Do not use estrogens and progestins if you are pregnant or breast-feeding. If you suspect you are pregnant, discontinue use immediately to avoid severely harming the fetus.
- Estrogens may increase blood glucose levels; if you are diabetic, your doctor may have to adjust your dosage of insulin or other antidiabetic drug.
- Progestins (alone) used for oral contraception have been associated with higher rates of ectopic (fallopian tube) pregnancy.
- These hormones may cause fluid retention, which can aggravate asthma, epilepsy, migraines, and heart and kidney disease.

POSSIBLE INTERACTIONS

Anticoagulants: estrogens and progestins may decrease the anticoagulant effect of these medicines.

E

Anti-infective drugs: may decrease the effectiveness of oral contraceptives by interfering with estrogen in the digestive system.

Barbiturates and rifampin: reduced effectiveness of estrogens and progestins.

Benzodiazepines and theophylline: oral contraceptives may alter the effectiveness of these drugs. Your doctor may have to adjust your dosage.

Beta blockers (usually heart medication): birth-control pills may interfere with some beta blockers.

Calcium supplements: oral contraceptives may increase calcium absorption.

Hydrocortisone and related cortisone drugs: estrogens and progestins may increase the anti-inflammatory effects of these drugs. Your doctor may lower the dosage of cortisones.

Tamoxifen: estrogen may decrease the effects of tamoxifen.

Tobacco (smoking): may increase the risk of cardiovascular side effects of estrogens, especially in women over 35.

Tricyclic antidepressants and maprotiline: estrogen may increase blood levels of these drugs.

Vitamin C: high doses of vitamin C may increase blood levels of estrogens or alter the body's response to them.

ESTROPIPATE

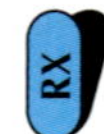

DRUG CLASS
Estrogens and Progestins

BRAND NAME
Ogen Tablets

GENERAL DESCRIPTION
Estropipate is an estrogen commonly prescribed in estrogen replacement therapy. It is used to treat symptoms of natural menopause and to prevent osteoporosis and atherosclerosis. Estropipate is also prescribed after surgical removal of the uterus or ovaries. For information about side effects and possible drug interactions, see ***Estrogens and Progestins.***

ETHINYL ESTRADIOL

DRUG CLASS
Estrogens and Progestins

BRAND NAMES
Desogen, Demulen, Loestrin FE, Lo/Ovral, Nordette, Ortho-Novum, Ovcon, Tri-Levlen, Triphasil

GENERAL DESCRIPTION
Ethinyl estradiol is an estrogen that is combined with a progestin, such as norethindrone, for use as an oral contraceptive. See ***Estrogens and Progestins*** for information about side effects and possible drug interactions.

ETHYNODIOL DIACETATE

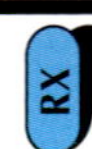

DRUG CLASS
Estrogens and Progestins

BRAND NAME
Demulen

GENERAL DESCRIPTION
Ethynodiol diacetate, a progestin combined with the estrogen ethinyl estradiol, is prescribed for use as an oral contraceptive. See ***Estrogens and Progestins*** for information about side effects and possible drug interactions.

ETODOLAC

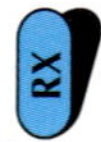

DRUG CLASS
Analgesics [Nonsteroidal Anti-Inflammatory Drugs (NSAIDs)]

BRAND NAME
Lodine

GENERAL DESCRIPTION
A newer NSAID, etodolac may be prescribed for acute and long-term management of osteoarthritis and pain. It is not generally recommended for rheumatoid arthritis. See ***Nonsteroidal Anti-Inflammatory Drugs (NSAIDs)*** for information about side effects and possible drug interactions.

EUCALYPTUS

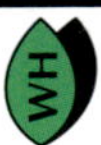

LATIN NAME
Eucalyptus globulus

GENERAL DESCRIPTION
Native to Australia and a favorite meal for koalas, the eucalyptus tree is sometimes called the Australian fever tree or gum tree. The oil extracted from eucalyptus leaves is an important ingredient in over-the-counter mouthwashes and decongestants. Herbalists include small amounts of the oil in several preparations, including gargles for sore throats, topical antiseptics for skin injuries, rubs for arthritis, and inhalants for asthma, bronchitis, and other respiratory conditions. The active ingredient in the eucalyptus leaf, a chemical called eucalyptol, is believed to be effective both in treating respiratory problems and, because of its antibacterial action, as a topical antiseptic.

TARGET AILMENTS
Apply externally for:
- arthritis, rheumatism, and minor cuts and scrapes.

Use as an inhalant in an extremely dilute form for:
- asthma, influenza, bronchitis, whooping cough, colds, and other respiratory illnesses.

PREPARATIONS
Over the counter:
Available in dry bulk, tinctures, and oils.

At home:
Inhalant: Put 1 to 3 drops of the oil in a bowl and add 1 pt boiling water; inhale steam until the vapors disappear.

Antiseptic: Dilute the oil with an equal amount of an alcohol-based topical antiseptic, and apply to cuts and other open wounds after you have washed them with soap.

Rub: Mix 1 to 5 drops eucalyptus oil with 1 cup olive oil.

▼SIDE EFFECTS

Not serious:
A skin rash can develop with external use. If it does, discontinue use.

SPECIAL INFORMATION
- WARNING: The oil of eucalyptus in concentrated form is poisonous if you ingest it. A teaspoonful can be fatal. Call your doctor immediately if you experience stomach upset or diarrhea with any dosage.

- Do not administer internally to children under two years of age. For older children and older adults, start with minimal doses.
- If you apply the oil to broken, irritated skin, use small amounts.
- Close your eyes when inhaling eucalyptus in any form because the fumes are very powerful, and be especially careful in protecting your eyes from any contact with the oils.

EUCOMMIA BARK

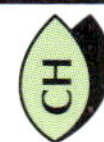

LATIN NAME
Eucommia ulmoides

GENERAL DESCRIPTION
Eucommia bark is used to strengthen the musculoskeletal system and to prevent miscarriages. Yellowish brown on the outside, it is dark purple inside. When broken, the bark should produce thin white threads. According to traditional Chinese medicine, the herb has acrid, sweet, and warm characteristics. It is harvested from trees at least 15 years old in several provinces of China.

TARGET AILMENTS
Take internally for:

- weak muscles and bones, especially in the back and knees, accompanied by poor circulation; low-back pain and soreness, accompanied by frequent urination.
- mild abdominal pain or slight vaginal bleeding during pregnancy, prevention of miscarriage and stabilization of pregnancy, back pain in pregnant women.
- dizziness and lightheadedness caused by high blood pressure.

PREPARATIONS
Eucommia bark is available in bulk or dried form at Chinese pharmacies, Asian markets, and some Western health food stores. It is sometimes possible to obtain it in pills or tablets. Herbalists recommend that you fry it in salt water, before you decoct it, when you use it as a tonic to strengthen the lower back and knees, and to treat fatigue and frequent urination.

Combinations: Eucommia bark is sometimes mixed with psoralea fruit, cornus, and cuscuta for impotence or urinary frequency and incontinence. It may be combined with Japanese teasel root, cuscuta, and mulberry mistletoe stems for low-back pain and stabilizing pregnancy. A preparation containing eucommia bark, Japanese teasel root, and Chinese yam is prescribed for pregnant women who have suffered habitual miscarriages. Consult a Chinese practitioner for advice about dosages and other herbal combinations.

SIDE EFFECTS
The herb has a mild sedative effect when taken in large doses.

SPECIAL INFORMATION

- Eucommia bark appears to have reduced high blood pressure in clinical trials, with the fried herb having a stronger effect than the dried herb.
- It seems to stimulate urination when tested in dogs, rats, and mice.

POSSIBLE INTERACTIONS
Some herbalists suggest that eucommia bark should not be taken at the same time as scrophularia.

EVENING PRIMROSE OIL

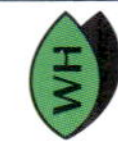

LATIN NAME
Oenothera biennis

GENERAL DESCRIPTION
Herbalists recommend the oil from the seeds of the plant known as evening primrose for a wide range of ailments that includes arthritis and premenstrual syndrome. Evening primrose supplements may also benefit brittle hair and fingernails, and may help to keep dry eyes lubricated. Native Americans and early settlers in North America used the oil to treat asthma, gastrointestinal ills, and bruises.

The therapeutic component of evening primrose oil, known as gamma-linolenic acid (GLA), is an essential fatty acid that the Western diet often lacks. GLA supports the body's production of hormones known as prostaglandins, which affect the body's hormone balance. When the body's supply of essential fatty acids such as GLA is deficient, the effects of premenstrual syndrome, diabetes, and other disorders may become more pronounced.

Evening primrose oil may also be useful in treating sore breasts in nursing mothers, through its anti-inflammatory action. In addition, recent studies suggest that evening primrose oil may have an anticlotting action. Some herbalists believe this may be helpful in treating coronary artery disease.

TARGET AILMENTS

- premenstrual syndrome, arthritis, dry eyes, hyperactivity in children, high blood pressure, eczema, brittle hair and fingernails. (Use internally.)

PREPARATIONS
Available in capsules and in liquid form. Use as directed.

SIDE EFFECTS
Too much evening primrose oil may cause headaches, skin rashes, and nausea; if this happens, either lower your dosage or discontinue use altogether.

SPECIAL INFORMATION

- Evening primrose supplements must be taken regularly for at least a month before their beneficial effects can be noticed.
- Consult a practitioner before using evening primrose oil medicinally for children.

EVODIA FRUIT

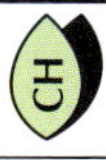

LATIN NAME
Evodia rutaecarpa

GENERAL DESCRIPTION
This extremely fragrant herb is prescribed for abdominal disorders and sometimes for its painkilling properties. Evodia fruit is characterized in traditional Chinese medicine as hot, acrid, and bitter. Grown in several Chinese provinces, the fruit is harvested between August and October, when it is brownish green in color and not fully ripe.

TARGET AILMENTS
Take internally or apply poultice externally for:

- diarrhea with undigested food, especially morning diarrhea; headaches with vomiting, and nausea accompanied by lack of appreciation of the taste of food; pain in the upper abdomen; hernia.

Apply poultice externally for:

- indigestion, high blood pressure, sores of the mouth or tongue.

PREPARATIONS
Evodia fruit is available in bulk or powdered form at Chinese pharmacies, Asian markets, and some Western health food stores.

Combinations: Evodia fruit is often mixed with other herbs to treat vomiting. These preparations frequently include fresh or dried ginger, pinellia root, or coptis. In addition, practitioners recommend that powdered evodia be combined with vinegar to make a poultice. These pastes are then placed on the navel to relieve indigestion, or on the soles of the feet to treat high blood pressure and sores of the mouth and tongue. Consult a Chinese practitioner for advice about dosages and other herbal combinations.

SIDE EFFECTS

Not serious:

An overdose of evodia fruit can cause the throat to become extremely dry.

Serious:

Large doses have led to visual disturbances and hallucinations.

SPECIAL INFORMATION

- WARNING: Herbalists consider evodia slightly toxic. They caution against long-term use and overdosage. They also believe that it can dry out body tissues.
- Practitioners often try to reduce side effects by giving patients a preparation of licorice before they take the evodia.
- In clinical tests, powdered evodia seems to have been helpful in treating eczema.

POSSIBLE INTERACTIONS

Some herbalists believe that evodia should not be used in combination with sage root.

EXPECTORANTS

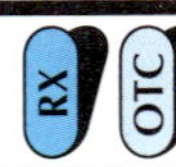

GENERAL DESCRIPTION

Expectorants help people cough up and remove thick and excessive mucus (also known as phlegm or sputum) from the lungs and upper respiratory tract, thus providing symptomatic relief from persistent coughs that frequently accompany the common cold or flu. These drugs work by reducing the stickiness and adhesiveness of mucus, making it easier to cough up and expel. Expectorants are particularly useful with dry coughs that are producing little, if any, phlegm. Eventually, as the phlegm is expelled, the respiratory tract becomes less congested and the need to cough is reduced. For information about a specific generic expectorant drug, see ***Guaifenesin.***

EYEBRIGHT

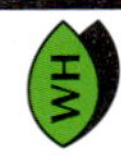

LATIN NAME

Euphrasia officinalis

GENERAL DESCRIPTION

Eyebright is an herb whose name suggests both its action and appearance. The red spots on its white or purple flowers seem to resemble bloodshot eyes. Moreover, its dried stems, leaves, and flowers have long been used as a tonic for irritated or infected eyes. Eyebright can be applied to eyes that are itching, red, and tearing from hay fever, other allergies, or colds. Herbalists also recommend it to alleviate the symptoms of conjunctivitis, and some advocates suggest that drinking eyebright tea can help to maintain good vision.

Eyebright teas are also used to diminish nasal congestion and coughs that accompany hay fever, colds, and sinusitis. The herb, indigenous to heaths and pastures throughout Great Britain and other parts of Europe, by now has become naturalized in the United States.

TARGET AILMENTS

Apply externally for:

- eye irritations including redness, itching, and tearing from hay fever, other allergies, or colds; conjunctivitis.

Take internally for:

- nasal congestion and coughs from colds, sinusitis, or allergies.

PREPARATIONS

Over the counter:

Available in bulk, capsules, and tinctures.

At home:

Tea: Pour 1 cup boiling water onto 2 tsp dried eyebright and steep for 10 minutes; drink three times daily.

Compress: Boil 1 to 2 tbsp of dried eyebright in 1 pt water for 10 minutes. After the water has cooled to a lukewarm temperature, strain the mixture to remove all parts of the herb, dip a sterile cloth in the liquid and wring it out, then put it over your eyes for 15 minutes several times daily.

Combinations to be taken orally: To treat respiratory and nasal congestion, eyebright is combined with goldenrod, elder flowers, or goldenseal. For hay fever that causes itchy or watery eyes, eyebright is mixed with ephedra. Consult an herbal practitioner for dosages.

SIDE EFFECTS

Not serious:

Eyebright may cause a skin rash or nausea. If this occurs, lessen your dose or stop taking completely.

SPECIAL INFORMATION

- Consult a practitioner before using eyebright to treat children.

FAMOTIDINE

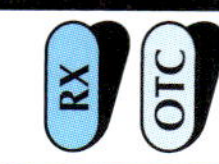

DRUG CLASS
Antiulcer Drugs [Histamine H_2 Blockers]

BRAND NAMES
Rx: Pepcid
OTC: Pepcid AC

GENERAL DESCRIPTION
Famotidine is used mainly to treat ulcers of the stomach and duodenum. It is also prescribed for Zollinger-Ellison syndrome, gastroesophageal reflux (in which stomach acid flows back into the esophagus), and other conditions involving the overproduction of stomach acid. It also used prevents upper gastrointestinal bleeding.

In the OTC form, famotidine is used not for ulcers but to relieve acid indigestion and heartburn. The OTC version, a lower dose than the prescription version, has milder side effects. The same drug interactions may apply, although none have been reported for the OTC drug.

Belonging to a subclass of antiulcer drugs known as histamine H_2 blockers, famotidine works by blocking the effects of the chemical histamine in the stomach, thereby reducing the secretion of the digestive juice hydrochloric acid. For more information on side effects and drug interactions, see ***Antiulcer Drugs.***

SIDE EFFECTS

Not serious:
Headaches, mild diarrhea, constipation, dizziness. Rare: skin rash, dry mouth or skin, fatigue, insomnia, loss of appetite, nausea, stomach pains, swelling of the eyelids. Contact your doctor if symptoms continue or become bothersome.

Serious:
Confusion, depression, anxiety, hair loss, hallucinations, muscle or joint pain, ringing in the ears, shortness of breath, tingling in fingers or toes, unusual bleeding or bruising, jaundice (yellowing of skin and eyes). If you experience any of these symptoms, call your doctor immediately.

SPECIAL INFORMATION
- Avoid while pregnant or nursing.
- Inform your doctor if you have a history of liver or kidney disease.
- This drug can interfere with skin allergy tests and cause false-negative results.
- You may need to avoid driving or potentially hazardous activities.
- Antacids can be taken with famotidine.

POSSIBLE INTERACTIONS

Alcohol, tobacco: may cause decreased effectiveness of famotidine.

Enteric-coated tablets: changes in stomach acidity may cause these medications to dissolve prematurely in the stomach; avoid taking them with famotidine.

Ketoconazole: decreased absorption of ketoconazole into the body.

FENNEL

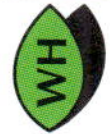

LATIN NAME
Foeniculum vulgare

GENERAL DESCRIPTION
The tiny fruits (seeds) of fennel have been used since ancient times to treat colic and to increase lactation in nursing mothers. Fennel may help digestion by relaxing the stomach and other digestive organs; it may also relieve diarrhea. In addition, it is believed that fennel may have effects upon the body similar to those of estrogen. Because it acts as a mild diuretic, fennel has been used to aid in flushing kidney stones from the body. And it acts as a soothing eyewash.

TARGET AILMENTS
Take internally for:
- digestive problems, gas, diarrhea.
- insufficient milk in nursing mothers.

Apply externally for:
- muscle pain and rheumatism.
- conjunctivitis.

PREPARATIONS
Over the counter:
Available in dry bulk, oil, and tinctures.

At home:
To help digestion, chew fresh fennel fruit.

Tea: Steep 2 tsp ground fennel in 1 cup boiling water for 10 minutes. Drink three times daily to aid digestion. For gas, drink a cup of the tea half an hour before eating. Use a weaker dosage when treating colic in children under age two.

SIDE EFFECTS

Not serious:
Fennel oil, used for inflamed joints, can cause a rash; discontinue if this occurs.

Serious:
Do not ingest the oil; it can cause nausea, vomiting, and seizures. Call your doctor if any of these symptoms develop.

SPECIAL INFORMATION
- Do not use fennel if you are pregnant or if you can't use birth-control pills or estrogen supplements.
- Do not take fennel if you have a history of alcoholism, hepatitis, liver disease, abnormal blood clotting, or estrogen-dependent breast tumors. Animal studies suggest that fennel may exacerbate liver damage.

FENUGREEK

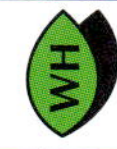

LATIN NAME
Trigonella foenum-graecum

GENERAL DESCRIPTION
Members of a legume family that includes beans and peas, fenugreek seeds have been used for centuries for digestive problems, skin injuries, sore throats, fever, muscle aches, and impotence. The seeds contain a large amount of mucilage, which becomes gelatinous when mixed with water; in this form it was thought to soothe irritated tissue. Some recent studies suggest that fenugreek has a mild anti-inflammatory effect. That may be why herbalists find it useful in treating boils, rashes, and other skin wounds, as well as arthritis. It also may be taken internally for sore throats and coughs.

TARGET AILMENTS
Take internally for:
- digestive disorders.
- sore throats and coughs.
- lactation problems of nursing mothers.
- high cholesterol or blood sugar.

Apply externally for:
- skin injuries, such as boils, rashes, cuts, or other wounds.
- pain caused by arthritis.

PREPARATIONS
Over the counter:
Available in bulk seeds, capsules, and tinctures.

At home:
Decoction: Mix 2 tsp ground fenugreek seeds in 1 cup water and simmer for 10 minutes; drink up to three times daily.

Gargle: Mix 1 tbsp ground seeds in 1 cup hot water; simmer for 10 minutes, then strain. Gargle three times daily, every three to four hours, for sore throat pain.

Poultice: Mix enough boiled seeds in 1 cup warm water to make a thick paste. Apply it directly to affected areas daily.

SIDE EFFECTS

Serious:
Fenugreek causes uterine contractions. Do not use it if you are pregnant.

F

SPECIAL INFORMATION
- Do not give to children under age two; for older children and adults, start treatment with low-strength doses.

FERRUM PHOSPHORICUM

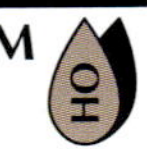

LATIN NAME
Ferrum phosphoricum

GENERAL DESCRIPTION
Ferrum phosphoricum, also called ferrum phos or iron phosphate, is a mineral compound of iron and phosphorus. Both elements are present in the body independently; phosphorus contributes to bone and muscle health, and iron aids the exchange of oxygen in the blood. Ferrum phos is derived from mixing solutions of iron sulfate, phosphate, and sodium acetate. The resulting iron phosphate is ground with large quantities of lactose (milk sugar) to render it nontoxic. Homeopathic practitioners consider ferrum phos good for patients who suffer from conditions with low energy and anemia.

TARGET AILMENTS
- Tickling, hacking coughs with chest pain, headaches, fevers that begin slowly, ear infections, incontinence, rheumatic joints, early menstrual periods accompanied by headaches, anemia, fatigue, nosebleeds, sore throat, vomiting, diarrhea, palpitations. (Take internally.)

PREPARATIONS
Ferrum phos is available in various potencies, in both liquid and tablet form, at selected stores and pharmacies. Consult your practitioner for more information.

SIDE EFFECTS
None expected.

FEVERFEW

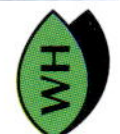

LATIN NAME
Chrysanthemum parthenium

GENERAL DESCRIPTION
Feverfew is a perennial with small, daisy-like blossoms and leaves that are medicinal. In the late 1970s, British researchers found feverfew leaves helpful in treating migraine headaches where other treatments had failed. They believe this relief is due to the chemical parthenolide, which blocks the release of inflammatory substances from the blood. The researchers consider these inflammatory elements, which affect the walls of the brain's blood vessels, to be key components in the onset of a migraine.

TARGET AILMENTS
- migraine headaches. (Take internally.)

PREPARATIONS
Over the counter:
Available in dry bulk, pills, capsules, and tinctures.

At home:
Chew two fresh or frozen leaves a day for migraines. If you find the leaves too bitter, substitute capsules or pills containing 85 mg of the leaf material, but fresh leaves are best for immediate results.

Tea: Steep 2 tsp dried herb in 1 cup boiling water for 5 to 10 minutes; drink two to three cups per day.

SIDE EFFECTS
Serious:
Chewing fresh or dried feverfew may cause internal mouth sores or abdominal pain. If these symptoms develop, discontinue use and notify your doctor.

SPECIAL INFORMATION
- Do not use feverfew if you are pregnant because it may stimulate uterine contractions.
- Feverfew may interfere with the blood's clotting ability; talk to your doctor before using if you have a clotting disorder or take anticoagulant medicine.
- You may need to take feverfew daily for two to three months before it has any effect.

FIELD MINT

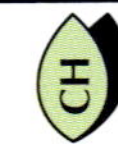

LATIN NAME
Mentha haplocalyx (or *Mentha arvensis*)

GENERAL DESCRIPTION
Chinese herbalists believe this fragrant mint speeds recovery in diseases such as measles by bringing rashes to the skin's surface. Field mint is also prescribed for a range of conditions that include gynecological problems and emotional disturbances. Characterized in Chinese medicine as an acrid, cool herb, field mint is cultivated throughout China.

TARGET AILMENTS
Take internally for:
- rashes in the early stages, sore throat, red eyes, headache.
- emotional instability.
- gynecological problems.
- childhood convulsions.

PREPARATIONS
You can buy field mint in its natural form at Chinese pharmacies, Asian, and Western groceries, and health food stores. It is also available in tablet form.

Combinations: A mixture with prunella is prescribed for inflammation of the eyes and swelling of the lymph nodes. A preparation prescribed for a sore, swollen throat combines field mint with platycodon and silkworm. Mixed with chrysanthemum flower *(Chrysanthemum morifolium)*, it is used to relieve headaches and other pains, as well as redness and swelling of the eyes. Practitioners warn against overcooking when preparing medicinal solutions of the mint; it is usually added to combinations five minutes before the cooking is finished. Consult your herbalist for further information on appropriate combinations and dosages.

SIDE EFFECTS
None expected.

SPECIAL INFORMATION
- Nursing mothers should not use this herb, since it may cause insufficient production of milk.

FLUOROQUINOLONES

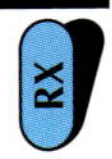

GENERIC NAMES
ciprofloxacin, ofloxacin.

GENERAL DESCRIPTION
Introduced in the 1980s, fluoroquinolones are broad-spectrum antibiotics. The drugs, which belong to a group known as quinolones, work by inhibiting the ability of bacteria to make DNA, thereby preventing the organisms' growth and reproduction. Because they enter into many parts of the body and are effective against a wide range of organisms, fluoroquinolones have been used to treat many kinds of infections, including those of the bones, joints, gastrointestinal tract, respiratory tract, skin, and urinary tract, as well as infections that are sexually transmitted. For more information about specific fluoroquinolones, see entries for the generic drugs listed above.

TARGET AILMENTS
- bronchitis (bacterial exacerbations).
- gonorrhea.
- pneumonia (bacterial), otitis media, sinusitis.
- prostatitis (bacterial).
- infections of the skin and soft tissue.
- urinary tract infections, pelvic inflammatory disease (PID).
- traveler's diarrhea.

SIDE EFFECTS

Not serious:
Mild central nervous system effects, including dizziness, lightheadedness, drowsiness, headache, nervousness, insomnia; minor gastrointestinal problems, such as pain or discomfort, diarrhea, nausea, and vomiting; photosensitivity (rare). Call your doctor if these symptoms persist or become bothersome.

Serious:
Central nervous system effects, including agitation, confusion, hallucinations, tremors, psychosis; allergic reactions (skin rash, itching or redness; swelling of face or neck; shortness of breath); fever or small ulcers on skin; bloody or cloudy urine; swelling of feet or legs; Stevens-Johnson syndrome (fever, skin blisters, or blisters and open sores on mucous membranes and genitals, weakness, joint pain). Call your doctor immediately if you have these reactions.

A rare condition known as pseudomembranous colitis may occur during or after the use of fluoroquinolones. Call your doctor at once if you experience abdominal or stomach cramps, severe pain and bloating, watery and severe diarrhea (may be bloody); fever, increased thirst; nausea or vomiting; tiredness or weakness; unusual weight loss. These symptoms may occur at any time while you are using fluoroquinolones, or they may strike weeks after you have stopped taking the drug.

SPECIAL INFORMATION
- Antibiotics kill not only harmful bacteria, but also "good" bacteria that keep unwanted fungi and intestinal organisms in check. Eating yogurt containing *Lactobacillus acidophilus* culture or taking acidophilus tablets may help restore the body's normal bacteria.
- Prolonged use of any antibiotic drug can lead to fungal infections, including candidiasis, or to bacterial infections such as pseudomembranous colitis.
- Pregnant and nursing women should not take fluoroquinolones because these drugs can cause arthropathy (abnormal development of joints) in the fetus and infant.
- Except in very limited cases, children and adolescents under the age of 18 should not use fluoroquinolones because of the risk of arthropathy. Some researchers say these drugs may be safe for use by adolescents who have completed their skeletal growth.
- Fluoroquinolones may cause sensitivity to the sun or to sunlamps. Limit your exposure while on these medications.
- Take the full course of your medicine.

POSSIBLE INTERACTIONS

Antacids, didanosine (antiviral), ferrous sulfate, laxatives containing magnesium, sucralfate (antiulcer), zinc: reduced fluoroquinolone effect. (See ***Ciprofloxacin*** and ***Ofloxacin*** for specific instructions on timing of these medications.)

Cimetidine (antiulcer) and probenecid (antigout): decreased elimination of fluoroquinolones, heightening risk of adverse effects and toxicity (especially with ofloxacin).

Warfarin (anticoagulant): increased anticoagulant effect.

FLUOXETINE

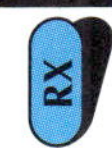

DRUG CLASS
Antidepressants [Selective Serotonin Reuptake Inhibitors (SSRIs)]

BRAND NAME
Prozac

GENERAL DESCRIPTION
Fluoxetine, a well-known antidepressant drug, is prescribed for control of a wide range of depressive illnesses. It is also used to treat alcohol dependence and obsessive-compulsive disorder.

Fluoxetine belongs to a subclass of antidepressants known as selective serotonin reuptake inhibitors (SSRIs) and works by restoring the neurotransmitter serotonin to normal levels in the brain. Although generally thought effective, fluoxetine may exacerbate suicidal tendencies in some people. Its use is considered controversial by some doctors. See ***Antidepressants*** for information on side effects and possible drug interactions.

SPECIAL INFORMATION
- Although fluoxetine benefits many of those who take it, a greater percentage of people experience side effects with this drug than with other antidepressants. If you have any questions about possible side effects, discuss them with your doctor.

FLURBIPROFEN

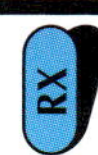

DRUG CLASS
Analgesics [Nonsteroidal Anti-Inflammatory Drugs (NSAIDs)]

BRAND NAME
Ansaid

GENERAL DESCRIPTION
Flurbiprofen is an NSAID useful for acute or long-term relief of the symptoms of rheumatoid arthritis and osteoarthritis. See ***Nonsteroidal Anti-Inflammatory Drugs (NSAIDs)*** for side effects and drug interaction information.

F

FUROSEMIDE

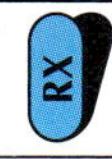

DRUG CLASS
Diuretics

BRAND NAME
Lasix Oral

GENERAL DESCRIPTION
The fast-acting and powerful diuretic furosemide has been prescribed since 1964 to treat high blood pressure (hypertension) and excess fluid retention. The drug acts by increasing urine production, thereby removing water from the body and reducing swelling and blood volume. In the process, however, salts containing sodium, potassium, calcium, and other vital minerals are also eliminated, sometimes leading to muscle cramps and serious cardiovascular side effects. For information about additional side effects and possible drug interactions, see ***Diuretics.***

SIDE EFFECTS

Not serious:
Increased risk of sunburn.

SPECIAL INFORMATION
- While taking this medicine you may become more photosensitive, meaning your skin will burn more readily when exposed to sunlight. To protect your skin, use a sunblocking lotion when outside and avoid prolonged exposure to the sun or sunlamps.

GANODERMA

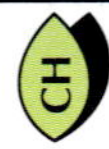

LATIN NAME
Ganoderma lucidum

GENERAL DESCRIPTION
A variety of mushroom also known as *ling zhi* in China and as *reishi* in the West, ganoderma grows in mountainous regions in China. It is a rare fungus that Chinese practitioners value highly for its multiple uses. Practitioners have traditionally used it to treat psychological disturbances as well as respiratory complaints and ulcers. In traditional Chinese medicine, where herbs are classified according to heating and cooling properties, ganoderma is categorized as neutral. Ganoderma has also been prescribed to boost patients' immune systems. It appears to help the body to resist a wide range of physical, biological, and environmental stresses.

TARGET AILMENTS
Take internally for:
- nervousness, insomnia, dizziness.
- asthma, allergy-related chronic bronchitis.
- weakened immune systems, tumors, ulcers, poor blood circulation, mushroom poisoning.

PREPARATIONS
Ganoderma can be found in bulk at Chinese pharmacies, Asian markets, and some Western health food stores (under the name *reishi*). It is also possible to obtain it in pill or tablet form, and in alcohol extracts. Consult a Chinese-medicine practitioner for information on dosages. Unlike most other Chinese herbs, ganoderma is not traditionally combined with other substances.

SIDE EFFECTS
Not serious:
Patients may experience dizziness, sore bones, itchy skin, increased bowel movements, hardened feces, and pimplelike eruptions when they use ganoderma. Stop using the herb immediately and see your doctor.

SPECIAL INFORMATION
- Ganoderma has proved useful in conjunction with conventional medical treatment of AIDS and cancer.
- In clinical studies, ganoderma seems to have reduced blood pressure in humans and animals.

GARLIC

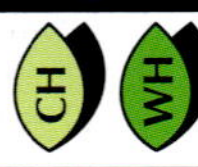

LATIN NAME
Allium sativum

GENERAL DESCRIPTION
Worn or carried as a protective talisman throughout the ages, and valued as a pungent culinary spice, the garlic bulb has gained recognition as a medicinal remedy in Chinese and Western cultures. It can be eaten raw or cooked, to release its therapeutic effects. Garlic's active ingredient is allicin, an amino acid derivative that is also responsible for the herb's pungent smell. In China this perennial herb is prescribed for colds and coughs, as well as for intestinal and digestive disorders. Chinese herbalists also believe that garlic can be used externally as an antibiotic, to relieve skin infections. In traditional Chinese medicine, garlic is characterized as acrid, bitter, and warm.

Western herbalists prescribe garlic for many of the same ailments as their Chinese counterparts. It is also thought to strengthen the cardiovascular system, by reducing cholesterol and lowering blood pressure.

TARGET AILMENTS
Chinese:
Take internally for:
- digestive disorders, diarrhea, food poisoning from shellfish, conditions that require an enema, colds, coughs, rheumatoid arthritis.

Apply externally for:
- hookworm, roundworm, ringworm of the scalp, carbuncles, swelling, pinworm, athlete's foot.

Western:
- colds, coughs, flu, high cholesterol, high blood pressure, atherosclerosis, digestive disorders, bladder infection, liver and gallbladder problems. (Take internally.)
- athlete's foot, ringworm of the body and scalp, minor skin infections. (Apply externally.)

PREPARATIONS
Over the counter:
Garlic is available as cloves and in tablet form.

At home:
Chinese: Nose drops: Combine 1 part crushed root with 10 parts water.

External treatment: Garlic is combined with sesame oil and applied externally to treat ringworm of the scalp, pinworm, carbuncles, swelling, athlete's foot, arthritis, and rheumatism.

Combinations: A mix of garlic and sugar water is sometimes prescribed for digestive disorders, diarrhea, colds, coughs, food poisoning from shellfish, and conditions that require an enema.

Western: Tincture: Combine 1 cup crushed cloves with 1 qt brandy. Shake daily for two weeks. Take up to 3 tbsp a day.

SIDE EFFECTS
Not serious:
People allergic to garlic may develop a rash from touching or eating the herb.

SPECIAL INFORMATION
- Consult your practitioner before using garlic if you are pregnant.
- Garlic has a blood clot-preventing agent. If you have a blood-clotting disorder, consult an herbalist or a licensed healthcare professional.
- Although no conclusive evidence has been found, a string of Western studies suggest that incorporating garlic into the daily diet may lower the risk of heart disease.
- Garlic is thought to function as an adjunct treatment for cardiovascular disease. Consult your practitioner before using it in this capacity.

GASTRODIA

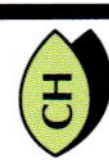

LATIN NAME
Gastrodia elata

GENERAL DESCRIPTION
The root of this member of the orchid family is prescribed by Chinese-medicine practitioners for conditions that they ascribe to disorders of the liver. A literal English translation would be "heavenly hemp." Look for a fat, solid, translucent, yellowish white root, probably imported from China's Sichuan, Yunnan, or Guizhou provinces. Gastrodia is categorized in traditional Chinese medicine as a sweet and neutral herb.

TARGET AILMENTS
- headaches, including migraines; dizziness; childhood convulsions; epilepsy. (Take internally.)

PREPARATIONS
Gastrodia is found in bulk or in tablets at Chinese pharmacies, Asian markets, and some Western health food stores.

Combinations: Mixed with gambir, skullcap, and achyranthes root, it is used for dizziness. Adding scorpion to that mixture creates a preparation for treating seizures. Herbalists prescribe a mix containing gastrodia, Asian ginseng, atractylodes (white), and silkworm for chronic childhood convulsions. Check with your practitioner for further information on combinations and dosages.

SIDE EFFECTS

None expected.

SPECIAL INFORMATION

- WARNING: Use the herb with caution and in consultation with your practitioner. In one laboratory experiment, rats injected daily with an alcohol extraction of gastrodia showed reduced activity and appetite. In another, rabbits injected with preparations of the herb became lethargic and lost their appetites; their heart rates increased and their EEGs altered.
- Preparations of the herb have halted seizures and inhibited the development of epilepsy-like symptoms in rabbits. Gastrodia, however, proved not as effective as phenobarbital.

GELSEMIUM

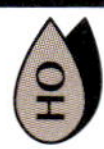

LATIN NAME

Gelsemium sempervirens

GENERAL DESCRIPTION

Sometimes called yellow jasmine, gelsemium is not really part of the jasmine family but is related to the plants ignatia and nux vomica. A climbing vine with trumpetlike yellow flowers, it is common to the woods and coastal shoreline of the southern United States. Taken in large doses, gelsemium causes paralysis of the motor nerves, impairing physical and mental functions like vision, balance, thought, and movement; ultimately, poisoning causes convulsions and death. Homeopathic physicians prescribe dilute solutions of gelsemium for ailments that are accompanied by symptoms like those of gelsemium poisoning. In its homeopathic form, *Gelsemium* is prepared from the fresh root, which is chopped, soaked in alcohol, strained, and diluted to the desired, highly dilute potencies.

For more information on homeopathic medicine, see page 1027.

TARGET AILMENTS

- anxiety; flu with aches, chills, and exhaustion; headache, beginning from the back of the head and moving forward; measles; sore throat; fever with chills that move up and down the spine, although the patient may not feel cold. (Take internally.)

PREPARATIONS

Gelsemium is available over the counter in various potencies, in both liquid and tablet form, from selected stores and pharmacies. Consult your homeopathic practitioner for more precise information.

SIDE EFFECTS

None expected.

GEMFIBROZIL

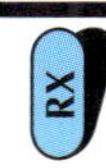

DRUG CLASS

Cholesterol-Reducing Drugs

BRAND NAME

Lopid

GENERAL DESCRIPTION

Introduced in 1976, gemfibrozil is used to lower cholesterol and triglyceride levels in the blood, thus reducing the risk of coronary artery disease. The drug seems to work by inhibiting production of triglycerides in the liver and accelerating removal of cholesterol from the body. For more information, see ***Cholesterol-Reducing Drugs.***

SIDE EFFECTS

Not serious:

Moderate increase in blood sugar levels; reduced libido in men.

Serious:

Fever, chills, sore throat, low-back and side pain, difficult or painful urination. Doubled risk of gallstone formation with long-term use.

SPECIAL INFORMATION

- This drug is usually taken twice a day, 30 minutes before the morning and evening meals.

POSSIBLE INTERACTIONS

Chenodiol and ursodiol: these two medications, prescribed to treat gallstones, have decreased effectiveness when taken with gemfibrozil.

Lovastatin: may lead to kidney failure when it is taken concurrently with gemfibrozil.

GENTIAN

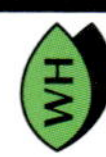

LATIN NAME

Gentiana lutea

GENERAL DESCRIPTION

Distinguished by oval leaves and orange blooms, gentian is believed to act as a general tonic, relieving exhaustion and helping the body rebuild its natural defenses against illness. The root of this herb has been used in different cultures for about 3,000 years to treat digestive disorders and to stimulate the appetite. It was introduced to Western herbalists by Native Americans who used the plant to alleviate back pains. Today, gentian is prescribed in Western countries primarily as a digestive aid. Because of its bitter properties, it stimulates the secretion of stomach acid and produces saliva. For this reason, contemporary herbalists frequently recommend ingesting this herb before or with large meals. Its most common form is in liqueurs, vermouths, and a variety of other bitter-tasting cocktails.

TARGET AILMENTS

- digestive disorders, loss of appetite, arthritis, exhaustion, weakness, irregular menstrual cycle. (Take internally.)

PREPARATIONS

Over the counter:

Gentian is available in bulk as dried roots, and in tincture.

At home:

Tea: Boil 1 oz gentian root with 1 cup water for 15 to 20 minutes. Drink 15 to 30 minutes before eating, to aid digestion.

Combinations: Use with ginger and cardamom for digestive disorders.

SIDE EFFECTS

Not serious:

Upset stomach, nausea, or vomiting may develop from taking gentian.

SPECIAL INFORMATION

- WARNING: Use only under the direction of an herbalist or a licensed healthcare professional if you are pregnant or have high blood pressure (hypertension), or chronic gastrointestinal conditions.
- Use low-strength preparations for children or for adults over 65. Do not give gentian to children under 2 years of age.

GENTIANA

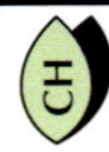

LATIN NAME
Gentiana scabra

GENERAL DESCRIPTION
Several varieties of this herb grow throughout China. *Gentiana scabra,* the most widely used, is a long, thick, yellow root, described as cold by Chinese herbalists. They prescribe the herb primarily for disorders of the liver and organs in the pelvic area. Gentiana tastes so bitter that herbalists use it as a standard for judging bitterness in plants.

TARGET AILMENTS
Use internally for:
- hepatitis, jaundice, and other liver disorders.
- sexually transmitted diseases, vaginal discharge, inflammation of the pelvis, pain or swelling in the genital area.
- convulsions.

PREPARATIONS
You can find gentiana in bulk at Chinese pharmacies, Asian markets, and some Western health food stores. While the Chinese variety is not available in pills or tablets, the European root can be obtained in that form.

Combinations: Chinese herbalists prescribe a preparation that contains gentiana, sophora root, and plantago seeds for genital itching and vaginal discharge. A combination of gentiana with cattle gallstone and gambir is given for convulsions, especially when the symptoms appear in children. Check with your practitioner for advice on other combinations and dosages.

SIDE EFFECTS
None expected.

SPECIAL INFORMATION
- WARNING: Chinese herbalists advise against the use of this root when diarrhea is among the symptoms.
- Gentiana is believed to have an antibiotic effect; it is also thought to be toxic to malarial parasites.

GINGER

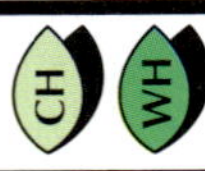

LATIN NAME
Zingiber officinale

GENERAL DESCRIPTION
Characterized by delicate yellow blooms rimmed with purple, ginger not only is a valued culinary seasoning but also is considered in many cultures a remedy for a range of ailments. Discovered by practitioners of traditional Ayurvedic (Hindu) medicine, the ginger root was originally thought of as a digestive aid. Today both Chinese and Western herbalists believe it relieves motion sickness and dizziness and improves digestion. Ginger is also believed to alleviate menstrual cramps. Its active constituents are gingerols, which soothe the abdomen and relieve excess gas.

In China, ginger, called *gan-jian,* is applied to first- and second-degree burns. It is described in traditional Chinese medicine as acrid and warm.

TARGET AILMENTS
Chinese:
- vomiting, abdominal pain, menstrual irregularity, coughs. (Take internally.)
- first- and second-degree burns. (Apply externally.)

Western:
- motion sickness, morning sickness, digestive disorders, menstrual cramps, colds, flu, arthritis, elevated cholesterol level, high blood pressure. (Take internally.)

PREPARATIONS
Over the counter:
Ginger is available as fresh or dried root, liquid extract, tablets, capsules, prepared tea.

At home:
Chinese: Traditional preparation: Wrap fresh ginger roots in five or six layers of rice paper. Bury under warm coals until the paper is blackened. Remove rice paper before using.

Rub: Treat first- and second-degree burns by rubbing fresh ginger juice, extracted from the root, on the wound.

Combinations: For vomiting, ginger is mixed with pinellia root; when there is also severe abdominal pain, the herb is combined with licorice or galanga. A preparation of ginger and chamomile is used to treat menstrual irregularity. For coughing and headaches, ginger is mixed with dried bamboo.

Western: Tea: Boil 1 oz dried ginger root in 1 cup water for 15 to 20 minutes.

SIDE EFFECTS
Not serious:
Heartburn may result from taking ginger.

SPECIAL INFORMATION
- Some Western studies show that ginger may help prevent heart disease and strokes by reducing internal blood clotting and lowering blood pressure.
- If you are pregnant, consult an herbalist or a licensed healthcare professional before using.

GINKGO

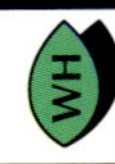

LATIN NAME
Ginkgo biloba

GENERAL DESCRIPTION
Chinese herbalists have used the fan-shaped leaves of the deciduous ginkgo tree for thousands of years to treat asthma, chilblains (an inflammation caused by exposure to cold), and swellings. Today, Western herbalists value ginkgo leaves for their action against vascular diseases that typically affect the elderly. One of ginkgo's most important benefits is its ability to increase vasodilation (expansion of blood vessels), and thereby improve blood flow in capillaries and arteries, especially in peripheral areas such as the lower legs and feet. It also appears to improve blood flow to the brain.

Herbalists believe that ginkgo may interfere with the development of blood clots and the processes that constrict bronchial tubes during an asthma attack. In addition it may help reduce retinal damage from macular degeneration, a cause of blindness particularly threatening for diabetics. And it may help reverse deafness caused by reduced blood flow to the nerves involved in hearing.

TARGET AILMENTS
- vertigo; Alzheimer's disease; tinnitus (ringing in the ears); phlebitis (inflammation of a vein); leg ulcers; cerebral atherosclerosis; diabetic vascular disease; Raynaud's syndrome; headaches; depression; lack of concentration or mental and emotional fatigue in the elderly; asthma; clotting disorders, including strokes and heart attacks. (Take ginkgo internally.)

PREPARATIONS
Ginkgo leaves are available in dry bulk, capsules, or tincture. You can find a standardized product known as ginkgo

biloba extract (GBE) in health food stores. Most herbalists recommend using only over-the-counter ginkgo products.

SIDE EFFECTS

Ginkgo can cause irritability, restlessness, diarrhea, nausea, and vomiting; if these symptoms develop, check with your practitioner to see if you should lower your dosage or stop taking ginkgo completely.

SPECIAL INFORMATION

- WARNING: Some people are unable to tolerate ginkgo even in small doses.
- Do not use if you have a clotting disorder, or if you are pregnant or nursing.
- Do not give ginkgo to children without a doctor's supervision.
- Use in medicinal amounts only in consultation with a healthcare professional.

GINSENG, AMERICAN

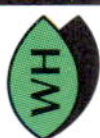

LATIN NAME

Panax quinquefolius

GENERAL DESCRIPTION

Native Americans believed American ginseng could alleviate painful childbirths and restore energy to the elderly. Found abundantly in the Cumberland Gap region of the southern Appalachians, American ginseng is identified by a single stalk crowned by delicate chartreuse blooms and crimson berries; its leaflets have sawlike teeth. The active ingredients of American ginseng are panaxosides, which are thought to calm the stomach and the brain and act as a mild stimulant to vital organs. American ginseng is milder than Asian ginseng and is often prescribed for people who consider Asian ginseng too potent. Both American and Asian ginseng are frequently used to treat the elderly.

TARGET AILMENTS

Take internally for:

- depression, fatigue, stress.
- colds, influenza, respiratory problems, inflammations, damaged immune systems.

PREPARATIONS

Over the counter:
Ginseng is available as fresh or dried root, root powder, capsules, tablets, prepared tea, freeze-dried root, cured rock candy.

At home:
Tea: Boil 1 oz fresh root with 1 cup water for 15 to 20 minutes. Drink up to 2 cups a day.

SIDE EFFECTS

Not serious:
Headaches, insomnia, anxiety, breast soreness, or skin rashes may develop.

Serious:
You may experience asthma attacks, increased blood pressure, heart palpitations, or postmenopausal uterine bleeding. Stop using ginseng and consult your doctor.

SPECIAL INFORMATION

- WARNING: Do not use American ginseng if you are also taking any antihistamine medications or other stimulants, such as caffeine, amphetamines, central nervous stimulants, or ephedra.
- American ginseng is considered an endangered species because of excessive harvesting.

GINSENG, ASIAN

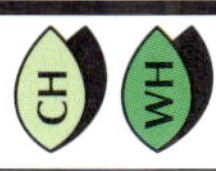

LATIN NAME

Panax ginseng

GENERAL DESCRIPTION

Ginseng means "the essence of the earth in the form of a man," and in fact the root's shape suggests the human form. Growing on mountain slopes in the northeastern provinces of China, Asian ginseng is considered the most potent and expensive form of ginseng.

With its yellow-green flowers and red berries, it looks similar to American ginseng, but the stalk is longer. Its active constituents are ginsenosides, substances that enhance pituitary-adrenal processes to strengthen the immune system and increase the body's ability to deal with fatigue and stress. It is described in traditional Chinese medicine as sweet, bitter, and warm.

TARGET AILMENTS

Chinese:
Take internally for:

- fatigue, weakness.
- symptoms of shock, profuse sweating, ice-cold extremities, shortness of breath, fever, thirst, irritability.
- diarrhea, vomiting, distention of the abdomen, anorexia.
- impotence.

Western:
Take internally for:

- depression, fatigue, stress.
- colds, influenza, respiratory problems, inflammations, damaged immune systems.

PREPARATIONS

Over the counter:
Ginseng is available as fresh or dried root, root powder, capsules, tablets, prepared tea, freeze-dried root, cured rock candy.

At home:
Chinese: Boil fresh roots in water for 3 to 7 minutes. Prick roots with needles. Dry roots in the sun and then soak in thick sugar 10 to 12 hours.

Combinations: Ginseng, atractylodes (white), and China root are used to treat anorexia, diarrhea, vomiting, and distention of the abdomen. For fever, thirst, and irritability, ginseng is prepared with Chinese foxglove cooked in wine and asparagus tuber. For impotence, ginseng is combined with deer antler.

Western: Tea: Boil 1 oz fresh root with 1 cup water for 15 to 20 minutes. Drink up to 2 cups a day.

SIDE EFFECTS

Not serious:
Headaches, insomnia, anxiety, breast soreness, or skin rashes may develop.

Serious:
Asthma attacks, increased blood pressure, heart palpitations, or postmenopausal uterine bleeding. Stop using ginseng and consult your doctor.

SPECIAL INFORMATION

- If you have any of the following conditions, use ginseng only under the direction of an herbalist or a licensed healthcare professional: pregnancy, insomnia, hay fever, fibrocystic breasts, asthma, emphysema, high blood pressure, blood-clotting problems, heart disorders, diabetes.

GINSENG, SIBERIAN

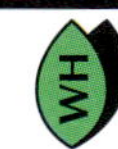

LATIN NAME

Eleutherococcus senticosus

GENERAL DESCRIPTION

Found in the Siberian regions of Russia and China, Siberian ginseng, also called eleuthero, affects the body in a manner similar to Asian and American ginseng, although these effects are more subtle and result in less-pronounced reactions. The active elements of Siberian ginseng are eleutherosides, which stimulate the immune system, increasing the body's resistance to disease, stress, and fatigue. Siberian ginseng has gained popularity as a Western herb because it does not cause the insomnia and anxiety that sometimes occur when Asian or American ginseng is used.

TARGET AILMENTS
Take internally for:

- depression, fatigue, stress.
- colds, influenza, respiratory problems, inflammations, damaged immune systems.

G

PREPARATIONS
Over the counter:
Ginseng is available as fresh or dried root, root powder, capsules, tablets, prepared tea, freeze-dried root, cured rock candy.

At home:
Tea: Boil 1 oz fresh root with 1 cup water for 15 to 20 minutes. Drink up to 2 cups a day.

SIDE EFFECTS

Not serious:
Headaches, insomnia, anxiety, breast soreness, skin rashes.

Serious:
Asthma attacks, increased blood pressure, heart palpitations, postmenopausal uterine bleeding.

SPECIAL INFORMATION

- Siberian ginseng gained popularity in Russia when an extract was mass-produced and used in a popular cola-like drink called Bodust, meaning "vigor."

GLIPIZIDE

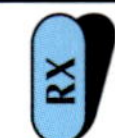

DRUG CLASS
Antidiabetic Drugs [Oral Hypoglycemics]

BRAND NAME
Glucotrol

GENERAL DESCRIPTION
Glipizide is used to treat a form of non-insulin-dependent (Type 2) diabetes that cannot be controlled by diet and exercise alone. The drug, introduced in 1972, stimulates the release of existing insulin in people whose bodies are capable of producing the hormone. See ***Oral Hypoglycemics*** for more information, including facts about side effects and possible drug interactions.

GLYBURIDE

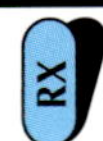

DRUG CLASS
Antidiabetic Drugs [Oral Hypoglycemics]

BRAND NAMES
DiaBeta, Glynase, Micronase

GENERAL DESCRIPTION
Glyburide, introduced in 1970, is used to treat a form of non-insulin-dependent (Type 2) diabetes that cannot be controlled by diet and exercise alone. The drug stimulates the release of existing insulin in people whose bodies are capable of producing the hormone. See ***Oral Hypoglycemics*** for more information, including facts about side effects and possible drug interactions.

GOLDENSEAL

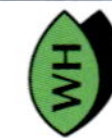

LATIN NAME
Hydrastis canadensis

GENERAL DESCRIPTION
Herbalists use the dried and powdered rhizomes and roots of goldenseal, a small perennial with white flowers and red berries, to treat several respiratory and skin infections. The herb acts as a stimulant and seems to affect the body's mucous membranes by drying up secretions, reducing inflammation, and fighting infection through the mild antimicrobial action of its active ingredient, berberine. Goldenseal also aids digestion by promoting the production of saliva, bile, and other digestive enzymes. In addition it may control postpartum bleeding by means of its astringent action.

TARGET AILMENTS

- infectious diarrhea, irritable bowel syndrome, colitis, ulcers, gastritis, gallstones, jaundice, sinusitis, laryngitis, sore throat, infected gums, ear infections, and vaginal yeast infections. (Take internally.)
- eczema, ringworm, contact dermatitis, athlete's foot, impetigo. (Use the herb externally.)

PREPARATIONS
Over the counter:
The dry root is available in bulk, capsules, and tincture.

At home:
Tea: Pour 1 cup boiling water onto 2 tsp goldenseal; steep for 10 to 15 minutes. Drink three times daily.

Douche: Simmer 1 tbsp powdered herb in 1 pt water for 10 minutes. The liquid should be as warm as is tolerable. Douche daily, up to two weeks.

Combinations: Use with meadowsweet and chamomile for stomach problems. For a skin wash, mix with distilled witch hazel; for ear infections, make drops using goldenseal and mullein. See your herbalist for exact instructions.

SIDE EFFECTS

Not serious:
In high doses, goldenseal can irritate the skin, mouth, throat, and vagina. It may also cause nausea and diarrhea. If any of these develop, stop taking immediately.

SPECIAL INFORMATION

- Do not use goldenseal if you are pregnant; it may stimulate the uterus.
- Do not use goldenseal without consulting a physician if you have had heart disease, diabetes, glaucoma, a stroke, or high blood pressure. It stimulates the heart muscle, and the result is increased blood pressure.
- Do not give goldenseal to children under two; for older children and older adults, start with small doses.
- Some herbalists consider this herb to be endangered; they recommend using goldenseal that is commercially and organically grown.

GOTU KOLA

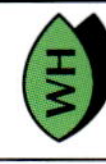

LATIN NAME
Centella asiatica

GENERAL DESCRIPTION
The gotu kola plant grows in marshy areas in many parts of the world. Its fan-shaped leaves contain the soothing agent known as asiaticoside. As a result they have been used to treat burns, skin grafts, and episiotomies (a surgical technique designed to prevent tearing of the vagina during childbirth). Gotu kola may also help heal outbreaks of psoriasis.

There is some evidence that in addition gotu kola may help decrease edema (the retention of fluid by the body) and promote blood circulation in the legs by strengthening the veins and capillaries. It may therefore be useful in treating phlebitis (inflammation of the leg veins).

TARGET AILMENTS

- poor circulation in the legs, edema. (Take internally.)
- Burns, cuts, and other skin injuries; psoriasis. (Use an external compress.)

PREPARATIONS

Over the counter:
Available in dry bulk, capsules, and tincture.

At home:
Tea: Use 1 to 2 tsp dried gotu kola per cup of boiling water; drink twice daily to improve circulation in the legs.

Compress: Soak a pad in gotu kola tea or in a tincture to help treat wounds or psoriasis. Start with a weak solution and increase the concentration of gotu kola if necessary.

SIDE EFFECTS

Not serious:
Gotu kola may cause a skin rash or headaches; in either case, lower your dosage or stop taking it.

SPECIAL INFORMATION

- Do not use gotu kola if you are pregnant or nursing, or using tranquilizers or sedatives, since gotu kola may have a narcotic effect.
- Do not give gotu kola to children under two. For older children and older adults, start with low-strength doses, and increase if necessary.

GRAINS-OF-PARADISE FRUIT

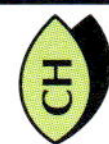

LATIN NAME
Amomum villosum (or *A. xanthioides*)

GENERAL DESCRIPTION
The fragrant, acrid-tasting grains-of-paradise fruit, a kind of cardamom, is prescribed for a variety of abdominal complaints. Grains-of-paradise fruit is considered a stimulant, and great value is placed on its aroma. Chinese herbalists may add it to fruits such as baked pears to reduce the production of mucus in the body. The choicest fruits are large, solid, and extremely aromatic. Classified in traditional Chinese medicine as an acrid, warm herb, grains-of-paradise fruit grows in the Chinese provinces of Guangdong and Guanxi and in several areas of Southeast Asia, where it is harvested in August and September.

TARGET AILMENTS
Take internally for:

- nausea and vomiting, abdominal pain, diarrhea, indigestion, gas, loss of appetite.
- morning sickness, pain, and discomfort during pregnancy.
- involuntary urination.

PREPARATIONS
Cardamom is available in bulk or powder from Chinese pharmacies, Asian markets, and some Western health food stores.

Combinations: Mixed with atractylodes (white) and codonopsis root, it is used to treat morning sickness. And for other types of discomfort during pregnancy, herbalists prescribe a mixture with mulberry mistletoe stems. It is generally added to combinations near the end of the cooking period, and should be crushed before it is used.

SIDE EFFECTS

None are expected if used precisely in the prescribed dosage.

SPECIAL INFORMATION

- Chinese practitioners avoid the use of cardamom in patients with what they call a yin deficiency, a condition marked by symptoms of heat such as fever, thirst, and sweating. Consult your practitioner for advice.
- The shell of the fruit is believed to have medicinal properties similar to but weaker than the fruit itself.

GUAIFENESIN

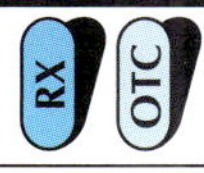

DRUG CLASS
Expectorants

BRAND NAMES
Rx: Duratuss G, Entex LA, Guaifed, Humibid DM, Humibid LA, Hycotuss, Vicotuss

OTC: Primatene Dual Action Formula, Robitussin-CF, Robitussin-DM, Triaminic Expectorant, Vicks DayQuil LiquiCaps, Vicks DayQuil Liquid

GENERAL DESCRIPTION
Guaifenesin is an expectorant drug, used to provide symptomatic relief from coughs, particularly those associated with the common cold or flu. The medication works by thinning and loosening mucus or phlegm from the upper respiratory tract, making it easier to cough up and expel the secretions. As the respiratory tract becomes less congested, the need to cough is reduced.

This drug is used in many over-the-counter and prescription cough preparations, often in combination with a decongestant, an antihistamine, or some other medication. Guaifenesin is available in tablet, capsule, or liquid form.

TARGET AILMENTS

- coughs due to the common cold, flu, and other minor upper respiratory conditions.

SIDE EFFECTS

Not serious:
Stomach pain, diarrhea, nausea, drowsiness, mild weakness (these effects are rare). Contact your doctor if these symptoms persist or become bothersome.

Serious:
Skin rash, persistent headache, vomiting, high fever. Contact your doctor at once.

SPECIAL INFORMATION

- If you are using the extended-release tablet form of this medication, swallow it whole; do not crush or chew the tablet before swallowing it.
- This medication is most effective when taken on an empty stomach.
- To help guaifenesin loosen mucus from the lungs, drink 8 to 10 glasses of fluid each day, including a glass of water after each dose.
- If you are pregnant or nursing, check with your doctor before using this medication.
- Do not give this medication to a child under the age of two without first consulting the child's pediatrician.
- Do not take this drug for persistent cough due to smoking, asthma, bronchitis, or emphysema.
- If your cough does not improve within seven days, see your doctor.

POSSIBLE INTERACTIONS

None expected.

GUANFACINE

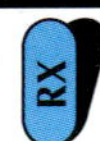

DRUG CLASS
Antihypertensive Drugs

BRAND NAME
Tenex

GENERAL DESCRIPTION
Introduced in 1980, guanfacine is used alone or in combination with a thiazide diuretic to help manage mild-to-moderate high blood pressure (hypertension). It decreases both systolic and diastolic blood pressure.

Guanfacine works by stimulating the alpha$_2$-adrenergic receptors in the brain, which causes a reduction in nerve impulses to the heart, kidneys, and arteries. With fewer of these impulses, the blood vessel walls relax and blood flows through them more easily, thus reducing heart rate and lowering blood pressure.

This drug does not cure high blood pressure, but it helps to control it. Because untreated hypertension can have serious consequences, you may need to take the medication for the rest of your life. Like other blood-pressure-lowering drugs, guanfacine is most effective when combined with regular exercise, stress reduction, weight loss, and a salt-restricted diet. For more information, see ***Antihypertensive Drugs.***

TARGET AILMENTS
- high blood pressure (hypertension).

SIDE EFFECTS

Not serious:
Drowsiness; dry mouth and nose; constipation; headache; dizziness; fatigue; insomnia; decreased sex drive; dry, itching, or burning eyes; nausea or vomiting. Call your doctor if these symptoms persist or are bothersome.

Serious:
Confusion, mental depression. Contact your doctor as soon as possible.

SPECIAL INFORMATION
- Do not take guanfacine if you have had an allergic reaction to this drug in the past.
- Tell your doctor if you are pregnant or planning a pregnancy; are nursing; have heart, kidney, or liver disease; have coronary insufficiency or cerebrovascular disease; or are suffering from depression.
- Tell your doctor if you are taking sedatives, hypnotics, or antidepressants, or are planning surgery requiring general anesthesia.
- Be sure to check with your doctor before taking any other medications, especially over-the-counter antihistamines; appetite-control pills; medicines for colds, coughs, sinus, or hay fever; pain pills; or muscle relaxants. Some of these medications may increase your blood pressure; others will result in excess drowsiness.
- Because guanfacine can act as a sedative, it may impair your mental alertness, judgment, and coordination. Until you know how the drug will affect you, be cautious about driving, using machines, or engaging in any potentially dangerous activity. To reduce daytime drowsiness, take the drug at bedtime.
- Be sure you always have an adequate supply of guanfacine to tide you over during holidays and vacations. You may want to carry a backup prescription for emergency use.
- Pay special attention to dental hygiene. Guanfacine can cause mouth dryness, which may increase the likelihood of dental disease. Check with your dentist or doctor if dry mouth continues for more than two weeks.
- It usually takes four to six weeks to know if guanfacine will control your high blood pressure. Do not abruptly stop taking the drug: You may experience severe withdrawal effects.

POSSIBLE INTERACTIONS

Alcohol and other central nervous system depressants, such as antihistamines and muscle relaxants: may increase drowsiness and guanfacine's blood-pressure-lowering effect.

Food: avoid excessive salt.

HAWTHORN

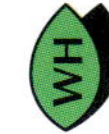

LATIN NAME
Crataegus laevigata (or *Crataegus oxyacantha*)

GENERAL DESCRIPTION
Herbalists use the flowers, fruit, and leaves of the hawthorn, a European shrub with thorny branches. They prescribe the herb as a mild heart tonic. It is thought to improve the flow of blood through the coronary blood vessels, lowering blood pressure. Hawthorn is also believed to increase the pumping force of the heart muscle and to eliminate arrhythmias. Some practitioners think hawthorn may have a calming effect on the nervous system, and they sometimes recommend it as a remedy for insomnia. Identified by crimson berries and blue-green leaves, hawthorn is also called the mayflower, because its delicate white flowers bloom primarily in May.

TARGET AILMENTS
Take internally in conjunction with conventional medical treatment for:
- high blood pressure, clogged arteries, heart palpitations, angina, inflammation of the heart muscle.

Take internally for:
- insomnia and nervous conditions.

Use as a gargle for:
- sore throat.

PREPARATIONS
Hawthorn is available as fluidextract, dried berries and leaves, capsules.

SIDE EFFECTS

Serious:
Taking large amounts of hawthorn may result in a dramatic drop in blood pressure, which in turn may cause you to feel faint.

SPECIAL INFORMATION
- WARNING: Use hawthorn as a heart tonic only if you have been diagnosed with angina, cardiac arrhythmias, or congestive heart failure, and only in consultation with a physician. Do not practice self-diagnosis.
- Children and pregnant or nursing women should use hawthorn only under the direction of a medical herbalist or a licensed healthcare professional.

HEPARIN

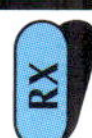

DRUG CLASS
Anticoagulant and Antiplatelet Drugs

GENERAL DESCRIPTION
Heparin, a very powerful drug, is the anticoagulant of choice when an instant effect is required. It works by inhibiting the formation of blood clots at various sites throughout the body. Heparin is administered by injection or intravenous infusion in a hospital, clinic setting, or at home by a trained healthcare professional. If you are receiving heparin at home, it is essential that the medicine be administered exactly as directed and that you have regular blood tests to determine how fast your blood is clotting. See ***Anticoagulant and Antiplatelet Drugs*** for additional information on side effects and drug interactions.

SIDE EFFECTS

Serious:
Heparin can cause hemorrhaging. Other serious symptoms include chest pain, severe headache, low blood pressure, rash, breathing problems, wheezing, runny nose, and tightness in the chest. Call your doctor if you experience any of these symptoms.

SPECIAL INFORMATION
- Because heparin is derived from animal tissue, individuals with a history of asthma or allergies should try a test dose before starting treatment.

HEPAR SULPHURIS

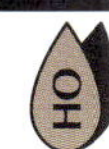

LATIN NAME
Hepar sulphuris calcareum

GENERAL DESCRIPTION
The flaky inner layer of oyster shells provides the calcium used in this homeopathic remedy, also called *Hepar sulph* and commonly known as calcium sulphide. Once an antidote for mercury poisoning, calcium sulphide is now used by homeopathic physicians to treat patients with conditions that tend to be infected, often producing pus. These disorders are accompanied by symptoms that include mental and physical hypersensitivity and an intolerance of pain and cold.

Finely ground oyster shell and sulphur are mixed together and then heated in an airtight container. The resulting powder is dissolved in hot hydrochloric acid, then combined with lactose (milk sugar) in a pharmaceutical process of dilution called trituration.

TARGET AILMENTS
- abscesses that are swollen and painful but have not yet opened; colds, sore throat, and earache; inflamed cuts and wounds that may be taking longer than normal to heal; aching joints; fits of coughing with chest pain, hoarseness, asthma, emphysema, croup; genital herpes; constipation.

PREPARATIONS
Hepar sulph is available over the counter in various potencies, in both liquid and tablet form, at selected stores and pharmacies. Consult your practitioner for more precise information.

SIDE EFFECTS
None expected.

HIBISCUS

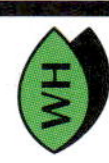

LATIN NAME
Hibiscus sabdariffa

GENERAL DESCRIPTION
Hibiscus, a widespread category of annuals whose lush, showy flowers are nearly synonymous with tropical beauty, includes more than 200 species of plants. Most of them are believed to have some medicinal properties; different species are used in Ayurvedic (Hindu), Chinese, and Western herbal medicines. *Hibiscus sabdariffa,* also known as roselle or Jamaica sorrel, is valued for its mild laxative effect and for its ability to increase urination, attributed to two diuretic ingredients, ascorbic acid and glycolic acid. Because it contains citric acid, a refrigerant, it is used as a cooling herb, providing relief during hot weather by increasing the flow of blood to the skin's surface and dilating the pores to cool the skin.

Hibiscus seeds, leaves, fruits, and roots are used in various folk remedies, and tea is made from the flowers, in particular, the calyx, the leaflike segment that makes up the outermost part of the flower. Its flowers are also used in jams and jellies, to impart a tart, refreshing taste.

TARGET AILMENTS

Take internally for:

- constipation, mild bladder infections, mild nausea.

Apply the herb or extract externally for:

- sunburn.

PREPARATIONS

Over the counter:
Fresh or dried hibiscus flowers and teas are available in health food stores.

At home:
Tea: Use 2 tsp crumbled, dried blossom or 1 tbsp fresh, chopped blossom per cup of boiling water; steep 10 minutes. Drink up to 3 cups per day. Iced hibiscus tea is also refreshing.

SIDE EFFECTS

Not serious:
You might notice a slightly dry sensation in the mouth because of the herb's astringent property.

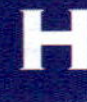

SPECIAL INFORMATION

- The tart flavor of hibiscus tea may clash with that of other strong-tasting herbs, such as chamomile or dandelion; mix with mint or rose hip tea instead.
- Because many types of hibiscus are sold, check with an herbal practitioner to determine if the species you are using is an appropriate treatment. Some species may not be recommended for pregnant women.

HISTAMINE H_2 BLOCKERS

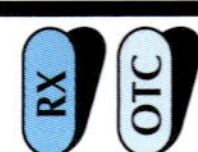

DRUG CLASS

Antiulcer Drugs

GENERIC NAMES

Rx: cimetidine, famotidine, nizatidine, ranitidine

OTC: cimetidine, famotidine, ranitidine

A subclass of antiulcer drugs, histamine H_2 blockers help reduce the secretion of certain digestive juices in the stomach. For more information, including facts about side effects and possible interactions with other medications, see ***Antiulcer Drugs***. For information about specific histamine H_2 blockers, see ***Cimetidine, Famotidine, Nizatidine,*** and ***Ranitidine.***

HONEYSUCKLE FLOWER

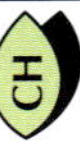

LATIN NAME

Lonicera japonica

GENERAL DESCRIPTION

This ornamental flower is prescribed for sores, swellings, fevers, colds, and flu. Chinese medicine practitioners use it as an antibiotic. In addition the flower is believed to have some value in the treatment of chronic conjunctivitis and other eye conditions. The best variety of the plant has several large, pale-yellow, unopened flowers. Considered a sweet, cold herb in traditional Chinese medicine, it grows throughout China and is harvested in May and June.

TARGET AILMENTS

Take honeysuckle flower internally for:

- sores and inflammations, particularly of the breast, throat, and eyes; heat rash; and boils.
- fevers, colds, flu; salmonella and other microbial infections.
- intestinal abscesses.
- painful urination and dysentery.

PREPARATIONS

You can find honeysuckle flowers in bulk at Asian markets and pharmacies and Western health food stores. The herb is also available in tablet form.

Combinations: The flowers, together with platycodon and great burdock fruit, form a mixture used to treat pain and swelling in the throat. A preparation with skullcap and coptis is prescribed for high fever. When skullcap alone is added to honeysuckle flowers, the blend is employed to discharge pus from boils. For advice on other combinations and dosages, consult a Chinese medicine practitioner.

SIDE EFFECTS

None expected.

SPECIAL INFORMATION

- Chinese medicine practitioners advise against using honeysuckle flower to treat sores exuding clear fluid; it should be used only in cases where there is a thick, yellow discharge. And they do not prescribe this herb for the type of diarrhea associated with stomach rather than intestinal problems.
- Test-tube studies indicate a possible antibiotic effect.
- In a laboratory test, honeysuckle flower seemed to lower the cholesterol levels in rats.
- Practitioners have found the stem of the honeysuckle, when prepared in a soup, also useful in clearing up abscesses and sores.

HOPS

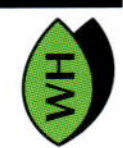

LATIN NAME

Humulus lupulus

GENERAL DESCRIPTION

A flavoring and preservative in beer since the ninth century, hops has a longer history as an herbal remedy. The plant is a perennial vine that grows to 20 feet; the medicinal part is found in tiny glandular hairs on the scaly, cone-shaped fruit. Chinese and European healers have valued the herb's sedative action and its ability to relieve muscle cramps. Today hops is still prescribed primarily as a sedative; the active ingredient is lupulinic acid, which depresses the central nervous system and induces sleep. Because of its bitterness, which stimulates gastric juices and decreases gas, hops is also prescribed as a digestive aid. And along with other ingredients in the hops fruit, zinc has astringent or binding effects on the body.

TARGET AILMENTS

Take internally for:

- insomnia, anxiety, tension headache; indigestion, depressed appetite.

Apply externally for:

- neuralgia, tension headache.

PREPARATIONS

Over the counter:
Available in commercial herbal remedies, as dried or fresh herbs, and in the form of capsules, powder, and tincture.

At home:
Tea: Use 2 tsp dried herb per cup of boiling water; steep 15 minutes. For insomnia, drink 1 cup at night; if a single dose doesn't bring sleep, or for general anxiety, take up to 3 cups a day. To soothe an acid stomach and aid digestion, drink the tea cold an hour before mealtimes or after a meal.

Poultice: Pour boiling water over 1 to 2 cups dried herbs to moisten, steep five minutes, and wrap in a cloth. Apply warm to the affected area for facial pain, neuralgia, or tension headache.

Hops pillow: Place freshly dried herbs in a pillowcase; dampen case with water to keep herbs from rustling.

Combinations: Used with valerian for stress, tension headache, or panic attacks. Used with passionflower or valerian for insomnia.

SIDE EFFECTS

Not serious:
Upset stomach, constipation, diarrhea, a skin rash, or irritation to the eyes from the spines of the fruits. Stop taking and call your doctor.

Serious:
Hops can cause sleepiness or worsen severe depression. Seek professional help.

SPECIAL INFORMATION

- For prolonged or daytime use, take hops under medical supervision.
- Do not take during the day if you operate heavy machinery or drive.
- Pregnant women and women with estrogen-dependent breast cancer should avoid hops; it may contain an estrogen-like chemical and has been known to induce menstruation.
- Use low-strength doses for adults over 65 years or children between 2 and 12 years old. Do not give to children under 2 years of age.

POSSIBLE INTERACTIONS

- Avoid overmedicating; use caution when taking hops with prescription sedatives or antianxiety medications.

HORSETAIL

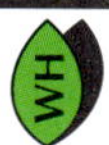

LATIN NAME
Equisetum arvense

GENERAL DESCRIPTION
Horsetail has been valued since ancient times for its ability to stem the flow of blood, bind tissues, and increase urine production. It is rich in silica, which helps mend broken bones and form collagen, an important constituent of bones and tissue. Herbalists today prescribe horsetail for urinary problems, wounds, benign prostate disorders, and the pain of rheumatism or arthritis. More closely related to ferns than to flowering plants, horsetail is a perennial with hollow stems and shoots that resemble asparagus. All the aboveground parts of the plant are used for medicinal purposes.

TARGET AILMENTS
Take internally for:
- bladder infections, cystitis, urethritis, prostatitis, kidney stones, stomach ulcers; broken bones or sprained tendons; strengthening nails, skin, and hair; pain of rheumatism or arthritis.

Apply externally for:
- sores, wounds, inflammations.

PREPARATIONS

Over the counter:
Available as dried or fresh herb, capsules, and tincture.

At home:
Tea: Steep 2 tsp dried herb or 1 tbsp fresh herb per cup of boiling water for 15 minutes. For bladder or kidney disorders, drink cold, up to four cups a day. To prevent kidney irritation, take two tablespoons at a time. Apply tea externally to wounds, sores, or mouth irritations.

Sitz bath: Simmer 3 to 4 oz of herb in 2 qt water for 5 minutes; steep 30 minutes and add to bathwater.

Combinations: Used with hydrangea for prostate problems.

SIDE EFFECTS

Not serious:
Upset stomach, diarrhea, increased urination. Discontinue and call your doctor.

Serious:
Pain in the kidneys or lower back, or upon urination, with nausea or vomiting may indicate kidney damage. Cardiac problems, including heart palpitations, may occur in cases of extreme overuse. Call your doctor immediately.

SPECIAL INFORMATION

- WARNING: Do not take internally for more than three consecutive days and do not exceed the recommended dosage; extended use may cause kidney or cardiac damage.
- Use only under a doctor's care. People with cardiac disease or high blood pressure should use horsetail with caution.
- Pregnant women should avoid horsetail. The herb's high selenium content can cause birth defects.
- The silica in horsetail, which aids in building cartilage, may help menopausal women offset the bone loss of osteoporosis, although this use has not been clinically tested in humans.
- Use low-strength doses for adults over 65 and children between 2 and 12 years old. Do not give horsetail to children under 2. Do not let children put the hollow stalks in their mouths; ingesting the juice can make your child ill.

HYDROCHLOROTHIAZIDE

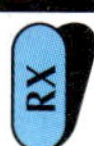

DRUG CLASS
Diuretics

BRAND NAMES
Dyazide, Maxzide-25

GENERAL DESCRIPTION
Introduced in 1959, hydrochlorothiazide is a nonpotassium-sparing diuretic used to treat high blood pressure (hypertension), diabetes insipidus (extreme thirst and excessive production of urine), and excess fluid retention.

This drug acts by promoting urine production. But increasing the flow of urine also has the effect of increasing the loss of potassium and other minerals from the body. This effect is particularly pronounced with hydrochlorothiazide. To prevent potassium loss, the drug is frequently combined with the potassium-sparing diuretic triamterene. (Unlike other diuretics, hydrochlorothiazide appears to decrease the body's loss of calcium.)

See ***Diuretics*** for information about other side effects and possible drug interactions. See ***Triamterene*** for information on a potassium-sparing diuretic often combined with this drug.

SPECIAL INFORMATION

- Because excess sodium loss appears more likely with hydrochlorothiazide than with some other diuretics, a higher risk of cardiovascular side effects is associated with this drug.
- Tell your doctor if you have gout; hydrochlorothiazide affects uric acid levels.
- Tell your doctor if you are allergic to sulfa drugs, such as sulfonamide antibiotics or sulfonylurea antidiabetics; hydrochlorothiazide is chemically related to these medications and may trigger similar reactions.

HYDROCODONE

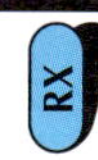

DRUG CLASS
Analgesics [Opioid Analgesics]

BRAND NAMES
Lorcet Plus, Lortab, Vicodin, Vicoprofen

GENERAL DESCRIPTION
Like other opioid analgesics, hydrocodone is often combined with aceta-

minophen for mild-to-moderate pain relief and cough suppression. A narcotic, hydrocodone may cause drowsiness and can be habit-forming. For information about side effects and possible drug interactions, see ***Opioid Analgesics.***

HYDROCORTISONE

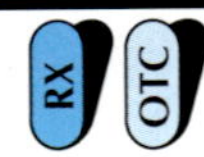

DRUG CLASS
Corticosteroids

BRAND NAMES
Rx: Hytone

OTC: Cortaid, Cortizone

GENERAL DESCRIPTION
Hydrocortisone cream is used for temporary relief of minor skin problems, including inflammation and rashes caused by eczema, poison ivy, poison oak, poison sumac, insect bites, psoriasis, soaps, detergents, cosmetics, and jewelry. The drug treats only the symptoms, not the underlying causes. See ***Corticosteroids*** for more information.

SPECIAL INFORMATION
- Hydrocortisone should not be used for rosacea, acne, viral skin infections such as herpes, or fungal infections such as athlete's foot.
- Do not use this medication near your eyes; with prolonged use, doing so can cause a number of problems, including glaucoma or cataracts.
- If you have diabetes, check with your doctor before using hydrocortisone.
- These creams may sting slightly when first applied.
- Do not use excessive quantities of this medication or bind dressings tightly over the treated area.

POSSIBLE INTERACTIONS
None expected.

HYDROXYZINE

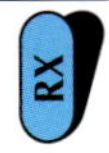

DRUG CLASS
Anti-Itch Drugs

BRAND NAME
Atarax

GENERAL DESCRIPTION
Introduced in 1953, hydroxyzine is an antihistamine that appears to depress the central nervous system. It also has antipruritic, or anti-itch, properties. This medication is used to treat tension, restlessness, and some types of anxiety, and to relieve itching due to allergic reactions. Hydroxyzine has also been prescribed for the treatment of motion sickness, as a sedative, and as an antinausea medication.

TARGET AILMENTS
- tension, restlessness, and some types of anxiety.
- itching due to allergic reactions.

SIDE EFFECTS
Not serious:
Primary side effects are dry mouth, drowsiness, and difficulty in urinating; these effects usually disappear after a few days or when dosage is reduced. Headaches, although rare, may also develop. Notify your doctor if these symptoms persist or become bothersome.

Serious:
Wheezing, chest tightness, and difficulty in breathing may be signs that you are having an adverse reaction to the drug. High doses of hydroxyzine may produce excessive drowsiness, unsteadiness, tremors, or convulsions. If these symptoms occur, call your doctor immediately.

SPECIAL INFORMATION
- Do not take if you have had an unusual or allergic reaction to this drug or to another antihistamine in the past.
- If you are pregnant, consult your doctor before using this medication.
- Hydroxyzine may pass into breast milk; avoid using it while nursing.
- Do not drink alcohol while using.
- To avoid stomach upset, try taking the medication with food or milk.
- To help relieve dry mouth (a common side effect), chew gum or suck on hard candy, and drink plenty of water.
- Because hydroxyzine can make you drowsy, avoid driving, operating hazardous machinery, or engaging in other potentially dangerous activities that require intense concentration.
- The body develops a tolerance to hydroxyzine after prolonged use, reducing the drug's effectiveness.
- Do not take hydroxyzine with any other prescription medication or over-the-counter drug without first consulting your doctor.

POSSIBLE INTERACTIONS
Attapulgite: a decrease in the effect of hydroxyzine.

Central nervous system depressants (such as alcohol, antidepressants, antipsychotics, hypnotics, narcotics, pain relievers, sedatives, sleep inducers, and tranquilizers): increased effects of both combined drugs.

Clozapine: may have a toxic effect on the central nervous system.

Nonprescription cold or allergy medications that contain antihistamines: increased drowsiness.

HYPERICUM

LATIN NAME
Hypericum perforatum

GENERAL DESCRIPTION
Also known as St.-John's-wort, hypericum grows in woodlands across Europe, Asia, and the United States, blooming with a profusion of yellow flowers from June to September. The flowers, if bruised, bleed a reddish juice. The dark-green leaves of the plant are dotted with oil-producing pores. According to ancient healing wisdom, because hypericum seemed to resemble skin, with its pores and its simulation of bleeding on injury, it was considered ideal for all manner of flesh wounds. *(See **St.-John's-wort.**)* In homeopathy, *Hypericum* is often prescribed for bodily injuries, among other conditions; but it is selected for the soothing effect it is said to have on injured nerves rather than for any traditional reason.

The entire plant is harvested for homeopathic use in summer, when its yellow flowers are in full bloom. It is pounded to a pulp and soaked in an alcohol solution before being weakened to the desired potencies through a vigorous dilution process.

TARGET AILMENTS
- backaches centered along the lower spine that may include shooting pains.
- bites and stings from animals and insects, especially when they have become inflamed or include nerve damage.
- cuts and wounds to nerve-rich parts of the body, like the fingers, toes, and lips, caused by accidents or surgery.
- dental pain caused by nerve inflammation.

PREPARATIONS
Hypericum is available over the counter in various strengths, in both liquid and tablet form, at selected stores and phar-

macies. Consult your practitioner for more precise information.

SIDE EFFECTS

None expected.

HYSSOP

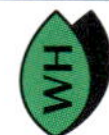

LATIN NAME
Hyssopus officinalis

GENERAL DESCRIPTION
After centuries of use in Europe, hyssop was such a popular remedy for coughs and other respiratory ills that European colonists brought it to North America. A shrub with white, pink, or blue flowers, hyssop is part of the mint family. It is used as an expectorant, digestive aid, sedative, and muscle relaxant. Volatile oils in the leaves and flowers, bitter tasting and with a strong camphorlike odor, help loosen mucus and stimulate coughing, and decrease gas. Hyssop is also used as an antiseptic; its oils may heal wounds and herpes simplex sores.

TARGET AILMENTS
Take internally for:
- coughs, common colds, bronchitis; indigestion, gas; anxiety, hysteria, petit mal (a form of epilepsy).

Apply externally for:
- cold sores, genital herpes sores, burns, wounds, skin irritations.

PREPARATIONS
Over the counter:
Available dried or fresh and as tincture.

At home:
Tea: Steep 2 tsp dried herb per cup of boiling water for 10 to 15 minutes. Drink three times a day for cough (add honey, sugar, or lemon to improve the flavor); gargle three times a day for sore throat. Apply to burns and wounds.

Compress: Steep 1 oz dried herb in 1 pt boiling water for 15 minutes; soak clean cloth in solution and apply warm to cold sores or genital herpes sores; place on the chest to relieve congestion.

Combinations: Used with white horehound and coltsfoot for coughs and bronchitis; with boneset, elder flower, and peppermint for cold symptoms; and with sage as a gargle for sore throats.

SIDE EFFECTS
Not serious:
Upset stomach or diarrhea. Discontinue use and call your doctor.

SPECIAL INFORMATION
- Use hyssop only under medical supervision if you use it for more than three consecutive days.
- Pregnant women should avoid hyssop; it was once used to induce abortion.
- Use low-strength preparations for adults over 65 or children between 2 and 12 years of age. Do not give to children under 2 years old.

IBUPROFEN

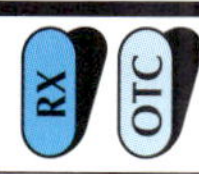

DRUG CLASS
Analgesics [Nonsteroidal Anti-Inflammatory Drugs (NSAIDs)]

BRAND NAMES
Rx: Children's Motrin Ibuprofen Suspension, various forms of Motrin for adults

OTC: Advil, Advil Cold and Sinus, Motrin IB, Nuprin

GENERAL DESCRIPTION
Introduced in 1969, ibuprofen was the first of two new arthritis and pain NSAIDs to become available for the OTC market in the 1980s and 1990s. The drug may be used to relieve the pain of headaches, menstrual cramps, muscle aches, minor aches and pains of the common cold, rheumatoid arthritis, and osteoarthritis. Ibuprofen also reduces inflammation and fever. For information about side effects and possible drug interactions, see ***Nonsteroidal Anti-Inflammatory Drugs (NSAIDs).***

SPECIAL INFORMATION
- Because ibuprofen can cause problems in the unborn child or with delivery, this drug should not be taken during the last three months of pregnancy unless directed by a physician.

IGNATIA

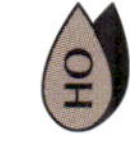

LATIN NAME
Ignatia amara

GENERAL DESCRIPTION
The beans of this plant, sometimes called St. Ignatius bean, are in fact seeds from the fruit of a small tree native to China and the Philippines. Seventeenth-century Spanish missionaries in the Philippines were introduced to the seeds by the locals, who wore them as amulets to ward off disease. Small doses of the seed can produce mild but unpleasant symptoms of poisoning, including increased salivation, pounding headache, cramps, giddiness, twitching, and trembling; large doses can be fatal. Homeopaths may prescribe *Ignatia,* a dilute solution of the seed, for ailments that include symptoms like those associated with mild poisoning.

For the homeopathic preparation, the seeds are collected and ground to a powder, then mixed with alcohol. When the powder is thoroughly saturated, the mixture is strained and diluted until it becomes a nontoxic substance.

TARGET AILMENTS
- anxiety; dry, tickling coughs; a sore throat that feels like there is a lump in it; painful tension headaches; indigestion; insomnia; irritable bowel syndrome; painful hemorrhoids; effects of grief, shock, or disappointment, or depression where the patient tends to sigh frequently. (Take internally.)

PREPARATIONS
Ignatia is available over the counter in various potencies, in both liquid and tablet form, at selected stores and pharmacies. Consult a homeopathic practitioner for more precise information.

SIDE EFFECTS

None expected.

INDAPAMIDE

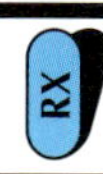

DRUG CLASS
Diuretics

BRAND NAME
Lozol

GENERAL DESCRIPTION
Indapamide is a relatively new diuretic prescribed to treat high blood pressure (hypertension) and excess fluid retention. Among the group of drugs known as nonpotassium-sparing diuretics, indapamide increases the loss of potassium and other minerals from the body as it promotes urine production. See ***Diuretics*** for more information, including other side effects and drug interactions.

H-I

SPECIAL INFORMATION
- Tell your doctor if you are allergic to sulfa drugs, such as sulfonamide antibiotics or sulfonylurea antidiabetics; indapamide is chemically related to these medications and may trigger similar reactions.

INSULIN

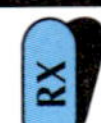

DRUG CLASS
Antidiabetic Drugs

BRAND NAMES
Humulin N, Humulin R, Humulin U, Humulin 50/50, Humulin 70/30, Iletin I NPH, Novolin 70/30

GENERAL DESCRIPTION
Insulin, a hormone naturally produced by the pancreas, helps regulate levels of glucose (blood sugar) in the body. The insulin used today in the treatment of diabetes is either manufactured semisynthetically or derived from beef or pork. The drug is injected directly beneath the skin of insulin-dependent (Type 1) diabetics, whose bodies are unable to produce the hormone on their own. Insulin is also used to treat some non-insulin-dependent (Type 2) diabetics experiencing a severe blood sugar imbalance. Such an imbalance can lead to ketoacidosis—in which a buildup of ketones (by-products of metabolism) causes the blood to become increasingly acidic—and possibly to a life-threatening diabetic coma.

TARGET AILMENTS
- insulin-dependent (Type 1) diabetes.
- non-insulin-dependent (Type 2) diabetes that is not properly controlled by diet, exercise, and weight reduction.
- severe blood sugar imbalances occurring in nondiabetics as a result of pregnancy, surgery, acute stress, or shock.

SIDE EFFECTS

Not serious:
Allergic reactions; a breakdown of fatty tissue at the site of the injection, which may cause a depression in the skin; an accumulation of fat under the skin as a result of an overdependence on the same site for injection.

Serious:
Diabetic coma or hyperglycemia (high blood sugar) from underdosing; hypoglycemia (low blood sugar) from overdosing. Call your doctor immediately if you experience intense itching (sometimes with hives or rash) or if you feel faint after a dose. See overdose and underdose symptoms below.

SPECIAL INFORMATION
- An overdose of insulin can result in low blood sugar (hypoglycemia). Symptoms include excessive hunger, cold sweats, shakiness, nervousness or anxiety, rapid pulse, headache, drowsiness, confusion, nausea, cool or pale skin. Keep hard candy or fruit juice handy to counteract hypoglycemia.
- An underdose of insulin can result in high blood sugar (hyperglycemia). Symptoms include drowsiness, dry mouth, fruity breath, increased frequency of urination, loss of appetite, stomach pain, nausea or vomiting, unusual thirst, trouble breathing, tiredness, flushed or dry skin. Hyperglycemia can lead to ketoacidosis or a life-threatening diabetic coma. Take a dose of insulin as soon as you realize you have missed one, or as soon as you begin to experience symptoms. Make advance preparations for a friend, colleague, or family member to administer the dose if you are unable.
- Insulin is considered safe for pregnant and nursing women, since the drug does not pass into breast milk.
- Strict adherence to a prescribed regimen of diet and exercise is essential to controlling the disease.
- Illness and exercise can alter your insulin requirements.
- Blood and urine should be monitored regularly for sugar and ketone levels. Do not change the brand or type of insulin you use or stop taking the drug without consulting your doctor.
- Be prepared for a diabetic emergency. Read about first aid for diabetics *(page 318)* and discuss a plan of action with your doctor, family members, friends, and co-workers.
- Smoking affects insulin requirements. If you stop smoking cigarettes or begin wearing a nicotine patch while taking insulin, your blood sugar level may change. You may need to adjust your dosage.
- Semisynthetic insulin is often prescribed for patients who are pregnant, allergic to other types of insulin, need the drug for only a short period (such as during surgery), or are newly diagnosed with diabetes. This type causes fewer allergic reactions than insulin derived from animals.

POSSIBLE INTERACTIONS
Insulin can interact with a number of other drugs. Check with your doctor or pharmacist before taking any other medications and be sure to read all labels for sugar content.

Alcohol, anabolic steroids, clofibrate, fenfluramine, guanethidine, MAO inhibitors, nonsteroidal anti-inflammatory drugs (NSAIDs), phenylbutazone, salicylates, sulfinpyrazone, tetracycline: these drugs decrease blood sugar levels and may affect insulin dosages.

Amphetamines, baclofen, corticosteroids, corticotropin (ACTH), danazol, dextrothyroxine, epinephrine, estrogens, ethacrynic acid, furosemide, glucagon, molindone, phenytoin, thiazide diuretics, thyroid hormones, and triamterene: may raise blood sugar levels, increasing the risk of hyperglycemia.

Beta-adrenergic blockers: may mask the symptoms of hypoglycemia when used concurrently with insulin.

IPECAC

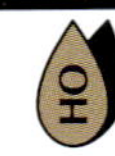

LATIN NAME
Ipecacuanha

GENERAL DESCRIPTION
The *Ipecacuanha* shrub, native to Central and South America, was named by Portuguese colonists, who called it "roadside sick-making plant" in recognition of its ability to induce vomiting. Varying doses of its root can produce a variety of symptoms that includes mild appetite stimulation, sweating, expectoration, vomiting, gastritis, inflammation of the lungs, and cardiac failure. Other health disorders can display symptoms similar to those of mild ipecac poisoning, and it is these symptoms that homeopathic practitioners hope to counteract when they prescribe ipecac.

The homeopathic remedy is made from the root, the most potent part of the plant. The root is dried and then ground into a coarse powder, which is diluted either in milk sugar as a dry substance or in a water-alcohol base. Both preparations are weakened to a nontoxic level.

For more information on homeopathic medicine, see page 1027.

TARGET AILMENTS
- persistent nausea, vomiting, motion sickness; menstrual problems; asthma; dry, irritating cough accompanied

by wheezing; diarrhea, flu with nausea, colic, gastroenteritis. (Take internally.)

PREPARATIONS
Ipecac is available over the counter in various potencies, in both liquid and tablet form, at selected stores and pharmacies. Consult your practitioner for more precise information.

SIDE EFFECTS
None expected.

IPRATROPIUM

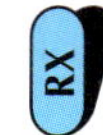

DRUG CLASS
Bronchodilators

BRAND NAME
Atrovent

GENERAL DESCRIPTION
Ipratropium is prescribed to prevent and to relieve the symptoms of chronic bronchitis and emphysema by opening up the bronchial tubes. Unlike many other bronchodilators, ipratropium is not used to treat acute bronchial asthma attacks because it is not a fast-acting medication. See ***Bronchodilators*** for information about side effects and possible drug interactions.

ISOCARBOXAZID

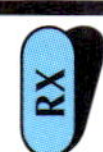

DRUG CLASS
Antidepressants [Monoamine Oxidase (MAO) Inhibitors]

BRAND NAME
Marplan

GENERAL DESCRIPTION
Isocarboxazid belongs to the subclass of antidepressants known as monoamine oxidase (MAO) inhibitors. Like other MAO inhibitors, this drug is used to treat depression when other antidepressant drugs have failed. See ***Monoamine Oxidase (MAO) Inhibitors*** for information about side effects, warnings, and possible drug interactions.

ISOSORBIDE DINITRATE

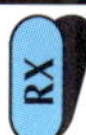

DRUG CLASS
Nitrates

BRAND NAME
Isordil

GENERAL DESCRIPTION
Like other drugs in its class, isosorbide dinitrate is used to control angina. In some cases it is also used as a complementary treatment for congestive heart failure. Isosorbide dinitrate, introduced in 1959, is available in a variety of forms; each is prescribed according to its therapeutic use. Sublingual tablets (those that are dissolved under the tongue) and chewable tablets are prescribed for immediate relief from angina, while standard and extended-use tablets are offered for long-term management of the condition. See ***Nitrates*** for information about side effects and possible drug interactions.

ISOSORBIDE MONONITRATE

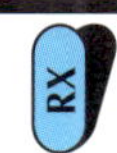

DRUG CLASS
Nitrates

BRAND NAMES
Imdur, Ismo, Monoket

GENERAL DESCRIPTION
Isosorbide mononitrate is used to prevent angina attacks. This medication relaxes smooth muscle of blood vessels, increasing the flow of blood, and oxygen, to the heart. Isosorbide mononitrate does not treat acute angina attacks. For more information, see ***Nitrates.***

SPECIAL INFORMATION

- Warning: An overdose of isosorbide mononitrate could be fatal. Contact a poison control center or seek emergency treatment if you have taken more than the prescribed amount.
- Isosorbide mononitrate must be taken on a precise, sometimes asymmetrical, schedule to avoid developing a tolerance to the drug.
- Take this drug with a half glass of liquid, with or without food.

ISRADIPINE

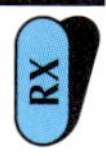

DRUG CLASS
Calcium Channel Blockers

BRAND NAME
DynaCirc

GENERAL DESCRIPTION
Like other calcium channel blockers, isradipine inhibits the passage of calcium into body cells, thus slowing the contraction of the heart and arteries, dilating the arteries, and lowering blood pressure. This drug is used primarily in the treatment of mild-to-moderate high blood pressure (hypertension), although in some cases it is prescribed to help manage angina. See ***Calcium Channel Blockers*** for information about side effects and possible drug interactions.

JUNIPER

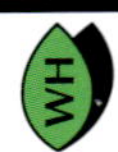

LATIN NAME
Juniperus communis

GENERAL DESCRIPTION
The berrylike juniper cone, a purple fruit, is produced by female varieties of an evergreen shrub that can grow 6 to 25 feet tall. Juniper is known for giving gin its tart bite. It also acts as a diuretic, since it includes among its components terpinen-4-ol, which increases the rate at which the kidneys filter body fluids. Because of this diuretic action, juniper is used to treat high blood pressure and premenstrual syndrome. Juniper oil is thought to have anti-inflammatory effects, considered useful for treating arthritis and gout. Juniper teas can be taken for digestive problems.

TARGET AILMENTS
Take internally for:
- bladder infections, cystitis, edema (water retention), digestive problems.
- menstrual irregularities and premenstrual syndrome.
- high blood pressure.

Apply externally for:
- arthritis.
- gout.

PREPARATIONS
Over the counter:
Available in whole berries, bulk, capsules, and tinctures.

At home:
Tea: Steep 1 tsp ground juniper berries in 1 cup boiling water for 10 to 20 minutes. Drink at least two times daily. Do not use for more than six weeks at a time.

SIDE EFFECTS

Not serious:
Individuals with hay fever may develop allergy symptoms such as nasal congestion when taking juniper. If this happens, stop taking the herb and call your doctor.

Serious:
Juniper in high doses can irritate and damage the kidneys and urinary tract. If you develop diarrhea, intestinal pain, kidney pain, blood in the urine, purplish urine, or a faster heartbeat, stop taking juniper immediately and see your doctor as soon as possible.

SPECIAL INFORMATION
- WARNING: Because it can irritate the kidneys and urinary tract, juniper is suitable for short-term use only.
- WARNING: Do not use juniper if you have a kidney infection or a history of kidney problems.
- Animal studies indicate that the herb prompts the uterus to contract, suggesting that it may also bring on menstrual periods.
- Pregnant women should not use juniper, because it may stimulate contraction of the uterus.

KALI BICHROMICUM

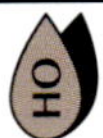

LATIN NAME
Kali bichromicum

GENERAL DESCRIPTION
Kali bichromicum is often called potassium bichromate; it is a chemical compound that may be acquired from chromium iron ore or by processing potassium chromate with one of a number of strong acids. A highly corrosive substance, it is used primarily in textile dyeing, in the staining of wood, and as a component in electric batteries. It is also a very powerful poison. Homeopathic practitioners believe *Kali bichromicum* works best for conditions that are accompanied by the symptom of pain in a distinct spot, where the ache is easily located with a fingertip.

For homeopathic use, this caustic chemical, also called *Kali bi,* is diluted to nontoxic levels with large amounts of milk sugar, a pharmaceutical process called trituration.

Like most homeopathic prescriptions, *Kali bi* was developed as a remedy by studying the reactions of healthy individuals to a series of undilute doses. The mental, emotional, and physical changes induced by *Kali bi* were then cataloged. When a homeopathic practitioner encounters a patient with a set of symptoms that matches the cataloged symptoms brought on by *Kali bi,* the practitioner then prescribes it in an extremely dilute form. It is presumed that in this highly dilute dosage, *Kali bi* can counter the symptoms that it induces when it is at full strength. For more information on homeopathic medicine, see page 1027.

TARGET AILMENTS
- acute bronchitis, colds in which there is a thick mucus discharge and a heavy cough that produces pain in the chest, croup, sinusitis and resulting headaches, indigestion, pains in the joints.

PREPARATIONS
Kali bichromicum is available over the counter in various potencies, in both liquid and tablet form, at selected stores and pharmacies. Consult your practitioner for more precise information.

SIDE EFFECTS
None expected.

KAVA

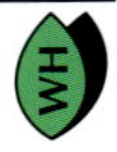

LATIN NAME
Piper methysticum

GENERAL DESCRIPTION
Drinking kava, a beverage brewed from the dried roots and rhizomes of an indigenous pepper plant, has been a feature of some South Pacific religious rituals for many centuries. Today kava is frequently prescribed, for that same euphoric effect, as an antidepressant; practitioners find it useful for treating anxiety and tension. Because of its diuretic action, it is also used to treat gout and rheumatism. In addition kava is believed to act as an antiseptic and anti-inflammatory agent in the urinary tract, making it suitable for treating urinary tract infections such as cystitis; it is also used for prostatitis (inflammation of the prostate gland) that may arise from bacteria traveling from the urethra.

Western herbalists recommend kava for its sedative properties, which do not seem to impair the user's mental alertness. The active ingredients, called kavalactones, act on the stem and other parts of the brain to yield kava's mild tranquilizing effect. While kava compounds do not seem to be addictive in the same way as alcohol or pharmaceutical drugs, the herb still must be used with caution.

TARGET AILMENTS
Take internally for:
- urinary disorders, prostate inflammations.
- gout, rheumatism.
- insomnia, depression, anxiety, muscle spasms.

PREPARATIONS
Available in dry bulk, capsules, and tinctures.

SIDE EFFECTS

Not serious:
Chronic use can cause a type of dermatitis that will clear up when you stop taking kava.

Serious:
Like most sedative substances, too much kava can cause intoxication or drowsiness. If this happens, lower your dosage or stop taking kava.

SPECIAL INFORMATION
- WARNING: Long-term, constant, large-dose use of kava has been associated with damage to the liver, skin, eyes, and even the spinal cord.
- Do not take this herb with alcohol or if you are also taking any antidepressant or anti-psychotic medicine. Kava can dangerously enhance the effects of those medications.
- Do not use kava if you are pregnant or breast-feeding.

KELP

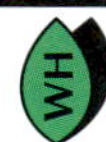

LATIN NAME
Fucus spp.

GENERAL DESCRIPTION
Extracts of iodine-rich kelp, one of many forms of seaweed, provided an effective goiter remedy for many years. Today some herbalists rely on another component of kelp's stemlike and leaflike parts, an agent known as sodium alginate. Because of its action, kelp is prescribed to aid in the treatment of heavy-metal environmental pollutants including barium and cadmium, and to prevent the body from absorbing strontium 90, a radioactive substance created in nuclear power plants.

Some practitioners of alternative medicine also recommend taking kelp supplements for thyroid disorders such as mild hypothyroidism (underactive thyroid).

TARGET AILMENTS
Take internally for:
- goiter, hypothyroidism, radiation exposure, heavy-metal environmental pollutants.

PREPARATIONS
Over the counter:
Available in dry bulk, capsules, and tinctures.

At home:
Infusion: Steep 2 to 3 tsp dried or powdered kelp in 1 cup boiling water for 10 minutes; drink three times daily.

SIDE EFFECTS
None expected.

SPECIAL INFORMATION
- WARNING: If you are already taking medication for hyperthyroidism (overactive thyroid), kelp supplements could worsen the condition.
- WARNING: Do not gather your own wild kelp for use; coastal colonies may be contaminated by offshore pollutants.
- WARNING: Check with your practitioner before using kelp if you have a history of thyroid problems or high blood pressure.

KETOCONAZOLE

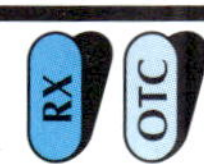

DRUG CLASS
Antifungal Drugs

BRAND NAMES
Rx: Nizoral

OTC: Nizoral AD

GENERAL DESCRIPTION
Ketoconazole, introduced in 1981, is a powerful antifungal medication that is used to treat a wide variety of skin, lung, and systemic fungal infections, including yeast infections (candidiasis) and ringworm (tinea). The drug works by preventing the growth and reproduction of fungal cells; in high concentrations, ketoconazole actually destroys fungal cells. This medication is available in cream, shampoo, oral suspension, or tablet form.

Ketoconazole is also an antiadrenal drug. Because it suppresses the excess production of adrenal corticosteroid hormones and testosterone, ketoconazole is occasionally used in the treatment of prostate cancer and Cushing's syndrome, in which the body produces excessive amounts of corticosteroid hormones. For more information, see ***Antifungal Drugs.***

TARGET AILMENTS
- fungal diseases of the lungs, including blastomycosis, coccidioidomycosis, histoplasmosis, and paracoccidioidomycosis.
- yeast infections (candidiasis) of the mouth, skin, and internal organs, such as thrush, peritonitis, pneumonia, and urinary tract infection.
- chromomycosis (a chronic, usually tropical skin infection).
- ringworm (tinea) of the body, skin, groin (jock itch), and feet (athlete's foot).
- seborrheic dermatitis; dandruff.
- Cushing's syndrome and prostate cancer (occasionally).

SIDE EFFECTS
Not serious:
Dizziness, drowsiness, headache, abdominal pain, diarrhea, mild nausea or vomiting, skin irritation (itching, stinging, increased risk of sunburn). Call your doctor if these symptoms persist or become bothersome.

Serious:
Signs of liver disease, including nausea, loss of appetite, dark urine, light-colored stools, jaundice (yellow eyes and skin); depression. Call your doctor if you experience any of these symptoms.

SPECIAL INFORMATION
- Do not take this drug if you have an active liver disease.
- Weigh the risks and benefits of this drug with your doctor if you have hypochlorhydria, a history of alcoholism, impaired liver function, or liver disease.
- Tell your doctor if you are allergic to other antifungal drugs or are taking any other medications.
- In some cases, this drug can be severely toxic to the liver; your doctor may want to perform periodic liver function tests.
- While you are taking this medicine, your skin may burn more readily when exposed to sunlight. To protect your skin, wear sunblock and avoid prolonged exposure to the sun and sunlamps.
- Avoid taking this drug if you are pregnant or nursing.
- High doses of this drug can suppress corticosteroid secretion in your body, reduce testosterone levels, decrease male libido, and cause breast enlargement or impotence in men, and menstrual irregularities in women.
- Take ketoconazole with food to increase absorption of the drug into the body and lessen stomach irritation.
- Some infections require that ketoconazole be taken for many months. If you are undergoing long-term treatment with this drug, be sure to contact your doctor for periodic evaluations and monitoring. Do not stop taking ketoconazole without consulting your doctor.

POSSIBLE INTERACTIONS
Alcohol and hepatoxic (liver) medications: increased risk of stomach ulceration and liver damage.

Antacids, histamine H_2 blockers, and other medications that reduce stomach acid: these medicines may counteract the effects of antifungal drugs by preventing their full absorption into the body.

Anticholinergics and omeprazole: may decrease the effectiveness of antifungal drugs.

Cyclosporine: ketoconazole may increase the absorption of cyclosporine to potentially toxic levels.

Didanosine: both ketoconazole and didanosine, when taken together, may be absorbed into the body less efficiently. Take these medications two hours apart.

Oral corticosteroids: ketoconazole may increase the blood levels of these drugs, which may lead to potentially fatal heart arrhythmias.

Phenytoin: blood levels of phenytoin may rise and those of the antifungal drug may decrease when these two medications are taken together.

Rifampin, isoniazid: may decrease blood levels, and thus the effectiveness, of ketoconazole.

Sucralfate: decreased absorption of ketoconazole. Take sucralfate two hours after ketoconazole.

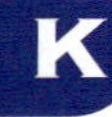

Theophylline: blood levels of this drug (which is used to treat asthma) may decrease when taken with antifungal drugs, possibly precipitating an asthma attack.

Warfarin: the anticoagulant effects of warfarin may increase when taken with an antifungal drug.

KETOROLAC

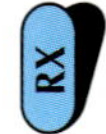

DRUG CLASS
Analgesics [Nonsteroidal Anti-Inflammatory Drugs (NSAIDs)]

BRAND NAME
Toradol

GENERAL DESCRIPTION
A new, nonnarcotic NSAID, ketorolac may be prescribed for short-term pain management, without the side effects of sedation or addiction. It is often used to relieve eye inflammation due to trauma and irritation. Unlike many other NSAIDs, ketorolac is not routinely used for treatment of arthritis. For information about side effects and possible drug interactions, see ***Nonsteroidal Anti-Inflammatory Drugs (NSAIDs).***

SPECIAL INFORMATION
- If NSAIDs upset your stomach, take them with food or milk.
- Do not use NSAIDs if you are allergic to them or to aspirin. NSAIDs may cause bronchoconstriction or anaphylaxis in aspirin-sensitive asthmatics.
- Avoid these drugs or consult your doctor before using them if you have asthma, peptic ulcer, enteritis, high blood pressure, bleeding problems, epilepsy, Parkinson's disease, or impaired liver or kidney function.
- Do not take more than the recommended dose and always seek emergency help in case of overdose. Possible symptoms include drowsiness, increased sweating, rapid heartbeat, abdominal pain, vomiting, nausea, gastrointestinal bleeding, and disorientation.
- NSAIDs are not recommended for pregnant women, especially during the last trimester, or for nursing mothers.

KOLA

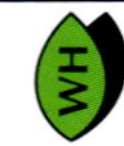

LATIN NAME
Cola vera (or *Cola nitada*)

GENERAL DESCRIPTION
The seed of the 40-foot kola tree, source of the world's most popular soft drink flavoring, is a stimulant that herbalists prescribe for overall mental fatigue or depression. It is in addition used to treat diarrhea caused by nervousness; headaches; motion sickness; and loss of appetite. Medical evidence suggests that the herb also may open the bronchial passages, helping asthmatics to breathe more easily. The effective ingredient in kola is caffeine; kola nuts contain more in proportion than coffee beans, although cola beverages generally contain considerably less caffeine than coffee.

Kola has a long history of medicinal use in West Africa. Brought to the Americas by slaves, it earned a reputation among 19th-century practitioners as a treatment for depression, diarrhea, pneumonia, migraine headaches, morning sickness, and typhoid fever.

TARGET AILMENTS
- depression, migraine headaches, poor appetite, diarrhea caused by nervousness, motion sickness, fluid retention, respiratory problems such as asthma. (Take internally.)

PREPARATIONS
Over the counter:
Available in dry bulk, capsules, and tinctures.

At home:
Soft drinks containing kola (or cola) syrups are probably the easiest way to use the herb medicinally, especially for children.

Decoction: Boil and simmer ½ tsp powdered seeds in 1 cup water for 10 minutes, and drink three times daily.

Combinations: For depression use kola mixed with any or all of the following: oats, damiana, and skullcap.

▼SIDE EFFECTS
Not serious:
Kola may be too strong a stimulant for individuals who are sensitive to caffeine. If you feel nervous or have trouble sleeping, decrease your dose or stop taking kola.

SPECIAL INFORMATION
- WARNING: Individuals with diabetes, insomnia, anxiety disorders, digestive disorders, chronic high blood pressure, high cholesterol, heart disease, or a history of strokes should not use kola.
- WARNING: Pregnant women should check with a practitioner before using kola, since it contains caffeine.

LACHESIS

LATIN NAME
Lachesis

GENERAL DESCRIPTION
The South American bushmaster snake grows to a length of seven feet and kills its prey, both animal and human, by constriction or by injection of its highly poisonous venom, known as lachesis, from which this homeopathic remedy is derived. Small doses of the venom can destroy red blood cells and impair the clotting of blood. Larger amounts of lachesis poison the heart. Homeopathic practitioners believe that the conditions best treated with *Lachesis* are those with symptoms similar to the ones induced by the venom. To prepare the homeopathic remedy, venom is extracted from the snake and diluted in large quantities of lactose (milk sugar).

Like most homeopathic prescriptions, *Lachesis* was developed as a remedy by observation of the reactions of healthy individuals to a series of undilute doses. The mental, emotional, and physical changes induced by *Lachesis* were then cataloged. When a homeopathic practitioner encounters a patient with a set of symptoms that matches the cataloged symptoms brought on by *Lachesis,* the practitioner then prescribes it in an extremely dilute form. It is presumed that in this highly dilute dosage, *Lachesis* can counter the symptoms that it induces when it is at full strength. For more information on homeopathic medicine, see page 1027.

TARGET AILMENTS
- choking coughs, croup, a constricted feeling in the throat, earaches that are worse during swallowing, left-sided sore throats, indigestion, throbbing headaches, especially those that appear during menopause, insomnia, hot flashes, heart arrhythmias, hemorrhoids, sciatica. (Take internally.)

PREPARATIONS
Lachesis is available over the counter in various potencies, in both liquid and tablet form, at selected stores and pharmacies. Consult your practitioner for more precise information.

SIDE EFFECTS
None expected.

LAVENDER

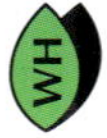

LATIN NAME
Lavandula officinalis

GENERAL DESCRIPTION
A fragrant herb that scents clothes and helps to drive away moths, lavender also has medicinal properties. Herbalists prescribe lavender tea and the essential oil of lavender, both made from the plant's blue-violet flowers, to treat common minor ailments such as insomnia, headaches, nausea, and flatulence. Years of anecdotal evidence suggest that lavender has a calming and soothing effect that relieves anxiety and promotes gastrointestinal relaxation. Its aroma is thought to stimulate mental processes and help alleviate depression, especially when it is used with other herbs. Like many aromatic essential oils, lavender oil has antiseptic qualities that may kill several types of disease-causing bacteria, and herbalists use it to treat skin ailments such as fungus, burns, wounds, eczema, and acne.

TARGET AILMENTS
Take internally for:
- insomnia, depression, or headache, especially when caused by stress.
- poor digestion, nausea, flatulence, colic.

Apply externally for:
- burns, wounds, eczema, acne, fungal infections such as candidiasis or ringworm.
- rheumatism.

PREPARATIONS
Over the counter:
Available in dried bulk, capsules, oils, and tinctures.

At home:
Tea: Steep 1 tsp dried flowers in 1 cup boiling water for 10 minutes; drink three times daily.

Oil: To relax, use a few drops of the essential oil in a bath; rub the oil on your skin to mitigate rheumatic pains, or use a few drops in a steam inhalation for coughs, colds, and flu.

Combinations: For depression, lavender can be used with rosemary, skullcap, or kola.

SPECIAL INFORMATION
- WARNING: Do not use oil of lavender internally.

LAXATIVES

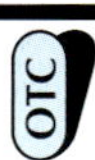

GENERIC NAMES
Bulk: calcium polycarbophil, methylcellulose, psyllium hydrophilic mucilloid

Stimulant: phenolphthalein, sennosides

Stool Softener: docusate

GENERAL DESCRIPTION
Laxatives are used for the temporary relief of occasional constipation and other bowel problems, and to prevent straining during bowel movements. The drugs can be taken orally in powder, liquid, granular, wafer, or pill form, or rectally as suppositories or enemas.

The bulk-forming types, considered the safest, work by absorbing water and expanding, thus increasing the moisture content of the stool to make passage easier. Increased bulk also encourages the bowels' motility. Stimulant laxatives are believed to promote evacuation by increasing peristalsis (waves of contractions) in the intestinal muscles. Stool softeners add to the bowels' liquid content, softening the stool. For more information, see entries for the individual generic drugs listed above.

TARGET AILMENTS
- constipation.
- diarrhea (bulk-forming types).
- irritable bowel syndrome, or spastic colon (bulk-forming types).
- straining during bowel movements following rectal surgery, heart attacks, childbirth, or when hemorrhoids are present.

SIDE EFFECTS
Not serious:
The dye in some laxatives can cause urine discoloration. In rare cases, the following additional side effects may occur: Suppositories may cause rectal irritation. Stimulant types may cause intestinal cramping, nausea, belching, or diarrhea. Stool softeners (liquid forms) may cause stomach cramps or throat irritation.

Serious:
Some laxatives can cause skin rashes. If you develop a rash, discontinue use and see your doctor. You should also call your doctor if the laxative fails to have the desired effect after one week of use, or if rectal bleeding or an infection develops from suppositories.

SPECIAL INFORMATION
- If you experience a sudden change in bowel habits that lasts longer than

two weeks, you should consult your doctor before using a laxative.

- If you are pregnant or nursing, consult your doctor before using any kind of laxative.
- Unless prescribed by your physician, laxatives should not be given to children under the age of six.
- Bulk-forming laxatives are best for geriatric patients with poorly functioning colons.
- Take bulk-forming laxatives with plenty of water or other liquid to avoid esophageal or throat obstruction.
- Laxatives can be habit-forming. Use them infrequently, at the lowest effective dosage, and for no longer than one week. Long-term use, particularly of stimulant laxatives, can cause physical dependence, resulting in loss of normal bowel function and chronic constipation.
- Do not use laxatives if you have symptoms of appendicitis, including abdominal pain, nausea, or vomiting, or if you think you may have an intestinal obstruction.
- If you have congestive heart failure or rectal bleeding of unknown cause, do not use laxatives without your doctor's consent.
- If you are diabetic, avoid sennosides and psyllium-type laxatives that contain large amounts of sugar; instead, use sugar-free types that contain the artificial sweetener aspartame.
- If you have hypertension or are on a low-sodium diet, avoid laxatives containing sodium.
- If you have difficulty swallowing—as with dysphagia—do not take bulk-forming laxatives, which can cause an esophageal obstruction.
- Chronic use of laxatives may cause excessive loss of potassium in the body.

POSSIBLE INTERACTIONS

Antacids, histamine H_2 blockers (cimetidine, famotidine, nizatidine, ranitidine), milk: if taken within an hour of some types of stimulant laxatives, these medications may cause gastric upset by dissolving the outer coating of the laxative too quickly.

Laxatives that may contain danthron, mineral oil, or phenolphthalein: increased absorption of these substances, increasing the possibility of toxic effects.

Oral anticoagulants, digitalis, salicylate, tetracycline: these drugs may be less effective when taken concurrently with bulk-forming laxatives. After taking any of these medications, wait two hours before taking a laxative.

LEDUM

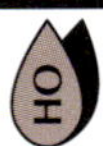

LATIN NAME
Ledum palustre

GENERAL DESCRIPTION
Ledum, sometimes called marsh tea, can be found in bogs across northern Europe, Canada, and the United States. The herb has an antiseptic smell, and its upper branches are covered with a coat of tiny brown hairs. These may have given ledum its name; in Greek, *ledos* means "woolly robe." Once used in Scandinavia for insect control, ledum has also served as a tea substitute and replaced hops in beer, although overconsumption has resulted in dizziness and a splitting headache—even before the hangover. Homeopathic practitioners consider dilute doses of *Ledum* helpful for conditions that may be accompanied by signs of infection or inflammation.

The homeopathic remedy is prepared from the whole plant, which is gathered, dried, and crushed to a powder. This is diluted to nontoxic levels in a water-alcohol mix.

Like most homeopathic prescriptions, *Ledum* was developed as a remedy by observation of the reactions of healthy individuals to a series of undilute doses. The mental, emotional, and physical changes induced by *Ledum* were then cataloged. When a homeopathic practitioner encounters a patient with a set of symptoms that matches the cataloged symptoms brought on by *Ledum,* the practitioner then prescribes it in an extremely dilute form. It is presumed that in this highly dilute dosage, *Ledum* can counter the symptoms that it induces when it is at full strength. For more information on homeopathic medicine, see page 1027.

TARGET AILMENTS
- animal bites or insect stings, bruises that have already discolored the skin, deep cuts or puncture wounds where there is danger of infection, gout, aching joints.

PREPARATIONS
Ledum is available over the counter in various potencies, in both liquid and tablet form, at selected stores and pharmacies. Consult your practitioner for more precise information.

SIDE EFFECTS
None expected.

LEMONGRASS

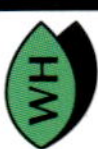

LATIN NAME
Cymbopogon citratus

GENERAL DESCRIPTION
Lemongrass, a tropical plant that can grow as high as five feet in dry soils, has uses that extend beyond its tangy role in Thai cuisine. Tea made from blades of lemongrass is a traditional Caribbean remedy for fevers, and Brazilians have a long history of using the herb for gastrointestinal and nervous disorders. Natives of the Amazon also hold that lemongrass is an effective contraceptive.

The results of a clinical study to pinpoint the herb's therapeutic properties suggest that myrcene, one of the active ingredients isolated in the essential oil of lemongrass, may serve as a site-specific painkiller, affecting particular parts of the body; herbalists differentiate this type from systemic painkillers such as aspirin. This analgesic action of myrcene may also explain the apparent sedative effect of lemongrass tea, a tart beverage long enjoyed in the Amazon region.

Some practitioners use the oil of lemongrass as a rub to treat circulatory problems and to enhance muscle tone by increasing the blood flow to the affected area.

TARGET AILMENTS
Take internally for:
- diarrhea and stomachache, headache, fever, influenza.

Apply externally for:
- athlete's foot, acne, circulatory problems.

PREPARATIONS
Over the counter:
Available in dried bulk.

At home:
Tea: Use 1 to 2 tsp fresh or dried blades in 1 cup boiling water and steep for 10 to 15 minutes; drink as often as needed until symptoms improve.

SIDE EFFECTS
None expected.

SPECIAL INFORMATION
- The oils from several closely related species of lemongrass are used to make citronella candles to repel insects.

LEVODOPA

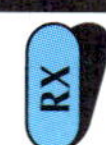

DRUG CLASS
Anti-Parkinsonism Drugs

BRAND NAME
Sinemet

GENERAL DESCRIPTION
Levodopa is used to treat the trembling, stiffness, indistinct speech, and other symptoms that characterize Parkinson's disease. In the brain, levodopa is converted into dopamine, a chemical necessary for proper transmission of the nerve impulses that control muscle movement. People with Parkinson's disease have a shortage of dopamine due to degeneration of the cells that produce the chemical.

Sinemet is a combination of levodopa and carbidopa, a chemical that prevents levodopa from breaking down in the system before reaching the brain. Carbidopa and levodopa may also be prescribed separately.

TARGET AILMENT
- Parkinson's disease.

SIDE EFFECTS

Not serious:
Headache, urine discoloration, loss of appetite, dry mouth and drooling, decreased attention span or intellectual functioning, mental confusion, insomnia, skin rash, drowsiness, fatigue. Consult your doctor if these symptoms persist or become bothersome.

Serious:
A sudden drop in blood pressure upon standing; uncontrollable movements of the hands, arms, legs, neck, face, eyelids, mouth, or tongue; double or blurred vision; marked changes in mood or mental state; irregular or rapid heartbeat; difficulty urinating; severe or persistent nausea or vomiting; weight change; bitter taste or burning sensation on tongue; stomach bleeding or ulcer. If you experience any of these symptoms, contact your doctor promptly.

SPECIAL INFORMATION
- Levodopa may interfere with normal fetal development; if you are pregnant, discuss the risk-to-benefit ratio with your doctor before using the drug. Do not take levodopa if you are nursing.
- Inform your doctor if you have a history of any of the following ailments: diabetes, epilepsy, urine retention, peptic ulcer, heart or lung disease, melanoma, glaucoma, asthma, psychosis, heart attack, kidney disease, liver disease. You should also tell your physician if you are planning surgery.
- If levodopa upsets your stomach, try taking it with food, although this will slow the drug's absorption.
- Levodopa may cause drowsiness; use caution when driving or operating machinery.
- It may take several weeks or months for the medication to reach maximum effectiveness.
- Laboratory tests that may be affected by levodopa include: complete blood cell counts, blood thyroxine levels, urine sugar or ketone tests.
- Dosages must be determined on an individual basis. Adjustments in quantity and dosing frequency are unavoidable.

POSSIBLE INTERACTIONS

Antacids, metoclopramide: increased levodopa effect.

Anticholinergics, methionine, papaverine, phenothiazines, phenytoin, pyridoxine, tricyclic antidepressants: decreased levodopa effect.

Some MAO inhibitors: may cause a severe rise in body temperature and blood pressure; these medications should be discontinued two to four weeks prior to your taking levodopa.

LEVONORGESTREL

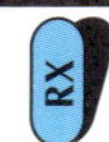

DRUG CLASS
Estrogens and Progestins

BRAND NAMES
Nordette, Tri-Levlen, Triphasil

GENERAL DESCRIPTION
Levonorgestrel is a synthetic progestin that is combined with the estrogen ethinyl estradiol for use as an oral contraceptive. It is available as tablets and as long-acting implants, which are inserted under the skin. See ***Estrogens and Progestins*** for information about side effects and possible drug interactions.

LEVOTHYROXINE

DRUG CLASS
Thyroid Hormones

BRAND NAMES
Levothyroid, Levoxine, Levoxyl, Synthroid

GENERAL DESCRIPTION
Introduced in 1953, synthetically produced levothyroxine is the drug of choice for thyroid replacement therapy because of its standard hormone content and predictable effect. Hormones produced by the thyroid gland regulate functions such as metabolism and protein synthesis, general body growth, and development of the bones and central nervous system. They also affect the heart rate. Thyroid hormone therapy usually must be maintained throughout the patient's life unless it is prescribed for a transient condition affecting thyroid function. Because these hormones are so critical to normal growth and development, children should be tested to ensure that their thyroid glands are functioning normally; those whose bodies are not producing sufficient quantities must be given supplemental thyroid hormones as soon as possible. Thyroid medications are sometimes used diagnostically to check for thyroid disease.

TARGET AILMENTS
- hypothyroidism (underactive or nonfunctioning thyroid) or as treatment following removal of thyroid gland.
- goiter (enlargement of thyroid).
- some types of thyroid cancer, for prevention and treatment, especially after radiation therapy to the neck.

SIDE EFFECTS

Not serious:
Rarely, except at beginning of treatment, changes in menstrual periods; clumsiness; coldness; constipation; dry, puffy skin; headache; sleepiness; tiredness; heart palpitations; weakness; muscle aches; weight gain. Call your doctor if these effects persist or are troublesome. (Some hair loss may occur in children during early treatment, but this condition is usually temporary.)

Serious:
Rarely, allergic reactions such as skin rash or hives, severe persistent and ongoing headache, changes in menstruation, changes in appetite, chest pain, irregular heartbeat, fever, hand tremors, irritability, leg cramps, nervousness, sensitivity to heat, sweating, weight loss. Contact your doctor, who may reduce the dosage.

SPECIAL INFORMATION

- Your doctor may tell you to continue using thyroid hormones while you're pregnant or nursing. Although small amounts of these hormones may cross the placenta or be present in breast milk, no studies have shown harm to the fetus or breast-feeding baby.
- Tell your doctor if you have cardiovascular disease, or if you have diabetes or other hormone problems, such as low pituitary gland secretions. Your doctor may decide not to use thyroid hormone or to lower the dosage.
- Absorption of levothyroxine through the digestive tract may be affected by food. Take on an empty stomach (one hour before or two hours after a meal).
- The dosage for older people and people with severe hypothyroidism or cardiovascular problems must be monitored closely. Dosages for older patients are usually lower than those prescribed for younger ones.
- In rare cases after long-term use at high dosages, levothyroxine may cause bone loss.

POSSIBLE INTERACTIONS

Anticoagulant and antiplatelet drugs (such as warfarin): increased anticlotting action. Your doctor may have to adjust the dosage of anticlotting drugs.

Antidepressants, including tricyclic antidepressants such as amitriptyline: increased action and side effects of both combined drugs, leading to heart-rhythm problems and other signs of excess stimulation.

Antidiabetic drugs (such as insulin): increased need for insulin or other diabetic drugs, perhaps leading to higher blood sugar levels. Your doctor may need to adjust your insulin dose.

Cholesterol-reducing drugs (such as cholestyramine): blocked or delayed absorption of thyroid hormones, decreasing their effectiveness. Take thyroid hormones one hour before or four to five hours after cholesterol-reducing drugs.

Heart-stimulating drugs (such as epinephrine or pseudoephedrine): increased effects of both combined drugs, potentially causing heart problems or increased chance of thyroid hormone overdose.

Other hormones (such as estrogen): may interfere with thyroid hormone action, necessitating higher doses.

LICORICE

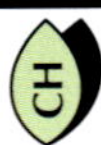

LATIN NAME

Glycyrrhiza uralensis

GENERAL DESCRIPTION

The licorice root is often used to flavor herbal formulas, but it has important medicinal properties of its own. Chinese herbalists prescribe it for several digestive and stomach problems and for coughs and colds. Licorice is also considered an anti-inflammatory medication, useful in treating skin diseases, and it is prescribed as well for ulcers. The best form of the herb is powdery, with a thin, unwrinkled, reddish brown outer skin and a white cross section. The raw form is characterized as neutral in traditional Chinese medicine; when fried in honey it is believed to be a warm herb.

TARGET AILMENTS

Take internally for:

- coughing and wheezing, asthma, sore throat.
- poor digestion, stomach and duodenal ulcers, abdominal pains and spasms.
- carbuncles and sores.

PREPARATIONS

Licorice can be purchased in bulk from Chinese pharmacies, Asian markets, and some Western health food stores, and is also available in tablet form.

Combinations: Mixed with ephedra stem and apricot seed, licorice is prescribed for coughing and wheezing. A preparation of licorice and mung bean is believed to be an antidote to aconite and several other toxins. And combined with honeysuckle flowers it is used to treat rashes or acne. For details on dosages and preparations, check with a Chinese medicine practitioner.

SIDE EFFECTS

Serious:

There is some evidence that licorice affects the body's balance between salt and potassium, retaining salt while depleting potassium. This can cause some people to retain fluid. You should probably take potassium supplements when using this herb. Consult a Chinese medicine practitioner for advice.

SPECIAL INFORMATION

- Individuals with edema (the retention of fluids in the body) and high blood pressure should avoid the herb.
- Practitioners speculate that an extract made from licorice may prevent tooth decay and gum disease.
- See also the species of licorice known as *Glycyrrhiza glabra,* regarded as a Western herb.

POSSIBLE INTERACTIONS

Euphorbia, genkwa flower, kan-sui root, sargassum seaweed, and polygala are considered incompatible with licorice.

LICORICE

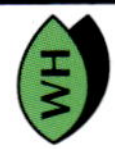

LATIN NAME

Glycyrrhiza glabra

GENERAL DESCRIPTION

Distinguished by tiny violet flowers that bloom in the summer, licorice is one of the most commonly used medicinal herbs. Its sweet taste, alleged to be 50 times sweeter than sugar, masks the bitterness in any herbal mixture. Chinese and Western herbalists use licorice root as a cough suppressant and maintain that it also soothes the mouth and throat. In addition they prescribe it for digestive disorders, believing that it acts as a mild laxative and prevents stomach ulcers by forming a protective coating on the stomach wall. Applying licorice as an external antibiotic, practitioners think it relieves skin irritations such as eczema and herpes sores.

TARGET AILMENTS

Take internally for:

- cough, sore throat, colic, constipation, heartburn, stomach ulcers, arthritis, hepatitis, cirrhosis.

Apply externally for:

- skin infections, eczema, herpes sores.

PREPARATIONS

Over the counter:

Licorice is available as dried root, liquid extract, and capsules.

At home:

Tea: Prepare by boiling 1 oz licorice root in 1 cup water for 15 to 20 minutes. Drink up to 2 cups daily.

Antibiotic: Sprinkle licorice powder directly on the infection or sore.

SIDE EFFECTS

Not serious:

You may experience upset stomach, diarrhea, headache, facial puffiness, ankle swelling, edema (fluid retention), grogginess, weakness.

SPECIAL INFORMATION
- WARNING: While licorice is safe in moderate, short-term doses, taken in large amounts over a long period it can affect the body's electrolyte balance, retaining sodium but depleting the body of potassium. This in turn can lead to high blood pressure and edema. Consult your practitioner for advice.
- Do not use licorice root if you have edema, high blood pressure, kidney disease, or glaucoma.
- Avoid the herb if you are pregnant. It causes increased production of aldosterone, a hormone that regulates the salt and water balance of the body, resulting in a rise of blood pressure.

LISINOPRIL

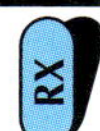

DRUG CLASS
Angiotensin-Converting Enzyme (ACE) Inhibitors

BRAND NAMES
Prinivil, Zestril

GENERAL DESCRIPTION
Introduced in 1988, the ACE inhibitor lisinopril relaxes arterial walls, thereby lowering blood pressure. It is used in the management of hypertension (mild-to-severe high blood pressure) and congestive heart failure. For increased blood-pressure-lowering action, lisinopril is sometimes combined with hydrochlorothiazide. See ***Angiotensin-Converting Enzyme (ACE) Inhibitors*** for information on side effects and possible drug interactions.

LIVE YEAST-CELL DERIVATIVE

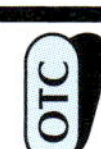

DRUG CLASS
Antihemorrhoid Drugs

BRAND NAME
Preparation H

GENERAL DESCRIPTION
Used in preparations for hemorrhoids, live yeast-cell derivative is tentatively classified as a wound healer. Though its safety and efficacy are only conditionally accepted by the FDA, live yeast-cell derivative is included in some hemorrhoid preparations because of two claims. The ingredient is purported to speed the healing of injured skin by stimulating the skin's intake of oxygen. Live yeast-cell derivative also may help in the building of connective tissue, one of the steps in wound healing.

TARGET AILMENTS
- burning and itching of the anorectal surface due to hemorrhoids.

SPECIAL INFORMATION
- In case of rectal bleeding or persistent itching, see your physician.

LOBELIA

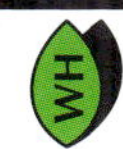

LATIN NAME
Lobelia inflata

GENERAL DESCRIPTION
Lobelia, sometimes called Indian tobacco, is prescribed for both respiratory ailments and external conditions, but it can be extremely toxic. Herbalists use the whole hairy plant, which grows up to three feet high and contains a milky sap; the seeds, however, are the most potent part. Two of lobelia's active ingredients, lobeline and isolobelanine, may give the plant the ability to act as a relaxant for the entire body even while it stimulates the respiratory system. Lobeline mildly mimics the effect of nicotine; this has prompted people who are trying to quit smoking to use it as a temporary substitute.

Because it is thought to relax overworked bronchial muscles and promote coughing, which helps to clear mucus from the lungs, lobelia is most widely used to treat respiratory illnesses such as asthma, bronchitis, pneumonia, and whooping cough. Lobelia compresses have also been used to treat skin injuries, fungus infections, and muscle sprains.

TARGET AILMENTS
Take internally for:
- pneumonia, asthma, bronchitis, smoking.

Apply externally for:
- bruises, insect bites, poison ivy, fungus infections including ringworm, sprains.

PREPARATIONS
Over the counter:
Available in dried bulk, capsules, and tinctures.

At home:
Tea: Steep ¼ to ½ tsp dried leaves in 1 cup boiling water for 10 to 15 minutes; drink three times daily.

Compress: Soak a piece of fabric in a lobelia infusion for several minutes; wring out and apply to affected area.

Combinations: For asthma, use with cayenne, skunk cabbage, and ginger.

▼SIDE EFFECTS
Serious:
WARNING: Symptoms of toxic doses of lobelia include vomiting, nausea, excessive salivation, diarrhea, hearing and vision problems, weakness, and mental confusion. If not treated promptly, acute cases of poisoning can bring on respiratory failure and even death. If you develop any side effects, call your doctor immediately.

SPECIAL INFORMATION
- WARNING: Use lobelia only in doses prescribed by your practitioner.
- If your practitioner prescribes lobelia for your child, monitor the child frequently for the development of any side effects.
- Do not use this herb if you are pregnant.

LOPERAMIDE

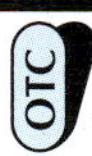

DRUG CLASS
Antidiarrheal Drugs

BRAND NAME
Imodium A-D

GENERAL DESCRIPTION
Introduced in 1977, loperamide is used primarily for symptomatic control of diarrhea and cramping. It should be taken on an empty stomach. See ***Antidiarrheal Drugs*** for more information and possible interactions.

SPECIAL INFORMATION
Do not use loperamide if:
- diarrhea is accompanied by high fever (101°F or higher).
- blood or mucus is present in stool.
- you have a rash or other allergic reaction to the drug.
- you are taking antibiotics or have a history of liver disease or colitis.
- you are pregnant or nursing a baby. Consult a doctor before using the drug.

LORACARBEF

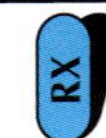

DRUG CLASS
Antibiotics [Carbacephems]

BRAND NAME
Lorabid

GENERAL DESCRIPTION
Loracarbef, introduced in 1992, is the first of the carbacephem antibiotics, a subclass of drugs that work in much the same way as penicillins and cephalosporins do to kill growing bacteria.

TARGET AILMENTS
- bacterial infections, such as bronchitis, otitis media, strep throat, some pneumonias, sinusitis, infections of the skin and soft tissue, and urinary tract infections.

SIDE EFFECTS

Not serious:
Nausea, abdominal pain, mild diarrhea, loss of appetite. Consult your doctor if these symptoms continue for more than two days or are bothersome.

Serious:
Severe itching, rash, or difficulty breathing (possibly indicating an anaphylactic reaction); severe diarrhea, severe abdominal pain, or stomach cramps. Call your doctor immediately; you may need to alter your current prescription or switch to a different medicine.

Other possible side effects that can become serious if they continue or are severe: dizziness, headache, drowsiness, insomnia, nervousness, and vaginal itching and discharge. Consult your doctor.

SPECIAL INFORMATION
- Tell your doctor if you are allergic to penicillins or cephalosporins; if so, you are likely to be allergic to loracarbef as well. Allergic reactions to these drugs can be life-threatening.
- Tell your doctor if your kidneys are impaired; you may require a smaller dose of loracarbef or you may need a different drug altogether.
- Take this drug one hour before or two hours after a meal.
- If this drug causes severe diarrhea, consult your doctor before taking any antidiarrheal medicine. For mild diarrhea, use only antidiarrheal preparations containing kaolin or attapulgite.
- To prevent reinfection, take the full course of your prescription, even if you feel better before you've taken all the medicine.
- Carbacephems kill not only harmful bacteria but also "good" intestinal bacteria that keep harmful fungi and intestinal bacteria in check. Eating yogurt containing *Lactobacillus acidophilus* culture or taking acidophilus tablets may help restore the body's normal bacteria.
- Prolonged use of any antibiotic can lead to fungal infections, including candidiasis, or to bacterial infections such as pseudomembranous colitis.
- Unless it is clearly needed, avoid taking loracarbef if you are pregnant or breast-feeding.

POSSIBLE INTERACTIONS

Probenecid: decreases the kidneys' ability to excrete loracarbef. Possible loracarbef toxicity.

NOTE: Carbacephems are a relatively new antibiotic subclass, and research into their interactions is ongoing. See entries for two similar antibiotic subclasses, ***Penicillins*** and ***Cephalosporins,*** for other possible drug interactions.

LORATADINE

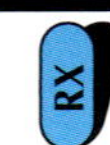

DRUG CLASS
Antihistamines

BRAND NAME
Claritin, Claritin-D

GENERAL DESCRIPTION
A newer, nonsedating antihistamine, loratadine is commonly prescribed for seasonal allergies. It generally doesn't cause the drowsiness, jitters, or dry mouth associated with drugs of its kind. See ***Antihistamines*** for additional side effects and interaction information.

SPECIAL INFORMATION
- If your liver is impaired, loratadine can build up in your body and provoke life-threatening heart problems. Depending on the severity of your liver condition, your doctor may prescribe a different antihistamine.

POSSIBLE INTERACTIONS

Azithromycin, cimetidine, clarithromycin, erythromycin, itraconazole, ketoconazole, ranitidine, theophylline, and troleandomycin: may interfere with the body's metabolism of loratadine, possibly causing life-threatening cardiac effects. Do not take loratadine in combination with any of these drugs.

LORAZEPAM

DRUG CLASS
Antianxiety Drugs [Benzodiazepines]

BRAND NAME
Ativan

GENERAL DESCRIPTION
Introduced as an injectable drug in 1963 and as a tablet in 1984, lorazepam is a benzodiazepine prescribed for the treatment of anxiety, severe nervous tension, and insomnia. In injection form, it is also used to relieve presurgery anxiety. See ***Benzodiazepines*** for information on side effects and possible drug interactions.

LOVASTATIN

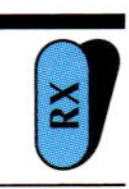

DRUG CLASS
Cholesterol-Reducing Drugs

BRAND NAME
Mevacor

GENERAL DESCRIPTION
Introduced in 1987, lovastatin is one of several HMG-CoA reductase inhibitors that lower the levels of cholesterol and other blood fats. These drugs work by blocking a liver enzyme needed in the production of cholesterol. For more information, see ***Cholesterol-Reducing Drugs.***

SIDE EFFECTS

Not serious:
Constipation, gas, decreased sex drive, insomnia.

Serious:
Fever, muscle aches, cramps, blurred vision.

SPECIAL INFORMATION
- Lovastatin works better when taken with food.
- If you become pregnant while taking this drug, stop using it immediately and inform your doctor.

POSSIBLE INTERACTIONS

Erythromycin, immunosuppressants, and niacin: severe muscle pain, kidney failure.

L

LYCIUM FRUIT

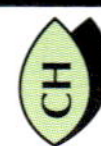

LATIN NAME
Lycium barbarum (or *Lycium chinense*)

GENERAL DESCRIPTION
Similar in appearance and action, the berries of both *Lycium barbarum* and *Lycium chinense* are large, soft, and red. The fruit is sometimes known as wolfberry. Ripening in the summer, lycium has thick flesh and small seeds. In traditional Chinese medical terms, the two herbs are classified as sweet and neutral. *Lycium chinense* appears largely in Hebei Province, while the more common *Lycium barbarum* grows in a number of Chinese provinces.

TARGET AILMENTS
Take internally for:
- night blindness, tinnitus (ringing in the ears), dizziness, and blurred vision.
- dry coughs.
- diabetes.
- sore back, knees, and legs.
- impotence and nocturnal emission.

PREPARATIONS
Lycium fruit can be obtained from Chinese pharmacies, Asian markets, and some Western health food stores, both fresh and in the form of tablets. Lycium fruit is usually added during the last five minutes of cooking.

Combinations: When mixed with cuscuta, eucommia bark, and Chinese foxglove root cooked in wine, lycium fruit is prescribed for impotence, dizziness, and tinnitus (ringing in the ears). Practitioners also use the fruit to treat consumptive coughs, when it is combined with ophiopogon tuber, anemarrhena, and fritillaria.

If used for chronic diarrhea, it should be toasted for maximum effectiveness. For further information on appropriate preparations and dosages, check with your herbal practitioner.

SPECIAL INFORMATION
- You should not take this herb if you suffer from an inflammatory ailment, weak digestion, or a tendency to become bloated.

LYCOPODIUM

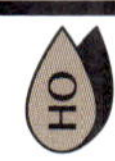

LATIN NAME
Lycopodium clavatum

GENERAL DESCRIPTION
Lycopodium, also known as club moss, grows in pastures and woodlands throughout Great Britain, northern Europe, and North America. Its spores contain a highly flammable pollen that was once used in fireworks and other pyrotechnics. Powder made from its ground-up spores has been used for internal complaints like diarrhea and dysentery since the 17th century. Homeopathic physicians use dilute doses of *Lycopodium* for complaints that are accompanied by symptoms of digestive upset, ailments that seem to develop on the right side of the body, a strong desire for sweets, anxiety, and symptoms that worsen in the early evening.

Pollen is extracted from the spores and diluted with milk sugar to create the homeopathic remedy. Like most homeopathic prescriptions, *Lycopodium* was developed as a remedy by observation of reactions of healthy individuals to a series of undilute doses. The mental, emotional, and physical changes induced by *Lycopodium* were than cataloged. When a homeopathic practitioner encounters a patient with a set of symptoms that matches the cataloged symptoms brought on by *Lycopodium,* the practitioner then prescribes it in an extremely dilute form. It is presumed that in this highly dilute dosage, *Lycopodium* can counter the symptoms that it induces when it is at full strength. For more information on homeopathic medicine, see page 1027.

TARGET AILMENTS
- backache with stiffness and soreness in the lower back, bedwetting, colds with stuffy nose, constipation, coughs with mucus present, cystitis, headache with throbbing pain that is at its worst between 4 and 8 p.m., gout, indigestion accompanied by abdominal cramps, gas, heartburn, joint pain, sciatica, right-sided sore throat, eczema.

PREPARATIONS
Lycopodium is available over the counter in various potencies, in both liquid and tablet form, at selected stores and pharmacies. Consult your homeopathic physician for more precise information.

▼SIDE EFFECTS
None expected.

L

MAGNESIUM HYDROXIDE

OTC

DRUG CLASS
Antacids

BRAND NAMES
Phillips' Milk of Magnesia, Rolaids, some types of Maalox and Mylanta

GENERAL DESCRIPTION
Magnesium hydroxide is a magnesium-containing antacid drug used to relieve symptoms of upset and sour stomach, acid indigestion, heartburn, and ulcers. The most common side effect is a laxative action or diarrhea. See ***Antacids*** for information about additional side effects and possible drug interactions.

SPECIAL INFORMATION
- Magnesium-containing antacids increase the risk of magnesium toxicity; do not take these drugs if you have kidney disease.

MAGNOLIA FLOWER

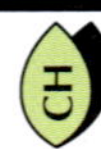

LATIN NAME
Magnolia liliflora (or *M. denudata*)

GENERAL DESCRIPTION
More accurately described as magnolia buds, this herb is the unopened magnolia flower. Chinese medicine practitioners prescribe it for blocked nasal and sinus passages. The best-quality buds are green and dry; they should include none of the stems or branches. The herb is characterized in traditional Chinese medicine as acrid and warm. Growing in several Chinese provinces, magnolia is harvested in early spring, before the flowers unfold.

TARGET AILMENTS
- nasal congestion, nasal discharge, sinus headaches, other sinus disorders. (Take internally.)

PREPARATIONS
Magnolia buds are available in bulk at Chinese pharmacies, Asian markets, and some Western health food stores.

Combinations: Magnolia flowers are mixed with xanthium, angelica *(Angelica dahurica),* and field mint to treat nasal congestion and sinus headaches, and with chrysanthemum flowers *(Chrysanthemum morifolium)* and siegesbeckia for frontal sinusitis. Consult an herbal practitioner for details of other mixtures and doses.

▼SIDE EFFECTS

Not serious:
Because of its hairy texture, the herb can irritate the throat. Rub the herb with cotton cloth or place it in cheesecloth before mixing it into a solution. In addition, overdoses can cause dizziness and red eyes.

MARSH MALLOW

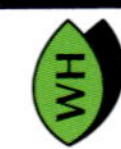

LATIN NAME
Althaea officinalis

GENERAL DESCRIPTION
For centuries, people in Europe and the Middle East have eaten wild-growing marsh mallow when their crops failed. Today it is still recognized as a wilderness forage food. Herbalists use the roots, and sometimes the leaves, of this downy, erect, five-foot-high perennial that grows in damp soils; they prescribe it for cuts and wounds, mouth sores, stomach distress, and other ailments. And teething, irritable babies and toddlers have traditionally found comfort in sucking on a root of marsh mallow.

The healing substance in marsh mallow is mucilage, a spongy root material that forms a gel when mixed with water and is especially soothing to inflamed mucous membranes. One study suggests that mucilage supports the immune system's white blood cells in their fight against invading microbes. Another trial, using animals, indicated that marsh mallow may help to lower blood sugar.

TARGET AILMENTS
Take marsh mallow internally for:
- sore throat, coughs, colds, flu, bronchitis, sinusitis.
- upset stomach, peptic ulcers, gastritis (stomach irritation), colitis (inflamed colon).
- cystitis, bladder infections, urethritis (inflammation of the urethra), kidney stones.

Apply marsh mallow externally for:
- abscesses, boils, skin ulcers, cuts, burns, scrapes, other wounds.
- varicose veins.
- dental abscesses and gingivitis.

PREPARATIONS
Over the counter:
Available in dried bulk, capsules, tincture.

At home:
Decoction: Simmer 1 to 2 tsp finely chopped or crushed root in 1 cup water for 10 to 15 minutes; drink three times daily. Use the decoction as a gargle for mouth problems.

Gel: Add just enough water to the finely chopped root to give it a gel-like consistency and use for skin problems.

SPECIAL INFORMATION
- The campfire candy named marshmallow contains none of the herb, although the marsh mallow plant was considered a delicacy by the Romans, who used it to make candy.
- Marsh mallow can be given in low doses to infants and children.

MEDROXYPROGESTERONE

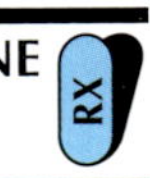

DRUG CLASS
Estrogens and Progestins

BRAND NAME
Premphase, Prempro, Provera

GENERAL DESCRIPTION
Medroxyprogesterone is a progestin used to treat menstrual problems that are caused by hormonal imbalance and to alleviate the side effects of estrogen in estrogen replacement therapy. The drug also induces uterine bleeding to allow the uterine lining to be shed. In injection form, medroxyprogesterone is sometimes used as a contraceptive, with one dose every three months. See ***Estrogens and Progestins*** for information about side effects and possible drug interactions.

MENTHOL

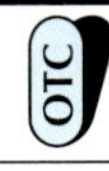

BRAND NAMES
Ben-Gay, Halls Mentho-Lyptus cough drops, N'Ice cough drops, Vicks VapoRub

GENERAL DESCRIPTION
Menthol, an aromatic oil from the peppermint plant, is a natural alcohol that is now usually produced synthetically. For centuries the drug has been used, either alone or in combination with other substances, in a wide variety of medicinal products, from rubs and liniments for

itchy skin and aching muscles to gargles and lozenges for mouth and throat irritations. Menthol has been shown effective in relieving the itching and pain of hemorrhoids and minor skin irritations. It is also a useful medication for soothing sore throat and suppressing coughs.

Menthol works by penetrating the skin or mucous membranes to calm nerve endings. It may also help kill some types of bacteria. The drug is available in many forms, including cough drops and lozenges, various topical preparations and rubs, and inhalants. Menthol is also used as an ingredient in mouthwashes, toothpastes, throat sprays, and foods such as candy and chewing gum.

TARGET AILMENTS

- itchy and painful skin.
- hemorrhoids (to relieve itching and pain).
- cough; minor sore throat and irritations of the throat.
- arthritis, muscle strain (often in combination with methyl salicylate and camphor).
- congestion associated with colds or allergies (often in combination with camphor and desoxyephedrine).
- cold sores (to soothe and relieve pain).

SIDE EFFECTS

Not serious:
Menthol may cause local irritation or a cooling sensation as part of its therapeutic action as a counterirritant. You need not call your doctor unless these symptoms become bothersome. To ease the symptoms, try using less of the drug.

Serious:
None expected; menthol, when used alone, is considered safe in the doses available. However, when combined with methyl salicylate (as in some ointments for relieving sore muscles), the medication may cause redness of skin. Discontinue use if redness develops. Also, when applied to the skin or mucous membranes, high concentrations of menthol or pure peppermint oil (which contains a high concentration of menthol) can cause serious irritation that may require medical attention.

SPECIAL INFORMATION

- Because instances of choking have been reported in very young children, menthol cough drops are not considered safe for children under five.
- Consult your doctor before using menthol liniments on children under the age of two.
- Because very little menthol is absorbed into the blood, low concentrations are generally considered safe for pregnant and nursing women. However, you should check with your doctor before using any medication that contains menthol.

MERCURIUS VIVUS

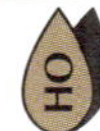

LATIN NAME
Mercurius vivus

GENERAL DESCRIPTION
One of the metallic chemical elements, mercury, also called quicksilver, was known in ancient Chinese and Hindu civilizations and has had a long history of medicinal use. Ingesting certain mercury compounds can cause increased perspiration and salivation; and so in ancient medicine mercury was used, along with bloodletting and purging, as a means of ridding the body of impurities. Undilute mercury is toxic, however, and severe symptoms of mercury poisoning may include nausea, inflammation of the digestive tract, and kidney failure.

Homeopathic practitioners prescribe *Merc vivus,* as the homeopathic preparation of mercury is called, for conditions accompanied by symptoms of shaking, hot and cold sweats, and restlessness. *Merc vivus* is made from the chemical element mercury by dilution with large quantities of milk sugar.

For more information on homeopathic medicine, see page 1027.

TARGET AILMENTS

- abscesses, especially dental or glandular; backache with burning, shooting pains in the lower back; chickenpox; colds with an exceptionally runny nose and pain in the nostrils; cystitis with slow urination; painful diarrhea; influenza; earache with discharge of pus; eye inflammation; indigestion; mouth ulcers; burning sore throat; toothache with increased salivation.

PREPARATIONS
Merc vivus is available over the counter in various potencies, in both liquid and tablet form, at selected stores and pharmacies. Consult a homeopathic physician for further information.

SIDE EFFECTS
None expected.

MESTRANOL

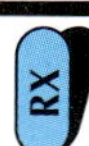

DRUG CLASS
Estrogens and Progestins

BRAND NAME
Ortho-Novum 1/50

GENERAL DESCRIPTION
Mestranol is an estrogen used in combination with the progestin norethindrone in oral contraceptives. See ***Estrogens and Progestins*** for information about side effects and possible drug interactions.

METHYL SALICYLATE

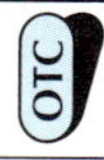

DRUG CLASS
Analgesics [Topical Analgesics]

BRAND NAME
Ben-Gay

GENERAL DESCRIPTION
Obtained from the leaves and bark of plants in the *Gaultheria,* birch, and poplar families, or produced synthetically, methyl salicylate is used as a topical medicine for relieving pain in muscles and joints. Sometimes called wintergreen oil, the substance works as a counterirritant; it stimulates skin receptors, providing temporary relief of aches and pains.

Methyl salicylate is available in a variety of gels, liniments, lotions, and ointments, usually in combination with menthol or camphor. The concentration of methyl salicylate in these products varies from 10 percent to 60 percent. Poisonous if ingested, methyl salicylate is relatively safe for external use.

TARGET AILMENTS

- minor muscle and joint aches and pains from arthritis, sprains, strains, and bruises (use only if skin is intact).

SIDE EFFECTS

Not serious:
Local skin redness or irritation. Discontinue use and contact your doctor if these effects become troublesome.

Serious:
Salicylate toxicity (dizziness, ringing in ears, nausea, vomiting), a rare condition caused by absorption through the skin into the blood. Discontinue use and contact your doctor.

SPECIAL INFORMATION
- Heat and humidity increase the absorption of methyl salicylate through the skin, thus increasing the risk of salicylate toxicity. Do not exercise vigorously in hot, humid weather after application or use a heating pad immediately after application.
- To reduce risk of irritation, avoid contact with eyes; mucous membranes; or broken, irritated skin.

METHYLCELLULOSE

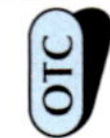

DRUG CLASS
Laxatives

BRAND NAME
Citrucel

GENERAL DESCRIPTION
Methylcellulose is a bulk-forming laxative used to temporarily relieve constipation and diarrhea and to prevent straining during bowel movements. This type of laxative may be especially beneficial to people on low-fiber diets, and patients with postpartum constipation, irritable bowel syndrome, diverticulitis, or hemorrhoids. See ***Laxatives*** for additional information.

METHYLPHENIDATE

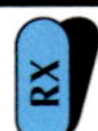

DRUG CLASS
Central Nervous System Stimulants

BRAND NAME
Ritalin

GENERAL DESCRIPTION
Methylphenidate is a mild central nervous system (CNS) stimulant that seems to work by activating the brainstem arousal system and cerebral cortex.

For some children with an attention deficit disorder, CNS stimulation decreases motor restlessness, increases attention span, and improves concentration. In adults, it can lead to increased motor activity and mental alertness, decreased fatigue, cheerier outlook, and mild euphoria.

Because methylphenidate is an amphetamine-like drug, it can be habit-forming, leading to marked tolerance and serious physical and psychological dependence. See ***Central Nervous System Stimulants*** for more information.

TARGET AILMENTS
- attention deficit disorders in children (formerly called hyperactivity, minimal brain dysfunction, or minimal brain damage).
- narcolepsy (uncontrollable spells of drowsiness or sleep).
- mild-to-moderate depression.
- apathy and withdrawal in the elderly.
- chronic pain (used with other drugs).

▼SIDE EFFECTS

Not serious:
Nervousness, trouble sleeping, loss of appetite, headache, dizziness, nausea, stomach pains, mild skin rash, unusual tiredness. See your doctor if symptoms persist.

Serious:
Severe skin rash or hives, irregular or fast heartbeat, chest pain, unusual bruising, blurred vision, joint pain, sore throat and fever, weight loss, mood or mental changes, abnormal behavior patterns, psychotic reactions. Contact your doctor immediately. Also see overdose symptoms below.

SPECIAL INFORMATION
- Seek immediate medical help for overdose. Signs of overdose include rapid, pounding, or irregular heartbeat; fever and sweating; confusion, convulsions, hallucinations, agitation, delirium, vomiting, dry mouth, trembling, muscle twitching, increased blood pressure, and loss of consciousness.
- Do not take if you have had an allergic reaction to this drug; have glaucoma or motor tics; or are suffering from severe tension, agitation, anxiety, or emotional depression.
- Before taking, tell your doctor if you have high blood pressure, epilepsy, angina, liver problems, or a history of alcoholism or drug dependence.
- Sleeping problems may be avoided if you take the last dose before 6 p.m.
- Although methylphenidate may be the primary agent in treating attention deficit disorders, its long-term effects are unknown. Your doctor may recommend occasional drug-free periods during treatment and discontinuance of the drug after puberty.

▼POSSIBLE INTERACTIONS

Anticholinergics, anticoagulants, anticonvulsants, and antidepressants (tricyclic): methylphenidate may increase the effects of these drugs.

Antihypertensives, guanethidine, minoxidil, and terazosin: methylphenidate may decrease the effects of these drugs.

Monoamine oxidase (MAO) inhibitors: methylphenidate should not be taken within two weeks of using MAO inhibitors. Concurrent use of the two drugs could cause dangerously high blood pressure and severe convulsions.

METOPROLOL

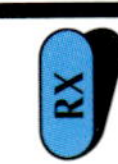

DRUG CLASS
Beta-Adrenergic Blockers

BRAND NAMES
Lopressor, Toprol

GENERAL DESCRIPTION
A cardioselective beta-blocking drug, metoprolol is prescribed to help manage hypertension (high blood pressure), angina, and myocardial infarction (heart attack). By blocking the action of certain parts of the nervous system, metoprolol slows the heart rate and relaxes blood vessels, thereby lowering blood pressure and easing the work load on the heart. See ***Beta-Adrenergic Blockers*** for more information about these drugs, including side effects and possible drug interactions.

MICONAZOLE

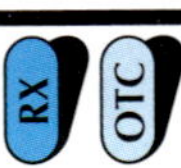

DRUG CLASS
Antifungal Drugs

BRAND NAMES
Rx: Monistat-Derm, Monistat Dual-Pak, Monistat 3 Vaginal Suppositories

OTC: Monistat 3, Monistat 7

GENERAL DESCRIPTION
Miconazole, available in topical and vaginal preparations, is used to treat a variety of fungal infections. See ***Antifungal Drugs*** for more information, including side effects and possible drug interactions. For information about other medications commonly used to treat vaginal yeast infections, see ***Vaginal Antifungal Drugs.***

SPECIAL INFORMATION
- Topical creams, lotions, and powders are applied directly to the skin to combat the fungi that cause body ringworm, jock itch, and athlete's foot. They can be used twice a day for up to one month.

- Vaginal creams and suppositories are inserted directly into the vagina, usually at bedtime, for a period of three to seven days.

MILK THISTLE

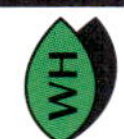

LATIN NAME
Silybum marianum

GENERAL DESCRIPTION
Milk thistle, a plant that reaches five feet in height and thrives both in the wild and in the garden, is used by herbalists to treat such liver disorders as cirrhosis and hepatitis. The active ingredient, silymarin, is found in the seeds. It is believed that silymarin prompts the manufacture of new, healthy liver cells without encouraging the growth of any malignant liver tissue that may be present. Silymarin, it is thought, also serves as an antioxidant, protecting liver cells from damage by free radicals, which are harmful by-products of many bodily processes including cellular metabolism. The use of silymarin by healthy people can increase by as much as one-third the liver's content of glutathione, a key substance in detoxifying many potentially damaging hormones, chemicals, and drugs.

Extracts of silymarin appear to neutralize toxins from the death cup mushroom, which can inflict lethal injury on the liver. Milk thistle also is believed to ease outbreaks of psoriasis, since these may worsen when the liver fails to neutralize certain toxins that circulate in the bloodstream.

TARGET AILMENTS
Take milk thistle internally for:
- liver problems, including cirrhosis and hepatitis.
- inflammation of the gallbladder duct.
- poisoning from ingestion of the death cup mushroom.
- psoriasis.

PREPARATIONS
Over the counter:
Available in dried bulk, capsules, extract.

At home:
Tea: Steep 1 tsp freshly ground seeds in 1 cup boiling water for 10 to 15 minutes, and drink three times daily. As an alternative to tea, eat 1 tsp of the freshly ground seeds. Milk thistle extract may be more effective than teas, since silymarin is only slightly soluble in water. See an herbalist for further information.

SIDE EFFECTS
Not serious:
Because taking milk thistle increases bile secretion, you may develop loose stools.

SPECIAL INFORMATION
- WARNING: If you think that you have a liver disorder, seek medical advice.

MISTLETOE

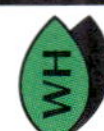

LATIN NAME
Viscum album

GENERAL DESCRIPTION
Mistletoe was sacred to the Celtic Druids of Europe, who depended on this parasitic, evergreen plant, found on the branches of deciduous trees, to guard them from evil. Today mistletoe is widely known as part of a Christmas kissing ritual. There is a great deal of controversy concerning mistletoe's medicinal value. Although the leaves are reputed to be an effective remedy for high blood pressure, the U.S. Food and Drug Administration has labeled this herb "unsafe" and does not approve of its use in treating any illnesses. The active constituents responsible for mistletoe's toxicity are proteins called viscotoxins, which slow and weaken the heartbeat and constrict blood vessels.

Mistletoe is believed to be a poisonous plant, to be used, if at all, only under the supervision of a healthcare professional.

TARGET AILMENTS
- high blood pressure, cancer. (In conjunction with conventional medical treatment.)

PREPARATIONS
Home remedies using mistletoe are not recommended. Check with an herbalist for other herbs that serve the same functions.

SIDE EFFECTS
Serious:
Symptoms of toxicity include nausea, vomiting, diarrhea, headache, decreased heart rate, hallucinations, muscle spasms, and convulsions.

SPECIAL INFORMATION
- WARNING: Mistletoe is a poisonous herb, potentially fatal. You should not take it unless instructed to do so by a healthcare professional.
- According to a string of studies conducted over the last 25 years in Germany, mistletoe impairs the growth of tumor cells in test tubes. No conclusions have been reached, although research is still being conducted to determine the herb's potential use in cancer chemotherapy.

MOMETASONE FUROATE

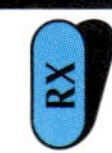

DRUG CLASS
Corticosteroids

BRAND NAME
Elocon

GENERAL DESCRIPTION
Mometasone furoate is a topical corticosteroid, commonly used for the temporary relief of inflammation and itchiness associated with various common skin diseases. The drug is available in cream, lotion, or ointment form and, when used sparingly for a brief period, has minimal side effects. See ***Corticosteroids*** for more information.

SPECIAL INFORMATION
- Do not use mometasone furoate if you are sensitive to this drug or to other corticosteroids.
- Mometasone furoate should not be used for treating acne, rosacea, or perioral dermatitis (lesions around the mouth and on the chin).
- Do not use this medication near your eyes; doing so can cause a number of problems, including glaucoma or cataracts with prolonged use.
- Unless your doctor advises otherwise, do not cover treated skin with a plastic bandage or other occlusive dressing.

POSSIBLE INTERACTIONS
None expected.

MONOAMINE OXIDASE (MAO) INHIBITORS

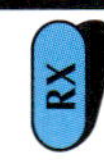

GENERIC NAMES
isocarboxazid, phenelzine, tranylcypromine

GENERAL DESCRIPTION
MAO inhibitors, a subclass of antidepressant drugs, are generally used when other medications have failed. They are

believed to work by stopping the breakdown of neurotransmitters in the brain, allowing these chemicals to maintain normal brain function. MAO inhibitors require more supervision by your doctor than do most drugs because they are known to have many side effects and adverse interactions with other drugs and even foods; they are not considered to be drugs of first choice in treating depression. For information about specific MAO inhibitors, see the entries for the generic drugs listed above; for information about other antidepressant medications, see ***Antidepressants.***

TARGET AILMENTS

- major depression, especially if the condition has not responded to other drugs.
- panic disorder (especially phenelzine).
- prevention of vascular headache (including migraine) or tension headache.

SIDE EFFECTS

Not serious:
Mild restlessness, insomnia, headache, shakiness or trembling, dizziness, weakness, blurred vision, drowsiness, decreased sexual ability, increased appetite, carbohydrate craving, weight gain or loss. Let your doctor know if these symptoms are bothersome. (Some of these effects may be alleviated if your doctor lowers the dosage.)

Serious:
Severe blood pressure changes, severe dizziness or lightheadedness when changing position. Infrequently: skin rash or bruising, diarrhea, swelling of lower body, excessive stimulation (pounding heartbeat, unusual excitement, nervousness). Rarely: yellow skin, fever, sore throat, Parkinson's-like symptoms (slurred speech, difficulty walking). Call your doctor immediately.

Seek medical help immediately if you experience severe headache, palpitations, or neck stiffness or soreness while taking MAO inhibitors. These could be signs of overdose.

SPECIAL INFORMATION

- Let your doctor know if you have diabetes, epilepsy, hyperthyroidism, or manic or suicidal tendencies, or if you have had a stroke.
- MAO inhibitors may suppress heart pain, thereby masking heart problems. Let your doctor know if you have any history of angina or other heart disease.
- MAO inhibitors react with many drugs and foods. Following are some of the substances you should avoid when taking these drugs: high-protein foods that are aged, fermented, or pickled, including (but not limited to) aged or processed cheeses; sour cream; alcohol, especially wine and beer (including alcohol-free wine and beer); pickled fish; dry sausages (salami); soy sauce; bean curd; yogurt; liver; figs; raisins; bananas; avocados; chocolate; papaya; meat tenderizers; and fava beans. Also avoid caffeine. WARNING: This is only a partial list. Talk to your doctor and pharmacist about other drugs and foods you should avoid.
- The full effects of MAO inhibitors may not be seen until after several weeks of therapy.
- Use these drugs during pregnancy or breast-feeding only if your doctor says that the benefits outweigh the risks.

POSSIBLE INTERACTIONS

Amphetamines and other stimulant drugs (including prescription and OTC cold or hay fever products): can cause a serious rise in blood pressure.

Anticoagulants (such as warfarin): increased anticoagulant effect.

Antihistamines: increased action of MAO inhibitors. Taking these drugs with MAO inhibitors may increase the side effects of antihistamines, especially drowsiness. Report any gastrointestinal problems to your doctor immediately; they could be signs of paralytic ileus (lack of intestinal activity), which requires emergency treatment.

Caffeine: severe heart-rhythm problems or high blood pressure.

Drugs: MAO inhibitors are known to interact with many drugs and may interact with others. Contact your doctor and pharmacist before taking any drug (prescription or OTC) while you are taking MAO inhibitors. Also tell your doctor about any medication you take one or two weeks before you start MAO therapy and one or two weeks after you stop.

Food: see Special Information, left.

Other antidepressants: taking these with or within a week of taking MAO inhibitors may cause an additive effect for either drug or both, possibly leading to serious side effects, including severe convulsions, changes in psychological states, severe hypertension, coma, and death.

Sedatives, including alcohol and barbiturates: high levels of sedation, very low blood pressure, possibly death.

MUGWORT LEAF

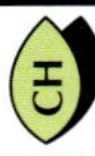

LATIN NAME

Artemisia argyi (or *A. vulgaris*)

GENERAL DESCRIPTION

The aromatic mugwort leaf is prescribed for a range of gynecological problems. In China, mugwort is harvested at the end of spring or in early summer, when the leaves are growing vigorously but flowers have not yet bloomed. Traditional Chinese medicine characterizes the herb as bitter, acrid, and warm. The best leaves are grayish white in color, with a thick, hairy texture.

TARGET AILMENTS

- excessive menstrual bleeding, menstrual cramps, uterine bleeding, vaginal pain and bleeding during pregnancy, threatened miscarriage. (Take internally.)

PREPARATIONS

Mugwort leaves are available in bulk at Chinese pharmacies, Asian markets, and some Western health food stores. The herb is also available in pills. The dried, aged, powdered herb can be rolled into a cigar-like cylinder, using tissue paper; one end is burned near the site of an injury to increase blood circulation and relieve pain. Acupuncturists sometimes use this technique instead of inserting needles.

Combinations: A mixture with gelatin is prescribed for vaginal bleeding and pain during pregnancy, or spotting between periods. Combining mugwort with dried ginger targets menstrual pain. And a preparation of mugwort leaves and kochia fruit is applied to itching lesions on the skin. For information on dosages and other preparations, check with an herbal practitioner.

SIDE EFFECTS

None expected.

SPECIAL INFORMATION

- Crushed fresh mugwort leaves were placed over warts in a clinical trial; some of the warts fell off within 10 days.
- The herb seems to indicate an antibiotic effect in test-tube studies.

MULLEIN

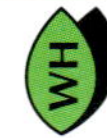

LATIN NAME
Verbascum thapsus

GENERAL DESCRIPTION
Mullein, a common roadside wildflower that may reach six feet in height, has large, velvety leaves and small, dense, yellow flowers. Owing to its astringent or binding action on tissue, it is useful in treating diarrhea and hemorrhoids. As an expectorant, it helps the body remove excess mucus from the lungs and is used to treat bronchitis and coughs. The dried leaves, flowers, and roots all serve as remedies.

TARGET AILMENTS
Take internally for:
- respiratory conditions such as bronchitis, coughs, colds, flu, asthma; gastrointestinal ailments such as stomach cramps, diarrhea.

Apply externally for:
- external ulcers, tumors, hemorrhoids.
- ear problems.

PREPARATIONS
Over the counter:
Mullein is available as tinctures and as dried leaves, flowers, or roots.

At home:
Tea: Steep 1 to 2 tsp dried leaves, flowers, or roots per cup of boiling water for 10 to 15 minutes. Drink as many as 3 cups a day.

Compress: Make a tea using vinegar, allow to cool; soak dry bandages in the tea, and apply to ulcers, tumors, or hemorrhoids.

Inhalant: Boil fresh leaves in water and inhale the steam to relieve coughs and congestion.

Combinations: Used with elder and red clover to ease painful coughing. Mixed with gumweed for asthma. Used as an extract in olive oil to apply to external ulcers, hemorrhoids, and tumors, and for ear problems. It also combines well with white horehound, coltsfoot, and lobelia for treating bronchitis.

SIDE EFFECTS
Not serious:
You may experience mild stomach upset or diarrhea. Use less mullein or discontinue using it altogether; consult your doctor when convenient.

SPECIAL INFORMATION
- WARNING: If you have a history of cancer, consult your doctor before taking this herb internally, since the tannin found in mullein is thought to have cancer-causing actions.
- WARNING: Although the leaves, flowers, and roots seem to cause no adverse effects, mullein seeds are toxic.
- WARNING: Do not take mullein if you are pregnant or nursing a baby.

MUPIROCIN

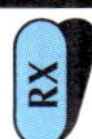

DRUG CLASS
Antibiotics [Topical Antibiotics]

BRAND NAME
Bactroban

GENERAL DESCRIPTION
Mupirocin is used to treat impetigo, a skin infection caused by certain strains of *Staphylococcus* and *Streptococcus* bacteria. This drug should not be applied to the eyes or mucous membranes. For side effects and other information, see ***Topical Antibiotics.***

MUSCLE RELAXANTS

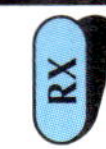

GENERAL DESCRIPTION
Muscle relaxants are a class of drugs that block messages from skeletal muscles to the brain. Some of these medications act at the site of the muscle, while others act at the brain or brainstem. They usually work by interfering with the body's response to various chemicals that transmit electrical impulses from the muscles to the brain. Drugs in this class are used for pain relief and for relaxing muscles in preparation for surgery. For information on specific muscle relaxants, see ***Carisoprodol*** and ***Cyclobenzaprine;*** for information on another drug that is used for this purpose, see ***Diazepam.***

MYRRH

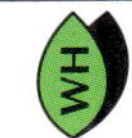

LATIN NAME
Commiphora molmol

GENERAL DESCRIPTION
Myrrh is a pale-yellow oil found in the bark of several species of shrubs native to northeast Africa and Arabia. The oil hardens into teardrop-shaped nuggets, called gum resin, which is powdered to make the healing herb. Myrrh fights infection by stimulating production of white blood cells and by a direct antibacterial action. This herb was used in biblical times for embalming, making perfume, and repelling insects and is still used as a fragrance in soaps, cosmetics, and perfumes.

TARGET AILMENTS
- mouth and throat infections, gum disease, pharyngitis. (Use as a mouthwash or gargle.)
- sinusitis, asthma, chest congestion, coughs, colds, boils. (Take internally.)
- wounds, abrasions. (Apply externally.)

PREPARATIONS
Over the counter:
Myrrh is available as tinctures and as an ingredient in commercial toothpastes. A powdered herb is made from the resin.

At home:
Mouthwash: Steep 1 tsp powdered herb and 1 tsp boric acid in 1 pt boiling water. Let stand 30 minutes and strain; use when cool.

Tea: Steep 1 to 2 tsp powdered herb per cup of boiling water for 10 to 15 minutes. Drink three times a day.

Combinations: With distilled witch hazel, applied externally.

SIDE EFFECTS
Not serious:
Myrrh may cause stomach upset or diarrhea. Use a smaller amount less frequently, or stop using.

Serious:
Large amounts may have violent laxative action and may cause sweating, nausea, vomiting, kidney problems, or accelerated heartbeat. Discontinue use and call your doctor.

SPECIAL INFORMATION
- WARNING: Any resin tends to be difficult to eliminate and can cause minor damage to the kidneys if taken internally for extended periods. Consult your physician or herbalist before using if you are pregnant or nursing, or have kidney disease. Do not exceed recommended doses and do not give to children younger than two years old.
- Preliminary studies indicate myrrh may prevent heart disease by reducing cholesterol and preventing the formation of blood clots.

NABUMETONE

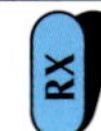

DRUG CLASS
Analgesics [Nonsteroidal Anti-Inflammatory Drugs (NSAIDs)]

BRAND NAME
Relafen

GENERAL DESCRIPTION
Introduced in 1984, nabumetone may be prescribed for the treatment of rheumatoid arthritis and osteoarthritis. Since it is a prodrug—a type of medication that exhibits pharmaceutical action only after the body changes it to another form—nabumetone must be metabolized by the liver to become effective. For information about side effects and other possible drug interactions, see ***Nonsteroidal Anti-Inflammatory Drugs (NSAIDs).***

POSSIBLE INTERACTIONS

Antipsychotic drugs (such as chlorpromazine and clozapine): decreased effects of these drugs.

Benzodiazepines (such as chlordiazepoxide, diazepam, and oxazepam): decreased effects of these drugs.

Tricyclic antidepressants (such as amitriptyline): decreased effects of these drugs.

N

NADOLOL

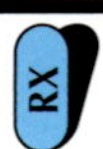

DRUG CLASS
Beta-Adrenergic Blockers

BRAND NAME
Corgard

GENERAL DESCRIPTION
Introduced in 1976, nadolol is a nonselective beta-blocking drug commonly prescribed in the management of high blood pressure (hypertension) and angina. By blocking the action of certain parts of the nervous system, the drug reduces the oxygen requirements and contraction force of the heart while also relaxing blood vessels, thereby lowering blood pressure and easing the work load of the heart. See ***Beta-Adrenergic Blockers*** for information about side effects and possible drug interactions.

NAPROXEN

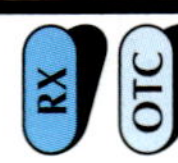

DRUG CLASS
Analgesics [Nonsteroidal Anti-Inflammatory Drugs (NSAIDs)]

BRAND NAMES
Rx: Anaprox DS, Napcalen, Naprøsyn

OTC: Aleve

GENERAL DESCRIPTION
Made available in the 1990s, naproxen is used to treat rheumatoid arthritis and osteoarthritis. Like other NSAIDs, this drug is used to relieve muscle, joint, and menstrual pain and to reduce fever. See ***Nonsteroidal Anti-Inflammatory Drugs (NSAIDs)*** for further information.

NATRUM MURIATICUM

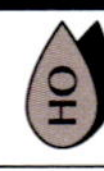

LATIN NAME
Natrum muriaticum

GENERAL DESCRIPTION
Natrum muriaticum is simply salt, or sodium chloride, a substance present in the natural world in quantities greater than any other except water. Essential to life and health, salt has been valued in human commerce throughout history. Roman soldiers were given a stipend, called a *salarium,* which they used to buy salt; from this we get the word "salary." Homeopaths prescribe dilute solutions of *Nat mur,* as they call it, for conditions that are coupled with symptoms of extreme thirst, emotional sensitivity, and a strong desire for salt.

Nat mur is prepared by adding pure sodium chloride to boiling water. Once the salt has dissolved, the solution is filtered and crystallized by evaporation. The final product is diluted in water to the desired potency.

For more information on homeopathic medicine, see page 1027.

TARGET AILMENTS
- backaches that are relieved by firm pressure; cold sores, especially in the corners of the mouth; colds with sneezing, watery eyes, and runny nose; constipation; fevers accompanied by weakness and chills; genital herpes; eczema; anemia; hay fever; migraine headaches; menstrual irregularity; indigestion; depression caused by grief, with a desire to be alone.

PREPARATIONS
Nat mur is available over the counter in various potencies, both in liquid and in tablet form. Consult a homeopathic physician for more information.

SIDE EFFECTS
None expected.

NEOMYCIN

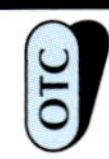

DRUG CLASS
Antibiotics [Topical Antibiotics]

BRAND NAME
Neosporin

GENERAL DESCRIPTION
Neomycin is an aminoglycoside, an antibiotic with a broad spectrum of activity and effectiveness. In oral forms the drug can be used to treat gastrointestinal infections, although it is rarely given orally because of the high risk of kidney and hearing damage. Neomycin is available over the counter as a topical ointment by itself, or in combination with polymyxin B and bacitracin. This combination is used on the skin to prevent infections in minor cuts, scrapes, and burns. For side effects and other information, see ***Topical Antibiotics.***

POSSIBLE INTERACTIONS

Other aminoglycosides: possible hypersensitivity reaction and toxicity leading to permanent deafness.

NEOMYCIN, POLYMYXIN B, AND HYDROCORTISONE

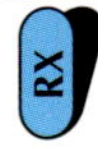

DRUG CLASS
Antibiotics [Topical Antibiotics]

GENERAL DESCRIPTION
This steroid-antibiotic combination is used to treat bacterial infections of the external ear canal. Other forms are used to treat inflammation of the skin or eyes where bacterial infection exists or is likely to occur. Don't use this drug in your ears if your eardrum is ruptured, and don't use it at all if you are sensitive to any of the ingredients. For side effects and other information, see ***Hydrocortisone*** and ***Topical Antibiotics.***

SPECIAL INFORMATION
- Do not use this combination if you are allergic to any of the component drugs, or if you have a fungal, viral, or herpes simplex infection.

NETTLE

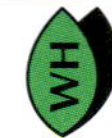

LATIN NAME
Urtica dioica

GENERAL DESCRIPTION
Notorious for the stinging needles along its leaves, nettle can be safely ingested when the irritant is tamed by boiling or drying. A tonic made from the leaves and stems is said to strengthen the body. Herbalists consider nettle a diuretic capable of removing toxins, and its iron and vitamin C may help prevent anemia. Nettle has an erect stem and serrated, dark-green, heart-shaped leaves.

TARGET AILMENTS
Take internally for:
- arthritis, gout, hay fever, premenstrual syndrome, vaginal yeast infections, excessive menstrual flow, hemorrhoids, eczema, diarrhea, chronic cystitis.

Use internally only under the supervision of a physician for:
- high blood pressure, congestive heart failure.

PREPARATIONS
Over the counter:
Nettle is available as tinctures, capsules, and dried leaves and stems.

At home:
Tea: Steep 1 to 2 tsp dried herb in 1 cup boiling water for 10 minutes. Drink up to 2 cups a day.

Juice: Add 2 tsp juice squeezed from nettle to a fresh vegetable or fruit drink.

Combinations: Nettle combines well with figwort and burdock to treat eczema; take orally as juice or tea.

SIDE EFFECTS
Not serious:
Large doses of nettle tea may cause stomach irritation, constipation, burning skin, or urinary suppression. Stop taking the herb and call your doctor.

SPECIAL INFORMATION
- WARNING: Do not use uncooked nettle. To do so may cause kidney damage and other symptoms of poisoning.
- WARNING: Nettle is a diuretic, and it may therefore remove potassium from the body. If you use it frequently, eat foods high in potassium, such as bananas and fresh vegetables.
- Do not give nettle to children younger than two years old.
- To harvest, wear gloves, long sleeves, and long pants to avoid nettle's sting.
- Do not take large doses of nettle if you are pregnant.

NICOTINE

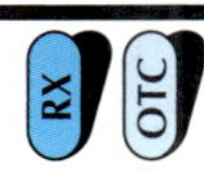

DRUG CLASS
Smoking Cessation Drugs

BRAND NAMES
Rx: Habitrol, Nicotrol, Zyban

OTC: Nicoderm, Nicorette, Nicotrol QD

GENERAL DESCRIPTION
Nicotine transdermal (skin) patches are designed to release a specific amount of nicotine through the skin and into the bloodstream every 24 hours. Nicotine gum and inhalers can be used as needed. The drug allows gradual nicotine withdrawal for people who want to stop smoking but find abrupt cessation difficult and physically painful. See ***Smoking Cessation Drugs*** for additional information.

TARGET AILMENTS
- smoking cessation.
- nicotine withdrawal.

SIDE EFFECTS
Not serious:
Mild, temporary irritation (redness, tingling, itchiness) at the patch site, fast heartbeat, increased appetite, mild headache, irritability, nervousness, coughing, dry mouth, mild dizziness or lightheadedness, muscle or joint pain, unusual dreams. Call your doctor if these symptoms persist or are bothersome.

Serious:
Chest pain, irregular heartbeat, allergic reactions (hives, rash, swelling). Check with your doctor. Also see signs of overdose below.

SPECIAL INFORMATION
- In order for nicotine replacement drugs to be safe and effective, stop smoking completely at the beginning of treatment.
- Extremely high doses of nicotine can produce toxic symptoms, even in heavy smokers; nicotine overdose can be fatal.
- Do not use more than one form of nicotine at one time.
- Call your doctor immediately if you have any of the following symptoms of toxic overdose: nausea, vomiting, abdominal cramps, diarrhea, dizziness, sweating, hearing or vision problems, confusion, weakness.
- Nicotine replacement products should not be used by nonsmokers or others who are not addicted to the drug.
- Do not use this drug if you have had an allergic reaction to it before. Consult your doctor if you have angina or an abnormal heart rhythm; have had a recent heart attack; or are pregnant, planning pregnancy, or nursing.
- Tell your doctor if you have diabetes, high blood pressure, skin disease, overactive thyroid, adrenaline-producing tumors, peptic ulcer, or liver or kidney disease, or if you get rashes from adhesive bandages or tape.
- Tell your doctor what other medications you take: Changes in nicotine levels may require dosage adjustments for other drugs, especially those affecting the nervous system.
- Nicotine can be very harmful to children and pets. Be sure to dispose of used patches carefully.
- Do not use nicotine replacement drugs for more than 12 to 20 weeks (depending on the system) if you have stopped smoking. Continued use can be harmful and addictive.

POSSIBLE INTERACTIONS
Bronchodilators, insulin, propoxyphene, and propranolol and other beta-adrenergic blockers: you may need decreased amounts of these drugs with smoking cessation.

NIFEDIPINE

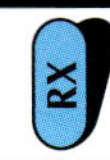

DRUG CLASS
Calcium Channel Blockers

BRAND NAMES
Adalat, Procardia XL

GENERAL DESCRIPTION
Used since 1972 to control high blood pressure, nifedipine inhibits the passage of calcium into certain body cells, retarding electrical stimulation of the heart, dilating the arteries, and slowing contraction of the heart and arteries. Nifedipine

is used to treat mild-to-moderate high blood pressure (hypertension) and to prevent angina. It is also sometimes used to treat Raynaud's syndrome.

Recent findings have prompted warnings from healthcare professionals about the safety of nifedipine, especially when taken in large doses of the short-acting form. Before using this drug, be sure to discuss this matter thoroughly with your doctor. If you are already taking nifedipine, do not stop the medication without first consulting your doctor. See ***Calcium Channel Blockers*** for information on side effects and drug interactions.

NITRATES

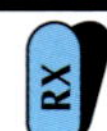

GENERIC NAMES
isosorbide dinitrate, isosorbide mononitrate, nitroglycerin

GENERAL DESCRIPTION
Used for decades to relieve chest pain associated with angina, nitrates relax and dilate the muscles of blood vessels. This dilation, which mostly affects the veins, relieves pressure on the heart by reducing its work load and its need for oxygen. In most cases, dilation also lowers blood pressure, especially systolic.

Nitrates come in a variety of forms; your medical condition will determine which form you receive. For example, sublingual tablets (those that are dissolved under the tongue) and chewable tablets, both of which are fast acting, are prescribed for the treatment of acute angina. Standard pills and skin patches are commonly used to prevent angina attacks. Other uses of nitrates include the treatment of some kinds of congestive heart failure.

TARGET AILMENTS
- acute angina pectoris.
- chronic angina pectoris.
- hypertension (nitroglycerin).
- congestive heart failure.
- heart attack (adjunct treatment).

SIDE EFFECTS

Not serious:
Headaches and lightheadedness when changing position (orthostatic hypotension), flushing of the face and neck, nausea or vomiting, restlessness, fast heartbeat. Call your doctor if these persist or become troublesome.

Serious:
In rare cases, nitrates may cause serious side effects. Call your doctor immediately if you experience any of the following symptoms while using these drugs: blurred vision; severe or prolonged headache; feelings of pressure in your head; fever; convulsions; dizziness or fainting; weakness or change in heartbeat; bluish tinge to lips, fingernails, or palms of hands; a skin rash not from an ointment or patch.

SPECIAL INFORMATION
- The safety of nitrates has not been established for pregnant or nursing women or for children; consult your doctor before using these drugs.
- Standard oral dosages should be taken on an empty stomach (either one hour before or two hours after meals) and with a full glass of water. This will improve absorption of the drug.
- Tolerance to nitrates may occur, requiring an adjustment (increase) of dosage over time to achieve the same therapeutic result. If tolerance becomes a problem for you, your doctor may advise that you take this medication intermittently, with a medication-free period each day. However, intermittent therapy can be done only so long as symptoms are under control and your doctor orders it.
- Discontinuation should be gradual to prevent rebound symptoms of angina.
- Tell your doctor if you have severe anemia, recent head trauma, glaucoma, an overactive thyroid, or a digestive absorption problem. Your doctor may decide not to use nitrates or to give you a smaller dose.
- Nitrates may cause the Zlatkis-Zak cholesterol test to show a lower-than-actual cholesterol level.

POSSIBLE INTERACTIONS

Alcohol: increased risk of orthostatic hypotension; do not drink while using nitrates.

Norepinephrine and histamine: decreased action of these medications.

Other cardiovascular medicines (including beta blockers, vasodilators, and other nitrates): use these drugs only under your doctor's direction; combining them with nitrates may cause a lowering of blood pressure and other side effects.

Stimulants (such as amphetamines, pseudoephedrine): decreased action of nitrates.

NITROFURANTOIN

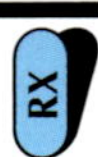

DRUG CLASS
Antibiotics

BRAND NAMES
Macrobid, Macrodantin

GENERAL DESCRIPTION
Used since 1953 to treat urinary tract infections, nitrofurantoin is a synthetic, broad-spectrum antibacterial agent. Its mode of action, unique among antibacterials, is to react chemically with bacterial enzymes, producing new substances that inactivate or alter vital proteins in the organism. Depending on the concentration of nitrofurantoin used, these changes either kill the organism outright or retard its growth. Because of its mode of action, bacterial resistance to this drug is rare.

Use of nitrofurantoin is limited to the prevention and treatment of urinary tract infections caused by susceptible bacteria, including *E. coli* and some species of *Enterococci* and *Staphylococci.* Nitrofurantoin does have potentially serious side effects that may require discontinuation of the drug.

TARGET AILMENTS
- urinary tract infections (prevention and treatment).

SIDE EFFECTS

Not serious:
Gastrointestinal upset (stomach pain, diarrhea, or nausea). Let your doctor know if these symptoms become troublesome. (A rusty or brownish color in the urine does not require a doctor's attention.)

Serious:
Pneumonitis (pneumonia symptoms, such as fever, cough, chest pain, difficulty in breathing). Less frequently: blood problems, such as reduced white cell count (manifested as sore throat and fever); tiredness or weakness; dizziness, drowsiness, headache; nerve problems (numbness, tingling, a burning sensation in the face or mouth); unusual muscle weakness. Rarely: allergic reactions, such as skin rash; pale skin; unusual tiredness or weakness; liver problems (jaundice). Call your doctor immediately if you experience any of these symptoms.

SPECIAL INFORMATION
- Take this medication with food or milk to reduce possible gastrointestinal effects.
- Nitrofurantoin should not be used by

N

women who are pregnant and near term or at delivery, or by women who are nursing. The drug can cross the placenta and affect the fetus. It also can enter breast milk in small amounts, possibly causing anemia in breast-feeding infants. Caution is advised for use during early pregnancy. Consult your doctor.
- Do not give nitrofurantoin to infants less than one month old; the drug may cause anemia.
- Nitrofurantoin may exacerbate peripheral neuropathy (a tingling sensation caused by a nervous system disorder), especially if you have G6PD deficiency (glucose enzyme), lung disease, or kidney problems.
- Antibiotics kill not only harmful bacteria but also "good" bacteria that keep unwanted fungi and intestinal organisms in check. Eating yogurt containing *Lactobacillus acidophilus* culture (or taking acidophilus tablets) may help restore normal bacteria.
- Prolonged use of any antibiotic can lead to fungal infections, including candidiasis, or to bacterial infections such as pseudomembranous colitis.

POSSIBLE INTERACTIONS

Nitrofurantoin may interact with a number of drugs that affect the blood, liver, or nervous system. Consult your doctor before taking any medication with nitrofurantoin.

Anticholinergic (atropine-like) drugs: increased nitrofurantoin effect.

Magnesium trisilicate antacids: reduced nitrofurantoin effect.

Nalidixic acid and quinolones: nitrofurantoin interferes with the action of these drugs.

Probenecid and sulfinpyrazone (antigout): increased levels and effectiveness of nitrofurantoin; risk of nitrofurantoin toxicity.

NITROGLYCERIN

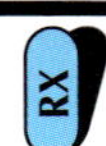

DRUG CLASS
Nitrates

BRAND NAMES
Minitran, Nitro-Dur, Nitrostat, Transderm-Nitro

GENERAL DESCRIPTION
Since 1847, nitroglycerin has been prescribed for cardiovascular disease. The drug is most commonly used to provide effective relief of acute chest pain. It is also offered as a preventive treatment for angina attacks and as a complementary treatment for congestive heart failure and heart attack.

Nitroglycerin comes in a variety of forms; each is prescribed according to its therapeutic use. For fast action, sublingual tablets (those that are dissolved under the tongue) or a spray form may be used. For long-term therapy, your doctor may prescribe standard tablets, ointment, or skin patches. See ***Nitrates*** for information about other side effects and possible drug interactions.

SIDE EFFECTS
Not serious:
Local skin irritation near application site of ointment or transdermal patch.

SPECIAL INFORMATION
- Keep sublingual tablets in the original container. After each use, replace the cap tightly to prevent loss of the drug's potency.

NIZATIDINE

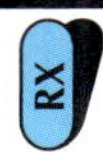

DRUG CLASS
Antiulcer Drugs [Histamine H_2 Blockers]

BRAND NAME
Axid

GENERAL DESCRIPTION
Nizatidine is used primarily to treat ulcers of the stomach and duodenum (upper intestine). It is also prescribed for Zollinger-Ellison syndrome, gastroesophageal reflux (in which stomach acid flows backward into the esophagus), and other conditions involving the overproduction of stomach acid. In some cases, nizatidine is used to prevent upper gastrointestinal bleeding.

Belonging to the subclass of antiulcer drugs known as histamine H_2 blockers, nizatidine works by blocking the effects of the chemical compound histamine in the stomach, thereby reducing the secretion of the digestive juice hydrochloric acid. For more information on side effects, possible drug interactions, and special information, see ***Antiulcer Drugs.***

SIDE EFFECTS
Not serious:
Drowsiness and increased sweating. Call your doctor if these symptoms persist or become bothersome.

SPECIAL INFORMATION
- Inform your doctor if you have a history of kidney or liver disease or are taking large doses of aspirin.
- If you are also using antacids for relief from ulcer pain, take the antacid at least two hours before or after taking nizatidine.
- If this drug causes dizziness or drowsiness, restrict your driving or your involvement in other potentially hazardous activities.

POSSIBLE INTERACTIONS

Alcohol, tobacco: increased stomach acidity, leading to decreased effectiveness of nizatidine.

Antacids containing aluminum and magnesium hydroxide: reduced effects of nizatidine; avoid taking antacids within two hours of taking nizatidine.

Aspirin: increased effect of aspirin if large doses of aspirin are being taken.

Enteric-coated tablets: changes in stomach acidity, causing these medications to dissolve prematurely in the stomach; avoid taking enteric-coated drugs with nizatidine.

Ketoconazole: increased ketoconazole effect.

NONSTEROIDAL ANTI-INFLAMMATORY DRUGS (NSAIDs)

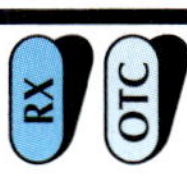

GENERIC NAMES
Rx: diclofenac, etodolac, flurbiprofen, ibuprofen, ketorolac, nabumetone, naproxen, oxaprozin; celecoxib, rofecoxib (Cox-2 Inhibitors)

OTC: ibuprofen, naproxen

GENERAL DESCRIPTION
NSAIDs are nonnarcotic analgesic drugs that reduce inflammation, especially from arthritis. These drugs are used by people who cannot take aspirin, or when aspirin or acetaminophen is not effective. In addition to reducing inflammation, NSAIDs relieve pain and reduce fever. For more information, see the entries for the generic drugs listed above.

TARGET AILMENTS
- inflammation, especially related to osteoarthritis and rheumatoid arthritis.
- pain, especially from inflammation, dental and other surgeries, menstruation, migraines.
- fever.

SIDE EFFECTS

Not serious:
Dizziness, drowsiness, headache, abdominal pain or cramps, constipation, diarrhea, heartburn, nausea. Consult your doctor if these symptoms persist.

Serious:
Anaphylactic reaction (hives, rash, intense itching, and trouble breathing). Seek emergency help.

Discontinue use and call your doctor immediately if you notice any of the following symptoms: chest pain or irregular heartbeat; diminished hearing or ringing in the ears; trouble breathing; fluid retention; black or tarry stools; blood in urine; photosensitivity; jaundice (indicated by bleeding, bruising, tiredness, tenderness in upper abdomen, and yellow eyes or skin).

SPECIAL INFORMATION

- If NSAIDs upset your stomach, take them with food or milk.
- Do not use NSAIDs if you are allergic to them or to aspirin. NSAIDs may cause bronchoconstriction or anaphylaxis in aspirin-sensitive asthmatics.
- Avoid these drugs or consult your doctor before using them if you have asthma, peptic ulcer, enteritis (intestinal inflammation), high blood pressure, bleeding problems, epilepsy, Parkinson's disease, or impaired liver or kidney function.
- Do not take more than the recommended dose and seek emergency help in case of overdose. Possible symptoms include drowsiness, increased sweating, rapid heartbeat, abdominal pain, vomiting, nausea, gastrointestinal bleeding, and disorientation.
- NSAIDs are not recommended for pregnant women, especially during the last trimester, or for nursing mothers.

N

POSSIBLE INTERACTIONS

Because NSAIDs interact with many substances, check with your doctor or pharmacist before taking in combination with other drugs. NSAIDs can affect liver and kidney function, thereby increasing the toxicity of other drugs.

Acetaminophen: increased risk of adverse liver or kidney effect.

Alcohol: possible bleeding and ulcers.

Antacids: decreased NSAID effect.

Anticoagulant drugs: increased anticoagulant effect, possible bleeding.

Anticonvulsant drugs (phenytoin): increased action of phenytoin.

Antidiabetic drugs and insulin: increased hypoglycemic effect.

Aspirin: increased risk of stomach problems.

Beta-adrenergic blockers: decreased antihypertensive effect.

Cimetidine: may increase or decrease the effect of the NSAID.

Colchicine: possibility of bleeding and ulcers when combined with certain NSAIDs.

Corticosteroids: possible bleeding and ulcers. Don't combine unless directed by your doctor.

Cyclosporine: increased risk of kidney damage.

Diuretics: reduced diuretic effect.

Methotrexate: increased toxicity of methotrexate; possibly fatal poisoning.

Probenecid: increased NSAID effect, possible NSAID toxicity.

Sulfonamides: possible sulfonamide toxicity.

Verapamil: increased toxicity.

NORETHINDRONE

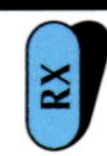

DRUG CLASS
Estrogens and Progestins

BRAND NAMES
Loestrin FE, Ortho-Novum, Ovcon

GENERAL DESCRIPTION
A progestin drug, norethindrone is prescribed in combination with an estrogen as an oral contraceptive. See ***Estrogens and Progestins*** for information about side effects and drug interactions.

NORETHINDRONE ACETATE

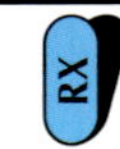

DRUG CLASS
Estrogens and Progestins

BRAND NAMES
Aygestin, Estrostep 21, Estrostep FE

GENERAL DESCRIPTION
Norethindrone acetate is a progestin that is used to treat abnormal uterine bleeding or lack of menstruation due to hormonal imbalance. It may also be combined with an estrogen, such as ethinyl estradiol, for use as an oral contraceptive. See ***Estrogens and Progestins*** for information about side effects and possible drug interactions.

NORGESTIMATE

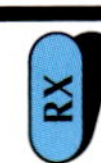

DRUG CLASS
Estrogens and Progestins

BRAND NAMES
Ortho Tri-Cyclen, Ortho-Cyclen

GENERAL DESCRIPTION
Norgestimate is a progestin that is combined with an estrogen, such as ethinyl estradiol, for use as an oral contraceptive. See ***Estrogens and Progestins*** for information about side effects and possible drug interactions.

NORGESTREL

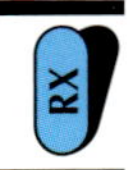

DRUG CLASS
Estrogens and Progestins

BRAND NAME
Lo/Ovral

GENERAL DESCRIPTION
A progestin used to induce uterine bleeding, norgestrel is combined with estrogen as an oral contraceptive. See ***Estrogens and Progestins*** for information about side effects and possible drug interactions.

NORTRIPTYLINE

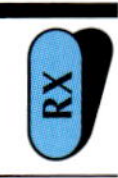

DRUG CLASS
Antidepressants
[Tricyclic Antidepressants (TCAs)]

BRAND NAME
Pamelor

GENERAL DESCRIPTION
In use for three decades, nortriptyline is prescribed for treatment of primary depression and panic attacks. It is also used in combination with other drugs to manage chronic pain. Like other tricyclic antidepressants, nortriptyline acts to restore normal levels of important brain chemicals such as serotonin and norepinephrine. See ***Antidepressants*** for information about side effects and possible drug interactions.

NOTOGINSENG ROOT

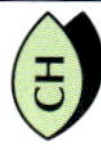

LATIN NAME
Panax notoginseng

GENERAL DESCRIPTION
Notoginseng root is used to stop bleeding, reduce swelling, and alleviate pain from injuries. Unlike Western medications, the root seems to halt the bleeding without making the blood clot, and to stop the clotting or hematoma without causing bleeding. Western practitioners of sports medicine frequently use this herb as a tonic to improve stamina. The best variety is large, solid, and dark brown, with thin skin. Also known as pseudoginseng root *(Panax pseudoginseng),* it is grown in several Chinese provinces and harvested in the fall or winter of the plant's third or seventh year, after the fruit is ripe. Chinese herbalists classify it as sweet, bitter, and warm.

TARGET AILMENTS
Take internally for:
- internal bleeding such as nosebleeds and blood in the stool and urine, coughing up blood.

Take both internally and externally for:
- bleeding from injuries; swelling and pain of fractures; falls; contusions and sprains, cuts, and gunshot wounds.

PREPARATIONS
Notoginseng root is available in bulk from Chinese pharmacies, Asian markets, and Western health food stores, where it is sold as loose, dried roots or in the form of tablets.

Combinations: Notoginseng can be made into a liniment for swelling and pain and is included in many injury tonics. It is also taken internally to heal injuries, cuts, and even gunshot wounds. A preparation containing notoginseng root and bletilla root is prescribed for vomiting, and for coughing up blood, nosebleeds, and blood in the urine. A mixture with dragon bone and gallnut from the Chinese sumac makes a poultice for bleeding caused by trauma. For information on appropriate preparations and doses, check with an herbal practitioner.

SIDE EFFECTS
Notoginseng may cause a miscarriage in at-risk pregnancies.

SPECIAL INFORMATION
- Pregnant women should avoid this herb.
- Powdered notoginseng has been used to treat individuals with coronary artery disease who complain primarily of chest pain. Many seemed to improve. Some also experienced reductions in blood pressure.
- In a small study, the herb appeared to reduce cholesterol levels.
- Notoginseng is sometimes used to treat acute attacks of Crohn's disease.

NUTMEG

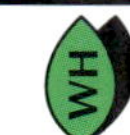

LATIN NAME
Myristica fragrans

GENERAL DESCRIPTION
As early as the seventh century, Arabs used nutmeg for digestive disorders, kidney problems, and lymphatic ailments. Today it is used principally as a spice in cooking and as a treatment for diarrhea, insomnia, indigestion, and flatulence. It relaxes muscles, sedates the body, and helps remove gas from the digestive tract. Early reports described hallucinogenic reactions to ingesting whole seeds, but these have not been substantiated. Nutmeg is native to a province of Indonesia once known as the Spice Islands, where it is still used as a culinary seasoning and medicinal herb. It comes from an evergreen tree that produces a fruit called the nutmeg apple. Nutmeg comes from the nut, which is removed and dried.

TARGET AILMENTS
- diarrhea, indigestion, loss of appetite, colic, flatulence, insomnia. (Take internally.)

PREPARATIONS
Nutmeg is available as a powder and tincture.

SIDE EFFECTS
Serious:
- Myristicin, a component of nutmeg, has narcotic properties. As little as a teaspoon of this substance can cause toxic symptoms in humans. Ingestion of 6 to 12 tsp or 1 to 2 oz of ground nutmeg can cause prolonged delirium, disorientation, and drunkenness.

SPECIAL INFORMATION
- WARNING: Women have suffered toxic reactions when attempting to use nutmeg to induce abortions. It is no longer thought to precipitate abortion.
- It is reported that in some Middle Eastern cultures, nutmeg is used in love potions as an aphrodisiac.

NUX VOMICA

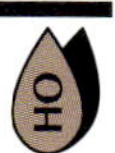

LATIN NAME
Nux vomica

GENERAL DESCRIPTION
Nux vomica, also known as poison nut, is a remedy made from seeds of an evergreen tree indigenous to parts of India, Thailand, China, and Australia. The seeds contain strychnine and have a bitter, unpleasant taste. Small doses of the seed stimulate the appetite, while somewhat larger doses decrease the appetite and cause motor dysfunction, including stiffness in the arms and legs and a staggered walk. Toxic doses can cause convulsions and death. *Nux vomica* is prescribed by homeopaths for ailments that occur from overindulgence in food, coffee, or alcohol, usually accompanied by irritability. To prepare the homeopathic remedy, poison-nut seeds are ground to a powder and then diluted with milk sugar to the desired potency.

For more information on homeopathic medicine, see page 1027.

TARGET AILMENTS
- colic and stomach cramps brought on by overeating, colds with sneezing and a stuffy nose, constipation resulting from physical inactivity, cystitis, headache with dizziness, fevers with chills, gas and gas pains, hangovers, indigestion, insomnia, irritable bowel syndrome, nausea (especially morning sickness), menstrual cramps with a heavy flow, sinusitis, stomach flu, vomiting brought on by overeating or eating rich foods, migraine headaches with painful vomiting.

PREPARATIONS
Nux vomica is available over the counter in various potencies, in both liquid and tablet form. Consult a homeopathic physician for more precise information.

SIDE EFFECTS
None expected.

N

OFLOXACIN

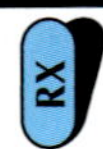

DRUG CLASS
Antibiotics [Fluoroquinolones]

BRAND NAME
Floxin

GENERAL DESCRIPTION
Introduced in 1984, ofloxacin is a synthetic fluoroquinolone that shares a wide range of uses with other drugs of its type. In addition to the ailments typically targeted by fluoroquinolones, ofloxacin is used to fight infections caused by *Chlamydia trachomatis* bacteria. See ***Fluoroquinolones*** for more information about uses, side effects, and possible drug interactions.

SPECIAL INFORMATION
- Take ofloxacin at least two hours before or two hours after taking antacids and similar drugs.

POSSIBLE INTERACTIONS

Theophyllines (asthma drugs): ofloxacin may inhibit metabolism of these drugs, increasing the risk of adverse effects and theophylline toxicity. (Generally, ofloxacin has less effect on theophylline metabolism than ciprofloxacin, another fluoroquinolone drug.)

OMEPRAZOLE

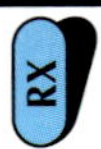

O

DRUG CLASS
Antiulcer Drugs

BRAND NAME
Prilosec

GENERAL DESCRIPTION
Omeprazole is used to treat several conditions associated with excessive production of stomach acid, such as ulcers of the stomach and duodenum (first portion of the small intestine), Zollinger-Ellison syndrome, multiple endocrine neoplasia, systemic mastocytosis, gastritis, gastroesophageal reflux (in which stomach acid flows backward into the esophagus), and gastrointestinal symptoms associated with the use of nonsteroidal anti-inflammatory drugs (NSAIDs) and aspirin. The drug works by inhibiting the action of enzymes in the acid-producing cells of the stomach lining. For more information on side effects and possible drug interactions, see ***Antiulcer Drugs.***

SIDE EFFECTS

Not serious:
Abdominal or stomach pain, skin rash or itching, headache, heartburn, dizziness, mild drowsiness, unusual tiredness, muscle pain, indigestion and gas, nausea and vomiting, diarrhea or loose stools, constipation. See your doctor if these symptoms persist or become bothersome.

Serious:
Mouth sores or ulcers, bloody or cloudy urine, difficult or painful urination, frequent urge to urinate, urinary tract infection, sore throat and fever, severe drowsiness, unusual bleeding or bruising, jaundice. If you experience these symptoms, contact your doctor at once.

SPECIAL INFORMATION
- While being treated with omeprazole, you may use antacids for relief of ulcer pain, but check with your doctor first.
- Inform your doctor if you have a history of liver disease, thyroid disease, Addison's disease, Cushing's syndrome, or any type of bone-marrow or blood cell disorder.
- Avoid taking omeprazole if you are pregnant or nursing.
- This drug may affect the results of some medical tests, including blood glucose levels and liver function tests. Inform the person giving you the test that you are taking this drug.
- Because this drug may cause dizziness or drowsiness, you may need to restrict your driving or your involvement in other potentially hazardous activities.

POSSIBLE INTERACTIONS

Alcohol, caffeine, spicy or highly seasoned foods, tobacco: decreased omeprazole effect.

Anticoagulants (such as warfarin), diazepam, phenytoin: increased effects of these drugs.

Iron, ketoconazole: decreased effects of these drugs.

OPHTHALMIC ANTIBIOTICS

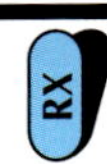

GENERIC NAMES
erythromycin, tobramycin

GENERAL DESCRIPTION
Ophthalmic antibiotics, available as ointments or eye drops, fight eye infections caused by bacteria. The generic drugs used in these eye medications may also come in the form of tablets, skin creams, or injectables for treating other, nonocular infections. However, you should never use these forms interchangeably; use each form only for its intended purpose. For more information, see the entries for the generic drugs listed above.

TARGET AILMENTS
- eye infections due to strains of strep, staph, *Hemophilus influenzae,* and other bacteria.

SIDE EFFECTS

Not serious:
Blurred vision, slight burning, or stinging that occurs momentarily upon each application.

Serious:
Eye irritation that develops and persists after using these drugs; itching, redness, or swelling. These may indicate an allergy or a superinfection. Discontinue use and call your doctor right away.

SPECIAL INFORMATION
- Tell your doctor if you have ever had an allergic reaction to these drugs. You may need a different treatment.
- Prolonged use of ophthalmic antibiotics may result in a superinfection in the eye, with symptoms of a worsening infection. Discontinue the antibiotic and call your doctor.
- Do not use these drugs if you are pregnant or breast-feeding unless they are clearly needed.

POSSIBLE INTERACTIONS

None expected for ophthalmic forms. However, since systemic absorption through the eyes can occur, you should tell your doctor about any other medicine you are using.

OPIOID ANALGESICS

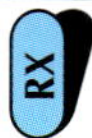

GENERIC NAMES
codeine, hydrocodone, oxycodone, propoxyphene

GENERAL DESCRIPTION
Opioid analgesics are narcotic drugs that act on the central nervous system (the spinal cord and brain) to alter the perception of pain. They are used to treat temporary moderate-to-severe pain and are often combined with nonnarcotic analgesics such as aspirin or acetaminophen. As narcotics, opioid analgesics may cause physical and psychological dependence, especially if used for long periods of time. See entries for generic drugs listed above for additional information.

TARGET AILMENTS
- moderate-to-severe pain, especially short-term pain from acute trauma or surgery.
- moderate-to-severe tension headaches.
- nonproductive cough in bronchial disorders (codeine, hydrocodone).

SIDE EFFECTS

Not serious:
Dry mouth, dizziness, fatigue, drowsiness, headache, nervousness, difficulty in urination, frequent urge to urinate, mild nausea, mild constipation. Consult your doctor if symptoms continue or are bothersome.

Serious:
Discontinue use and call your doctor if your symptoms include: slow or shallow breathing; somnolence; skin rash, hives or itching, or facial swelling; decrease in blood pressure or heart rate; fast heartbeat with increased sweating and shortness of breath; severe constipation, nausea, stomach pain, or vomiting.

Propoxyphene only: reduced liver function (brownish urine or whitish stool) or jaundice.

SPECIAL INFORMATION
- Opioid analgesics can lead to addiction, both physical and psychological.
- Tell your doctor if you notice the following withdrawal symptoms after you stop taking an opioid drug: fever, runny nose, or sneezing; diarrhea; goose flesh; unusually large pupils; nervousness or irritability; fast heartbeat.
- Seek emergency medical care if you overdose on opioid analgesics. Symptoms of overdose include pinpoint pupils; slow, shallow, or troubled breathing, and slow heartbeat; extreme dizziness or weakness; confusion; convulsions.
- These drugs are not recommended if you are pregnant or breast-feeding.
- Before taking these drugs, tell your physician if you have kidney or liver impairment, asthma, breathing problems, glaucoma, a stomach ulcer, a history of convulsions or drug abuse, inflammatory bowel disease, gallbladder disease, hypothyroidism, a bladder obstruction, or prostate problems.
- Do not drive or operate machinery until you know how the drug you are taking affects you.
- Do not drink alcoholic beverages while you are taking these drugs.
- Some opioid analgesic drugs also contain a nonnarcotic analgesic, such as aspirin or acetaminophen. Before taking any other medication, read the label carefully to avoid accidental overdose.

POSSIBLE INTERACTIONS

Anticholinergic drugs: opioid drugs may increase the effects of these drugs; risk of severe constipation and urinary retention (difficulty in urination with frequent urge to urinate).

Antidepressants [especially monoamine oxidase (MAO) inhibitors]: increased sedative effect and serious toxicity.

Antidiarrheal drugs: risk of severe constipation.

Antihypertensives, diuretics: may lower blood pressure causing orthostatic hypotension (dizziness related to change in body position).

Central nervous system depressants and drugs with sedative effects (such as alcohol, antihistamines, benzodiazepines, and other opioid drugs): increased sedative effects; risk of coma.

Metoclopramide: opioids render this drug less effective.

Nonnarcotic analgesics: see ***Aspirin*** and ***Acetaminophen.***

ORAL HYPOGLYCEMICS

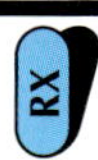

DRUG CLASS
Antidiabetic Drugs

GENERIC NAMES
glipizide, glyburide

GENERAL DESCRIPTION
A subclass of antidiabetic drugs, oral hypoglycemics (also known as sulfonylureas) are used to treat a form of non-insulin-dependent (Type 2) diabetes that cannot be controlled by diet and exercise alone. Oral hypoglycemic drugs stimulate the release of existing insulin in people whose bodies are capable of producing insulin. These drugs do not lower blood sugar on their own but can work effectively when used in conjunction with a prescribed diet and exercise program. For information on specific oral hypoglycemics, see entries for the generic drugs listed above. For information about other medications used to treat diabetes, see ***Antidiabetic Drugs*** and ***Insulin.***

TARGET AILMENTS
- non-insulin-dependent (Type 2) diabetes.

SIDE EFFECTS

Not serious:
Constipation, diarrhea, nausea, vomiting, stomach pain, indigestion, dizziness, mild drowsiness, headache, heartburn, appetite changes, skin allergies, weakness, tingling of hands and feet.

Serious:
Sore throat, unusual bleeding or bruising, water retention (edema), weight gain, yellowing of the skin or eyes (jaundice), abnormally light-colored stools, low-grade fever, fatigue, chills. Contact your doctor immediately. Also see overdose symptoms below.

SPECIAL INFORMATION
- An overdose of these drugs can result in hypoglycemia (abnormally small concentrations of sugar in the blood). Signs of hypoglycemia include excessive hunger, cold sweats, shakiness, nervousness or anxiety, rapid pulse, headache, drowsiness, confusion, nausea, and cool, pale skin. Keep hard candy or fruit juice handy to raise your blood sugar level and counteract hypoglycemia. Call your doctor.
- Tell your doctor if you are allergic to other sulfa drugs; you may also be allergic to oral hypoglycemics.

O

- Avoid oral antidiabetic drugs if you are pregnant or nursing; abnormal blood sugar levels have been associated with birth defects in laboratory animals. Injectable insulin is more effective than oral medications at maintaining close-to-normal blood sugar concentrations in women who are pregnant or nursing.
- People who are elderly, debilitated, or malnourished, as well as those with adrenal, thyroid, pituitary, kidney, or liver problems, have an increased susceptibility to the hypoglycemic action of antidiabetic drugs and should use them with caution.
- Do not stop taking this medication without your doctor's approval.
- Mild stress may reduce the effectiveness of oral hypoglycemics.
- Some studies have shown that the use of oral hypoglycemic drugs to control diabetes is more likely to lead to fatal heart problems than the use of diet alone or diet in conjunction with insulin. Your doctor can help determine the best course of treatment.
- These drugs may cause photosensitivity; avoid prolonged exposure to the sun and sunlamps.
- It is important to self-monitor your glucose level when taking these drugs.
- Strict adherence to your prescribed regimen of diet and exercise is required for these medications to be effective.

POSSIBLE INTERACTIONS

Oral hypoglycemics may interact with a number of other drugs. Check with your doctor or pharmacist before taking any medication, and be sure to read all labels for sugar content.

Alcohol, aspirin, and other salicylates: avoid these substances while taking oral hypoglycemics.

Beta-adrenergic blockers, bumetanide, diazoxide, estrogens, ethacrynic acid, oral contraceptives, phenytoin, rifampin: decreased effects of oral hypoglycemics.

Cimetidine, clofibrate, fenfluramine, monoamine oxidase (MAO) inhibitors, phenylbutazone, ranitidine: increased effects of oral hypoglycemics.

OXAPROZIN

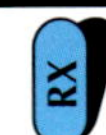

DRUG CLASS
Analgesics [Nonsteroidal Anti-Inflammatory Drugs (NSAIDs)]

BRAND NAME
Daypro

GENERAL DESCRIPTION
Introduced in 1992, oxaprozin is an NSAID used in the treatment of osteoarthritis and rheumatoid arthritis. See ***Nonsteroidal Anti-Inflammatory Drugs (NSAIDs)*** for further information.

OXYCODONE

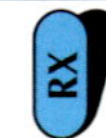

DRUG CLASS
Analgesics [Opioid Analgesics]

BRAND NAMES
Percocet, Percodan, Roxicet, Roxicodone

GENERAL DESCRIPTION
A narcotic pain reliever, oxycodone is prescribed for moderate-to-severe pain relief, often in combination with acetaminophen or aspirin. See ***Opioid Analgesics*** for information about side effects and possible drug interactions.

OXYMETAZOLINE

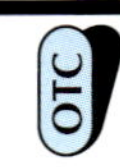

DRUG CLASS
Decongestants

BRAND NAME
Afrin

GENERAL DESCRIPTION
Used as an active ingredient in over-the-counter nose sprays, oxymetazoline relieves nasal congestion due to colds, allergies, or sinusitis by constricting blood vessels in nasal passages. Its best use is as a short-term (several days) decongestant. While short-term use as directed on the label usually produces minimal side effects, long-term use or overuse may result in rebound congestion or absorption into the bloodstream, producing central nervous system effects similar to those of oral decongestants (dizziness, headache, insomnia, nervousness, high blood pressure, heart-rhythm problems). For more information, see ***Decongestants.***

POSSIBLE INTERACTIONS

Tricyclic antidepressants (such as amitriptyline): increased serious central nervous system side effects if oxymetazoline is absorbed into the bloodstream.

PAROXETINE

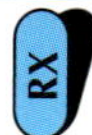

DRUG CLASS
Antidepressants [Selective Serotonin Reuptake Inhibitors (SSRIs)]

BRAND NAME
Paxil

GENERAL DESCRIPTION
Paroxetine belongs to a subclass of antidepressants known as selective serotonin reuptake inhibitors (SSRIs), but it is chemically unrelated to other similar-acting drugs used to treat depressive illness. Although this drug has not been shown to be habit-forming, long-term studies have not been completed on its addictive potential. See ***Antidepressants*** for information on side effects and possible drug interactions.

PARSLEY

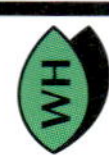

LATIN NAME
Petroselinum crispum

GENERAL DESCRIPTION
The feathery leaves of parsley, added to salads and cooked foods or used as a decorative garnish, are also a source of chlorophyll and vitamins C and A, as well as a versatile herbal remedy. Because of its ability to ease muscle spasms or cramps, parsley is used as a digestive aid. Parsley is also considered an expectorant to be taken for coughs and asthma. And it is prescribed as a diuretic and mild laxative. Native to the eastern Mediterranean area, parsley is now cultivated around the world. One of the first herbs to appear in the spring, the plant develops tiny chartreuse flowers on an umbrella-shaped canopy.

TARGET AILMENTS
- indigestion, congestion from coughs and colds, asthma, irregular menstruation, premenstrual syndrome, fever. (Take internally.)
- high blood pressure, congestive heart failure. (Take internally under the supervision of your physician.)

PREPARATIONS
Over the counter:
Available as tinctures and as fresh or dried leaves, seeds, stems, and roots.

At home:
Tea: Steep 1 to 2 tsp dried leaves or roots per cup of boiling water for 5 to 10 minutes in a closed container. Drink up to 3 cups a day. Or steep chopped fresh leaves and stems in hot water.

Nutrition and diet: Eat raw, green leaves as a breath freshener.

SIDE EFFECTS
None expected.

SPECIAL INFORMATION
- WARNING: Pregnant and nursing women should not take parsley juice or oil in medicinal doses, because it may stimulate uterine contractions. A few sprigs served as garnish will probably not cause any harm if eaten.
- WARNING: If you use this herb frequently as a medicine, you should increase your intake of foods high in potassium, such as bananas and fresh vegetables, because diuretics deplete the body of potassium.
- Do not give medicinal doses to children younger than two years old.
- Only experienced field botanists should pick wild parsley, because of its resemblance to toxic plants.

PASSIONFLOWER

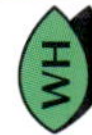

LATIN NAME
Passiflora incarnata

GENERAL DESCRIPTION
Passionflower, a long, climbing vine native to North America, was so named by Spanish explorers who saw in the ornate design of its flowers the crown of thorns, nails, and other elements of the "passion," or suffering, of Christ. Native Americans in the southeastern United States, particularly the Cherokee, used the pleasant-tasting herb in healing; it soon became popular in Europe, in part for its Christian symbolism. Today, passionflower is thought to have a calming effect on the central nervous system. Modern herbalists recommend it as a sedative, as a digestive aid, and as a pain reliever. Because it dilates blood vessels, it is also being tested as a heart disease preventive.

TARGET AILMENTS
- insomnia, anxiety, tension, neuralgia, shingles, persistent hiccups, menstrual cramps, hyperactivity in children, the seizures of Parkinson's disease, epilepsy, asthma, whooping cough, and addictive disorders—to aid withdrawal. (Take internally.)

PREPARATIONS
Over the counter:
Available in commercial homeopathic or herbal remedies and as dried or fresh leaves, capsules, and tincture.

At home:
Tea: Steep 2 tsp dried herb per cup of boiling water for 15 minutes. For insomnia, drink 1 cup in the evening.

Tincture: 1 dropperful in warm water, up to four times a day, for anxiety in adults and in children weighing more than 100 pounds. For hyperactivity in smaller children, use 3 to 10 drops (depending on the child's weight and the advice of a trained practitioner) in water every 30 minutes, not to exceed 50 drops per four-hour period. Give to children only under medical supervision.

Combinations: For insomnia, used with valerian, hops, Jamaican dogwood, or chamomile.

SIDE EFFECTS
Not serious:
Upset stomach, nausea, vomiting, diarrhea. Discontinue and call your doctor.

Serious:
Sleepiness may occur.

SPECIAL INFORMATION
- WARNING: Because passionflower can cause sleepiness, do not take this herb during the day if you operate heavy machinery or drive.
- Always use passionflower under medical supervision.
- Many herbalists recommend using only professionally prepared remedies; another species, *Passiflora caerulea,* contains cyanide, and there is some fear that this may be used instead.
- Pregnant women should avoid passionflower, since it may stimulate the uterine muscles.
- Use low-strength preparations for adults over 65 or children between 2 and 12 years old. Do not give to children under 2 years of age.
- Passionflower is sometimes substituted for prescription sedatives in people who are addicted to drugs or alcohol.
- Homeopathic uses may differ from herbal uses; for more information, consult a licensed homeopath.

POSSIBLE INTERACTIONS
- Use caution when taking passionflower with prescription sedatives and anti-anxiety medications to avoid overmedication.

PAU D'ARCO

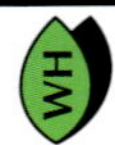

LATIN NAME
Tabebuia impetiginosa

GENERAL DESCRIPTION
Pau d'arco is the name of both a tree and a medicinal extract from the tree's bark or heartwood. The extract is believed to be effective against bacterial, fungal, viral, and parasitic infections, and is also considered an anti-inflammatory agent. It is thought to destroy microorganisms by increasing the supply of oxygen to cells. For centuries before modern science isolated some 20 of its chemical ingredients, pau d'arco was used as a folk remedy. The pau d'arco tree, also called the trumpet tree, is native to Central and South America and the West Indies; it can reach a height of 125 feet.

TARGET AILMENTS
- bacterial, fungal, viral, and parasitic infections; indigestion. (Take internally.)

PREPARATIONS
Over the counter:
Pau d'arco is available as capsules, tinctures, and dried bark.

At home:
Decoction: Boil 1 tbsp bark in 2 to 3 cups water for 10 to 15 minutes. Drink 2 to 8 cups a day.

SIDE EFFECTS
None expected.

PECTIN

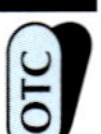

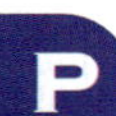

BRAND NAMES
Kaopectate, Luden's cough drops

GENERAL DESCRIPTION
Pectin, a fruit extract, has been used for centuries to help jell fruit preserves and as an ingredient in numerous other foods and medicines. It is generally believed to be a safe ingredient for medications, although experts disagree over its effectiveness in some products.

Pectin is recognized as a safe and effective demulcent, or soother, for the membranes of the mouth and throat. It also has been shown to form a protective coating over sore or ulcerated areas in the mouth and throat, helping to relieve pain by preventing further stimulation of nerve endings in these areas. Pectin is sometimes used in cough drops, lozenges, mouth rinses, gargles, and sprays. (It has not been shown effective against cold sores.) To work, pectin must be applied in sufficient quantities and thickness to form a solid or semisolid coating over the affected area.

Because of its protectant action and its ability to absorb liquids, pectin also serves as a safe and effective antidiarrheal agent.

TARGET AILMENTS
- mouth and throat irritations.
- diarrhea and intestinal cramps.

SIDE EFFECTS
Not serious:
When it is taken in an antidiarrheal medication, pectin can sometimes cause constipation.

Serious:
None expected, although an overdose of this medication may lead to an inability to defecate. Call your doctor.

SPECIAL INFORMATION
- When taken in an antidiarrheal medication, pectin may interfere with the absorption of other drugs. For this reason, you should exercise caution in combining it with other oral medicines. Take pectin at least two hours before or after other drugs.

POSSIBLE INTERACTIONS
Digitalis preparations, such as digoxin: pectin may interfere with the absorption of digitalis preparations, decreasing their effectiveness. Make sure that you take the different medications at least two hours apart.

PENICILLINS

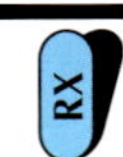

GENERIC NAMES
amoxicillin, amoxicillin and clavulanate, penicillin V

GENERAL DESCRIPTION
A subclass of antibiotic drugs, penicillins act by killing sensitive strains of growing bacteria. Penicillins are ineffective against fungi, viruses, and parasites.

When discovered in 1928, "penicillin" referred to a single drug. Today, more than 20 penicillins—some derived from molds or bacteria, others produced synthetically—are used to treat a wide range of bacterial infections. Penicillins work by attacking a bacterium's cell wall. Because body cells have a membrane but no cell wall, the drugs can selectively destroy invading bacteria without harming body tissues. See entries for the generic drugs listed above for more information.

TARGET AILMENTS
- Each generic drug listed above targets a different spectrum of disease organisms, including *Escherichia coli, Hemophilus influenzae,* as well as the streptococcal, staphylococcal, and gonorrheal bacteria. These organisms are responsible for a number of disorders, including otitis media, sinusitis, infections of the skin and soft tissues, pharyngitis, pneumonia, and genitourinary tract infections.

SIDE EFFECTS
Not serious:
Mild nausea, mild diarrhea, oral candidiasis (sore mouth or tongue), vaginal candidiasis. Tell your doctor when convenient.

Serious:
Allergic reaction (skin rash, hives, intense itching, or difficulty breathing). Severe allergic reactions (anaphylactic shock) can be life-threatening; call your doctor, 911, or your emergency number immediately.

Unusual bruising or bleeding, sore throat with fever, severe abdominal pain with diarrhea, seizures: Call your doctor immediately.

SPECIAL INFORMATION
- Take the full course of your prescription, even if you feel better before finishing the medicine; otherwise, the infection may return.
- Most penicillins are better absorbed if taken on an empty stomach. However, amoxicillin, amoxicillin and clavulanate, and penicillin V work equally well whether taken on a full or on an empty stomach.
- Tell your doctor if you are allergic to cephalosporins; you may also be allergic to penicillins.
- Let your doctor know if you have impaired kidneys, gastrointestinal disease, or a history of bleeding disorders. Your doctor may need to adjust your dosage, monitor you more closely, or prescribe a different drug.
- Penicillins also kill "good" intestinal bacteria that keep harmful fungi and intestinal bacteria in check. Eating yogurt containing *Lactobacillus acidophilus* culture or taking acidophilus tablets may help restore the body's normal bacteria.

- Prolonged use of any antibiotic drug can lead to fungal infections, including candidiasis, or to bacterial infections such as pseudomembranous colitis.
- Taking amoxicillin when you have mononucleosis may produce a skin rash.
- Penicillin may cause false-positive results in tests for glucose and protein in urine.
- If possible, avoid taking penicillins if you are pregnant or breast-feeding.

POSSIBLE INTERACTIONS

Allopurinol: may cause a skin rash.

Bacteriostatic drugs (chloramphenicol, erythromycins, sulfonamides, tetracyclines): these medicines can interfere with the bacteria-killing action of all penicillins.

Disulfiram: do not combine with amoxicillin and clavulanate.

Estrogen (oral contraceptives): decreased efficacy of contraceptives when taken with penicillin V.

Probenecid: decreases the kidneys' ability to excrete penicillins. Possible penicillin toxicity. However, probenecid is sometimes prescribed in combination with penicillin when the treatment of severe infections requires that high levels of penicillin remain in the body.

PENICILLIN V

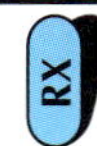

DRUG CLASS
Antibiotics [Penicillins]

BRAND NAMES
Betapen-VK, Penicillin VK, Veetids

GENERAL DESCRIPTION
Introduced in 1953, penicillin V is commonly used to treat otitis media and other infections of the respiratory tract, and skin infections. It may be prescribed to prevent endocarditis and rheumatic fever. This type of penicillin is not used to treat severe infections. For more information on side effects, interactions, and the possibility of anaphylactic shock, see ***Penicillins.***

POSSIBLE INTERACTIONS

Estrogen (oral contraceptives): decreased effectiveness in preventing pregnancy.

PENNYROYAL

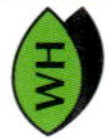

LATIN NAME
Mentha pulegium

GENERAL DESCRIPTION
Pennyroyal, a plant with smooth oval leaves, has been used since ancient times as a cough remedy and digestive aid, as well as a flea repellent. The strong aroma of its infusion acts as a decongestant and possibly as an expectorant, helping to remove excess mucus from the lungs; it is therefore useful for coughs. While the dried herb is safe in recommended doses, the oil of the pennyroyal plant should not be ingested, since even small amounts of it are toxic.

TARGET AILMENTS
- colds, coughs, premenstrual syndrome, menstrual cramps, gas, indigestion, anxiety. (Use internally.)
- fleas on pets. (Use as you would commercial flea powder.)

PREPARATIONS
Over the counter:
Pennyroyal is available as tinctures and as dried leaves and flowers.

At home:
Tea: Steep 1 to 2 tsp dried leaves in 1 cup boiling water for 10 to 15 minutes. Drink up to 2 cups a day. Or mix 1 tbsp dried herb with 1 cup warm water.

SIDE EFFECTS
None expected if used precisely as directed.

SPECIAL INFORMATION
- WARNING: Present-day practitioners advise against taking pennyroyal oil in any amount, because of its toxicity.
- Do not exceed the recommended dose of the herb and do not take for longer than a week at a time.
- Pennyroyal stimulates uterine contractions and should not be used during pregnancy.
- In the past pennyroyal has been used to induce abortion because of its ability to stimulate menstruation and strengthen uterine contractions; but it should never be used for that purpose, since it may cause serious complications, such as hemorrhage or convulsions. The amount needed to abort a fetus is close to a lethal dose.
- Do not give to children younger than two years of age.

PENTOXIFYLLINE

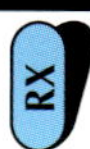

DRUG CLASS
Blood Viscosity-Reducing Agents

BRAND NAME
Trental

GENERAL DESCRIPTION
Since 1972, pentoxifylline (also known as oxypentifylline) has been used to relieve painful leg cramps and intermittent claudication (blood-vessel spasms) associated with peripheral vascular disease, a chronic blood-vessel disorder that primarily affects the legs. The cramping, which usually occurs during walking, is the result of leg muscles' becoming deprived of oxygen. Pentoxifylline eases the pain by improving blood flow to the small vessels in the legs, thus increasing the supply of oxygen to the leg muscles.

As the first real "blood thinner," pentoxifylline works by reducing blood viscosity (thickness), increasing the flexibility of oxygen-carrying red blood cells, and preventing the formation of red blood cells and platelets. When taken at the recommended dosages, the drug usually produces no side effects. See ***Blood Viscosity-Reducing Agents*** for additional information.

TARGET AILMENT
- intermittent claudication (blocked blood vessels in the legs) associated with peripheral vascular disease.

SIDE EFFECTS
Not serious:
Headache, dizziness, tremors, indigestion, nausea, vomiting. Contact your doctor if these symptoms persist or are bothersome.

Serious:
Chest pains, irregular heart rhythms. Contact your doctor promptly.

SPECIAL INFORMATION
- In managing peripheral vascular disease, pentoxifylline should be part of an overall treatment that includes physical exercise and a low-fat diet.
- Do not take pentoxifylline if you have had an allergic reaction to this drug in the past.
- Before taking pentoxifylline, tell your doctor if you smoke tobacco, are taking any antihypertensive drugs, or are allergic to caffeine, theobromine, theophylline, or other xanthine drugs.
- Before taking this drug, tell your physician if you have angina or cere-

bral artherosclerosis, kidney or liver disease, low blood pressure, or any condition (such as a stroke) in which there is a risk of bleeding.
- Do not use pentoxifylline during the first three months of pregnancy or while nursing.
- Do not stop using this drug on your own: It takes several weeks for pentoxifylline to work, and at least three months to assess its full effectiveness in preventing or easing leg pains.
- Pentoxifylline should be taken with meals or with antacids to lessen the chance of stomach upset. Tablets should be swallowed whole.
- Do not smoke tobacco. Nicotine constricts blood vessels and may make your condition worse.

POSSIBLE INTERACTIONS

Alcohol and antihypertensive drugs: may increase blood pressure-lowering effects of both medications.

Anticoagulants: pentoxifylline also inhibits blood clotting; concurrent use may increase the risk of unwanted bleeding.

Caffeine and nicotine: may decrease the effectiveness of pentoxifylline.

PEPPERMINT

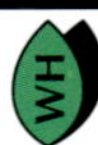

LATIN NAME
Mentha piperita

GENERAL DESCRIPTION
Peppermint plants, which reach a height of two feet or more, have stems with a purplish cast; long, serrated leaves; and a familiar minty aroma. This pleasant-tasting herb has been used as a remedy for indigestion since the era of ancient Egypt. Menthol, the principal active ingredient of peppermint, stimulates the stomach lining, thereby reducing the amount of time food spends in the stomach. It also relaxes the muscles of the digestive system. Peppermint can be grown easily from root cuttings; but if it is not confined, it tends to spread rapidly.

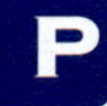

TARGET AILMENTS
- Cramps (including menstrual), stomach pain, gas, nausea associated with migraine headaches, morning sickness, travel sickness, insomnia, anxiety, fever, colds, flu. (Take internally.)
- Itching and inflammation. (Apply a few drops externally.)

PREPARATIONS
Over the counter:
Peppermint is available as commercial tea, tinctures, and fresh or dried leaves and flowers.

At home:
Tea: Drink commercial brands, or steep 1 to 2 heaping tsp dried herb per cup of boiling water for 10 minutes. Drink up to 3 cups a day.

Bath: Fill a cloth bag with several handfuls of dried or fresh herb and let hot water run over it.

Combinations: For colds and flu, peppermint may be used as a tea or tincture with boneset, elder flower, and yarrow.

SIDE EFFECTS
None expected.

SPECIAL INFORMATION
- WARNING: Do not ingest pure menthol or pure peppermint; these substances are extremely toxic. Pure peppermint may cause cardiac arrhythmias, and pure menthol can be fatal in a dose as small as a teaspoon.
- Do not use peppermint if you are having an acute gallstone attack or if you have a hiatal hernia.
- Give only very dilute preparations to children younger than two years old and only under the supervision of a doctor or an herbalist.
- Pregnant women with morning sickness should use a dilute tea rather than a more potent infusion. Peppermint should not be used by women who have a history of miscarriage.

PHENELZINE

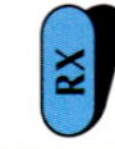

DRUG CLASS
Antidepressants [Monoamine Oxidase (MAO) Inhibitors]

BRAND NAME
Nardil

GENERAL DESCRIPTION
Introduced in 1961, phenelzine—like other medications in the subclass of antidepressants known as MAO inhibitors—is used to treat depression, anxiety, and phobias when other antidepressant drugs have failed. See ***Monoamine Oxidase (MAO) Inhibitors*** for information about side effects, warnings, and possible drug interactions.

PHENOL

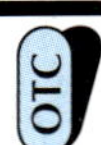

DRUG CLASS
Antiseptics

BRAND NAME
Anbesol

GENERAL DESCRIPTION
Phenol was discovered in 1834 as a component of coal tar (hence its other name, carbolic acid). Used alone, phenol is extremely toxic and potentially fatal, so this antiseptic is used only in small amounts and in combination with other chemicals. These preparations are used to inhibit the growth of bacteria and to reduce the chance of infection in minor scrapes, cuts, and burns. Sometimes phenol is included in preparations used to treat poison ivy rashes and insect bites, or to relieve the pain associated with toothaches, teething, fever blisters, and other soreness of the gums, mouth, and throat. Combined with certain other drugs, such as benzocaine, phenol has an analgesic or local anesthetic effect, which makes it useful in temporarily reducing pain and itching when applied directly on the skin.

TARGET AILMENTS
- minor cuts, scrapes, and burns (used as a first-aid antiseptic).
- local infections (to limit the development and spread of infection).
- pain and soreness of gums and mouth caused by braces or dentures, toothache or teething, sore throat, canker sores, and fever blisters (cold sores).
- pain and itching due to insect bites or poison ivy.

SIDE EFFECTS
Not serious:
When used according to package label instructions, products containing phenol are considered safe and effective and very rarely produce side effects.

Serious:
If irritation, pain, redness, rash, swelling, or fever develops, discontinue use and contact your doctor promptly. Overuse or overapplication of this drug can lead to serious, potentially life-threatening side effects. See the warnings below for more information.

SPECIAL INFORMATION
- This drug is potentially fatal if swallowed; keep away from children.
- Do not use phenol if you are allergic to local anesthetics containing benzocaine.

- Do not swallow this drug or use it near the eyes.
- Do not use on children under age two or for diaper rash, as this medication is easily absorbed into the skin.
- Do not apply topical preparations over large areas of skin, and never cover the treated area with a bandage or dressing.
- Do not use for longer than seven days; if the irritation has not improved within that period, see your doctor or dentist.
- If you are pregnant or nursing, check with your doctor before using this drug.
- To treat a teething baby, use only the recommended amount. Do not overdose.
- If you have an infection or many sores in your mouth, check with your doctor or dentist before using oral preparations containing phenol.

POSSIBLE INTERACTIONS

Phenol preparations have not been shown to interact with any specific drugs. However, before using these medications, be sure to inform your doctor, dentist, or pharmacist of any other prescription or nonprescription drug you are taking.

PHENOLPHTHALEIN

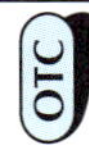

DRUG CLASS
Laxatives

BRAND NAMES
Correctol, some types of Ex-Lax

GENERAL DESCRIPTION
Phenolphthalein is a stimulant type of laxative used to relieve constipation. See ***Laxatives*** for additional information about side effects and possible drug interactions.

SIDE EFFECTS

Not serious:
Rectal irritation, pink or red urine or feces, belching, cramps, nausea, diarrhea. If these symptoms become bothersome, call your doctor.

Serious:
In rare cases, phenolphthalein may cause an allergic reaction, most often displayed on the skin in the form of increased pigmentation, eruptions, rashes, burning, and itching. Other rare side effects include irritability, confusion, skin rash, breathing difficulty, burning sensation when urinating, kidney problems, respiratory problems, and heart-rhythm problems that could lead to cardiac arrest. Discontinue the drug and call your doctor immediately.

SPECIAL INFORMATION
- Overdose or prolonged use or misuse of this drug may result in an electrolyte imbalance. Symptoms include irregular heartbeat, confusion, unusual tiredness or weakness, and muscle cramps.
- Do not use phenolphthalein or any other stimulant type of laxative if you think you may have an intestinal obstruction.

PHENYL-PROPANOLAMINE

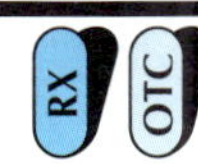

DRUG CLASS
Decongestants

BRAND NAMES
Rx: Duratuss, Entex LA, Zefrex LA

OTC: Alka-Seltzer Plus, Comtrex Liqui-Gel, Dexatrim (diet aid), Dimetapp (for adults and children), Robitussin-CF, Tavist-D, Triaminic DM Syrup, Triaminic Expectorant, Triaminicol Multi-Symptom Relief, Triaminic Syrup, Tylenol Cold (effervescent formula)

GENERAL DESCRIPTION
A nasal decongestant sometimes used as an appetite suppressant, phenylpropanolamine is widely used in over-the-counter cold and allergy products. This medication is banned for use during athletic competition. See ***Decongestants*** for information about other side effects and possible drug interactions.

SIDE EFFECTS

Serious:
In rare cases, phenylpropanolamine has been associated with serious cardiovascular, central nervous system, and psychological effects such as stroke, irregular heart rhythms, high blood pressure, hallucinations, and seizures. These effects may be more likely in individuals who take high dosages or who have an underlying cardiovascular or psychological illness.

PHENYTOIN

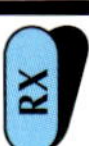

DRUG CLASS
Anticonvulsant Drugs

BRAND NAME
Dilantin

GENERAL DESCRIPTION
Introduced in 1938, phenytoin is one of several hydantoin anticonvulsant drugs used primarily in the suppression and control of epileptic seizures. This drug, formerly known as diphenylhydantoin, is used to treat all types of epilepsy except absence (petit mal) seizures. It may be used alone or in combination with other anticonvulsants. For more information, see ***Anticonvulsant Drugs.***

TARGET AILMENTS
- epileptic seizures, except absence (petit mal) type.
- prevention and treatment of seizures during and following neurosurgery.
- relief of pain in trigeminal neuralgia (tic douloureux). May be used alone or with carbamazepine.

SIDE EFFECTS

Not serious:
Mild sluggishness and fatigue, diarrhea, excessive growth of facial and body hair, enlargement of jaw, widening of nose tip, thickening of lips, swollen breasts (in males), muscle twitching, nausea and vomiting, headache, dizziness, insomnia. Consult your doctor if these effects persist or are bothersome.

Serious:
Gum overgrowth, bleeding or tender gums, fever, enlarged glands in underarms or neck, mood changes, increase in seizures, muscle pain or weakness, excitability or nervousness, severe skin rash, joint pain and swelling, blurred or double vision, elevated blood sugar, bone-marrow depression (sore throat, weakness, fever, abnormal bruising or bleeding), discolored urine, drug-induced hepatitis or nephritis. Contact your doctor immediately. Also see overdose symptoms below.

SPECIAL INFORMATION
- Seek immediate medical help for overdose. Overdose signs include: double or blurred vision; jerky or rolling eye movements; slurred speech or stuttering; severe clumsiness, unsteadiness, confusion, and trembling; and staggering walk.
- Do not use phenytoin if you have had an allergic reaction to this drug

or to any of the hydantoin drugs in the past.
- Tell your doctor if you: are taking any other drugs (prescription or over the counter); have diabetes, heart disease, or low blood pressure; have a history of impaired liver function or liver disease; or may soon have surgery under general anesthesia.
- Using phenytoin during pregnancy increases the risk of birth defects ("fetal hydantoin syndrome"). Be sure to tell your doctor if you are pregnant or planning to become pregnant soon.
- Since phenytoin can cause gum problems (bleeding, tenderness, abnormal growth), good oral hygiene is essential: Be sure to brush and floss your teeth and massage your gums regularly and carefully. You should also see your dentist every three months to have your teeth cleaned.
- Phenytoin may affect complete blood cell counts; blood cholesterol, calcium, glucose, thyroid hormone, and other levels; and liver function tests.
- Do not abruptly discontinue this drug or switch to another brand or generic unless advised by your physician.

POSSIBLE INTERACTIONS

Phenytoin interacts with a vast number of drugs, only a few of which are described here. Be sure to check with your physician before taking any other medication.

Alcohol, antidepressants (tricyclic), antacids, antihistamines, central nervous system depressants, diazoxide, and rifampin: decreased effectiveness of phenytoin in controlling epileptic seizures.

Anticoagulants, drugs for high blood pressure, sedatives, propranolol and other beta-adrenergic blockers, caffeine, corticosteroids, cyclosporine, doxycycline, and oral contraceptives: phenytoin may increase or decrease the effects of these drugs.

Cimetidine, sulfonamides, and valproic acid: increased effects of phenytoin and increased risk of severe side effects.

PHOSPHORUS

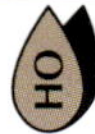

LATIN NAME

Phosphorus

GENERAL DESCRIPTION

The chemical element phosphorus can be found in the cellular fluid of all living tissue. Phosphorus plays a vital role in the activity of the body's cells, most importantly in the transfer of genetic information. Many phosphorus compounds are used commercially in toothpaste, fertilizer, and laundry detergent. Phosphorus poisoning causes irritation of the mucous membranes and inflammation of tissue; over time, it can destroy bone. As a homeopathic remedy, minute doses are prescribed by practitioners for conditions accompanied by symptoms of fatigue and nervousness, with a tendency to bleed easily and an unquenchable thirst for cold water. Pure *Phosphorus* is diluted in large quantities of milk sugar to prepare the homeopathic remedy.

Like most homeopathic prescriptions, *Phosphorus* was developed as a remedy by observation of the reactions of healthy individuals to a series of undilute doses. The mental, emotional, and physical changes induced by *Phosphorus* were then cataloged. When a homeopathic practitioner encounters a patient with a set of symptoms that matches the cataloged symptoms brought on by *Phosphorus,* the practitioner then prescribes it in an extremely dilute form. It is presumed that in this highly dilute dosage, *phosphorus* can counter the symptoms that it induces when it is at full strength.

TARGET AILMENTS

- bronchitis, pneumonia, coughs with congestion and burning pains in the chest, high fever, visual problems resulting from eyestrain, gastritis, nosebleeds, indigestion accompanied by vomiting or pain, stomach ulcers, kidney infections, nasal polyps, hepatitis, anemia, hemorrhages, diarrhea, menstrual problems, food poisoning. (Take internally.)

PREPARATIONS

Phosphorus is available over the counter in various potencies, in both liquid and tablet form, at selected stores and pharmacies. Consult your homeopathic physician for further information.

SIDE EFFECTS

None expected.

PLANTAIN

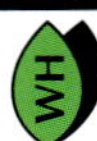

LATIN NAME

Plantago major

GENERAL DESCRIPTION

A perennial weed, plantain bears leaves that grow low to the ground and a spiked stalk with inconspicuous flowers. It is as useful to the herbalist as it is annoying to the homeowner trying to grow an attractive lawn. Due to its astringent or binding properties, it can aid in the treatment of diarrhea and hemorrhoids. Plantain also helps the body remove excess mucus from the lungs and soothes inflamed and sore membranes, making it useful for treating coughs and mild bronchitis. And its antimicrobial and anti-inflammatory actions help in healing skin wounds.

TARGET AILMENTS

- diarrhea, jaundice, neuralgia, kidney and bladder infection, urinary incontinence, thrush, hemorrhoids, loss of appetite. (Take internally.)
- external tumors and ulcers; itching, burning, or inflamed skin; cuts; snake and insect bites. (Apply externally.)

PREPARATIONS

Over the counter:
Plantain is available as tinctures, powdered seeds, dried leaves, seeds, and aboveground parts.

At home:
Tea: Steep 2 tsp dried herb per cup of boiling water for 10 minutes. Drink 3 to 4 cups a day.

Decoction: Simmer 1 oz seeds in 1½ pt water until reduced to 1 pt. Sweeten with honey. Take 1 tbsp three to four times a day.

Powdered seeds: Take 1 tsp dissolved in juice three times a day as a laxative.

Dressing: Use the tincture as a dressing for cuts, wounds, bruises, and bites.

Combinations: A liniment made from plantain juice (or tea) and rose oil can be used externally for gout.

SIDE EFFECTS

None expected.

SPECIAL INFORMATION

- A piece of cotton may be soaked with plantain juice or tincture and applied to a tooth to control toothache until you get to a dentist.

POLYGONUM

LATIN NAME
Polygonum multiflorum (root)

GENERAL DESCRIPTION
Polygonum is also known as fleece-flower root, and frequently called fo-ti by sellers, users, and practitioners. It is prescribed for a wide variety of disorders that include such disparate conditions as signs of premature aging and symptoms of malaria. The herb usually appears heavy, solid, and reddish brown. In traditional Chinese medicine it is classified as bitter, sweet, astringent, and slightly warm.

TARGET AILMENTS
Take internally for:
- dizziness and blurred vision.
- insomnia.
- prematurely gray hair.
- nocturnal emission.
- vaginal discharge.
- carbuncles, sores, abscesses, scrofula (a form of tuberculosis in the neck), goiter, and neck lumps.
- constipation.
- sore knees and back.
- malaria (the chronic, weakened condition, not the acute stages).

PREPARATIONS
Polygonum is available at Chinese pharmacies, Asian markets, and some Western health food stores. You can also find it in pill form.

Combinations: With lycium fruit, psorolea fruit, and cuscuta it is prescribed for sore knees and back, dizziness, and premature aging. A preparation containing polygonum, scrophularia, and forsythia fruit is prescribed for scrofula, abscesses, and other swellings. And a combination with Asian ginseng, dong quai, and tangerine peel is recommended for chronic malarial symptoms. For information on dosages and additional preparations, check with a Chinese medicine practitioner.

SIDE EFFECTS
Not serious:
Some patients have noticed flushing of the face and increased frequency of bowel movements, diarrhea, and mild abdominal pain.

SPECIAL INFORMATION
- Practitioners do not prescribe the herb for patients with phlegm or diarrhea.
- Malaria patients, in a study, were treated with a preparation of polygonum and licorice root, which seemed to have some effect in reducing their symptoms.
- In test-tube studies, the root seems to have an antibiotic effect.

POSSIBLE INTERACTIONS
Some traditional sources suggest that you should not take this herb with onions, chives, or garlic.

POLYMYXIN B

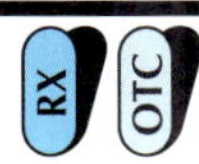

DRUG CLASS
Antibiotics [Topical Antibiotics]

BRAND NAME
Rx: Neosporin

OTC: Neosporin

GENERAL DESCRIPTION
Over-the-counter forms of polymyxin B, combined with bacitracin and neomycin, are used topically to prevent infections in minor cuts, scrapes, and burns. The prescription form, also in combination with bacitracin and neomycin, is an eye drop used to treat eye infections. See ***Topical Antibiotics*** for side effects and other information.

POTASSIUM CHLORIDE

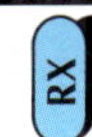

DRUG CLASS
Diuretics [Adjunct Therapy]

BRAND NAMES
K-Dur, Klor-Con 10, Micro-K 10, Slow-K

GENERAL DESCRIPTION
Potassium chloride is a mineral supplement prescribed for the prevention and treatment of potassium depletion. Such depletion usually results from the use of drugs known as nonpotassium-sparing diuretics, which promote the excretion of minerals through increased urine flow. For more information, see ***Diuretics.***

SIDE EFFECTS
Not serious:
Gastrointestinal upset. (To help alleviate this discomfort, take the medication with meals.)

Serious:
Black stools (a symptom of gastrointestinal bleeding), severe vomiting.

Excessive doses of potassium chloride can lead to high potassium levels in the blood, causing heart-rhythm problems and mental confusion. If you experience an irregular heartbeat or feel confused, call your doctor immediately. Elevated potassium levels in the blood can also cause muscle cramps, a less serious side effect but one that also warrants consultation with your doctor.

SPECIAL INFORMATION
- Inform your doctor if you have stomach ulcers; potassium chloride can cause stomach irritation.
- Do not use this drug if you are taking potassium-sparing diuretics or salt substitutes.

POSSIBLE INTERACTIONS
Angiotensin-converting enzyme (ACE) inhibitors: increased potassium chloride levels.

Digoxin: increased digoxin levels.

Potassium-sparing diuretics (such as amiloride or triamterene): increased potassium chloride levels.

PRAVASTATIN

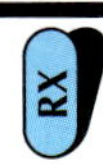

DRUG CLASS
Cholesterol-Reducing Drugs

BRAND NAME
Pravachol

GENERAL DESCRIPTION
Introduced in 1986, pravastatin is an HMG-CoA reductase inhibitor, a type of drug that alters blood levels of cholesterol and other fats. It works by blocking a liver enzyme needed in the production of cholesterol. Pravastatin may also increase the blood level of high-density lipoproteins (HDLs), the so-called good cholesterol that seems to protect against heart disease. For more information, see ***Cholesterol-Reducing Drugs.***

SIDE EFFECTS
Not serious:
Constipation, gas.

Serious:
Fever, muscle aches, cramps, blurred vision.

SPECIAL INFORMATION

- If you become pregnant while taking this drug, stop using it immediately and inform your doctor.

POSSIBLE INTERACTIONS

Erythromycin, immunosuppressants, and niacin: may cause severe muscle pain or kidney failure if used with pravastatin.

Gemfibrozil: may affect the absorption and excretion of pravastatin; do not take concurrently.

PREDNISONE

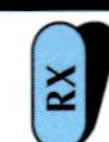

DRUG CLASS
Corticosteroids

BRAND NAME
Deltasone

GENERAL DESCRIPTION
Introduced in 1955, prednisone is a powerful medication used to treat a wide variety of disorders, including ulcerative colitis, Crohn's disease, serious skin problems, severe allergies (such as hay fever and asthma), and rheumatic disorders (including bursitis, tendonitis, and arthritis). Prednisone is also used to speed recovery from acute attacks of multiple sclerosis; to prevent rejection of transplanted organs; as replacement therapy in adrenocortical deficiency; and in some cancer cases. See ***Corticosteroids*** for more information.

POSSIBLE INTERACTIONS

Aminoglutethimide, antacids, barbiturates, phenytoin, and rifampin: decreased effectiveness of corticosteroids.

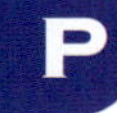

Diuretics: decreased effectiveness of both combined drugs.

Growth hormones, isoniazid, potassium supplements, and salicylates: corticosteroids may decrease the effectiveness of these drugs.

Oral anticoagulants: corticosteroids may increase or decrease the effectiveness of oral anticoagulants.

Vaccines (live virus, other immunizations): corticosteroids may make you more susceptible to the injected virus.

PROCHLORPERAZINE

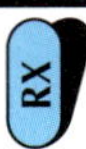

DRUG CLASS
Antinausea Drugs

BRAND NAME
Compazine

GENERAL DESCRIPTION
Prochlorperazine, introduced in 1956, is one of a group of drugs called phenothiazines. These drugs control nausea and vomiting by blocking stimulation of the area of the brain that controls vomiting. This drug must be used with care, as its antiemetic action can mask signs of overdosage of other drugs and obscure symptoms of other diseases, such as intestinal obstructions, Reye's syndrome, and brain tumor. See ***Antinausea Drugs*** for additional information.

TARGET AILMENTS
- nausea and vomiting.

SIDE EFFECTS

Not serious:
Drowsiness, dizziness, blurred vision; dry mouth, nasal congestion, constipation; impaired urination, pink- or purple-colored urine; decreased sex drive, menstrual irregularities, swollen breasts. See your doctor if these symptoms persist or are bothersome.

Serious:
Jaundice, muscle spasms of the face and neck, extreme restlessness or agitation, tremors, disorientation, fainting, skin rashes. Contact your doctor immediately.

SPECIAL INFORMATION
- Do not take prochlorperazine if you have had an allergic reaction to it in the past or if you have a blood or bone-marrow disease, Parkinson's disease, breast cancer, or any liver or kidney disease.
- Tell your doctor if you: are planning surgery within two months; have diabetes, asthma, glaucoma, emphysema, or heart disease; have a history of lupus erythematosus, prostate problems, or seizure disorders; or are pregnant or nursing.
- Prochlorperazine interacts with many other drugs. Be sure to tell your doctor if you are taking any prescribed or over-the-counter medications.
- This drug has many different side effects. Report any unusual symptoms to your physician.
- If you are too nauseated to swallow tablets, capsules, or syrup, you can ask for prochlorperazine in suppository or injection form.
- The drug may cause unusual sensitivity to the sun or to sunlamps.
- Prochlorperazine can cause a decrease in white blood cell count, an increase in liver enzymes and bilirubin, and false-positive pregnancy test results.
- Prochlorperazine should not be given to children under age two or who weigh less than 20 pounds. Children with acute illnesses, such as measles, chickenpox, or flulike infections, are very susceptible to adverse reactions to this drug.

POSSIBLE INTERACTIONS

Prochlorperazine interacts unfavorably with many OTC cold, cough, and allergy medications, and with many prescription drugs. Ask your pharmacist or physician for assistance.

Alcohol, barbiturates, tranquilizers, narcotics, sedatives: increased sedative and depressive effects.

Antacids (containing aluminum or magnesium), benztropine, trihexyphenidyl: decreased prochlorperazine effect.

Atropine-like drugs: prochlorperazine can increase the effects of these drugs, possibly leading to nervous system toxicity.

Guanethidine: decreased guanethidine effect.

Propranolol: increased effects of both drugs.

PROMETHAZINE

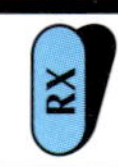

DRUG CLASS
Antihistamines

BRAND NAME
Phenergan

GENERAL DESCRIPTION
Promethazine is a sedating antihistamine that can cause the following side effects: dryness of the nose, throat, or mouth; reduced sweating; increased heart rate; dilated pupils; clumsiness; flushing; and shortness of breath. Promethazine is prescribed for allergies as well as for motion sickness, nausea related to anesthesia, and pain control following surgery. See ***Antihistamines*** for additional side effects and drug interaction information.

PROPOXYPHENE

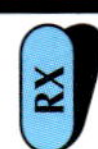

DRUG CLASS
Analgesics [Opioid Analgesics]

BRAND NAMES
Darvocet-N 100, Propacet 100

GENERAL DESCRIPTION
A narcotic prescribed for mild-to-moderate pain relief, propoxyphene is frequently combined with acetaminophen. It is less likely to cause dependence and severe withdrawal symptoms than other opiate drugs. See ***Opioid Analgesics*** for additional information on side effects and possible drug interactions.

SPECIAL INFORMATION
- Rarely, propoxyphene can cause jaundice and reduced liver function, which may include such symptoms as weakness, loss of appetite, and nausea.
- Combining propoxyphene with alcohol, tranquilizers, sedatives, muscle relaxants, or antidepressants can lead to death. Do not combine these drugs without your doctor's knowledge.

POSSIBLE INTERACTIONS
Amphetamines: risk of convulsions if a patient taking amphetamines takes an overdose of propoxyphene.

Anticoagulants: may increase the effects of some anticoagulants.

Carbamazepine: may increase the effects of carbamazepine, leading to an increased risk of toxicity.

Cimetidine: possible central nervous system toxicity.

Smoking cessation drugs, such as nicotine patches or chewing gum: may increase the effects of propoxyphene.

Tobacco: may decrease the effects of propoxyphene.

PROPRANOLOL

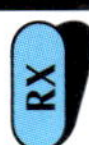

DRUG CLASS
Beta-Adrenergic Blockers

BRAND NAMES
Inderal, Inderal LA

GENERAL DESCRIPTION
A nonselective beta-blocking drug, propranolol is prescribed to help manage high blood pressure (hypertension), heart-rhythm disorders, angina, tremors, and myocardial infarction (heart attack). Other uses include the prevention of migraine headaches.

By blocking the action of certain parts of the nervous system, propranolol reduces the oxygen requirements and contraction force of the heart while also relaxing blood vessels, thereby lowering blood pressure and easing the heart's work load. The drug also affects the movement of nerve impulses in the heart, helping to control some heart-rhythm problems. Since propranolol has a stronger effect on the central nervous system than other beta-adrenergic blockers, it is more likely to cause tiredness or dizziness. See ***Beta-Adrenergic Blockers*** for more information about these drugs, including side effects and possible drug interactions.

PSEUDOEPHEDRINE

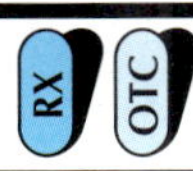

DRUG CLASS
Decongestants

BRAND NAMES
Rx: Allegra-D, Claritin-D

OTC: Actifed, Advil Cold and Sinus, Comtrex Multi-Symptom Cold Reliever Tablets or Liquid, Contac, Drixoral, NyQuil, Sudafed, Tavist-D, TheraFlu, Triaminic Nite Light, Triaminic Sore Throat Formula, Tylenol Allergy Sinus, Tylenol Cold (adults and children), Tylenol Sinus

GENERAL DESCRIPTION
Pseudoephedrine is a synthetic decongestant drug modeled on the ephedrine found in plants of the *Ephedra* genus. The drug is used to treat congestion of the nasal, sinus, and Eustachian passages caused by colds, allergies, or related respiratory problems. Pseudoephedrine is banned for use during athletic competition. See ***Decongestants*** for information about side effects and other possible drug interactions.

SPECIAL INFORMATION
- Some preparations that contain pseudoephedrine also contain antihistamines, which can cause other side effects, including drowsiness. See ***Antihistamines*** for further information.

POSSIBLE INTERACTIONS
Levodopa (anti-Parkinsonism drug): increased risk of heart-rhythm problems.

Thyroid hormones: increased effects of both combined drugs. Your doctor may have to adjust the dosage of both medications.

PSYLLIUM

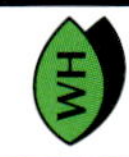

LATIN NAME
Plantago psyllium

GENERAL DESCRIPTION
For centuries, traditional Chinese and Ayurvedic (Hindu) physicians have used psyllium to treat diarrhea, constipation, hemorrhoids, and urinary problems. The ground-up seeds, rich in fiber, make a safe, gentle, bulk-forming laxative and are the active ingredient in many commercial laxative products. Both diarrhea and constipation may be treated, because the herb absorbs excess fluid in the intestinal tract and increases stool volume. Recently it has been suggested that psyllium may help prevent heart disease by clearing excess cholesterol from the body. This 18-inch-tall herb produces white flowers and abundant, small, brown seed pods.

TARGET AILMENTS
- ulcers, colitis, constipation, hemorrhoidal irritation, diarrhea. (Take internally.)

PREPARATIONS
Over the counter:
Psyllium is available as whole seeds, ground or powdered seeds, and in various commercial bulk-forming laxative preparations.

At home:
Drink: Mix 1 tsp ground seeds or powder in 1 cup cool liquid. Drink 2 to 3 cups a day.

Seeds: Take 1 tsp seeds with water at mealtimes.

SIDE EFFECTS
Not serious:
Psyllium can cause allergic reactions in people who have allergies to dust or grasses. Call your doctor if bothersome.

Serious:
Severe allergic reactions are rare; if you have difficulty breathing, seek emergency help.

SPECIAL INFORMATION
- WARNING: You must drink 8 to 10 glasses of water throughout the day when taking psyllium as a laxative, to prevent blockage of the intestines.
- Start using this herb gradually, so your body can adjust to the increase in fiber.
- Do not use psyllium to treat ulcers or colitis without consulting your doctor.
- Do not use this herb if you have a bowel obstruction or intestinal or esophageal narrowing.
- Oral medication should be taken away from psyllium as the herb may delay the absorption of the other medication.
- Do not give this herb to children younger than two years of age. Consult your pediatrician if your infant or child is constipated.
- Pregnant women should avoid psyllium and all laxatives, because they stimulate the lower pelvis near the uterus.

PSYLLIUM HYDROPHILIC MUCILLOID

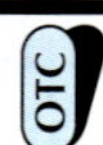

DRUG CLASS
Laxatives

BRAND NAME
Metamucil

GENERAL DESCRIPTION
Psyllium hydrophilic mucilloid is a bulk-forming laxative used to relieve chronic constipation. It also helps relieve chronic, watery diarrhea. This type of laxative may be especially beneficial to people on low-fiber diets and to those with irritable bowel syndrome (spastic colon), diverticulitis, or hemorrhoids. See ***Laxatives*** for information about other side effects and possible drug interactions.

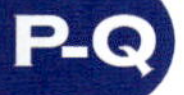

SIDE EFFECTS

Serious:
In rare cases, people with respiratory problems may have adverse reactions to inhaled particles from powder preparations.

SPECIAL INFORMATION
- When taking this laxative, be sure to drink plenty of water or other fluid to avoid obstruction of the throat and esophagus. Taking this medication without enough liquid may cause choking.
- This laxative is slow-acting; you may not experience its effects for 12 to 72 hours after taking it.

PULSATILLA

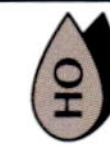

LATIN NAME
Pulsatilla nigricans

GENERAL DESCRIPTION
Common to meadowlands in northern and central Europe, the pulsatilla, or windflower, contains a caustic substance, and chewing the plant may cause blisters in the mouth and throat. Homeopathic physicians often prescribe *Pulsatilla* to patients with conditions accompanied by a thick yellow or white discharge. For homeopathic use, *Pulsatilla* is collected when in full bloom and pounded to a pulp. The pulp is steeped in an alcohol-and-water solution and then strained and diluted.

Like most homeopathic prescriptions, pulsatilla was developed as a remedy by observation of the reactions of healthy individuals to a series of undilute doses. The mental, emotional, and physical changes induced by *Pulsatilla* were then cataloged. When a homeopathic practitioner encounters a patient with a set of symptoms that matches the cataloged symptoms brought on by *pulsatilla,* the practitioner then prescribes it in an extremely dilute form. It is presumed that in this highly dilute dosage, *Pulsatilla* can counter the symptoms that it induces when it is at full strength.

TARGET AILMENTS
- bedwetting, breast infections, chickenpox; conjunctivitis; coughs that cause a rattling sound in the chest and interfere with sleep; headaches in the forehead; eye inflammation, if the eyes ache and there is a thick discharge; fever with chills; hay fever; incontinence; indigestion from rich, fatty foods; aching joints that improve with movement and cold compresses; urethritis in men; late menstrual periods; endometriosis, otitis media (middle ear infection); sciatica; sinusitis; varicose veins; depression with excessive weeping.

PREPARATIONS
Pulsatilla is available over the counter in various potencies, both in liquid and in tablet form, at selected stores and pharmacies. Consult your homeopathic physician for more precise information.

SIDE EFFECTS
None expected.

QUINAPRIL

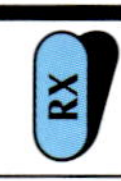

DRUG CLASS
Angiotensin-Converting Enzyme (ACE) Inhibitors

BRAND NAME
Accupril

GENERAL DESCRIPTION
Quinapril is prescribed to treat hypertension (mild-to-moderate high blood pressure) and congestive heart failure. Like other ACE inhibitors, this drug works by relaxing the artery walls, thereby lowering blood pressure. See ***Angiotensin-Converting Enzyme (ACE) Inhibitors*** for information on side effects and other possible drug interactions.

POSSIBLE INTERACTIONS
Drugs that interact with magnesium, such as tetracycline and diuretics: because of its high magnesium content, quinapril may reduce the body's absorption of these medications.

RAMIPRIL

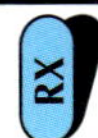

DRUG CLASS
Angiotensin-Converting Enzyme (ACE) Inhibitors

BRAND NAME
Altace

GENERAL DESCRIPTION
Because it relaxes arterial walls and lowers blood pressure, the ACE inhibitor ramipril is prescribed for mild-to-severe high blood pressure (hypertension). See ***Angiotensin-Converting Enzyme (ACE) Inhibitors*** for information on side effects and possible drug interactions.

RANITIDINE

DRUG CLASS
Antiulcer Drugs [Histamine H_2 Blockers]

BRAND NAMES
Rx: Tritec, Zantac 150, Zantac 300
OTC: Zantac 75

GENERAL DESCRIPTION
Ranitidine is used primarily to treat ulcers of the stomach and duodenum (upper intestine). It is also prescribed for Zollinger-Ellison syndrome, gastroesophageal reflux (in which stomach acid flows backward into the esophagus), and other conditions involving the overproduction of stomach acid. In some cases, ranitidine is used to prevent upper gastrointestinal bleeding.

Belonging to the subclass of antiulcer drugs known as histamine H_2 blockers, ranitidine works by blocking the effects of the chemical compound histamine in the stomach, thereby reducing the secretion of the digestive juice hydrochloric acid. For more information on side effects and possible drug interactions, see ***Antiulcer Drugs.***

SIDE EFFECTS

Not serious:
Constipation, diarrhea, dizziness, drowsiness, headache, nausea or vomiting, skin rash. Less common: blurred vision, joint or muscle pain, hair loss, decreased libido, decreased sexual ability, swelling of breasts or breast soreness (in women or men). Call your doctor if these symptoms persist or become bothersome.

Serious:
Allergic reaction (burning, redness, or swelling of the skin). Rare: irregular heartbeat, tightness in the chest, confusion, fever, sore throat, unusual bleeding or bruising, unusual tiredness or weakness. Call your doctor immediately if you experience these symptoms.

SPECIAL INFORMATION
- You may need to take this drug for several days before experiencing any relief from stomach pain.
- Tell your doctor if you have a history of kidney or liver disease.
- If you are also using antacids for relief from ulcer pain, take the antacid at least two hours before or after taking ranitidine.
- Because this drug may cause dizziness or drowsiness, you may need to restrict your driving or involvement in potentially hazardous activities.
- Avoid this drug if you are pregnant or nursing.
- Ranitidine may cause a false-positive result in urine protein tests.

POSSIBLE INTERACTIONS

Alcohol: significantly increased concentration of alcohol in the blood.

Antacids: decreased absorption of ranitidine into the body; avoid taking antacids within two hours of ranitidine.

Diazepam: inhibited absorption of diazepam into the body.

Glipizide, glyburide, theophylline: increased effects of these drugs.

Warfarin: decreased elimination of warfarin from the body, possibly resulting in bleeding complications.

RED CLOVER

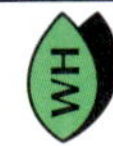

LATIN NAME
Trifolium pratense

GENERAL DESCRIPTION
The perennial plant known as red clover grows as high as two feet. Its medicinal parts are the red or purple ball-shaped flowers, which are gathered between May and September. Red clover has been used medicinally in many parts of the world. It was prescribed as an expectorant in China, and as a cure for asthma in Russia. Other cultures have used it to treat skin sores and eye irritations, and as a diuretic. Herbalists today prescribe red clover for skin ailments, indigestion, and coughs. It is an anti-inflammatory agent and also, as an expectorant, helps remove excess mucus from the lungs. In addition, the herb appears to act like the female hormone estrogen; it is believed that it might help women with menopausal symptoms.

TARGET AILMENTS
Take internally for:
- coughs, bronchitis, whooping cough, indigestion, menopausal symptoms.

Use internally and externally for:
- skin problems such as eczema and psoriasis.

PREPARATIONS

Over the counter:
Red clover is available in dried bulk and tincture.

At home:
Infusion: Steep 1 to 3 tsp dried flower tops in 1 cup boiling water for 10 to 15 minutes. Drink up to 3 cups a day.

Compress: Soak a clean cloth in the infusion and apply to the skin.

SIDE EFFECTS

Serious:
Overdoses of red clover may cause stomachaches or diarrhea. Discontinue if you experience these symptoms.

SPECIAL INFORMATION
- WARNING: Do not use red clover if you are pregnant, because of its estrogen-like behavior.
- WARNING: Avoid the herb if you have estrogen-dependent cancer or a history of heart disease, stroke, or thrombophlebitis.
- Do not use red clover if you are taking blood thinning medicine. The herb's blood thinning properties will poteniate the medication.
- If you are taking birth-control pills, consult your doctor before using red clover.
- Do not give the herb to children under 2 years of age. Older children and people over 65 should start with a low dose and increase as needed.
- Red clover contains four antitumor compounds among its chemical components, and some herbalists believe it may find use in combination with more powerful drugs to treat cancers that are not aggravated by estrogen.

RED RASPBERRY

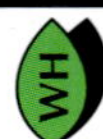

LATIN NAME
Rubus idaeus

GENERAL DESCRIPTION
The berry of this biennial bush is commonly used in gourmet desserts, but herbalists value the leaves. These have high concentrations of tannin, a chemical that herbalists believe is effective in treating diarrhea, nausea, vomiting, and morning sickness in pregnancy. It is also thought that tannin, an astringent substance, helps prevent miscarriages and, during labor, strengthens contractions, checks hemorrhaging, and reduces labor pains; you should not, however, use red raspberry for this purpose at home. Red raspberry leaves are included in several herbal pregnancy formulas sold in the United States. The herb is also used as a gargle for sore throats.

TARGET AILMENTS
- morning sickness, threatened miscarriage, problems arising during labor, diarrhea, mouth ulcers, bleeding gums. (Take internally.)

PREPARATIONS
Over the counter:
Red raspberry is available as dried leaves or berries, and as a tincture.

At home:
Infusion: Use 1 to 2 tsp dried leaves or berries per cup of boiling water. Steep for 10 to 15 minutes. Drink cold and as desired. During pregnancy and with the consent of your physician, drink up to 3 cups daily. For children, dilute the infusion with more water.

SIDE EFFECTS
Not serious:
Red raspberry may cause stomach upset or diarrhea if you exceed the recommended dose.

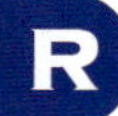

SPECIAL INFORMATION
- Pregnant women should take red raspberry only with the consent and supervision of a physician.
- Animal tests suggest that red raspberry may reduce levels of glucose (blood sugar) in animals, and hence may help in the management of diabetes.

RHUS TOXICODENDRON

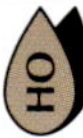

LATIN NAME
Rhus toxicodendron

GENERAL DESCRIPTION
This vinelike shrub, also known as poison ivy, grows throughout North America and is well known for the itchy, red rash its oil can cause on the skin. The medicinal history of its leaves and stalk began in the late 18th century, when it was used to treat conditions such as paralysis and rheumatism. The effects of its undilute form can range from a rash to nausea, fever, delirium, swollen glands, and ulcers in the oral cavity. For this reason, homeopathic practitioners use *Rhus toxicodendron,* or *Rhus tox,* as it is also called, to treat conditions that may be accompanied by a fever, restlessness, and swollen glands.

Rhus tox is prepared from plants gathered at night, when the oil is said to be in its most potent state. The leaves and stalks are pounded to a pulp and mixed with alcohol, then strained and diluted.

Like most homeopathic prescriptions, *Rhus tox* was developed as a remedy by studying the reactions of healthy individuals to a series of undilute doses. The mental, emotional, and physical changes induced by *Rhus tox* were then cataloged. When a homeopathic practitioner encounters a patient with a set of symptoms that matches the cataloged symptoms brought on by *Rhus tox,* the practitioner then prescribes it in an extremely dilute form. It is presumed that in this highly dilute dosage, *Rhus tox* can counter the symptoms that it induces when it is at full strength. For more information on homeopathic medicine, see page 1027.

TARGET AILMENTS
- arthritis with stiffness that is worse in the morning and better from motion; backache with stiffness along the spine; bursitis; carpal tunnel syndrome; eye inflammation with swelling and itching, and with sticky matter between the eyelids; genital herpes; hamstring injury; influenza with painful joints; headaches; hives that itch, sting, and intensify after scratching; joint and back pains brought on by overexertion; impetigo; poison ivy; sprains with stiffness; toothaches.

PREPARATIONS
Rhus tox is available over the counter in various potencies, both in liquid and in tablet form, at selected stores and pharmacies. Consult your homeopathic physician for more precise information.

SIDE EFFECTS
None expected.

ROFECOXIB

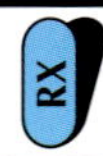

DRUG CLASS
Nonsteroidal Anti-Inflammatory Drug (NSAIDs) [COX-2 Inhibitors]

BRAND NAME
Vioxx

GENERAL DESCRIPTION
Rofecoxib is used to treat osteoarthritis (degenerative joint disease), acute pain in adults, and painful menstrual cycles. It is a type of nonsteroidal anti-inflammatory drug (NSAID) that selectively inhibits the COX-2 enzyme active at sites of inflammation. Rofecoxib does not inhibit the COX-1 enzyme present in the stomach. Because of this selectivity for COX-2, it is less likely to cause ulcers and stomach bleeding than nonselective NSAIDs. For additional information, see ***COX-2 Inhibitors.***

ROSE HIP

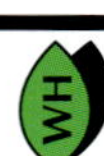

LATIN NAME
Rosa spp.

GENERAL DESCRIPTION
In the 1930s, herbalists discovered vitamin C in fresh rose hips—the cherry-sized, bright red fruits that remain after the rose petals have fallen off. Since then, scientists have found that rose hips also contain flavonoids, which increase the body's utilization of the vitamin. For these reasons, herbalists prescribe rose hips for colds and flu. Between 45 and 90 percent of the vitamin is lost, however, when the herb is dried. Beware when buying prepackaged rose hip teas, jams, extracts, purées, and soups; while often consumed for their natural vitamin C, they may actually contain very small amounts of it.

TARGET AILMENTS
- colds and flu. (Take internally.)

PREPARATIONS
Over the counter:
Rose hips are available as dried bulk and in tincture.

At home:
Infusion: Use 2 to 3 tsp dried, chopped hips per cup of boiling water. Steep for 10 minutes. Drink hot or warm, as desired.

Jam: Collect the hips after the first frost and do not use any that have been sprayed with insecticide. Place in a heavy, stainless steel pan and simmer until tender, using 1 cup water to 1 lb rose hips. Rub through a fine sieve. Weigh the pulp and add 1 lb heated sugar for each lb pulp. Simmer until thick.

SIDE EFFECTS
Not serious:
High doses of vitamin C may cause diarrhea and may slightly strain the kidneys.

SPECIAL INFORMATION
- If you have a kidney infection, consult your doctor before taking large quantities of rose hips.
- Do not use x potency dilutions of this remedy if you are severely sensitive to poison ivy.

ROSEMARY

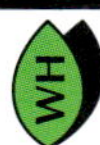

LATIN NAME
Rosmarinus officinalis

GENERAL DESCRIPTION
The evergreen perennial known as rosemary has a plethora of uses in addition to serving as a culinary spice. Herbalists believe that its leaves stimulate the circulatory and nervous systems and therefore serve as an antidepressant. Rosemary leaves also are thought to contain antispasmodic chemicals that relax the smooth muscle lining of the digestive tract. In addition they are used to treat muscle pain. In recent years, rosemary has developed a reputation for antibacterial and antifungal action, and herbalists recommend that the leaves be used externally for skin infections. Rosemary is also prescribed as a gargle for bad breath. Before refrigeration was invented, crushed rosemary leaves were wrapped around meats to prevent them from becoming rancid, and to give them a pleasant fragrance and flavor.

TARGET AILMENTS
Take internally for:
- indigestion, upper-respiratory infections that require a decongestant, tension, muscle pain, sprains, rheumatism, neuralgia.

Apply externally, as an antiseptic, for:
- skin infections.

PREPARATIONS
Over the counter:
Rosemary is available as dried bulk, in tincture, and as two types of oil, one for internal use and the other for external application.

At home:
Infusion: Use 1 tsp crushed leaves per cup of boiling water. Steep 10 to 15 minutes. To settle the stomach or clear a stuffy nose, drink 3 cups a day. For children younger than two years, dilute the infusion with more water.

SIDE EFFECTS
Not serious:
Rosemary oil for internal use may cause mild stomach, kidney, and intestinal irritation, even in small doses. If you experience any of these discomforts, consult your physician.

Serious:
Rosemary oil, taken internally in large amounts, can be poisonous. Keep to the prescribed dosage.

SPECIAL INFORMATION
- WARNING: Do not confuse rosemary oil for internal use with that applied externally. Never ingest the external variety.
- Pregnant women should avoid rosemary. It may stimulate the uterus.
- Some herbalists suggest putting rosemary leaves in baths for relaxation and even rubbing them on the head to redress premature baldness.
- Recent studies indicate that rosemary may contain antioxidant chemicals that may help to prevent food poisoning and to fight tumors.

RUTA

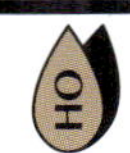

LATIN NAME
Ruta graveolens

GENERAL DESCRIPTION
Native to southern Europe, ruta spread across the continent in the wake of the Romans, who valued it for its medicinal properties. *Ruta* comes from the Greek *reuo,* meaning "to set free," an allusion to its historical popularity as a cure for numerous complaints, including headaches, coughs, and croup. Through centuries of use, this small shrub, sometimes called rue or rue bitterwort, has spread to herb gardens worldwide.

In large doses, *Ruta* has toxic properties, but homeopathic physicians prescribe minute doses to treat conditions or injuries that may be accompanied by symptoms of weakness or a bruised sensation. The plant is collected for homeopathic use just before blossoming; it is pounded to a pulp and pressed for its juice, which is then diluted in a water-and-alcohol base.

Like most homeopathic prescriptions, *Ruta* was developed as a remedy by studying the reactions of healthy individuals to a series of undilute doses. The mental, emotional, and physical changes induced by *Ruta* were then cataloged. When a homeopathic practitioner encounters a patient with a set of symptoms that matches the cataloged symptoms brought on by *Ruta,* the practitioner then prescribes it in an extremely dilute form. It is presumed that in this highly dilute dosage, *Ruta* can counter the symptoms that it induces when it is at full strength. For more information on homeopathic medicine, see page 1027.

TARGET AILMENTS
- carpal tunnel syndrome; eyestrain caused by overwork, and accompanied by heat and pain; sciatica; groin strain; sprains with pain and a bruised sensation; tennis elbow; injuries of tendons and cartilage.

PREPARATIONS
Ruta is available over the counter in various potencies, in both liquid and tablet form, at selected stores and pharmacies. Consult your homeopathic physician for further information.

SIDE EFFECTS
None expected.

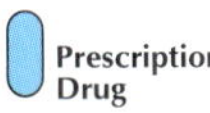

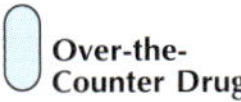

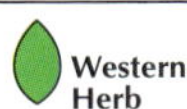

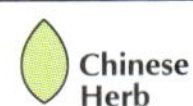

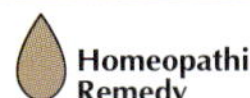

SAFFLOWER FLOWER

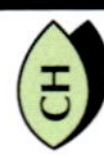

LATIN NAME
Carthamus tinctorius

GENERAL DESCRIPTION
The Chinese name of this herb, *hóng huā,* means "red flower," and herbalists prescribe safflower flower for several conditions related to the flow of blood through the body. It is harvested in several Chinese provinces throughout June and July, when the color of the flowers changes from yellow to red; traditionalists prefer picking safflower flower on the morning of a cloudy day, before the dew has dried. In addition to their fresh red color, the best safflower flowers have long petals and feel soft. According to traditional Chinese medicine, the herb is characterized as acrid and warm.

TARGET AILMENTS
Take internally for:
- delayed menstruation, poor blood circulation, blood clots, stabbing chest pain.

Apply externally for:
- burns, bruises, and other injuries to the skin.

Use both internally and externally for:
- sores and carbuncles, measles in its early stages.

PREPARATIONS
Dried safflower flower is available in bulk at Chinese pharmacies, Asian markets, and some Western health food stores. You can also obtain it in tablet form. It is frequently sold in liniments for treating bruises and injuries.

Combinations: Safflower flower is mixed with cnidium root *(Ligusticum chuanxiong)* for chest pain. It is combined with dong quai and sappan wood to make a preparation for treating the pain and swelling associated with trauma. A mixture with Chinese foxglove root, red peony root, and forsythia fruit is prescribed for pain, redness, and swelling of the eyes. Safflower flowers and groomwell root are combined into a decoction and taken internally or used externally to treat boils, carbuncles, and childhood measles. For information on dosages and additional preparations, check with a Chinese medicine practitioner.

SIDE EFFECTS
None expected.

SPECIAL INFORMATION
- Do not use safflower flowers if you are pregnant, because there is evidence that the herb stimulates the uterus.

SAFFRON

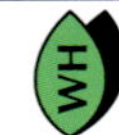

LATIN NAME
Crocus sativus

GENERAL DESCRIPTION
Saffron is one of the most expensive herbs, with prices ranging from $55 to $250 an ounce. The price is high because the valuable components are not the leaves or the violet petals but the three tiny, orange, antenna-like stigmas inside the flower of this member of the crocus family. An ingredient of the stigmas known as crocetin is the active agent. To produce one ounce of saffron, you would need to harvest almost 5,000 flowers. Even if you have that energy, you should never try to harvest your own saffron; you might use the wrong kind of crocus. Herbalists prescribe saffron primarily in conjunction with the conventional treatment for high blood pressure and heart disease. Laboratory studies have indicated that injections of crocetin may decrease cholesterol levels in animals. Some herbalists believe that saffron may increase the amount of oxygen in the blood; the oxygen, in turn, may slow the growth of artery-clogging plaque deposits.

Crocetin is also thought to stimulate the uterus and the digestive process, and so practitioners also recommend saffron for digestion and to promote menstruation.

TARGET AILMENTS
- high cholesterol, high blood pressure, atherosclerosis, indigestion, delayed menstruation. (Take internally.)

PREPARATIONS
Over the counter:
Saffron is available as dried powder and dried stigmas.

At home:
Infusion: Place 12 to 15 stigmas in 1 cup boiling water. Steep 10 minutes. Drink up to 1 cup a day.

SIDE EFFECTS
None expected.

SPECIAL INFORMATION
- WARNING: In large amounts, saffron is highly toxic. Take the herb only in the recommended dosage, in consultation with your practitioner.
- Do not use saffron to induce an abortion. Women have died as a result of taking an overdose, in an attempt to end their pregnancies.
- Do not give saffron to children under 2 years of age. For older children and adults over 65, begin with low-strength preparations and increase gradually.

SAGE

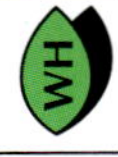

LATIN NAME
Salvia officinalis

GENERAL DESCRIPTION
The scientific name of sage, *Salvia,* derives from the Latin for "to save," which underscores the herb's early reputation as a cure-all. Modern herbalists are more specific. They believe that sage contains an aromatic oil that reduces excessive perspiration and the night sweats associated with such diseases as tuberculosis. In addition, the oil, which is antiseptic, combines with another component, the astringent tannin, to relieve sore throats or gums. This savory herb, whose gray-green, oval leaves are familiar to most gardeners, has also been used to cleanse wounds, stem lactation in nursing mothers, aid digestion, and preserve meat.

TARGET AILMENTS
Take internally for:
- indigestion, gas, nausea, and to stem lactation or reduce the night sweats of menopause.

Use as a mouthwash or gargle for:
- mouth and throat infections, inflammations, and ulcers, including canker sores, bleeding gums, sore throats, and tonsillitis.

Apply externally for:
- bacterial infections in wounds; insect bites.

PREPARATIONS
Over the counter:
Available as tinctures, prepared tea, or dried or fresh leaves.

At home:
Infusion: Steep 2 to 3 tsp leaves per cup of boiling water for 10 minutes. Drink 3 cups a day, hot or cold, or use

as a wash for bacterial infections in wounds.

Compress: Soak a clean cloth in the infusion and apply to insect bites.

Tincture: Take 1 to 1½ tsp three times daily with water or juice.

Mouthwash: Add 3 tsp leaves to 1 pt water, bring to a boil, and let stand covered for 15 minutes. Gargle the warm liquid three times daily.

Fresh: Apply fresh sage leaves to minor cuts or scrapes before washing and bandaging.

SIDE EFFECTS

Not serious:
Drinking the tea may inflame the lips and mouth lining.

SPECIAL INFORMATION
- WARNING: Sage contains the toxic chemical thujone, which can lead to convulsions if taken in high doses. However, the heat of cooking or preparing an infusion reduces toxicity. Sage oil should not be ingested.
- Because it may cause convulsions, sage is best avoided by persons with epilepsy.
- Do not take sage if you are pregnant or nursing.
- Use dilute preparations for children under 12 and adults over 65.

ST.-JOHN'S-WORT

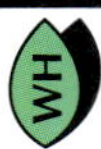

LATIN NAME
Hypericum perforatum

GENERAL DESCRIPTION
Herbalists now know that the flowers of the plant called St.-John's-wort, used for centuries to heal wounds, contain hypericin, a substance with germicidal, anti-inflammatory, and antidepressant properties. These blooms also hold high concentrations of chemicals known as flavonoids, which are thought to boost the immune system. The plant (*wort* means "plant" in Old English) was named for St. John the Baptist, because its blood-red flowers are said to bloom on the anniversary of his execution. A woody perennial, its leaves are dotted with glands that produce a red oil when pinched.

TARGET AILMENTS
Use externally for:
- wounds, including cuts, abrasions, burns; scar tissue.

Take internally, in consultation with an herbalist or a doctor for:
- depression.

PREPARATIONS
Over the counter:
Available as dried leaves and flowers, tinctures, extract, oil, ointment, capsules, and prepared tea.

At home:
Tea: Add 1 to 2 tsp dried herb to 1 cup boiling water; steep for 15 minutes. Drink up to 3 cups a day.

Oil: Use a commercial preparation, or make by soaking the flowers in almond or olive oil until the oil turns bright red.

Ointment: Use a commercial preparation, or make by warming the leaves in hot petroleum jelly or a mixture of beeswax and almond oil.

Fresh: Apply crushed leaves and flowers to cleaned wounds.

Tincture: Add ¼ to 1 tsp to an 8-oz glass of water and drink daily.

SIDE EFFECTS

Serious:
High blood pressure, headaches, stiff neck, nausea, and vomiting. In the fair-skinned, it can exacerbate sunburn and cause blistering after sun exposure.

SPECIAL INFORMATION
- Consult a doctor or an herbalist before using St.-John's-wort. If you are taking any antidepressant medications, take St.-John's-wort only with your physician's consent.
- Do not take St.-John's-wort if you are pregnant.

SALMETEROL

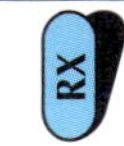

DRUG CLASS
Bronchodilators

BRAND NAME
Serevent

GENERAL DESCRIPTION
Used principally as a treatment for chronic asthma, salmeterol causes the bronchial smooth muscles to relax, relieving spasms and opening the airways. If taken regularly, this drug helps relieve symptoms of asthma, including asthma induced by exercise. Salmeterol, available as an aerosol inhaler and as a powdered inhalant, may be used in conjunction with short-acting inhaled bronchodilators or with inhaled or oral steroids. For side effects and drug interactions, see ***Bronchodilators.***

SPECIAL INFORMATION
- WARNING: Do not take salmeterol if you have an irregular heart rhythm or if you have taken a monoamine oxidase (MAO) inhibitor within the past two weeks.
- WARNING: Do not take salmeterol for an acute asthma attack or if your asthma is getting worse; use a short-acting bronchodilator or oral steroids instead.

SARGASSUM SEAWEED

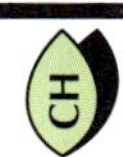

LATIN NAME
Sargassum pallidum

GENERAL DESCRIPTION
More commonly known as seaweed, sargassum is collected from the coastal provinces of China, and from other coastlines around the world. Its high content of the element iodine makes it effective in treating a variety of ailments related to the thyroid gland. It also promotes urination and is traditionally prescribed for the pain of hernia. In traditional Chinese medicine sargassum is characterized as a cold, salty herb.

TARGET AILMENTS
Take internally for:
- nodules in the neck, which include goiter (a thyroid problem) and other thyroid disorders; scrofula (a form of tuberculosis).
- inadequate urination; edema (retention of fluids in the body); pain from hernia; swollen, painful testes.

PREPARATIONS
Sargassum is available in bulk at Chinese pharmacies, Asian markets, and Western health food stores.

Combinations: A mixture of sargassum, silkworm, prunella, and scrophularia is used for goiter and scrofula. The same symptoms can also be treated with a preparation of sargassum and licorice; some traditional texts suggest that these two herbs are incompatible, although animal experiments have shown no adverse reactions. A combination of sargassum and water chestnut is prescribed for the lung disease silicosis. For information on dosages and other preparations, consult a Chinese medicine practitioner.

SIDE EFFECTS
None expected.

SPECIAL INFORMATION
- Sargassum's ability to stimulate the excretion of fluids from the body makes it useful for individuals trying to lose weight; but the herb is not appropriate for all weight-loss patients, because its impact on the thyroid gland affects the metabolism rate. Consult a Chinese medicine practitioner before using this herb.
- In laboratory tests, extracts of the herb inhibited the growth of fungi.

SASSAFRAS

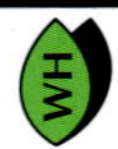

LATIN NAME
Sassafras albidum

GENERAL DESCRIPTION
The root bark of this native American tree yields a tea with not only a pleasant taste but also a wide reputation as a tonic. It contains a volatile oil once prized as a flavoring for root beer and other beverages. Laboratory tests in the 1960s, however, revealed that the main component of the oil, safrole, is carcinogenic in rats and mice, and the U.S. Food and Drug Administration has prohibited the internal use of sassafras containing safrole. Until the ban, the herb was widely used for a variety of ailments, including colic, rheumatism, and poison ivy. The essential oil of the root bark has recently been found to have mild antiseptic action and is still used to combat external infections.

TARGET AILMENTS
The only approved applications are external.
Use as liniment for:
- rheumatism.

Use a compress for:
- skin irritations such as acne, boils, poison ivy, and poison oak.

S

PREPARATIONS
Over the counter:
Sassafras is available as an essential oil and tincture and as fresh or dried root bark, although internal use is prohibited.

At home:
Liniment: Mix 1 oz each of the tinctures of sassafras, prickly ash, cayenne, myrrh, and camphor with 3 oz water; shake well, and apply to areas afflicted by rheumatism.

SIDE EFFECTS
None expected if used externally.

SAW PALMETTO

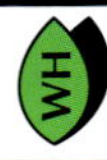

LATIN NAME
Serenoa repens

GENERAL DESCRIPTION
An extract made from the berries of this shrub is used to treat and strengthen the male reproductive system. It is particularly recommended for benign enlargement of the prostate gland. This disorder is indicated by urination difficulties and can lead to bladder infections and kidney problems. Common among men over 50, the condition is thought to be caused by an accumulation of a testosterone derivative called dihydrotestosterone, which saw palmetto appears to block the production of. The herb has also been used as an expectorant, diuretic, tonic, antiseptic, sedative, and digestive aid. It is native to the sandy coast of the southeastern United States, where the plant reaches a height of about 10 feet.

TARGET AILMENTS
- benign prostatic hyperplasia (enlargement of the prostate gland); nasal congestion; asthma and bronchitis; coughs due to colds; sore throats; sinus ailments. (Use internally.)

PREPARATIONS
Over the counter:
Available as fresh or dried berries and in powder or capsule form. Gel capsules are preferable to tea or tincture, because the active ingredients of the herb are fat soluble and do not dissolve well in water.

At home:
Infusion: If you have fresh berries, prepare by steeping ½ to 1 tsp berries per cup of boiling water for 10 minutes. Drink 6 oz, two or three times a day.

Decoction: Add ½ to 1 tsp dried berries to 1 cup water, bring to a boil, and simmer for 5 minutes. Drink three times daily.

Tincture: Drink 15 to 60 drops in water two or three times daily.

SIDE EFFECTS
None expected.

SPECIAL INFORMATION
- WARNING: Do not substitute saw palmetto for medical treatment. Although saw palmetto is thought to be effective for treating an enlarged prostate, it has no known effect against prostate cancer. Because the symptoms of prostate enlargement and prostate cancer are similar, men should see a doctor when they have urological symptoms such as urine retention, dribbling, and passage of blood in the urine.
- Do not use saw palmetto if you are pregnant.

SCALLION

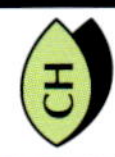

LATIN NAME
Allium Pstulosum

GENERAL DESCRIPTION
The white bulb and green parts of scallions, or spring onions, are prescribed to improve digestion and help regulate the metabolism rate. They affect the body in a manner similar to garlic but are often preferred because of their less powerful odor. Traditional Chinese medicine characterizes the herb as acrid and warm.

TARGET AILMENTS
Take internally for:
- chills and fevers, nasal congestion, abdominal pain and distention.

Apply externally for:
- sores and abscesses.

PREPARATIONS
Over the counter:
Scallions are available at Chinese pharmacies as well as at Asian and Western food markets. You can also obtain tablets containing the herb.

At home:
Tea: Chop two to five scallions and steep in a cup of boiling water. Top the brew with honey and drink at the first signs of chills and fever.

Poultice: Mix scallions with honey, wrap in a cloth, and apply to sores and abscesses.

Combinations: The herb is prepared with soybeans for chills, fever, and nasal congestion. For more information on appropriate preparations and doses, check with a Chinese medicine practitioner.

SIDE EFFECTS
None expected.

SPECIAL INFORMATION

- Do not use scallions if you are sweating profusely, since the herb promotes sweating.
- In a clinical trial, a combination of scallions, pinellia root, and ginger juice, given as an enema, seemed useful in treating acute mastitis (breast inflammation).
- The essential oils of scallions seemed to inhibit the spread of staphylococcus, streptococcus, and other types of bacteria in trials with diseased persons.

SCHISANDRA

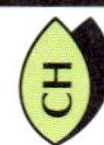

LATIN NAME

Schisandra chinensis

GENERAL DESCRIPTION

The fruit of schisandra, a member of the magnolia family, is valued for its medicinal properties. Look for shiny, purplish red fruit that is thick, fleshy, and oily. Chinese medicine practitioners prescribe it for a variety of disorders as varied as allergic skin reactions, insomnia, and hepatitis. Western herbalists often use it as a tonic to help the body resist physical, biological, and environmental stresses. Traditional Chinese medicine characterizes the fruit as sour and slightly warm.

TARGET AILMENTS

Take internally for:

- chronic coughs and wheezing, asthma.
- allergic skin reactions.
- excessive sweating, insomnia, irritability, forgetfulness, dream-disturbed sleep, general lethargy.
- irregular heartbeat with coughing and thirst, palpitations, shortness of breath.
- hepatitis—to improve liver functions.
- nocturnal emission, vaginal discharge, frequent urination.
- skin irritations.

PREPARATIONS

Dried schisandra fruit is available at Chinese pharmacies, Asian markets, and some Western health food stores. The fruit also comes in tablet form. It is sometimes prepared in wine as a tonic. In 160 proof alcohol, it makes a medicinal wine for itchiness and other irritations of the skin.

Combinations: Schisandra is mixed with zizyphus and Chinese foxglove root to treat insomnia, irritability, and forgetfulness. When combined with Asian ginseng and ophiopogon tuber, it is prescribed for shortness of breath accompanied by coughing and thirst, and for irregular heartbeat or palpitations. Other combinations are used to treat the chronic coughing of tuberculosis. For additional information, consult a Chinese medicine practitioner.

SIDE EFFECTS

Not serious:

Schisandra occasionally causes heartburn. Overdoses can also lead to restlessness, insomnia, or difficulties in breathing.

SPECIAL INFORMATION

- The herb is not recommended for use in the early stages of coughs or rashes.
- In tests with health volunteers, preparations of schisandra seemed to improve visual acuity.
- In one clinical trial, a preparation of schisandra fruit seemed useful in treating patients with infectious hepatitis.

SELECTIVE SEROTONIN REUPTAKE INHIBITORS (SSRIs)

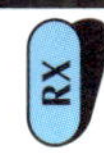

DRUG CLASS

Antidepressants

GENERIC NAMES

fluoxetine, paroxetine, sertraline

GENERAL DESCRIPTION

Drugs in this subclass of antidepressant medications work by restoring the neurotransmitter serotonin to normal levels in the brain. This group includes the widely used drug fluoxetine, which is better known by the brand name Prozac. See ***Antidepressants*** for information about side effects and possible drug interactions.

SPECIAL INFORMATION

- The severity of any side effects may decrease with time (after two weeks) or with lowered dosages. If you have any questions about potential side effects, discuss them with your doctor.

SENNA

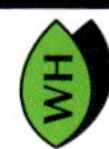

LATIN NAME

Cassia senna

GENERAL DESCRIPTION

Senna is a powerful laxative that should not be taken lightly. This woody shrub contains colon-stimulating chemicals known as anthraquinones, which in high doses act as cathartics, or extremely strong laxatives. Both leaves and seedpods are used medicinally, although the pods are milder. Anthraquinones, derived from senna and other herbs, are among the ingredients of many commercial laxatives. The medicinal use of senna dates to ancient civilizations; it was introduced into European medicine by Arab healers in the ninth century. The herb grows primarily in India and Egypt.

TARGET AILMENTS

- constipation. (Take internally.)

PREPARATIONS

Over the counter:

Available in prepared tea bags, syrups, and tablets, as well as in the form of dried leaves and seedpods.

At home:

Infusion: Steep 1 to 2 tsp dried leaves per cup of cold water and let sit overnight. Drink cold, ½ cup a day, in the morning or at night for a maximum of three days. If desired, offset the bitter taste by adding anise, peppermint, fennel, lemon, or a sweetener.

Decoction: Simmer four chopped pods in 1 cup warm water for 5 to 10 minutes; drink as above.

Tincture: Take ½ to 1 tsp in juice or water once a day in the morning or at night for no more than three days.

SIDE EFFECTS

Not serious:

Mild gastrointestinal cramps (can be offset by drinking cold); skin rash.

Serious:

Large doses can cause diarrhea, nausea, severe stomach cramps, or dehydration. Discontinue use and call your doctor immediately.

SPECIAL INFORMATION

- WARNING: Avoid senna if you are pregnant, nursing, or have gastrointestinal ailments such as ulcers, colitis, or hemorrhoids.
- WARNING: Long-term use of senna can deplete electrolytes, particularly potassium, so you should consult

your physician before taking senna if you are also taking any heart medications.
- Because of senna's strength, try milder laxatives first, such as fiber-rich foods; consider also a gentler anthraquinone.
- Overdependence on senna can result in lazy bowel syndrome; use this herb for no more than three days.

SENNOSIDES

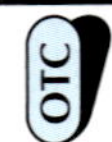

DRUG CLASS
Laxatives

BRAND NAME
Ex-Lax Gentle Natural Laxative Pills

GENERAL DESCRIPTION
A stimulant type of laxative, sennosides is used to relieve constipation. See ***Laxatives*** for additional information about side effects and possible drug interactions.

SPECIAL INFORMATION
- An overdose or prolonged use of this drug may result in an electrolyte imbalance. Symptoms include irregular heartbeat, confusion, unusual tiredness or weakness, and muscle cramps.
- Do not use sennosides or any other stimulant type of laxative if you think you may have an intestinal obstruction.

SEPIA

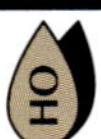

LATIN NAME
Sepia

GENERAL DESCRIPTION
The cuttlefish is a soft-bodied mollusk with eight arms that is closely related to the squid and octopus; it propels itself by squirting jets of water from special organs in its body. When threatened, it releases spurts of dark ink called sepia that cloud the water and camouflage its retreat. Sepia has been used for artistic purposes, although its ingestion, such as when a painter licks the brush, can bring about unpleasant side effects. Homeopathic physicians prescribe *Sepia* to patients with conditions whose symptoms include apathy, moodiness, and weakness. The cuttlefish ink is collected for the homeopathic preparation and diluted with large quantities of milk sugar for final use.

Like most homeopathic prescriptions, *Sepia* was developed as a remedy by observation of the reactions of healthy individuals to a series of undilute doses. The mental, emotional, and physical changes induced by *Sepia* were then cataloged. When a homeopathic practitioner encounters a patient with a set of symptoms that matches the cataloged symptoms brought on by the herb, the practitioner then prescribes it in an extremely dilute form. It is presumed that in this highly dilute dosage, *Sepia* can counter the symptoms that it induces when it is at full strength. For more information on homeopathic medicine, see page 1027.

TARGET AILMENTS
- backaches and weakness in the small of the back, violent fits of coughing, cold sores and fever blisters around the mouth, exhaustion, genital herpes, hair loss, gas, headaches with throbbing pain, sinusitis, urinary incontinence, menopausal hot flashes, menstrual cramps with intense, bearing-down pain, nausea resulting from motion sickness or during pregnancy, brown spots on the skin.

PREPARATIONS
Sepia is available over the counter in various potencies, in both liquid and tablet form, at selected stores and pharmacies. Consult your homeopathic physician for further information.

▼SIDE EFFECTS

None expected.

SERTRALINE

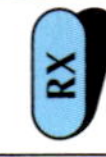

DRUG CLASS
Antidepressants [Selective Serotonin Reuptake Inhibitors (SSRIs)]

BRAND NAME
Zoloft

GENERAL DESCRIPTION
Introduced in 1986, sertraline belongs to a subclass of antidepressants known as selective serotonin reuptake inhibitors (SSRIs) and works by restoring levels of serotonin, an important brain chemical. This medication is prescribed for treatment of depression and obsessive-compulsive disorder. See ***Antidepressants*** for information about side effects and possible drug interactions.

SESAME OIL

LATIN NAME
Sesamum indicum

GENERAL DESCRIPTION
The oil is prepared from large, round, black sesame seeds, which have a sweet taste. Chinese medicine practitioners often prescribe the oil, sometimes called *hu ma you,* for constipation. They also use the sesame seeds as a laxative. Traditional Chinese medicine characterizes sesame oil as sweet and neutral.

TARGET AILMENTS
- constipation; certain types of blurred vision, tinnitus (ringing in the ears), and dizziness; recuperation after severe illness—to help restore the vitality that serious illness depletes. (Take internally.)

PREPARATIONS
Sesame seeds or oil is available at Chinese pharmacies, Asian markets, and Western health food stores. The seeds are also available in tablet form. A tablespoonful of the oil by itself in the evening is considered effective for constipation.

Combinations: Sesame oil is also mixed with therapeutic oils that contain other medicinally useful herbs. One remedy for constipation combines the seeds with chicken eggs; another formula mixes sesame seeds, dong quai, and biota seeds. Chinese medicine practitioners prescribe a combination of sesame seeds and white mulberry leaf for dizziness, blurred vision, tinnitus (ringing in the ears), and headaches. For information on dosages and other preparations, check with a Chinese medicine practitioner.

▼SIDE EFFECTS

None expected.

SPECIAL INFORMATION
- WARNING: Do not use this herb if you have diarrhea.

SHARK LIVER OIL

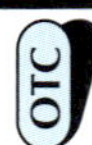

DRUG CLASS
Antihemorrhoid Drugs

BRAND NAME
Preparation H

GENERAL DESCRIPTION
A brown fatty oil, rich in vitamin A, shark liver oil is a skin protectant, a chemically inactive substance that provides a physical barrier between the skin and the environment. Shark liver oil is used only in combination with other skin protectants, such as cocoa butter, lanolin, petrolatum, and glycerin. In hemorrhoid medications, shark liver oil coats the skin in the anorectal area, protecting it against rough, chafing bowel movements. Like other skin protectants, this oil helps prevent loss of moisture for temporary relief of skin irritation and burning associated with hemorrhoids.

TARGET AILMENTS
- burning and itching of the anorectal surface due to hemorrhoids.

SPECIAL INFORMATION
- In case of rectal bleeding or persistent itching, see your physician.

SHEEP SORREL

LATIN NAME
Rumex acetosella

GENERAL DESCRIPTION
Herbalists use the leaves, roots, stems, and flowers of sheep sorrel, a common, native European weed. They believe the herb possesses astringent properties that are helpful for mild ulcerative conditions, such as mouth and throat ulcers. A topical wash of sheep sorrel is also recommended for itchy skin rashes. And the juice of the fresh plant is said to help urinary conditions. Recently sheep sorrel has been used in treating the side effects of chemotherapy. Its mechanism of action is not well understood.

TARGET AILMENTS
Take internally for:
- constipation; diarrhea; cysts; mouth, throat, and stomach ulcers; excessive menstruation.

Apply externally for:
- itchy skin rashes such as hives and poison ivy; mild skin abrasions.

PREPARATIONS
Over the counter:
Available as tinctures, capsules, and prepared tea, or as fresh or dried plant parts (leaves, root, flowers, stems) in combination with other herbs. Capsules may harm the kidneys, so the fresh or dried plant is preferred.

At home:
Infusion: Steep leaves or stems for 5 minutes, or roots for 10 minutes, in hot (not boiling) water and drink two or three times a day.

Tincture: Stir 30 drops into a glass of water and drink 4 glasses (120 drops) daily.

SIDE EFFECTS
Not serious:
Some patients may experience nausea, tingling tongue, severe headache.

Serious:
WARNING: Large doses can be toxic because sheep sorrel contains high levels of oxalic acid, which can cause kidney stones, worsen existing kidney ailments, and otherwise irritate the kidneys.

SPECIAL INFORMATION
- WARNING: If you have kidney problems, do not take sheep sorrel.

SHIITAKE

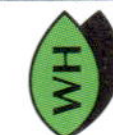

LATIN NAME
Lentinus edodes

GENERAL DESCRIPTION
The shiitake mushroom, a tasty, meaty-flavored fungus that grows on the trunks of dead trees, has long been a staple of Chinese cuisine. And in both China and Japan, shiitake mushrooms have been used for hundreds of years as cancer-fighting agents. Today Chinese herbalists also use the mushroom as a medicine to lower blood cholesterol. The fungus contains cortinelin, a strong antibacterial agent that kills many disease-causing germs. A sulfide component of shiitake mushrooms also has antibiotic properties. Moreover these mushrooms contain a polysaccharide complex called lentinan, which studies indicate may be effective in stimulating the immune system. Herbalists think that this chemical may eventually prove useful in shrinking cancerous tumors; they base this hope on the fact that lentinan has slowed the growth of malignancies in several animal studies.

TARGET AILMENTS
Take internally for:
- high blood cholesterol.
- depressed immune system disorders, chronic fatigue syndrome, and possibly, some forms of cancer. (Use only in consultation with a doctor.)

PREPARATIONS
Over the counter:
Available dried or in capsules.

At home:
Tea: Cover a handful of dried shiitakes with boiling water; soak 10 to 30 minutes. Strain the liquid and drink the tea; you can use the mushrooms in cooking.

Food: After soaking mushrooms in boiling water, eat one a day (many recipes are available) to maintain good health. Chinese medicine practitioners recommend eating two to four ounces of shiitake mushrooms two or three times a week for general health benefits.

SIDE EFFECTS
None expected.

SPECIAL INFORMATION
- Shiitake mushrooms are rich in protein, in vitamins B_1, B_2, B_{12}, niacin, and in pantothenic acid.

SILDENAFIL

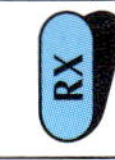

DRUG CLASS
Anti-Impotence Drugs

BRAND NAME
Viagra

GENERAL DESCRIPTION
Sildenafil is the first oral drug approved to treat impotence. In many cases, impotence is caused by a decreased blood flow to the penis. Sildenafil maintains that blood flow and prolongs the erection by delaying the breakdown of a chemical that ordinarily relaxes the smooth muscle in the penis. This drug can prolong an erection following sexual stimulation, but it cannot initiate erection in the absence of sexual arousal.

S

SIDE EFFECTS

Not serious:
Headache, flushing, stomach upset, nasal stuffiness, diarrhea.

Serious:
Dizziness, fainting, painful or prolonged erection, rash, edema (swollen feet or ankles), vision problems, light sensitivity, chest pain, seizures. Call your doctor immediately.

SPECIAL INFORMATION

- WARNING: Do not take sildenafil if you are taking any nitrate medications. The combination could be fatal.
- WARNING: Use sildenafil with caution if you have a cardiovascular disease; increased sexual activity associated with sildenafil has caused cardiac arrest, heart attacks, brain hemorrhages, and other serious cardiovascular events in men with heart conditions.
- Men with liver disease, severe kidney disease, and over age 65 should be started on low doses of this drug.
- Consult your doctor before taking any other prescription or over-the-counter drugs. The effects of either or both medications could be altered.

POSSIBLE INTERACTIONS

Nitrates, either short- or long-acting and including nitrate patches: dangerously low blood pressure levels, perhaps causing death.

SILICA

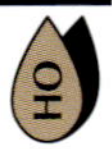

LATIN NAME

Silica

GENERAL DESCRIPTION

Silica, also called flint, is a mineral that is present in the human body in only trace amounts but is vital to the development of bones, the flexibility of cartilage, and the health of the skin and connective tissues. Many industrial operations rely on silica, including the manufacture of concrete, paper, glass, and enamelware. Flint's medicinal use is limited to homeopathy. Minute doses are prescribed for patients with conditions accompanied by excessive sweating, weakness, and extreme sensitivity to cold. For homeopathic use, silica powder is mixed with sodium carbonate through a pharmaceutical process of dry substance dilution.

Like most homeopathic prescriptions, *Silica* was developed as a remedy by observation of the reactions of healthy individuals to a series of undilute doses. The mental, emotional, and physical changes induced by *Silica* were then cataloged. When a homeopathic practitioner encounters a patient with a set of symptoms that matches the cataloged symptoms brought on by *Silica,* the practitioner then prescribes it in an extremely dilute form. It is presumed that in this highly dilute dosage, *Silica* can counter the symptoms that it induces when it is at full strength. For more information on homeopathic medicine, see page 1027.

TARGET AILMENTS

- athlete's foot, constipation resulting from large stools, wounds that are inflamed due to foreign matter, earache with decreased hearing and a stopped-up sensation, fingernails that have white spots and split easily, headaches beginning in the back of the head and spreading forward to the eyes, abscesses, swollen glands in the neck, gum infections, hemorrhoids, breast cysts.

PREPARATIONS

Silica is available over the counter in various potencies, in both liquid and tablet form, at selected stores and pharmacies. Consult your homeopathic physician for further information.

SIDE EFFECTS

None expected.

SIMETHICONE

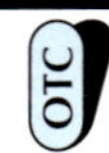

DRUG CLASS

Antigas

BRAND NAMES

Tums Antigas/Antacid formula; some types of Mylanta; Mylanta Gas; some types of Maalox

GENERAL DESCRIPTION

Simethicone is an antigas drug used to relieve the pain, cramping, bloating, intestinal pressure, and "full" sensation that accompany flatulence, or gas. Gas can build up in the gastrointestinal tract as a result of excessive swallowing of air or from eating foods the body does not tolerate well.

The defoaming properties of simethicone act in the gastrointestinal tract to disperse gas bubbles and to prevent their formation. The drug changes the surface tension of small gas bubbles in the stomach, causing them to coalesce and form larger ones. These larger bubbles are more easily expelled through belching or passing flatus. Simethicone is often combined with antacids for the dual relief of gas and heartburn.

TARGET AILMENTS

- symptoms of gas: bloating, abdominal cramps, intestinal pressure, and fullness; postoperative gaseous distention.

SIDE EFFECTS

Not serious:
Simethicone is nontoxic; when used as indicated, the drug produces no side effects. A possible adverse effect could include excessive expulsion of gas in belching or flatus.

SPECIAL INFORMATION

- Do not take this drug if you have kidney disease.
- The adult dosages of this drug are not recommended for treating infant colic. Infant drops are available, but check with your pediatrician for guidance on their use.
- Tablets should be chewed thoroughly before swallowing.
- Do not take this medication for more than two weeks, and do not exceed the recommended dosage.

POSSIBLE INTERACTIONS

- Although unlikely, this drug may interact with some medications. Check with your doctor before using a product containing simethicone if you are taking other drugs.

SIMVASTATIN

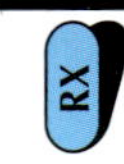

DRUG CLASS

Cholesterol-Reducing Drugs

BRAND NAME

Zocor

GENERAL DESCRIPTION

Introduced in 1986, simvastatin is an HMG-CoA reductase inhibitor, a type of drug that alters the blood levels of cholesterol and other fats. These drugs work by blocking a liver enzyme needed in the production of cholesterol. Simvastatin may also increase the blood level of high-density lipoproteins (HDLs), the so-called good cholesterol that seems to protect against heart disease. See ***Cholesterol-Reducing Drugs.***

SIDE EFFECTS

Not serious:
Constipation, gas.

Serious:
Fever, muscle aches, cramps.

SPECIAL INFORMATION
- If you become pregnant while taking this drug, stop using it immediately and inform your doctor.

POSSIBLE INTERACTIONS

Erythromycin, immunosuppressants, and niacin: severe muscle pain or kidney failure.

Gemfibrozil: may affect the absorption and excretion of simvastatin; do not take concurrently.

SKULLCAP

LATIN NAME
Scutellaria baicalensis

GENERAL DESCRIPTION
Chinese herbalists prescribe the long, thick, skinless yellow root of skullcap for a wide range of disorders. In traditional Chinese medicine skullcap is characterized as bitter and cold.

TARGET AILMENTS
Take internally for:
- diarrhea, dysentery.
- upper-respiratory infections with fever.
- urinary tract infections, jaundice, hepatitis.
- nervous tension, irritability, headache, insomnia, epilepsy and other seizures.
- red face or eyes.
- coughing up or vomiting blood, nosebleeds, blood in the stool.
- abdominal pain and vaginal bleeding, threatened miscarriage during pregnancy, premenstrual stress.

PREPARATIONS
Skullcap root is available in bulk from Chinese pharmacies, Asian markets, and Western health food stores. You can also obtain the herb as pills.

The root is usually decocted. Before decocting, it can be fried dry for use in pregnancy and to treat diarrhea and infections of the urinary tract, or cooked in wine for upper-respiratory infections and redness of the face and eyes.

Combinations: A mixture with coptis is prescribed for high fever and irritability. Skullcap root mixed with anemarrhena is thought to alleviate chronic coughs. For further information on preparations and doses, consult a Chinese medicine practitioner.

SIDE EFFECTS

None expected.

SPECIAL INFORMATION
- Before using skullcap to treat diarrhea or problems of pregnancy, check with a Chinese medicine practitioner.
- The root seemed to have a diuretic effect in laboratory tests on healthy animals and humans.
- Skullcap has been shown to have broad antimicrobial effect in the laboratory.

POSSIBLE INTERACTIONS

Some sources in traditional Chinese medicine suggest that skullcap counteracts the effects of moutan and veratrum.

SKULLCAP

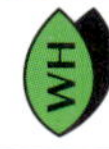

LATIN NAME
Scutellaria lateriflora

GENERAL DESCRIPTION
The leaves and blue flowers of this two-foot-tall perennial are used as an ingredient in many over-the-counter herbal sleep remedies. Some researchers, especially in Europe and Asia, report that skullcap contains chemicals that calm the nervous system. Chinese medicine physicians believe that skullcap is effective for treating hepatitis, a serious liver disease. In the United States, however, skullcap is considered controversial and even useless by many medical authorities, at least partly because of its early—and unearned—reputation for curing rabies, for which it garnered the now archaic name of mad dog weed. Its current name comes from an elongated, caplike appendage on the upper lip of the flower.

TARGET AILMENTS
Take internally for:
- nervous tension, headaches and muscle aches caused by tension, insomnia, convulsions, drug or alcohol withdrawal.
- symptoms of premenstrual syndrome aggravated or caused by stress.

PREPARATIONS

Over the counter:
Available as prepared tea, tinctures, dried leaves, capsules.

At home:
Tea: Pour a cup of boiling water over 2 tsp dried leaves and steep for 10 to 15 minutes; drink this amount up to three times daily.

Tincture: Take ½ to 1 tsp per 8-oz glass of warm water.

SIDE EFFECTS

Not serious:
Stomach upset or diarrhea. Reduce intake or stop using it.

SPECIAL INFORMATION
- WARNING: Skullcap may cause drowsiness. Do not operate a car or heavy machinery after taking it.
- WARNING: Large amounts of the tincture may cause confusion, giddiness, twitching, and possibly, convulsions.
- Use skullcap in medicinal amounts only under professional supervision.
- Two Japanese animal studies showed that skullcap increases levels of the "good" kind of cholesterol, raising the possibility that skullcap may one day be useful in preventing heart disease and strokes.

SLIPPERY ELM

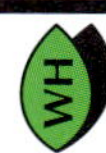

LATIN NAME
Ulmus fulva

GENERAL DESCRIPTION
The U.S. Food and Drug Administration calls slippery elm a good demulcent, or soothing agent. Herbalists recommend its use externally to ease wounds and skin problems, and internally to soothe sore throats, coughing, and diarrhea and other gastrointestinal disorders. Slippery elm's active ingredient is found in the white inner bark, whose mucilaginous cells expand into a spongy mass when mixed with water. Elm trees were prized in the 18th and 19th centuries by American settlers, for whom slippery elm was a valuable cure. They soaked it in water and applied it to wounds, where it dried into a natural bandage. In addition, they wrapped it around meats and other perishable foods to prevent spoilage. Mixed with water, it made a soothing gruel for children and sick people. While lozenges,

powder, and other elm products are still available in health food stores, the great elm forests once common throughout the East Coast of the United States have been ravaged by Dutch elm disease.

TARGET AILMENTS
Apply externally for:
- wounds, cuts, abrasions.

Take internally for:
- coughing, sore throats, digestive complaints.

Use externally and internally for:
- gynecological problems.

PREPARATIONS
Over the counter:
Available as capsules, tea, powder.

At home:
Poultice: For wounds that have been thoroughly cleaned with soap and water, moisten powdered bark with enough water to make a paste; apply to wound and allow to dry. This forms a natural bandage that delivers soothing agents to the wound.

Tea: Add 2 tsp powder to a cup of boiling water; simmer for 15 minutes. Drink up to 3 cups a day for throat, digestive, and gynecological problems.

Food: Mix slippery elm powder with water or milk until it has the consistency of a thin porridge.

SIDE EFFECTS
Some people may be allergic to the powdered bark. If you experience any problems, stop using it. Consult your doctor before taking doses that are larger than recommended.

SPECIAL INFORMATION
- Consult your doctor if your symptoms do not improve significantly within two weeks.

SMOKING CESSATION DRUGS

GENERIC NAMES
bupropion, nicotine

GENERAL DESCRIPTION
Smoking cessation drugs are used to reduce nicotine craving and withdrawal effects in people who want to stop smoking. By slowly reducing nicotine intake with nicotine replacements, or by changing the brain chemistry with bupropion, these products can reduce smoking-withdrawal effects, such as irritability, nervousness, drowsiness, fatigue, headache, and nicotine craving. There is no evidence that these drugs work unless the smoker participates in a medically supervised stop-smoking program. For more information, see ***Nicotine*** and ***Bupropion.***

SODIUM BICARBONATE AND CITRIC ACID

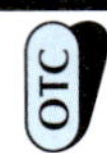

DRUG CLASS
Antacids

BRAND NAME
Alka-Seltzer

GENERAL DESCRIPTION
The combination of sodium bicarbonate and citric acid is used to relieve symptoms of upset and sour stomach, acid indigestion, and heartburn. The drug is absorbed quickly and easily into the body. If taken by itself for a long time, sodium bicarbonate may cause systemic alkalosis, a condition in which the blood becomes less acidic than normal. This can adversely affect the blood and kidneys. Citric acid is added to sodium bicarbonate to add acidity to the stomach and help correct the imbalance. See ***Antacids*** for information about additional side effects and possible drug interactions.

SPECIAL INFORMATION
- Do not take antacids containing sodium if you have high blood pressure, congestive heart failure, cirrhosis, renal failure, or edema, or if you are on a low-sodium diet; the high sodium content of the drugs may exacerbate these problems.

SPEARMINT

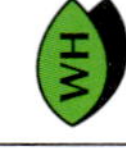

LATIN NAME
Mentha spicata

GENERAL DESCRIPTION
Spearmint has been valued since ancient times to promote digestion, heal wounds, and relieve colds and congestion. When the lance-shaped, serrated leaves are crushed or boiled, they release carvone, a chemical similar to but milder than the menthol found in peppermint, a close relative. Modern herbalists suggest using spearmint externally for itching and inflammation, and internally for digestive ailments, colds, and insomnia.

This perennial, fast-spreading plant, which has distinctive whorls of small white, pink, or lilac flowers, is praised in an Egyptian papyrus deemed the world's oldest surviving medical text. Spearmint was used by the Greeks and Romans for ailments from hiccups to leprosy. Chinese and Ayurvedic (Hindu) physicians have used it for centuries to treat indigestion, colds, coughs, and fever. Many herbalists prescribe spearmint and peppermint interchangeably as medicines, although the latter is considered more potent.

TARGET AILMENTS
Take internally for:
- upset stomach, stomach spasms, flatulence, heartburn, stomach cramps, morning sickness during pregnancy.
- nasal, sinus, and chest congestion; colds; headache; sore mouth or throat.

Take internally and apply externally for:
- muscle pains, external infections, chapped hands.

PREPARATIONS
Over the counter:
Available as capsules, prepared tea, fresh or dried leaves, tinctures, oil.

At home:
Tea: Boil 1 to 2 tsp dried herb or several fresh leaves per cup of water; steep 10 minutes. Drink up to 3 cups a day.

Tincture: Add ¼ to 1 tsp to an 8-oz glass of water and drink up to three glasses a day.

Herbal bath: Fill a cloth bag with a few handfuls of dried or fresh spearmint leaves and add to running bathwater.

SIDE EFFECTS
None expected.

SPECIAL INFORMATION
- Spearmint oil (carvone) may cause stomach upset if ingested. The oil is recommended for external use only.
- For children under two, dilute spearmint tea or tincture with water.

SUCRALFATE

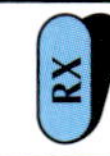

DRUG CLASS
Antiulcer Drugs

BRAND NAME
Carafate

GENERAL DESCRIPTION
Sucralfate is used primarily in the treatment and prevention of ulcers of the stomach and duodenum (first portion of the small intestine). It is also sometimes used to treat gastroesophageal reflux and gastrointestinal symptoms associated with the use of nonsteroidal anti-inflammatory drugs (NSAIDs) and aspirin.

The precise mechanisms by which sucralfate works are not clearly understood. However, the drug is believed to inhibit the digestive action of pepsin, one of the stomach's digestive juices. Sucralfate may also form a coating over ulcers, protecting them from the erosive effect of another digestive fluid, hydrochloric acid. Although sucralfate is often used alone, it is sometimes prescribed in conjunction with antacids for pain relief. For more information on side effects and other possible drug interactions, see ***Antiulcer Drugs.***

SIDE EFFECTS
Not serious:
Constipation, mild back pain. Rare: diarrhea, nausea, vomiting, stomach cramping, dry mouth, rash, itching, dizziness, drowsiness. See your doctor if these symptoms continue or become bothersome.

Serious:
None expected.

SPECIAL INFORMATION
- Sucralfate may interfere with the absorption of vitamins A, D, E, and K; if you are taking vitamin supplements, wait an hour before taking a dose of sucralfate.
- If you are also using antacids for relief from ulcer pain, take the antacid at least 30 minutes before or after taking sucralfate.
- Because this drug may cause dizziness or drowsiness, you may need to restrict your driving or your involvement in other potentially hazardous activities.
- If you have had kidney or liver disease or any diseases that have caused obstruction of the gastrointestinal tract, weigh carefully the risks and benefits of using this drug.

POSSIBLE INTERACTIONS
Aluminum-containing antidiarrheal drugs, aspirin buffered with aluminum, and aluminum-containing vaginal douches: increased absorption of aluminum into the body, possibly to toxic levels.

Vitamins A, D, E, and K: decreased absorption of these vitamins.

SULFAMETHOXAZOLE AND TRIMETHOPRIM

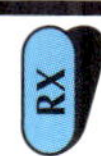

DRUG CLASS
Antibiotics [Sulfonamides in Combination]

BRAND NAME
Bactrim, Cotrim, Septra

GENERAL DESCRIPTION
Sulfamethoxazole, a sulfonamide antibiotic, is often combined with the antibiotic drug trimethoprim to increase the effectiveness of both medications. This combination is sometimes known as cotrimoxazole or TMP-SMZ. Both component drugs work by interfering with the ability of certain disease-causing bacteria to synthesize folic acid, thereby inhibiting the organisms' growth. For more information, see ***Sulfonamides in Combination.***

TARGET AILMENTS
- bronchitis (caused by *Hemophilus influenzae* or *Streptococcus pneumoniae*).
- urinary tract infections.
- enterocolitis (caused by certain species of *Shigella*).
- acute otitis media (in children).
- prevention and treatment of pneumonia *(Pneumocystis carinii)* in people with compromised immune systems (including AIDS patients).
- traveler's diarrhea.
- numerous other infections.

SIDE EFFECTS
Not serious:
Gastrointestinal problems (including diarrhea and nausea), headache or dizziness, photosensitivity. Let your doctor know if these symptoms become troublesome.

Serious:
Allergic reactions (fever, itching skin rash). Less frequently: blood abnormalities causing fever, sore throat, unusual bleeding, bruising, tiredness, or weakness; liver problems, including jaundice; Stevens-Johnson syndrome (fever, skin blisters or blisters and open sores on mucous membranes and genitals, weakness, joint pain). Rarely: urinary problems resulting in burning with urination, back pain; goiter; bluish fingernails, skin, or lips; difficulty in breathing. Call your doctor immediately.

SPECIAL INFORMATION
- Pregnant and nursing women should avoid using this combination since it may interfere with folic acid metabolism in the fetus and infant, especially near birth.
- Cotrimoxazole may cause sensitivity to the sun or sunlamps. Limit your exposure while on this drug.
- Cross-sensitivity reactions: If you are sensitive to thiazide diuretics, PABA, local anesthetics (benzocaine), or oral antidiabetic medicines, you may also have sensitivity to cotrimoxazole. Advise your doctor of your sensitivity.
- Many people are sensitive to these drugs, so be sure to tell your doctor if you have severe allergies or bronchial asthma.
- To prevent reinfection, complete the full course of your medication.
- When taking these drugs, drink plenty of fluids to prevent formation of crystals in the urine.

POSSIBLE INTERACTIONS
This combination can interact with a number of drugs, especially those that affect the liver or blood. Consult your doctor before taking any other medication.

Anticoagulants (warfarin), anticonvulsants (hydantoin), oral antidiabetics, phenylbutazone (NSAID), or sulfinpyrazone (antigout): may interfere with action or metabolism of these drugs and could result in increased effects or toxicity. Your doctor may need to adjust the dosage.

Birth-control pills containing estrogen: may result in decreased contraceptive effectiveness and increased breakthrough bleeding.

Cyclosporine: decreased effectiveness of cyclosporine.

Digoxin: decreased digoxin effects.

Methotrexate: increased methotrexate effects.

SULFONAMIDES IN COMBINATION

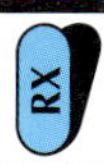

GENERAL DESCRIPTION
Sulfonamides, a subclass of antibiotics, are synthetic derivatives of a compound that interferes with the ability of bacteria to produce folic acid, necessary for cell growth and development. While this doesn't immediately kill bacteria, it inhibits their growth and aids the body in its fight against infection. These drugs are often used in combinations to enhance the effectiveness of other medications and to offset possible bacterial resistance to sulfonamides. For information about a specific sulfonamide, see ***Sulfamethoxazole and Trimethoprim.***

SPECIAL INFORMATION

- Antibiotics affect not only harmful bacteria, but also "good" bacteria that keep unwanted fungi and intestinal organisms in check. Eating yogurt containing *Lactobacillus acidophilus* culture or taking acidophilus tablets may help restore the body's normal bacteria.
- Prolonged use of any antibiotic drug can lead to fungal infections, including candidiasis, or to serious bacterial infections such as pseudomembranous colitis.

SULFONYLUREAS

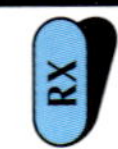

GENERAL DESCRIPTION

Sulfonylureas form a subclass of antidiabetic drugs also known as oral hypoglycemics. For more information about medications used to treat diabetes, see ***Antidiabetic Drugs, Insulin,*** and ***Oral Hypoglycemics.***

SULPHUR

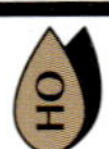

LATIN NAME

Sulphur

GENERAL DESCRIPTION

The chemical element sulphur, or more commonly sulfur, is present in all living tissue. It was known to ancient societies, and in the Bible it is called brimstone. Among the various conditions to which it has been applied as a medication, for some 2,000 years, are skin disorders such as scabies. Commercially, sulfur is used in the production of dyes, fungicides, and gunpowder. Homeopathic physicians may prescribe dilute doses of the remedy *Sulphur* to treat conditions accompanied by irritability, intense itching, burning pains, and offensive odors. The homeopathic remedy is made from pure sulfur powder that is diluted with either milk sugar or a water-and-alcohol solution.

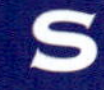

Like most homeopathic prescriptions, *Sulphur* was developed as a remedy by observation of the reactions of healthy individuals to a series of undilute doses. The mental, emotional, and physical changes induced by *Sulphur* were then cataloged. When a homeopathic practitioner encounters a patient with a set of symptoms that matches the cataloged symptoms brought on by *Sulphur,* the practitioner then prescribes it in an extremely dilute form. It is presumed that in this highly dilute dosage, *Sulphur* can counter the symptoms that it induces when it is at full strength. For more information on homeopathic medicine, see page 1027.

TARGET AILMENTS

- asthma that is worse at night and is accompanied by rattling mucus, cough with chest pain, morning diarrhea, eye inflammation, bursitis, headaches with burning pain, indigestion, joint pain, anal itching with redness, burning vaginal discharge, eczema with intense itching and burning.

PREPARATIONS

Sulphur is available over the counter in various potencies, in both liquid and tablet form, at selected stores and pharmacies. Consult your homeopathic physician for further information.

SIDE EFFECTS

None expected.

SUMATRIPTAN

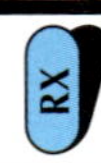

DRUG CLASS

Antimigraine Drugs

BRAND NAME

Imitrex

GENERAL DESCRIPTION

Introduced in 1993, sumatriptan is an antimigraine drug used to treat classic migraine headaches (those preceded by the warning sensation known as an aura) as well as common migraines (those without an aura). The drug—originally sold only in injectable form but now also available as a tablet and as a nasal spray—provides fast relief from the intense pain associated with these types of headaches.

Sumatriptan, a vasoconstrictor, works by narrowing dilated blood vessels and reducing the amount of blood flowing through them. Swollen cranial blood vessels are believed to be a major cause of migraine headaches. Sumatriptan may also act as an anti-inflammatory, which appears to further reduce the swelling. In addition, the medication relieves the nausea, vomiting, and intense light and sound sensitivity that frequently accompany migraines.

TARGET AILMENTS

- migraine headaches.

SIDE EFFECTS

Not serious:

Tightness in the chest, jaw, or neck immediately after the drug is injected; pain, redness, or burning at the injection site; nausea or vomiting; dizziness or fainting; drowsiness; flushing, tingling, or numbness; confusion; excessive thirst; frequent urination. If these effects continue for more than an hour, contact your doctor.

Serious:

Continuing pain or tightness in the chest; swelling of the face, lips, or eyelids; wheezing, changes in heart rate or blood pressure; skin rash; difficulty in swallowing or breathing. If you notice these symptoms, call your doctor immediately.

SPECIAL INFORMATION

- Do not use this drug if you have ever had an allergic reaction to it.
- Do not use sumatriptan for the treatment of hemiplegic (restricted to one side of the head) or basilar (restricted to the base of the skull) migraine.
- Do not use this drug if you have uncontrolled high blood pressure (hypertension) or Prinzmetal's angina, or if you have had a heart attack or stroke.
- Inform your doctor and use this drug with caution if you are pregnant or nursing; or if you have liver, kidney, or heart disease; coronary artery disease; heart arrhythmia; Raynaud's syndrome; or epilepsy; or are taking high blood pressure medications or other prescription or over-the-counter drugs, especially other migraine-relieving medications.
- Take at the first sign of a migraine. If your first dose fails to relieve your migraine, do not take a second one without first checking with your doctor.

POSSIBLE INTERACTIONS

Alcohol: may cause excess sedation and make headaches worse.

Ergotamine: may increase the effects of sumatriptan. Allow at least 24 hours between taking ergotamine and sumatriptan.

Lithium, MAO inhibitors, antidepressants: may result in excessive quantities of the neurotransmitter serotonin in the brain.

TAMOXIFEN

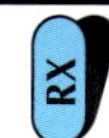

DRUG CLASS
Anticancer Drugs

BRAND NAME
Nolvadex

GENERAL DESCRIPTION
Tamoxifen is an antiestrogen drug used to prevent or delay the recurrence of breast cancer after primary therapy, including breast surgery, radiation therapy, and chemotherapy. The drug may be given in conjunction with chemotherapy treatments after surgery or used alone to treat metastatic breast cancer.

TARGET AILMENTS
- breast cancer (in women and men, although male breast cancer is rare).

SIDE EFFECTS

Not serious:
Hot flashes, nausea, vomiting, skin rash, menstrual irregularities, genital itching, increased flaring pain in tumor or bone, and impotence and loss of libido in men. Consult your doctor if these effects continue or are bothersome.

Serious:
Changes in vaginal bleeding or discharge; confusion. Call your doctor promptly. Rarely, these risks may be associated with use of this drug: thrombotic events, including pulmonary embolism (shortness of breath), deep vein thrombosis, or superficial phlebitis; liver damage (no symptoms); retinopathy, cataracts, corneal changes; abnormally high blood calcium levels (confusion); endometrial cancer, endometrial polyps, or endometrial hyperplasia (abnormal vaginal bleeding, pain or pressure in pelvis, change in vaginal discharge); low white blood cell count (fever, infections) or low platelet count (bleeding). Call your doctor promptly.

SPECIAL INFORMATION
- Do not use tamoxifen if you have had a serious adverse reaction to it.
- Tell your doctor if you have ever had thrombophlebitis, pulmonary embolism, impaired liver function, cataracts, a blood cell or bone-marrow disorder, or abnormally high blood calcium levels. Your doctor may lower your dose of tamoxifen or prescribe a different drug.
- This drug may decrease your blood cell counts, so use with caution if you have significantly low levels of white blood cells or platelets.
- Maintain routine gynecologic care while taking tamoxifen. Report abnormal vaginal bleeding to your doctor.
- Do not use hormonal contraceptives with tamoxifen because they decrease tamoxifen's effects.
- Do not use tamoxifen during pregnancy or breast-feeding, or become pregnant while using this drug.

POSSIBLE INTERACTIONS

Antacids and some antiulcer drugs (cimetidine, famotidine, and ranitidine): prematurely dissolve tamoxifen's enteric coating. Take these medications one to two hours before taking tamoxifen.

Anticancer drugs (bleomycin, daunorubicin, doxorubicin, fluorouracil, hydroxyurea, methotrexate, mitotane, mitoxantrone, procarbazine, and vincristine): increased risk of thromboembolism.

Anticoagulants (such as warfarin): increased anticoagulant effect.

Estrogen or oral contraceptives: decreased tamoxifen effect.

TANGERINE PEEL

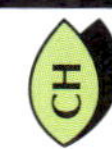

LATIN NAME
Citrus reticulata

GENERAL DESCRIPTION
Sometimes called mandarin orange peel, this herb is prescribed for digestive disorders. Chinese medicine practitioners believe that the peel gets better as it ages, and its Chinese name, *chén pí,* can be translated into English as "aged peel." The best samples of the fruit are thin-skinned, pliable, oily, and fragrant. Chinese herbalists characterize the herb as acrid, bitter, and warm.

TARGET AILMENTS
- indigestion, gas; a feeling of swelling, bloatedness, or fullness in the abdomen; nausea and vomiting; loose stools; bringing up phlegm. (Take internally.)

PREPARATIONS
Tangerine peel is available at any Chinese pharmacy or Asian food market, as well as at Western health food stores. It is also available as pills.

Combinations: In a preparation with Asian ginseng, tangerine peel is used as a digestive stimulant. Chinese herbalists prescribe a mixture of tangerine peel, ripe bitter orange, and aucklandia for abdominal distention, fullness, and pain. And a preparation containing tangerine peel and pinellia root is used to treat a stifling feeling in the chest that makes deep breathing difficult, together with an excess of phlegm. For further information on appropriate preparations and doses, check with an herbal practitioner.

SIDE EFFECTS
None expected.

SPECIAL INFORMATION
- Do not use this herb if you have a dry cough or an excessively red tongue, or if you are spitting up blood.
- A mixture of aged tangerine peel and licorice has been used in a clinical study to treat mastitis (inflammation of the breast).
- Herbalists use the red part of tangerine peel (when dried, some parts are orange and others red) to control vomiting and belching.
- Chinese practitioners also prescribe young, or green, tangerine peel for breast and side pain and for hernia pain. The green peel has recently been used to raise blood pressure when it is too low.

TEA TREE OIL

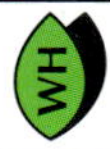

LATIN NAME
Melaleuca spp.

GENERAL DESCRIPTION
The first Europeans to reach Australia made tea from the leaves of what then became known as the tea tree, which should not be confused with the common tea plant. For centuries before the Europeans arrived, native Australians were using the leaves of this tree as an antiseptic. Eventually the Europeans learned to use the leaves' volatile oil to treat cuts, abrasions, burns, insect bites, and other minor skin ailments. Modern studies show that the strong germicidal activity of tea tree oil is caused primarily by a single ingredient, terpineol. The oil, which smells like nutmeg, is extracted from the leaves by steam distillation. During World War II, tea tree oil was added to machine oils to reduce infections in the hands of workers during metal fabrication. The oils of some species of *Melaleuca* may irritate the skin and are not used.

TARGET AILMENTS
Apply externally for:
- cuts, abrasions, insect bites, acne seen

in teenagers, fungal infections such as athlete's foot, and other skin ailments.
- minor vaginal infections. (Use as a douche.)
- flea shampoos for pets.

PREPARATIONS
Over the counter:
Available as oil and also as an additive to health and beauty products such as toothpaste, soap, and shampoo.

At home:
Apply fresh leaves directly to wounds.

SIDE EFFECTS
Not serious:
Local skin and vaginal irritation may develop in sensitive individuals. Let your doctor know if it persists.

SPECIAL INFORMATION
- People with sensitive skin should dilute tea tree oil with a bland oil, such as vegetable oil.

TEMAZEPAM

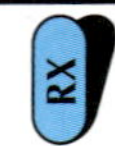

DRUG CLASS
Antianxiety Drugs [Benzodiazepines]

BRAND NAME
Restoril

GENERAL DESCRIPTION
A mild sedative-hypnotic, temazepam is prescribed for the short-term treatment of insomnia. See ***Benzodiazepines*** for information on side effects and possible drug interactions.

SPECIAL INFORMATION
- Do not use this drug unless you can allow yourself seven or eight hours of sleep every night for the duration of the treatment. If you don't give the medication time to wear off, you may experience temporary amnesia, perhaps lasting several hours.

TERAZOSIN

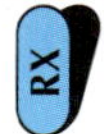

DRUG CLASS
Alpha$_1$-Adrenergic Blockers

BRAND NAME
Hytrin

GENERAL DESCRIPTION
Introduced in 1987, terazosin is one of several alpha-adrenergic blocking agents used in the treatment of high blood pressure (hypertension). It can be used alone or in combination with other drugs, depending on the degree of hypertension. For more information, see ***Alpha$_1$-Adrenergic Blockers.***

SIDE EFFECTS
Not serious:
Although rare, a slight (two- to three-pound) weight gain is possible with use of this drug.

SPECIAL INFORMATION
- You should not take terazosin if you have ever had an allergic or unusual reaction to it, or to doxazosin or prazosin.

TERBUTALINE

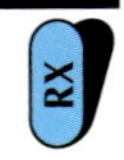

DRUG CLASS
Bronchodilators

BRAND NAMES
Brethaire, Brethine, Bricanyl

GENERAL DESCRIPTION
Introduced in 1974, terbutaline is prescribed to relieve the symptoms of bronchial asthma and the asthmalike symptoms of chronic bronchitis and emphysema. The drug may also be used to inhibit premature labor. See ***Bronchodilators*** for information about side effects and possible drug interactions.

TERCONAZOLE

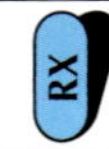

DRUG CLASS
Antifungal Drugs [Vaginal Antifungal Drugs]

BRAND NAME
Terazol

GENERAL DESCRIPTION
The antifungal drug terconazole is available in vaginal creams and suppositories for the treatment of vaginal yeast infections (candidiasis). A common side effect of terconazole is headache, which afflicts about one-fourth of the women who use the medication. For more information about this drug, including other side effects as well as possible drug interactions, see ***Antifungal Drugs*** and ***Vaginal Antifungal Drugs.***

TETRACYCLINE

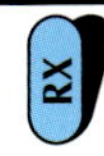

DRUG CLASS
Antibiotics [Tetracyclines]

BRAND NAME
Sumycin

GENERAL DESCRIPTION
Introduced in 1953, tetracycline is an antibiotic drug produced or derived from a strain of bacteria known as *Streptomyces aureofaciens* and used to treat a wide range of bacteria-caused diseases. Like most other drugs of its type, tetracycline should be taken on an empty stomach. See ***Tetracyclines*** for information about side effects and possible drug interactions.

TETRACYCLINES

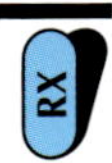

GENERIC NAMES
doxycycline, tetracycline

GENERAL DESCRIPTION
Tetracyclines are natural or semisynthetic antibiotics developed from a particular strain of bacteria. The drugs work by inhibiting protein synthesis in certain disease-causing bacteria, including many that cause sexually transmitted diseases. Tetracyclines are also useful in treating many mosquito- and tick-borne diseases, such as Rocky Mountain spotted fever.

Tetracyclines are important for combating bacterial strains resistant to penicillin, or for use by patients who are sensitive or allergic to penicillin or other antibiotics. They are also useful for treating serious acne, which can cause lesions and scarring. Although their full actions in treating acne are not known, tetracyclines reduce concentrations of fatty acids in oil-gland secretions, suppress inflammation, and kill susceptible bacteria on the skin. These effects probably combine to reduce acne lesions. For more information, see the entries for the generic drugs listed above.

TARGET AILMENTS

- some sexually transmitted diseases, including syphilis, gonorrhea, and chlamydia.
- urinary tract infections.
- acne vulgaris (characterized by lesions and cysts).
- mosquito-borne diseases, such as malaria, and tick-borne diseases, such as Rocky Mountain spotted fever and Lyme disease.
- infections of the skin and soft tissue.
- prevention and treatment of chronic bronchitis and pneumonia.
- sinusitis.
- certain peptic ulcers.

SIDE EFFECTS

Not serious:
Lightheadedness, dizziness, gastrointestinal upsets (cramps, burning sensation in stomach, diarrhea, nausea, vomiting), photosensitivity. Less frequently: fungal infection of the mouth, genital, or rectal area; darkening or discoloration of the tongue. Let your doctor know if these symptoms persist or become troublesome.

Serious:
Discoloration of the teeth in infants or children, serious photosensitivity, apparent symptoms of diabetes (noticeable increase in volume of urine or frequency of urination, increased thirst, unusual tiredness or weakness). Rarely: liver or pancreas toxicity (yellowing of skin, abdominal pain, nausea, vomiting). Call your doctor immediately.

SPECIAL INFORMATION

- Tetracyclines kill not only harmful bacteria, but also "good" bacteria that keep unwanted fungi and intestinal organisms in check. Eating yogurt containing *Lactobacillus acidophilus* culture (or taking acidophilus tablets) may help restore the body's normal bacteria.
- Prolonged use of any antibiotic drug can lead to fungal infections, including candidiasis, or to bacterial infections such as pseudomembranous colitis.
- Tetracyclines should not be taken by pregnant or nursing women or by children under nine years of age. The drugs may cause permanent discoloration of teeth, underdevelopment of tooth enamel, and skeletal growth problems in the fetus, in nursing infants, and in young children who take them.
- Tetracyclines may cause liver toxicity or renal problems in some individuals.
- Do not take these drugs with milk or dairy products. Take tetracyclines one to two hours before or two to three hours after consuming dairy products.
- Never take outdated tetracyclines or those that have changed in color, taste, or appearance; they may break down into toxic substances in the body.
- These drugs may cause increased sensitivity to the sun or to sunlamps. Limit your exposure while on these medications.
- Most tetracyclines (except doxycycline) should be taken on an empty stomach.

POSSIBLE INTERACTIONS

Tell your doctor if you are taking lithium, insulin, digoxin, or an anticoagulant drug. Your dosage of these drugs may need to be adjusted.

Antacids, bicarbonate of soda, calcium, iron, laxatives, magnesium supplements: decreased absorption of tetracyclines. Take tetracyclines one to two hours before or two to three hours after taking any of these products.

Cholesterol-reducing drugs, such as cholestyramine: reduced absorption and effectiveness of tetracyclines. Allow several hours to pass between doses of tetracyclines and these drugs.

Cimetidine (antiulcer): may decrease absorption of tetracycline.

Estrogen-containing contraceptives or medications: reduced birth-control effect; possible pregnancy or breakthrough bleeding.

Penicillins: may interfere with tetracyclines, reducing effect of both drugs.

THEOPHYLLINE

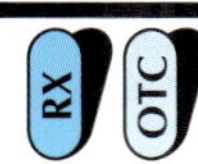

DRUG CLASS

Bronchodilators

BRAND NAMES

Rx: Slo-Bid, Theo-Dur

OTC: Primatene Dual Action Formula, Primatene Tablets

GENERAL DESCRIPTION

Introduced in 1900, theophylline is an antiasthmatic drug that acts by relaxing the muscles in the bronchial tubes as well as the blood vessels in the lungs. It is prescribed for symptoms of acute bronchial asthma, chronic bronchitis, and emphysema, and to help prevent bronchial-asthma episodes. Theophylline may be combined with other drugs such as ephedrine to provide additional relief of asthma symptoms, and with mild sedatives to relieve anxiety from asthma attacks. For information about side effects and possible drug interactions, see ***Bronchodilators.***

THYROID HORMONES

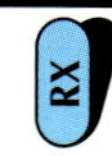

GENERIC NAMES

levothyroxine, thyroid USP

GENERAL DESCRIPTION

Thyroid hormones are naturally or synthetically produced drugs—usually given orally—that are used to replace or supplement the normal secretions of the thyroid gland. Most preparations contain a mixture of several different thyroid hormones in varying ratios.

Hormones produced by the thyroid gland regulate functions such as metabolism and protein synthesis, general body growth, and development of the bones and central nervous system. They also affect the heart rate. Thyroid hormone therapy usually must be maintained throughout the patient's life unless it is prescribed for a transient condition that may affect thyroid function.

Because these hormones are so critical to normal growth and development, children should be tested to ensure that their thyroid glands are functioning normally; those whose bodies are not producing sufficient quantities must be given supplemental thyroid hormones as soon as possible. Thyroid medications are sometimes used diagnostically to check for thyroid disease.

TARGET AILMENTS

- hypothyroidism (underactive or nonfunctioning thyroid) or as treatment following removal of thyroid gland.
- goiter (enlargement of thyroid).
- some types of thyroid cancer, especially after radiation therapy to the neck.

SIDE EFFECTS

Not serious:
Rarely, except at beginning of treatment, changes in menstrual periods, clumsiness, coldness, constipation, dry puffy skin, headache, sleepiness, tiredness, heart palpitations, weakness, muscle aches, weight gain. Call your doctor if these effects persist or are troublesome. (Some hair loss may occur in children during early treatment, but this condition is usually temporary.)

T

Serious:
Rarely, allergic reactions such as skin rash or hives, severe persistent and ongoing headache, changes in menstrual periods, changes in appetite, chest pain, irregular heartbeat, fever, hand tremors, irritability, leg cramps, nervousness, sensitivity to heat, sweating, weight loss. Contact your doctor, who may reduce the dosage.

SPECIAL INFORMATION
- Your doctor may tell you to continue using thyroid hormones while you're pregnant or nursing. Although small amounts of these hormones may cross the placenta or be present in breast milk, no studies have shown harm to the fetus or breast-feeding baby.
- Tell your doctor if you have cardiovascular disease, or diabetes or other hormone problems such as low pituitary gland secretions. Your doctor may decide not to use thyroid hormones or to lower the dosage.

POSSIBLE INTERACTIONS

Anticoagulant and antiplatelet drugs (such as warfarin): increased anticlotting action. Your doctor may have to adjust the dosage of anticlotting drugs.

Antidepressants, including tricyclic antidepressants such as amitriptyline: increased action and side effects of both combined drugs, leading to heart-rhythm problems and other signs of excess stimulation.

Antidiabetic drugs (such as insulin): increased need for insulin or other diabetic drugs, perhaps leading to higher blood sugar levels. Your doctor may need to adjust your insulin dose.

Cholesterol-reducing drugs (such as cholestyramine): blocked or delayed absorption of thyroid hormones, decreasing their effectiveness. Take thyroid hormones one hour before or four to five hours after cholesterol-reducing drugs.

Heart-stimulating drugs (such as epinephrine or pseudoephedrine): increased effects of both combined drugs, potentially causing heart problems or increased chance of thyroid hormone overdose.

Other hormones (such as estrogen): may interfere with thyroid hormone action, requiring higher doses.

THYROID USP

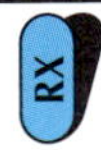

DRUG CLASS
Thyroid Hormones

BRAND NAME
Armour Thyroid

GENERAL DESCRIPTION
Thyroid USP is a natural form of thyroid hormones obtained from the thyroid glands of domestic animals. It is not the most widely used drug for treating hypothyroidism (underactive thyroid) because it doesn't have a predictable hormone content; however, your doctor may prescribe it for you. Although USP (United States Pharmacology) standards for thyroid were recently revised, it is still difficult to determine these ratios, and the standards have not been fully implemented. See ***Thyroid Hormones*** for information on side effects and possible interactions.

TIMOLOL

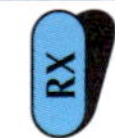

DRUG CLASS
Beta-Adrenergic Blockers

BRAND NAME
Blocadren, Timoptic (ophthalmic)

GENERAL DESCRIPTION
In oral form, the nonselective beta-blocking drug timolol is prescribed to help manage high blood pressure (hypertension), heart attack (myocardial infarction), and migraine headaches. In ophthalmic, or eye drop, form, the drug is used to control glaucoma and to prevent increased eye pressure during eye surgery. See ***Beta-Adrenergic Blockers*** for information about the side effects and possible drug interactions of non-ophthalmic forms of these drugs.

SIDE EFFECTS (ophthalmic only)

Not serious:
Itching, stinging, or watering of the eye. Contact your doctor for advice if these effects are prolonged or bothersome.

Serious:
Redness of the eyes or inside the eyelids, blepharitis (inflammation of the eyelid), conjunctivitis, keratitis (severe swelling, irritation, or inflammation of the cornea), droopy upper eyelid, double or blurred vision, or other change in vision. Tell your doctor about these symptoms.

TOBRAMYCIN

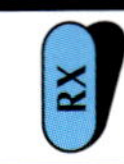

DRUG CLASS
Antibiotics [Ophthalmic Antibiotics]

BRAND NAME
Tobrex

GENERAL DESCRIPTION
Tobramycin is an aminoglycoside antibiotic drug that works by killing bacteria. Tobramycin is administered by injection to treat severe systemic infections. When used for the eyes in solution or ointment form, tobramycin has fewer side effects and possible drug interactions than the injectable forms used for systemic problems. For more information, see ***Ophthalmic Antibiotics.***

SPECIAL INFORMATION
- Tobramycin may slow the healing of corneal wounds.

TOLNAFTATE

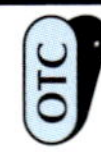

DRUG CLASS
Antifungal Drugs

BRAND NAME
Tinactin

GENERAL DESCRIPTION
Tolnaftate, available in topical aerosol, powder, cream, gel, or solution form, is used to treat several types of superficial fungal infections. It can also help prevent the development of some types of athlete's foot. Tolnaftate is not an effective treatment for bacterial or yeast infections (candidiasis). For more information, see ***Antifungal Drugs.***

TARGET AILMENTS
- jock itch.
- body ringworm.
- white-brown skin patches (a ringworm infection also known as tinea versicolor).
- athlete's foot.

SIDE EFFECTS

Not serious:
Skin may become slightly irritated at the site of application. If this becomes bothersome, discontinue use and consult your doctor.

Serious:
None expected.

SPECIAL INFORMATION
- Do not use on children under age two or for diaper rash without consulting your doctor.
- Contact your doctor if your symptoms worsen or do not improve within 10 days.
- Do not allow medication to come in contact with your eyes.
- Because it lacks antibacterial properties, tolnaftate is most effective for the dry, scaly type of athlete's foot.
- Although it may sting slightly when first applied, tolnaftate can be applied to broken skin.
- To prevent reinfection of fungal infections involving the feet or genitals, wear cotton rather than synthetic-fiber socks or underwear during treatment.
- Avoid wearing tight underwear if you have jock itch.

POSSIBLE INTERACTIONS
None expected.

TOPICAL ANTIBIOTICS

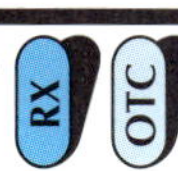

GENERIC NAMES
Rx: chlorhexidine (for gums); mupirocin (for skin); combination of neomycin, polymyxin B, and hydrocortisone (antibiotic-corticosteroid for ears)

OTC: bacitracin, neomycin, polymyxin B

GENERAL DESCRIPTION
Topical antibiotics are used to prevent or clear up bacterial infections of the skin, ears, or gums. They should never be used interchangeably; drugs for the skin, for example, should not be applied to the ears or mouth. Each drug is effective against a specific group of bacteria. For self-treatment of minor skin wounds, it may therefore be useful to choose an over-the-counter product that combines two or more antibacterial ingredients.

Over-the-counter topical antibiotics are available in an ointment base that helps close and soothe wounds. In general, though, OTC drugs are used to guard against possible infections. Once a skin infection is under way, your doctor may prescribe a stronger medication.

See the entries for the generic drugs for more information.

TARGET AILMENTS
- minor cuts, scrapes, and burns (bacitracin, neomycin, polymyxin B, to prevent bacterial infection).
- gingivitis (chlorhexidine).
- impetigo (mupirocin).
- external ear canal infections (neomycin, polymyxin B, and hydrocortisone in combination).

SIDE EFFECTS

Not serious:
Chlorhexidine: stained teeth, increased tartar, irritation on the inside of the mouth, temporary changes in your sense of taste. Call your doctor if these symptoms become bothersome.

Serious:
Bacitracin, mupirocin, neomycin, and polymyxin B: allergic reaction (itching, stinging, rash, redness, or swelling at the application site). Call your doctor immediately.

Chlorhexidine: anaphylactic reaction (nasal congestion, difficulty in breathing, rash, hives, facial swelling). Seek medical help immediately.

Neomycin: kidney damage or hearing loss may result if extensive systemic absorption of neomycin occurs via application over large areas of the body or through prolonged use. Call your doctor immediately.

SPECIAL INFORMATION
- Check with your doctor if you notice no improvement after using these medications for two or three days.
- Prolonged use of a prescription topical antibiotic may result in fungal superinfection.
- The use of topical antibiotics increases the risk of kidney damage or hearing loss in people with impaired kidney function who are already taking nephrotoxic (kidney damaging) medicines.
- If you are allergic to a topical antibiotic, you should not use that drug.
- If you are pregnant or nursing, check with your doctor before using.

POSSIBLE INTERACTIONS
Aminoglycosides: possible hypersensitivity reaction and toxicity, leading to permanent deafness if combined with neomycin, which is also an aminoglycoside.

For other possible interactions, see the entries for the generic drugs listed above.

TRANYLCYPROMINE

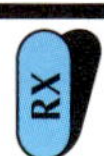

DRUG CLASS
Antidepressants [Monoamine Oxidase (MAO) Inhibitors]

BRAND NAME
Parnate

GENERAL DESCRIPTION
Tranylcypromine, like other medications in the subclass of antidepressants that is known as monoamine oxidase (MAO) inhibitors, is used to treat depression, anxiety, and phobias when other antidepressant drugs have failed. See ***Monoamine Oxidase (MAO) Inhibitors*** for information on side effects, warnings, and possible drug interactions.

TRETINOIN

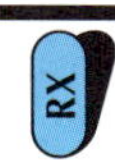

DRUG CLASS
Antiacne Drugs

BRAND NAME
Avita, Retin-A (in various formulations)

GENERAL DESCRIPTION
Tretinoin, a derivative of vitamin A, is used topically to treat skin conditions such as acne. It is sometimes used in conjunction with other drugs, including benzoyl peroxide or antibiotics, to treat severe acne, although you should not combine it with other acne medications without your doctor's knowledge.

Although the exact mechanism by which tretinoin works has not been established, it is classified as a cell stimulant. The drug also appears to weaken the attachment of certain skin cells to each other. These actions cause skin and other cells to slough off the body's surface, possibly preventing plugs that block skin pores. Mild inflammation often accompanies its use.

Tretinoin does not cure acne; your skin will return to its pretherapy state within three to six weeks after you stop taking the drug. Its effectiveness in reversing skin damage caused by exposure to ultraviolet radiation has not been confirmed.

TARGET AILMENTS
- acne (used alone or in combination with other drugs).
- skin disorders such as keratinization, keratosis, and flat warts.

SIDE EFFECTS

Not serious:
Warming or reddening of the skin, mild stinging or peeling of the skin. Consult your doctor if these symptoms become excessive. However, mild inflammation and peeling of the skin may represent the normal action of the drug and may lessen with time.

Serious:
Crusting, blistering, swelling, and darkening or lightening of the skin; severe reddening or burning of the skin. Consult your doctor, who may tell you to stop using the drug or to use it less often, depending on the severity of the symptoms. Rarely, when absorbed through the skin, tretinoin may cause toxicity symptoms, including dizziness, headache, nausea, diarrhea, and ringing in the ears. Contact your doctor immediately if you have these symptoms.

SPECIAL INFORMATION

- To avoid irritation, be careful not to get any tretinoin in your eyes, mouth, nose, or other mucous membranes.
- Tretinoin may cause increased sensitivity to the sun and to ultraviolet radiation. Wear a sunscreen or cover affected skin when outdoors, and do not use a sunlamp.
- Acne may appear to worsen for up to a week after tretinoin is applied, because lesions just under the skin are made more prominent by the drug.
- You may wear nonmedicated cosmetics, but be sure to wash your skin thoroughly to remove any cosmetics before applying tretinoin.
- Tretinoin may cause increased sensitivity to cold or wind.

POSSIBLE INTERACTIONS

Benzoyl peroxide: do not use with tretinoin except under a doctor's direction, because the two medications may be incompatible.

Medicated, abrasive, or peeling acne products (such as benzoyl peroxide or medicated soaps); perfumes or astringents containing alcohol: may cause excessive irritation or drying of the skin. Consult your doctor before using these products.

Medicated cosmetics: may cause excessive irritation of the skin.

Minoxidil (topical for hair growth, especially in bald men or women): tretinoin increases the absorption of minoxidil and may increase its side effects, which include low blood pressure, heart-rhythm problems, and impotence. Let your doctor know if you are using minoxidil.

TRIAMCINOLONE

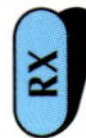

DRUG CLASS
Corticosteroids

BRAND NAMES
Azmacort, Nasacort

GENERAL DESCRIPTION
Triamcinolone is a potent adrenal corticosteroid, available in nasal spray and oral inhaler forms. The drug, introduced in 1985, is normally prescribed when a person's medical condition does not respond to other treatments. Oral inhalant forms of triamcinolone are used to treat bronchial asthma; they are intended to prevent, not relieve, acute asthma attacks. Previous use of other oral or inhalant bronchodilators may increase the effectiveness of triamcinolone.

In nasal spray form, triamcinolone is used to treat allergic rhinitis (nasal inflammation). It is also used for severe seasonal or perennial hay fever when decongestants are inadequate (although clearing your nasal passages with a decongestant spray before using triamcinolone may improve the drug's effectiveness). Some systemic absorption may occur with long-term use of triamcinolone. See ***Corticosteroids*** for more information.

SIDE EFFECTS

Not serious:
White patches in mouth, throat, or nose; throat irritation; stuffy or runny nose, and burning or dryness inside the nose. See your doctor if these symptoms persist or if there is no improvement in your condition in three weeks.

Serious:
None expected with low-dose, short-term use.

TRIAMTERENE

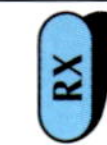

DRUG CLASS
Diuretics

BRAND NAMES
Dyazide, Maxzide

GENERAL DESCRIPTION
Triamterene, among the drugs known as potassium-sparing diuretics, is prescribed for high blood pressure (hypertension), congestive heart failure, and kidney and liver problems associated with fluid retention. Because it prevents the excess excretion of potassium from the body, triamterene is frequently used in combination with nonpotassium-sparing diuretics, such as hydrochlorothiazide. See ***Diuretics*** for more information, including side effects and possible drug interactions. For information about a nonpotassium-sparing diuretic often used in combination with this drug, see ***Hydrochlorothiazide.***

SIDE EFFECTS

Not serious:
Increased risk of sunburn.

SPECIAL INFORMATION

- Because triamterene inhibits potassium excretion, you should not take potassium supplements (including salt substitutes) while on this medication. Excess potassium can lead to heart-rhythm problems.
- While you are taking this medicine, your skin may burn more readily when exposed to sunlight. To protect your skin, use a sunblocking lotion when outside and avoid prolonged exposure to the sun and sunlamps.

TRIAZOLAM

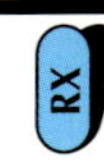

DRUG CLASS
Antianxiety Drugs [Benzodiazepines]

BRAND NAME
Halcion

GENERAL DESCRIPTION
A mild sedative-hypnotic, triazolam is prescribed for the treatment of insomnia. Triazolam is more likely than most other benzodiazepines to cause short-term amnesia if you have to wake up and be alert before the drug's effects have worn off. See ***Benzodiazepines*** for more information on side effects and possible drug interactions.

POSSIBLE INTERACTIONS

Erythromycin: increased triazolam effect.

Isoniazid: increased triazolam effect and possible toxicity.

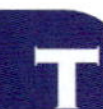

TRICYCLIC ANTIDEPRESSANTS (TCAs)

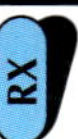

DRUG CLASS
Antidepressants

GENERIC NAMES
amitriptyline, doxepin, nortriptyline

GENERAL DESCRIPTION
An important group of antidepressant drugs, tricyclic antidepressants (TCAs) are widely used to treat depressive illnesses and, less often, in the treatment of ulcers. See ***Antidepressants*** for information about side effects and other possible drug interactions.

SPECIAL INFORMATION
- Before taking these drugs, let your doctor know if you are suffering from glaucoma, urinary retention, epilepsy, or hyperthyroidism.

POSSIBLE INTERACTIONS

Cimetidine (antiulcer): increased TCA effects.

Clonidine (blood pressure medication): may cause a dangerous increase in blood pressure.

Haloperidol (antipsychotic), oral contraceptives, phenothiazines (antipsychotic), levodopa (anti-Parkinsonism): decreased levels of TCAs.

Tobacco (smoking): increased elimination of TCAs from the body, lessening their effectiveness.

TRIMETHOPRIM

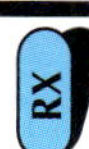

GENERAL DESCRIPTION
Trimethoprim is a generic antibiotic drug often used in combination with sulfamethoxazole. For more information, see ***Sulfamethoxazole and Trimethoprim.***

TRIPROLIDINE

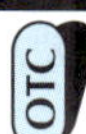

DRUG CLASS
Antihistamines

BRAND NAME
Actifed

GENERAL DESCRIPTION
Triprolidine is an antihistamine with mild sedative effects. See ***Antihistamines.***

TURMERIC

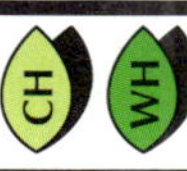

LATIN NAME
Curcuma longa

GENERAL DESCRIPTION
The turmeric root, an ingredient of Indian curries for thousands of years, also has medicinal properties. Today in Ayurvedic (Hindu) medicine, turmeric is used for several purposes, including as a digestive aid. One of its active ingredients, curcumin, induces the flow of bile, which in turn breaks down fats. Curcumin is also an anti-inflammatory agent and thus relieves the aches and pains associated with arthritis.

Turmeric also contains a volatile oil, which functions as an external antibiotic, preventing bacterial infection in wounds. In traditional Chinese medicine turmeric is categorized as acrid, bitter, and warm. The turmeric plant is recognized by spongy, orange bulbs and yellow trumpet-shaped flowers.

TARGET AILMENTS
Chinese:
Take internally for:
- shoulder pain, menstrual cramps, pain after childbirth, menstrual irregularity.

Apply externally for:
- skin infections.

Western:
Take internally for:
- digestive disorders, fever, chest congestion, menstrual irregularity, aches and pains of arthritis.

Apply externally for:
- pain and swelling caused by trauma.

PREPARATIONS
Over the counter:
Turmeric is available as powdered root, capsules, and liquid extract.

At home:
Chinese:
Combinations: For shoulder pain, turmeric is mixed with cinnamon twig and astragalus. Menstrual cramps and pain after childbirth may be alleviated with a combination of turmeric and cinnamon bark; for menstrual irregularity the herb is combined with dong quai. Turmeric is mixed with sesame or salad oil and applied externally to swollen areas.

Western:
Decoction: Steep 1 tsp turmeric powder in 1 cup milk for 15 to 20 minutes. Drink up to 3 cups a day.

SIDE EFFECTS

Not serious:
Possible heartburn or upset stomach. Reduce dosage or discontinue use and consult your practitioner.

SPECIAL INFORMATION
- If you are pregnant, consult your practitioner before using.
- One animal study indicated that the herb reduces fertility. If you are trying to conceive or if you have a history of fertility problems, consult your practitioner before using.
- If you have a blood-clotting disorder consult your practitioner before using. Turmeric is thought to have an anticlotting effect on the body.
- Use low-strength preparations for children, or adults over 65. Do not give to children under 2 years of age.

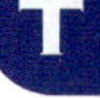

USNEA

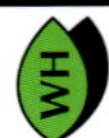

LATIN NAME
Usnea spp.

GENERAL DESCRIPTION
Usnea, or larch moss, refers to a group of lichens, which are plants made up of algae and fungi that grow together in an interdependent relationship. Larch moss is found hanging from the larch and many other trees in the Northern Hemisphere. Sometimes called old-man's-beard for its shaggy appearance, it frequently appears in fruit orchards. The active ingredient, usnic acid, seems to have an antibiotic effect against the Gram-positive class of bacteria, which includes, for example, streptococcus. It may also be effective against some fungi and protozoans.

Usnea is believed to work by disrupting the cell metabolism of bacteria and other simple organisms, although it does not damage human cells. Herbalists consider it an immune system stimulant and a muscle relaxant. Some species of usnea, including at least four found in the western United States, are also used as herbal remedies and serve as food for some animals and people.

TARGET AILMENTS
Take internally for:
- colds, influenza, sore throats, respiratory infections.
- gastrointestinal irritations.

Apply externally for:
- skin ulcers and fungal infections such as athlete's foot.
- urinary tract infections such as urethritis and cystitis, vaginal infections. (Use as a douche.)

PREPARATIONS
Over the counter:
The dried herb is available in bulk, powder, or tincture.

At home:
Tea: Steep 2 to 3 tsp dried lichen or 1 to 2 tsp of powder in 1 cup boiling water. Take three times daily.

SIDE EFFECTS
Not serious:
If digestive disorders arise, reduce dosage. Call your doctor if these symptoms persist.

SPECIAL INFORMATION
- WARNING: Pregnant women should avoid using this herb, because it may stimulate uterine contractions.
- Dilute tincture before ingesting; high concentrations may cause digestive problems.
- Do not use for more than three consecutive weeks.

UVA URSI

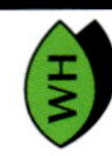

LATIN NAME
Arctostaphylos uva-ursi

GENERAL DESCRIPTION
The leaves of the uva ursi shrub have been used worldwide for urinary problems for at least 1,000 years. The leaves contain arbutin, which is converted in the urinary tract to hydroquinone, a widely used antiseptic. They also contain tannin, an astringent useful in treating wounds, and allantoin, which soothes and accelerates the healing of tissue. Uva ursi, which literally means "bearberry," is an ingredient in most herbal teas that are taken for urinary problems. This woody, mat-forming, evergreen shrub, which appears throughout the Northern Hemisphere, prefers poor, gravelly soil and rarely grows more than a few inches tall.

TARGET AILMENTS
Take internally for:
- mild urinary tract infections, such as urethritis and cystitis, high blood pressure, menstrual bloating.

Apply externally for:
- minor skin problems such as cuts and abrasions.

PREPARATIONS
Over the counter:
Uva ursi is available in the form of dried leaves; as a tincture; and as a tea, alone or in combination with other ingredients.

At home:
Tea: Simmer in hot water for 5 to 10 minutes, and allow to stand for 12 to 24 hours. To counteract the effect of the tannin content, add peppermint or chamomile. Drink three cups a day.

Compress: Make a tea; strain and discard the herb. Soak a pad in the tea and apply.

SIDE EFFECTS
Not serious:
Taking uva ursi may result in the production of dark-green urine; this is harmless. In addition stomach upset may be caused by the herb's high tannin content.

Serious:
Ringing in the ears, nausea, and convulsions were reported in a 1949 study involving very high doses of isolated hydroquinone. Prescribed doses of the whole herb are considered safe, but in case of side effects, discontinue taking until you contact your doctor.

SPECIAL INFORMATION
- Uva ursi's disinfectant properties work only in an alkaline environment. When taking this herb, avoid acidic foods, such as most fruit juices, sauerkraut, and vitamin C.
- Because hydroquinone is toxic in high doses, use uva ursi only in recommended amounts.
- Pregnant women should not use uva ursi, because it may stimulate uterine contractions.

VAGINAL ANTIFUNGAL DRUGS

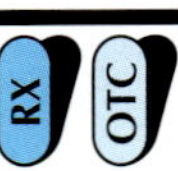

DRUG CLASS
Antifungal Drugs

GENERIC NAMES
Rx: clotrimazole, miconazole, terconazole

OTC: clotrimazole, miconazole

GENERAL DESCRIPTION
Vaginal antifungal drugs are commonly prescribed in the treatment of vaginal yeast infections. These medications work by damaging the membranes of fungal cells and inhibiting the enzyme activity essential for the cells' growth and reproduction. The drugs are available in the form of vaginal creams and suppositories. For more information, see entries for the generic drugs listed above. Also see ***Antifungal Drugs.***

TARGET AILMENTS
- yeast infections (candidiasis) of the vulva and vagina.

SIDE EFFECTS
Not serious:
Headaches, mild abdominal or stomach cramps; in rare cases, irritation to the sexual partner's penis.

Serious:
If you experience vaginal burning, itching, or discharge; or skin rash, hives, or other skin irritation, discontinue the medication and contact your doctor.

SPECIAL INFORMATION

- If you are pregnant or nursing, do not use a vaginal antifungal medication without consulting your doctor.
- Do not use these medications if you have a fever above 100°F; abdominal, shoulder, or back pain; or a malodorous vaginal discharge.
- Be sure to use these medications for the prescribed amount of time, even during menstruation or if your symptoms abate.
- If you are using a vaginal cream, protect clothing from possible soiling by wearing panty liners or sanitary napkins.
- Avoid possible reinfection by wearing cotton rather than synthetic-fiber underwear.
- Refrain from sexual activity during treatment to avoid possible transmission and reinfection. Also, some vaginal antifungal preparations contain a vegetable oil base that might weaken latex condoms, diaphragms, or cervical caps.
- If your male partner has any penile discomfort, burning, irritation, or itchiness, he may require simultaneous treatment for infection. He should consult his doctor.
- Douching may or may not be advised while using this medication; consult your doctor.
- If your symptoms do not show improvement within three to seven days, consult your doctor.
- If your symptoms return within two months, see your doctor; you may be pregnant or have a serious disorder, such as diabetes or an HIV infection.

POSSIBLE INTERACTIONS

None expected.

VALERIAN

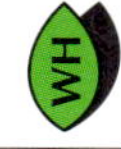

LATIN NAME

Valeriana officinalis

GENERAL DESCRIPTION

Valerian root has been used for more than 1,000 years for its calming qualities, and recent research has confirmed its efficacy and safety as a mild tranquilizer and sleep aid. For sufferers of insomnia, valerian has been found to hasten the onset of sleep, improve sleep quality, and reduce nighttime awakenings. Unlike barbiturates or benzodiazepines, prescribed amounts leave no morning grogginess and do not interfere with the vivid dreaming sleep known as REM sleep. It is not habit-forming and produces no withdrawal symptoms when discontinued. The plant is a hardy perennial that reaches a height of about five feet. As the roots dry, they develop an unpleasant odor compared by one herbalist to that of dirty socks. Most people add sugar or honey to make valerian tea more palatable.

TARGET AILMENTS

Take internally for:

- insomnia, anxiety, nervousness, anxiety-induced heart palpitations.
- headache.
- intestinal pains.
- menstrual cramps.

PREPARATIONS

Over the counter:
Valerian is widely available dried or as capsules, tinctures, and teas.

At home:
Steep 2 tsp dried, chopped root in 1 cup boiling water. Let stand 8 to 12 hours. Drink 1 cup before bed.

SIDE EFFECTS

Not serious:
A mild headache or upset stomach may develop. Reduce dosage, and let your doctor know if it persists.

Serious:
More severe headache, restlessness, nausea, morning grogginess, or blurred vision may be caused by using too much valerian. Contact your doctor, who will probably tell you to take less or to stop using the herb.

SPECIAL INFORMATION

- Do not take valerian with conventional tranquilizers or sedatives, because of possible additive effects.
- Paradoxically, valerian may produce excitability in some people.
- Since it has sedative effects, be careful about driving until you know how the herb affects you.

VALPROIC ACID

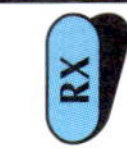

DRUG CLASS

Anticonvulsant Drugs

BRAND NAME

Depakote

GENERAL DESCRIPTION

Introduced in 1967, valproic acid is used in the control of epileptic seizures, primarily the simple and complex absence types (petit mal). It is also used alone or as an adjunct to other anticonvulsant drugs to treat other types of epilepsy. For more information, see ***Anticonvulsant Drugs.***

TARGET AILMENTS

- epileptic seizures, absence types.
- epileptic seizures, other types.
- prevention and treatment of bipolar disorder (manic-depression).

SIDE EFFECTS

Not serious:
Some of the more common side effects experienced include: loss of appetite, indigestion, mild nausea, vomiting and diarrhea, unusual weight loss or gain, skin rash, trembling arms and hands, change in menstrual periods, lethargy, drowsiness, dizziness, unsteadiness, emotional changes. Call your physician if these or other side effects persist or are bothersome.

Serious:
Bizarre behavior, hallucinations, unusual bleeding or bruising, yellow eyes or skin, severe stomach cramps, double vision, spots in front of your eyes, jerky or rolling eye movements, swelling of the face, continual nausea or vomiting. Seek medical care immediately. Also see overdose symptoms below.

SPECIAL INFORMATION

- Valproic acid overdose can be fatal: Seek emergency help. Overdose symptoms include restlessness, hand tremors, hallucinations, and deep coma.
- Do not use valproic acid if you have had an allergic reaction to this drug, an active liver disease or significant liver function impairment, or a bleeding disorder.
- Tell your physician if you are taking anticoagulants, other anticonvulsants, or any other drugs (prescription or over the counter), especially those that depress the central nervous system, such as antihistamines, antidepressants, tranquilizers, barbiturates, narcotics, sedatives, pain medication, sleeping pills, or muscle relaxants.
- Before using this drug, tell your doctor if you have a history of brain, blood, liver, or kidney disease; are pregnant or planning pregnancy; or are anticipating surgery or dental extraction.
- You can take valproic acid with food to reduce stomach upset. To prevent

irritation of the mouth or throat, swallow the tablets or capsules whole, without chewing or breaking them.
- Older adults are more likely to develop side effects from this drug and should be treated with smaller dosages.
- Blood cell counts may show decreased white cells and platelets.
- Valproic acid may affect some laboratory tests, including liver function tests. Be sure to tell any healthcare practitioner who gives you a lab test that you are taking this medication.
- Do not stop taking this drug or switch brands without checking with your physician.

POSSIBLE INTERACTIONS

Alcohol, antidepressants, barbiturates, sedatives, tranquilizers, and other depressant drugs: increased depressive and sedative effects.

Anticoagulant and antiplatelet drugs, including aspirin: increased risk of bleeding.

Phenytoin and other anticonvulsants: concurrent use of phenytoin or another anticonvulsant with valproic acid may increase the risk of breakthrough seizures.

VALSARTAN

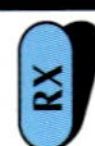

DRUG CLASS
Antihypertensive Drugs

BRAND NAME
Diovan

GENERAL DESCRIPTION
Valsartan is one drug in a new class of blood pressure medications known as angiotensin II receptor antagonists. These drugs inhibit the angiotensin II hormone from causing blood vessels to constrict, improving blood flow and lowering blood pressure. Valsartan may be used alone or in combination with other antihypertensive drugs. For more information, see ***Antihypertensive Drugs.***

TARGET AILMENTS
- high blood pressure (hypertension).

SIDE EFFECTS

Not serious:
Headache, dizziness, fever, sore throat, upper respiratory infections, cough, cold, diarrhea, fatigue. Call your doctor if these symptoms persist or become bothersome.

SPECIAL INFORMATION
- This drug can harm the development of an unborn child; do not take valsartan if you are pregnant. If you are nursing, consult with your doctor before taking this drug.
- Valsartan should be used with caution if you have kidney or liver disease.
- Valsartan should be combined with exercise, stress reduction, weight loss, and a salt-restricted diet to best control blood pressure.

VERAPAMIL

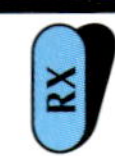

DRUG CLASS
Calcium Channel Blockers

BRAND NAMES
Calan SR, Isoptin SR, Verelan

GENERAL DESCRIPTION
A calcium channel blocker introduced in 1967, verapamil is prescribed for high blood pressure, angina, and heart-rhythm problems. The drug works by blocking the passage of calcium into body cells, thus slowing the contraction of the heart and arteries, dilating the arteries, and lowering blood pressure. Verapamil is sometimes used to control cluster headaches and panic attacks. See ***Calcium Channel Blockers*** for information on side effects and possible drug interactions.

WARFARIN

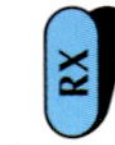

DRUG CLASS
Anticoagulant and Antiplatelet Drugs

BRAND NAME
Coumadin

GENERAL DESCRIPTION
Warfarin, introduced in 1941, is a powerful anticoagulant. It inhibits blood clotting by blocking the action of vitamin K, a central ingredient in the production of four essential blood-clotting factors. Warfarin is administered orally and can be extremely dangerous if not used properly. It is essential that you have periodic blood tests to monitor clotting time. See ***Anticoagulant and Antiplatelet Drugs*** for important information on serious side effects, such as hemorrhaging, and drug interactions.

SIDE EFFECTS

Not serious:
Minor bleeding, mild skin rash.

POSSIBLE INTERACTIONS

Alcohol, aspirin, and other salicylates: avoid these when taking warfarin.

Vitamin K: counteracts warfarin. Avoid eating large quantities of foods rich in vitamin K, including leafy green vegetables, dairy products, bacon, beef liver, cabbage, cauliflower, and fish.

WHITE WILLOW

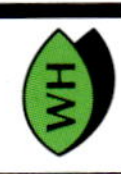

LATIN NAME
Salix alba

GENERAL DESCRIPTION
White willow, like other willows, is a natural source of salicin, a precursor of modern aspirin, and indeed it has been used for centuries worldwide as a pain reliever. Although all parts of the plant contain some salicin, the best source is the mature bark, either fresh or dried. Like other salicin-producing plants, white willow also reduces fever and inflammation, probably by suppressing the action of prostaglandins (hormone-like substances), which are produced by the body in response to injuries.

In addition to salicin, willow bark contains other compounds that the body metabolizes to salicylic acid. For this reason willow bark acts more slowly and over a longer period of time than aspirin does.

TARGET AILMENTS
Take internally for:
- gout, minor muscle strains, menstrual cramps, headache, fever, aches and pains, pain and inflammation of arthritis.

Apply externally for:
- sores and burns, pain and inflammation of arthritis.

PREPARATIONS

Over the counter:
Available as dried bark, tincture, tea, and capsules.

At home:
Tea: Steep 1 to 2 tsp of powdered bark

in 1 cup boiling water for eight hours; strain. Drink up to 3 cups a day. The bitter taste can be improved by mixing with honey and lemon or another herbal tea.

SIDE EFFECTS

Not serious:
Upset stomach, nausea, or ringing in the ears may result. Lower the dosage or stop using white willow; call your doctor if symptoms persist.

SPECIAL INFORMATION

- WARNING: Children under the age of 16 should not use white willow if they have a cold, influenza, or other viral illness. Using salicylates may cause Reye's syndrome, a potentially fatal condition.
- Individuals with ulcers or other stomach problems should use white willow with caution, because it can worsen stomach ills.
- If you are taking blood thinning medications, use white willow only with the consent of your physician.

POSSIBLE INTERACTIONS

Do not mix white willow with other salicylates, such as aspirin or wintergreen oil, because of the potential for additive side effects.

WILD YAM

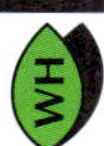

LATIN NAME

Dioscorea villosa

GENERAL DESCRIPTION

Used during the 18th and 19th centuries as a remedy for menstrual pain and complications associated with childbearing, wild yam is a perennial vine that entwines itself around fences and bushes. It is recognized by a slender reddish brown stem and drooping yellow flowers that bloom during the summer. Wild yam extract, taken from the root, contains an alkaloid substance that relaxes the muscles of the entire abdominal region. Consequently, it is prescribed to alleviate menstrual cramps and to relieve the nausea and muscle tension associated with pregnancy. Wild yam also contains steroidal saponins, believed to act as anti-inflammatory agents, and used to reduce the swelling caused by rheumatoid arthritis.

TARGET AILMENTS

- menstrual cramps, nausea due to pregnancy, morning sickness, urinary tract disorders, intestinal colic, rheumatoid arthritis. (Take internally.)

PREPARATIONS

Over the counter:
Wild yam is available as dried root, tincture, or capsules.

At home:
Tea: Boil 1 oz wild yam root with 1 cup water for 15 to 20 minutes. Drink three times daily.

Combinations: For intestinal colic, wild yam is combined with calamus, chamomile, and ginger. Rheumatoid arthritis is treated with a mix of wild yam and black cohosh. Herbalists use a combination of wild yam and cramp bark for menstrual cramps.

SPECIAL INFORMATION

- Wild yam is sometimes prescribed by herbalists for its supposed progesterone-like properties for women undergoing menopause. There is still a great deal of controversy, however, as to the effectiveness of this treatment. You should consult a practitioner before using wild yam as a progesterone supplement.

YARROW

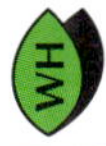

LATIN NAME

Achillea millefolium

GENERAL DESCRIPTION

Yarrow has been used to heal wounds since ancient times; the Greek hero of the Trojan War, Achilles, is said to have stopped the bleeding of his warriors' wounds by applying the crushed leaves of yarrow. Modern investigation has revealed many chemicals in yarrow that have anti-inflammatory and pain-relieving effects. The leaves, stems, and flower tops contain more than 10 different active ingredients, including salicylic acid, menthol, and camphor. Two major constituents, achilletin and achilleine, are thought to help blood coagulate, while thujone (also found in chamomile) has mild sedative properties. Because yarrow may have diuretic properties, it is sometimes used to treat menstrual bloating and high blood pressure. The somewhat bitter taste of yarrow tea can be relieved by adding sweeteners or other herbs. A naturalized, three-foot-tall perennial from Eurasia, yarrow is widely planted in flower and herb gardens and found growing wild in most areas of the United States.

TARGET AILMENTS

Take internally for:

- fever, digestive disorders, menstrual cramps, colds, flu, high blood pressure.

Apply externally for:

- minor wounds, bleeding.
- vaginal irritations. (Use as a douche.)

PREPARATIONS

Over the counter:
Available as dried herb or tea.

At home:
Tea: Steep 1 to 2 tsp of dried herb in 1 cup boiling water for 10 to 15 minutes. Drink up to 3 cups a day.

SIDE EFFECTS

Not serious:
Rash, nausea, or diarrhea may result from taking yarrow. Stop using the herb and consult your doctor.

SPECIAL INFORMATION

- If you are allergic to ragweed, you may develop a rash from ingesting yarrow.
- Do not take yarrow internally if you are pregnant.

ZOLPIDEM

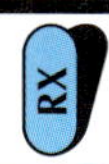

DRUG CLASS

Anti-Insomnia Drugs

BRAND NAME

Ambien

GENERAL DESCRIPTION

Zolpidem, introduced in 1993, is the most commonly prescribed drug for the short-term (7 to 10 days) management of sleeping problems in adults. Its major advantages include a low incidence of adverse effects, rapid absorption and elimination, and minimal interference with normal sleep patterns, which includes the rapid eye movement (REM) stage.

A nonbenzodiazepine medication, zolpidem works by binding to a specific receptor in the brain to simulate normal sleep processes. Most users report few side effects, and little or no hangover effects, memory loss, or "rebound" insomnia when not using the drug. For

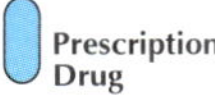
Prescription Drug
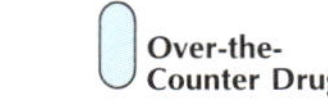
Over-the-Counter Drug
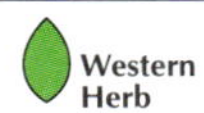
Western Herb
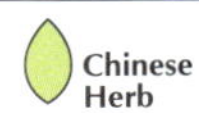
Chinese Herb
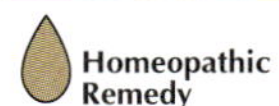
Homeopathic Remedy

more information, see ***Anti-Insomnia Drugs.***

TARGET AILMENTS
- insomnia.

SIDE EFFECTS

Not serious:
Daytime drowsiness, dizziness, lightheadedness, blurred vision, dry mouth, memory problems, abdominal or gastric pain, diarrhea, nausea, vomiting, headache, unusual dreams, malaise. See your doctor if these symptoms persist or are bothersome.

Serious:
Clumsiness, confusion, unsteadiness and falling, mental depression, skin rash, agitation, irritability, wheezing or difficulty in breathing, hallucinations, increased insomnia. Contact your doctor as soon as possible.

SPECIAL INFORMATION
- Do not take zolpidem if you have had an allergic reaction to the drug in the past. Before taking zolpidem, tell your doctor if any of the following conditions apply: you are pregnant, plan to become pregnant, or are nursing; you have a kidney or liver disease; you have sleep apnea; you have asthma, bronchitis, emphysema, or other chronic lung disease; you have a history of mental depression or disorder; you have a history of alcoholism or drug dependence.
- Zolpidem is most rapidly absorbed when taken on an empty stomach (at least two hours after eating).
- Because zolpidem works so fast, it should be taken just before bedtime.
- Take zolpidem only if you have time to get a full night's sleep (seven or eight hours). Otherwise, the drug will not have time to wear off, and you may experience hangover effects, including drowsiness and memory problems.
- Older adults may be more sensitive to the drug's effects and side effects and may require a smaller dosage.
- Until you know how you react to zolpidem, do not drive, operate machinery, or do anything requiring unimpaired coordination and clear vision.
- Long-term use of zolpidem may result in dependence. Withdrawal symptoms may occur when you stop taking the drug.

POSSIBLE INTERACTIONS

Alcohol and other central nervous system depressants (anesthetics, antidepressants, antihistamines, barbiturates, benzodiazepines, monoamine oxidase (MAO) inhibitors, muscle relaxants, narcotics or prescription pain medicines, tranquilizers): increased anti-insomniac and depressant effect.

Caffeine and nicotine: these are stimulants that can interfere with zolpidem's anti-insomniac effects.

ABOUT HERBAL PREPARATIONS 

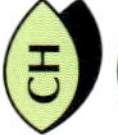
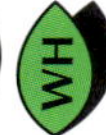

HERBAL RECIPES

Preparing herbs for therapeutic use is typically more art than science, and recipes abound. Homemade preparations will differ in strength from those sold in stores, and even these will vary from store to store. So you may find that the dose labeled on an over-the-counter remedy is different from that given in a recipe for home preparation.

The three basic herbal preparations for taking internally are decoctions, tinctures, and teas, also known as infusions. They can be made from the fresh or dried plant. The amount of herb used and the time of preparation may vary, depending on the particular plant. Preparations for external use include compresses and poultices—for care of wounds and relief of strained muscles—and infused oils, creams, and ointments, which alleviate skin ailments.

Some herbs work best when taken together with others. Chinese herbs, for example, are almost always used in combinations; since mixing herbs is a tricky business, you should check with your Chinese herbal practitioner for these dosages.

TEAS/INFUSIONS

An herbal **tea,** or **infusion,** is made with the leaves, flowers, or soft stems of a plant. To make a tea, measure 1 to 2 tsp dried herb directly in a cup or into a tea ball. Triple the amount if you're using fresh herbs. Pour 1 cup hot water, just off the boil, over the herb and let it sit (steep) for 10 to 20 minutes. Strain before drinking. If you need to mask a bitter taste, add sugar, lemon, or honey.

The leaves and flowers are not boiled, because boiling disperses too many of their volatile constituents. You can make larger quantities, using ½ to 1 oz dried herb (1 to 2 oz fresh) for every 2 cups water.

Another option is to buy herbal tea bags from an herb store. Note that prepackaged tea bags are less potent than fresh bulk herbs sold in herb stores or prepared at home. Herbal teas lose their medicinal value after a few hours when exposed to the air, but if stored in a tightly sealed glass jar and refrigerated, the teas will last up to three days.

DECOCTIONS

A **decoction** is a water extract made from the root, bark, and sometimes twigs, berries, or seeds of a plant. Unlike the less dense plant parts that are prepared as teas, these woody plant materials require boiling before their active constituents can be extracted. To make a decoction, break or cut into pieces 1 tbsp dried herb, or 2 to 3 tbsp fresh herb, and put into a saucepan; glass, ceramic, or enameled pans are best. Pour 2 cups cold water over the herb, bring to a boil, and simmer for 10 to 15 minutes. Strain the solid matter from the liquid. You can drink the decoction hot or cold. As with teas, it's best to make fresh batches as you need them, but you can store larger quantities in the refrigerator in a tightly covered glass jar for two to three days.

TINCTURES

Tinctures use alcohol to make a more concentrated extract than teas and decoctions. The recipes vary in the proportion of herb and alcohol and in the preparation time, but a fairly standard recipe calls for 4 oz of ground or chopped dried herb and 2 cups of at least 100 proof vodka. The alcohol should cover the herb completely, so use more if necessary. If you're using fresh herbs, double the amount of herb and alcohol. Put the herb in an opaque jar or bottle that can be sealed tightly, pour the vodka over it, cover, and store the mixture in a warm place, about 80°F, but out of direct sunlight. Do not leave the jar

HERB SAFETY

Use herbs with caution at all times. Be especially careful if you have allergies, are sensitive to drugs, are taking drugs for a chronic illness, or are older than 65 or younger than 12 years of age. Start with the lowest dose appropriate for you to help ensure against adverse reactions. Herbs are best absorbed on an empty stomach; if nausea occurs, take them with meals or immediately afterward. If you consistently develop nausea, diarrhea, or headache within two hours of taking an herb, discontinue its use. Call your practitioner if the symptoms are prolonged. Herbs can interact with drugs, so check with your physician before you start taking herbs. Pregnant and breast-feeding women are advised not to ingest medicinal amounts of herbs without first consulting their obstetrician.

Many herbalists recommend purchasing herbs as a safer practice than harvesting your own plants. You can buy dried and fresh herbs, herbal capsules, tinctures, teas, tablets, ointments, and oils at herb stores, at some health food stores and pharmacies, and through mail order. Obtain herbs and herb preparations from a reputable source to guard against frauds such as substitution or adulteration of an herb with a different, cheaper plant. Whether dried, fresh, powdered, or in liquid extract, all herbs lose their potency after time, so look for a source that provides the freshest possible product.

ABOUT HERBAL PREPARATIONS

on good furniture or other surfaces that could corrode if the jar leaks. Shake the jar twice a day for two weeks. After two weeks, decant the liquid into another opaque jar or dark bottle, and store it in a cool place away from direct sunlight, to avoid weakening the tincture. The usual dose ranges from 10 to 30 drops taken straight or mixed with water or syrup, two to four times daily. The alcohol in tinctures gives them a shelf life of at least two years, but tinctures made from fresh herbs may not last as long as those made from dried herbs. Tinctures are a basic ingredient in other preparations such as herbal compresses and ointments, and can be added to baths.

Rum, gin, and brandy are also good solvents. Never use methyl alcohol, rubbing alcohol, or industrial alcohol to make a tincture, because these forms are extremely toxic. Pregnant women, children, diabetics, and others who need to avoid alcohol can use tinctures prepared with apple cider vinegar or glycerin instead of distilled spirits. Another option is to remove alcohol from a tincture by putting the tincture dose in a cup and adding 2 tbsp of almost boiling water. By the time the mixture cools, most of the alcohol will have evaporated.

SYRUPS

Used to relieve coughing or to mask the flavor of a tincture, **syrups** are prepared by combining in a saucepan 1 lb sugar and 1 cup water. Bring to a boil and let simmer until all the crystals are dissolved, stirring constantly. Let the syrup cool and store it in a dark bottle in the refrigerator. Add syrup to a tincture as needed to make it palatable.

COMPRESSES

To make a hot **compress,** also known as a fomentation, soak a soft cotton or linen cloth in a hot infusion or decoction. Wring the cloth and place it against the injured area. Repeat the process as the compress cools. For headaches, make a cold compress using a cold infusion.

POULTICES

A **poultice** is used like a compress, but the herb itself is applied to the skin. Pour a small amount of boiling water over chopped or crushed fresh herbs. Let sit two to five minutes, then squeeze out the water. You can also use dried herbs boiled for three to five minutes, or powders mixed with enough water to make a paste. To apply the poultice, place gauze or a thin strip of cotton over the affected area, and spread the herb directly on the gauze. Cover the herb with a second piece of gauze or plastic wrap. Hold the poultice in place with gauze or cotton strips, and leave it in place for an hour. Repeat, depending on the condition.

OILS

Herbal **oils** are used for massage and in creams and ointments. You can purchase **essential oils,** made by a complex distillation process. These highly concentrated oils are so potent that the dosage is measured in drops. When essential oils are applied to the skin, they usually are first mixed with a carrier oil such as almond or sunflower oil. **Infused oils** are used in the same way as essential oils but can be prepared at home. The two ways of making infused oil are called cold infusion and hot infusion; the method you use depends on the herb.

Use the hot infusion for roots and the dense, woody leaves of herbs like rosemary. Gently heat 1 to 2 oz dried herb (double or triple this for fresh herb) in a double boiler with 2 cups olive, sunflower, or almond oil. Make sure you have enough oil to completely cover the herbs. Watch carefully, because overheating will make the oil rancid and medicinally useless. Simply warm the oil; do not let it boil or smoke. After two hours, strain the mixture. To strain, pour the mixture through a cloth or into a sieve lined with cheesecloth. Store in a glass bottle and seal tightly.

For flowers and soft leaves, use the cold-infusion method. Cut up the dried herb, pack it in a clear jar, and cover it with oil. Seal the jar and set it in the sun for two days. Then place it in a well-lighted room out of direct sunlight for two to three weeks, shaking the jar daily. Filter by pouring through cheesecloth. Store the infused oil in a dark glass jar. For a more concentrated infusion, repeat the process one more time with the infused oil and more of the dried herb.

CREAMS

A **cream** is an oil-and-water mixture that is easily absorbed in the skin and relieves dry, flaking skin; insect bites; or sunburn. For a simple herbal cream, mix 10 drops of the desired essential oil with 2½ oz of a pure vegetable face cream that you can buy at a health food store.

OINTMENTS

Ointments are waterless, waxy or oily salves that form a protective layer over the skin, guarding it from moisture that can cause such skin irritations as diaper rash or chafing. To prepare an ointment, combine in a saucepan 4 parts petroleum jelly and 1 part herb. Simmer on very low heat for one hour. Do not overheat; simply warm the petroleum jelly. Strain the liquid using fine gauze. Pour the ointment into a glass jar; allow it to cool and resolidify before sealing. The herbs can be flowers, leaves, or roots, either fresh or dried. If you use fresh herbs, simmer them long enough to evaporate the water; otherwise the water in the plant will turn the ointment rancid.

POWDERS

Herbal **powders** are ground from dried herbs, and are sprinkled on food and in drinks, mixed with water to make a poultice, or used to make capsules.

CAPSULES

Capsules can be made at home using standard capsule cases (size 00) that hold about ¼ to ½ tsp of the powdered herb. Scoop the powder into each half of the case and fit the two halves together. Store in an opaque jar. ■

ABOUT HOMEOPATHIC REMEDIES

Homeopathic treatment should not be confused with any other type of medicinal care. Its guiding principles are unlike those for herbal therapies or conventional drugs, and the testing, prescribing, and rules of use for homeopathic remedies have been developed for this form of treatment alone. If you choose homeopathy, follow its precepts precisely, and do not substitute other substances or drugs for the ones recommended by your practitioner.

PROVINGS

Most homeopathic remedies are prepared from herbal and plant extracts, many of which are poisonous. The toxicity of these extracts, or "mother tinctures," is what makes them homeopathically valuable; a substance that, undiluted, can induce a certain group of symptoms in a healthy person is believed capable, in a highly dilute form, of curing similar symptoms in a person who is sick. Tests to determine which substance is best for treating a specific set of symptoms have been carried out for years. These trials—known as provings—are conducted with healthy individuals, who are given undiluted or lightly diluted doses of a mother tincture. Mental, emotional, and physical symptoms brought on by this intentional, but not fatal, poisoning are recorded and compiled to create a full picture of the symptoms caused by the substance. The extract is then diluted to the desired homeopathic potency. Since the early 19th century, more than 2,000 remedies have been "proved" in this manner.

POTENCIES

The potency of a homeopathic remedy is based on the dilution ratio: the ratio of active substance to inactive base.

RULES OF USE

A few basic rules apply to the use of homeopathic remedies. When administering a remedy, only the patient should touch the pills. If tablets are spilled, throw them away. In both cases, homeopaths believe that such pills become contaminated and do not have the full intended effect. Pills should be allowed to dissolve on or under the tongue unless a hard, chewable pill has been prescribed. Practitioners recommend that the mouth be clean of flavors 15 minutes before and after taking a remedy. Strong flavors and aromas, including camphor, coffee, and heavily scented perfumes, should be avoided for the duration of treatment.

Dilution ratios are expressed either decimally, by a factor of 10, or centesimally, by a factor of 100. Decimal ratios are labeled with an *x* and indicate that the remedy consists of 1 part mother tincture mixed with 9 parts of a water-and-alcohol base; centesimal ratios, labeled with a *c*, consist of 1 part mother tincture and 99 parts base. Further dilutions are represented by a number in front of the *x* or *c*. For example, a remedy labeled 30c has first been mixed 1 part to 99; then, 1 part of the resulting mixture is diluted again with 99 parts of the base, and this process is repeated for a total of 30 times.

Most homeopaths feel that, since all remedies are highly diluted, it would be impossible to overdose on homeopathic drugs; the number of pills required for a toxic effect would simply be too high to consume at once.

Practitioners also believe that if a remedy does not seem to be working, increasing the number of pills will not help. If a remedy is not having the desired effect, stop taking it and return to your homeopathic practitioner for another prescription.

SELECTING A REMEDY

Symptom analysis is the key to any successful prescription. If, for example, a patient has a high fever, flushed face, and delirium during sleep, the homeopathic practitioner may prescribe ***Belladonna,*** because its symptom picture matches those that the patient is experiencing.

If the correct remedy has been prescribed, healing usually begins immediately or within a few days. Sometimes the symptoms temporarily worsen—a situation homeopaths call an "aggravation." If the first remedy does not relieve the symptoms, your homeopathic practitioner will study your symptoms again; perhaps symptoms were missed, which might indicate another remedy. Your practitioner may then prescribe a second one; this process will continue until the correctly matched remedy is found.

Once your symptoms begin to disappear, stop taking the remedy. According to some, homeopathy is like jump-starting a car; once a healing process has been initiated, your body can finish the work.

Most practitioners follow classical homeopathy, in which only one remedy is prescribed at a time. However, new over-the-counter combinations may be useful for some acute conditions. For chronic conditions or for treatments that demand personal attention, a single remedy at a time under a homeopath's supervision is usually recommended.

Two people suffering from the same disorder, such as the flu, may not receive the same prescription. Sickness can elicit different mental, emotional, and physical symptoms from different people, and symptom-based homeopathic prescribing is extremely individualized.

Remedies are available in a variety of forms. Tablets can include soft, easily dissolved pills; hard, chewable pills; and tiny, round pills known as globules. There are also powders, wafers, and liquids in an alcohol base. ■

EATING FOR HEALTH

CONTENTS

Basic Nutrition 1030

The Food Guide Pyramid 1031

Essential Vitamins and Minerals 1032

BASIC NUTRITION

Eating a balanced diet is a major factor in a healthy lifestyle. Your body requires more than 40 nutrients for energy, growth, and tissue maintenance. As the most plentiful component in the body, water is also crucial to survival. It is the medium for such bodily fluids as blood and lymph, and it transports nutrients into cells and carries waste products and toxins out.

Carbohydrates, proteins, and fats—a group known as macronutrients or "energy nutrients"—provide fuel in the form of calories. Carbohydrates, the body's main energy source, are divided into two types: Simple carbohydrates are sugars; complex carbohydrates include starches, such as those found in potatoes and bread.

Proteins support tissue growth and repair, and help produce antibodies, hormones, and enzymes—which are essential for all chemical reactions in the body. Dietary protein sources include meat, fish, dairy products, poultry, dried beans, nuts, and eggs.

Dietary fat protects internal organs, provides energy, insulates against cold, and helps the body absorb certain vitamins. There are three kinds of fats: saturated, found in meat, dairy food, and coconut oil; monounsaturated, in olive, peanut, and canola oils; and polyunsaturated, in corn, cottonseed, safflower, soy, and sunflower oils.

Your diet also supplies the important micronutrients we call vitamins and minerals. They are needed only in trace amounts, but the absence or deficiency of just one vitamin or mineral can cause major illness. Your body also needs a supply of dietary fiber, the indigestible portion of plant foods. A high-fiber diet reduces the risks of various gastrointestinal problems and promotes cardiovascular health.

Science is continually making discoveries about nutrients and their effects on health. As a result, the Food and Nutrition Board of the National Research Council, National Academy of Sciences, routinely revises its recommended dietary allowances (RDA)—also known as the recommended daily allowances—for essential nutrients. In general, most Americans eat far more fat, protein, cholesterol, sugar, and salt than they need. The official dietary guidelines, established jointly by the U.S. Departments of Agriculture and Health and Human Services, include seven basic recommendations:

- **Eat a variety of foods.** This will help ensure you get enough calories, protein, and fiber, as well as the vitamins, minerals, and other nutrients you need.
- **Control your weight.** Keep within recommended weight limits for your age, sex, and build. Obesity is defined as being 20 percent above normal weight.
- **Eat a low-fat, low-cholesterol diet.** Ideally, no more than 30 percent of your daily calories should come from fat, and no more than 10 percent should come from saturated fat. Choose polyunsaturated fats over saturated fats when possible.
- **Eat plenty of vegetables, fruits, and grains.** They are rich in nutrients, fiber, and complex carbohydrates, but low in fat. More than half of your daily calories should come from carbohydrates, and 80 percent of those calories should come from complex carbohydrates.
- **Eat sugar in moderation.** Sugar is high in calories and promotes tooth decay.
- **Use salt in moderation.** Too much salt increases the risk of developing ***high blood pressure.*** Prepared foods are notoriously high in salt or other forms of sodium, so read labels carefully.
- **If you drink alcohol, do so in moderation.** Alcohol provides calories but no nutrients, and too much is harmful. "Moderation" generally means one drink for women or two drinks for men daily.

If you consistently eat a well-balanced diet of fresh fruits, vegetables, grains, and some animal protein, you probably don't require a nutritional supplement. Multinutrient supplements offer insurance for those times when eating well is a challenge—and can be indispensable during pregnancy and times of disease, injury, and extreme stress or physical exertion. Always take supplements in moderation; they are safe in doses at or below RDAs, but higher doses may be harmful and should be taken only under a doctor's or registered dietitian's guidance. ■

THE FOOD GUIDE PYRAMID

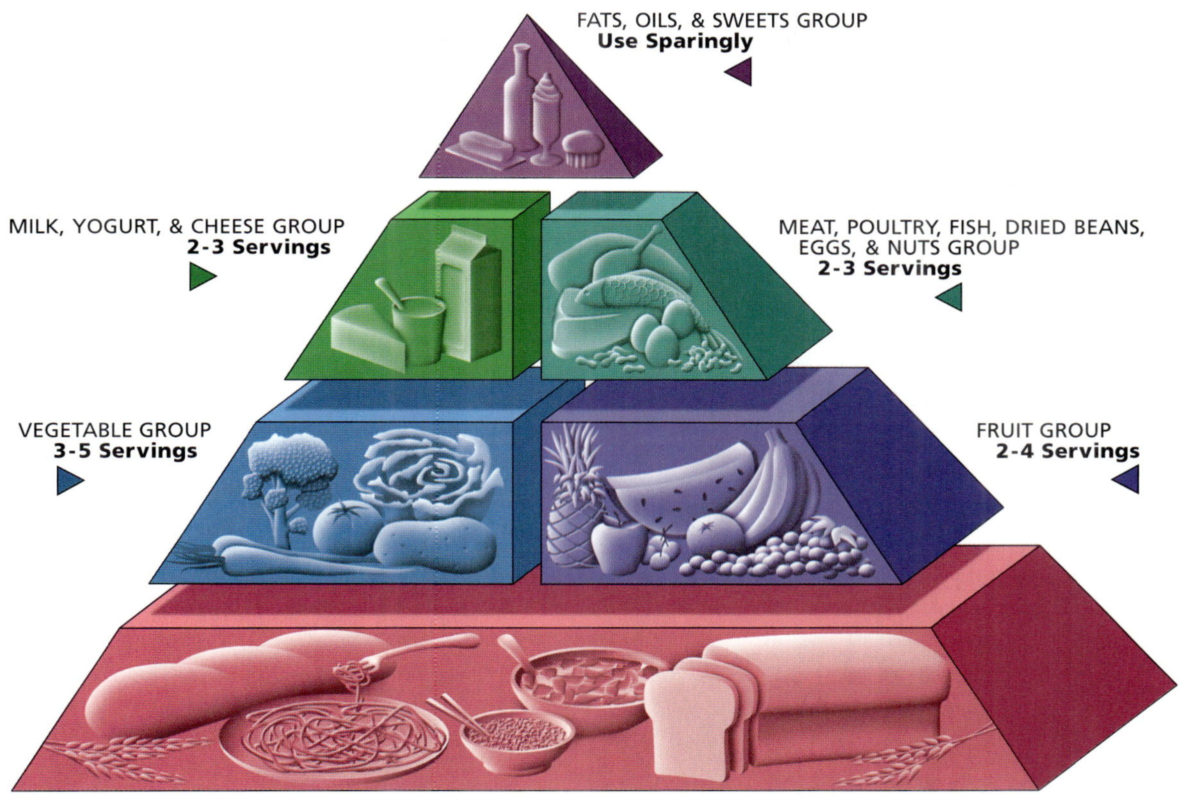

The Food Guide Pyramid—developed on the advice of nutritional scientists—makes healthy eating easier by showing how much of each type of food you should eat for good nutrition. Each of the groups provides some of the nutrients you need each day; no one group provides them all. Variety within and among groups is key.

The foundation of the pyramid is grain-based foods, which provide complex carbohydrates, vitamins, minerals, and fiber. On the next level are fruits and vegetables, which are rich in vitamins, minerals, and fiber but low in fat. The next two groups are critical sources of protein, calcium, iron, zinc, and other nutrients, but many of these foods are also high in fat and cholesterol. Fats, oils, and sweets occupy the tip of the pyramid and should be eaten sparingly.

The pyramid suggests a range of daily servings for each group. Your actual needs depend on your daily caloric requirements. Experts recommend about 1,600 calories for older adults and sedentary women; 2,200 calories for children, teenage girls, active women, and sedentary men; and 2,800 calories for teenage boys, active men, and very active women.

One vegetable serving equals 1 cup of raw leafy greens, ½ cup of other vegetables, or ¾ cup of vegetable juice. One serving from the fruit group is equal to one apple, orange, or banana; ½ cup of chopped, cooked, or canned fruit; or ¾ cup of fruit juice. One grain serving equals one slice of bread; half a bun, bagel, or muffin; 1 oz of dry cereal; or ½ cup of cooked cereal, rice, or pasta. One dairy serving equals 1 cup of milk or yogurt, 1½ oz of natural cheese, or 2 oz of processed cheese. One serving from the meat group equals 2 to 3 oz of cooked lean meat, poultry, or fish. You can substitute one egg, ½ cup of cooked dried beans, or 2 tbsp of peanut butter for each ounce of lean meat. ■

ESSENTIAL VITAMINS AND MINERALS

Your body requires vitamins and minerals to function properly. Known as micronutrients because they are needed in minute amounts, vitamins and minerals contribute to virtually every biochemical process in your body. With a few exceptions, the body does not manufacture micronutrients and so must obtain them from food. Thirteen vitamins and some twenty minerals, most of which are described below, are considered essential for human health. The Food and Nutrition Board of the National Research Council, National Academy of Sciences, has determined a recommended dietary allowance (RDA)—an appropriate range of intake with built-in margins to allow for variations in individual nutritional needs. Essential nutrients that do not yet have RDAs are assigned a safe and adequate daily intake or an estimated minimum daily requirement (EMDR).

Taking vitamins or minerals in excess can upset the natural balance of nutrients. The four fat-soluble vitamins—A, D, E, and K—can be retained in your body and can be toxic in high amounts. The rest are water-soluble and are unlikely to be toxic, since excess amounts are excreted in the urine.

VITAMINS

BIOTIN (VITAMIN B_7, VITAMIN H)

EMDR: 30 mcg to 100 mcg

Along with other B vitamins, biotin helps convert food to energy and is required for the synthesis of carbohydrates, proteins, and fatty acids. Biotin is especially important for healthy hair, skin, and nails.

Among the types of food that are good dietary sources of biotin are cheese, kidneys, salmon, soybeans, sunflower seeds, nuts, broccoli, and sweet potatoes. Biotin deficiency is rare, and supplements are unnecessary. People can become biotin deficient through long-term use of ***antibiotics*** or by regularly eating raw egg whites, which contain avidin, a protein that blocks the body's absorption of biotin.

Because breast milk contains little biotin, infants who are breast-fed can suffer biotin deficiency, although this is uncommon. Signs of biotin deficiency include a scaly, oily skin rash; hair loss; nausea; vomiting; muscle pain; loss of appetite; a red, inflamed tongue; and fatigue. Research has not revealed a toxic level for biotin.

FOLIC ACID (VITAMIN B_9)

RDA: men, 200 mcg; women, 180 mcg; women of childbearing age, 400 mcg

Healthy hair, skin, nails, nerves, mucous membranes, and blood all depend on folic acid—sometimes called vitamin B_9, folacin, or folate. A critical component of RNA and DNA—the genetic material that controls the growth and repair of all cells—folic acid supports immune function and may help deter ***atherosclerosis*** as well as some ***cancers*** of the mucous membranes.

Sources of folic acid include liver, kidneys, avocados, beans, beets, celery, eggs, fish, green leafy vegetables, nuts, seeds, peas, orange juice, and fortified breakfast cereals. A healthy diet should provide adequate folic acid, but the need increases during pregnancy, with injury, with some diseases—especially cancer—and with long-term use of drugs such as ***aspirin*** and oral contraceptives. Supplements taken during pregnancy may help deter the birth defects spina bifida and cleft palate. For this reason, experts now recommend that all women of childbearing age consume 400 mcg daily. High doses of folic acid are not toxic but may mask the symptoms of vitamin B_{12} deficiency. Therefore, it's best to increase folic acid intake through diet or a multivitamin that contains low-dose folic acid, rather than through individual supplements, which have to be prescribed by a doctor.

Extreme vitamin B_9 deficiency may cause megaloblastic ***anemia,*** a disease characterized by red blood cells that are too few in number and malformed. Symptoms include pallor; fatigue; loss of appetite; insomnia; diarrhea; and a red, inflamed tongue. Those who are most susceptible to folic acid deficiency include alcoholics, people with gastrointestinal diseases, adolescents who subsist mainly on junk food, women taking oral contraceptives, and pregnant women who are not taking supplements.

NIACIN (VITAMIN B_3)

RDA: men, 19 mg; women, 15 mg; pregnant women, 17 mg

Niacin contributes to more than 50 vital bodily processes: It helps convert food into energy; build red blood cells; synthesize hormones, fatty acids, and steroids; maintain skin, nerves, and blood vessels; support the gastrointestinal tract; stabilize mental health; and detoxify certain drugs and chemicals in the body. In addition, it helps insulin regulate blood sugar levels.

Niacin is also a powerful drug, capable of lowering blood cholesterol and triglycerides, dilating blood vessels to improve circulation, and alleviating ***depression, insomnia,*** and hyperactivity.

Niacin-rich foods include liver, poultry, lean meats, fish, nuts, peanut butter, and enriched flour. If you get enough protein, you are probably receiving adequate niacin as well. If adequate vitamin B_6 is present, the body can also produce niacin from the amino acid tryptophan, which is found in milk, eggs, and cheese. Signs of niacin deficiency include indigestion; diarrhea; muscle weakness; loss of appetite; ***dermatitis*** that is worsened by exposure to sunlight; mouth sores; a red, inflamed tongue; ***headaches; irritability; anxiety;*** or ***depression.*** Pregnant or breast-feeding women, the elderly, alcoholics, and people with hyperthyroidism are most likely to be niacin deficient. Extreme deficiency results in pellagra, characterized by ***diarrhea, dermatitis,*** and mental illness. Pellagra was common until the discovery that niacin was a cure; the disease is now virtually nonexistent in the U.S. thanks to niacin-enriched flour and other foods. Multivitamin supplements can raise niacin levels safely. Vitamin B_3 is toxic in high amounts, so megadoses should be taken only under a doctor's supervision. Nausea is the first symptom, which often prevents further intake; continued overuse may cause a rash, itchy skin, and liver damage.

VITAMIN A (BETA CAROTENE, RETINOL)

RDA: men, 5,000 IU (or 3 mg beta carotene); women, 4,000 IU (or 2.4 mg beta carotene)

The first vitamin ever discovered, vitamin A is essential for good vision—especially in dim light—and for healthy skin, hair, and mucous membranes of the nose, throat, respiratory system, and digestive system. This vitamin is also necessary for the proper growth and development of bones and teeth. It stimulates wound healing and is used to treat some skin disorders. Beta carotene, the precursor to vitamin A, is a carotenoid, a type of pigment found in plants. Your skin stores beta carotene and your body metabolizes it to produce vitamin A as needed. Excess beta carotene, along with other carotenoids such as alpha carotene, acts as an antioxidant and supports immune function, so it increases your resistance to ***infection;*** it may help prevent some ***cancers*** and vision problems such as night blindness. Beta carotene may also help lower cholesterol levels and reduce the risk of ***heart disease.***

Vitamin A is present in orange and yellow vegetables and fruits; dark-green leafy vegetables such as collard and mustard greens and kale; whole milk, cream, and butter; and organ meats such as liver. Because it is fat-soluble, vitamin A is stored in the body long-term and supplements are generally not recommended. Too much vitamin A can cause ***headaches, vision problems, nausea, vomiting,*** dry and flaking skin, or an enlarged liver or spleen. Other names for vitamin A are retinol, retinene, retinoic acid, and retinyl palmitate.

VITAMIN B COMPLEX

RDA: See individual vitamin entries

As its name implies, vitamin B complex is a combination, or mixture, of eight essential vitamins. Although each is chemically distinct, the B vitamins coexist in many of the same foods and often work together to bolster metabolism, maintain healthy skin and muscle tone, enhance immune and nervous system function, and promote cell growth and division—including that of the red blood cells that help prevent ***anemia.*** Together they may also combat ***stress, depression,*** and cardiovascular disease.

Foods rich in B-complex vitamins include liver and other organ meats, fish, poultry, brewer's yeast, eggs, beans and peas, dark-green leafy vegetables, whole-grain cereals, and dairy products. B vitamins, which are water-soluble, are dispersed throughout the body and must be replenished daily; any excess is excreted in urine. People susceptible to vitamin B deficiency include pregnant women, nursing mothers, vegetarians, alcoholics, "sugar-holics," the elderly, and people with malabsorption conditions or who take certain ***antibiotics*** long-term; the symptoms include oily and scaly skin, upset stomach, ***headaches, anxiety,*** moodiness, and ***heart arrhythmias.*** A deficiency of one B vitamin usually means that intake of all B vitamins is low. If your doctor suggests you need more B vitamins, take a daily multivitamin or B-complex supplement rather than individual B-vitamin supplements. Most B vitamins are nontoxic unless taken in excessively large amounts.

VITAMIN B_1 (THIAMINE)

RDA: men, 1.5 mg; women, 1.1 mg

Thiamine is sometimes called the "energy vitamin" because it is needed to metabolize carbohydrates, fats, and proteins, and it helps convert excess glucose into stored fat. Vitamin B_1 also ensures proper nerve-

ESSENTIAL VITAMINS AND MINERALS

impulse transmission and contributes to maintaining normal appetite, muscle tone, and mental health. In the 1930s thiamine was discovered to be the cure for the crippling and potentially fatal disease beriberi. Now that rice, flour, and bread are generally enriched with thiamine, beriberi is relatively rare.

A diet that regularly includes lean pork, milk, whole grains, peas, beans, peanuts, or soybeans generally provides enough thiamine. Athletes, laborers, pregnant women, and other people who burn great amounts of energy may require more than the adult RDA of thiamine. Mild deficiency may cause ***fatigue,*** loss of appetite, ***nausea,*** moodiness, confusion, ***anemia,*** and possibly ***heart arrhythmias.*** Alcohol suppresses thiamine absorption; for this reason and because of typically poor diets, alcoholics are likely to be deficient in thiamine and other nutrients. To increase thiamine levels, try changing your diet or taking a multivitamin instead of thiamine supplements. Large doses up to 100 mg of thiamine may alleviate itching from insect bites; otherwise, megasupplements are not known to be either harmful or helpful.

VITAMIN B_2 (RIBOFLAVIN)

RDA: men, 1.7 mg; women, 1.3 mg; pregnant women, 1.6 mg

Like other members of the vitamin B complex, riboflavin helps produce energy from carbohydrates, fats, and proteins. Riboflavin also promotes healthy skin, hair, nails, and mucous membranes; aids the production of red blood cells, corticosteroids, and thyroid hormones; and is required for the proper function of the nerves, eyes, and adrenal glands. It is often used to treat ***acne, anemia, cataracts,*** and ***depression.***

A well-balanced diet provides most people with adequate riboflavin, although athletes and others who need a great deal of energy may require more than the RDA. Lean organ meats, enriched bread and flour, cheese, yogurt, eggs, almonds, soybean products such as tofu, and green leafy vegetables—especially broccoli—are good sources. Store these foods in the dark, because vitamin B_2 breaks down in sunlight. Alcoholics and elderly people are susceptible to riboflavin deficiency: The signs include oily, scaly skin rash; sores, especially on the lips and corners of the mouth; a swollen, red, painful tongue; sensitivity to light; and burning or red, itchy eyes. Although vitamin B_2 supplements are available, they provide far more riboflavin than anyone needs. Diet changes are better, or you should take a multivitamin supplement. It is best to take the supplements with food, which increases their absorption tremendously compared with tablets alone.

VITAMIN B_5 (PANTOTHENIC ACID)

EMDR: 4 mg to 7 mg

The Greek term *pan* in pantothenic acid means "everywhere," indicating this vitamin's abundance. Along with other B vitamins, pantothenic acid is required for converting food to energy; building red blood cells; making bile; and synthesizing fats, adrenal gland steroids, antibodies, and acetylcholine and other neurotransmitters—chemicals that permit nerve transmission. Pantothenic acid in dexpanthenol lotions and creams relieves the pain of ***burns,*** cuts, and abrasions; reduces skin inflammation; and speeds wound healing.

Vitamin B_5 is abundant in organ meats, dark turkey meat, salmon, wheat bran, brewer's yeast, brown rice, lentils, nuts, beans, corn, peas, sweet potatoes, and eggs. Excess pantothenic acid may cause ***diarrhea.*** A deficiency in this vitamin does not seem to occur naturally in humans and is likely only with extreme starvation. A pantothenic acid supplement, calcium pantothenate, is available.

VITAMIN B_6 (PYRIDOXINE)

RDA: men, 2 mg; women, 1.6 mg; pregnant women, 2.2 mg

Vitamin B_6 encompasses a family of compounds that includes pyridoxine, pyridoxamine, and pyridoxal. This vitamin supports immune function, nerve-impulse transmission (especially in the brain), energy metabolism, and red blood cell synthesis. Prescribed as a drug, vitamin B_6 can sometimes alleviate ***carpal tunnel syndrome,*** infant seizures, and ***premenstrual syndrome.***

A healthy diet provides enough vitamin B_6 for most people. Brown rice, lean meats, poultry, fish, bananas, avocados, whole grains, corn, and nuts are rich in vitamin B_6. People most likely to be at risk for vitamin B_6 deficiency include anyone with a malabsorption problem such as ***lactose intolerance*** or ***celiac disease; diabetic*** or elderly people; and women who are pregnant, nursing, or taking oral contraceptives. Severe deficiency is rare. Mild deficiency may cause ***acne*** and inflamed skin, ***insomnia,*** muscle weakness, ***nausea, irritability, depression,*** and ***fatigue.*** A daily multivitamin supplement is usually recommended to boost low vita-

min B_6 levels. Taking too much or too little vitamin B_6 can impair nerve function and mental health. If high levels (2,000 mg to 5,000 mg) are taken for several months, vitamin B_6 can become habit-forming and may induce sleepiness as well as tingling, numb hands and feet. These symptoms will most likely disappear when the vitamin B_6 intake is reduced, and there is usually no permanent damage.

VITAMIN B_{12} (COBALAMIN)

RDA: adults, 2 mcg; pregnant women, 2.2 mcg

Vitamin B_{12} is the largest and most complex family of the B vitamins; it includes several chemical compounds known as cobalamins. Cyanocobalamin, the most stable form, is the one most likely to be found in supplements. Like other B vitamins, B_{12} is important for converting fats, carbohydrates, and protein into energy, and assisting in the synthesis of red blood cells. It is critical for producing the genetic materials RNA and DNA, as well as myelin, a fatty substance that forms a protective sheath around nerves. Unlike other B vitamins, vitamin B_{12} needs several hours to be absorbed in the digestive tract. Excess vitamin B_{12} is excreted in urine, even though a backup supply can be stored for several years in the liver.

Vitamin B_{12} is not produced by plants but is supplied through animal products such as organ meats, fish, eggs, and dairy products. Dietary deficiency is uncommon and usually limited to alcoholics, strict vegetarians, and pregnant or nursing women—who should take supplements. More often, deficiency stems from an inability to absorb the vitamin, a problem that may occur for years before symptoms show; it tends to affect the elderly, those who have had stomach surgery, or people who have a disease of malabsorption, such as ***colitis.***

Lack of ***calcium, vitamin B_6,*** or ***iron*** may also interfere with the normal absorption of B_{12}. Signs of vitamin B_{12} deficiency include a sore tongue, weakness, weight loss, body odor, back pains, and tingling arms and legs. Severe deficiency leads to pernicious ***anemia,*** causing ***fatigue,*** a tendency to bleed, lemon yellow pallor, ***abdominal pain,*** stiff arms and legs, irritability, and ***depression.***

Without treatment, pernicious anemia can lead to permanent nerve damage and possibly death; the disease can be controlled, although not cured, with regular B_{12} injections. Vitamin B_{12} is considered nontoxic, even when taken at several times the RDA.

VITAMIN C (ASCORBIC ACID)

RDA: adults, 60 mg; pregnant women, 70 mg

Vitamin C is well known for its ability to prevent and treat scurvy, a disease that causes swollen and bleeding gums, aching bones and muscles, and in some cases even death. Connective tissue throughout the body is made of collagen, which depends on vitamin C for its production. In this role, vitamin C helps heal wounds, burns, bruises, and broken bones. As a powerful antioxidant and immune system booster, vitamin C may alleviate the pain of rheumatoid ***arthritis,*** protect against ***atherosclerosis*** and ***heart disease,*** and help prevent some forms of ***cancer,*** and has the reputed potential (yet unproved) to prevent the ***common cold.*** More than the RDA may be needed under conditions of physical or emotional ***stress.***

Sources of vitamin C include citrus fruits, rose hips, bell peppers, strawberries, broccoli, cantaloupes, tomatoes, and leafy greens. Vitamin C breaks down faster than any other vitamin, so it is best to eat fruits and vegetables when fresh, and to cook them minimally or not at all. Slight vitamin C deficiency is rather common, although severe deficiencies are rare in the United States today. Symptoms of deficiency include weight loss, fatigue, bleeding gums, easy bruising, reduced resistance to colds and other infections, and slow-healing wounds and fractures.

Because it is water-soluble, excess vitamin C is excreted in the urine, so large amounts of it may usually be taken without fear of toxicity. Doses larger than 1,000 mg a day have been suggested for preventing cancer, infections including the common cold, and other ailments. In some people, large doses may induce such side effects as ***nausea, diarrhea,*** reduced selenium and copper absorption, excessive iron absorption, increased kidney stone formation, and false-positive reaction to ***diabetes*** tests.

VITAMIN D (CHOLECALCIFEROL, ERGOCALCIFEROL)

RDA: adults, 200 IU (5 mcg); children, adolescents and pregnant women, 400 IU (10 mcg)

Vitamin D not only promotes healthy bones and teeth by regulating the absorption and balance of ***calcium*** and ***phosphorus,*** but also fosters normal muscle contraction and nerve function. Vitamin D prevents rickets, a disease of calcium-deprived bone that results in bowlegs, knock-knees, and other bone defects. Vitamin

ESSENTIAL VITAMINS AND MINERALS

D supplements may help treat ***psoriasis*** and slow or even reverse some ***cancers,*** such as myeloid ***leukemia.***

Fatty fish such as herring, salmon, and tuna, followed by dairy products, are the richest natural sources of this nutrient. Few other foods naturally contain vitamin D, but 10 minutes in midday summer sun enables the body to produce about 200 IU of it. Milk, breakfast cereals, and infant formulas are fortified with vitamin D. In adults, vitamin D deficiency can cause nervousness and ***diarrhea, insomnia,*** muscle twitches, and bone weakening, and it may worsen ***osteoporosis.*** Too much vitamin D raises the calcium level in the blood, which in turn may induce ***headaches, nausea,*** loss of appetite, excessive thirst, muscle weakness, and even heart, liver, or kidney damage as ***calcium*** deposits accumulate in soft tissue. Vitamin D is fat-soluble; excess amounts of it are stored in the body. Because of its potentially toxic effects, vitamin D should not be taken in supplements of more than 400 IU daily unless prescribed by a doctor.

VITAMIN E

RDA: women, 12 IU (8 mg); men and pregnant or nursing women, 15 IU (10 mg)

Vitamin E encompasses a family of compounds called tocopherols, of which alpha-tocopherol is the most common. It is required for proper function of the immune system, endocrine system, and sex glands. As a powerful antioxidant, it prevents unstable molecules known as free radicals from damaging cells and tissues. In this capacity, vitamin E deters ***atherosclerosis,*** accelerates wound healing, protects lung tissue from inhaled pollutants, may reduce risk for ***heart disease,*** and may prevent premature skin aging. Researchers suspect that vitamin E has other beneficial effects ranging from preventing ***cancer*** and ***cataracts*** to alleviating rheumatoid ***arthritis*** and a skin disorder associated with ***lupus.***

Most people get enough vitamin E through diet and don't need supplements. Vegetable oils, nuts, dark-green leafy vegetables, organ meats, seafood, eggs, and avocados are rich food sources. Symptoms of vitamin E deficiency, such as fluid retention and hemolytic ***anemia,*** are rare in adults but are sometimes seen in premature infants. Because of its many suggested therapeutic roles, vitamin E is popular as an oral supplement and an ingredient of skin-care products. Although it is fat-soluble, vitamin E is considered nontoxic, because it does no harm except in extremely high doses.

VITAMIN K (MENADIONE, PHYTONADIONE)

RDA: men, 80 mcg; women, 65 mcg

Vitamin K is needed in a small but critical amount to form essential proteins, mainly for blood clotting but also for kidney function and bone metabolism. Vitamin K exists in two natural forms that require some dietary fat for absorption.

Bacteria living in the intestines produce about half the body's needs; the rest comes from diet. Good food sources include spinach, cabbage, broccoli, turnip greens, or other leafy vegetables; beef liver; green tea; cheese; and oats. Vitamin K deficiency is extremely rare in adults but may occur in newborns until their intestinal bacteria begin producing the vitamin. To enhance a newborn's blood-clotting ability, the mother may take vitamin K supplements before delivery, and infants usually receive them after birth. Otherwise, supplements are neither necessary nor recommended. Megadoses higher than 500 mcg can be toxic or cause allergic reaction, and must be prescribed by a doctor. Large doses of ***vitamin E*** may interfere with vitamin K's blood-clotting effects.

MINERALS

CALCIUM

RDA: adults, 800 mg; pregnant women and young adults, 1,200 mg

Calcium, the most abundant mineral in the body, is essential for the growth and maintenance of bones and teeth. It enables muscles, including your heart, to contract; it is essential for normal blood clotting, proper nerve-impulse transmission, and connective-tissue maintenance. It helps keep blood pressure normal and may reduce the risk of ***heart disease;*** taken with ***vitamin D,*** it may help lessen the risk of ***colorectal cancer.*** It helps prevent rickets in children and ***osteoporosis*** in adults.

Good sources include dairy products, dark-green leafy vegetables, sardines, salmon, and almonds. Calcium is needed in varying amounts by different people. Too much calcium can lead to ***constipation*** and to calcium deposits in soft tissue, causing damage to the heart, liver, or kidneys. For calcium to be properly absorbed, the body must have sufficient levels of ***vitamin D*** and of hydrochloric acid in the stomach, and a balance of other minerals, including ***magnesium*** and ***phosphorus.*** A sedentary lifestyle and consuming too much

alcohol, dietary fiber, and fat can interfere with calcium absorption; too much protein and caffeine results in calcium being excreted in urine. Supplemental calcium is available in many forms; the form that is best absorbed by the body is calcium citrate-malate.

CHLORIDE

EMDR: adults, 750 mg

A natural salt of the mineral chlorine, chloride works with ***sodium*** and ***potassium*** to help maintain the proper distribution and pH of all bodily fluids and encourage healthy nerve and muscle function. Independently, chloride contributes to digestion and waste elimination. It is a key component of hydrochloric acid, one of the gastric juices that digest food.

A diet of unprocessed natural foods provides more than enough chloride for human health. Just a pinch of table salt contains about 250 mg, one-third of the RDA. Chloride deficiency is extremely rare and is usually due to illness. Excessive ***vomiting*** can reduce the stomach's chloride level, upsetting its pH balance and causing sweating, ***diarrhea,*** loss of appetite, slow and shallow breathing, listlessness, and ***muscle cramps.*** Although toxic in large amounts, excess chloride is excreted in urine, preventing potentially dangerous accumulation.

CHROMIUM

EMDR: adults, 50 mcg to 200 mcg

As a component of a natural substance called glucose tolerance factor, chromium works with insulin to regulate the body's use of sugar and is essential to fatty-acid metabolism. Its contribution to metabolism makes chromium a helpful supplement in weight-loss programs. Additional evidence suggests that chromium may help deter ***atherosclerosis*** and reduce risk of cardiovascular disease. Inadequate chromium can result in alcohol intolerance, elevate blood sugar levels, and possibly induce ***diabetes***-like symptoms such as tingling in the extremities and reduced muscle coordination.

Trace amounts of chromium are found in many foods, including brewer's yeast, liver, lean meats, poultry, molasses, whole grains, eggs, and cheese. Chromium is not absorbed well, so the body must take in far more than it actually uses. Most people do not get enough dietary chromium and some may benefit from a multinutrient supplement, such as chromium citrate or chromium picolinate. Supplemental chromium may be used to treat some cases of adult-onset ***diabetes,*** to reduce insulin requirements of some diabetic children, and to relieve symptoms of ***hypoglycemia.*** Taken regularly in supplements greater than 1,000 mcg, however, chromium inhibits insulin's activity and can be toxic.

COBALT

RDA/EMDR: not established

The mineral cobalt is a constituent of cobalamin (***vitamin B_{12});*** Cobalt helps form red blood cells and maintain nerve tissue. Consuming large amounts of inorganic cobalt stimulates growth of the thyroid gland and may lead to the overproduction of red blood cells, a disorder known as polycythemia.

To be biologically useful, cobalt must be obtained from foods such as liver, kidneys, milk, oysters, clams, or sea vegetables, or from vitamin B12 supplements. Inorganic cobalt has no nutritional value but is sometimes added to beer as an antifoaming agent.

COPPER

EMDR: adults, 1.5 mg to 3 mg

Copper is indispensable to human health. Its many functions include the following: helping to form hemoglobin in the blood; facilitating the absorption and use of iron so red blood cells can transport oxygen to tissues; assisting in the regulation of blood pressure and heart rate; strengthening blood vessels, bones, tendons, and nerves; promoting fertility; and ensuring normal skin and hair pigmentation. Some evidence suggests that copper helps prevent cardiovascular problems such as ***high blood pressure*** and ***heart arrhythmias*** and that it may help treat ***arthritis*** and ***scoliosis.*** Copper may also protect tissue from damage by free radicals, support the body's immune function, and contribute to preventing ***cancer.***

Most adults get enough copper from a normal, varied diet. Seafood and organ meats are the richest sources; blackstrap molasses, nuts, seeds, green vegetables, black pepper, cocoa, and water passed through copper pipes also contain significant quantities. Supplemental copper should be taken only on a doctor's advice. Common supplemental forms are copper aspartate, copper citrate, and copper picolinate. Excess calcium and zinc will interfere with copper absorption, but a true copper deficiency is rare and tends to be limited to people either with certain inherited diseases that inhibit copper absorption, such as albinism, or with acquired malabsorption ailments, such as ***Crohn's***

disease and ***celiac disease.*** The deficiency may also occur in infants who are not breast-fed and some premature babies. Symptoms of copper deficiency include brittle, discolored hair; skeletal defects; ***anemia; high blood pressure; heart arrhythmias;*** and ***infertility.*** Taking more than 10 mg of copper daily can bring on nausea, vomiting, muscle pain, and stomachaches. Women who are pregnant or taking birth-control pills are susceptible to excess blood levels of copper. Some research suggests that high levels of copper and iron may play a role in hyperactivity and autism.

FLUORIDE

EMDR: adults, 1.5 mg to 4 mg

Fluoride, a natural form of the mineral fluorine, is required for healthy teeth and bones. It helps form the tough enamel that protects teeth from decay and cavities, and increases bone strength and stability. Since the 1950s, many U.S. cities have added fluoride to municipal drinking water at a ratio of about 1 part per million (ppm), or 1 mg per liter. Many believe this practice is responsible for the 40 to 70 percent reduction in tooth decay that dentists have since observed. Fluoride's decay-reducing effects are strongest if children are exposed to the mineral while their teeth are forming. Fluoride toothpaste is helpful, but it is not nearly as effective as regularly ingested fluoride.

Fluoridated water provides most individuals with at least 1 mg of fluoride daily; other dietary sources are dried seaweed, seafood—especially sardines and salmon—cheese, meat, and tea. Nursing babies and children who do not regularly drink fluoridated water should be given supplements, but only as prescribed by a dentist or doctor, because excess fluoride can have adverse effects: At levels of 2 ppm to 8 ppm, the teeth may soften and discolor; at over 8 ppm, fluoride toxicity can depress growth, harden ligaments and tendons, make bones brittle, and induce degeneration of major body systems; 50 ppm may cause fatal poisoning. The low fluoride levels in fluoridated drinking water, however, pose no harmful effects to health.

IODINE

RDA: adults, 150 mcg; pregnant women, 175 mcg

Iodine was one of the first minerals recognized as essential to human health. For centuries, it has been known to prevent and treat ***goiter***—enlargement of the thyroid gland. As part of several thyroid hormones, iodine strongly influences nutrient metabolism; nerve and muscle function; skin, hair, tooth, and nail condition; and physical and mental development. Iodine may also help convert beta carotene into ***vitamin A,*** and it is an effective antiseptic and water sterilizer.

Kelp, seafood, and vegetables grown in iodine-rich soils are excellent sources of this mineral. More than half of all the salt consumed in the U.S. is iodized, supplying sufficient iodine in a regular diet. Supplements are usually unnecessary, but pregnant women should have sufficient intake for themselves and their babies to prevent potential mental retardation or cretinism, a form of dwarfism in infants. Iodine deficiency is now uncommon; besides goiter, its effects include weight gain, ***hair loss,*** listlessness, ***insomnia,*** and some forms of mental retardation. Most excess iodine is excreted by the kidneys, but extremely high intake may cause nervousness, hyperactivity, ***headache,*** rashes, a metallic taste in the mouth, and goiter—in this case due to thyroid hyperactivity.

IRON

RDA: adults, 10 mg; premenopausal women, 15 mg; pregnant women, 30 mg

Iron is found in hemoglobin, the protein in red blood cells that transports oxygen from the lungs to body tissues. It is also a component of myoglobin, a protein that provides extra fuel to muscles during exertion.

Dietary iron exists in two forms: heme iron, found in red meat, chicken, seafood, and other animal products; and nonheme iron, found in dark-green vegetables, whole grains, nuts, dried fruit, and other plant foods. Many flour-based food products are fortified with iron. Heme iron is easier to absorb, but eating foods containing nonheme iron along with foods that have heme iron or ***vitamin C*** will maximize iron absorption.

Coffee, tea, soy-based foods, ***antacids,*** and ***tetracycline*** inhibit iron absorption, as do excessive amounts of ***calcium, zinc,*** and ***manganese.*** Lack of iron deprives body tissues of oxygen and may cause iron deficiency ***anemia;*** warning signs include ***fatigue,*** paleness, ***dizziness,*** sensitivity to cold, listlessness, ***irritability,*** poor concentration, and heart palpitations. Because iron strengthens immune function, iron deficiency also may increase susceptibility to infection. Women need more iron before menopause than after, because menstruation causes iron loss each month. People who have special iron intake needs include menstruating or pregnant

women, children under two years of age, vegetarians, anyone with bleeding conditions such as ***hemorrhoids*** or bleeding ***stomach ulcers,*** and anyone taking the medications listed above.

On a doctor's recommendation, adults can augment their iron intake by means of a multinutrient supplement; straight iron supplements should be taken only under a doctor's supervision. Excess iron inhibits absorption of ***phosphorus,*** interferes with immune function, and may increase your risk of developing ***cancer, cirrhosis,*** or ***heart attack.*** Symptoms of iron toxicity include ***diarrhea, vomiting, headache, dizziness, fatigue,*** stomach cramps, and weak pulse. Though uncommon, severe iron poisoning can result in coma, heart failure, and death. Children should never be given adult iron supplements, which can easily poison them. If your pediatrician recommends an iron supplement, make sure it is a specific, child-formulated variety.

MAGNESIUM

RDA: men, 350 mg; women, 280 mg; pregnant women, 320 mg

Magnesium contributes to health in many ways. Along with ***calcium*** and ***phosphorus,*** it is a main ingredient of bone. A proper balance of calcium and magnesium is essential for healthy bones and teeth, reduces the risk of developing ***osteoporosis,*** and may minimize the effects of existing osteoporosis. Calcium and magnesium also help regulate muscle activity: While calcium stimulates contraction, magnesium induces relaxation. Magnesium is essential for metabolism—converting food to energy—and for building proteins. Adequate blood levels of magnesium protect the body from cardiovascular disease, ***heart arrhythmias,*** and possibly, ***stroke*** due to blood clotting in the brain.

On average, people get enough (or nearly enough) magnesium in their diet. Fish, green leafy vegetables, milk, nuts, seeds, and whole grains are good sources. Many over-the-counter ***antacids, laxatives,*** and ***analgesics*** contain magnesium, but these medications should not be used as magnesium supplements. A multinutrient supplement is a relatively safe way to augment your magnesium intake. Take specific magnesium supplements only under a doctor's supervision. Of the supplemental forms, magnesium citrate-malate is the easiest to absorb, while magnesium glycinate is least likely to cause ***diarrhea*** at high doses.

The body's need for magnesium increases with stress or illness. Administered as a supplement, magnesium may successfully treat ***insomnia, muscle cramps, premenstrual syndrome,*** and cardiovascular problems including ***high blood pressure, angina*** due to coronary artery spasm, and pain and cramping due to insufficient blood flow to the legs. Studies indicate that giving magnesium immediately to a ***heart attack*** patient greatly increases the chance of survival.

The body processes magnesium efficiently; the kidneys conserve it as needed and excrete any excess amounts, so the incidences of both severe deficiency and toxicity are rare. These conditions are dangerous when they do occur, however. Magnesium deficiency may cause ***nausea, vomiting,*** listlessness, ***muscle weakness,*** tremor, disorientation, and heart palpitations. Toxicity can induce ***diarrhea, fatigue, muscle weakness,*** and in extreme cases, severely depressed heart rate and blood pressure, shallow breathing, loss of reflexes, coma, and possibly, death. People who abuse ***laxatives*** or experience kidney failure are most vulnerable to magnesium poisoning.

MANGANESE

EMDR: 2.5 mg to 5 mg

Manganese is essential for the proper formation and maintenance of bone, cartilage, and connective tissue; it contributes to the synthesis of proteins and genetic material; it helps produce energy from foods; it acts as an antioxidant; and it assists in normal blood clotting.

Most people get enough manganese through diet alone; for example, a breakfast of orange juice, a 1-oz serving of bran cereal, and a banana provides just over 2.5 mg of manganese. Other food sources include brown rice, nuts, seeds, wheat germ, beans, whole grains, peas, and strawberries. Manganese citrate, a supplement, may help repair damaged tendons and ligaments. Excess dietary manganese is not considered toxic, and manganese deficiency is extremely rare.

MOLYBDENUM

EMDR: adults, 75 mcg to 250 mcg

The obscure mineral molybdenum is an enzyme component. It helps generate energy, process waste for excretion, mobilize stored ***iron*** for the body's use, and detoxify sulfites—chemicals used as food preservatives. As such, molybdenum is essential to normal development, particularly of the nervous system. It is also an ingredient of tooth enamel and may help prevent tooth decay.

ESSENTIAL VITAMINS AND MINERALS

Molybdenum is present in peas, beans, cereals, pastas, leafy vegetables, yeast, milk, and organ meats. People generally get enough through diet; deficiency is virtually nonexistent. Toxicity is also rare in humans. Molybdenum is available in supplement form as molybdenum picolinate; however, prolonged intake of more than 10 mg daily can cause goutlike symptoms such as joint pain and swelling.

PHOSPHORUS

RDA: adults over 25 years old, 800 mg; young adults and pregnant women, 1,200 mg

Phosphorus is the second most plentiful mineral in the body and is found in every cell. Like ***calcium,*** phosphorus is essential for bone formation and maintenance; more than 75 percent of the body's phosphorus is contained in bones and teeth. Phosphorus stimulates muscle contraction and contributes to tissue growth and repair, energy production, nerve-impulse transmission, and heart and kidney function.

Phosphorus exists to some degree in nearly all foods, especially meats, poultry, eggs, fish, nuts, dairy products, whole grains, and soft drinks. Deficiency is rare—most people take in far more phosphorus than they need—but may be induced by long-term use of ***antacids*** or ***anticonvulsant drugs*** that contain ***aluminum hydroxide.*** Symptoms of phosphorus deficiency include general weakness, loss of appetite, bone pain, and increased susceptibility to bone fracture. Excess phosphorus in the bloodstream promotes calcium loss, which may weaken bones. Extreme phosphorus toxicity is rare, except in the event of ***kidney disease.***

POTASSIUM

EMDR: adults, 2,000 mg

Potassium is the third most abundant mineral in the body, after ***calcium*** and ***phosphorus.*** It works closely with ***sodium*** and ***chloride*** to maintain fluid distribution and pH balance and to augment nerve-impulse transmission, muscle contraction, and regulation of heartbeat and blood pressure. Potassium is also required for protein synthesis, carbohydrate metabolism, and insulin secretion by the pancreas. Studies suggest that people who regularly eat potassium-rich foods are less likely to develop ***atherosclerosis, heart disease,*** and ***high blood pressure,*** or to die of a ***stroke.***

Dietary sources include lean meats, raw vegetables, and fruits—especially citrus fruits, bananas, and avocados—and potatoes. Many Americans may get only marginal amounts of potassium, but supplements, such as potassium aspartate, are best taken only under a doctor's guidance. Marginal potassium deficiency causes no symptoms but may increase the risk of developing ***high blood pressure*** or aggravate existing ***heart disease.*** More severe deficiency can result in ***nausea, vomiting, diarrhea, muscle cramps*** and ***muscle weakness,*** poor reflexes, poor concentration, ***heart arrhythmias,*** and rarely, death due to heart failure. Acute potassium toxicity may have similar effects, including possible heart failure. However, acute toxicity is rarely linked to diet and tends to occur only in the event of kidney failure.

SELENIUM

RDA: men, 70 mcg; women, 55 mcg; pregnant women, 65 mcg

An antioxidant, selenium protects cells and tissues from damage wrought by free radicals. Because its antioxidant effects complement those of ***vitamin E,*** the two are said to potentiate, or reinforce, each other. Selenium also supports immune function and neutralizes certain poisonous substances such as cadmium, mercury, and arsenic that may be ingested or inhaled. Although its full therapeutic value is unknown, adequate selenium levels may help combat ***arthritis,*** deter ***heart disease,*** and prevent ***cancer.***

Whole grains, asparagus, garlic, eggs, and mushrooms are typically good sources, as are lean meats and seafood. Very little selenium is required for good health, and most people get adequate amounts through diet alone. High-dose supplements such as selenium citrate and selenium picolinate should be taken only if prescribed by a doctor. Selenium can be toxic in extremely high doses, causing ***hair loss,*** nail problems, accelerated tooth decay, and swelling of the fingers, among other symptoms. Some multinutrients contain selenium, but always in small, safe amounts.

SODIUM

EMDR: adults, 500 mg

All bodily fluids—including blood, tears, and perspiration—contain sodium. Together with ***potassium*** and ***chloride,*** sodium maintains fluid distribution and pH balance; with potassium, sodium also helps control muscle contraction and nerve function.

Most of the sodium in American diets is from table salt. Among many other sources are processed foods, soft drinks, meats, shellfish, condiments, snack foods, food additives, and over-the-counter ***laxatives.*** Americans generally consume far too much sodium. A single teaspoon of salt contains 2,000 mg—four times the daily minimum—but average daily consumption in the U.S. ranges from 3,000 mg to 7,000 mg.

Keeping sodium intake within reasonable limits is critical for long-term health. When sodium levels are persistently elevated, the body loses ***potassium*** and retains water, making blood pressure rise. Adopting a low-sodium diet can reduce ***high blood pressure*** and correct a potassium deficiency. Overexertion can induce temporary sodium deficiency, characterized by ***nausea,*** dehydration, ***muscle cramps,*** and other symptoms of heatstroke *(see* ***Emergencies/First Aid: Heatstroke and Heat Exhaustion****).* Drinking several glasses of water with a pinch of salt added replaces the sodium and eases the symptoms.

SULFUR

RDA/EMDR: not established

Accounting for some 10 percent of the body's mineral content, sulfur is part of every cell, especially in the protein-rich tissues of hair, nails, muscle, and skin. It assists in metabolism as a part of ***vitamin B_1, biotin,*** and ***vitamin B_5;*** helps regulate blood sugar levels as a constituent of insulin; and helps regulate blood clotting. Sulfur is also known to convert some toxic substances into nontoxic ones that can then be excreted and therefore is used to treat poisoning from aluminum, cadmium, lead, and mercury.

Any diet that provides sufficient protein is also providing adequate sulfur. Meat, fish, poultry, eggs, dairy products, peas, and beans are rich in both nutrients. Neither sulfur deficiency nor toxicity occurs naturally in humans. Inorganic sulfur ingested in large amounts can be harmful, but excess organic sulfur from food is readily excreted.

VANADIUM

RDA/EMDR: not established

Vanadium is a trace mineral whose role in human nutrition is little known, but possibly essential. Limited evidence suggests that vanadium lowers blood sugar levels in some people and inhibits tumor development, and therefore may protect against ***diabetes*** and some forms of ***cancer.*** It also appears to contribute to cholesterol metabolism and hormone production. Vanadium exists in whole grains, nuts, root vegetables, liver, fish, and vegetable oils. Because vanadium deficiency symptoms are unknown, researchers assume that humans require only a small amount, which diet apparently provides.

ZINC

RDA: adults, 15 mg; pregnant women, 30 mg

The mineral zinc is integral to the synthesis of RNA and DNA, the genetic material that controls cell growth, division, and function. In various proteins, enzymes, hormones, and hormonelike substances called prostaglandins, zinc contributes to many bodily processes, including bone development and growth; cell respiration; energy metabolism; wound healing; the liver's ability to remove toxic substances such as alcohol from the body; immune function; and the regulation of heart rate and blood pressure. An adequate zinc intake enhances the ability to taste, promotes healthy skin and hair, enhances reproductive functions, and may improve short-term memory and attention span. As an anti-inflammatory agent, zinc is sometimes used to treat ***acne,*** rheumatoid ***arthritis,*** and prostatitis. Taking supplemental zinc may boost resistance to ***infection,*** especially in the elderly, and stimulate wound healing.

Zinc is most easily obtained from lean meat and seafood, but it is also found in eggs, soybeans, peanuts, wheat bran, cheese, oysters, and other foods. Many American diets are slightly low in zinc. Young children, pregnant women, vegetarians, and elderly people are most susceptible to zinc deficiency. Loss of taste is usually the first warning; other symptoms are ***hair loss*** or discoloration, white streaks on the nails, ***dermatitis,*** loss of appetite, ***fatigue,*** and poor wound healing. In children, zinc deficiency can retard growth and stunt sexual development in boys. On the other hand, ingesting extreme amounts of zinc daily can impair immune function and cause ***nausea, headaches, vomiting,*** dehydration, stomachaches, poor muscle coordination, ***fatigue,*** and possibly kidney failure. Experts recommend increasing zinc levels by increasing the zinc-rich foods in your diet or by taking a multinutrient supplement that includes zinc chelate, zinc picolinate, or zinc aspartate, the three most easily absorbed forms. If zinc is used for more than three to six months to treat a chronic condition, it is essential to consult a nutritionist to avoid creating a mineral imbalance. Zinc ointment, which contains zinc oxide, is the most common topical form, useful in skin disorders, burns, and other wounds. ■

A VISUAL DIAGNOSTIC GUIDE

The photographs on the following pages show the visible symptoms of a variety of conditions, ranging from childhood illnesses and benign skin disorders to more serious diseases such as cancer. This section is intended to help you distinguish among different conditions that look similar and are often confused with one another. Keep in mind that symptoms can vary greatly in appearance, depending on such factors as the severity of an individual case; always consult your doctor for a proper diagnosis. For more information on many of the disorders included here, refer to the appropriate entries in the Ailments and Options section of the book.

CONTENTS

Children's Problems 1044
Mouth Problems 1045
Skin Growths 1046
Rashes, Insect Bites, and Skin Discolorations 1048
Eye Problems 1051

CHILDREN'S PROBLEMS

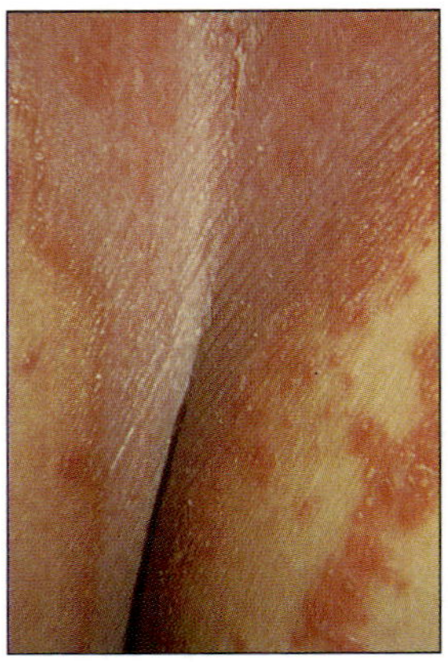

CANDIDIASIS

Often confused with ***diaper rash,*** candidiasis is a type of yeast infection that may appear on the buttocks and genital area of infants. In most cases, the characteristic bright red spots come together to form a rash with a scalloped border. See also ***Yeast Infections.***

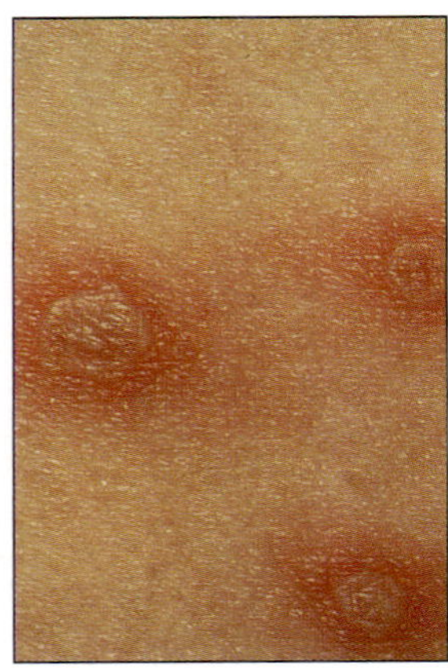

CHICKENPOX

A highly contagious childhood disease, chickenpox usually begins with an itchy red rash that then develops into small fluid-filled blisters *(above);* the blisters eventually rupture and become crusty. The rash first appears on the torso, then spreads to the face.

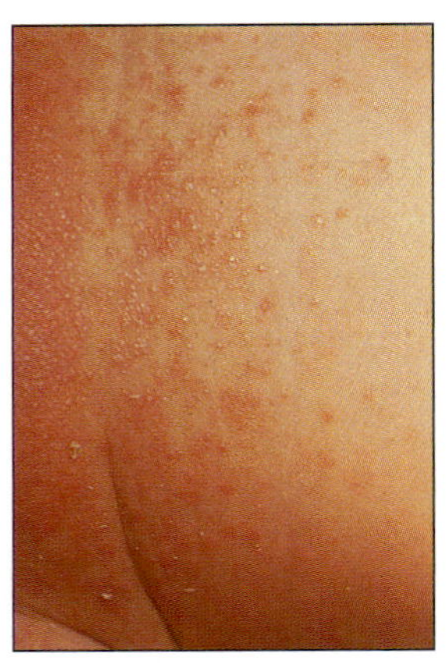

DIAPER RASH

Infants often develop a rash in the area covered by a diaper. The rash can vary from slight redness to severe inflammation *(above).* Diaper rash is caused by exposure to moisture, heat, urine, and feces. Excessive bathing can also contribute to the problem.

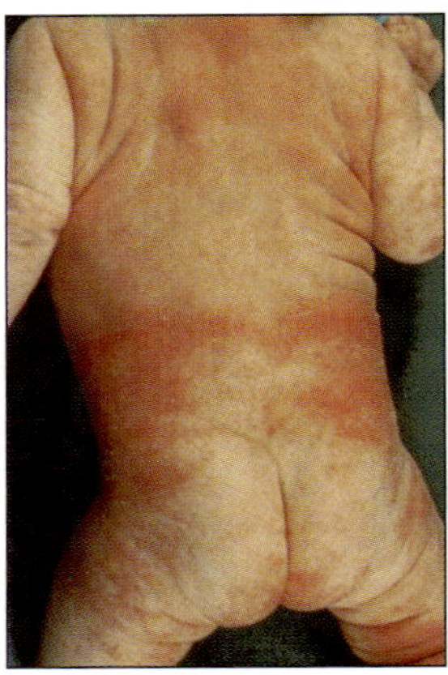

INFANTILE ECZEMA

This form of eczema usually occurs in infants during their first year. The condition is characterized by extremely dry skin that appears as a red, rough, patchy rash, usually on the cheeks, forehead, and elbows. In severe cases the rash can cover the entire body.

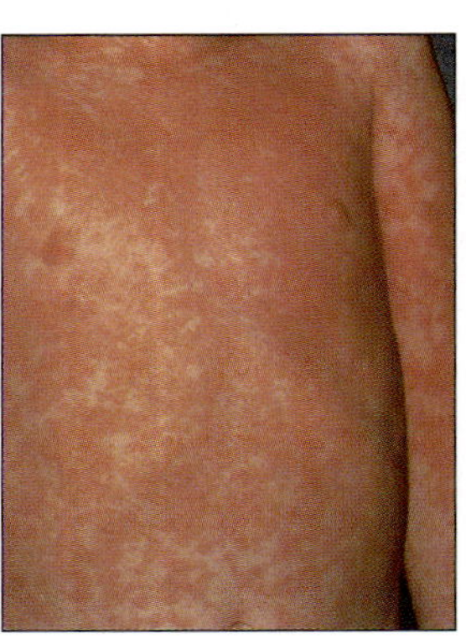

MEASLES

This highly contagious childhood disease is characterized by flat, dark pink spots that form blotches on the skin. The blotches first appear on the forehead and behind the ears, rapidly spreading to the torso, arms, and legs. It may be confused with ***German measles.***

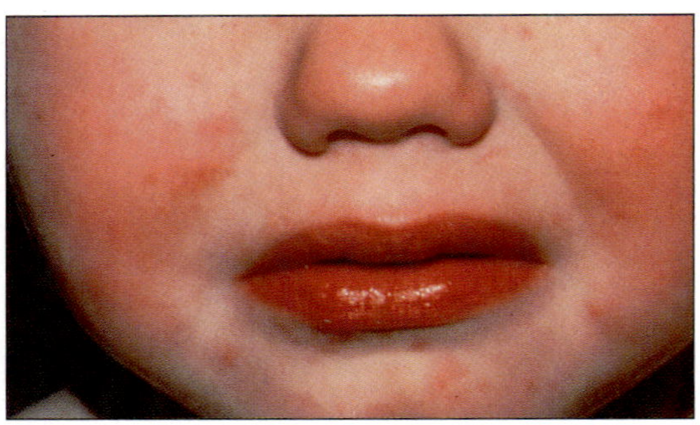

GERMAN MEASLES

Often confused with ***measles,*** German measles (or rubella) is less severe. As with measles, the rash appears first on the face and then spreads to the rest of the body, and is accompanied by fever, swollen lymph nodes, upper respiratory tract infection, and joint pain. The rash consists of tiny, light red spots that come together to form an evenly colored patch.

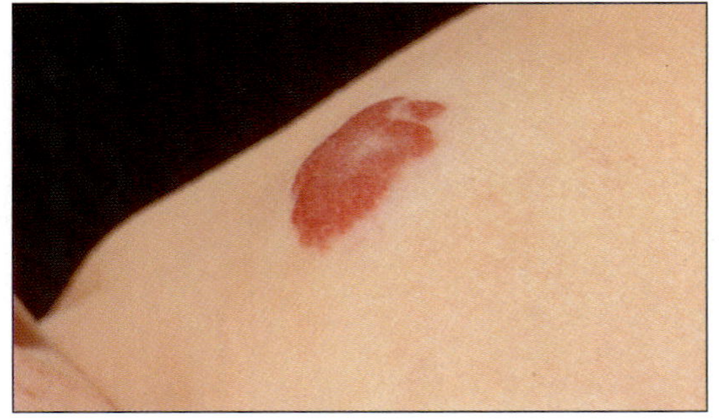

STRAWBERRY NEVUS

The raised, bright red patch of a strawberry nevus usually appears within the first few months of a child's life; in rare cases, it may be present at birth. This benign skin growth is more common in girls and can occur anywhere on the body, but typically appears on the scalp, face, back, or chest. It will eventually shrink and fade, usually between the ages of three and nine.

MOUTH PROBLEMS

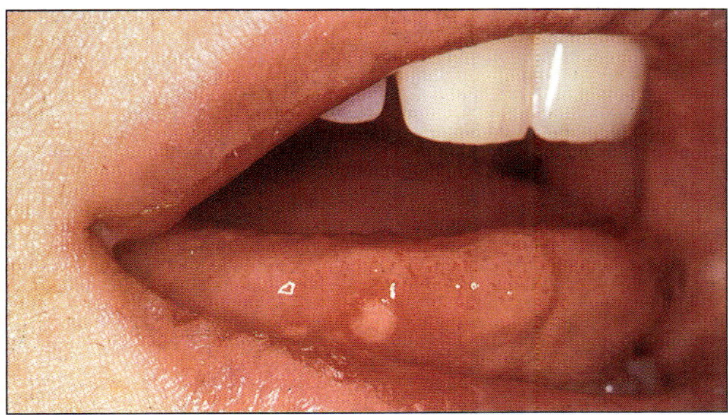

CANKER SORE

Mouth ulcers that occur on the inside surface of the mouth are called canker sores. They can appear on the inside of the cheeks or lips, on the tongue, or at the base of the gums. The sores are painful, typically have a white or yellow center with a red border, and often appear in clusters. They are most common in children and young adults.

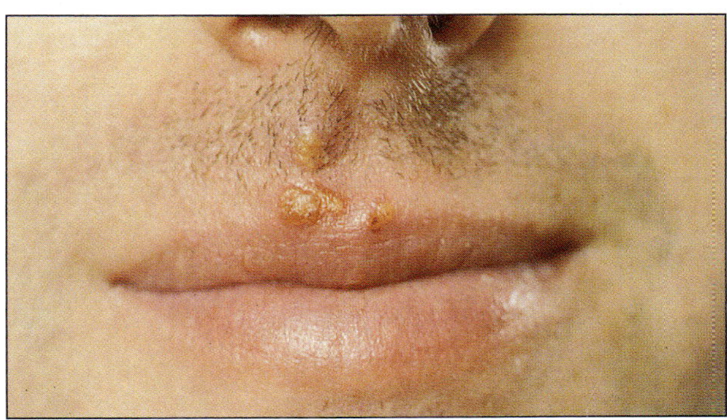

COLD SORE

Herpes simplex, a contagious viral infection, is usually found on the face, particularly around the nose and mouth. The first symptom is typically a burning, itching sensation around the lips; later, small fluid-filled blisters will form. The blisters are painful and may come together to form a larger blister.

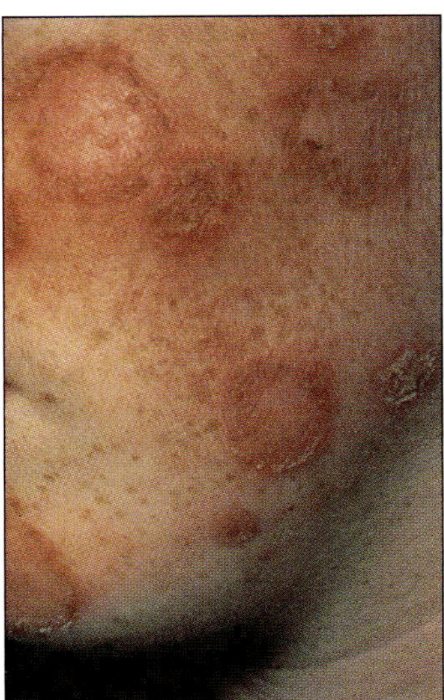

IMPETIGO

A contagious bacterial infection more common in children but sometimes seen in adults, impetigo usually occurs on the face, particularly around the mouth and nose. Water-filled blisters will gradually spread and rupture, creating a thick yellow crust.

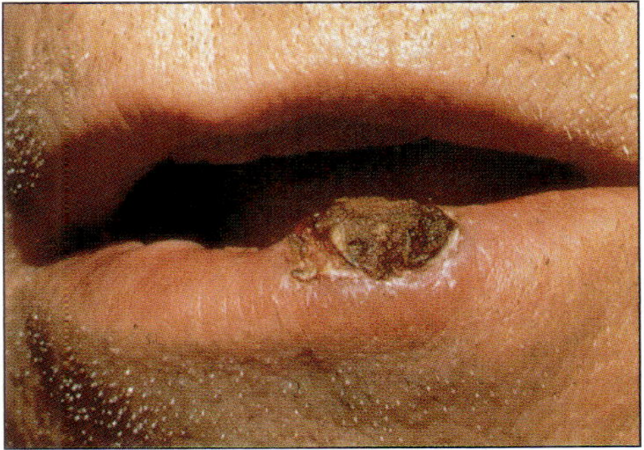

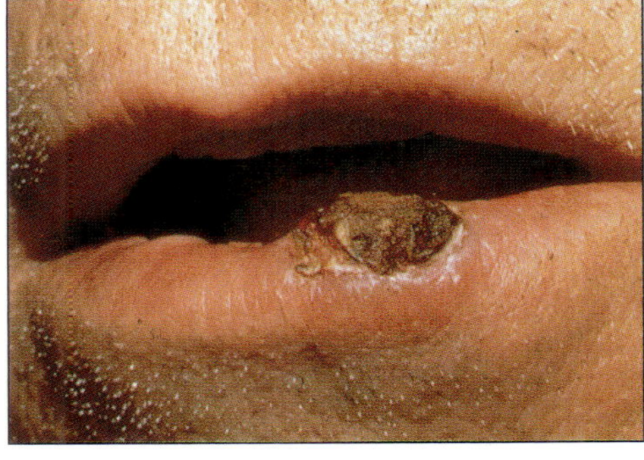

ORAL CANCER

Squamous cell carcinoma—the most common type of cancer affecting the mouth—often appears on the outside of the lip but may also occur on any tissue inside the mouth. More frequent in people over 60, the cancer begins as a small, painless ulcer that eventually develops into a rough, raised sore. At the relative y advanced stage shown at left, the sore can be confused with a wart.

ORAL THRUSH

Most common in infants and the elderly, oral thrush is a ***yeast infection*** that results when illness or the use of antibiotics disturbs the balance of naturally occurring microorganisms in the mouth. A raised, creamy white patch resembling cottage cheese usually appears on the inside of the cheek. With treatment, the infection typically clears up within 5 to 10 days.

SKIN GROWTHS

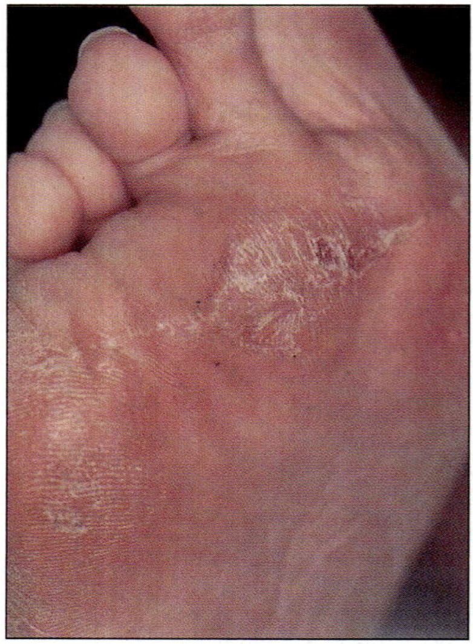

CALLUS

Caused by constant friction against the skin, calluses consist of a raised patch of hard, dead skin. They typically appear on the ball of the foot, on the palm of the hand, on fingers, or over a bunion. If they become painful or exceedingly thick or if they tear, consult your doctor. Calluses on the sole of the foot can sometimes be confused with ***plantar warts.***

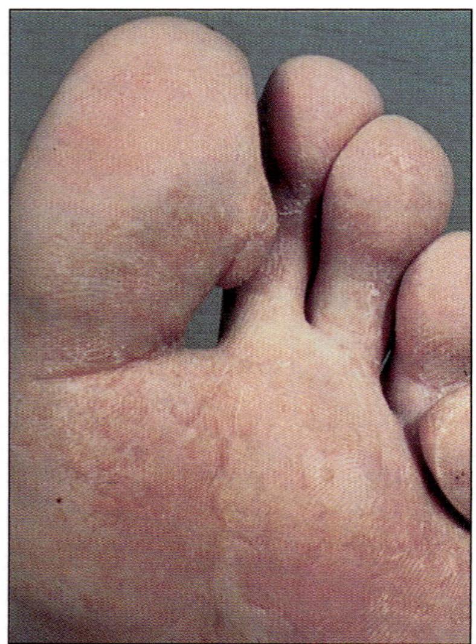

CORN

Smaller than calluses, corns are caused by pressure and friction on or between the toes. Hard corns are commonly found on the upper surface of the toes or on the outside of a little toe. Soft corns appear where moisture is trapped between the toes. Often painful, corns can be chemically or surgically removed.

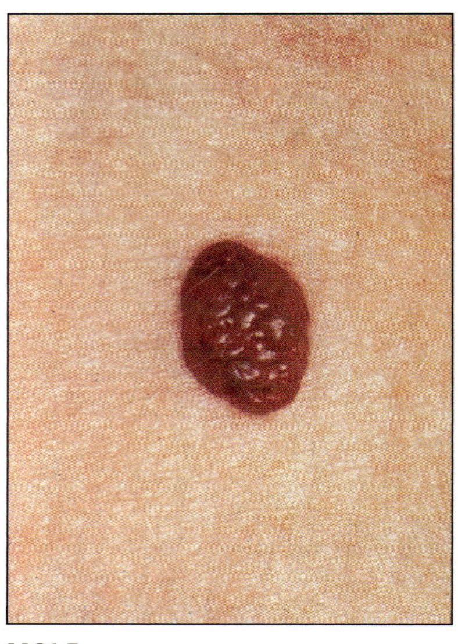

MOLE

Sometimes confused with melanoma, moles are benign growths that come in a wide variety of shapes and sizes. They can develop at any age and on any part of the body. Most tend to be dark and circular in shape, and can be smooth and flat, or raised and wrinkled. If any change in color or size occurs or if a mole starts to bleed, call your doctor.

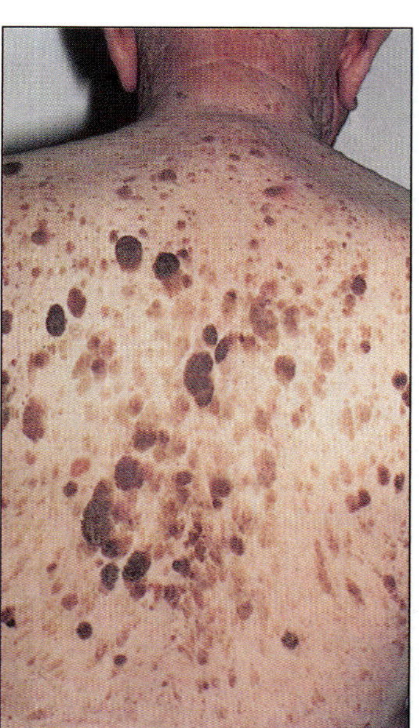

SEBORRHEIC KERATOSIS

This benign skin condition consists of dark, oval, wartlike growths that range in size from one-third to one inch across; the growths typically occur in large numbers, are slightly raised, and may have a pasted-on, waxy appearance. Most often seen among the elderly, they usually occur on the face, neck, scalp, chest, and back. They can be frozen off or surgically removed by a doctor.

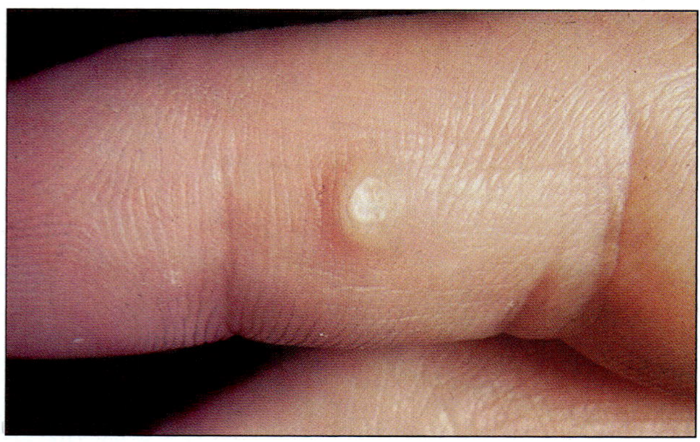

COMMON WART

Typically found on the hands and feet either singly or in clusters, common warts vary in size but average a quarter inch in diameter. The flesh-colored bumps tend to be circular, feel hard, and are rough to the touch. They pose no health risks and will eventually disappear, but they can also be removed with over-the-counter medications.

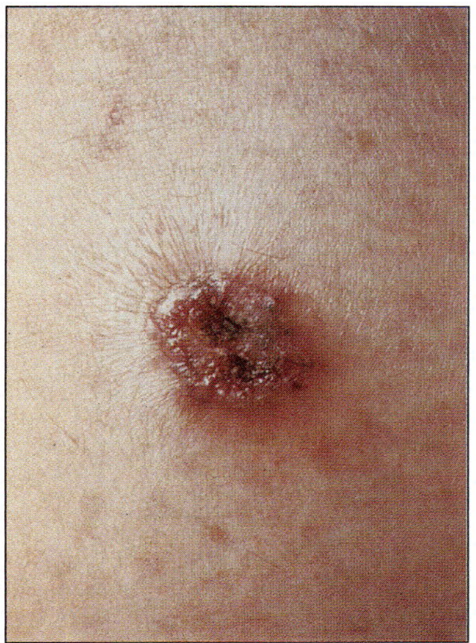

SKIN CANCER

Basal Cell Carcinoma
The most common of the three types of skin cancer, basal cell carcinoma is a malignancy that grows slowly and rarely spreads to other organs. A small bump—typically in areas routinely exposed to the sun—develops a central crater that eventually erodes, crusts, and bleeds. This type of cancer is most common in fair-skinned people over 40.

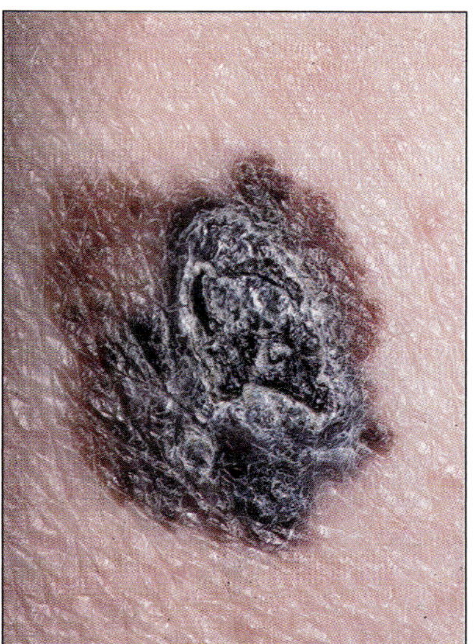

SKIN CANCER

Melanoma
The most serious form of skin cancer, melanoma may develop from an existing mole with an irregular border or in an area where there was no previous mole. The dark spot can become inflamed and change shape, color, size, and elevation. If any of these conditions develops or if the growth bleeds spontaneously, call your doctor immediately.

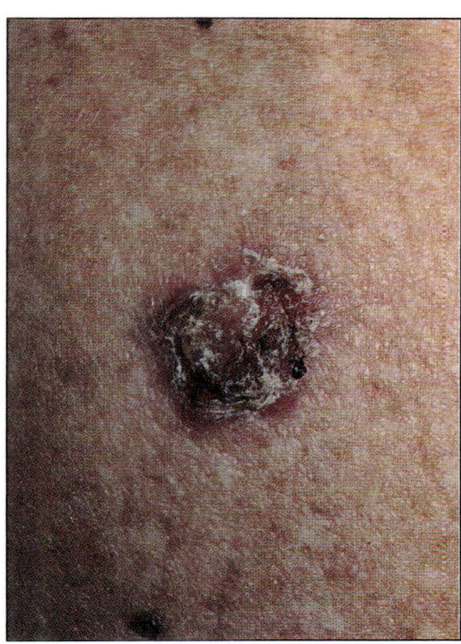

SKIN CANCER

Squamous Cell Carcinoma
Continual overexposure to the sun is the most frequent cause of this cancer; fair-skinned people over 60 are the most susceptible. The tumor typically appears as a hard lump with a scaly, crusted surface. Growths develop most often on the lips, ears, hands, neck, and arms. More aggressive than basal cell carcinoma, this cancer can spread to internal organs.

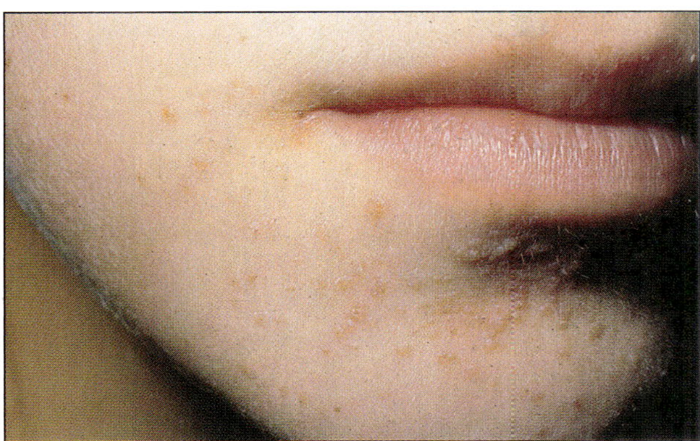

FLAT WARTS

Children and young adults are the most likely to develop flat warts, which often occur in clusters of 10 to 30. The warts are slightly raised, smooth, and tan or flesh-colored; they are often barely visible. Flat warts typically appear on the neck, face, wrists, backs of the hands, and knees. In children, they most often appear on the face.

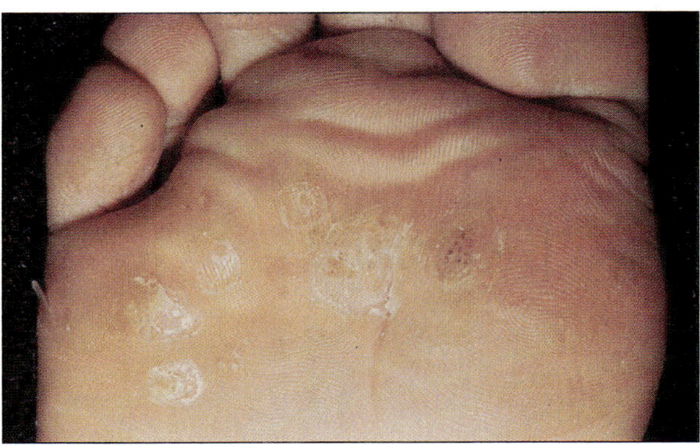

PLANTAR WARTS

Caused by the common wart virus, plantar warts appear on the sole of the foot, usually at pressure points such as the heel. They begin as small, painful warts that become flattened and pressed into the skin. The soft core of the wart is surrounded by a hard calluslike ring that may be peppered with tiny blood clots that appear as black dots.

RASHES, INSECT BITES, AND SKIN DISCOLORATIONS

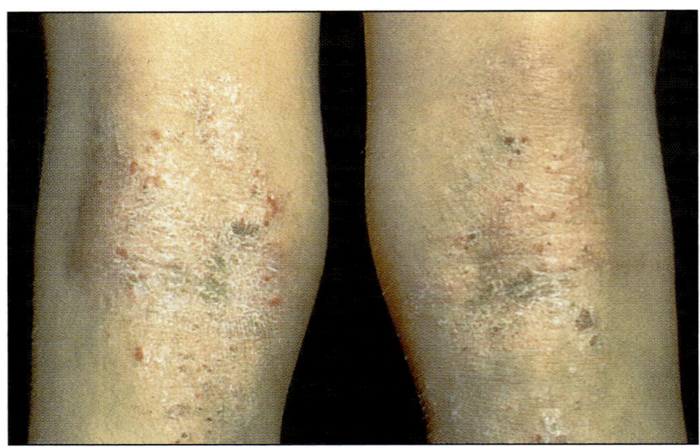

ATOPIC DERMATITIS

Also known as eczema, this type of dermatitis is most common in infants and young children. It usually appears in the inner crease of the elbows and the knees, and begins as an itchy rash with small red pimples that leak; the rash may spread into thick, scaly patches. People with inherited allergies are more likely to develop atopic dermatitis.

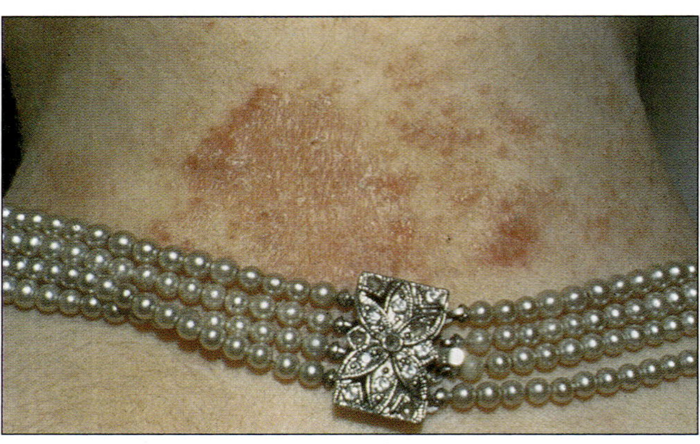

CONTACT DERMATITIS

This rash results from contact with various substances, including certain types of plants, cosmetics, jewelry, medications, and detergents. Symptoms include small bumps or blisters that develop—over a period of weeks or months—into a red rash. The rash is usually very itchy, and skin may flake in affected areas.

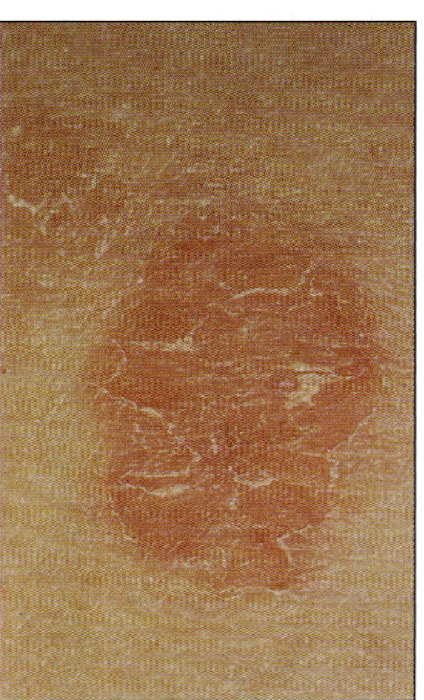

NUMMULAR DERMATITIS

Most often occurring in adults, nummular dermatitis consists of itchy, scaly, circular patches appearing anywhere on the body but usually on the forearms and the shins. It can be confused with the fungal infection ringworm, which has almost identical symptoms. The cause of nummular dermatitis is unknown.

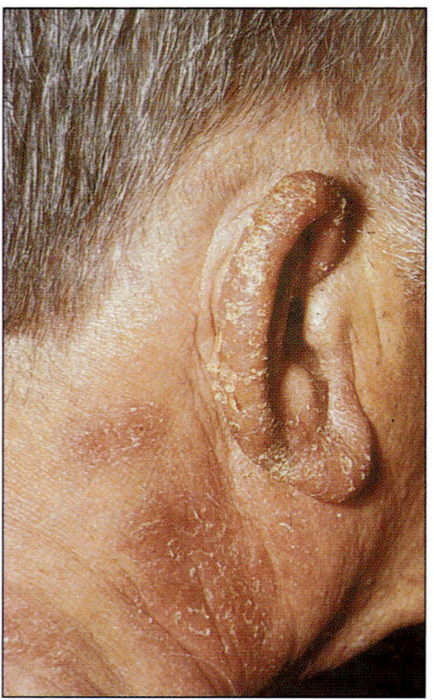

SEBORRHEIC DERMATITIS

Usually developing during periods of stress, seborrheic dermatitis appears on the face, scalp, chest, back, eyelids, and outer surface of the ears. The rash is marked by yellow crusts and dry or greasy scales, and is often accompanied by chronic itching. Lower humidity during the winter can make the condition worse.

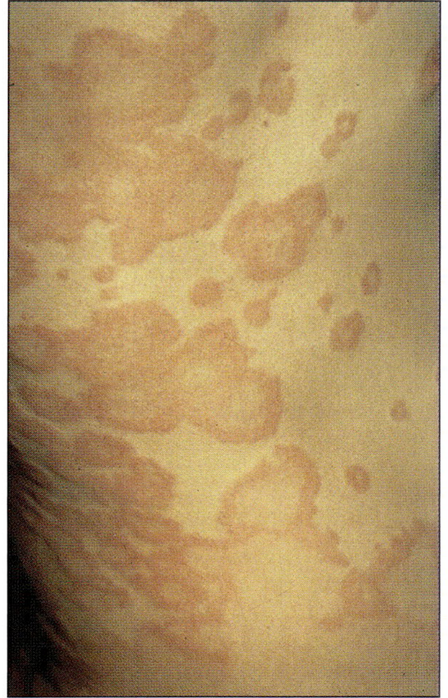

HIVES

Often an allergic reaction to certain foods and drugs or airborne irritants such as pollen, hives can also result from an illness or even from emotional stress. The rash—consisting of itchy, raised welts with pale centers and red borders—can occur anywhere on the body. In advanced stages, separate rashes can grow together to create larger patches.

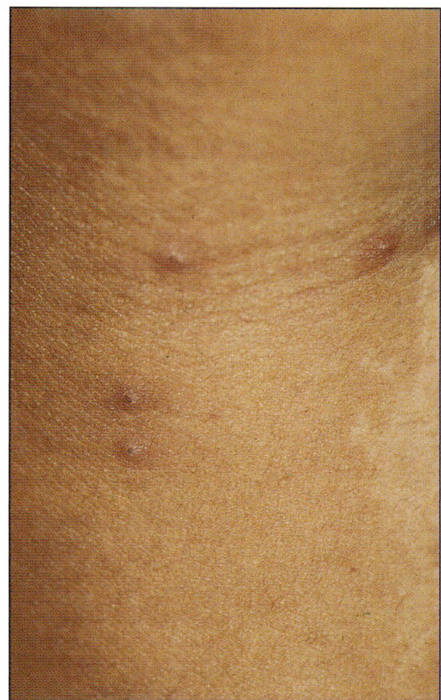

INSECT BITE

When an insect bites, it injects venom into the skin, causing inflammation. Depending on the type of insect and on the individual, the reaction can range from small, itchy red bumps *(above)* to a large, puffy swelling; the bite may subside quickly or last for several days. The most likely culprits are fleas, mosquitoes, gnats, bedbugs, and lice. See also ***Insect and Spider Bites.***

LYME DISEASE

The bite of a tick carrying Lyme disease first appears as a tiny red dot, which gradually expands to form a red rash up to eight inches or more across. Lyme disease is accompanied by flulike symptoms—fever, headache, muscle ache, and joint inflammation—that may take as long as a week to develop. Call your doctor; Lyme disease can have serious consequences if left untreated.

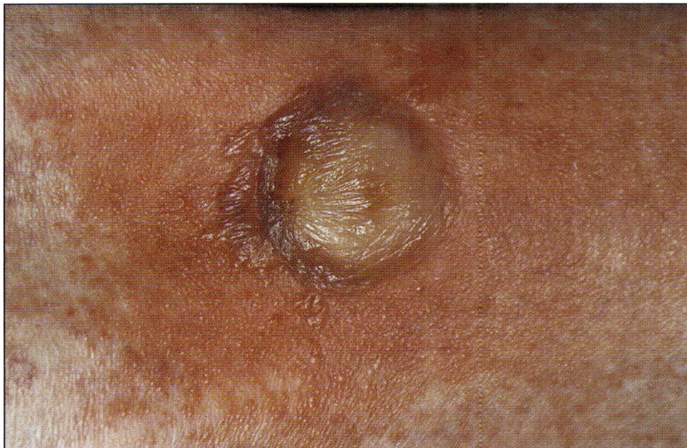

SPIDER BITE

Brown Recluse

Venom from the bite of a brown recluse spider causes mild stinging and local redness, followed by intense pain about four hours later. A fluid-filled blister *(left)* forms within days, eventually rubbing off and leaving an ulcerated sore. Other symptoms include nausea, vomiting, fever, and joint pain. Seek treatment immediately. See also ***Insect and Spider Bites.***

RASHES, INSECT BITES, AND SKIN DISCOLORATIONS

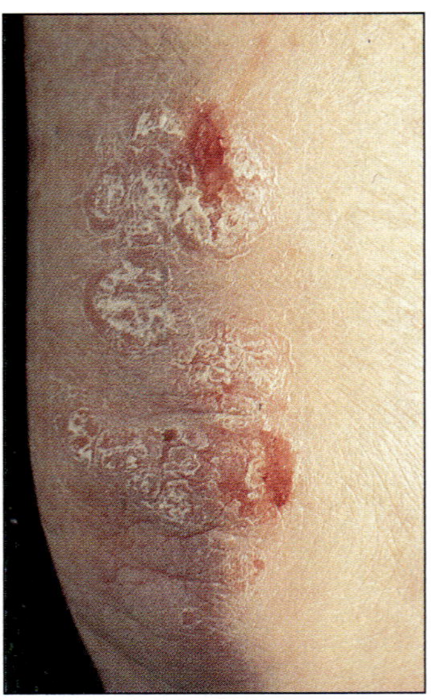

PSORIASIS

Usually occurring around the knees, elbows, and scalp, psoriasis is characterized by thick, silvery scales. There may be some itching but usually only a vague feeling of discomfort. Emotional stress and poor health can contribute to an outbreak of psoriasis; heredity is also a factor. Psoriasis is most common between the ages of 10 and 40.

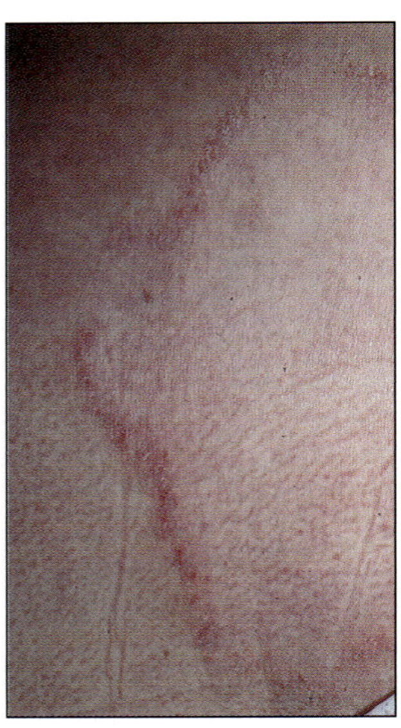

RINGWORM

A contagious fungal infection, ringworm starts out as a small red patch and eventually grows into a ring-shaped, scaly, itchy rash; the center of the rash remains clear as the ring spreads *(left)*. Typical sites include the groin, feet, scalp, and torso. Ringworm is most common in children and can be contracted from infected domestic animals and other infected children. See ***Infections*** for information about treatment. (The name refers to the infection's appearance; the condition is not caused by any kind of worm.)

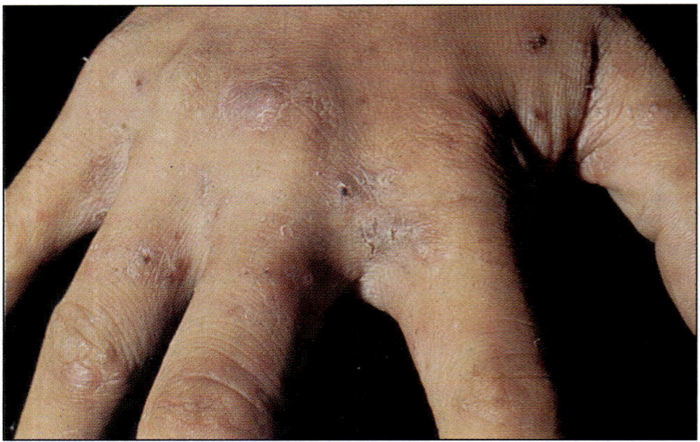

SCABIES

Most often afflicting children and young adults, scabies is contagious; it is contracted from small mites that burrow under the skin and lay eggs. Tiny swellings—typically around the lower abdomen and back and in the webs of the fingers—develop into red bumps that are extremely itchy. Scratching causes the bumps to become more inflamed, scaly, and red.

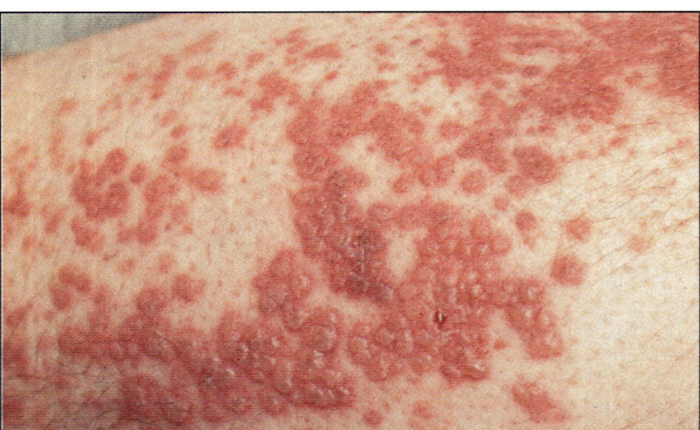

SHINGLES

Localized over one side of the body, shingles is the result of the herpes zoster virus; its most common victims are people over 50. Symptoms begin with a tingling sensation, followed by severe pain, and eventually a raised red rash consisting of small, fluid-filled blisters. The blisters will dry out and crust over, then slough off, leaving small scars.

EYE PROBLEMS

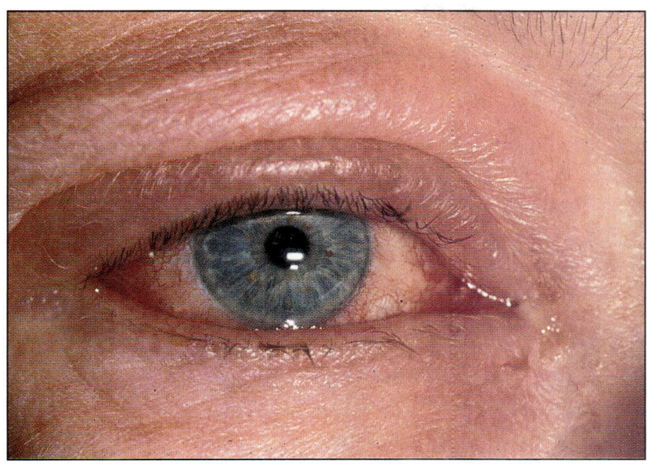

CONJUNCTIVITIS

Also known as pinkeye, conjunctivitis is a contagious infection, usually bacterial, that causes inflammation of the conjunctiva—the eye's mucous membrane. Symptoms include itchiness, swelling, and redness of the eyelid, and a thick discharge causing the eye to look bloodshot. Conjunctivitis is most common in children and adults who have allergies.

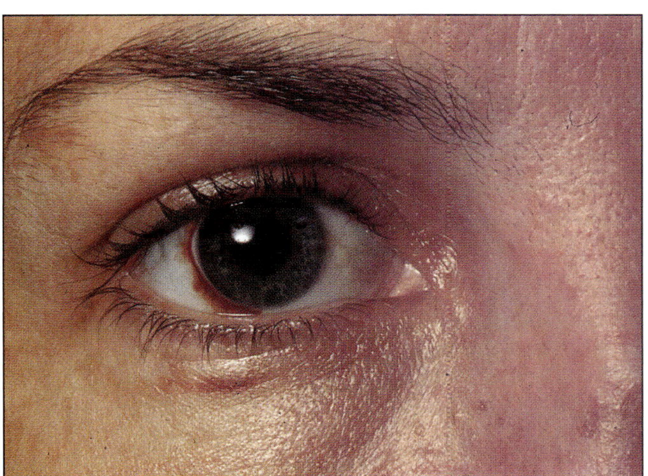

SUBCONJUNCTIVAL HEMORRHAGE

Usually resulting from an injury to the eye or a severe bout of coughing or sneezing that causes small blood vessels to leak, subconjunctival hemorrhages appear as one or more irregular red spots in the white of the eye. They are harmless and generally disappear within two or three weeks. Call your doctor if the hemorrhages cause any discomfort or if they recur.

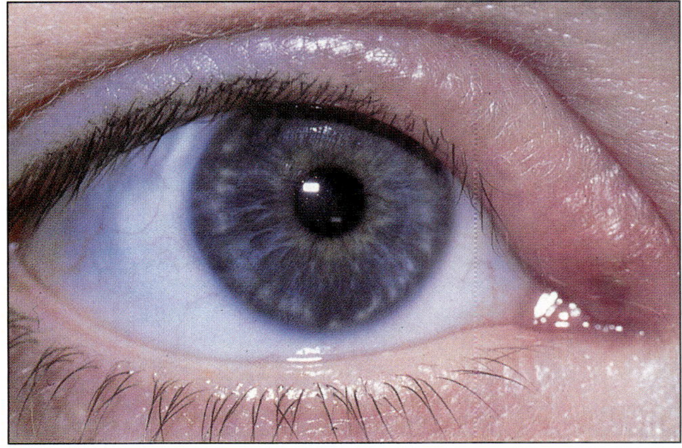

STY

A sty results from a bacterial infection at the root of an eyelash, typically at the inner corner of the eye. It causes the follicle of the eyelash to become inflamed *(left);* a pus-filled bump will form and then rupture. A sty can be painful, but it typically clears up on its own within a week.

ATLAS OF THE BODY

CONTENTS

The Muscular System 1054

The Skeletal System 1056

The Torso 1058

The Digestive System 1059

The Circulatory and Respiratory Systems 1060

The Urinary/Reproductive Systems 1062

The Nervous System 1064

The Endocrine/Immune Systems 1065

The Senses 1066

THE MUSCULAR SYSTEM

Muscles are parallel bundles of interlocking fibers that contract in response to signals from nerves. The body's more than 600 named muscles vary from less than a quarter inch to about a foot in length. There are three main types. Striated muscles, which are tethered to bones, ligaments, tendons, and other muscles, carry out voluntary movements. Smooth muscles, found in such hollow organs as the blad-

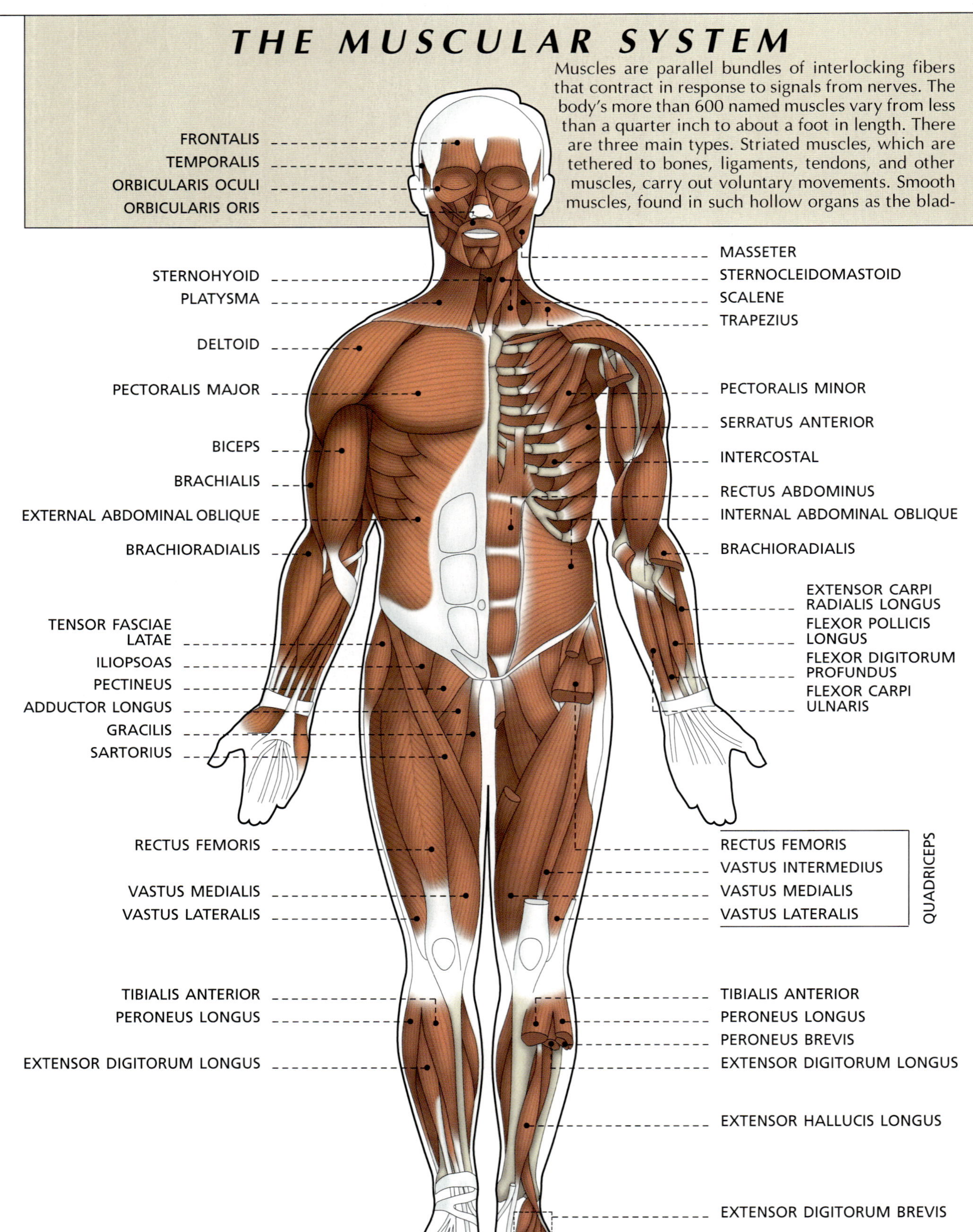

der, intestines, and blood vessels, aid in digestion, circulation, and other involuntary functions. Cardiac muscle is striated like skeletal muscles but operates without conscious control. Some muscles, including those of the hands, are designed to contract and relax quickly, while others—such as the muscles of the back and neck that control posture—perform over longer periods of time.

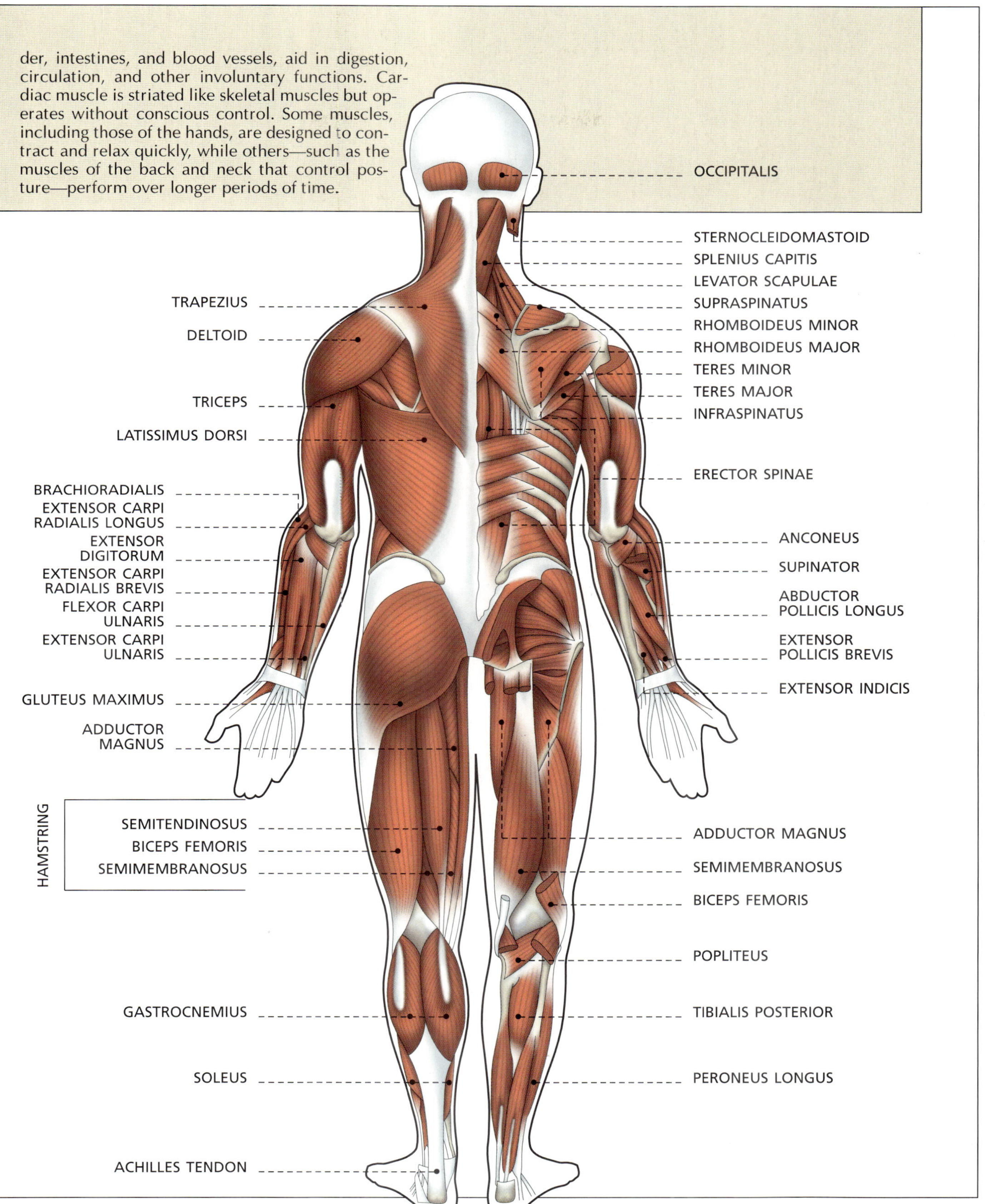

THE SKELETAL SYSTEM

The 206 bones of the human skeleton provide the body's structural framework. They also work with muscles to make movement possible. Some bones, such as the skull and ribs, protect vital organs. Bones are ever-changing masses of hardened living tissue that includes calcium and other essential minerals. The soft marrow core of certain large bones produces blood cells and essential clotting agents

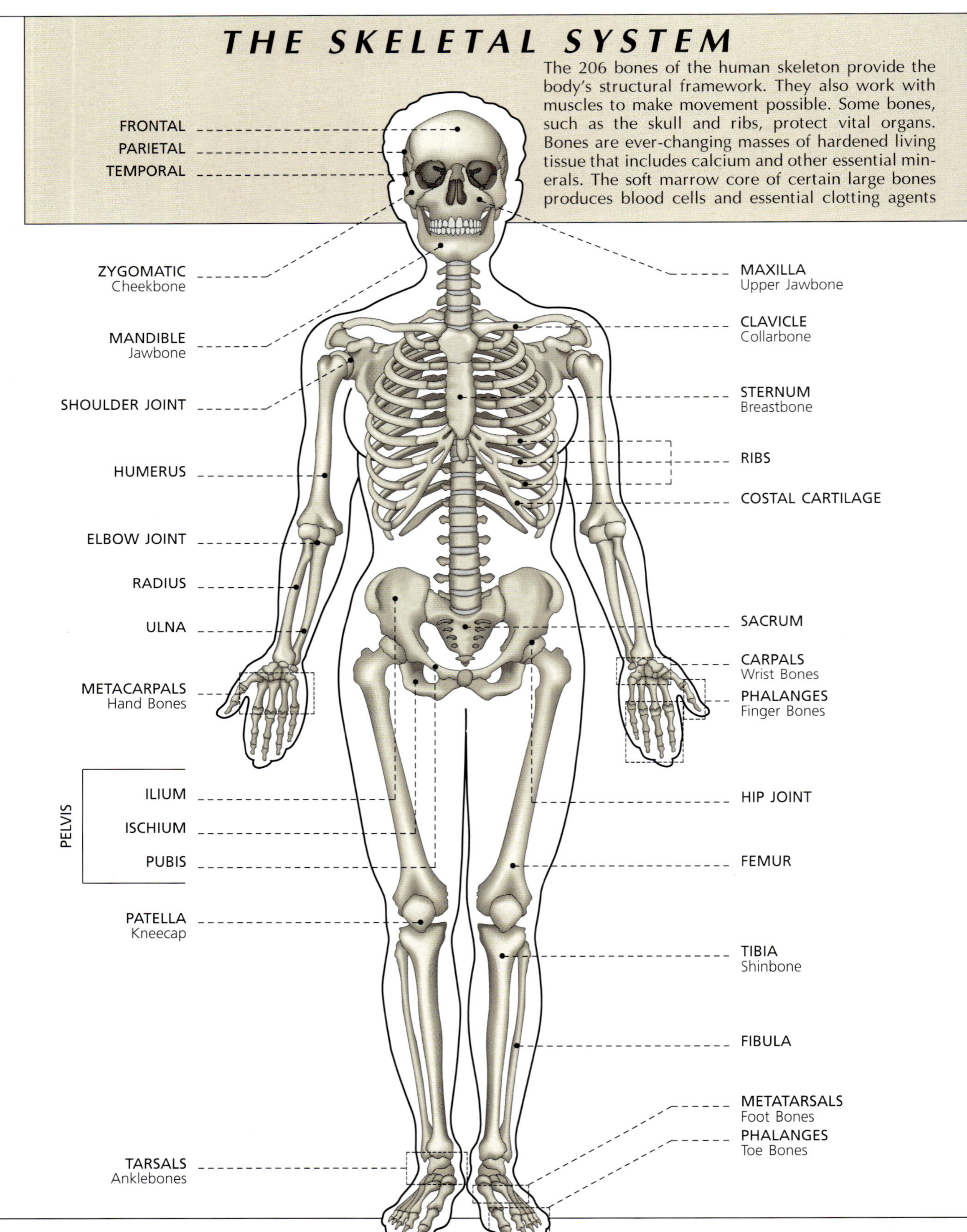

called platelets. Two or more bones come together at junctures called joints. Bands of connective tissue known as ligaments hold joints together; dense strands of tissue called tendons join bones to muscle. The ends of bones are covered by cartilage, a tough, elastic material that absorbs shock and reduces joint wear and tear.

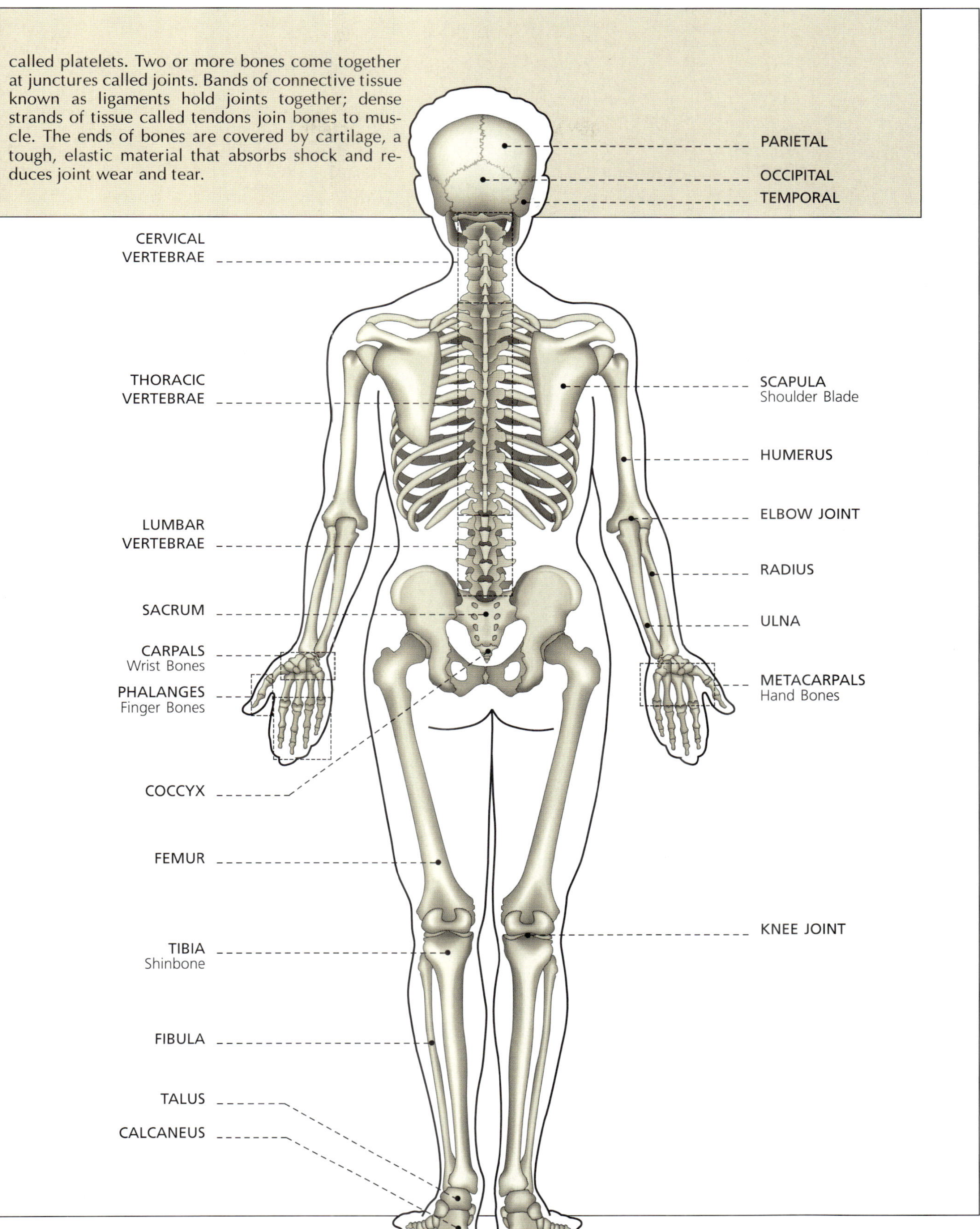

THE TORSO

Almost all of the body's vital organs reside in the torso, the cylindrical middle section that is often referred to as the trunk. The torso also serves as the center for a number of important bodily systems, including the respiratory, circulatory, digestive, and reproductive systems.

The chest, or upper part of the torso, houses the heart and lungs, which are protected by the long, narrow bones of the rib cage. The diaphragm, a thin, dome-shaped sheet of muscle, separates the chest from the abdomen, or lower part of the torso, and it plays a vital role in breathing, helping the lungs to expand and contract. The abdomen holds a number of vital organs, including the stomach, liver, kidneys, intestines, gallbladder, and spleen.

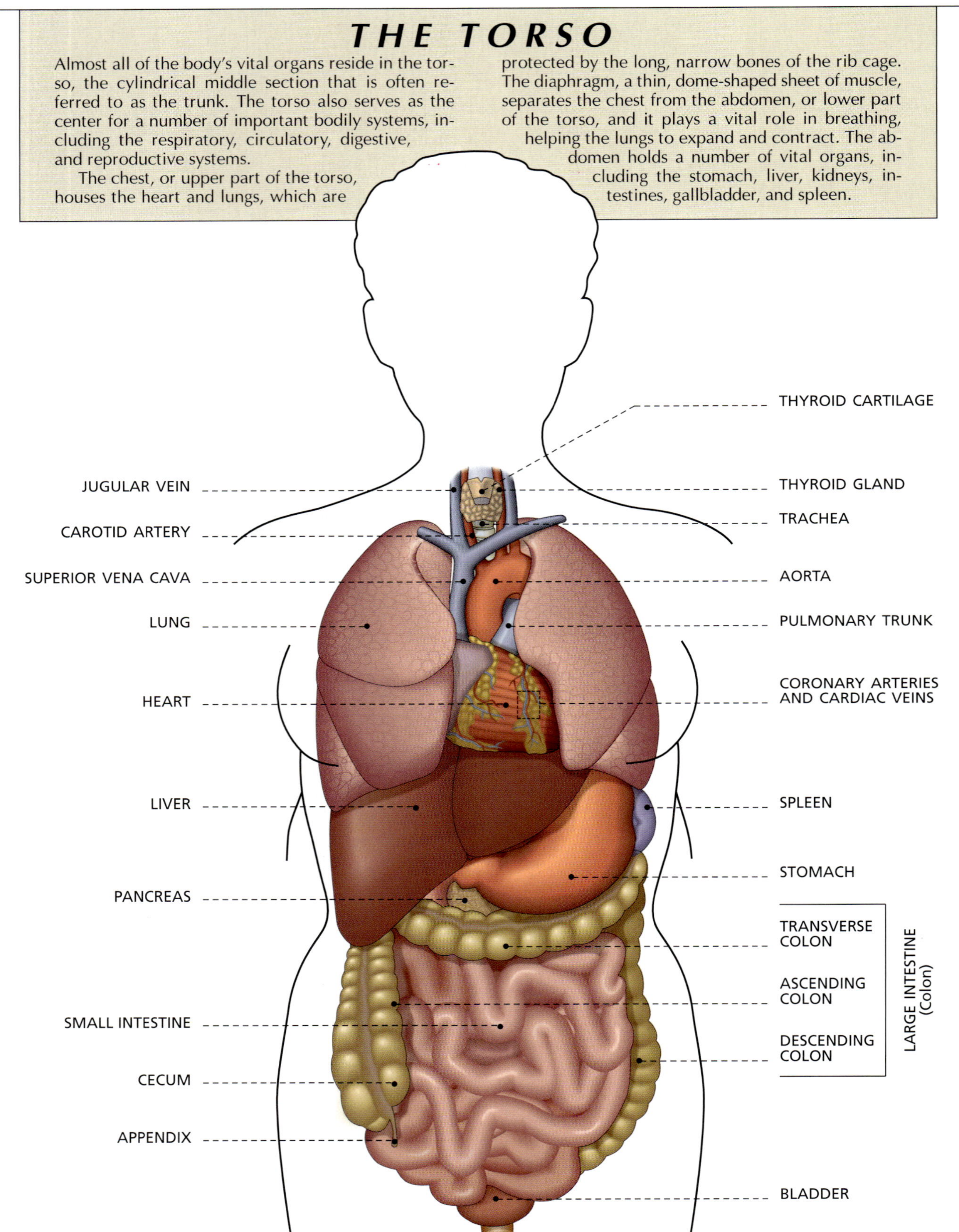

THE DIGESTIVE SYSTEM

Food begins its journey through the digestive tract in the mouth. Teeth grind and tear food into smaller bits, while saliva liquefies the material and breaks down some carbohydrates. The tongue and other muscles push food to the esophagus, which then delivers it to the stomach. Broken down further, the food moves to the duodenum, the upper portion of the small intestine, and is bathed in fat-dissolving bile from the liver and gallbladder, and digestive juices from the pancreas. The last stage of digestion occurs in the small intestine, where nutrients are absorbed into the bloodstream. Undigested material moves into the large intestine for removal of excess water, is stored briefly in the rectum, then passes from the body through the anus.

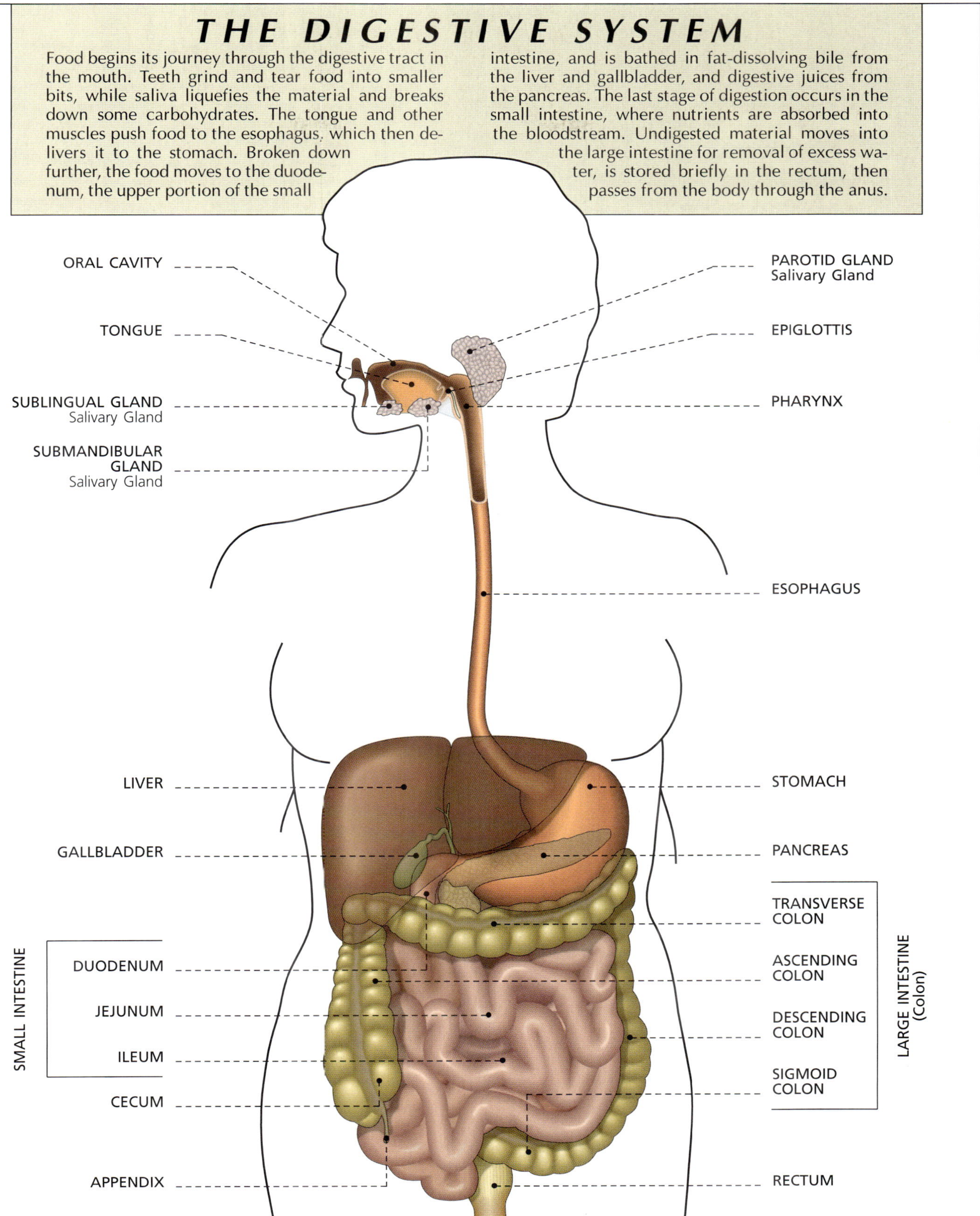

THE CIRCULATORY AND

The vital job of delivering oxygen fuel to the body and removing carbon dioxide waste involves a close partnership between the respiratory and circulatory systems. The actual point of contact between the two lies deep within the lungs, where airways and tiny blood vessels meet.

Air entering the nose and mouth travels down past the larynx (voice box), into the trachea

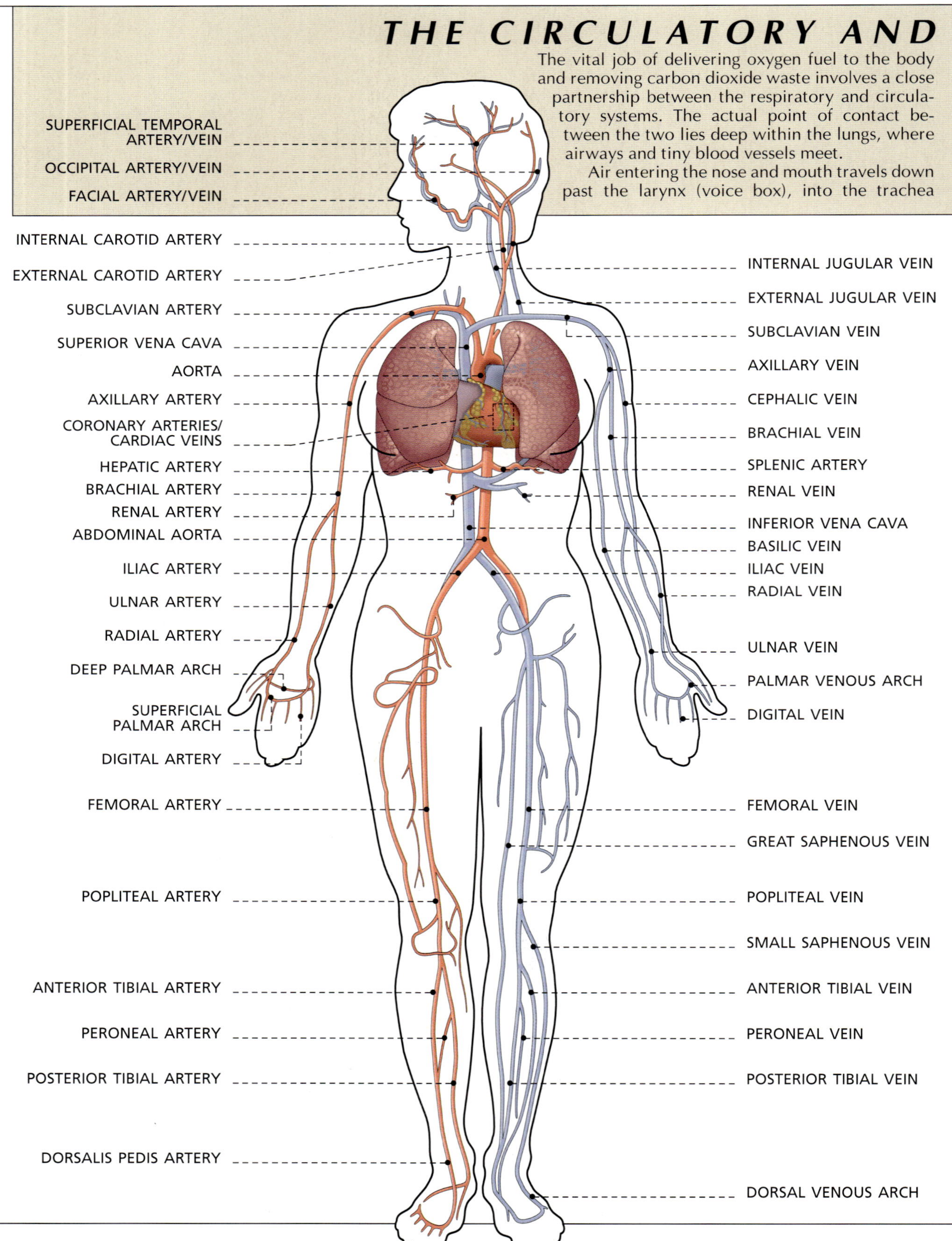

RESPIRATORY SYSTEMS

(windpipe), through branching tubes called the bronchi and bronchioles, and into the lungs; the airways further branch out into millions of thin-walled sacs called alveoli. Here, inhaled air comes in close contact with webs of surrounding capillaries, allowing blood to exchange carbon dioxide for oxygen through diffusion.

Blood travels through the body via an elaborate network of interconnected vessels. Driving the system is the heart—a muscular, double-sided pump whose rhythmic contractions propel blood into the lungs and, through the aorta, to the rest of the body. Arteries carry blood away from the heart, and veins return "spent" blood back to begin the cycle anew.

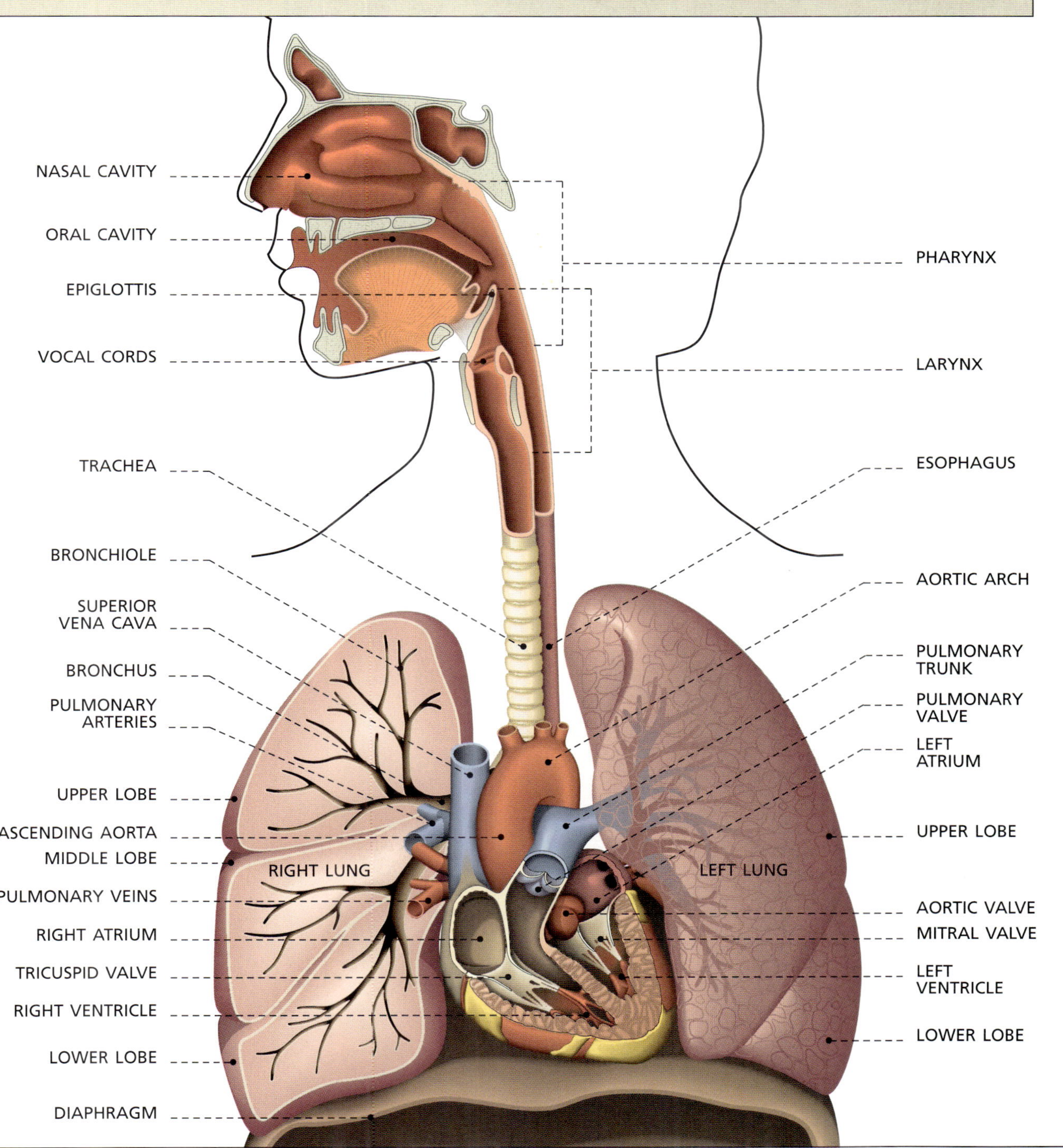

URINARY/REPRODUCTIVE SYSTEMS
FEMALE

The basic mechanisms of the male and female urinary systems are the same. The kidneys act as filters that cleanse the blood and absorb essential fluids back into the bloodstream. Waste material drains through the ureters to the bladder for temporary storage, then exits the body through the urethra.

In the female reproductive system, the ovaries release mature eggs into the fallopian tubes. If an egg is fertilized by a sperm cell, it travels to the uterus and attaches to the uterine lining, where the fetus will develop. The vagina serves as a conduit for entering sperm and as a passageway for the baby during birth. If an egg is not fertilized, the uterus sheds its lining in the process known as menstruation.

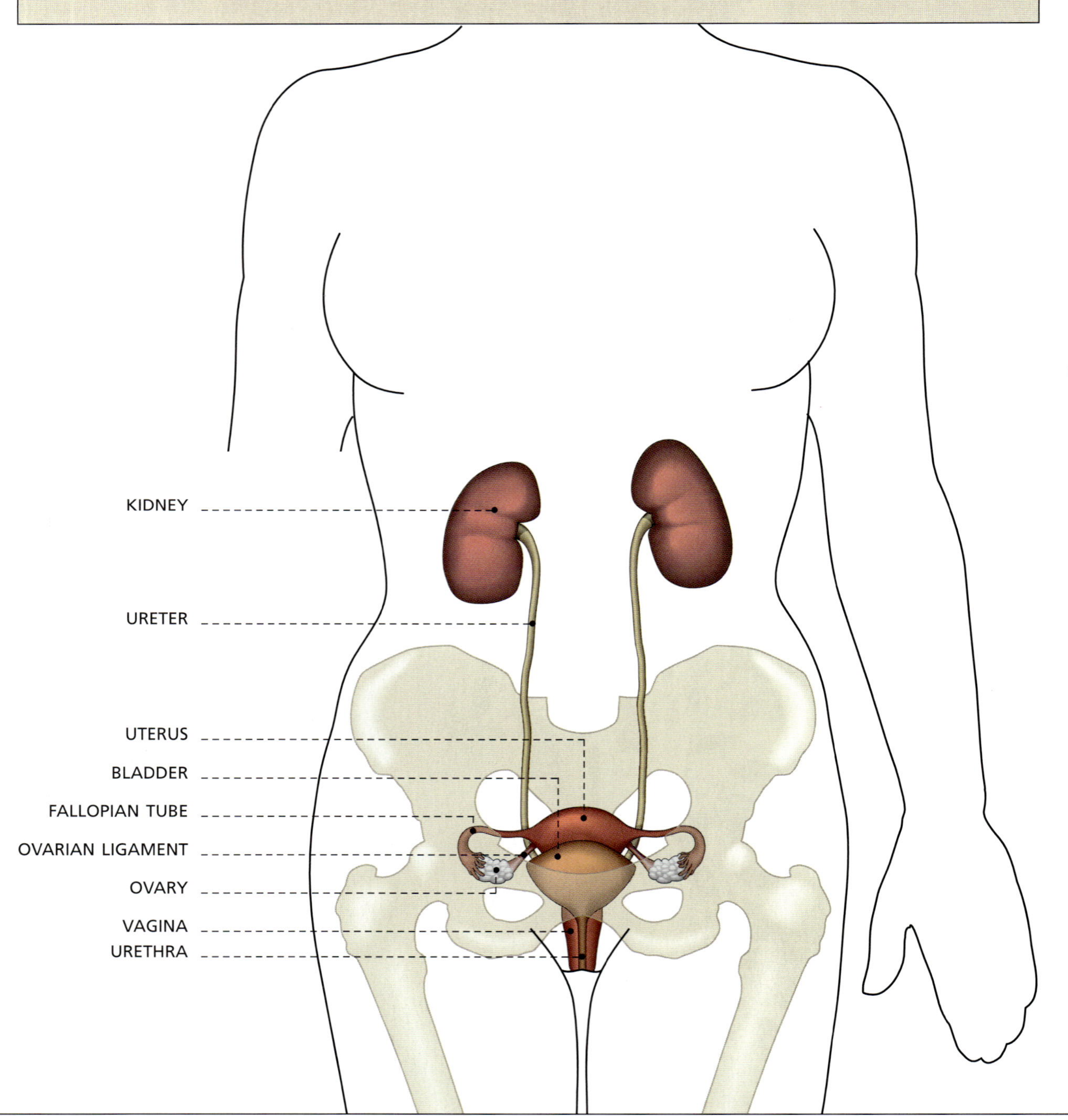

URINARY/REPRODUCTIVE SYSTEMS
MALE

The only difference in the male urinary system is that the urethra also plays a role in the reproductive system, providing a channel for sperm. Sperm cells are manufactured in the testes, or testicles, which hang outside the abdominal cavity in the scrotum. (The temperature inside the body is too high for sperm production.) From the testes, sperm enter a system of ducts and mix with the secretions from a number of accessory glands, most notably the prostate, forming the fluid called semen. When a man is sexually stimulated, blood rushes in to the penis and fills up rows of spongy columns, causing the organ to become erect. Contractions of muscles located at the base of the penis bring on ejaculation, or the sudden discharge of semen through the urethra.

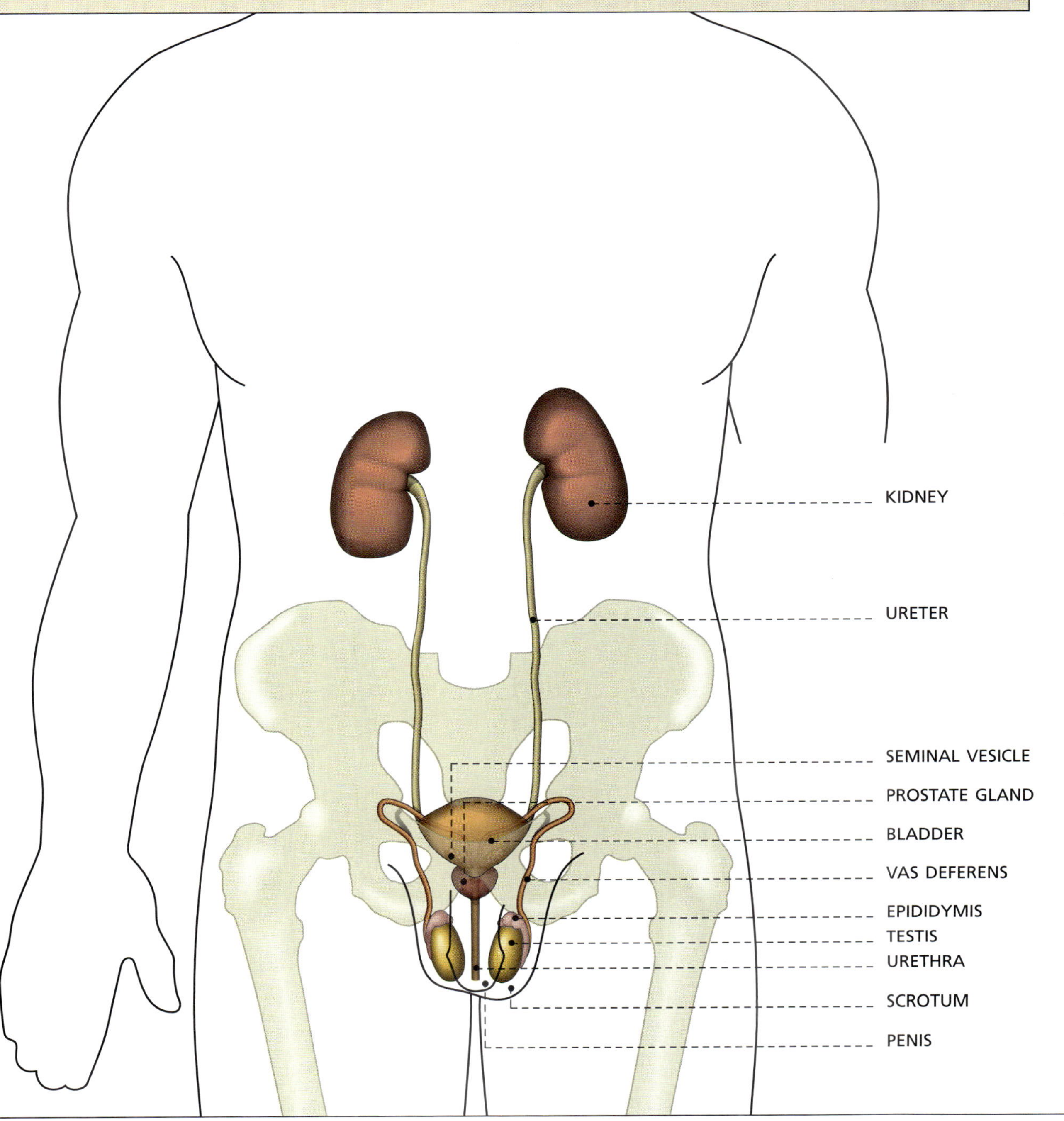

THE NERVOUS SYSTEM

Using a complex "language" of chemicals and electrical impulses, the nervous system regulates movement, thought, emotion, sensation, and many key body functions. Signals pass between nerve cells, or neurons, which often are joined end to end to form fibrous structures called nerves. In the peripheral nervous system, nerves pick up impulses from sensory receptors throughout the body, then pass these messages along to the spinal cord and brain, known collectively as the central nervous system. Neurons in the brain process this flood of information and issue command messages in response, which speed along peripheral nerves to spark movement in muscles and switch glands on or off.

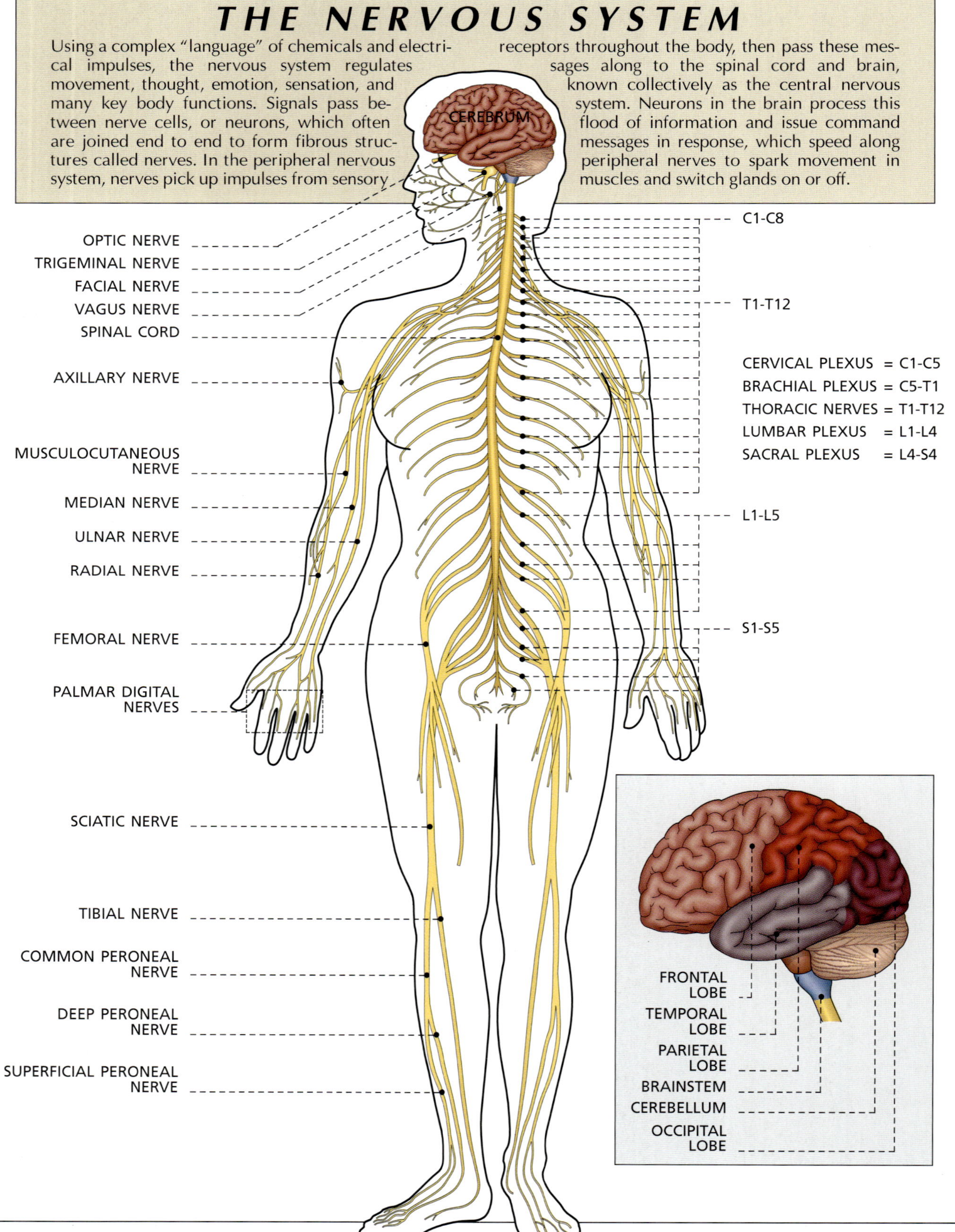

THE ENDOCRINE/IMMUNE SYSTEMS

The endocrine system consists of glands that perform specialized tasks by secreting chemical "messengers" called hormones. The pituitary gland plays a key role, stimulating other endocrine glands to release hormones into the bloodstream, where they trigger various responses. The thyroid gland, for example, controls metabolism, and the adrenal glands, among other things, secrete hormones that help us to respond to stress.

The immune system includes an assortment of cells, glands, and vessels that help in defending the body against bacteria, viruses, and other invaders. The spleen, thymus, and lymph nodes and vessels produce, store, and transport immune cells and other elements of this defense, such as antibodies.

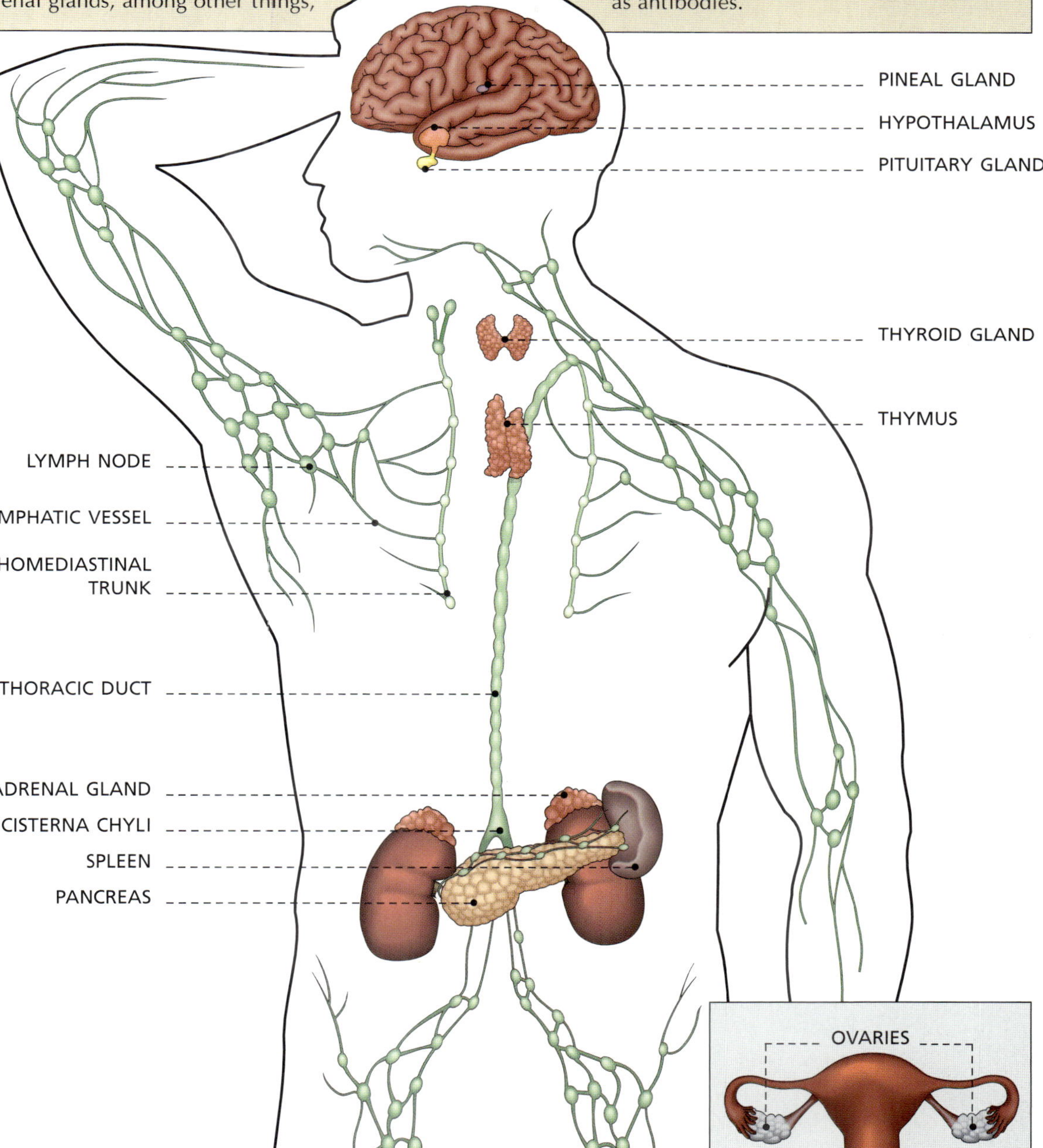

THE SENSES

Five separate systems function as the body's sensory switchboard, constantly receiving and processing torrents of stimuli from the external world. Signals from the eyes, nose, ears, skin, and taste buds travel along nerves to the brain, where they are rendered into the sensations we describe as sight, smell, hearing, touch, and taste.

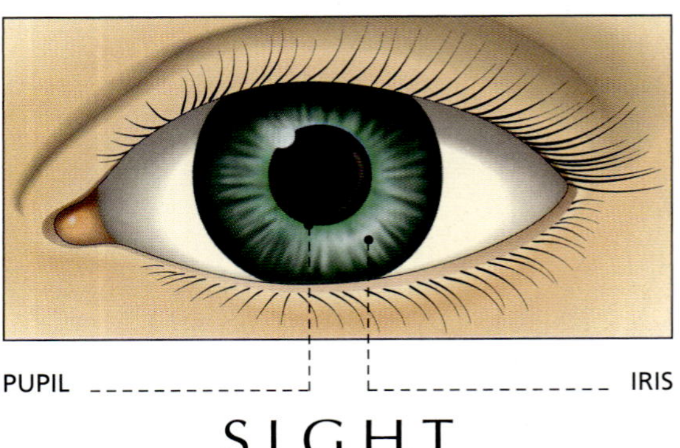

SIGHT

Light striking the eye passes first through the cornea and is directed into the pupil, an opening in the ringlike structure of the iris, which gives our eyes their color and regulates the pupil's size. The lens inverts the image and projects it onto the retina at the back of the eyeball. Specialized cells in the retina convert the image to electrical impulses and send them through the optic nerve to the brain.

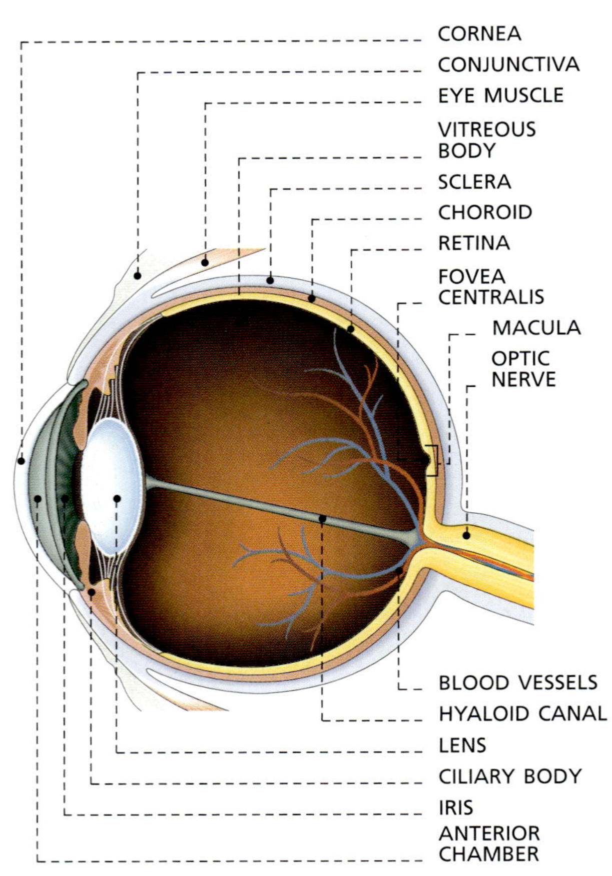

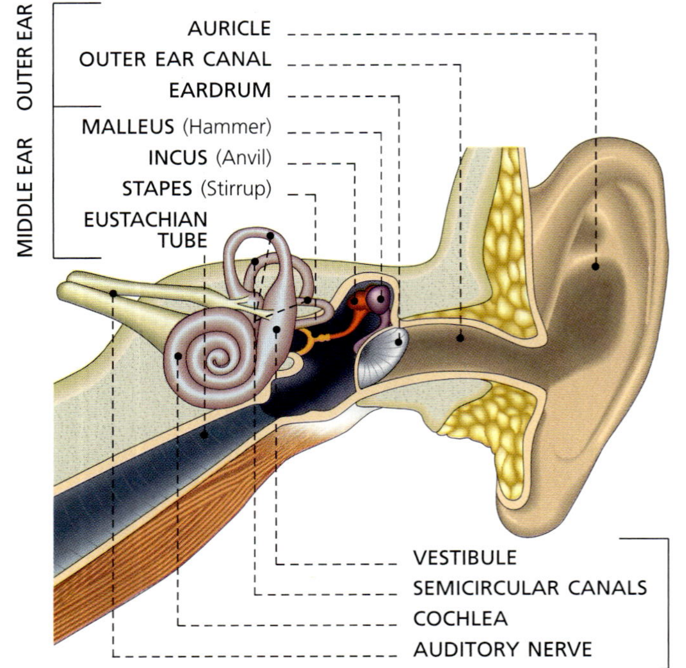

HEARING

Sound waves captured by the flexible outer ear are directed through the outer ear canal to the eardrum, a thin, flexible membrane. Vibrations from the eardrum pass through the tiny bones of the middle ear and into a spiral structure known as the cochlea. Small hairs within the cochlea translate the vibrations into electrical signals, which are then sent along the auditory nerve to the brain.

TASTE

After partially dissolving in saliva, food seeps into the taste buds—specialized cells on the upper surface of the tongue—through tiny openings. Deep within each bud are hairlike receptors designed to detect a certain taste. "Sweet" buds lie at the tip of the tongue, salty in the front, bitter at the back, and sour along the edges. All flavors are derived from these four basic tastes.

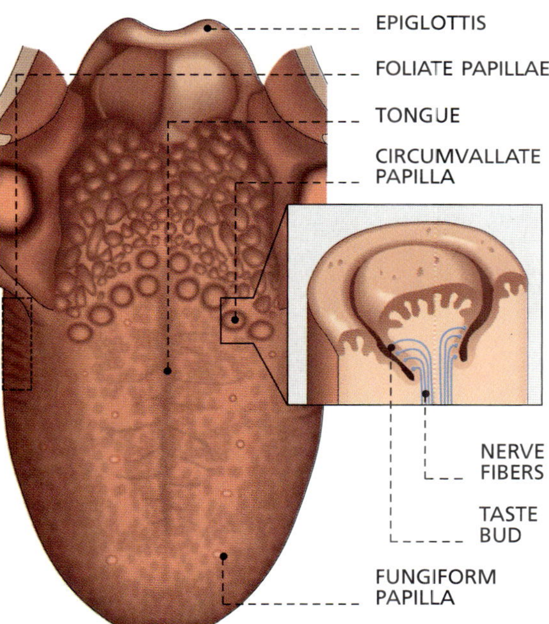

SMELL

Along the upper part of the nasal cavity lie millions of specialized cells that are tipped with hairlike olfactory receptors. When certain molecules from the air enter the nose, they hook up with specific receptors, stimulating olfactory nerves to transmit signals to the olfactory bulbs, which in turn forward information to the brain for interpretation.

TOUCH

Specialized nerves under the surface of the skin transmit the sensation of touch. Several sets of nerves, embedded at different levels, are associated with the various types of touch. Receptors near the surface, for example, detect slight pressure and moderate temperature changes, while deeper nerves sense vibration. Impulses from these receptors travel to the brain along the branching pathways of the nervous system.

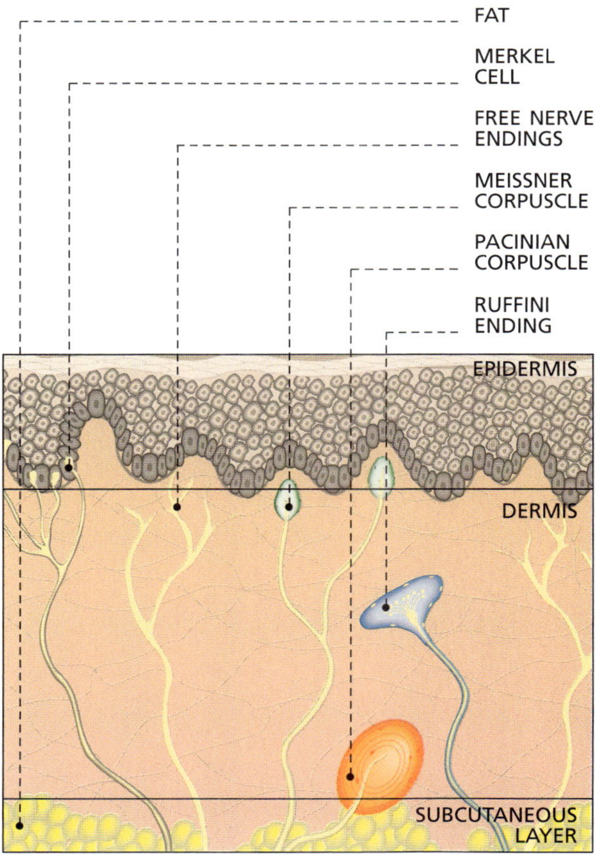

APPENDIX

CONTENTS

Abbreviations 1070

Key to Professional Titles. 1070

Health Associations and Organizations 1071

Gallery of Acupressure Techniques 1076

Gallery of Yoga Positions. 1085

ABBREVIATIONS

cal calorie
gal gallon
in inch
F Fahrenheit
IU international units, measurement used for fat-soluble vitamins
lb pound
mcg microgram
mg milligram
oz ounce
pt pint
qt quart
spp. various species, often used with botanical names of herbs to indicate that more than one species of a plant may be used medicinally
tbsp tablespoon
tsp teaspoon
c in homeopathic dosages, indicating a dilution ratio of 1 part to 99 parts
x in homeopathic dosages, indicating a dilution ratio of 1 part to 9 parts

KEY TO PROFESSIONAL TITLES

CA Certified Acupuncturist
DC Doctor of Chiropractic
DDS Doctor of Dental Surgery
DHANP Diplomate of Homeopathic Academy of Naturopathic Physicians
Dipl Ac Diplomate of Acupuncture
Dipl CH Diplomate of Chinese Herbology
NCCAOM National Certification Commission for Acupuncture and Oriental Medicine
DH Doctor of Homeopathy
DO Doctor of Osteopathy
DSc Doctor of Science
EdD Doctor of Education
FAAAI Fellow of the American Academy of Allergy and Immunology
FAAN Fellow of the American Academy of Neurology
FAAO Fellow of the American Academy of Ophthalmology
FAAO Fellow of the American Academy of Osteopathy
FAAOS Fellow of the American Academy of Orthopaedic Surgeons
FAAP Fellow of the American Academy of Pediatrics
FACCP Fellow of the American College of Chest Physicians
FACE Fellow of the American College of Endocrinology
FACP Fellow of the American College of Physicians
FACS Fellow of the American College of Surgeons
FAOSSM Fellow of the American Orthopaedic Society for Sports Medicine
FICC Fellow of the International College of Chiropractors
FNAAOM Fellow of the National Academy of Acupuncture and Oriental Medicine
JD Doctor of Jurisprudence
LAc Licensed Acupuncturist
LCSW Licensed Clinical Social Worker
MA Master of Arts
MACP Master of the American College of Physicians
MALS Master of Arts in Library Sciences
MBA Master of Business Administration
MD Doctor of Medicine
MD(H) Licensed Homeopathic Physician
MNIMH Member of the National Institutes of Medical Herbalists (British)
MPH Master of Public Health; Master Practitioner of Homeopathy
MS Master of Science
MSPH Master of Science in Public Health
ND Doctor of Naturopathy
OMD Oriental Medical Doctor
PhD Doctor of Philosophy
PT Physical Therapist
RN Registered Nurse
RPh Registered Pharmacist

HEALTH ASSOCIATIONS AND ORGANIZATIONS 

GENERAL

American Board of Medical Specialties
1007 Church Street, Suite 404
Evanston, IL 60201-5913
phone: (800) 776-CERT
website: www.abms.org
(Will tell you if your physician is board certified.)

American Holistic Medical Association
6728 Old McLean Village Drive
McLean, VA 22101
website: www.holisticmedicine.org
(Will provide national referral directory for a fee; send written request.)

Centers for Disease Control and Prevention (CDC)
1600 Clifton Road
Atlanta, GA 30333
phone: (800) 311-3534
website: www.cdc.gov

National Health Information Center (NHIC)
PO Box 1133
Washington, DC 20013-1133
phone: (800) 336-4797
website: www.nhic-nt.health.org
(Referrals to health agencies that provide public information.)

National Hospice Organization (NHO)
1700 Diagonal Road, Suite 300
Alexandria, VA 22314
phone: (800) 658-8898
website: www.nho.org
(Hospice is care for terminally ill people and their families, primarily at home.)

National Library of Medicine
8600 Rockville Pike
Bethesda, MD 20894
phone: (888) 346-3656
website: www.nlm.nih.gov
(Medical and scientific books and journals.)

ACUPUNCTURE AND CHINESE MEDICINE

National Acupuncture and Oriental Medicine Alliance
14637 Starr Road, SE
Olalla, WA 98359
phone: (253) 851-6896
website: www.acuall.org

National Certification Commission for Acupuncture and Oriental Medicine (NCCAOM)
11 Canal Center Plaza, Suite 300
Alexandria, VA 22314
phone: (703) 548-9004
website: www.nccaom.org

AGING

National Institute on Aging (NIA) Information Center
PO Box 8057
Gaithersburg, MD 20898-8057
phone: (800) 222-2225
website: www.nih.gov/nia

AYURVEDIC MEDICINE

The Ayurvedic Institute
11311 Menaul Boulevard, NE
Albuquerque, NM 87112
phone: (505) 291-9698
website: www.ayurveda.com

BODY WORK

American Massage Therapy Association (AMTA)
820 Davis Street, Suite 100
Evanston, IL 60201-4444
phone: (847) 864-0123
website: www.amtamassage.org

Aston-Patterning
PO Box 3568
Incline Village, NV 89450-3568
phone: (775) 831-8228
website: www.astonpatterning.com

Feldenkrais Guild of North America
3611 SW Hood Avenue, Suite 100
Portland, OR 97201
phone: (800) 775-2118
website: www.feldenkrais.com

International Institute of Reflexology, Inc.
5650 First Avenue North
PO Box 12642
St. Petersburg, FL 33733-2642
phone: (727) 343-4811
website: www.reflexology-usa.net

American Society for the Alexander Technique
401 East Market Street
Charlottesville, VA 22902
phone: (800) 473-0620
website: www.alexandertech.org

The Rolf Institute of Structural Integration
205 Canyon Boulevard
Boulder, CO 80302
phone: (800) 530-8875
website: www.rolf.org

CANCER

American Cancer Society
1599 Clifton Road, NE
Atlanta, GA 30329-4251
phone: (800) ACS-2345
website: www.cancer.org

CancerCare Inc., National Office
275 7th Avenue
New York, NY 10001
phone: (800) 813-HOPE
website: www.cancercare.org

Candlelighters Childhood Cancer Foundation
3910 Warner Street
Kensington, MD 20895
phone: (800) 366-CCCF
website: www.candlelighters.org

The Leukemia & Lymphoma Society,
1311 Mamaroneck Avenue
White Plains, NY 10605
Information Resource Center:
(800) 955-4572
website: www.leukemia-lymphoma.org

National Alliance of Breast Cancer Organizations (NABCO)
9 East 37th Street, 10th Floor
New York, NY 10016
phone: (888) 80-NABCO
website: www.nabco.org

National Brain Tumor Foundation
414 13th Street, Suite 700
Oakland, CA 94612-2603
phone: (800) 934-CURE
website: www.braintumor.org

National Cancer Institute Cancer Information Service (CIS)
phone: (800) 4CANCER
TTY/TDD: (800) 332-8615
website: cis.nci.nih.gov

The Skin Cancer Foundation
PO Box 561
New York, NY 10156
phone: (800) SKIN490
website: www.skincancer.org

HEALTH ASSOCIATIONS AND ORGANIZATIONS

CHILDREN'S HEALTH

American Academy of Pediatrics (AAP)
141 Northwest Point Boulevard
Elk Grove Village, IL 60007-1098
phone: (847) 228-5005
website: www.aap.org

National Reye's Syndrome Foundation
PO Box 829
Bryan, OH 43506-0829
phone: (800) 233-7993
website: www.bright.net

CHIROPRACTIC

American Chiropractic Association
1701 Clarendon Boulevard
Arlington, VA 22209
phone: (800) 986-4636
website: www.amerchiro.org

DENTAL PROBLEMS

American Dental Association (ADA)
211 E. Chicago Avenue
Chicago, IL 60611
phone: (312) 440-2500
website: www.ada.org

DIGESTION/GASTROINTESTINAL PROBLEMS

Celiac Sprue Association, USA
PO Box 31700
Omaha, NE 68131-0700
phone: (402) 558-0600
website: www.csaceliacs.org

Crohn's & Colitis Foundation of America (CCFA)
386 Park Avenue South, 17th Floor
New York, NY 10016-8804
phone: (800) 932-2423
website: www.ccfa.org

Digestive Disease National Coalition
507 Capitol Court, Suite 200
Washington, DC 20002
phone: (202) 544-7497
E-mail: ddirks@aol.com

Gluten Intolerance Group of North America
15110 10th Avenue, SW, Suite A
Seattle, WA 98166
phone: (206) 246-6652
website: www.gluten.net

National Digestive Diseases Information Clearinghouse (NDDIC)
2 Information Way
Bethesda, MD 20892-3570
website: www.niddk.nih.gov/health/digest/nddic.htm

United Ostomy Association, Inc. (UOA)
19772 MacArthur Boulevard, Suite 200
Irvine, CA 92612-2405
phone: (800) 826-0826
website: www.uoa.org

EAR, NOSE, AND THROAT PROBLEMS

American Academy of Otolaryngology-Head and Neck Surgery
1 Prince Street
Alexandria, VA 22314-3357
phone: (703) 836-4444
TTY/TDD: (703) 519-1585
website: www.entnet.org

American Tinnitus Association
PO Box 5
Portland, OR 97207-0005
phone: (800) 634-8978
website: www.ata.org

ENDOCRINE PROBLEMS

American Diabetes Association
Attention: Customer Service
1701 North Beauregard Street
Alexandria, VA 22311
phone: (800) DIABETES
website: www.diabetes.org

Juvenile Diabetes Foundation International (JDFI)
120 Wall Street, 19th Floor
New York, NY 10005-4001
phone: (800) JDF-CURE
website: www.jdf.org

National Diabetes Information Clearinghouse (NDIC)
1 Information Way
Bethesda, MD 20892-3560
phone: (301) 654-3327
website: www.niddk.nih.gov/health/diabetes/ndic.htm

Thyroid Foundation of America Inc.
Ruth Sleeper Hall, RSL 350
40 Parkman Street
Boston, MA 02114-2698
phone: (800) 832-8321
website: www.tsh.org

ENVIRONMENTAL ILLNESS

American Academy of Environmental Medicine (AAEM)
American Financial Center
7701 East Kellogg, Suite 625
Wichita, KS 67207-1705
phone: (316) 684-5500
website: www.aaem.com

National Coalition Against the Misuse of Pesticides (NCAMP)
701 E Street, SE, Suite 200
Washington, DC 20003
phone: (202) 543-5450
website: www.ncamp.org

National Institute of Environmental Health Science (NIEHS)
PO Box 12233
Research Triangle Park, NC 27709
website: www.niehs.nih.gov

EYE PROBLEMS

American Academy of Ophthalmology
PO Box 7424
San Francisco, CA 94120-7424
phone: (415) 561-8500
website: www.eyenet.org

National Eye Institute (NEI)
2020 Vision Place
Bethesda, MD 20892-3655
phone: (301) 496-5248
website: www.nei.nih.gov

Prevent Blindness America
500 E. Remington Road
Schaumburg, IL 60173
phone: (800) 331-2020
(Ask for the Information Center.)
website: www.preventblindness.org

FITNESS

American Council on Exercise (ACE)
5820 Oberlin Drive, Suite 102
San Diego, CA 92121-3787
phone: (800) 825-3636
website: www.acefitness.org

HEART AND CIRCULATORY PROBLEMS

American Board of Chelation Therapy
1407B N. Wells Street, Suite B
Chicago, IL 60610
phone: (800) 356-2228
(For information or referrals, send a self-addressed, stamped envelope.)

American Heart Association
National Center
7272 Greenville Avenue
Dallas, TX 75231-4596
phone: (800) AHA-USA1
website: www.americanheart.org

National Heart, Lung, and Blood Institute (NHLBI) Information Center
PO Box 30105
Bethesda, MD 20824-0105
phone: (800) 575-WELL
website: www.nhlbi.nih.gov

National Stroke Association
9707 East Easter Lane
Englewood, CO 80112-5112
phone: (303) 649-9299;
(800) STROKES (hot line)
website: www.stroke.org

American Stroke Association
A Division of American Heart Association
7272 Greenville Avenue
Dallas, TX 75231
phone: (888) 4-STROKE
website: www.strokeassociation.org

HEMATOLOGICAL/HEPATOLOGICAL

American Liver Foundation
75 Maiden Lane, Suite 603
New York, NY 10038
phone: (800) GO-LIVER
website: www.liverfoundation.org

The Sickle Cell Disease Association of America
200 Corporate Point, Suite 495
Culver City, CA 90230-7633
phone: (800) 421-8453
website: www.sicklecelldisease.org

HERBS

Herb Research Foundation
1007 Pearl Street, Suite 200
Boulder, CO 80302
phone: (800) 748-2617
website: www.herbs.org

HOMEOPATHY

National Center for Homeopathy
801 N. Fairfax Street, Suite 306
Alexandria, VA 22314
phone: (703) 548-7790
website: www.homeopathic.org

IMMUNE DISORDERS

AIDS, Medicine & Miracles
Suite 330, 1201 East Colfax Avenue
Denver, CO 80218
phone: (800) 875-8770
website: www.inspirational.org/~amm

AIDS Clinical Trials Information Service (ACTIS)
PO Box 6421
Rockville, MD 20849-6421
phone: (800) TRIALS-A
TTY/TDD: (800) 243-7012
website: www.actis.org

American Academy of Allergy, Asthma & Immunology (AAAAI)
611 E. Wells Street
Milwaukee, WI 53202
phone: (800) 822-2762
website: www.aaaai.org

CDC National HIV/AIDS Hotline
phone: (800) 342-AIDS
Spanish access: (800) 344-SIDA
TTY/TDD: (800) AIDS-TTY

CDC National Prevention Information Network (NPIN)
8401 Colesville Road, Suite 200
Silver Spring, MD 20910
phone: (800) 458-5231
TTY/TDD: (800) 243-7012
website: www.cdcnpin.org

CFIDS Association of America
PO Box 220398
Charlotte, NC 28222-0398
phone: (800) 442-3437
website: www.cfids.org
(Chronic fatigue and immune dysfunction syndromes.)

HIV/AIDS Treatment Information Service (ATIS)
PO Box 6303
Rockville, MD 20849-6303
phone: (800) 448-0440
TTY/TDD: (888) 480-3739
website: www.hivatis.org

Lupus Foundation of America (LFA)
1300 Piccard Drive, Suite 200
Rockville, MD 20850-4303
phone: (800) 558-0121
Spanish access: (800) 558-0231
website: www.lupus.org

National Institute of Allergy and Infectious Diseases (NIAID)
Office of Communications and Public Liaison (OCPL)
Building 31, Room 7A-50
31 Center Drive, MSC 2520
Bethesda, MD 20892-2520
phone: (301) 496-5717
website: www.niaid.nih.gov

LUNG DISEASE

American Lung Association
1740 Broadway
New York, NY 10019-4374
phone: (800) LUNG-USA
website: www.lungusa.org

MAGNETIC FIELD THERAPY

Bio-Electro-Magnetics Institute
2490 West Moana Lane
Reno, NV 89509-7801
phone/fax: (775) 827-9099
E-mail:dzimmerz889@aol.com
(Will provide information about magnetic field therapy for a fee; send written request.)

Enviro-Tech Products
17171 Southeast 29th Street
Choctaw, OK 73020
phone: (800) 445-1962
fax: (405) 390-8934

MENTAL HEALTH

American Psychiatric Association
Division of Public Affairs
1400 K Street, NW
Washington, DC 20005
phone: (888) 357-7924
website: www.psych.org

Children and Adults with Attention Deficit Disorders (CHADD)
8181 Professional Place, Suite 201
Landover, MD 20785
phone: (800) 233-4050
website: www.chadd.org

Depression & Related Affective Disorders Association (DRADA)
Meyer 3-181
600 North Wolfe Street
Baltimore, MD 21287-7381
phone: (410) 955-4647;
(202) 955-5800
website: www.med.jhu.edu/drada/index.html

HEALTH ASSOCIATIONS AND ORGANIZATIONS

National Association of Anorexia Nervosa and Associated Disorders (ANAD)
PO Box 7
Highland Park, IL 60035
phone: (847) 831-3438
website: www.anad.org

National Institute of Mental Health (NIMH)
6001 Executive Boulevard
Bethesda, MD 20892-9663
Information Resources and Inquiries Branch phone: (301) 443-4513
website: www.nimh.nih.gov

NIMH Anxiety Disorders Information Line
phone: (888) 8-ANXIETY

NIMH Depression Information Line
phone: (800) 421-4211

National Mental Health Association (NMHA)
Information Center
1021 Prince Street
Alexandria, VA 22314-2971
phone: (800) 969-NMHA
website: www.nmha.org

MIND/BODY MEDICINE

Association for Applied Psychophysiology and Biofeedback (AAPB)
10200 W. 44th Avenue, Suite 304
Wheat Ridge, CO 80033-2840
website: www.aapb.org
(Send a self-addressed, stamped envelope for further information about biofeedback.)

MUSCULOSKELETAL PROBLEMS

American Academy of Physical Medicine and Rehabilitation
1 IBM Plaza, Suite 2500
Chicago, IL 60611-3604
phone: (312) 464-9700
website: www.aapmr.org

Arthritis Foundation
1330 West Peachtree Street
Atlanta, GA 30309
phone: (800) 283-7800
website: www.arthritis.org

National Osteoporosis Foundation (NOF)
1232 22nd Street, NW
Washington, DC 20037-1292
phone: (202) 223-2226
website: www.nof.org

Scoliosis Association, Inc.
PO Box 811705
Boca Raton, FL 33481-1705
phone: (800) 800-0669
website: www.scoliosis-assoc.org

NATUROPATHIC MEDICINE

American Association of Naturopathic Physicians
601 Valley Street, Suite 105
Seattle, WA 98109
phone: (206) 298-0126
website: www.naturopathic.org

NEUROLOGICAL PROBLEMS

Alzheimer's Association
919 N. Michigan Avenue, Suite 1000
Chicago, IL 60611-1676
phone: (800) 272-3900
website: www.alz.org

American Parkinson Disease Association (APDA)
1250 Hylan Boulevard, Suite 4B
Staten Island, NY 10305-1946
phone: (800) 223-2732
Information and Referral Center: (888) 400-2732
website: www.apdaparkinson.com

The Amyotrophic Lateral Sclerosis Association (ALSA)
27001 Agoura Road, Suite 150
Calabasas Hills, CA 91301-5104
phone: (800) 782-4747
website: www.alsa.org

The Epilepsy Foundation, National Office
4351 Garden City Drive
Landover, MD 20785
phone: (800) EFA-1000
website: www.efa.org

The Multiple Sclerosis Foundation (MSF)
6350 N. Andrews Avenue
Ft. Lauderdale, FL 33309
phone: (800) 441-7055
website: www.msfacts.org

National Headache Foundation
428 West St. James Place, 2nd Floor
Chicago, IL 60614-2750
phone: (888) NHF-5552
website: www.headaches.org

Parkinson's Disease Foundation (PDF)
William Black Medical Building
Columbia-Presbyterian Medical Center
710 W. 168th Street
New York, NY 10032-9982
phone: (800) 457-6676
website: www.pdf.org

NUTRITION AND DIET

American Dietetic Association National Center for Nutrition and Dietetics (NCND)
216 W. Jackson Boulevard, Suite 800
Chicago, IL 60606-6995
ADA's Consumer Nutrition Hotline: (800) 366-1655
phone: (312) 899-0040
website: www.eatright.org/ncnd.html

Nutrition for Optimal Health Association, Inc.
PO Box 380
Winnetka, IL 60093
phone: (708) 786-5326

OSTEOPATHY

American Osteopathic Association (AOA)
142 East Ontario Street
Chicago, IL 60611
phone: (800) 621-1773
website: www.aoa-net.org

SEXUAL HEALTH

CDC National Prevention Information Network (NPIN)
8401 Colesville Road, Suite 200
Silver Spring, MD 20910
phone: (800) 458-5231
TTY/TDD: (800) 243-7012
website: www.cdcnpin.org

CDC National STD Hotline
phone: (800) 227-8922

Couple to Couple League International, Inc.
PO Box 111184
Cincinnati, OH 45211-1184
phone: (513) 471-2000
website: www.ccli.org
(Natural family planning.)

Impotence Institute of America
PO Box 410
Bowie, MD 20718-0410
phone: (800) 669-1603
website: www.impotenceworld.org

National Herpes Hotline
phone: (919) 361-8488

Planned Parenthood Federation of America, Inc.
810 Seventh Avenue
New York, NY 10019
phone: (800) 230-PLAN for referrals; (800) 669-0156 for publications
website: www.plannedparenthood.org

RESOLVE
1310 Broadway
Somerville, MA 02144-1731
phone: (617) 623-0744 (HelpLine)
website: www.resolve,org
(Women's and men's infertility.)

SKIN

American Academy of Dermatology (AAD)
930 N. Meacham Road
Schaumburg, IL 60173
phone: (888) 462-DERM
website: www.aad.com
(For information about skin disorders, send a self-addressed, stamped envelope.)

SUBSTANCE ABUSE

Alcoholics Anonymous (AA)
PO Box 459
Grand Central Station
New York, NY 10163
phone: (212) 870-3400
website: www.aa.org

Narcotics Anonymous
World Service Office
PO Box 9999
Van Nuys, CA 91409
phone: (818) 773-9999
website: www.na.org

National Institute on Alcohol Abuse and Alcoholism (NIAAA)
6000 Executive Boulevard
Willco Building
Bethesda, MD 20892-7003
phone: (301) 443-3860
website: www.niaaa.nih.gov

Rational Recovery Systems
PO Box 800
Lotus, CA 95651
phone: (800) 303-2873
voice/fax: (530) 622-4296
website: www.rational.org/recovery

Smokenders
9617 NW Golden Avenue
Vancouver, WA 98665
phone: (800) 828-HELP
website: www.smokenders.com

Women for Sobriety Inc.
PO Box 618
Quakertown, PA 18951-0618
phone/fax: (215) 536-8026
website: www.womenforsobriety.com
(For information, send a self-addressed, stamped envelope.)

URINARY TRACT PROBLEMS

National Kidney and Urologic Diseases Information Clearinghouse (NKUDIC)
3 Information Way
Bethesda, MD 20892-3590
phone: (301) 654-4415
website: www.niddk.nih.gov/health/kidney/nkudic.htm

National Kidney Foundation, Inc.
30 E. 33rd Street, Suite 1100
New York, NY 10016
phone: (800) 622-9010
website: www.kidney.org

WOMEN'S HEALTH

American College of Obstetricians and Gynecologists (ACOG), Resource Center
PO Box 96920
Washington, DC 20090-6920
website: www.acog.org
(For patient education brochures, send a self-addressed, stamped business envelope and specify topic of interest.)

Human Development Resource Council, Inc.
3941 Holcomb Bridge Road, Suite 300
Norcross, GA 30092
phone: (770) 447-1598
website: www.hdrc.org

March of Dimes Birth Defects Foundation
1275 Mamaroneck Avenue
White Plains, NY 10605
phone: (888) MODIMES
TTY/TDD: (914) 997-4764
website: www.modimes.org

National Women's Health Network (NWHN)
514 10th Street, NW, Suite 400
Washington, DC 20004
phone: (202) 347-1140
Health Information Line:
(202) 628-7814
website:www.womenshealthnetwork.org

Project Rachel
PO Box 07477
Milwaukee, WI 53207-0477
phone: (800) 5WE-CARE
website: www.multimaxx.com/project-rachel
(Referral to a local office for post-abortion trauma.)

YOGA

International Association of Yoga Therapists
Yoga Research and Education Center
PO Box 1386
Lower Lake, CA 95457
phone: (707) 928-9898
website: www.yrec.org
(Send self-addressed, stamped envelope for an educational brochure on finding a yoga teacher.)

MISCELLANEOUS

American Academy of Neural Therapy, Inc.
410 East Denny Way, Suite 18
Seattle, WA 98122
phone: (206) 749-9967
website: www.neuraltherapy.com

American Apitherapy Society (AAS)
5390 Grande Road
Hillsboro, OH 45133
phone: (937) 364-1108
website: www.apitherapy.org/aas

GALLERY OF ACUPRESSURE TECHNIQUES

The principal acupressure points discussed in this book are grouped here according to traditional acupressure meridians—the invisible channels that are believed to carry energy through the body. The name of each meridian indicates the organ associated with bodily functions that are thought to be affected when point sites along that channel are stimulated.

The purpose of this gallery is to help you locate acupressure point sites on the body and to show you, in general, the proper stimulation techniques. Individual entries in the Ailments and Options section contain more specific information, such as how long to apply pressure to a given point. As a rule, you should use light touching instead of pressure on a weak back or other area that is injured or unusually sensitive. Also be aware that certain points should be avoided altogether during pregnancy.

Applying pressure to carefully chosen point sites on the body may help relieve symptoms associated with some medical disorders. But remember: Acupressure is not a substitute for a physician's medical advice. For more information, see the sources listed under "Acupressure and Acupuncture" in the Bibliography.

BLADDER

BLADDER 10

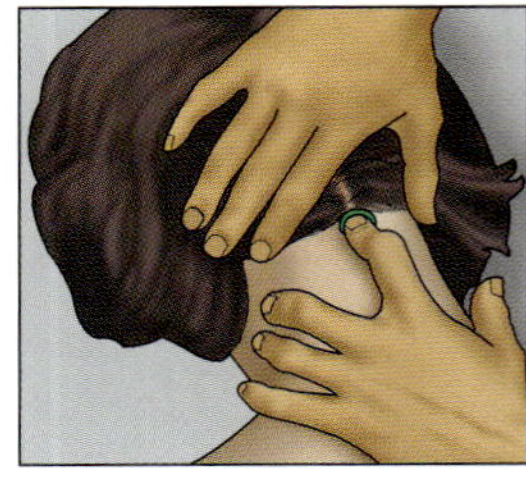

Locate the ropy muscles one-half inch below the base of the skull. Press inward using the thumb or a finger.

BLADDER 13

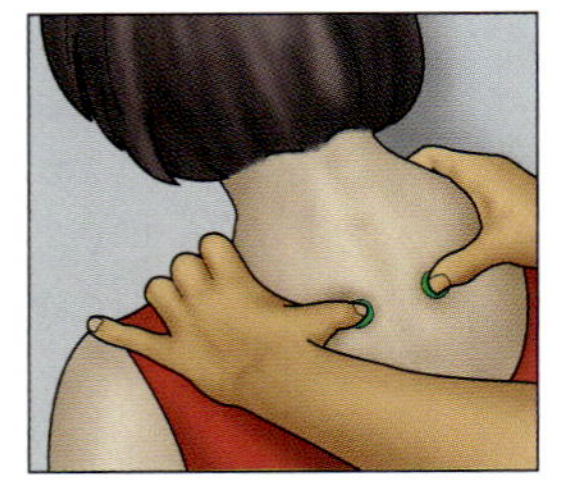

Use your thumbs or fingers to press into the muscles one-half inch outward from either side of the spine and one finger width below the upper tip of the shoulder blade.

BLADDER 23

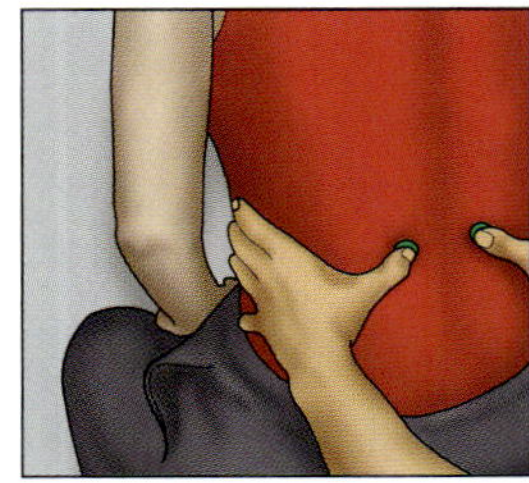

This point site is level with the space between the second and third lumbar vertebrae. Find BL 23 by aligning your thumbs or fingers about an inch outward from either side of the spine, just behind the navel, then press inward.

BLADDER 25

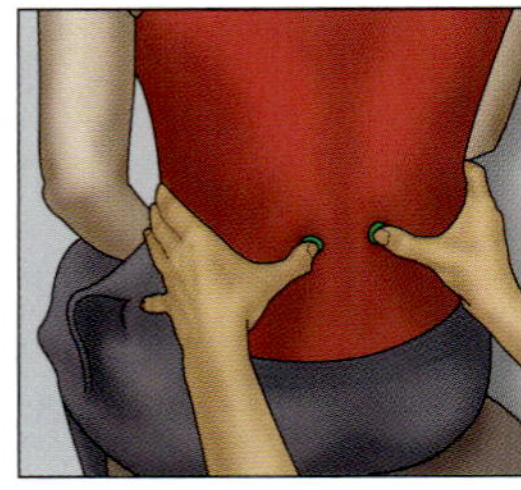

With your thumbs or fingers, press into the muscles about an inch outward from either side of the spine, about midway between BL 23 *(left)* and the bottom of the spine. The point is level with the fourth and fifth lumbar vertebrae.

BLADDER 32

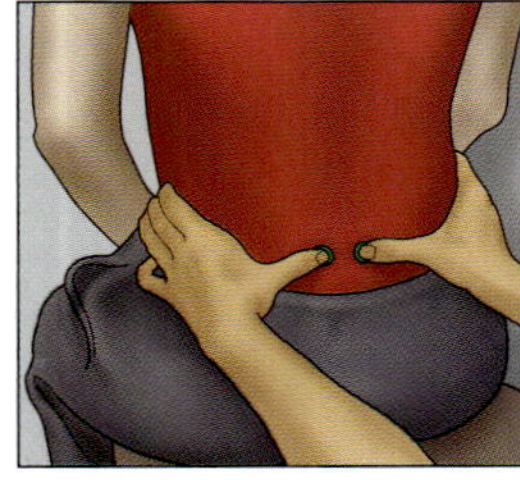

At the base of the spine, directly above the tailbone, use your thumbs or fingers to press into the muscles one-half inch outward from either side of the spine.

BLADDER 40

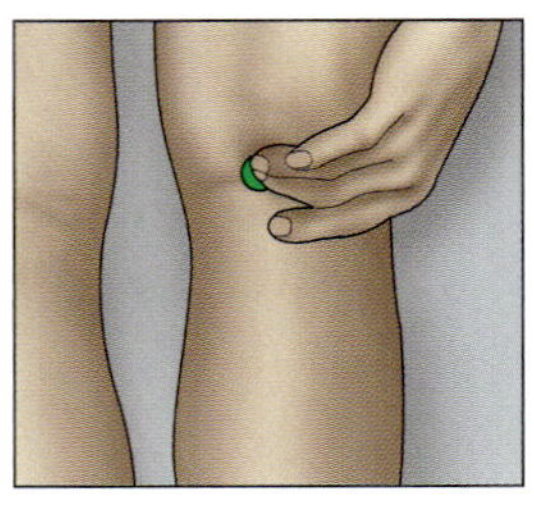

With your leg slightly bent, find the fold on the back of your knee where the knee bends. Use your middle finger to press inward on the fold, between the two tendons.

CONCEPTION VESSEL

CONCEPTION VESSEL 4

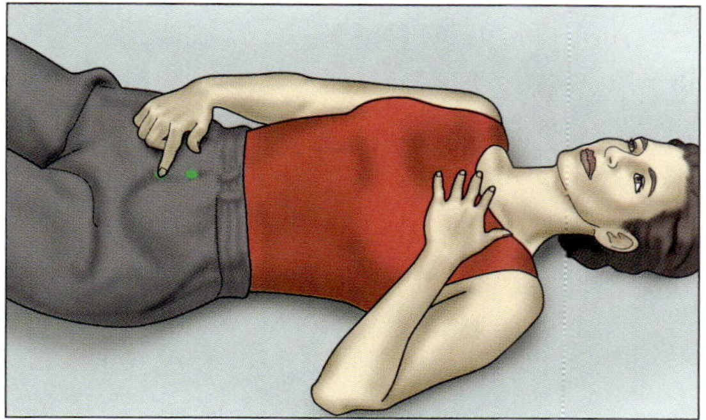

Locate this point, which lies just below CV 6, by measuring four finger widths down from the navel on the midline of the abdomen. With your index finger, gradually press as deep as possible on the point site.

CONCEPTION VESSEL 6

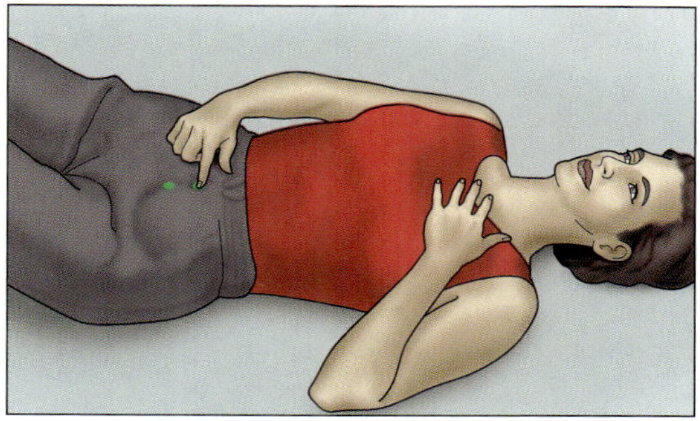

Measure three finger widths below the navel (or about one finger width up from CV 4), then press inward on this point as far as you can, using your index finger. Inhale slowly and deeply, relaxing as you exhale.

CONCEPTION VESSEL 12

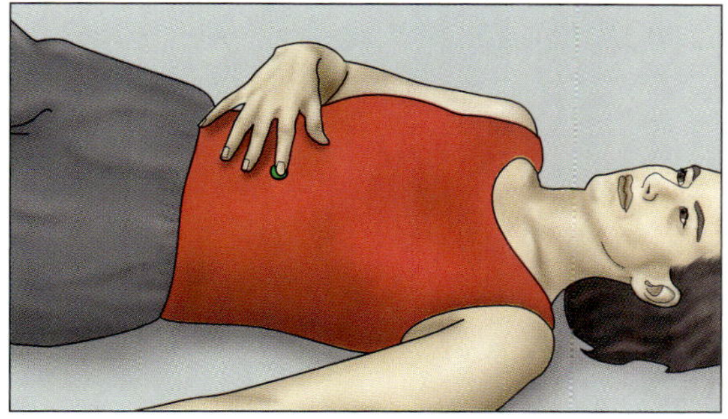

This point lies four thumb widths above the navel along the midline of the belly, about halfway between the navel and the bottom of the breastbone. Press softly inward, using your index finger.

CONCEPTION VESSEL 17

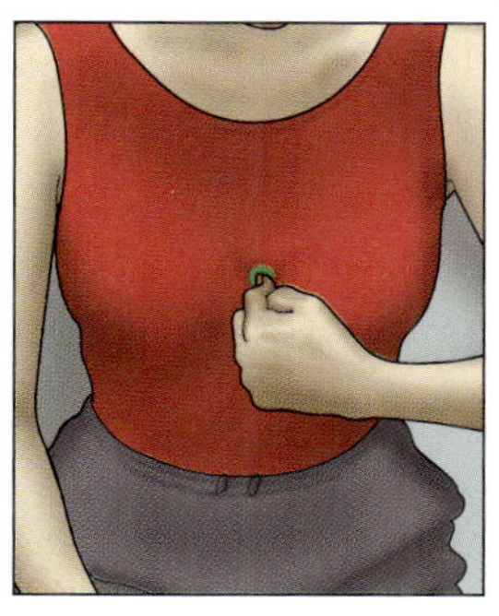

Place your index finger in the center of your chest, midway between the nipples, and press lightly.

CONCEPTION VESSEL 22

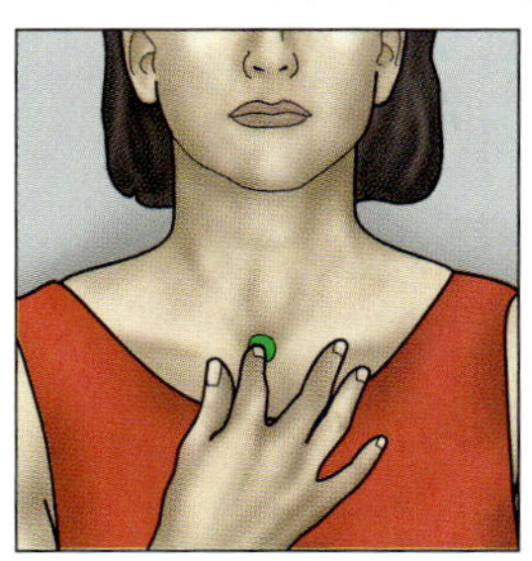

This point lies directly below the Adam's apple, midway between the collarbones in the large hollow at the base of the throat. Place the tip of your index or middle finger on the point site and press downward lightly.

GALLERY OF ACUPRESSURE TECHNIQUES

GALL BLADDER

GALL BLADDER 2

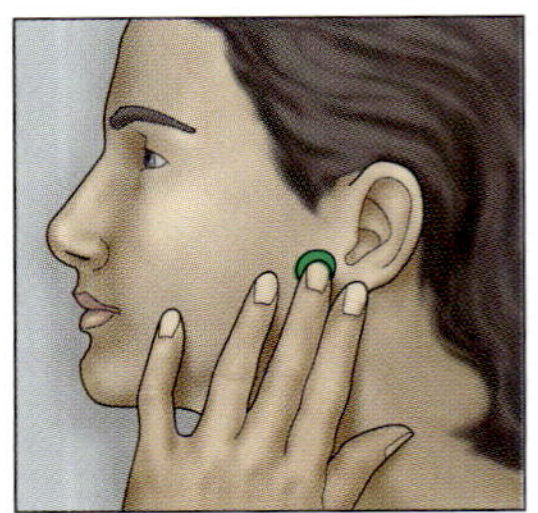

Open your mouth and, feeling along the jawbone, locate the depression directly in front of your ears. Place the tips of your middle fingers about one-half inch below the base of the depression. Close your mouth and press steadily on the point.

GALL BLADDER 20

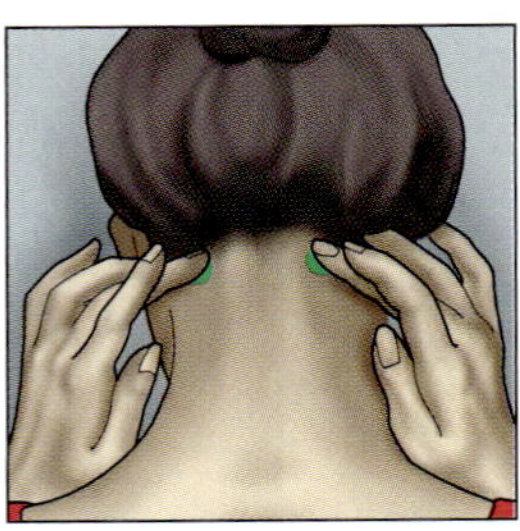

Place the tips of your middle fingers in the hollows at the base of your skull, about two inches apart on either side of the spine. Press firmly.

GALL BLADDER 21

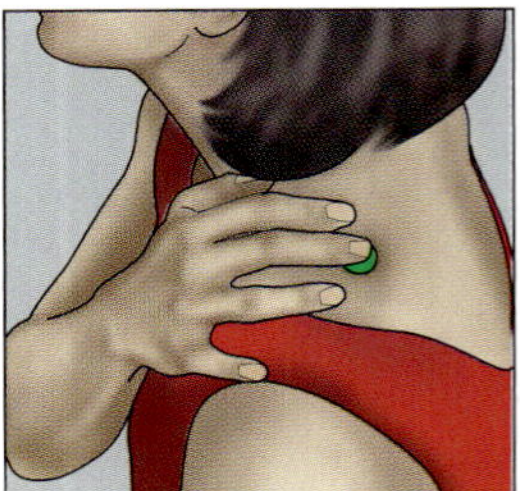

Apply pressure with your right middle finger to the highest point on your left shoulder muscle, one or two inches out from the base of the neck. Repeat on the other side. (Use light pressure if you are pregnant.)

GALL BLADDER 34

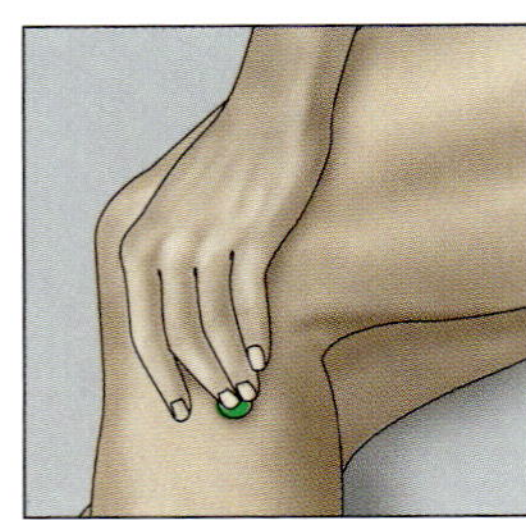

While seated with legs bent, locate the bony indentation on your lower leg just below and to the outside of the kneecap. Apply firm pressure to the point with your finger or thumb.

GALL BLADDER 39

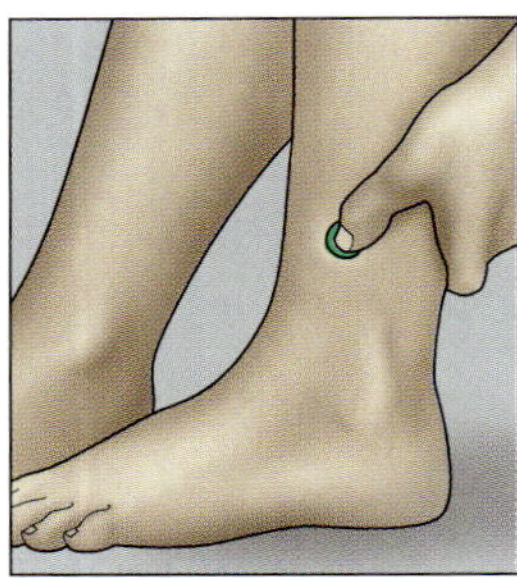

To find this point, measure four finger widths above the outside anklebone, in front of the fibula, on the lower leg. Apply pressure with the tip of your finger or thumb.

GOVERNING VESSEL

GOVERNING VESSEL 4

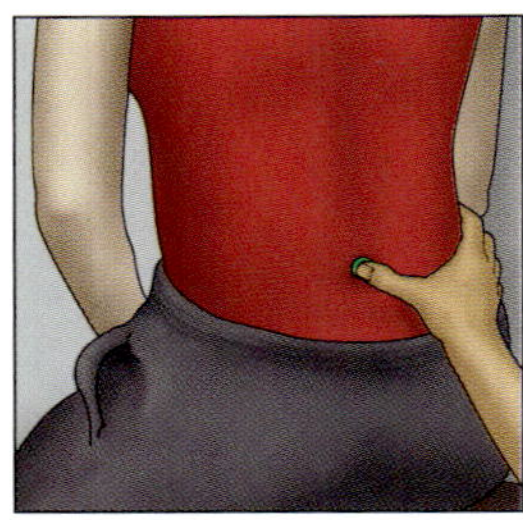

Press hard with your thumb on the midline of the spine, directly behind the navel. The point is located between the second and third lumbar vertebrae.

GOVERNING VESSEL 14

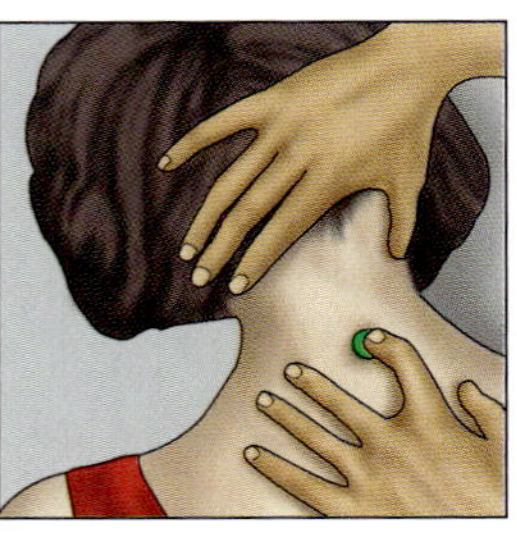

Tilt your head forward and locate the seventh cervical vertebra, the most prominent bone on the back of your neck. Have a helper use the thumb or index finger to press hard between this bone and the first thoracic vertebra below it.

GOVERNING VESSEL CONTINUED

GOVERNING VESSEL 20

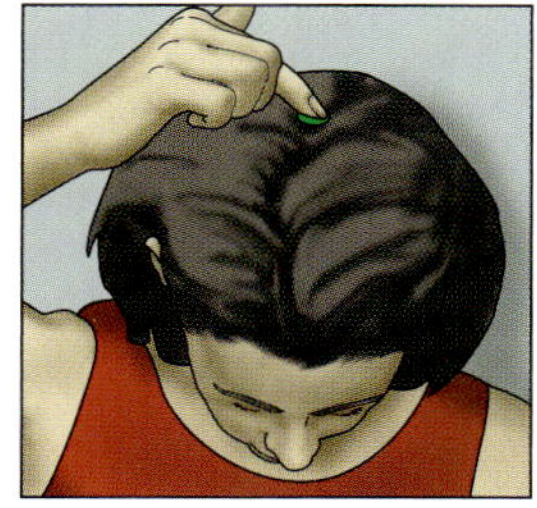

This point is located on the flat spot at the top of the head, midway along an imaginary line connecting the upper part of the ears. Apply pressure with your thumb or index finger. (Do not press this point if you have high blood pressure.)

GOVERNING VESSEL 24.5

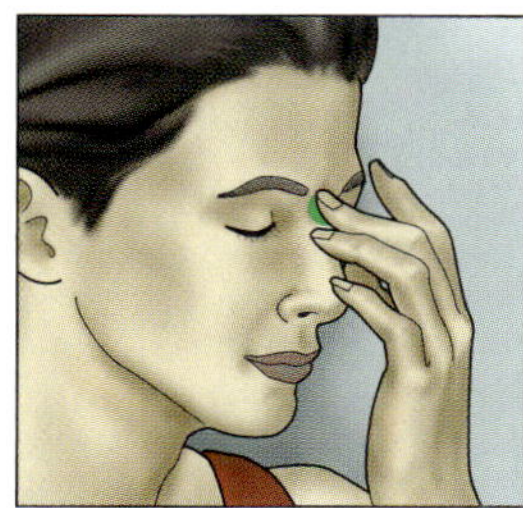

Place the tip of your middle finger at the top of the bridge of the nose, between your eyebrows. Press lightly.

GOVERNING VESSEL 25

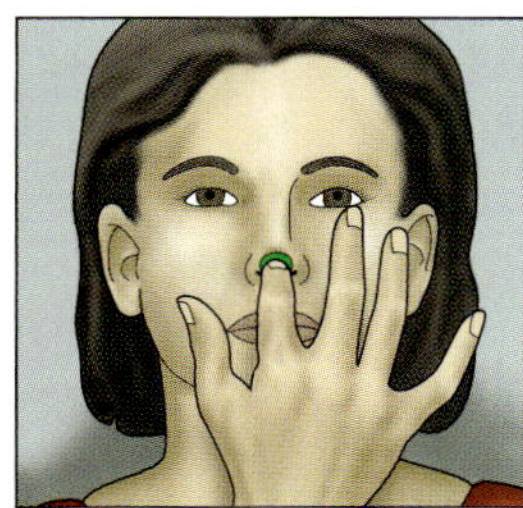

Lightly press the tip of your nose with the end of your finger.

HEART

HEART 3

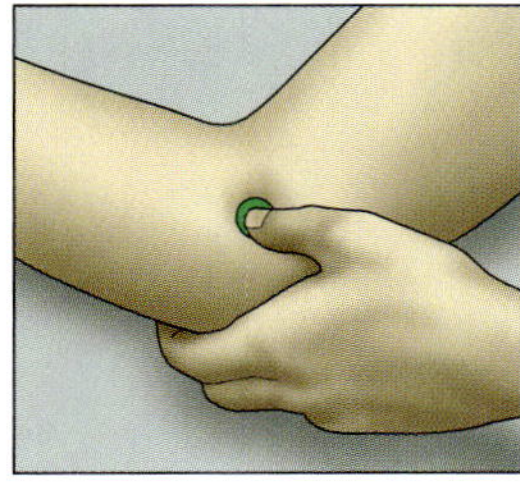

On the inside of the upper arm, use your thumb to apply pressure next to the tendon in the indentation near the inside elbow crease, in line with the little finger.

HEART 7

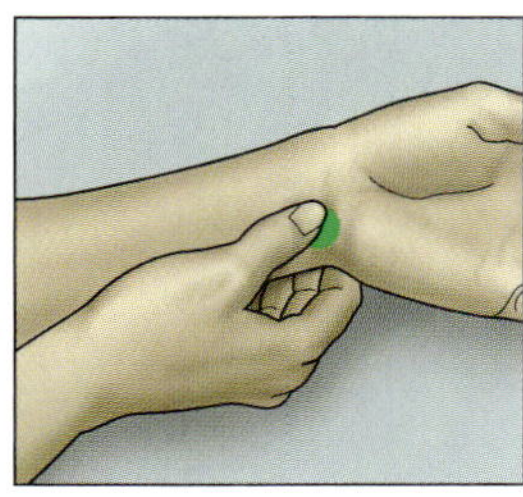

This point is located on the crease along the inside of the wrist, directly in line with the little finger. Squeeze firmly, using the thumb and index finger of your other hand.

KIDNEY

KIDNEY 1

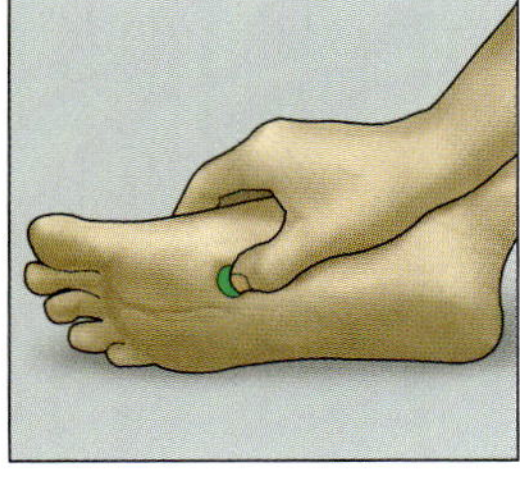

Use one or both thumbs to press just behind the ball of the foot, in the slight indentation of the back of the large pad that corresponds to the big toe. (Do not use this point if you have low blood pressure.)

KIDNEY 3

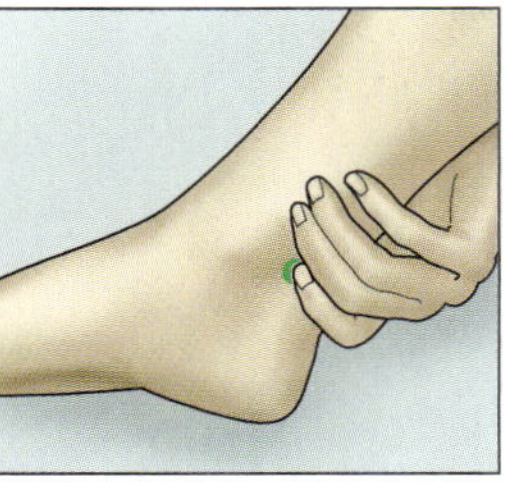

This point lies midway between the inside anklebone and the Achilles tendon at the back of the ankle. Apply pressure with your thumb or index finger. (Avoid using this point after the third month of pregnancy.)

GALLERY OF ACUPRESSURE TECHNIQUES

LARGE INTESTINE

LARGE INTESTINE 4

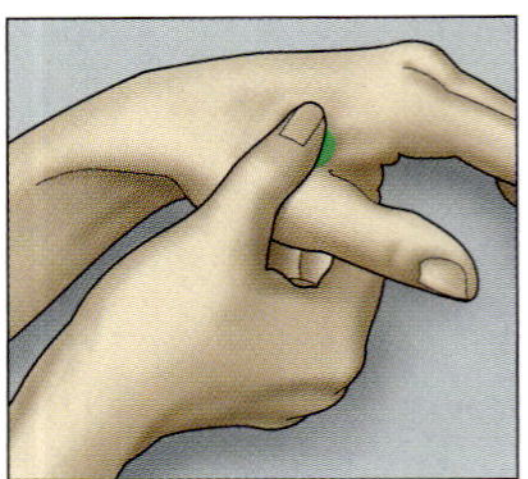

Use the thumb and index finger of your right hand to squeeze the webbing between the thumb and index finger of your left hand. Switch hands and repeat. (Do not apply pressure to this point if you are pregnant.)

LARGE INTESTINE 10

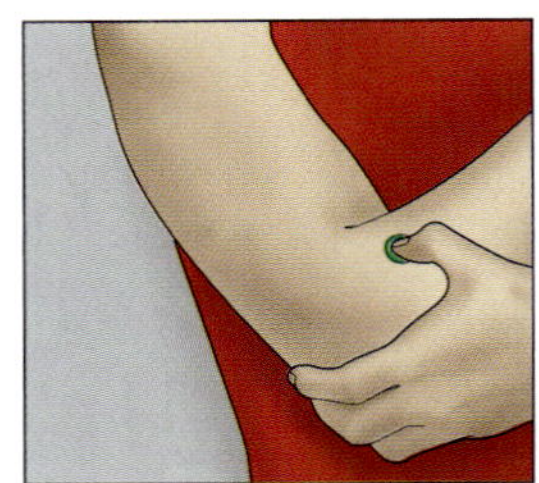

With your arm bent and palm down, measure two thumb widths below the edge of the elbow crease. The point site lies in the groove between the muscles on the outside of the arm. Press hard with your thumb, then repeat on the other arm.

LARGE INTESTINE 11

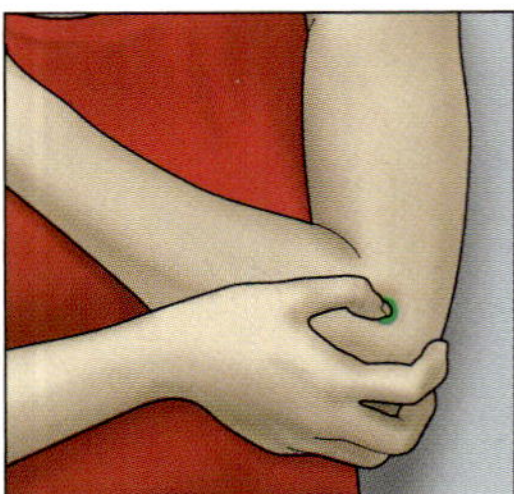

With your arm bent, use your thumb to press deeply on the outer edge of the elbow crease. Repeat on the other arm.

LARGE INTESTINE 20

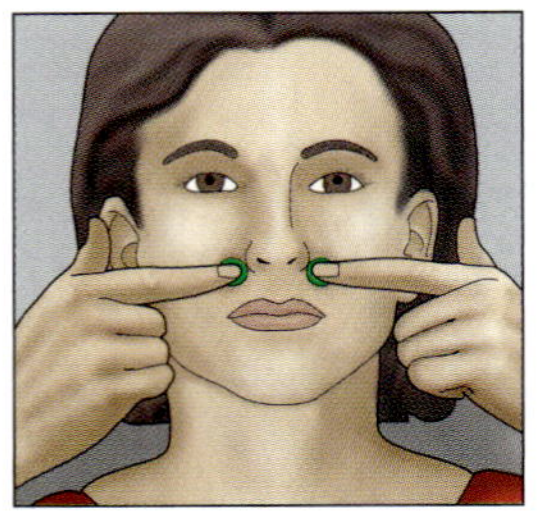

Using your index or middle fingers, press hard on the outer edge of the nostrils at the base of the nose.

LIVER

LIVER 2

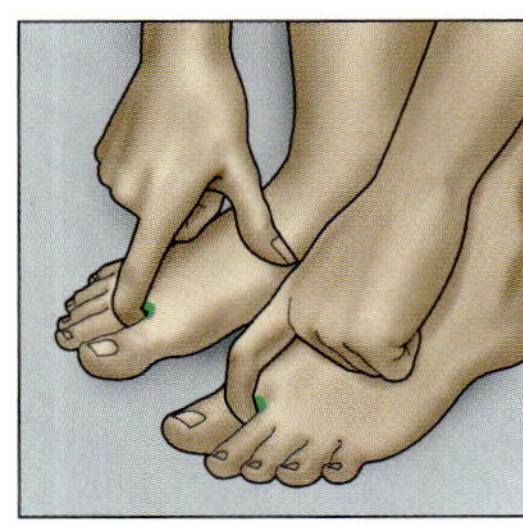

On the top of each foot, use your index finger to press into the webbing between the big toe and second toe.

LIVER 3

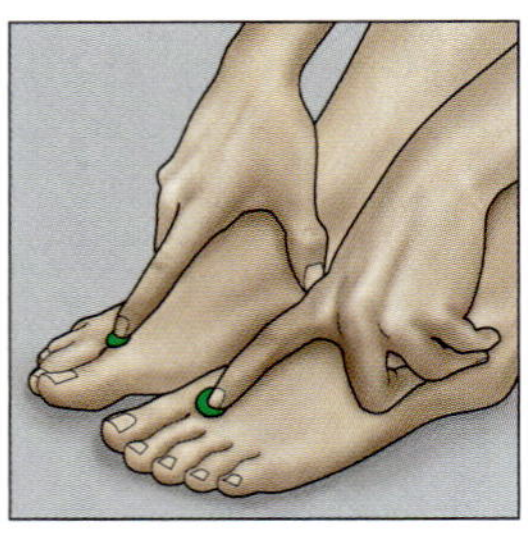

Place your index fingers next to the large knuckle of each big toe, then press into the groove on top of the foot between the big toe and second toe.

LIVER 8

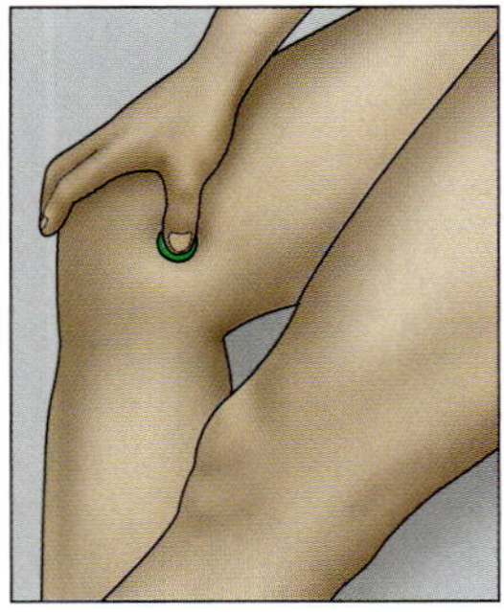

Bend the right knee and place your right thumb just above the knee crease on the inside of the leg. The point lies just below the knee joint (swing your leg a few times to help locate it). Press, then repeat on the other leg.

LUNG

LUNG 1

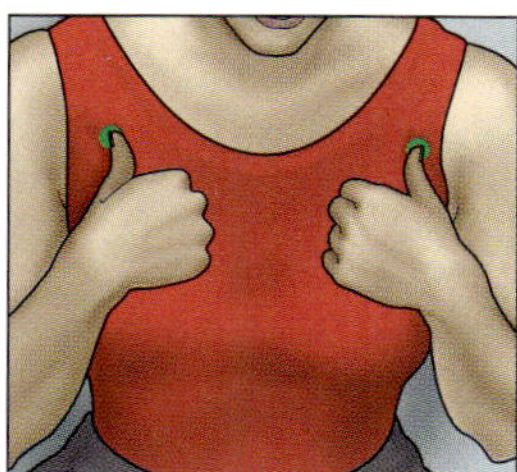

Place the thumb or index finger of each hand about one-half inch below the large hollow under the collarbone, on the outer part of the chest near the shoulder. Apply pressure gently.

LUNG 5

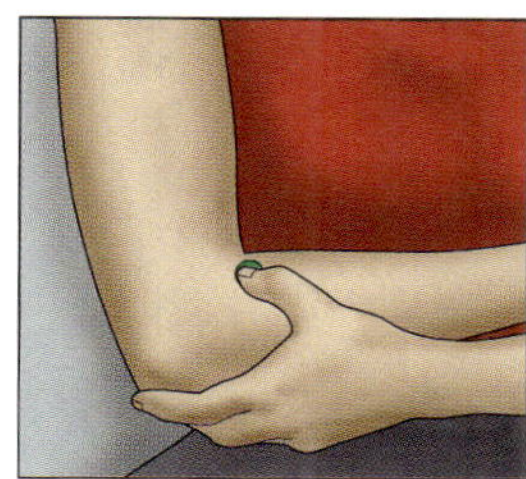

Bend your right elbow and make a fist. Place your left thumb on the outside crease (thumb side) of the elbow alongside the taut tendon and press firmly. Repeat on the other arm.

LUNG 7

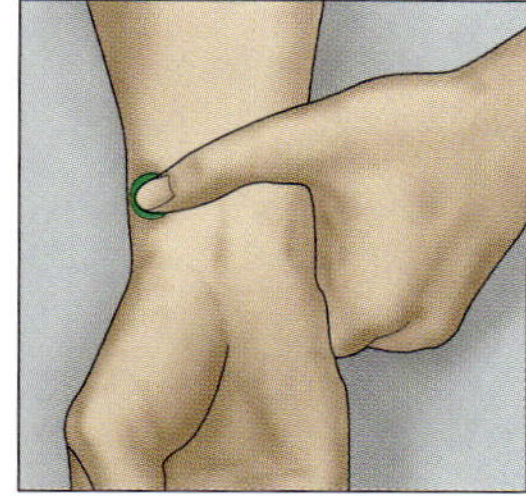

On the thumb side of the inner forearm, measure two finger widths above the crease in the wrist. Apply steady, firm pressure to the point site with your thumb, then repeat on the other arm.

LUNG 10

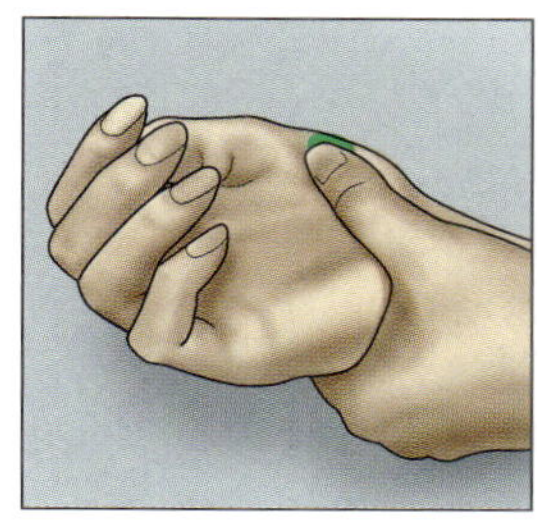

On the palm side of the hand, locate this point at the center of the pad at the base of the thumb. Apply pressure with your other thumb while taking several deep breaths.

PERICARDIUM

PERICARDIUM 3

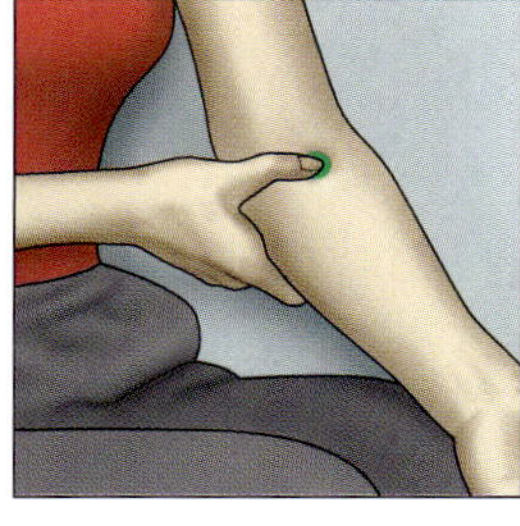

Locate the point along the biceps tendon at the elbow crease, in a direct line with your ring finger. Use your thumb to apply firm pressure, then repeat on the other arm.

PERICARDIUM 6

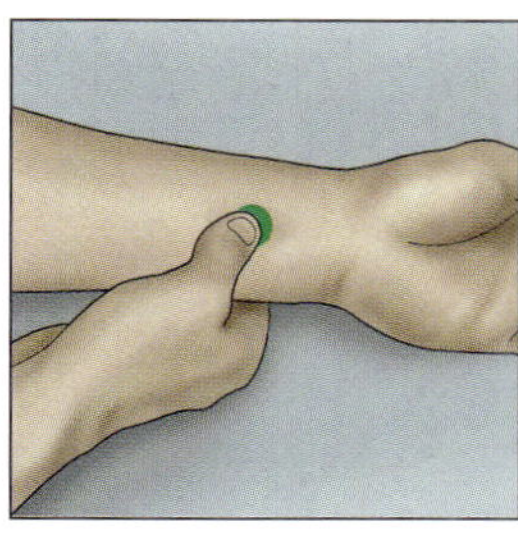

To find this point, measure two finger widths above the center of the wrist crease on the inside of your arm. With your thumb, press between the two bones of the forearm. Repeat on the other arm.

SMALL INTESTINE

SMALL INTESTINE 3

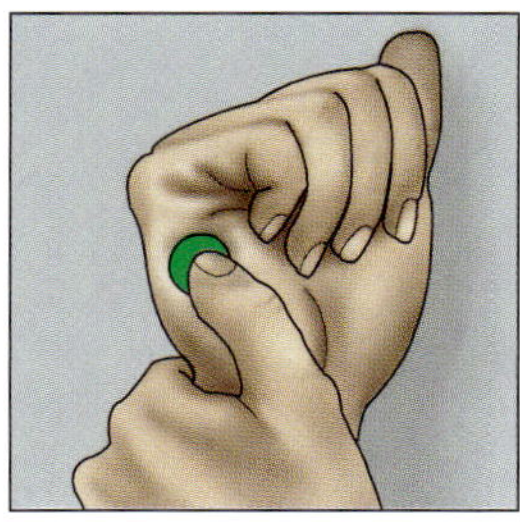

Make a loose fist, then twist your wrist to view the side of your little finger. Using your thumb, apply pressure to the side of your palm just below the knuckle of the little finger, between the bone and muscle.

SMALL INTESTINE 17

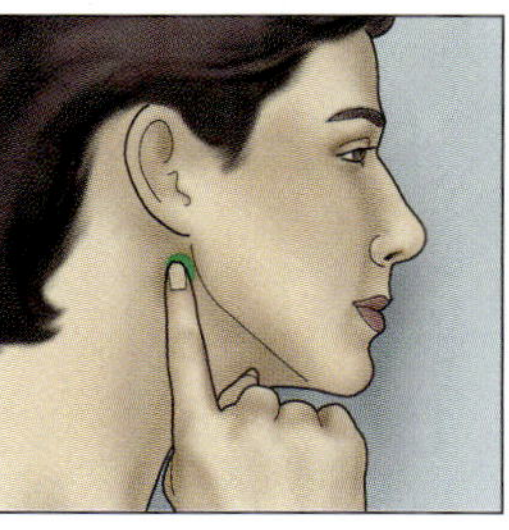

Place your index fingers just below your earlobes, in the indentations at the back of the jawbone. Apply light pressure while breathing deeply.

GALLERY OF ACUPRESSURE TECHNIQUES

SPLEEN

SPLEEN 3

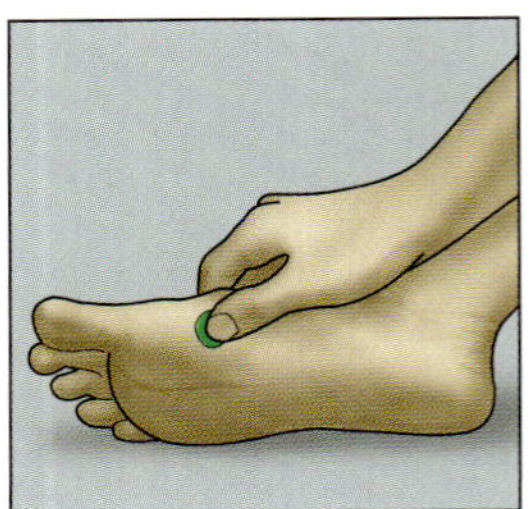

Locate the indentation on the inside of the foot, just behind the bulge made by the large joint of the big toe. Maintain steady pressure on the point site with your thumb. Repeat on the other foot.

SPLEEN 4

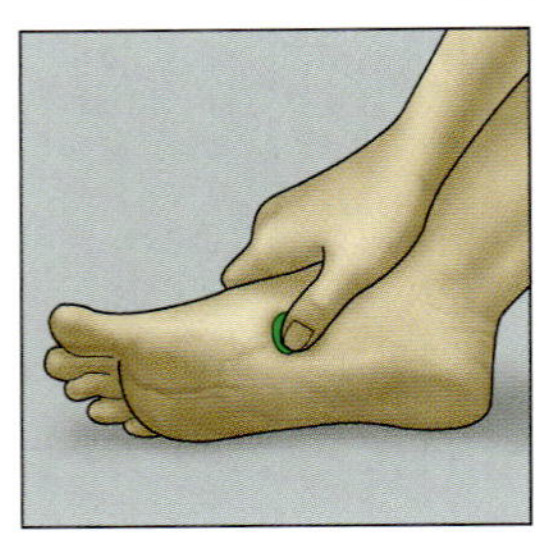

On the inside arch of your foot, measure one thumb width back from the ball of the foot. Apply pressure to this point with your thumb, and then repeat on the other foot.

SPLEEN 6

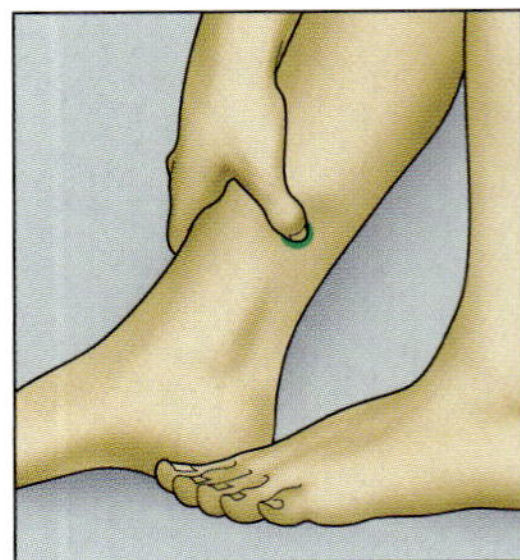

Measure four finger widths up from the top of the right inside anklebone. With your thumb, press near the edge of the shinbone. Repeat on the other leg. (Do not use this point if you are pregnant.)

SPLEEN 8

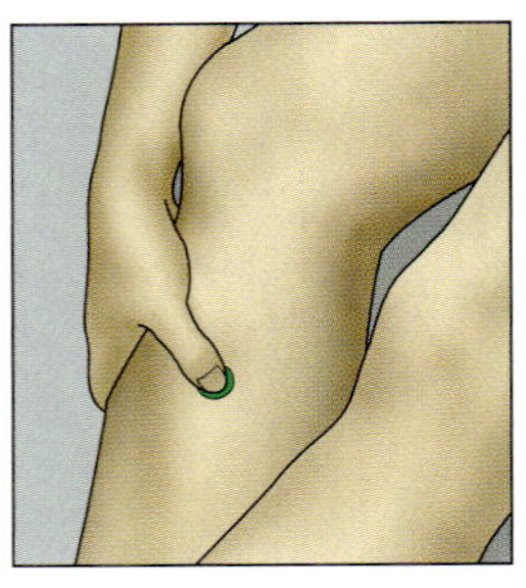

On the inside of the lower leg, locate the depression four finger widths below the knee on the inside of your leg. Press firmly between your calf muscle and your leg bone.

SPLEEN 9

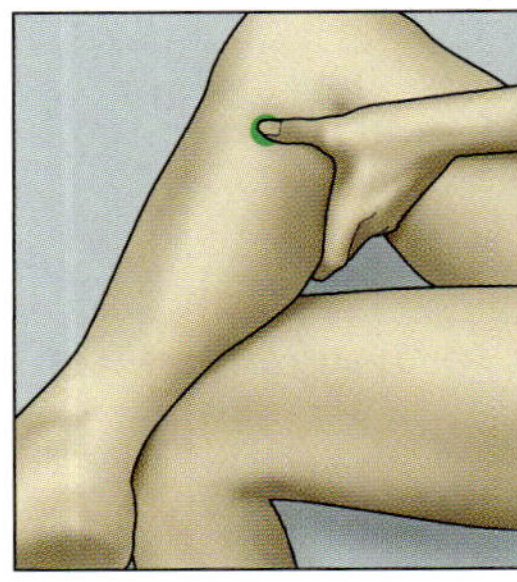

Place your thumb in the depression between the tibia and calf muscle on the inside of your leg, just below the knee joint. Press under the large bulge of the bone.

SPLEEN 10

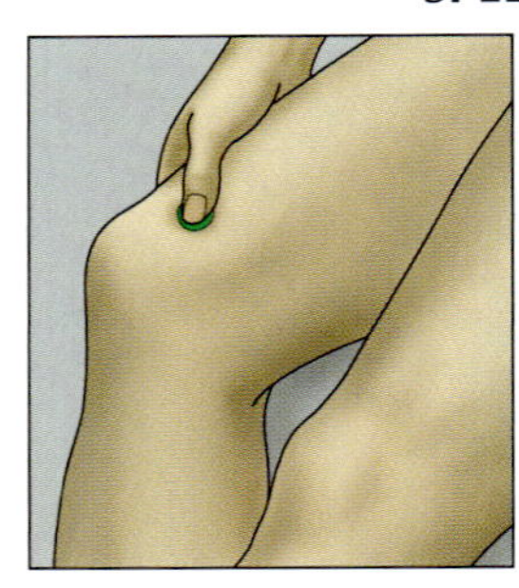

Bend your knee slightly to find this point, located two thumb widths up from the top of your knee, in line with the inner edge of the kneecap. Press on the bulge of the muscle with your thumb.

SPLEEN 12

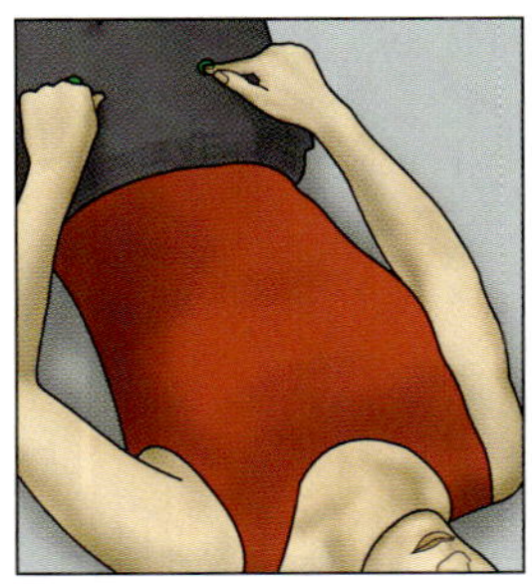

In the pelvic area, use your fingertips to press the middle of the crease where the leg joins the trunk of the body.

STOMACH

STOMACH 2

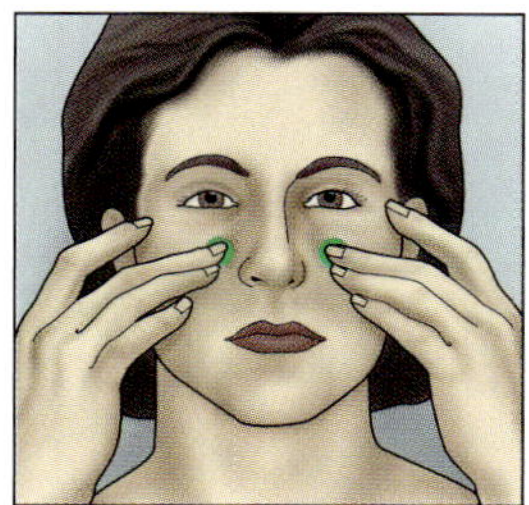

Measure one finger width below the lower ridge of the eye sockets, in line with the pupils. Press into the indentation of the cheeks.

STOMACH 3

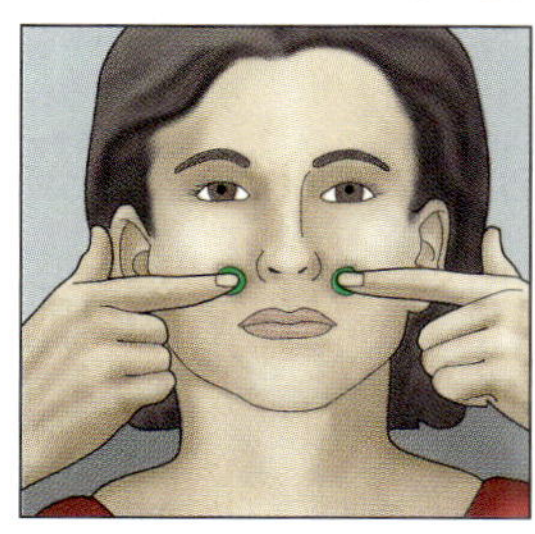

Place your index fingers at the bottom of your cheekbones, directly under the pupils of your eyes, then press firmly.

STOMACH 7

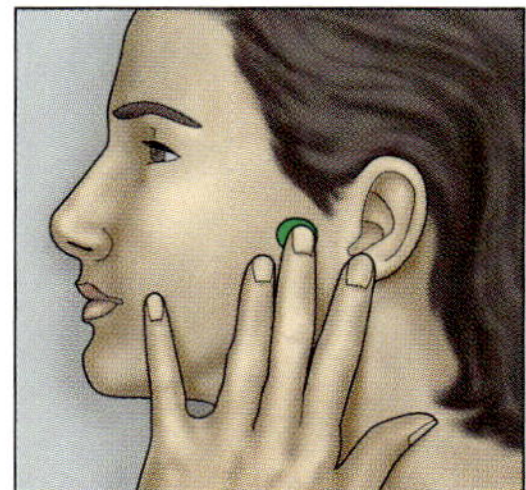

With your middle fingers, feel on either side of your jaw about one thumb width in front of your ears. Apply pressure to the point site in the slight indentation along the upper jawline.

STOMACH 25

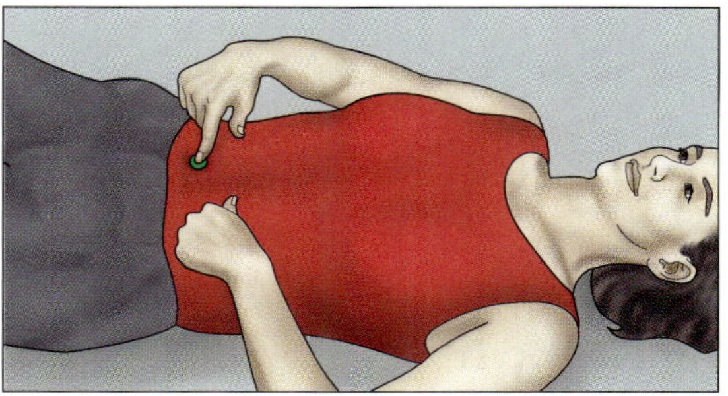

Place the index fingers of both hands two finger widths from your navel on either side. Press down firmly and breathe deeply.

STOMACH 36

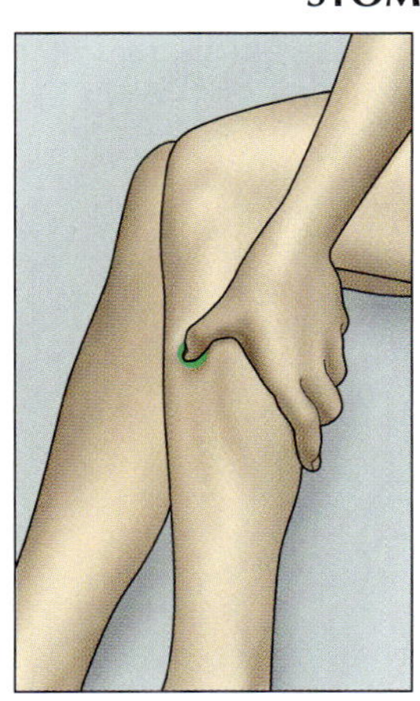

To find this point, measure four finger widths below the kneecap just outside the shinbone. To verify the location, flex ycur foot; you should feel a muscle bulge at the point site. Apply steady pressure with a finger or thumb, then repeat on the other leg.

STOMACH 44

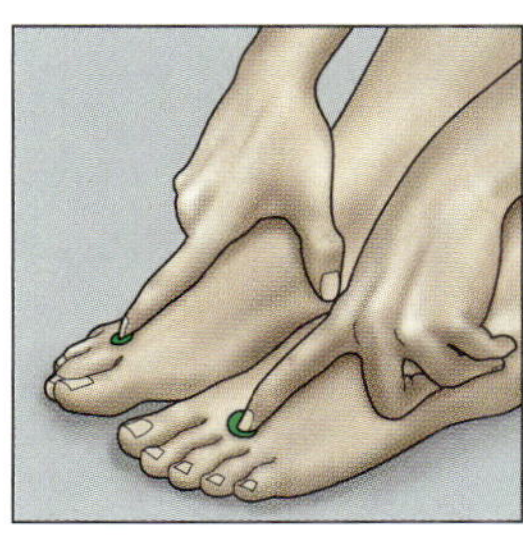

Using your index fingers, press lightly on the webbing between the second and third toes of each foot.

GALLERY OF ACUPRESSURE TECHNIQUES

TRIPLE WARMER

TRIPLE WARMER 3

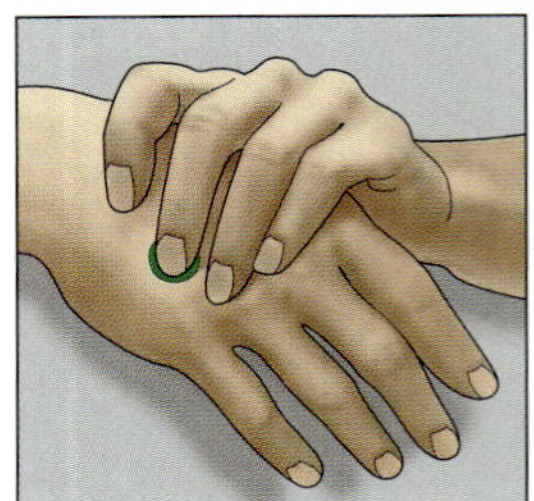

On the back of the hand, press firmly into the furrow just below the fourth and fifth knuckles (between the ring and little fingers). Repeat on the other hand.

TRIPLE WARMER 5

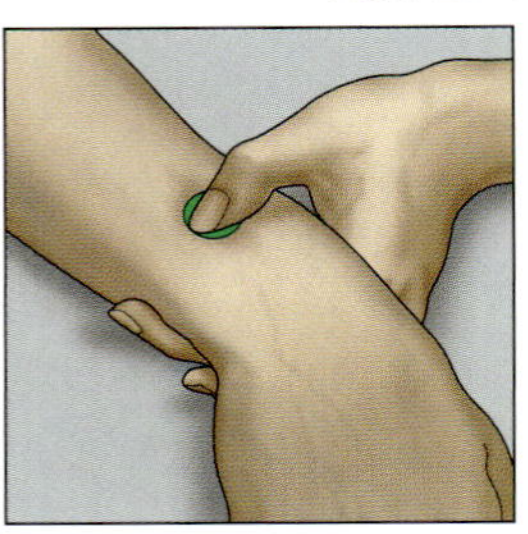

Center your thumb on the top of your forearm, two thumb widths from the wrist joint, and press firmly. Repeat on the other arm.

TRIPLE WARMER 6

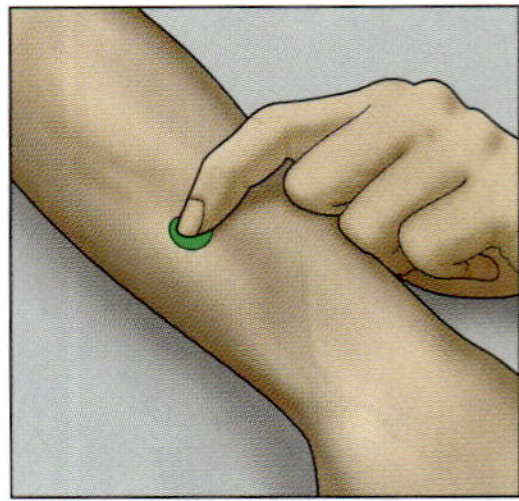

Measure about three finger widths from the wrist on the top of the forearm, then press this point with your thumb or index finger. Repeat on the other arm.

TRIPLE WARMER 17

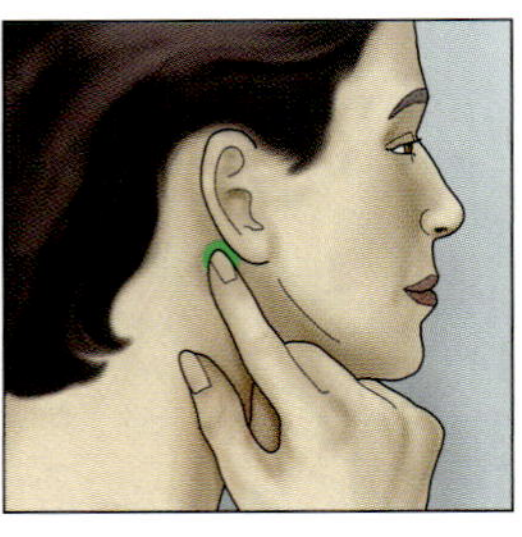

Using the tips of your index or middle fingers, find the hollows behind the earlobes where the ears meet the jawbone. Press lightly and breathe deeply.

MISCELLANEOUS

HICCUP 1

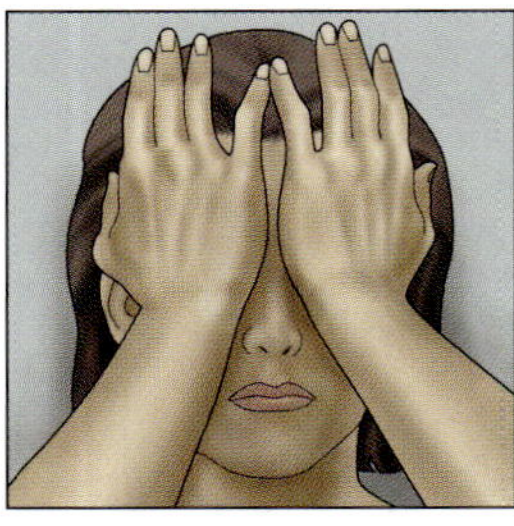

To stop an attack of hiccups, place the palms of your hands over both eyes, with the heels resting on your cheekbones. Gently massage around the eyes by pressing the pads below your thumbs inward toward your palms, then follow the instructions for **Governing Vessel 25.**

GALLERY OF YOGA POSITIONS

Following is an alphabetical directory of most of the yoga positions mentioned in this book. Each illustration shows a position as it should look when fully executed; the accompanying text explains the various steps involved along the way. See individual ailment entries for the recommended time each position should be held.

Done properly, yoga can help you stay fit and may also aid in the treatment of certain medical disorders. Taking a yoga class can help you learn to form the positions correctly. To avoid injury, however, you must keep a few important points in mind: When getting into a position, take slow, deep breaths. Always inhale as you move parts of your body upward and exhale as you move downward. In the Abdominal Massage, for example, exhale as you bend from the hips, then inhale as you raise your torso. Breathing instructions accompany movements that are not up or down. Never strain or force the stretch and always take a moment to breathe deeply before easing out of a position.

YOGA

ABDOMINAL MASSAGE

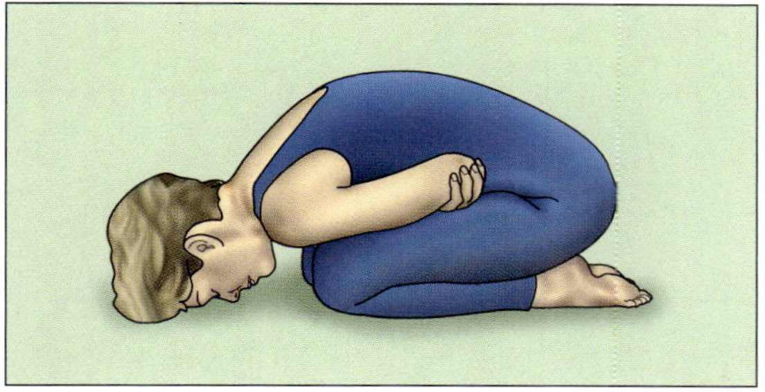

Kneel upright and fold your arms, placing your left fist on the right side of your belly and right hand over your left elbow. Bend at the hips and lower your forehead toward the floor. Hold. Raise your torso slowly, then switch arm positions and repeat.

BOAT

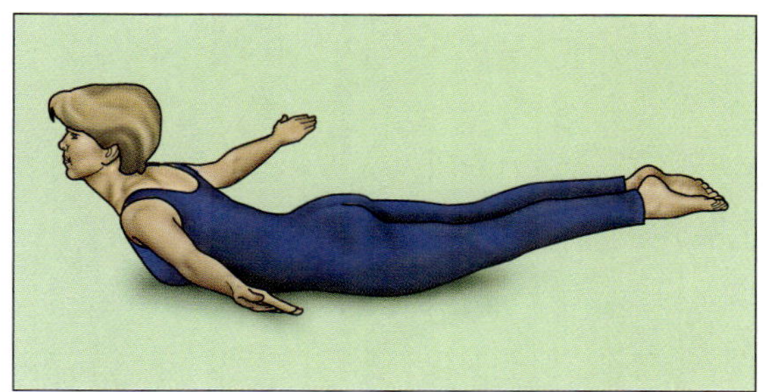

Lie on your stomach with your arms at your sides, palms down. Slightly squeeze your buttocks and lift your head, chest, arms, and legs off the floor. Stretch and hold your arms behind you. Hold. Relax back onto the floor.

BOW

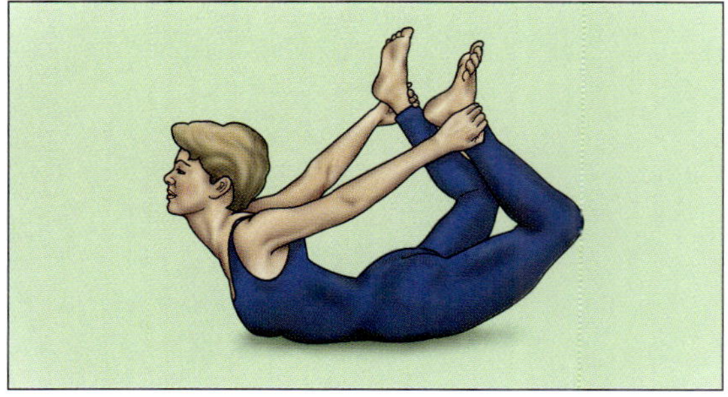

Lie on your stomach and grasp both ankles. While inhaling, slightly squeeze your buttocks and slowly raise your head, chest, and thighs off the floor, pressing your ankles backward. Hold and breathe slowly, then release.

BRIDGE

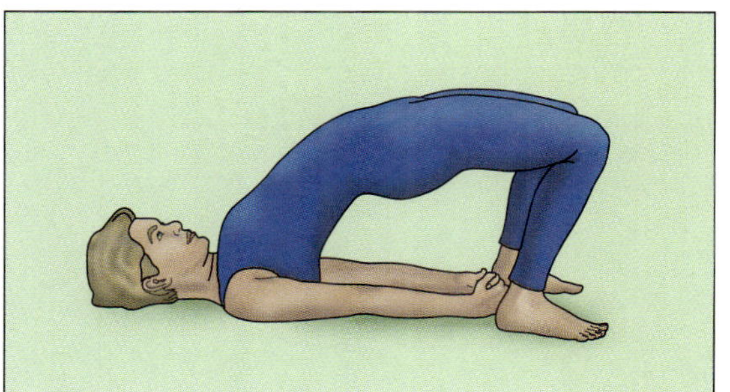

Lie on your back, knees bent, palms on the floor. Tense your buttocks and slowly raise your pelvis. Clasp your hands, arching as you press your shoulders to the floor. Hold this position, then unclasp your hands and slowly lower your pelvis to the floor.

GALLERY OF YOGA POSITIONS

YOGA

C

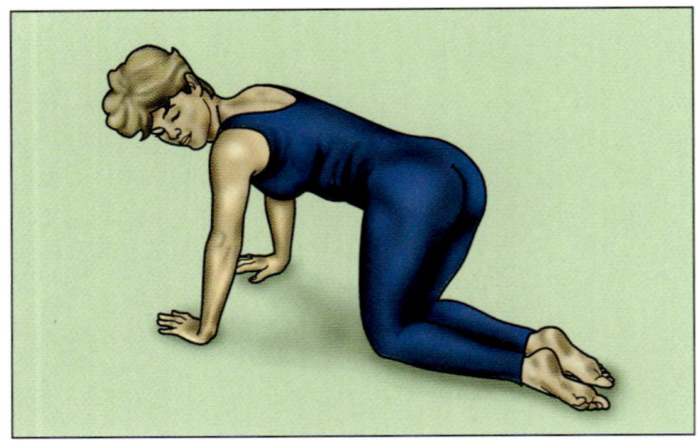

On your hands and knees, exhale and swing your head and buttocks as far to the left as you can. Inhale as you slowly straighten your back, and then do the same movement to the right.

CAMEL

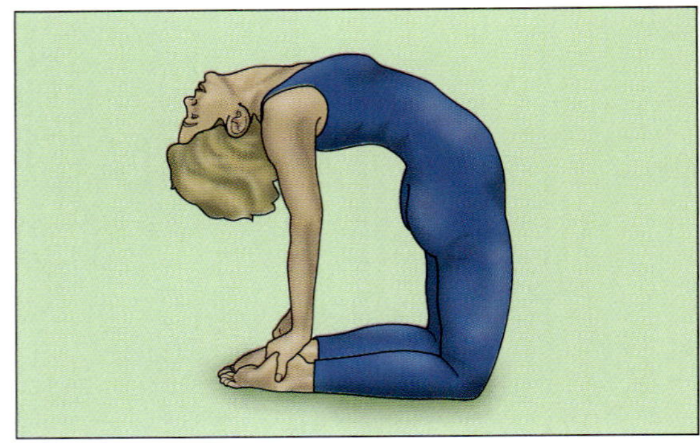

From an upright kneeling position, bend your head backward. Exhale and arch your back, placing your right hand on your right heel, left hand on left heel. Hold. Then slowly straighten up, placing your hands on your lower back and raising your torso, then your head. Breathe evenly. Relax and sit back on your heels.

CAT

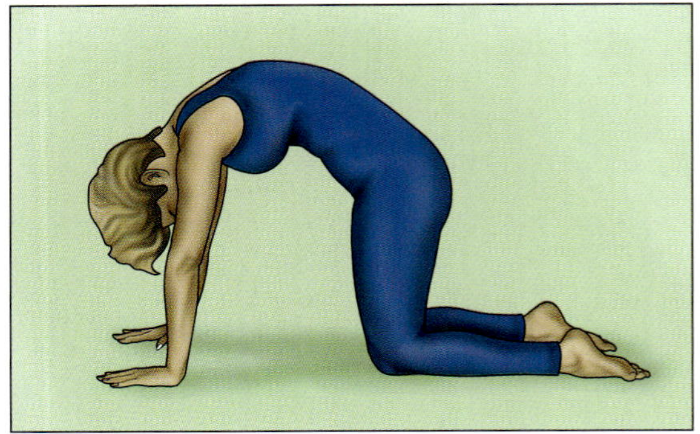

On your hands and knees, exhale as you arch your back, stretching your shoulder, neck, and back muscles. Inhale and bring yourself back to the horizontal.

CHILD

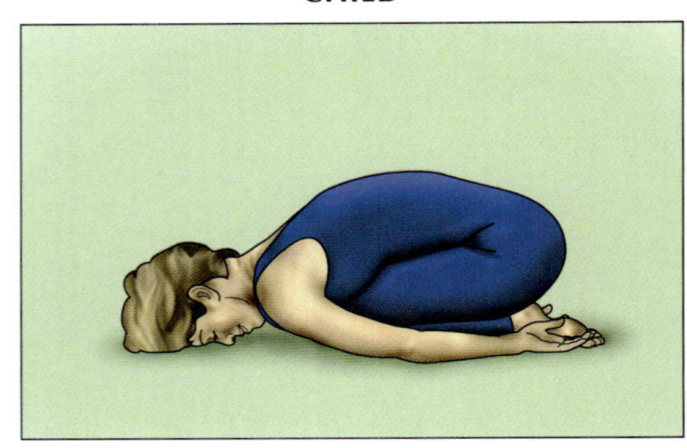

Sit on your heels, knees together. With your arms at your sides, palms up, bend from the hips and extend your upper body over your knees, bringing your forehead toward the floor. Hold. Then slowly sit up.

YOGA

COBRA

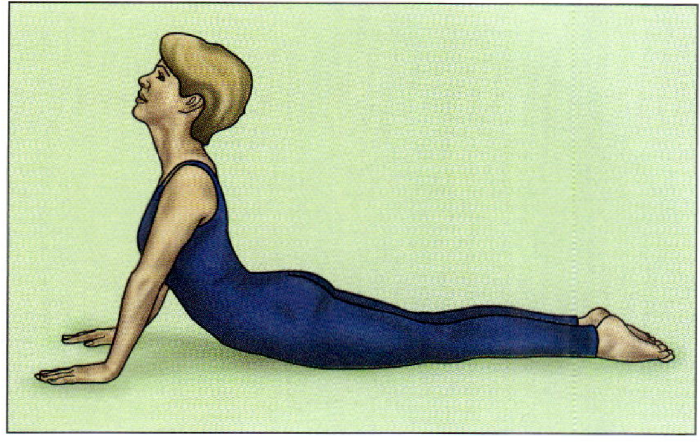

Place both forearms on the floor, hands directly under your shoulders. Press your pelvis and palms against the floor as you slowly straighten your arms and arch your back until your abdomen is off the ground. Hold. Relax and slowly uncurl, lowering your torso back to the floor.

COBRA (HALF)

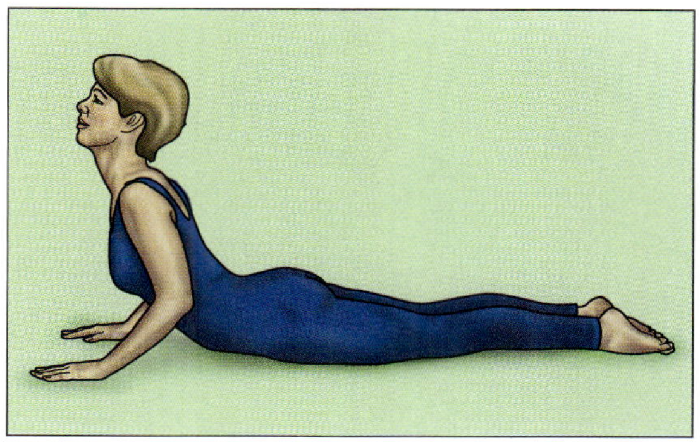

Begin as you would for the Cobra. Press your pelvis and palms against the floor to raise your chest. Keep your arms bent as you arch your back, stopping just before your navel comes off the floor. Hold. Lower your torso to release.

CORPSE

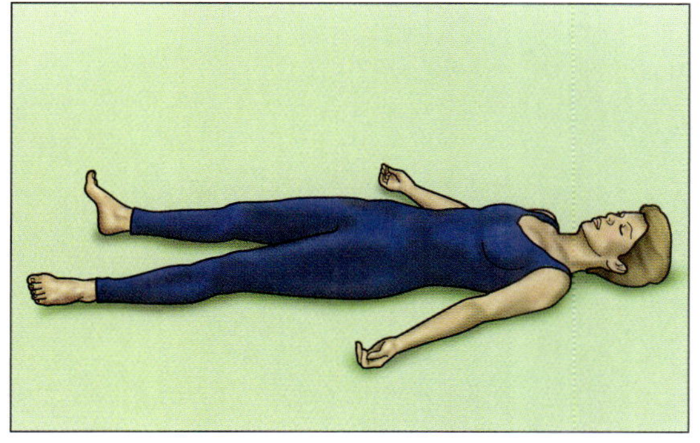

Lie on your back, with your feet about 18 inches apart and turned out slightly. Place your hands about 6 inches from your hips, palms up. Close your eyes and breathe deeply for at least 5 minutes.

DOG

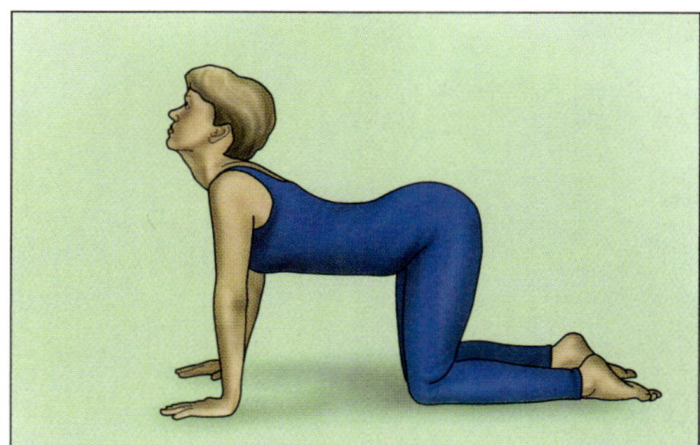

While on your hands and knees, inhale as you dip your back, bringing your head and buttocks up. Exhale as you return your back to the horizontal.

GALLERY OF YOGA POSITIONS

YOGA

HEAD TO KNEE

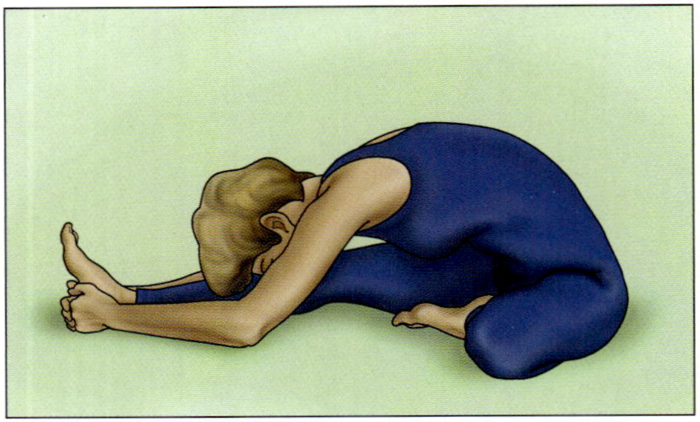

Sit with your right leg out, the sole of your left foot against your right thigh. Raise your arms overhead, then bend forward from the hips and clasp your right foot, ankle, or leg with both hands, pressing your forehead toward your knee. Bend your knee as needed. Hold. Release and repeat on the other side.

HERO

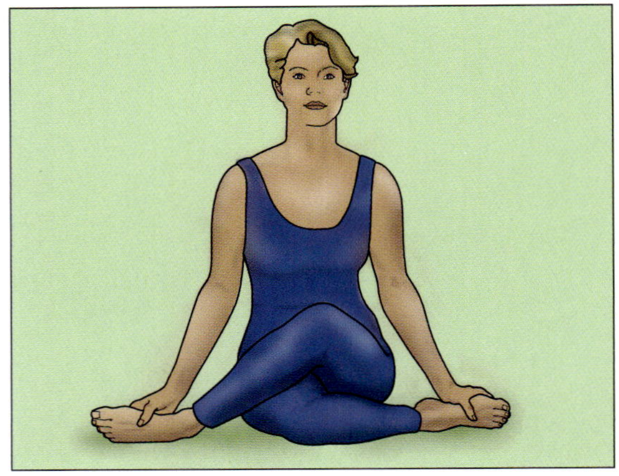

While on hands and knees, cross your left knee in front of your right knee. Keep your knees in place as you sit back between your heels. With your back straight, place your palms on the soles of your feet. Slowly bend forward as far as you can, and hold. Slowly release, and repeat on the other side.

KNEE DOWN TWIST

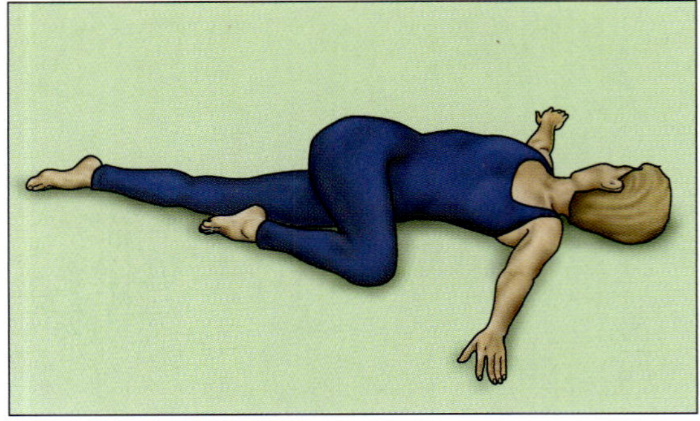

Lie on your back with your arms out. Inhale and place your right foot on your left knee. Exhale, then turn your head to the right and bring your right knee toward the floor to your left. Hold. Release slowly, then repeat on the other side.

LOCUST (FULL)

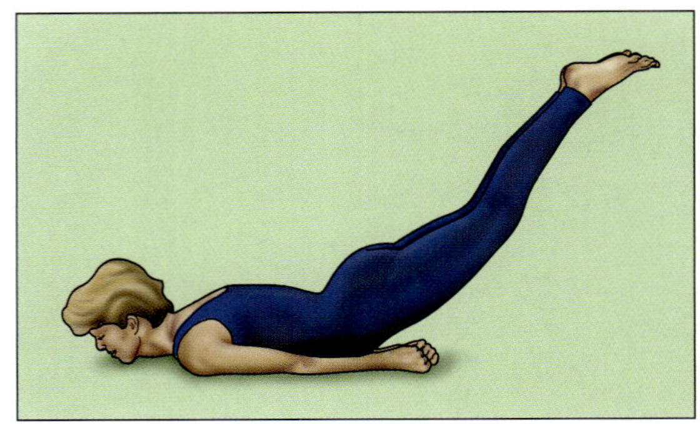

Lie on your stomach, chin to floor, arms under your body. Squeeze your buttocks as you press down with your arms and hands. Raise your legs, keeping them straight as you press outward through the toes and heels. Hold, then release slowly.

YOGA

LOTUS (HALF)

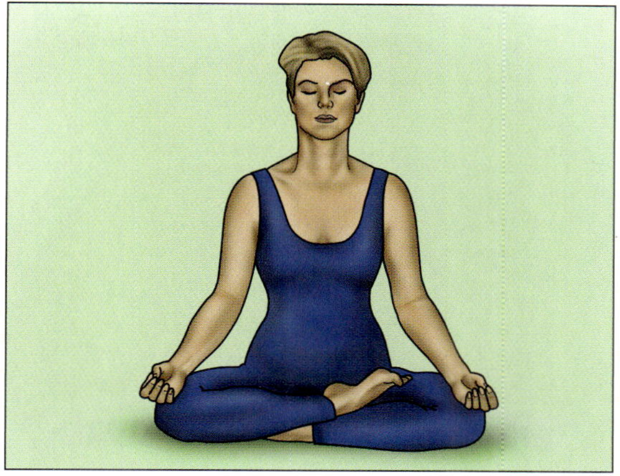

Sit with your legs in a V, spine straight. Bend one leg and bring the foot close to your body. Bend the other leg and place the foot high on the opposite thigh. (For full Lotus, place each foot on the opposite thigh.)

MOUNTAIN

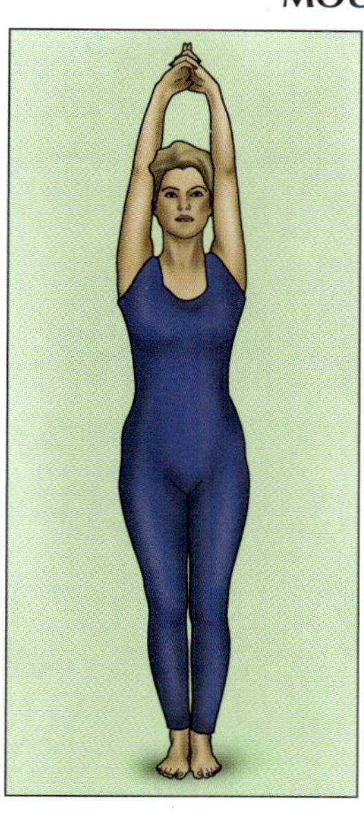

Stand with your feet together. Inhale and raise your arms straight out from your sides, then join them over your head. Keep your legs and back straight and your shoulders relaxed. If you can't bring your hands together comfortably, then hold your arms straight up. Hold. To release, exhale and slowly lower your arms.

PIGEON

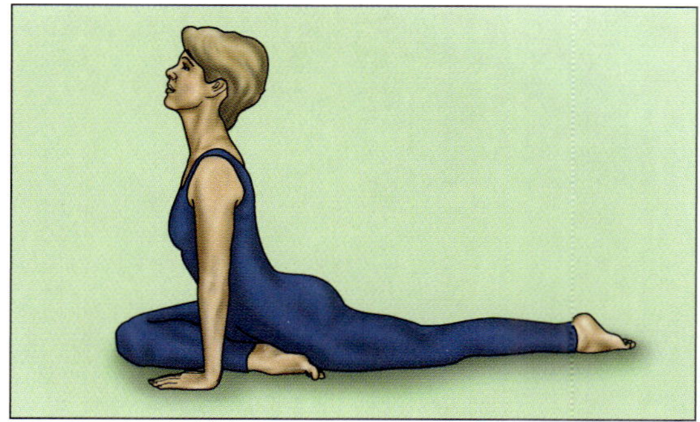

From a kneeling position, slide your left leg straight behind you and place your right knee between your hands. Inhale and stretch up through your torso while arching your back slightly. Release, then repeat on the other side.

PLOW

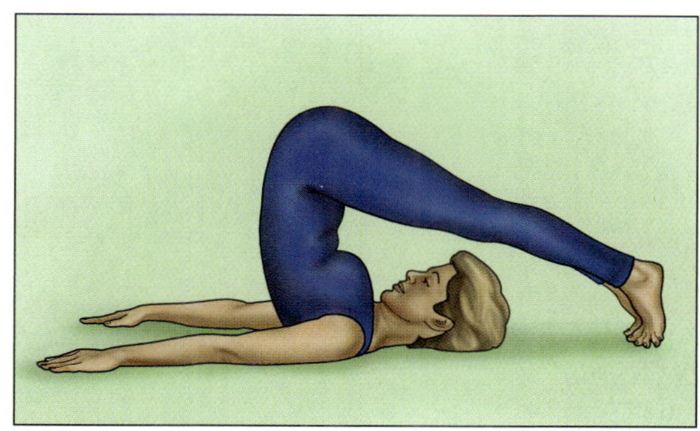

While on your back, inhale and raise both legs, using your hands to support your hips. Exhale as you try to touch the floor behind you with your toes. Stretch your arms on the floor. Hold. To release, place your hands back on your hips, slowly raise your legs up, and then lower your torso and legs back to the floor.

GALLERY OF YOGA POSITIONS

YOGA

POSTERIOR STRETCH

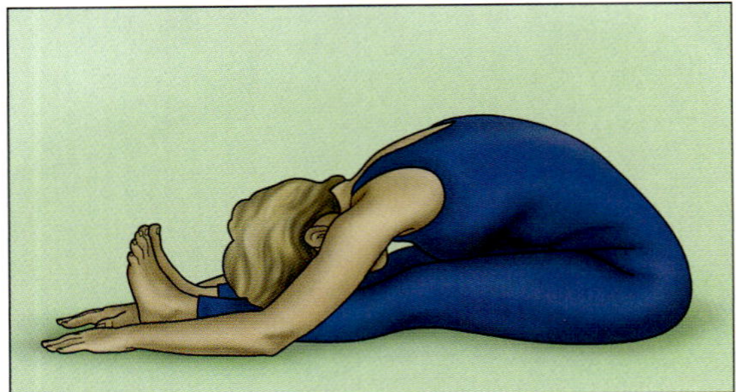

Sit with legs extended and feet together. Raise your arms overhead, then bend forward from the hips and place your hands on your feet, ankles, lower legs, or on the floor beside your feet. Move your head as close to your toes as possible. Hold. Slowly raise your torso as you inhale.

SEATED ANGLE

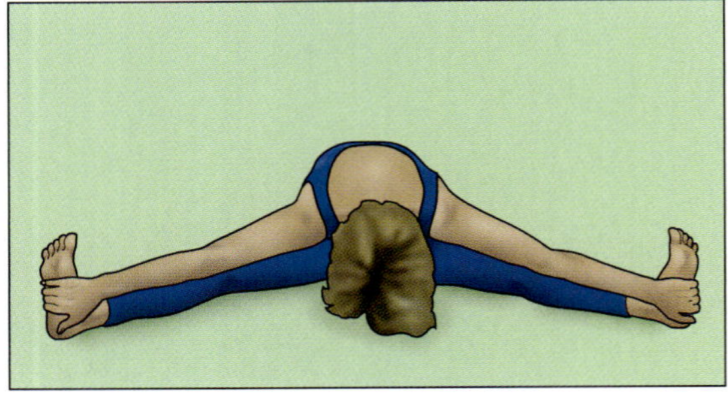

Sit with your legs in a V. Raise your arms over your head. Bending from the hips, extend your arms and grab your legs or feet. Move your head toward the floor. Hold. Release by lifting your arms back over your head, then slowly raise your torso.

RAG DOLL

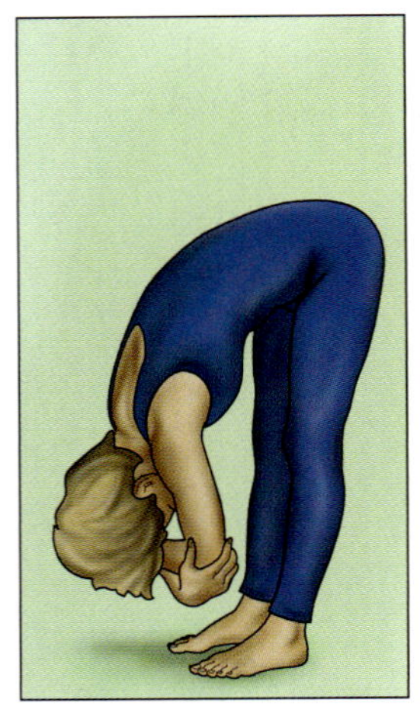

Standing with arms at your sides, exhale and bend forward from the hips, letting the top of your head drop toward the floor. Cup your elbows in your palms and breathe deeply. Relax and hold. Slowly stand up, bringing your head up last.

SHOULDER CRUNCH

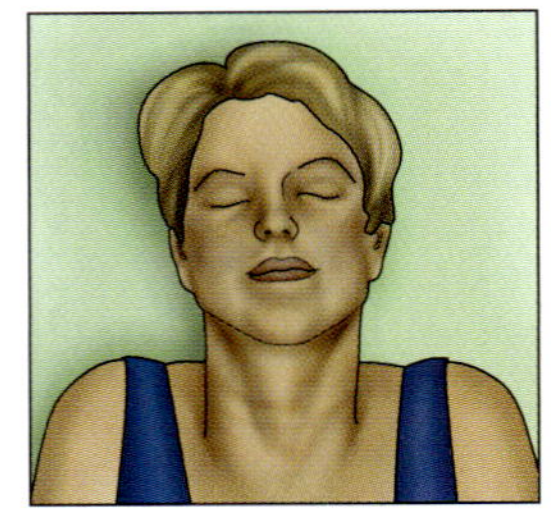

Straighten your back and relax your neck. Slowly lift your right shoulder, then lower it. Repeat with your left shoulder. Lift both shoulders together and slowly bring them down as you exhale.

SHOULDER STAND

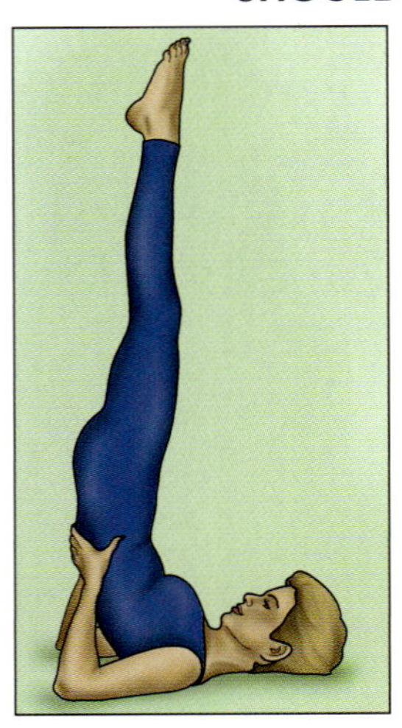

Lie on your back, hands at your sides, and lift both legs until they are at a right angle to your back. Supporting your hips with your hands, push your back and legs upward until they are vertical. Hold. Slowly lower your legs to release.

YOGA

SHOULDER STAND (HALF)

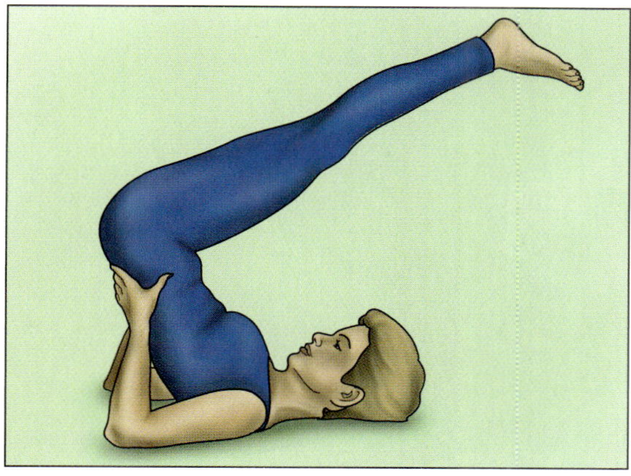

Lie on your back, hands at your sides, and lift both legs until they are at a right angle to your back. Supporting your hips with your hands, inhale and extend your legs, maintaining the same angle. Breathe deeply and hold. Lower your legs to release.

SPINAL

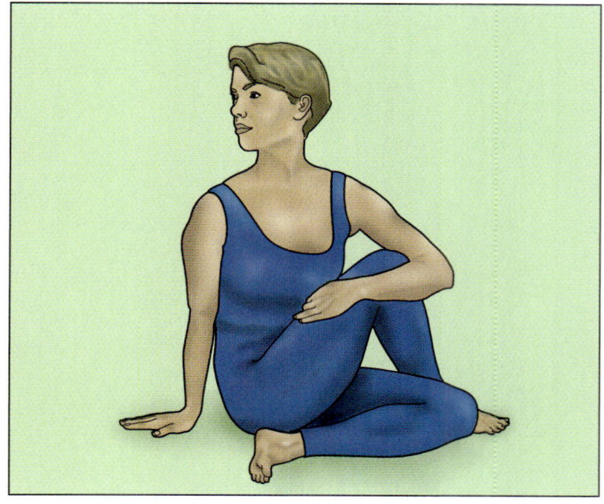

While sitting, place your right foot outside the left knee. Grasp your right knee with your left arm and place your right hand on the floor behind you. Inhale, then exhale as you twist your torso slowly as far as you can to the right. Hold. Release by lifting your right arm and untwisting your torso. Repeat on the other side.

SPHINX

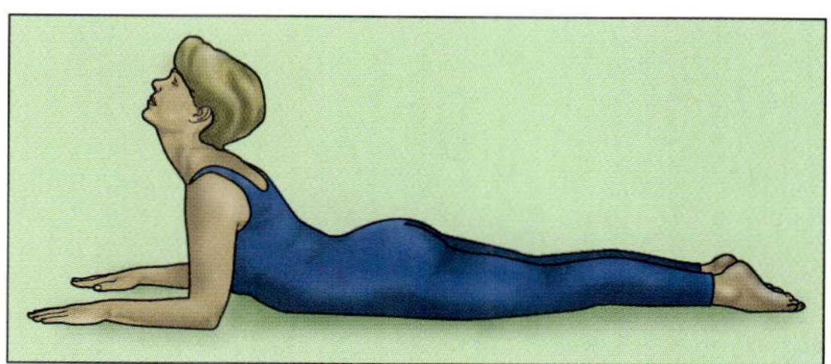

Lie on your stomach and place both forearms on the floor, palms down and elbows directly under your shoulders. Push your chest away from the floor as far as comfortably possible and look upward slightly. Hold. Lower your torso to release.

SPIDER

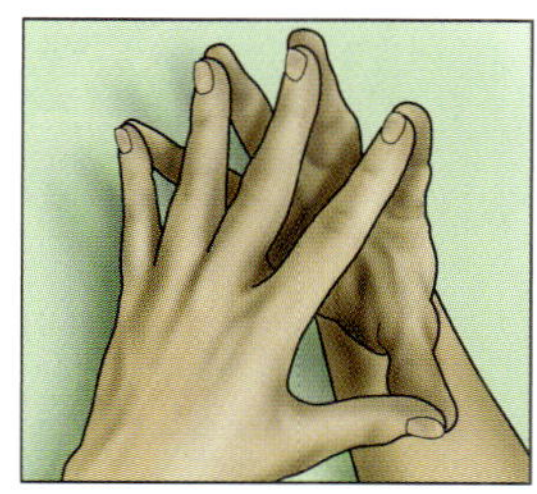

1. Press your fingertips together firmly, holding your palms two to three inches apart.

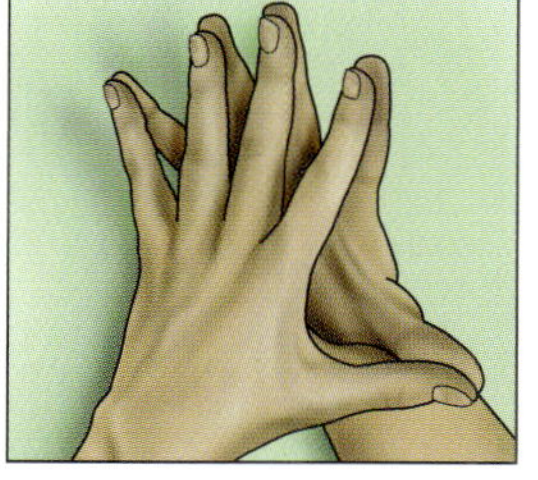

2. Keep your fingertips together while pushing your palms toward each other, then release back to the first position. Repeat the push-up motion quickly 20 to 25 times.

GALLERY OF YOGA POSITIONS

YOGA

STANDING ANGLE

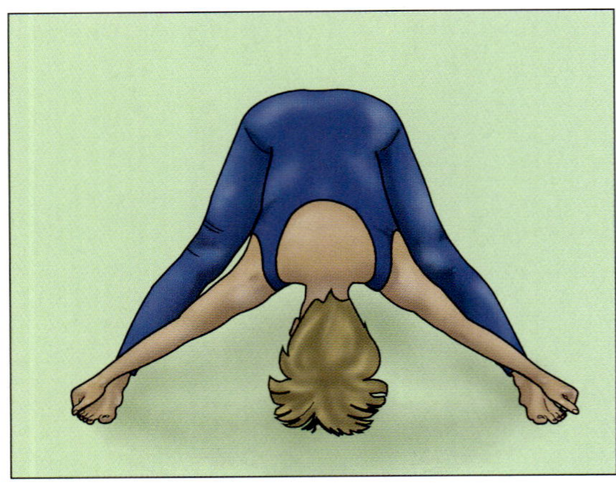

Inhale and step wide to your right with arms outstretched. Exhaling, bend forward at the hips and grasp your feet, ankles, or legs, moving the top of your head toward the floor. Hold. Rise slowly, keeping your back straight.

STANDING YOGA MUDRA

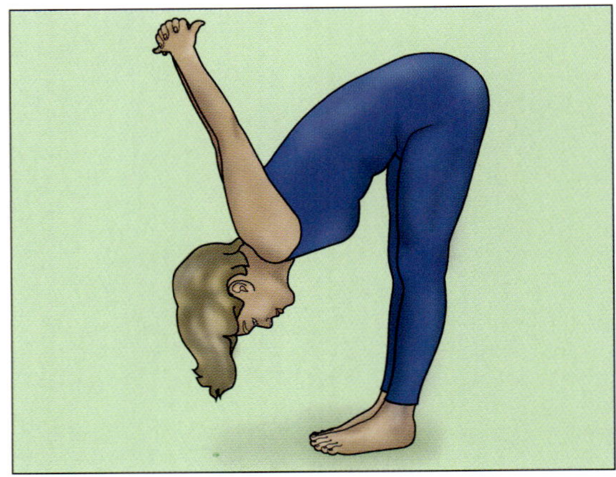

Stand with your arms at your sides. Inhale, raise your arms in front of you, then exhale and sweep them behind your back, squeezing the shoulder blades. Interlace your fingers and bend forward as you lift your arms and drop your head down. Hold for 20 seconds, then inhale and raise your torso and drop your arms to release.

TREE

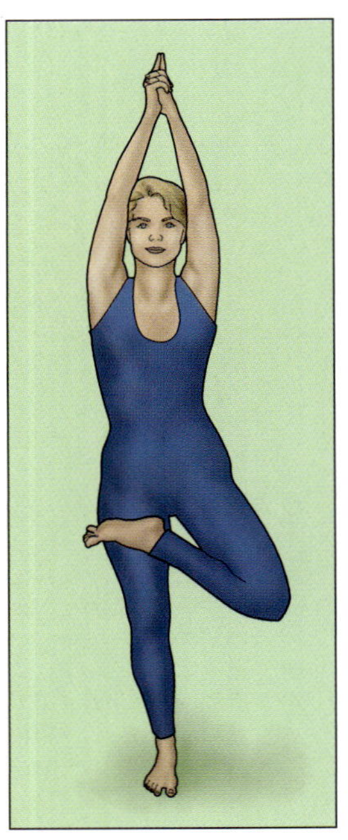

Stand with your feet hip-width apart. Balance on your left foot and use your hands to lift your right foot to the top of the left thigh. If balancing is difficult, place your right foot lower on your left thigh or on your calf instead. Place your palms together at heart level and raise your hands overhead; point the index fingers and interlace the others. Press your bent knee down and back without tilting your pelvis. Bring your hands back down to heart level; lower your leg and arms. Repeat on the other side.

TRIANGLE

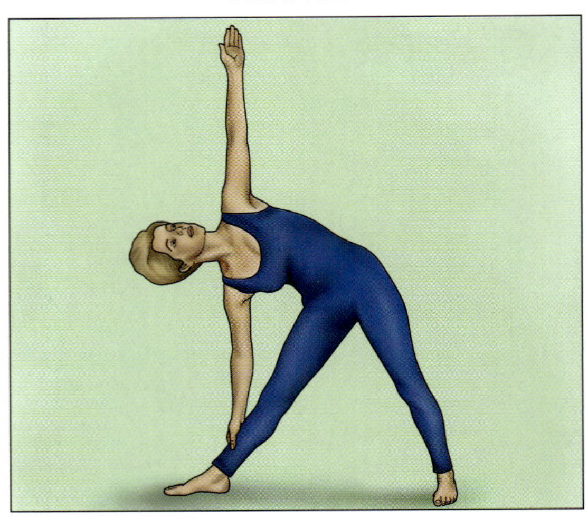

With arms parallel to the floor and feet apart, turn your right toes out and left toes forward. Bend to the right, moving your left arm up and right arm to the right leg. Look up at your raised palm; if you have neck pain or injury, look down. Hold. Return to the starting position and repeat on the other side.

YOGA

UPWARD DOG

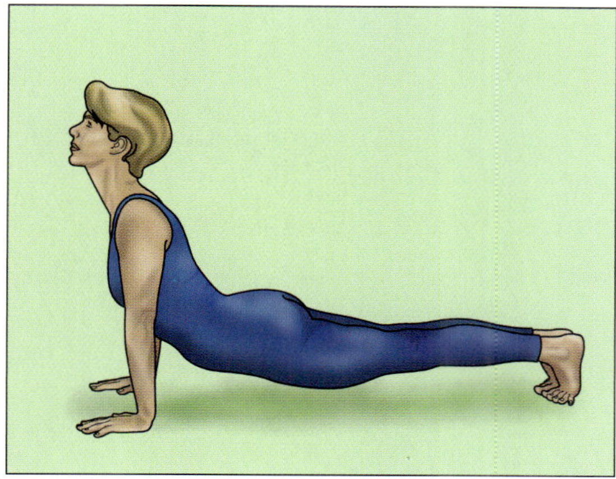

Lie facedown, palms at chest level and elbows close to the body. Spread your fingers, keeping the index fingers forward. Pressing your hands and toes into the floor, lift your torso, hips, and knees off the floor, arching your back slightly. Hold. Return to starting position.

WARRIOR 1

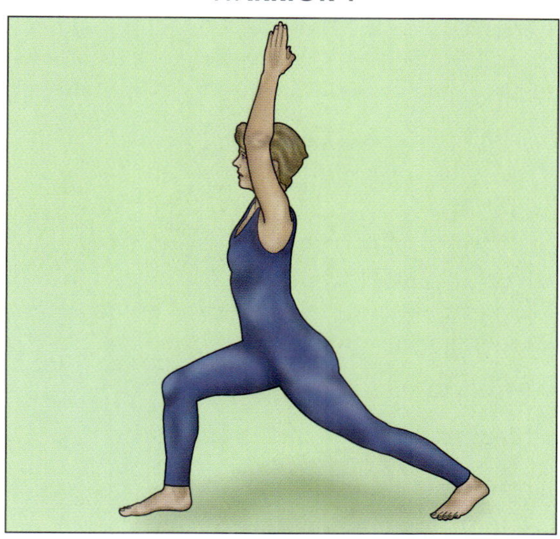

Stand with your feet hip-width apart. Raise your arms overhead, palms together. Lunge forward with your right foot, keeping the knee directly above the ankle. Press your left heel down and left hip forward. Arch your back slightly. Hold. Step forward and lower your arms to come out. Repeat on the other side.

WARRIOR 2

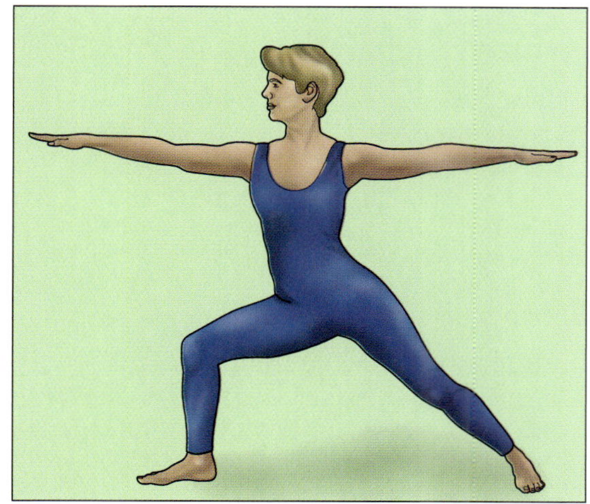

With arms parallel to the floor and feet apart, turn your right toes out and left toes forward. Bend your right knee and bring it above your right ankle, keeping hips forward. Look over your right hand. Hold. Return to the starting position, then repeat on the opposite side.

YOGA MUDRA

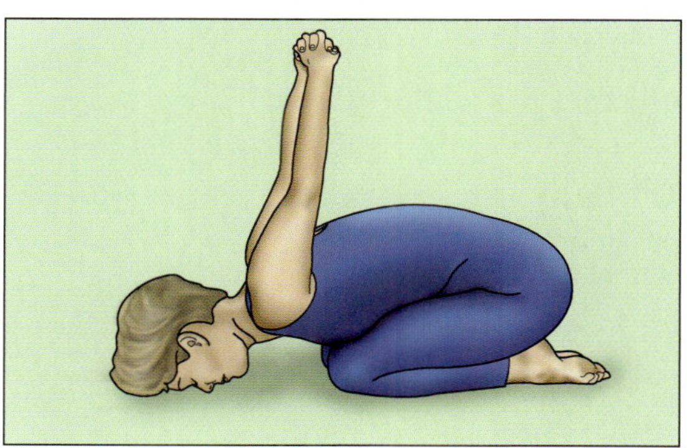

Sit on your heels, knees together, then follow the arm motion and stretch for Standing Yoga Mudra. Move the top of your forehead to the floor and stretch your arms overhead. Breathe deeply and move the front of your forehead to the floor. Hold. Exhale, bringing your arms back down. Inhale and slowly raise your torso.

GLOSSARY

This glossary is intended as a general reference to terms that are used frequently throughout the volume. For other definitions, see the Dictionary of Conventional Medicine and Alternative Therapies, and the Index of Conventional and Natural Medicines. Cross references to other glossary entries are indicated by bold italic type.

A

Acute: sudden, brief, and severe; not ***chronic.***

Adrenal gland: a small gland located just above each kidney that produces ***epinephrine, norepinephrine,*** and ***steroid*** hormones.

Adrenaline: see ***Epinephrine.***

Allergen: any substance, even apparently harmless ones such as pollen, dust, or certain foods and medications, that can trigger an inappropriate immune response, or allergy, in susceptible people. See also ***Antigen.***

Amino acid: a class of organic chemical compounds that combine to build proteins; 20 basic amino acids in various combinations make up all the proteins in the human body.

Anesthetic: an agent that produces anesthesia, or insensibility to pain.

Angiogram: an x-ray of blood vessels or lymphatic vessels after the injection of a radiopaque substance (one through which x-rays cannot pass), which shows up white on an x-ray.

Antibody: any of numerous proteins produced by the human immune system that defend against invading ***antigens.***

Antigen: any substance able to provoke an immune response in the human body.

Antioxidant: a compound, such as vitamin E, that is able to counteract the damage done by oxidation in cells or tissue. See also ***Free radical.***

Artery: a vessel that carries blood away from the heart to other tissues in the body.

Astringent: any substance or agent that causes tissues to contract or that inhibits secretion of fluids such as mucus or blood.

Autoimmune disorder: a disease that results when the immune system attacks the body's own tissues, as in rheumatoid arthritis.

B

Bacteria: one-celled organisms, some of which are capable of causing infection.

Benign: not ***malignant;*** not life-threatening.

Biopsy: removal of a sample of tissue from the body for the purpose of diagnostic study.

C

Calcification: abnormal deposition of calcium and magnesium salts in tissue.

Capillary: the smallest type of blood vessel; some are just big enough for blood cells to pass through only one at a time.

Carbohydrate: any of various organic compounds, including sugars and starches, that contain carbon and hydrogen and that constitute an important class of food for humans.

Carcinogen: any agent that causes cancer.

Carotenoid: any of the group of red and yellow pigments in plants that are thought to protect against cancer; one type of carotenoid is converted to vitamin A in the body.

Cartilage: dense, pliable connective tissue found in the joints, nose, and ears, and at the ends of some bones.

Catheterization: the insertion of a hollow tube into a body cavity or passage to drain off or inject fluids, or for the purpose of examination.

Chemotherapy: treatment of disease by the use of chemical agents; usually refers to drugs used in treating cancer.

Cholesterol: a fatty substance produced by the human liver and present in foods of animal origin; high levels of cholesterol in the blood are associated with increased risk of heart disease.

Cholinergic: resembling acetylcholine in action. Acetylcholine is a ***neurotransmitter*** that inhibits heart rate and stimulates the release of certain hormones.

Chromosome: a structure in a cell nucleus that consists of genes. In humans, 23 pairs of chromosomes, each pair containing one chromosome from each parent, carry the entire genetic code.

Chronic: of long duration; recurring; not ***acute.***

Collagen: fibrous protein in connective tissue.

Compress: a cloth covering used to apply pressure to a wound or body part, or to supply heat, cold, moisture, or other treatment.

Computed tomography (CT): also called computerized axial tomography (CAT); a scanning method that uses computerized x-ray images to provide a three-dimensional picture of an internal part of the body.

Congenital: existing at birth.

Contraception: birth control; deliberate prevention of the conception of offspring by any of various means.

Cortisone: a ***steroid*** hormone that is used to treat many autoimmune or inflammatory diseases, including rheumatoid arthritis.

CT scan: see ***Computed tomography.***

Cyst: a closed sac that forms in tissue or a body cavity.

D

Decoction: an extract obtained by boiling.

Dehydration: loss of water from the body.

Diaphragm: the muscular partition between the abdominal cavity and the chest cavity; a birth-control device inserted in the vagina to prevent contact between sperm and egg.

Dilate: to widen, stretch, or expand.

Disease: malfunctioning of the body or any part of the body resulting from any number of influences, including genetic errors, toxins, ***infections,*** nutritional deficiencies, and environmental factors.

DNA: deoxyribonucleic acid, the basic genetic material in humans.

Dopamine: a ***neurotransmitter*** involved in muscle activation.

Drug class: a group of pharmacological agents that are chemically related, similar in action, or both. Drugs within a class generally behave the same way, generate the same kinds of side effects, and interact with other drugs similarly.

E

Electrocardiogram (ECG or EKG): a graphic record of electrical activity within the heart; typically used to diagnose various heart conditions or to confirm a diagnosis of heart attack.

Electroencephalogram (EEG): a graphic record made by an instrument that measures the electrical activity of the brain and records it as patterns of fluctuating waves.

Electrolyte: sodium, potassium, magnesium, or chloride, all of which can conduct electrical impulses. Electrolytes also play an essential role in controlling the ***pH*** balance of body fluids.

Electromyogram (EMG): a graphic record of electrical activity associated with muscle function.

Enzyme: any of numerous proteins, produced by living cells, that serve as catalysts for specific functions in the body, such as digestion.

Epiglottis: a small flap of cartilage that covers the windpipe behind the tongue; ***inflammation*** of the epiglottis is known as epiglottitis, a rare but serious condition whose symptoms can resemble those of tonsillitis or pharyngitis.

Epinephrine: a stress-related hormone produced in the ***adrenal glands*** that increases heart rate, carbohydrate metabolism, and blood pressure; also known as adrenaline.

Ergonomics: also called human engineering, an applied science concerned with working conditions and equipment designed for comfort and safety.

Estrogen: a hormone found in greater quantities in females, in whom it is responsible for the development of the breasts and other female sexual characteristics as well as the maturation of eggs; synthetic forms of estrogen are used in some cancer treatments and other therapies.

Extract: a solution that contains the essential or active constituents of a plant material or other substance.

F

Fast: to abstain from all or some foods.

Fat: any of several organic substances that make up most of the fatty tissue of plants and animals; a major class of food. See also ***Fatty acid*** and ***Triglyceride.***

Fatty acid: one of the substances that make up fats. Fatty acids are either saturated, monounsaturated, or polyunsaturated.

Fiber: the wholly or partially indigestible structural part of plants; indigestible fiber speeds the passage of food through the intestines.

Flavonoid: any of a group of plant pigments found in many foods that are thought to help protect the body from disease.

Fomentation: an herbal preparation or water applied warm to a wound or affected area, often using a piece of soft cloth or linen.

Free radical: an atom or molecule produced as a by-product of oxidation (the cellular process of "burning" fuel) that bears an unpaired electron and is potentially harmful to the body. Free radicals are neutralized in the body by ***antioxidants.***

Fungus: any of a group of parasitic lower organisms, including molds and yeasts, that can infect tissues in the human body.

G

Gene: the basic unit of heredity; a length of ***DNA*** that provides the coded instructions for the production of a specific protein.

Generic drug: a medication sold without an indicated brand name and not protected by trademark.

Gland: an organ that produces a hormone or other secretion.

H

Hemoglobin: the iron-containing pigment in red blood cells that transports oxygen from the lungs to the body's tissues.

Herb: in general, a plant or part of a plant that is used for medical treatment, flavoring, or other purposes.

High-density lipoprotein (HDL): a component of blood that is involved in cholesterol transport and that is associated with a lowered risk of developing atherosclerosis; the so-called good cholesterol.

Histamine: a chemical released in the body during an allergic reaction, causing ***inflammation;*** also used in medical treatment, especially to dilate capillaries.

Hormone: one of a large class of chemicals that are secreted by ***glands*** and some organs. Hormones travel throughout the body and regulate the activities of systems, tissues, organs, and glands. They play an important role in regulating functions such as growth, reproduction, digestion, and fighting ***infection.***

Hyper-: a prefix usually meaning excess.

Hypo-: as opposed to hyper-, a prefix usually meaning deficient.

I

Immunization: the creation of an immunity, especially through use of a vaccine.

Incubation: the time between ***infection***

by a ***pathogen*** and the appearance of disease symptoms.

Infection: invasion of the body by agents that cause disease or tissue damage.

Inflammation: a by-product of the immune response, a reaction of tissue to injury or ***infection,*** characterized by redness, pain, swelling, heat, and sometimes impaired function.

Infusion: an extract, as of a plant, made by soaking or steeping, usually in water; sometimes referred to as a tea.

Insulin: a hormone involved in the metabolism of carbohydrates and used in the treatment of diabetes.

Intravenous (IV): within or administered by injection into a vein.

L

Ligament: a fibrous band of tissue that connects the ends of bones or holds organs in place.

Lipoprotein: see ***High-density lipoprotein; Low-density lipoprotein; Very-low-density lipoprotein.***

Low-density lipoprotein (LDL): a component of blood that carries cholesterol and is associated with an increased risk of atherosclerosis; the so-called bad cholesterol.

Lumbar puncture: a puncture made through a protective membrane of the spinal cord in order to withdraw cerebrospinal fluid for diagnostic examination; also used to inject dye or to administer medication.

M

Magnetic resonance imaging (MRI): a noninvasive diagnostic procedure using radio waves and magnetic fields to provide a highly detailed map of an interior structure of the body, such as the brain.

Malignant: tending to become worse; harmful; of a tumor, cancerous.

Mammography: x-ray examination of a breast, usually for the detection of tumors.

Megadose: a dose much larger than the usual amount, as of a vitamin.

Metabolism: the physical and chemical processes of an organism that are necessary to maintain life.

Metastasis: the spread of cancer cells from one site to other parts of the body.

Midbrain: the uppermost of the three segments of the brainstem, primarily serving as an intermediary between the rest of the brain and the spinal cord.

Mineral: in nutrition, any of various inorganic elements or compounds, such as iron or calcium, that are essential to the human body; along with ***vitamins,*** known as micronutrients.

Mucus: a slippery, viscous secretion of mucous membranes that protects and moistens their surfaces.

Mutation: a change in the genetic code of an organism.

N

Neurological: concerning the nervous system.

Neurotransmitter: any of various substances that transmit impulses across the gap from a neuron to another neuron, or through the blood stream.

Norepinephrine: also called noradrenaline, a ***neurotransmitter;*** an adrenal hormone that constricts blood vessels and raises blood pressure.

O

Omega-3 fatty acid: a polyunsaturated ***fatty acid*** found in fish and plants that may help lower cholesterol and ***triglyceride*** levels in the blood.

Over-the-counter (OTC) drug: any medication legally sold without being prescribed by a doctor.

P

Parasite: an organism, such as a tapeworm, that lives on or in a host organism of another kind and derives benefit from the host's body.

Pathogen: any disease-causing agent, such as a virus or bacterium.

pH: a measure of the acidity or alkalinity of a substance using a scale from 0 (most acidic) to 14 (most alkaline), with 7 indicating neutrality.

Photosensitivity: oversensitivity of the skin to sunlight or other radiant energy, sometimes following exposure to sensitizing chemicals or drugs, resulting in accelerated burning of the skin by ultraviolet (UV) light; possible effects range from itching and swelling to skin cancer.

Pituitary gland: a structure in the brain that controls most of the other glands in the body and that influences most basic functions through the release of ***hormones.***

Plaque: an abnormal patch on the skin or other organ or tissue, often occurring on the arterial linings in atherosclerosis.

Platelet: a cell fragment in the blood that is essential in blood clotting.

Polyp: an abnormal tissue growth arising from a mucous membrane.

Positron emission tomography (PET): a noninvasive diagnostic technique that traces emissions from an injected radioactive substance to generate images of activity at specific brain receptors.

Poultice: a mass of crushed herbs that is applied, often warm and moist, directly to an affected area.

Progesterone: a hormone involved in the preparation for and maintenance of pregnancy; progesterone is also used to treat some gynecological conditions.

Progestin: any chemical agent that acts like progesterone.

Protein: any of numerous complex molecules made of ***amino acids.*** Proteins are the fundamental components of the body and are essential to all biological processes.

Psychoactive: of a drug or other substance, having significant effects on the brain.

Psychosomatic: involving both mind and body; of physical symptoms, caused by emotional or mental factors.

R

Recommended dietary allowance (RDA): in the United States, the amount of an essential nutrient that is recommended on a daily basis to maintain health in various age groups and categories, as determined by a board of nutrition experts; used in labeling of foods.

Red blood cell: a ***hemoglobin***-containing blood cell that carries oxygen from the lungs to body tissues.

Remission: a period or state during which the symptoms of a disease subside or decrease.

S

Sebaceous gland: a type of gland in the skin that secretes an oily substance that lubricates skin and hair.

Sedative: a drug or other agent that works to calm anxiety.

Serotonin: a ***neurotransmitter*** involved in the processes of sleep and memory, as well as other neurological functions.

Sitz bath: a shallow bath; a therapeutic immersion of the thighs and hips in warm water, sometimes with another substance in solution.

Sonogram: an image produced by reflected sound waves. See also ***Ultrasound.***

Spinal tap: see ***Lumbar puncture.***

Steroid: any of numerous organic compounds, including ***cortisone, estrogen,*** and testosterone, each of which has many effects on the body.

Stress test: a heart-function test that involves monitoring during physical exertion.

Superinfection: a second ***infection*** that develops during the course of an original infection.

Supplement: nutritionally, a substance such as a vitamin pill, fiber solution, or herbal extract that is consumed in addition to food in order to complete or enhance the diet.

Symptom: an abnormal function, sensation, or appearance experienced by an individual.

Syndrome: a group of symptoms that characterize a specific condition.

Systemic: affecting the entire body.

T

Tendon: a tough, inelastic tissue that connects muscle to another structure, usually bone.

Thalamus: part of the brain through which nearly all sensory input passes to the cerebral cortex.

Thymus: a lymphoid organ in the chest where certain cells of the immune system develop.

Thyroid gland: a gland in the neck that secretes hormones involved in the regulation of growth and metabolic rate.

Tincture: a solution composed of a medicinal material and alcohol or alcohol and water; sometimes made with glycerin or vinegar instead of alcohol.

Toxin: a poison produced by an organism, such as the substance released by certain bacteria that causes tetanus.

Triglyceride: a complex molecule, made of ***fatty acids,*** which is the main component of dietary and body fat.

Tumor: abnormal tissue growth, either ***benign*** or ***malignant.***

U-V

Ultrasound: diagnostic or therapeutic use of high-frequency sound waves, especially to examine fetuses or internal structures.

Vascular: relating to or supplied with vessels that conduct fluids, such as blood or lymph.

Vein: a blood vessel that carries blood toward the heart.

Vertebra: any of the bony segments that make up the spinal column.

Very-low-density lipoprotein (VLDL): a fatty protein that carries cholesterol in the blood and is associated with increased risk of atherosclerosis.

Virus: a simple pathogenic microorganism that invades living cells and uses cellular mechanisms to create multiple copies of itself.

Vitamin: any of many organic substances that are vital in small amounts to the normal functioning of the body. Vitamins are found in food, produced by the body, and manufactured synthetically; along with ***minerals,*** they are known as micronutrients.

W-X-Y

White blood cell: any of a group of blood cells that have no ***hemoglobin*** and migrate into tissues to fight ***infection*** and digest cell debris.

X-ray: a form of radiation similar to light but capable of penetrating many solids and of ionizing gases; an image made by using x-rays.

Yeast infection: a fungal ***infection*** in mucous tissue or skin. Vaginal yeast infections can be a side effect of taking antibiotics or other kinds of drugs. See also ***Superinfection.***

BIBLIOGRAPHY

GENERAL

BOOKS

Alternative Medicine: Expanding Medical Horizons. A Report to the National Institutes of Health on Alternative Medical Systems and Practices in the United States (#017-040-00537-7). Washington, D.C.: U.S. Government Printing Office, 1994.

Apple, Michael, MD. *Symptoms and Early Warning Signs.* New York: Dutton, 1994.

Arnot, Robert. *The Best Medicine: How to Choose the Top Doctors, the Top Hospitals, the Top Treatments.* New York: Addison-Wesley, 1993.

A Barefoot Doctor's Manual: The American Translation of the Official Chinese Paramedical Manual. Philadelphia: Running Press, 1990.

Beinfield, Harriet, and Efrem Korngold. *Between Heaven and Earth: A Guide to Chinese Medicine.* New York: Ballantine Books, 1991.

Burroughs, Hugh, and Mark Kastner. *Alternative Healing.* La Mesa, Calif.: Halcyon, 1993.

Burton Goldberg Group. *Alternative Medicine: The Definitive Guide.* Puyallup, Wash.: Future Medicine, 1993.

Butler, Kurt. *A Consumer's Guide to Alternative Medicine.* Buffalo, N.Y.: Prometheus Books, 1992.

Clayman, Charles B., MD, ed. *The American Medical Association Family Medical Guide* (3d ed.). New York: Random House, 1994.

Clayman, Charles B., and Raymond H. Curry, eds. *American Medical Association Guide to Your Family's Symptoms.* New York: Random House, 1992.

Columbia University College of Physicians and Surgeons Complete Home Medical Guide. New York: Crown, 1994.

Dossey, Larry. *Space, Time, and Medicine.* Boulder, Colo.: Shambhala, 1982.

The Editors of Consumer Guide. *Family Medical and Health Guide.* Lincolnwood, Ill.: Publications International, 1991.

The Editors of *Prevention* Magazine Health Books:

The Complete Book of Natural and Medicinal Cures. Emmaus, Pa.: Rodale Press, 1994.

The Prevention How-to Dictionary of Healing Remedies and Techniques. Emmaus, Pa.: Rodale Press, 1992.

Prevention's Giant Book of Health Facts. Emmaus, Pa.: Rodale Press, 1991.

The Editors of Time-Life Books. *Journey through the Mind and Body* (series). Alexandria, Va.: Time-Life Books, 1994.

Elkins, Rita. *The Complete Home Health Advisor.* Pleasant Grove, Utah: Woodland Health Books, 1994.

Encyclopedia of Associations (Vol. 1, pt. 2). Washington, D.C.: Gale Research, 1993.

Feinstein, Alice, and the Editors of *Prevention* Magazine Health Books. *Symptoms, Their Causes, and Cures: How to Understand and Treat 265 Health Concerns.* Emmaus, Pa.: Rodale Press, 1994.

Fugh-Berman, Adriane, MD. *Alternative Medicine: What Works.* Tucson, Ariz.: Odonian Press, in press.

Giller, Robert, MD, and Kathy Matthews. *Natural Prescriptions.* New York: Ballantine Books, 1995.

Glanze, Walter D., ed. *The Mosby Medical Encyclopedia* (rev. ed.). New York: Plume, 1992.

Griffith, H. Winter, MD. *Complete Guide to Symptoms, Illness, and Surgery.* New York: Body Press/Perigee Books, 1989.

Health and Wellness Confidential. New York: Boardroom Classics, 1986.

Hoffman, Matthew, and William LeGro. *Disease Free: How to Prevent, Treat and Cure More than 150 Illnesses and Conditions.* Emmaus, Pa.: Rodale Press, 1993.

Hurst, J. W., ed. *Medicine for the Practicing Physician* (3d ed.). Boston: Butterworth-Heinemann, 1992.

Inlander, Charles, et al. *Good Operations, Bad Operations.* New York: Viking, 1993.

Janiger, Oscar, and Philip Goldberg. *A Different Kind of Healing.* New York: Jeremy P. Tarcher/Putnam, 1993.

Kaptchuk, Ted. *The Web That Has No Weaver: Understanding Chinese Medicine.* New York: Congdon and Weed, 1983.

Kiester, Edwin, Jr., ed. *Better Homes and Gardens New Family Medical Guide.* Des Moines: Meredith, 1989.

Kircheimer, Sid, and the Editors of *Prevention* Magazine Health Books. *The Doctors Book of Home Remedies II.* Emmaus, Pa.: Rodale Books, 1993.

Larson, David E., MD, ed. *Mayo Clinic Family Health Book.* New York: William Morrow, 1990.

Lerner, Michael. *Choices in Healing.* Cambridge, Mass.: MIT Press, 1994.

Lesko, Matthew. *What to Do When You Can't Afford Health Care.* Kensington, Md.: Information USA, 1993.

Lever, Ruth, MD. *The Consumer's Guide to Treating Common Illnesses.* New York: Simon & Schuster, 1990.

The Macmillan Visual Dictionary. New York: Macmillan, 1992.

Margolis, Simon, MD, ed. *Johns Hopkins Symptoms and Remedies.* New York: Rebus, 1995.

Marieb, Elaine N. *Essentials of Human Anatomy and Physiology* (4th ed.). Redwood City, Calif.: Benjamin/Cummings, 1994.

Marshall Cavendish Encyclopedia of Family Health. North Bellmore, N.Y.: Marshall Cavendish, 1991.

Mayell, Mark. *Natural Health First-Aid Guide.* New York: Pocket Books, 1994.

Mills, Simon, and Steven Finando. *Alternatives in Healing.* New York: New American Library, 1989.

Monte, Tom. *World Medicine: The East West Guide to Healing Your Body.* New York: Jeremy P. Tarcher/Perigee Books, 1993.

Mosby's Medical, Nursing, and Allied Health Dictionary (4th ed.). New York: Mosby-Year Book, 1994.

Murphy, Michael. *The Future of the Body: Explorations into the Further Evolution of Human Nature.* Los Angeles: Jeremy P. Tarcher, 1992.

Murray, Michael T., and Joseph E. Pizzorno. *An Encyclopedia of Natural Medicine.* Rocklin, Calif.: Prima, 1991.

Netter, Frank H. *Atlas of Human Anatomy.* Summit, N.J.: Ciba-Geigy, 1989.

The New Good Housekeeping Family Health and Medical Guide. New York: Hearst Books, 1989.

The Official American Board of Medical Specialties Directory of Board Certified Medical Specialists, 1995 (27th ed.). New Providence, N.J.: Reed Reference, 1995.

Olshevsky, Moshe, et al. *The Manual of Natural Therapy: A Practical Guide to Alternative Medicine.* New York: Citadel Press, 1993.

Professional Guide to Diseases. Springhouse, Pa.: Springhouse, 1995.

Reader's Digest Association. *The Good Health Fact Book.* Pleasantville, N.Y.: Reader's Digest Association, 1992.

Reader's Digest Association. *Reader's Digest Family Guide to Natural Medicine.* Pleasantville, N.Y.: Reader's Digest Association, 1993.

Rees, Alan M., ed. *The Consumer Health Information Source Book* (4th ed.). Phoenix: Oryx Press, 1994.

Rose, Stuart R., MD. *1994 International Travel Health Guide* (5th ed.). Northampton, Mass.: Travel Medicine, 1994.

Rosenfeld, Isadore, MD:

The Best Treatment. New York: Simon & Schuster, 1991.

Doctor, What Should I Eat? New York: Random House, 1995.

Symptoms. New York: Simon & Schuster, 1989.

Shtasel, Philip. *Medical Tests and Diagnostic Procedures.* New York: Harper & Row, 1990.

Signs and Symptoms Handbook. Springhouse, Pa.: Springhouse, 1988.

Simons, Anne, MD, Bobbie Hasselbring, and Michael Castleman. *Before You Call the Doctor: Safe, Effective Self-Care for over 300 Medical Problems.* New York: Fawcett Columbine, 1992.

Slabey, Frank. *Gross Anatomy in the Practice of Medicine.* Philadelphia: Lea and Febiger, 1994.

Smyth, Angela. *The Complete Home Healer: Your Guide to Every Treatment Available for over 300 of the Most Common Health Problems.* San Francisco: HarperCollins, 1994.

Stedman's Medical Dictionary (25th ed.). Baltimore: Williams and Wilkins, 1990.

Taber's Cyclopedic Medical Dictionary. Philadelphia: F. A. Davis, 1993.

Taylor, R. B., ed. *Family Medicine: Principles and Practice.* New York: Springer-Verlag, 1994.

Tierney, Lawrence M. *Current Medical Diagnosis and Treatment.* Norwalk, Conn.: Appleton & Lange, 1994.

Tkac, Debora (ed.), and the Editors of *Prevention* Magazine Health Books:

The Doctors Book of Home Remedies: Thousands of Tips and Techniques Anyone Can Use to Heal Everyday Health Problems. Emmaus, Pa.: Rodale Press, 1990.

Everyday Health Tips: 2000 Practical Hints for Better Health and Happiness. Emmaus, Pa.: Rodale Press, 1988.

Ullman, Dana. *The One-Minute or So Healer.* New York: Jeremy P. Tarcher/Perigee Books, 1991.

Van Straten, Michael. *The Complete Natural-Health Consultant.* New York: Prentice Hall, 1987.

Vickers, Andrew:

Complementary Medicine and Disability. London: Chapman and Hall, 1993.

Examining Complementary Medicine: The Sceptical Holist. London: Chapman and Hall, in preparation.

Vickery, Donald M., MD, and James F. Fries, MD. *Take Care of Yourself: The Complete Guide to Medical Self-Care.* Reading, Mass.: Addison-Wesley, 1994.

Weil, Andrew, MD:

Health and Healing. Boston: Houghton Mifflin, 1995.

Natural Health, Natural Medicine. Boston: Houghton Mifflin, 1995.

Spontaneous Healing: How to Discover and Enhance Your

Body's Natural Ability to Maintain and Heal Itself. New York: Knopf, 1995.

Wilen, Joan, and Lydia Wilen. *Live and Be Well.* New York: Harper Perennial, 1992.

Woodburne, Russell, and William E. Burkel. *Essentials of Human Anatomy* (9th ed.). New York: Oxford University Press, 1994.

Wyngaarden J. B., et al., eds. *Cecil Textbook of Medicine* (20th ed.). Philadelphia: W. B. Saunders, 1995.

Zwicky, John F., et al. *Reader's Guide to Alternative Health Methods.* Milwaukee: American Medical Association, 1993.

PERIODICALS

Barasch, Douglas. "The Mainstreaming of Alternative Medicine." *New York Times Magazine,* October 4, 1992.

Boodman, Sandra G. "What Do the Certificates on Your Doctor's Wall Really Mean?" *Washington Post,* July 12, 1994.

Gallo, Nick. "Alternative Medicine: Is It for You?" *Better Homes and Gardens,* May 1995.

Hamilton, Linda. "Colds . . . Headache . . . Heartburn: Easy Remedies for Everyday Miseries." *Family Circle,* January 10, 1995.

"Health Report." *Time,* December 5, 1994.

King, Jennifer. "Starting Out: A Consumer's Guide to Getting the Most from Holistic Health Care." *1994-1995 Holistic Health Directory.*

OTHER SOURCES

Folkenberg, Judy, ed. *NIH Healthline.* Bethesda, Md.: National Institutes of Health.

Friedman, Rodney, ed. "The University of California at Berkeley Wellness Letter: The Newsletter of Nutrition, Fitness, and Stress Management." New York: Healthletter Associates.

"Personal Health Guide: Put Prevention into Practice." Booklet. U.S. Department of Health and Human Services, June 1994.

ACUPRESSURE

BOOKS

Bauer, Cathryn. *Acupressure for Everybody.* New York: Henry Holt, 1991.

Chan, Pedro. *Finger Acupressure.* New York: Ballantine Books, 1985.

Gach, Michael Reed. *Acupressure's Potent Points: A Guide to Self-Care for Common Ailments.* New York: Bantam Books, 1990.

Jarmey, Chris, and John Tindall. *Acupressure for Common Ailments.* New York: Simon & Schuster, 1991.

AGING ISSUES

BOOKS

Griffith, H. Winter, MD. *Complete Guide to Symptoms, Illness and Surgery for People over 50.* New York: Putnam, 1992.

Margolis, Simon, MD, and Hamilton Moses, III, MD, eds. *The Johns Hopkins Medical Handbook: The 100 Major Medical Disorders of People over the Age of 50.* New York: Rebus, 1992.

AROMATHERAPY

BOOKS

Davis, Patricia. *Aromatherapy: An A-Z.* Essex, England: C. W. Daniel, 1992.

Ryman, Danielle. *Aromatherapy: The Complete Guide to Plant and Flower Essences for Health and Beauty.* New York: Bantam Books, 1993.

Valnet, Jean. *The Practice of Aromatherapy.* Rochester, Vt.: Healing Arts Press, 1990.

Worwood, Valerie Ann. *The Complete Book of Essential Oils and Aromatherapy.* San Rafael, Calif.: New World Library, 1991.

BODY WORK

BOOKS

Beck, Mark. *The Theory and Practice of Therapeutic Massage* (2d ed.). Albany, N.Y.: Milady, 1994.

Byers, Dwight. *Better Health with Foot Reflexology.* St. Petersburg, Fla.: Ingham, 1987.

Egoscue, Peter. *The Egoscue Method of Health through Motion.* New York: HarperCollins, 1992.

Kunz, Kevin, and Barbara Kunz. *The Complete Guide to Foot Reflexology* (rev. ed.). Albuquerque, N.Mex.: Reflexology Research, 1993.

Lidell, Lucy, et al. *The Book of Massage: Complete Step-by-Step Guide to Eastern and Western Techniques.* New York: Fireside Books, 1984.

Norman, Laura. *Feet First: A Guide to Foot Reflexology.* New York: Simon & Schuster, 1988.

Ohashi, Wataru. *Do-It-Yourself Shiatsu.* New York: Viking Penguin, 1992.

Shaw, Eva. *60 Second Shiatzu: The Natural Way to Energize, Erase Pain, and Conquer Tension in One Minute.* New York: Henry

Holt, 1995.
Tappan, Frances. *Healing Massage Technique: Holistic, Classical and Emerging Methods.* Norwalk, Conn.: Appleton & Lange, 1988.

CANCER

BOOKS

Bombeck, Erma. *I Want to Grow Hair, I Want to Grow Up, I Want to Go to Boise.* New York: Harper & Row, 1989.
Caring for the Terminally Ill Patient at Home. Philadelphia: University of Pennsylvania Cancer Center, 1986.
Dollinger, Malin, Ernest Rosenbaum, and Greg Cable. *Everyone's Guide to Cancer Therapy.* New York: Somerville House Books, 1991.
Dreher, Henry. *Your Defense against Cancer: The Complete Guide to Cancer Prevention.* New York: Harper & Row, 1988.
Greenspan, Ezra. *What Every Woman and Her Doctor Could Discuss about Ovarian Cancer: A Medical Oncologist's Perspective.* New York: Chemotherapy Foundation, 1990.
Lerner, Michael. *Choices in Healing: Integrating the Best of Conventional and Complementary Approaches to Cancer.* Cambridge, Mass.: MIT Press, 1994.
Rosenberg, Steven, and John Barry. *The Transformed Cell: Unlocking the Mysteries of Cancer.* New York: Putnam, 1992.
Weissman, David E., et al. *Handbook of Cancer Pain Management* (4th ed.). Madison: Medical College of Wisconsin, and the University of Wisconsin Medical School in conjunction with the Wisconsin Cancer Pain Initiative, 1994.

PERIODICALS

Adler, T. "Study Reaffirms Tamoxifen's Dark Side." *Science News,* June 4, 1994.
Altman, Lawrence, MD. "Stomach Microbe Offers Clues to Cancer as Well as Ulcers." *New York Times,* February 22, 1994.
"Birch Used to Shrink Melanoma in Mice." *New York Times,* March 28, 1995.
Blakeslee, Sandra. "Discoveries on the Makings of a Suntan Reveal How Cancer Lurks in the Wings." *New York Times,* December 7, 1994.
Brody, Jane:
"Disputing Four Studies, New Research Supports Chest X-Rays as Cancer Screen." *New York Times,* November 30, 1994.
"Hormone Replacement Study Answers Questions, but Not All." *New York Times,* January 18, 1995.
"New Therapy for Menopause Reduces Risk." *New York Times,* November 18, 1994.
"Prostate Patients 'Learn to Hope by Sharing.' " *New York Times,* December 14, 1994.
Brownlee, Shannon. "The Smoke Next Door." *U.S. News & World Report,* June 20, 1994.
"Cancer Gene Found to Play Nonhereditary Role as Well." *New York Times,* April 4, 1995.
"Cancer: Pare Protein to Spare the Kidneys." *Science News,* August 6, 1994.
Cowley, Geoffrey. "A Varied but Brutal Disease." *Newsweek,* May 30, 1994.
Fackelmann, Kathy:
"Antioxidant Vitamins Fail to Prevent Polyps." *Science News,* July 23, 1994.
"Immune Trait Ups Cervical Cancer Risk." *Science News,* April 30, 1994.
"Sizing Up a Smoker's Risk of Lung Cancer." *Science News,* April 16, 1994.
"Veggies May Cut Nonsmoker Lung Cancer Risk." *Science News,* January 8, 1994.
Fisher, Lawrence. "Enzyme May Offer Target to Tumors." *New York Times,* April 12, 1994.
Garnick, Marc. "The Dilemmas of Prostate Cancer." *Scientific American,* April 1994.
Gorman, Christine. "The Doctor's Crystal Ball." *Time,* April 10, 1995.
Hall, Stephen. "Cancer." *Health,* March/April 1994.
Hilts, Philip J.:
"Less-Drastic Alternative to Mastectomy Is Offered." *New York Times,* January 14, 1994.
"Two Studies Find No Breast-Implant Tie to Connective-Tissue Illness." *New York Times,* October 26, 1994.
Kolata, Gina:
"Data on Risks Create Debate about Drug to Prevent Breast Cancer." *New York Times,* March 16, 1994.
"Study Finds Hope in Immune Therapy for Cancer." *New York Times,* March 23, 1994.
"Study Finds No Implant-Disease Links." *New York Times,* June 16, 1994.
"Tests to Assess Risks for Cancer Raising Questions." *New York Times,* March 27, 1995.
Lamm, Donald L., et al. "Megadose Vitamins in Bladder Cancer: A Double-Blind Clinical Trial." *Journal of Urology,* January 1994.
Lane, William, MD. "Medical Application of Whole Shark Cartilage." *Natural Health,* August/September 1994.
Leary, Warren. "Studies Raise Doubts about Need to Lower Home Radon Levels." *New*

York Times, September 6, 1994.

"Link of Radon to Lung Cancer Looks Loopy." *Science News,* March 19, 1994.

McCarty, Mary. "Doctors Wave Wand for Detailed Views of Brains' Workings." *Washington Times,* December 11, 1994.

"Mammograms and Age." *New York Times,* Health section, January 11, 1995.

Maugh, Thomas. "Pancreatic Cancer Is Treated by Freezing: Technique Has Already Been Used on Liver, Prostate." *Washington Post,* Health section, November 22, 1994.

"Meat's Risk for Cancer: Just Bologna? . . . Not When It's Prostate Cancer." *Science News,* February 19, 1994.

Montgomery, Pam. "The Re-Emergence of Essiac, a Native American Cancer Remedy." *American Herb Association Quarterly Newsletter,* Spring 1994.

"New Clue to Prostate Cancer Spread." *Science,* May 12, 1995.

Pennisi, Elizabeth:

"P16's Cancer Role Debated and Verified." *Science News,* September 3, 1994.

"Quest for Genes That Stop Cancer Spread." *Science News,* April 2, 1994.

"A Plate of Protection: Nutrients May Lower Stomach Cancer Risk." *Prevention,* January 1994.

Raloff, Janet:

"Menstrual Cycles May Affect Cancer Risk." *Science News,* January 7, 1995.

"Sorting Out Cancer IQs in Browned Meat." *Science News,* January 8, 1994.

"Studies Spark New Tamoxifen Controversy." *Science News,* February 26, 1994.

"The Sausage Cure." *Discover,* November 1994.

Schmitz, Anthony. "The Kindest Cut." *Health,* January/February 1994.

"Selenium Study Finds No Anti-Cancer Role." *New York Times,* April 18, 1995.

Service, Robert F. "Stalking the Start of Colon Cancer." *Science,* March 18, 1994.

"U.S. Warns about Drug for Cancer." *New York Times,* April 9, 1994.

"Vegetarian Diet Prevents Cancer and Heart Disease." *Natural Health,* August/September 1994.

"Women Smokers Appear to Run Higher Risk." *New York Times,* January 4, 1994.

OTHER SOURCES

"Cancer Pain Can Be Relieved: A Guide for Patients and Families." Madison: Wisconsin Cancer Pain Initiative, 1988.

"Chemotherapy: Your Weapon against Cancer." New York: Chemotherapy Foundation, 1991.

"Managing Cancer Pain." Silver Spring, Md.: Cancer Pain Guideline, AHCPR Publication #94-0595, March 1994.

Office of Technology Assessment. "Unconventional Cancer Treatments" (OTA-H-405). Washington, D.C.: U.S. Goverment Printing Office, 1990.

Parker, Gwendolyn. "First-Ever Prostate Cancer Prevention Trial." *Advance.* Richmond: Massey Cancer Center, Virginia Commonwealth University, Winter 1995.

"Silicone Implant Litigation Update." Dow Chemical, February 10, 1995.

CHILDREN'S HEALTH

BOOKS

Austin, Phylis, Agatha Thrash, and Calvin Thrash. *Natural Healthcare for Your Child.* Sunfield, Mich.: Family Health Publications, 1990.

Betz, Cecily Lynn, et al. *Family Centered Nursing Care of Children.* Philadelphia: W. B. Saunders, 1994.

Columbia University. *Complete Guide to Early Child Care.* New York: Crown, 1990.

Eisenberg, Arlene, Heidi E. Murkoff, and Sandee E. Hathaway. *What to Expect the First Year.* New York: Workman, 1989.

Foley, Denise, et al. *Doctors Book of Home Remedies for Children.* Emmaus, Pa.: Rodale Press, 1994.

Franck, Irene, and David Brownstone. *The Parent's Desk Reference.* New York: Prentice Hall, 1991.

Griffith, H. Winter. *Complete Guide to Pediatric Symptoms, Illness and Medications.* Los Angeles: Body Press, 1989.

Inlander, Charles B., and J. Lynne Dodson. *Take This Book to the Pediatrician with You.* Allentown, Pa.: People's Medical Society, 1992.

Kelly, Marguerite, and Ella Parsons. *The Mother's Almanac II.* New York: Doubleday, 1989.

Pantell, Robert H., James F. Fries, and Donald Vickery. *Taking Care of Your Child* (4th ed.). New York: Addison-Wesley, 1993.

Schmitt, Barton. *Your Child's Health.* New York: Bantam Books, 1991.

Spock, Benjamin. *Dr. Spock's Baby and Child Care* (6th ed.). New York: Pocket Books, 1992.

Stanway, Andrew. *The Natural Family Doctor.* New York: Simon &

Schuster, 1987.
Stoppard, Miriam. *Baby and Child A to Z Medical Handbook.* Tucson, Ariz.: Body Press, 1986.

PERIODICALS

Brody, Jane. "The Real Problem with Children's Scalp Ills." *New York Times,* November 9, 1994.
Carey, William B. "The Effectiveness of Parent Counseling in Managing Colic." *Pediatrics,* September 1994.
Creager, Ellen. "Here's How to Cope with Baby's Colic, Colds, and Diarrhea." *Knight-Ridder/Tribune News Service,* January 18, 1994.
Newson, C. "Getting to the Root of the Problem: Many Parents Worried by Repeated Insecticidal Treatments for Head Lice Are Fighting Back with Age-Old Methods." *Time Educational Supplement,* October 28, 1994.
Oliver, P. "Making Sense of . . . Head Lice." *Nursing Times,* June 1, 1994.
Pellman, H. "Infestations That Itch: Head Lice and Scabies." *Pediatrics for Parents,* March 1994.
"Treating Children's Croup with Steroids." *Child Health Alert,* September 1994.
Watson, Barbara, and Stuart Starr. "Varicella Vaccine for Healthy Children." *Lancet,* April 16, 1994.

OTHER SOURCES

"Brief Currents: Infectious Diseases in Children." Pediatric Report's Child's Health Newsletter, November 1993.
"Can Anything Be Done about Colic?" Pediatric Report's Child's Health Newsletter, October 1993.
"Child Health Guide: Put Prevention into Practice" (booklet.) U.S. Department of Health and Human Services, June 1994.
"Colic: Learning How to Deal with Your Baby's Crying." American Academy of Family Physicians, 1993.

DENTAL PROBLEMS

BOOK

Proffit, William R., and Raymond P. White, Jr. *Surgical-Orthodontic Treatment.* St. Louis: Mosby-Year Book, 1991.

PERIODICALS

Ciancio, S. G. "Expanded and Future Uses of Mouthrinses." *Journal of American Dental Association,* August 1994.
Gray, R. J. M., and C. A. Hall. "Physiotherapy in the Treatment of TMJ Disorders." *British Dental Journal,* April 9, 1994.

DIGESTION AND GASTRO-INTESTINAL PROBLEMS

PERIODICALS

Aurisicchio, L. N., and C. S. Pitchumoni. "Lactose Intolerance: Recognizing the Link between Diet and Discomfort." *Postgraduate Medicine,* January 1994.
Brody, Jane. "New Exercise Benefits for the Elderly: Walking Reduces Risk of GI Hemorrhage." *New York Times,* August 24, 1994.
Catassi, C., et al. "Coeliac Disease in the Year 2000: Exploring the Iceberg." *Lancet,* January 22, 1994.
Colburn, Don. "Exercise Helps Elderly Avoid Bleeding in Gut." *Washington Post,* September 13, 1994.
"Complicated Pain Relief: Health Risks When Taking NSAIDs." *Newsletter of the People's Medical Society,* August 1994.
Fackelmann, Kathy. "Seniors Gain Gut Protection: Moderate Exercise Reduces Risk of Intestinal Bleeding in Senior Citizens." *Science News,* September 3, 1994.
Frey, Charles. "Abdominal Hernia Repair." *Journal of the American Medical Association,* July 20, 1994.
"Gastrointestinal Hemorrhage and Use of NSAIDs." *American Family Physician,* July 1994.
"Hemorrhoids: What Helps—and What Doesn't." *Consumer Reports on Health,* February 1994.
Pauker, Stephan, and Richard Kopelman. "A Masked Marauder: Appendicitis." *New England Journal of Medicine,* June 2, 1994.
"Screening for Gastric Damage Caused by NSAIDs." *American Family Physician,* October 1994.
Sena, M. M., M. L. Stoddard, and S. Pashko. "Use of Nonantacid Antiulcer Agents in the Treatment of Heartburn and Dyspepsia" (abstract). *Clinical Therapeutics,* January/February 1994.
Sturgess, Richard. "Wheat Peptide Challenge in Celiac Disease." *Lancet,* March 26, 1994.

DRUGS

BOOKS

Edelson, Edward. *The ABCs of Prescription Drugs.* New York: Ivy Books, 1987.

Griffith, H. Winter, MD. *Complete Guide to Prescription and Non-Prescription Drugs.* New York: Putnam, 1994.

Katzung, Bertram. *Basic and Clinical Pharmacology* (6th ed.). Norwalk, Conn.: Appleton & Lange, 1995.

Long, James W., MD, and James J. Rybacki. *The Essential Guide to Prescription Drugs.* New York: Harper/Perennial, 1994.

McEvoy, Gerald K., ed. *American Hospital Formulary Service Drug Information 1995.* Bethesda, Md.: American Society of Hospital Pharmacists, 1994.

Melmon, Kenneth, Howard Morrelli, et al. *Melmon and Morrelli's Clinical Pharmacology: Basic Principles in Therapeutics* (3d ed.). New York: Pergamon Press, 1991.

Oppenheim, Mike. *100 Drugs That Work.* Chicago: Contemporary Books, 1994.

Physician's Desk Reference (49th ed.). Montvale, N.J.: Medical Economics Data, 1995.

Physician's Desk Reference for Non-Prescription Drugs (15th ed.). Montvale, N.J.: Medical Economics Data, 1995.

Physician's Desk Reference Guide to Drug Interactions, Side Effects, Indications (49th ed.). Montvale, N.J.: Medical Economics Data, 1995.

Physician's Drug Handbook (5th ed.). Springhouse, Pa.: Springhouse, 1993.

Rathgeber, Mark. *Drug Consultant and Interaction Guide.* St. Louis: G. W. Manning, 1992.

Schein, Jeffrey R. *The Consumer's Guide to Drug Interactions.* New York: Collier Books, 1993.

Silverman, Harold, ed. *The Pill Book* (6th ed.). New York: Bantam Books, 1994.

Sonberg, Lynn. *The Pill Guide.* New York: Berkeley Books, 1992.

United States Pharmacopeia Drug Information, Volume I: Drug Information for the Health Care Professional. Rockville, Md.: United States Pharmacopeial Convention, 1995.

Winter, Ruth. *A Consumer's Dictionary of Medicines.* New York: Crown, 1993.

Zimmerman, David R. *Zimmerman's Complete Guide to Nonprescription Drugs.* Washington, D.C.: Visible Ink Press, 1993.

EAR, NOSE, AND THROAT PROBLEMS

PERIODICALS

Banquero, F., and E. Loza. "Antibiotic Resistance of Microorganisms Involved in Ear, Nose and Throat Infections." *Pediatric Infectious Disease Journal,* 1994, Vol. 13, pp. S9-S14.

Brooks, Adrienne C. "Middle Ear Infections in Children." *Science News,* November 19, 1994.

Klein, J. O. "Current Issues in Upper Respiratory Tract Infections in Infants and Children: Rationale for Antibacterial Therapy." *Pediatric Infectious Disease Journal,* 1994, Vol. 13, pp. S5-S8.

Lund, V. J. "Bacterial Sinusitis: Etiology and Surgical Management." *Pediatric Infectious Disease Journal,* 1994, Vol. 13, pp. S58-S63.

Pichichero, M. E. "Assessing the Treatment Alternatives for Acute Otitis Media." *Pediatric Infectious Disease Journal,* 1994, Vol. 13, pp. S27-S34.

Theiss, Barbara, and Peter Theiss. "Natural Immune Boosters." *Mothering,* Winter 1994.

Willensky, Diana. "How It Works: The Ear." *American Health,* September 1994.

Willett, L. R., J. L. Carson, and J. W. Williams. "Current Diagnosis and Management of Sinusitis." *Journal of General Internal Medicine,* 1994, Vol. 9, pp. 38-45.

Wilson, J. "Current Approaches to Sinusitis." *Practitioner,* 1994, Vol. 238, pp. 467-472.

EMERGENCIES AND FIRST AID

BOOKS

American Medical Association. *Pocket Guide to Emergency First Aid.* New York: Random House, 1993.

Handal, K. *The American Red Cross First Aid and Safety Handbook.* Boston: Little, Brown, 1992.

Ho, M. T., and C. E. Saunders, eds. *Current Emergency Diagnosis and Treatment.* Norwalk, Conn.: Appleton & Lange, 1990.

Parcel, G. S., and C. E. Rinear. *Basic Emergency Care of the Sick and Injured* (4th ed.). St. Louis: Times Mirror, 1990.

Rosenberg, Stephen N. *The Johnson and Johnson First Aid Book.* New York: Warner Books, 1985.

ENDOCRINE PROBLEMS

BOOK

Surks, Martin. *The Thyroid Book.* Yonkers, N.Y.: Consumer Reports Books, 1993.

PERIODICAL

"Common Class of Viruses Implicated as Cause of Type 1 Diabetes." *Washington Post,* November 26, 1994.

EYE PROBLEMS

BOOKS

Anshel, Jeffrey, MD. *Healthy Eyes, Better Vision: Everyday Eyecare for the Whole Family.* Los Angeles: Body Press, 1990.

Gillis, James P., Robert G. Martin, and Donald R. Sanders. *Sutureless Cataract Surgery: An Evolution toward Minimally Invasive Technique.* Thorofare, N.J.: Slack, 1992.

PERIODICALS

Schumer, Robert A., MD, and Steven M. Podos, MD. "The Nerve of Glaucoma." *Archives of Opthalmology,* January 1994.

Seddon, Johanna M., MD, and Charles H. Hennekens, MD. "Vitamins, Minerals, and Macular Degeneration." *Archives of Opthalmology,* February 1994.

HEART AND CIRCULATORY PROBLEMS

BOOKS

Clayman, Charles B., MD, ed. *The American Medical Association: Your Heart.* Pleasantville, N.Y.: Reader's Digest Association, 1989.

McGoon, Michael D., MD, ed. *The Mayo Clinic Heart Book.* New York: William Morrow, 1993.

PERIODICALS

Baker, David W., et al. "Management of Heart Failure: I. Pharmacologic Treatment." *Journal of the American Medical Association,* November 2, 1994.

Brody, Jane. "Heart Diseases Are Persisting in Study's Second Generation." *New York Times,* January 5, 1994.

Dracup, Kathleen, et al. "Management of Heart Failure: II. Counseling, Education, and Lifestyle Modifications." *Journal of the American Medical Association,* November 9, 1994.

Hankinson, Susan E., and M. J. Stampfer. "All That Glitters Is Not Beta Carotene" (editorial). *Journal of the American Medical Association,* November 9, 1994.

Kolata, Gina:
"Novel Bypass Method: A Dose of New Genes." *New York Times,* December 13, 1994.
"Study Finds Cholesterol-Lowering Drug May Save Lives." *New York Times,* November 17, 1994.

Mirbod, S. M., et al. "Prevalence of Raynaud's Phenomenon in Different Groups of Workers Operating Hand-Held Vibrating Tools." *International Archives of Occupational and Environmental Health,* 1994, Vol. 66, pp. 13-22.

Morris, Dexter L., Stephan B. Kritchevsky, and C. E. Davis. "Serum Carotenoids and Coronary Heart Disease." *Journal of the American Medical Association,* November 9, 1994.

"Occasional, Not Daily, Drinkers Show Low Death Rates in Study." *New York Times,* November 17, 1994.

Winslow, Ron. "Guidelines for Treating Angina Offer More Consistency of Cardiac Condition." *Wall Street Journal,* March 16, 1994.

HEMATOLOGICAL PROBLEMS

PERIODICAL

Samuel-Reid, Joy H. "Common Problems in Sickle Cell Disease." *American Family Physician,* May 1, 1994.

OTHER SOURCE

U.S. Department of Health and Human Services. "Sickle Cell Disease in Newborns and Infants: A Guide for Parents." Rockville, Md.: Agency for Health Care Policy and Research, 1993.

HERBS

BOOKS

Bensky, Dan, and Randall Barolet. *Chinese Herbal Medicine: Formulas and Strategies.* Seattle: Eastland Press, 1990.

Bensky, Dan, and Andrew Gamble. *Chinese Herbal Medicine: Materia Medica.* Seattle: Eastland Press, 1993.

Buchman, Dian Dincin. *Herbal Medicine: The Natural Way to Get Well and Stay Well.* New York: Gramercy, 1979.

Castleman, Michael. *The Healing Herbs: The Ultimate Guide to the Curative Power of Nature's Medicines.* Emmaus, Pa.: Rodale Press, 1991.

Coon, Nelson. *Using Plants for Healing.* Emmaus, Pa.: Rodale Press, 1979.

Duke, James A. *CRC Handbook of Medicinal Herbs.* Boca Raton, Fla.: CRC Press, 1985.

Foster, Steven, and Yue Chonxi. *Herbal Emissaries.* Rochester, Vt.: Healing Arts Press, 1992.

Herbal Encyclopedia: The Comprehensive Family Resource for Safeguarding Health and Preventing Illness. Boston: Houghton Mifflin, 1991.

Hoffmann, David. *The New Holistic Herbal.* New York: Barnes & Noble, 1995.

Hoffmann, David, ed. *The Herbal Handbook: A User's Guide to Medical Herbalism.* Rochester, Vt.: Healing Arts Press, 1987.
Hsu, Hong-Yen:
Chinese Herb Medicine and Therapy (rev. ed.). New Canaan, Conn.: Keats, 1994.
How to Treat Yourself with Chinese Herbs. New Canaan, Conn.: Keats, 1993.
Hutchens, Alma R. *A Handbook of Native American Herbs.* Boston: Shambhala, 1992.
Kloss, Jethro. *Back to Eden: A Human Interest Story of Health and Restoration to Be Found in Herb, Root, and Bark* (2d ed.). Loma Linda, Calif.: Back to Eden Books, 1988.
Kowalchik, Claire, and William Hylton. *Rodale's Illustrated Encyclopedia of Herbs.* Emmaus, Pa.: Rodale Press, 1987.
Lu, Henry C. *Chinese Herbal Cures.* New York: Sterling, 1991.
Lucas, Richard. *Miracle Medicine Herbs.* New York: Parker/Simon & Schuster, 1991.
Mabey, Richard. *The New Age Herbalist.* New York: Collier Books, 1988.
McIntyre, Abbe. *Herbs for Common Ailments.* New York: Fireside Books, 1992.
Martin, Corinne. *Earthmagic: Finding and Using Medicinal Herbs.* Woodstock, Vt.: Countryman Press, 1991.
Mindell, Earl. *Earl Mindell's Herb Bible.* New York: Simon & Schuster, 1992.
Murray, Michael T.:
The Healing Power of Herbs: The Enlightened Person's Guide to the Wonders of Medicinal Plants. Rocklin, Calif.: Prima, 1992.
Natural Alternatives to Over-the-Counter and Prescription Drugs. New York: William Morrow, 1994.
Ody, Penelope. *The Complete Medicinal Herbal.* New York: Dorling Kindersley, 1993.
Polunin, Miriam. *The Natural Pharmacy: An Illustrated Guide to Natural Medicine.* New York: Collier Books/Dorling Kindersley, 1992.
Reid, D. P. *Chinese Herbal Medicine.* Boston: Shambhala, 1987.
Santillo, Humbart. *Natural Healing with Herbs.* Prescott Valley, Ariz.: Hohm Press, 1993.
Thomas, Lalitha. *Ten Essential Herbs.* Prescott Valley, Ariz.: Hohm Press, 1992.
Tierra, Lesley. *The Herbs of Life: Health and Healing Using Western and Chinese Techniques.* Freedom, Calif.: Crossing Press, 1992.
Tierra, Michael:
Planetary Herbology. Twin Lakes, Wis.: Lotus Press, 1988.
Way of Herbs. Santa Cruz, Calif.: Pocket Books, 1990.
Tyler, Varro E.:
Herbs of Choice: The Therapeutic Use of Phytomedicinals. New York: Pharmaceutical Products Press, 1994.
The Honest Herbal: A Sensible Guide to the Use of Herbs and Related Remedies (3d ed.) New York: Pharmaceutical Products Press, 1993.
Weiner, Michael A. *The Herbal Bible.* San Rafael, Calif.: Quantum Books, 1992.
Weiner, Michael, and Janet Weiner. *Herbs That Heal: Prescription for Herbal Healing.* San Rafael, Calif.: Quantum Books, 1994.
Werbach, Melvyn R., and Michael T. Murray. *Botanical Influences on Illness.* Tarzana, Calif.: Third Line Press, 1994.
Wren, R. C. *Potter's New Cyclopaedia of Botanical Drugs and Preparations.* Essex, England: C. W. Daniel, 1988.

PERIODICAL

Brown, J. S., and S. A. Marcy. "The Use of Botanicals for Health Purposes by Members of a Prepaid Health Plan." *Research in Nursing & Health,* October 1991.

HOMEOPATHY

BOOKS

Buegel, Dale, Blair Lewis, and Dennis Chernin. *Homeopathic Remedies for Health Professionals and Lay People.* Honesdale, Pa.: Himalayan International Institute of Yoga Science and Philosophy in the U.S.A., 1991.
Castro, Miranda. *The Complete Homeopathy Handbook,* New York: St. Martin's Press, 1990.
Cook, Trevor M. *Homeopathic Medicine Today.* New Canaan, Conn.: Keats, 1989.
Cummings, Stephen, and Dana Ullman. *Everybody's Guide to Homeopathic Medicines.* Los Angeles: Jeremy P. Tarcher, 1991.
Hayfield, Robin. *Homeopathy for Common Ailments.* Berkeley, Calif.: Frog, 1993.
Lockie, Andrew, MD. *The Family Guide to Homeopathy.* New York: Fireside Books, 1993.
Panos, M., and J. Heimlich. *Homeopathic Medicine at Home.* Los Angeles: Jeremy P. Tarcher, 1980.
Tyler, M. C. *Homeopathic Drug Pictures.* Essex, England: C. W. Daniel, 1987.
Ullman, Dana. *Discovering Homeopathy.* Berkeley, Calif.: North Atlantic Books, 1991.
Vithoulkas, George. *The Science of Homeopathy.* New York: Grove Press, 1980.
Weiner, Michael, and Kathleen Gross. *Complete Book of*

Homeopathy. Garden City Park, N.Y.: Avery, 1989.

PERIODICAL

Jacobs, Jennifer, et al. "Treatment of Acute Childhood Diarrhea with Homeopathic Medicine: A Randomized Clinical Trial in Nicaragua." *Pediatrics,* May 1994.

IMMUNE DISORDERS

BOOKS

Crook, William, MD. *Chronic Fatigue Syndrome and the Yeast Connection.* Jackson, Tenn.: Professional Books, 1992.

Edelson, Edward. *The Immune System.* New York: Chelsea House, 1989.

Feiden, Karyn. *Hope and Help for Chronic Fatigue Syndrome.* New York: Prentice Hall, 1990.

Heinerman, John. *Double the Power of Your Immune System.* New York: Parker, 1991.

Hoffman, Ronald, MD. *Tired All the Time.* New York: Poseidon Press, 1993.

Horowitz, Mark, MD, and Marietta Abrams-Brill. *Living with Lupus.* New York: Plume, 1994.

Lark, Susan M., MD. *Dr. Susan Lark's Chronic Fatigue Self-Help Book.* Berkeley, Calif.: Celestial Arts, 1995.

Sussman, Lesley. *Relief from Hay Fever and Other Airborne Allergies.* New York: Dell Medical Library, 1992.

Thom, Dick W. *Surviving the Nineties: Coping with Food Intolerances.* Portland, Ore.: Better Impressions, 1991.

PERIODICALS

"Fail to Snooze, Immune Cells Lose." *Science News,* January 7, 1995.

Fettner, Ann Guidici. "DHEA Gets Respect." *Harvard Health Letter,* July 1994.

Foster, Daniel. "Quiet Resistance." *Cooking Light,* March 1995.

Langer, Stephen, MD, and James Scheer. "Chronic Fatigue Syndrome: Coping Naturally." *Energy Times,* January/February 1995.

"Postherpetic Neuralgia: Preventive Measures." *HealthFacts,* December 1994.

Stone, Arthur, et al. "Daily Events Are Associated with a Secretory Immune Response to an Oral Antigen in Men." *Health Psychology,* 1994, Vol. 13, no. 5.

OTHER SOURCES

"Hopkins Research Links Chronic Fatigue and Blood Pressure." Press release. Johns Hopkins Children's Center, March 9, 1995.

"Study Shows Bacterial DNA Can Cause Lupus in Mice: Result Implicates Bacterial Infection in Human Lupus." Press release. Duke University, March 6, 1995.

INFECTIONS

BOOKS

Bell, David S., MD. *Curing Fatigue: A Step-by-Step Plan to Uncover and Eliminate the Causes of Chronic Fatigue.* Emmaus, Pa.: Rodale Press, 1993.

Lark, Susan M., MD. *Chronic Fatigue and Tiredness.* Los Altos, Calif.: Westchester, 1993.

PERIODICALS

"Cold Comfort: Chicken Soup . . . and Alcohol?" *Consumer Reports on Health,* February 1994.

"Guide to OTC Cold Products: Guidelines for Patients." *Nursing,* September 1994.

Hamlin, Suzanne. "Take 2 Bowls of Garlic Pasta, Then Call Me in the Morning." *New York Times,* January 25, 1995.

Heinerman, John. "Stinking Rose Gives Sweet Relief, Naturally: Garlic's Antibiotic Properties May Help Prevent, Shorten Colds and Flu Misery." *Health News & Review,* Winter 1994.

Hemila, H. "Does Vitamin C Alleviate the Symptoms of the Common Cold?" (abstract). *Scandinavian Journal of Infectious Diseases,* March 21, 1994.

"Is It a Cold or the Flu That's Bugging You?" *Washington Post,* March 21, 1995.

Kantor, F. S. "Disarming Lyme Disease." *Scientific American,* September 1994.

Langer, Stephan. "Optimal Nutrition to Fight Colds and Flu." *Better Nutrition for Today's Living,* February 1994.

Levy, Joseph. "Newborn Jaundice." *Parents Magazine,* July 1994.

Lewis, R. "Getting Lyme Disease to Take a Hike." *FDA Consumer,* June 1994.

"Lingering Lyme Disease." *Science News,* January 7, 1995.

McCaleb, Rob. "Herbal Remedies That Won't Leave You Out in the Cold." *Better Nutrition for Today's Living,* October 1994.

Middleton, D. B. "Tick-Borne Infections: What Starts as a Tiny Bite May Have a Serious Outcome." *Postgraduate Medicine,* April 1994.

Moore, Patrick S., and Claire V. Broome. "Cerebrospinal Meningitis Epidemics." *Scientific American,* November 1994.

Pfister, H. W., et al. "Lyme Borreliosis: Basic Science and Clinical Aspects." *Lancet,* April 23, 1994.

Sabe, K. S., and J. F. Reinhardt. "Rocky Mountain Spotted Fever versus Lyme Disease" (letter). *Southern Medical Journal,* 1995, Vol. 88, p. 248.

Schemo, Diana Jean. "Prolonged Lyme Treatments Posing Risks, Experts Warn." *New York Times,* January 4, 1994.

Sigal, L. H. "Persisting Complaints Attributed to Chronic Lyme Disease: Possible Mechanisms and Implications for Management." *American Journal of Medicine,* April 1994.

"The Value of Early Treatment of Deer Tick Bites for the Prevention of Lyme Disease" AMA Specialty Journal Abstracts. *Journal of the American Medical Association,* January 12, 1994.

"Viruses." *National Geographic,* July 1994.

OTHER SOURCES

Home Health Handbook. "Lyme Disease." Pittsburgh: International Masters Publishers, 1992.

Miller, L. E. "Lyme Disease Treatment Categories." Notes from 6th Annual Lyme Disease Scientific Conference, Atlantic City, N.J., May 5-6, 1993.

"Rocky Mountain Spotted Fever." Mimeograph. New York State Department of Health, December 9, 1994.

LUNG AND RESPIRATORY PROBLEMS

BOOK

Breathe Easy: Self-Help for Respiratory Ailments. Emmaus, Pa.: Rodale Press, 1994.

PERIODICALS

Altman, Lawrence K.: "Scientists Say Gene Is Linked to Asthma." *New York Times,* June 7, 1994.

"Surgery Found to Help Emphysema Patients." *New York Times,* April 28, 1994.

Sue, D. Y. "Community-Acquired Pneumonia in Adults." *Western Journal of Medicine,* 1994, Vol. 161, pp. 383-389.

Willensky, Diana. "How It Works: Lungs." *American Health,* April 1994.

MEN'S HEALTH

BOOKS

Lafavore, Michael. *Men's Health Advisor.* Emmaus, Pa.: Rodale Press, 1992.

Oppenheim, Michael. *The Man's Health Book.* Englewood Cliffs, N.J.: Prentice Hall, 1994.

PERIODICALS

Boyd, S. D., and P. Narayan. "Management of Benign Prostatic Hyperplasia." *Western Journal of Medicine,* February 1994.

Bruskewitz, R. C. "Benign Prostatic Hyperplasia" (editorial). *Journal of Urology,* June 1994.

Goluboff, E. T., and C. A. Olsson. "Urologists on a Tightrope: Coping with a Changing Economy." *Journal of Urology,* January 1-4, 1994.

Guess, H. A. "The Natural History of Benign Prostatic Hyperplasia: Implications for Patient Care and Clinical Trial Design." *European Urology,* June 1994.

Hill, S. J. "New Use for Alpha Blockers: Benign Prostatic Hyperplasia." *American Family Physician,* 1994, Vol. 49, pp. 1885-1888.

Roberts, R. G. "BPH: New Guidelines Based on Symptoms and Patient Preference: The Agency for Health Care Policy and Research." *Geriatrics,* July 1994.

Stoner, E. "Three-Year Safety and Efficacy Data on the Use of Finasteride in the Treatment of BPH." *Urology,* March 1994.

MENTAL HEALTH

BOOKS

Goldman, H. H., ed. *Review of General Psychiatry* (4th ed.). Norwalk, Conn.: Appleton & Lange, 1995.

Goodwin, Fredrick K., and Kay Redfield Jamison. *Manic-Depressive Illness.* New York: Oxford University Press, 1990.

Hartmann, Thom. *Attention Deficit Disorder: A Different Perception.* Penn Valley, Calif.: Underwood-Miller, 1993.

Kaplan, Harold I., MD, Benjamin J. Sadock, MD, and Jack A. Grebb, MD. *Synopsis of Psychiatry: Behavioral Sciences Clinical Psychiatry.* Baltimore: Williams and Wilkins, 1994.

Koziol, Leonard F., Chris E. Stout, and Douglas H. Ruben. *Handbook of Childhood Impulse Disorders and ADHD: Theory and Practice.* Springfield, Ill.: Charles C. Thomas, 1993.

Rosenthal, Norman E., MD. *Winter Blues: Seasonal Affective Disorder.* New York: Guilford Press, 1993.

Werbach, Melvyn R. *Nutritional Influence on Mental Illness.* Tarzana, Calif.: Third Line Press, 1991.

PERIODICALS

American Psychiatric Association. "Practice Guideline for the Treatment of Patients with Bipolar Disorder." *Ameri-*

can Journal of Psychiatry, December 1994.

"An Appetizing New Use for a Cancer Drug." *American Journal of Nursing,* April 1994.

Biley, F. C. "Effects of Noise in Hospitals." *British Journal of Nursing,* 1994, Vol. 3, pp. 110-113.

Brody, Jane. "Scientists Find Ways to Reset Biological Clocks in Dim Winter." *New York Times,* September 21, 1994.

Carpenter, W. T., Jr., and R. W. Buchanan. "Schizophrenia." *New England Journal of Medicine,* 1994, Vol. 330, pp. 681-689.

Conger, R. D., et al. "Economic Stress, Coercive Family Process, and Developmental Problems of Adolescents." *Child Development,* March 1994.

Fishman, Rachelle H. B. "Treating Depression." *Lancet,* November 5, 1994.

Green, Bonnie L. "Psychosocial Research in Traumatic Stress: An Update." *Journal of Traumatic Stress,* 1994, Vol. 7, no. 3, pp. 341-357.

Haugli, L., et al. "Health, Sleep, and Mood Perceptions Reported by Airline Crews Flying Short and Long Hauls." *Aviation, Space, and Environmental Medicine,* 1994, Vol. 65, pp. 17-34.

Huber, J. H., et al. "National and State Spending on Speciality Alcoholism Treatment: 1979 and 1989." *American Journal of Public Health,* October 1994.

Lark, Susan M., MD. "Strike Back at High Anxiety: Natural Ways to Stay Calm in Stressful Times." *Vegetarian Times,* February 1994.

Lepola, U. "Alcohol and Depression in Panic Disorder." *Acta Psychiatrica Scandinavica Supplementum,* 1994, Vol. 377, pp. 33-35.

Marder, S. R., and R. C. Meibach. "Risperidone in the Treatment of Schizophrenia." *American Journal of Psychiatry,* June 1994.

Marriott, P. F., et al. "Seasonality in Panic Disorder." *Journal of Affective Disorder,* June 1994.

"Melatonin Is Helpful for Insomnia, Jet Lag." *Better Nutrition for Today's Living,* September 1994.

Montano, C. Brendan, MD. "Recognition and Treatment of Depression in a Primary Care Setting." *Journal of Clinical Psychiatry,* December 1994.

Oldenburg, Don. "Focus Is in the Eye of the Beholder: Is a Controversial Technique That Heals Trauma Victims Too Good to Be True?" *Washington Post,* April 12, 1994.

Pollack, M. H., et al. "Cognitive Behavior Therapy for Treatment-Refractory Panic Disorder." *Journal of Clinical Psychiatry,* May 1994.

Shaffer, David. "Attention Deficit Disorder in Adults." *American Journal of Psychiatry,* May 1994.

Southwick, S. M., et al. "Psychobiologic Research in Post-Traumatic Stress Disorder." *Psychiatric Clinics of North America,* June 1994.

Spiegel, D. A., et al. "Does Cognitive Behavior Therapy Assist Slow-Taper Alprazolam Discontinuation in Panic Disorder?" *American Journal of Psychiatry,* June 1994.

Sutherland, S. M., and J. R. Davidson. "Pharmacotherapy for Post-Traumatic Stress Disorder," *Psychiatric Clinics of North America,* June 1994.

Terman, Michael, and Jiuan Su Terman. "Treatment of Seasonal Affective Disorder with a High-Output Negative Ionizer." *Journal of Alternative and Complementary Medicine,* January 1995.

Wharton, Ralph N., and Ronald R. Fieve. "The Use of Lithium in the Affective Psychoses." Sesquicentennial Anniversary Supplement, 1844-1994: IV; Developments in Somatic Treatment. *American Journal of Psychiatry,* June 1994.

OTHER SOURCE

Brunner, Philip R. "Attention Deficit Disorder and Specific Learning Disability: A Handbook for Parents." Kaiser-Permanente, Southern California Permanente Medical Group, no date.

MIND/BODY MEDICINE

BOOKS

Basmajian, J. V., ed. *Biofeedback: Principles and Practice for Clinicians.* Baltimore: Williams and Wilkins, 1984.

Bell, Lorna, and Eudora Seyfer. *Gentle Yoga.* Berkeley, Calif.: Celestial Arts, 1987.

Benson, Herbert:

The Relaxation Response. Avenal, N.J.: Random House Value, 1992.

The Wellness Book. New York: Simon & Schuster, 1993.

Blumenfeld, Larry. *The Big Book of Relaxation.* Rosalyn, N.Y.: The Relaxation Company, 1994.

Bricklin, Mark, et al. *Positive Living and Health: The Complete Guide to Brain/Body Healing and Mental Empowerment.* Emmaus, Pa.: Rodale Press, 1990.

Epstein, Gerald. *Healing Visualizations: Creating Health through*

Imagery. New York: Bantam Books, 1989.

Erickson, Milton, Seymour Hershman, and Irving I. Secter. *The Practical Application of Medical and Dental Hypnosis.* New York: Brunner Mazel, 1991.

Goleman, Daniel, and Joel Gurin, eds. *Mind Body Medicine: How to Use Your Mind for Better Health.* Yonkers, N.Y.: Consumer Reports Books, 1993.

Lidell, Lucy, et al. *The Sivananda Companion to Yoga.* New York: Simon & Schuster, 1983.

Loehr, James E., and Jeffrey A. Migdow, MD. *Take a Deep Breath.* New York: Villard Books, 1986.

Monro, Robin, R. Nagarathna, and R. H. Nagendra. *Yoga for Common Ailments.* New York: Simon & Schuster, 1990.

Moyers, Bill. *Healing and the Mind.* New York: Doubleday, 1993.

Zi, Nancy. *The Art of Breathing.* Glendale, Calif.: Vivi Books, 1994.

MUSCULOSKELETAL PROBLEMS

BOOKS

Appenzeller, O., ed. *Sports Medicine: Fitness, Training, Injuries* (3d ed.). Baltimore: Urban & Schwarzenberg, 1988.

Bradford, D. S., et al. *Moe's Textbook of Scoliosis and Other Spine Deformities* (3d ed.) Philadelphia: W. B. Saunders, 1994.

Brewer, Earl J., and Kathy Cochran Angel. *The Arthritis Sourcebook.* Chicago: Contemporary Books, 1993.

Crouch, Tammy, and Michael Madden. *Carpal Tunnel Syndrome and Overuse Injuries: Prevention, Treatment, Recovery.* Berkeley, Calif.: North Atlantic Books, 1992.

Foot Owner's Manual. San Bruno, Calif.: Krames Communications, 1984.

Fries, James F., MD. *Arthritis: A Comprehensive Guide* (3d ed.). Reading, Mass.: Addison-Wesley, 1990.

Griffith, H. Winter, MD. *Complete Guide to Sports Injuries: How to Treat Fractures, Bruises, Sprains, Strains, Dislocations and Head Injuries.* Tuscon, Ariz.: Body Press, 1986.

Guten, Gary N., MD. *Play Healthy, Stay Healthy: Your Guide to Managing and Treating 40 Common Sports Injuries.* Champaign, Ill.: Leisure Press, 1991.

Harries, M., et al., eds. *Oxford Textbook of Sports Medicine.* New York: Oxford University Press, 1994.

Hochschuler, Stephen, MD. *Back in Shape.* Boston: Houghton Mifflin, 1991.

Kantrowitz, Fred G., MD. *Taking Control of Arthritis.* New York: HarperCollins, 1990.

Ward, Robert C., ed. *Foundations for Osteopathic Medicine.* Baltimore: Williams and Wilkins/Waverly Press, in press.

Zimmerman, Julie. *The Almanac of Back Pain Treatments.* Brunswick, Maine: Biddle, 1991.

PERIODICALS

"Are Diagnostic Tests for Neck Pain Useless?" *The Back Letter,* May 1994.

Barry, M., and J. R. Jenner. "Pain in Neck, Shoulder, and Arm" (abstract). *British Medical Journal,* January 21, 1995.

Bentley, G., and S. T. Donell. "Scoliosis in Childhood and Its Management." *British Journal of Rheumatology,* 1994, Vol. 33, no. 5, pp. 486-494.

Clark, H. Vondell, et al. "Carotidynia." *American Family Physician,* October 1994.

"Common Whiplash Treatment Discredited." *The Back Letter,* May 1994.

Dvorak, John C. "Mouse Shoulder: A New Ailment." *PC Magazine,* December 6, 1994.

Hill, Larry, and Glen Hastings. "Carotidynia: A Pain Syndrome." *Journal of Family Practice,* July 1994.

Jeffrey, Isaac. "Dislocation on Location." *Field & Stream,* February 1994.

Krstulovich, Diane. "When Structure Equals Function: Osteopathic Physicians Treat the Whole Patient." *Vegetarian Times,* June 1994.

Roth, James. "Endoscopic Carpal Tunnel Release" (abstract). *Journal of the American Medical Association,* September 14, 1994.

Rovner, Sandy. "Back to Basics with Backs." *Washington Post,* December 13, 1994.

Winter, R. B. "The Pendulum Has Swung Too Far: Bracing for Adolescent Scoliosis in the 1990s." *Orthopedic Clinics of North America,* 1994, Vol. 25, no. 2, pp. 195-204.

NEUROLOGICAL PROBLEMS

BOOKS

Bair, Frank E., ed. *Alzheimer's, Stroke, and 29 Other Neurological Disorders Sourcebook.* Detroit: Omnigraphics, 1993.

Devinsky, Orrin, MD. *A Guide to Understanding and Living with Epilepsy.* Philadelphia: F. A. Davis, 1994.

PERIODICALS

"Apo E: Caught inside the Nerve Cell." *Science News,* August 13, 1994.
Austin, Elizabeth. "Migraine Mania." *Shape,* December 1994.
Baker, Beth. "Outsmarting Alzheimer's." *American Association of Retired Persons Bulletin,* October 1994.
Barinaga, Marcia. "Possible New Test Found for Alzheimer's Disease." *Science,* November 11, 1994.
Blakeslee, Sandra. "Substance Hailed as Tool to Fight Neurodegenerative Disease." *New York Times,* January 31, 1995.
Brownlee, Shannon. "Hopeful Hunt for an Alzheimer's Cure." *U.S. News & World Report,* November 21, 1994.
Bulkeley, William M. "E-Mail Medicine." *Wall Street Journal,* February 27, 1995.
"Can Alternative Medicine Help My Headache?" *U.S.A. Weekend,* December 30, 1994-January 1, 1995.
Davies, Karen N., et al. "A Study of the Nutritional Status of Elderly Patients with Parkinson's." *Age and Ageing,* March 1994.
"Diet and Parkinson's: A Review." *Nutrition Research Newsletter,* April 1994.
"Environmental and Genetic Factors in Parkinson's Disease." *American Family Physician,* January 1994.
Fenwick, P. "The Behavioral Treatment of Epilepsy Generation and Inhibition of Seizures." *Neurologic Clinics,* February 1994.
Gorman, Christine. "An Eye on Alzheimer's." *Time,* November 21, 1994.
Hewitt, Bill, et al. "Into the Twilight." *People,* November 21, 1994.
"Implants in Monkeys Aid Alzheimer's Researchers." *Wall Street Journal,* November 8, 1994.
Kaiser, Jocelyn. "Alzheimer's: Could There Be a Zinc Link?" *Science,* September 2, 1994.
Kolata, Gina. "A Simpler Test for Alzheimer's Is Reported." *New York Times,* November 11, 1994.
Limousin, Patricia, et al. "Effect on Parkinsonian Signs and Symptoms of Bilateral Subthalamic Nucleus Stimulation." *Lancet,* January 14, 1995.
McFarling, Usha Lee. "Beating Pain without Pills or Surgery." *Natural Health,* January/February 1995.
"Many Diets Touted for MS, but No Proven Winners." *Environmental Nutrition,* March 1994.
Munson, Marty, and Greg Gutfeld. "Hormones from Heaven: Can Estrogen Tame Alzheimer's Disease?" *Prevention,* April 1994.
Schapiro, R. T. "Symptom Management in Multiple Sclerosis." *Annals of Neurology,* 1994, Vol. 36, supplement, pp. S123-S129.
Seligmann, Jean, and Karen Springen. "Progress on Alzheimer's." *Newsweek,* November 21, 1994.
Smith, Susan Male. "New 7:1 Diet May Offer Better Odds for Parkinson's Patients." *Environmental Nutrition,* May 1994.
Stipp, David. "Pupil-Dilation Test Appears Promising for the Detection of Alzheimer's Disease." *Wall Street Journal,* November 11, 1994.
Stoneham, Laurie. "Progress in Treating Progressive Multiple Sclerosis." *Living with Multiple Sclerosis,* September 1994.

OTHER SOURCES

"Cephalon Initiates Phase II Clinical Trials of Myotrophin for the Treatment of ALS." Press release. Cephalon, 1993.
"Zinc Is Implicated in the Formation of Alzheimer's Lesions." Press release. Washington, D.C.: Society for Neuroscience, September 1, 1994.

NUTRITION AND DIET

BOOKS

Aihara, Cornellia, and Herman Aihara. *Natural Healing from Head to Toe: Traditional Macrobiotic Remedies.* Garden City Park, N.Y.: Avery, 1994.
Balch, James, and Phyllis Balch. *Prescription for Nutritional Healing.* Garden City Park, N.Y.: Avery, 1990.
Barnard, Neal. *Food for Life: How the New Four Food Groups Can Save Your Life.* New York: Crown, 1993.
Carper, Jean. *The Food Pharmacy.* New York: Bantam Books, 1988.
Griffith, H. Winter. *Complete Guide to Vitamins, Minerals, Nutrients, and Supplements.* Tucson, Ariz.: Fisher Books, 1988.
Hausman, Patricia, and Judith Benn Hurley. *The Healing Foods.* Emmaus, Pa.: Rodale Press, 1989.
Health Media of America and Elizabeth Somer. *The Essential Guide to Vitamins and Minerals.* New York: HarperPerennial, 1992.
Hendler, Sheldon Saul, MD. *The*

Doctors Vitamin and Mineral Encyclopedia. New York: Fireside Books, 1990.

Herbert, Victor. *Total Nutrition: The Only Guide You'll Ever Need —From the Mount Sinai School of Medicine.* New York: St. Martin, 1994.

Herbert, Victor, and Stephen Barrett. *Modern Nutrition in Health and Disease* (Vol. 2, 8th ed.). Edited by M. E. Shils, J. A. Olson, and M. Shike. Philadelphia: Lea and Fabiger, 1994.

Krause, Marie, and Kathleen Mahan. *Food, Nutrition, and Diet Therapy* (7th ed.). Philadelphia: W. B. Saunders, 1984.

Margen, Sheldon, and the Editors of the Univeristy of California at Berkeley Wellness Letter. *The Wellness Encyclopedia of Food and Nutrition.* New York: Rebus, 1992.

Mindell, Earl. *Earl Mindell's Vitamin Bible.* New York: Warner Books, 1991.

Rosenbaum, Michael E., and Dominick Bosco. *Super Supplements.* New York: Signet Books, 1989.

Ulene, Art, MD, and Val Ulene, MD. *The Vitamin Strategy.* Berkeley, Calif.: Ulysses Press, 1994.

Werbach, Melvyn R., MD: *Healing through Nutrition.* New York: HarperCollins, 1993. *Nutritional Influences on Illness* (2d ed.). Taranza, Calif.: Third Line Press, 1993.

Winter, Ruth. *A Consumer's Guide to Medicines in Food.* New York: Crown Trade Paperbacks, 1995.

PERIODICALS

Herbert, Victor, and Tracy Stopler Kasdan. "Misleading Nutrition Claims and Their Gurus." *Nutrition Today,* May/June 1994.

Webb, Denise. "Vitamins, Minerals, Potions and Pills." *American Health,* July/August 1995.

SEXUAL HEALTH

BOOKS

Baum, Neil, *ECNETOPMI-Impotence: It's Reversible.* Van Buren, Ark.: Southwest Impotency Center, 1993.

Novotny, Pamela Patrick. *What Women Should Know about Chronic Infections and Sexually Transmitted Diseases.* New York: Dell, 1991.

PERIODICALS

Agarwal, S. K., and A. F. Haney. "Does Recommending Timed Intercourse Really Help the Infertile Couple?" *Obstetrics & Gynecology,* August 1994.

Dean, N. L., and R. G. Edwards. "Oocyte Donation: Implications for Fertility Treatment in the Nineties." *Current Opinion in Obstetrics & Gynecology,* April 1994.

Goldstein, I. "Impotence" (editorial). *Journal of Urology,* June 1994.

Morales, A. "Impotence" (editorial). *Journal of Urology,* May 1994.

Nachtsheim, D. "Treating Impotence" (letter). *Western Journal of Medicine,* February 1994.

Naz, R. K., and A. C. Menge. "Antisperm Antibodies: Origin, Regulation, and Sperm Reactivity in Human Infertility." *Fertility and Sterility,* June 1994.

Nessel, M. A. "Yohimbine and Pentoxifylline in the Treatment of Erectile Dysfunction" (letter). *American Journal of Psychiatry,* March 1994.

Yavetz, H., et al. "Retrograde Ejaculation." *Human Reproduction,* March 1994.

OTHER SOURCE

Clark, Kay. "Talking with Your Partner about Herpes" (pamphlet). Santa Cruz, Calif.: Network Publications, 1984.

SKIN AND HAIR PROBLEMS

BOOK

Kotler, Robert. *Chemical Rejuvenation of the Face.* St. Louis: Mosby-Year Book, 1992.

PERIODICALS

Ballo, Frances. "Fracture Blisters." *Journal of the American Academy of Dermatology,* June 1994.

Fletcher, Jacqui. "Pressure Sore Prevention." *Nursing Times,* June 15-21, 1994.

Lontz, Werner, et al. "Pigment Cell Transplantation for Treatment of Vitiligo." *Journal of the American Academy of Dermatology,* April 1994.

Lyons, Paula. "The Most Dangerous Medicine." *Ladies Home Journal,* June 1994.

Marks, Robin. "Sunburn and Melanoma: How Strong Is the Evidence." *British Medical Journal,* January 8, 1994.

"A New Season Brings Dangers of Scalding." *Washington Post,* September 20, 1994.

"Nurse-Aid Management of Burns." *British Journal of Nursing,* 1994, Vol. 9, no. 3.

Olsson, Mats, et al. "Vitiligo: Repigmentation with Cultured Melanocytes." *Acta Dermato-Venereologica,* May 1994.

Picaquadio, Daniel, et al. "Obesity and Female Androgenic Alopecia: A Cause and Effect?" *Journal of the American Academy of Dermatology,* June 1994.

Sargent, Susie, and Jena Martin. "Scabies Outbreak in a Day Care Center." *Supplement to*

Pediactrics, December 1994.
Savin, Ronald, et al. "Terbinafine and Tinea Pedis." *Journal of the American Academy of Dermatology,* April 1994.
"Short Shadow Rule for Avoiding Sunburn." *Medical Update,* August 1994.
Wang, Sue-Jane, et al. "Increased Risk of Type I Diabetes in Relatives of Patients with Alopecia Areata." *American Journal of Medical Genetics,* July 1, 1994.
Winslow, Elizabeth. "Mattresses That Spell Pressure R-E-L-I-E-F." *American Journal of Nursing,* September 1994.

SUBSTANCE ABUSE

BOOK

Covington, Stephanie. *A Woman's Way through the 12-Steps.* San Francisico: Hazelden, 1994.

PERIODICALS

Burman, S. "The Disease Concept of Alcoholism: Its Impact on Women's Treatment." *Journal of Substance-Abuse Treatment,* 1994, Vol. 11, pp. 121-126.
Califano, Joseph A., Jr. "It's Drugs, Stupid." *New York Times Magazine,* January 29, 1995.
Comings, D. E. "Genetic Factors in Substance Abuse Based on Studies of Tourette Syndrome and ADHD Probands and Relatives." *Drug and Alcohol Dependence,* 1994, Vol. 35, pp. 1-16.
Ennett, S. T., et al. "Long-Term Evaluation of Drug Abuse Resistance Education." *Addictive Behavior,* March-April 1994.
Kendler, K. S., et al. "A Twin-Family Study of Alcoholism in Women." *American Journal of Psychiatry,* May 1994.
Lieb, R. J., and N. P. Young. "A Case-Specific Approach to the Treatment of Alcoholism: The Application of Control Mastery Theory to Alcoholics Anonymous and Professional Practice." *Journal of Substance-Abuse Treatment,* January-February 1994.
Maltzman, I. "Why Alcoholism Is a Disease." *Journal of Psychoactive Drugs,* January-March 1994.
Mann, K. "Alcoholism: Still an Inferior Disease?" (editorial). *Addiction,* 1994, Vol. 89, pp. 5-7.
Moos, R. H. "Why Do Some People Recover from Alcohol Dependence, whereas Others Continue to Drink and Become Worse over Time?" *Addiction,* 1994, Vol. 89, pp. 31-34.
Mulford, H. A. "What If Alcoholism Had Not Been Invented? The Dynamics of American Alcohol Mythology." *Addiction,* May 1994.
"Reasons for Tobacco Use and Symptoms of Nicotine Withdrawal." *Journal of the American Medical Association,* December 7, 1994.
Sherman, Carl. "Kicking Butts." *Psychology Today,* September/October 1994.
"Smoking Cessation Aided by a Variety of Methods." *Menninger Letter,* May 1995.
"Treatment of Alcoholism." *Journal of Substance-Abuse Treatment,* March-April 1994.
Wing, D. M. "Understanding Alcoholism Relapse: A Case Study Illustrating the Integration of Two Theories." *Nurse Practitioner,* April 1994.

URINARY TRACT PROBLEMS

BOOK

Corriere J. N., ed. *Essentials of Urology.* New York: Churchill Livingstone, 1986.

PERIODICALS

Avorn, Jerry, MD, et al. "Reduction of Bacteriuria and Pyuria after Ingestion of Cranberry Juice." *Journal of the American Medical Association,* March 9, 1994.
Fleet, James C. "New Support for a Folk Remedy: Cranberry Juice Reduces Bacteriuria and Pyuria in Elderly Women." *Nutrition Reviews,* May 1994.

WOMEN'S HEALTH

BOOKS

Breast Diseases (2d ed.). Philadelphia: Lippincott, 1991.
Carlson, Karen J., and Stephanie A. Eisenstat, eds. *Primary Care of Women.* St. Louis: Mosby, 1995.
Current Obstetric and Gynecologic Diagnosis and Treatment (8th ed.). Norwalk, Conn.: Appleton & Lange, 1994.
Dalton, Katherina. *Once a Month* (4th ed.). Claremont, Calif.: Hunter House, 1990.
Eisenberg, Arlene, Heidi Eisenberg Murkoff, and Sandee Eisenberg Hathaway. *What to Expect When You're Expecting.* New York: Workman, 1991.
Foley, Denise, and Eileen Nechas. *Women's Encyclopedia of Health and Emotional Healing.* Emmaus, Pa.: Rodale Press, 1993.
Gaby, Alan. *Preventing and Reversing Osteoporosis: Every Woman's Essential Guide.* Rocklin, Calif.: Prima, 1993.
Gynecology: Well-Woman Care. Norwalk, Conn.: Appleton & Lange, 1990.
Hudson, Tori. *Gynecology and*

Naturopathic Medicine: A Treatment Manual. Olympia, Wash.: C. K. E. Publications, 1993.

Northrup, Christiane, MD. *Women's Bodies, Women's Wisdom: Creating Physical and Emotional Health and Healing.* New York: Bantam Books, 1994.

Perry, Susan, and Katherine O'Hanlan, MD. *Natural Menopause: The Complete Guide to a Woman's Most Misunderstood Passage.* New York: Addison-Wesley, 1992.

Shephard, Bruce, MD, and Carroll A. Shephard. *The Complete Guide to Women's Health.* New York: Plume, 1990.

Stoppard, Miriam. *Everywoman's Medical Handbook.* New York: Ballantine Books, 1988.

Women: How to Understand Your Symptoms. New York: Random House, 1986.

PERIODICALS

Bachman, Gloria A. "The Changes Before 'the Change.' " *Postgraduate Medicine,* March 1994.

"Consensus Development Conference: Diagnosis, Prophylaxis, and Treatment of Osteoporosis." *American Journal of Medicine,* June 1994.

Curtis, Nigel, Barbara Chan, and Michael Levin. "Toxic Shock Syndrome Toxin-Secreting Staphylococcus Aureus in Kawasaki Syndrome." *Lancet,* January 29, 1994.

Oldenhave, Anna. "Pathogenesis of Climacteric Complaints: Ready for the Change?" *Lancet,* March 12, 1994.

"Safety of Some Calcium Supplements Questioned." *Nutrition Reviews,* March 1994.

MISCELLANEOUS

BOOKS

Harkless, Lawrence, and Steven Krych. *Handbook of Common Foot Problems.* New York: Churchill Livingstone, 1990.

Harte, John, et al. *Toxics A to Z: A Guide to Everyday Pollution Hazards.* Berkeley: University of California Press, 1991.

McGee, Charles T., and Effie Chow. *Miracle Healing from China: Qigong.* Coeur D'Alene, Idaho: Medi Press, 1994.

PERIODICALS

Broccolo-Philbin, Anne. "Don't Make Waves." *Current Health,* December 2, 1994.

Claes, Goran, and Christer Drott. "Hyperhidrosis." *Lancet,* January 29, 1994.

"Curing the Ills of Summer." Health Tips. *Mother Earth News,* June-July 1994.

Drewnowski, Adam. "Body Weight and Dieting in Adolescence: Impact of Socialeconomic Status." *International Journal of Eating Disorders,* 1994, Vol. 16, pp. 61-65.

French, Simone, et al. "Weight Concerns, Dieting and Smoking Initiation among Adolescents." *American Journal of Public Health,* November 1994.

French, Simone, and Robert Jeffery. "Consequences of Dieting to Lose Weight: Effect on Physical and Mental Health." *Health Psychology,* 1994, Vol. 13, pp. 195-212.

Judge, Gillian. "Cures for Holiday Health Hazards." *McCall's,* December 1994.

Kolata, Gina. "Metabolism Found to Adjust for Body's Natural Weight." *New York Times,* March 9, 1995.

Kuehnel, Robert, and Thomas Warden. "Binge Eating, Weight Cycling." *International Journal of Eating Disorders,* 1994, Vol. 15, pp. 321-332.

Melinyk, Mary Grace, and Estelle Weinstein. "Preventing Obesity in Black Women." *Journal of the American Diabetic Association,* May 1994.

Munson, Marty, et al. "Antinausea Trick." *Prevention,* June 1994.

O'Keeffe, S. T., et al. "Iron Status and Restless Legs Syndrome in the Elderly." *Age and Ageing,* May 1994.

Panton, Ormond, and Rhona Panton. "Laparoscopic Hernia Repair." *American Journal of Surgery,* May 1994.

Prager, Ellen J. "Seasickness: A Sacrifice to Neptune." *Sea Frontiers,* August 1994.

Reisman, R. E. "Insect Stings." *New England Journal of Medicine,* August 25, 1994.

Schwartz, John. "A Genetic Signal Gone Awry May Nourish Obesity." *Washington Post,* December 1, 1994.

"A Soothing Shock: A Little Electricity Helps Ease Nausea." *Prevention,* January 1994.

Stevens, June, et al. "Attitudes toward Body Size and Dieting: Differences between Elderly Black and White Women." *American Journal of Public Health,* August 1994.

"Study Scorns Over-Control of a Fat Child." *New York Times,* November 10, 1994.

Vgontzas, Alenxdros. "Sleep Apnea and Sleep Disruption in Obese Patients." *Archives of Internal Medicine,* August 8, 1994.

"Why Are You Dizzy?" *Health News,* June 1994.

WHERE TO FIND MORE INFORMATION ELECTRONICALLY

FAX INFORMATION SERVICES

CancerFax
National Cancer Institute
(301) 402-5874;
(800) 624-2511

CDC Fax Information Service
Centers for Disease Control
(888) 232-3299

Mental Health FAX4U
National Institute of Mental Health
(301) 443-5158

CD-ROMs

A number of medical CD-ROMS are available, including:

- Cancerlit
- The Family Doctor
- Health Index on InfoTrac
- Health Reference Center
- Mayo Clinic Family Health Book
- Mayo Clinic Family Pharmacist
- MDX Health Digest
- MEDLINE
- PharmAssist: The Family Guide to Health and Medicine
- Physician's Data Query
- Physician's Desk Reference on CD-ROM
- The Pill Book
- USP DI, Volume II, Advice for the Patient

INTERNET WEBSITES

Please note that many of the Health Associations and Organizations listed on pages 1071-1075 also have internet websites.

The Alternative Medicine Homepage
www.pitt.edu/~cbw/altm.html

AltHealth Search
www.althealthsearch.com

AMED: Allied and Complementary Medicine Database
www.bl.uk/services/stb/amed.html

American Medical Association Health Insight
www.ama-assn.org/consumer.htm

Ask Noah (New York Online Access to Health)
www.noah.cuny.edu/qksearch.html

Go Ask Alice!, Columbia University
www.goaskalice.columbia.edu/1424.html

Healthfinder
www.healthfinder.gov

Healthworld Online
www.healthy.net

LaurusHealth.com
laurushealth.com

MedHelp International
www.medhelp.org

Medical Matrix Database
www.medmatrix.org

Medinex
www.medinex.com

MEDLINE Plus, National Library of Medicine
www.nlm.nih.gov/medlineplus/

National Center for Complementary and Alternative Medicine
nccam.nih.gov

PDR.net for Consumers
www.pdr.net/consumer

Support Links
www.americanhealthvalue.com/healthy_links.html

Top Seven Alternative Medicine Sites
www.topseven.com/altmed.htm

CANCER

Center for Alternative Medicine Research in Cancer, University of Texas
www.sph.uth.tmc.edu/utcam/default.htm

CancerNet, National Cancer Institute
cancernet.nci.nih.gov

DRUG DATABASES

Consumer Drug Information Database
www.fda.gov/cder/drug/default.htm

USP DI, Volume II, Advice for the Patient: Drug Information in Lay Language
health.phillynews.com/pharmacy/search.asp

PharmInfoNet Drug Database
pharminfo.com/drugdb/db_mnu.html

REFERENCE

MEDLINE, National Library of Medicine
www.nlm.nih.gov/databases/freemedl.html

The On-line Medical Dictionary
www.graylab.ac.uk/omd/index.html

MISCELLANEOUS

Mental Health Net
mentalhelp.net

National Organization for Rare Disorders Inc. (NORD)
www.rarediseases.org

The National Women's Health Information Center (NWHIC)
www.4women.gov

Pediatric Database
www.icondata.com/health/pedbase

Yahoo Search Service
dir.yahoo.com/health/index.html

INDEX

Page numbers in italics refer to illustrations or illustrated text.

A

Abana (Ayurvedic remedy), 126
Abdominal pains: *chart*, 84-87; acupressure for, *650*; in pregnancy, 688
Abdominal thrusts, *54*, *55*
Abrasions, 304, 305
Abscesses, *773*, *774*, *775*; appendix, 138, 139; diverticula, *331*; teeth, 362-363, 372-373, 836, *837*; tonsillar, 834-835
Accupril (quinapril), 998
ACE (angiotensin-converting enzyme) inhibitors, 890-891; interactions with, 915, 931, 939, 995
Acetaminophen, 884, 889; in combinations, 927, 942, 959-960, 987, 988, 997; interactions with, 984
Acetohexamide, 319
Acetylcarnitine, 112
Acetylcholine, 660, 661, 937, 1034
Aches and pains, *chart*, 88-89
Achillea millefolium (yarrow), 1023; in combinations, 911, 918, 934, 941
Achilleine, 1023
Achilles tendonitis, 128-129
Achilletin, 1023
Acne, 90-93
Acne neonatorum; acne infantum, 91
Aconite, 884
Acorus calamus (sweet flag), 475
Acquired immune deficiency syndrome (AIDS), 96-101
Acromioclavicular joint (AC) separation, 158, 159, 160
Actein, 908
Actifed (pseudoephedrine, triprolidine), 997, 1019
Actinic keratoses, 758, 794
Acupressure, 20, *22-23*, *1076-1084*; Bladder 10 (BL 10), *246*, *1076*; Bladder 13 (BL 13), *1076*; Bladder 23 (BL 23), *1076*; Bladder 25 (BL 25), *1076*; Bladder 32 (BL 32), *1076*; Bladder 40 (BL 40), *1076*; Conception Vessel 4 (CV 4), *592*, *1077*; Conception Vessel 6 (CV 6), *290*, *596*, *1077*; Conception Vessel 12 (CV 12), *1077*; Conception Vessel 17 (CV 17), *303*, *1077*; Conception Vessel 22 (CV 22), *1077*; Gall Bladder 2 (GB 2), *445*, *1078*; Gall Bladder 20 (GB 20), *246*, *438*, *650*, *832*, *1078*; Gall Bladder 21 (GB 21), 233, *246*, *650*, *1078*; Gall Bladder 34 (GB 34), *1078*; Gall Bladder 39 (GB 39), *1078*; Governing Vessel 4 (GV 4), *1078*; Governing Vessel 14 (GV 14), *1078*; Governing Vessel 20 (GV 20), *1079*; Governing Vessel 24.5 (GV 24.5), *434*, *438*, *1079*; Governing Vessel 25 (GV 25), *477*, *1079*; Heart 3 (HE 3), *1079*; Heart 7 (HE 7), *112*, *137*, *829*, *1079*; Hiccup 1 (palm pressure), *477*, *1084*; Kidney 1 (KI 1), *1079*; Kidney 3 (KI 3), *112*, *650*, *832*, *1079*; Large Intestine 4 (LI 4), *92*, *290*, *431*, *434*, *438*, *596*, *625*,*650*, *756*, *763*, *768*, *808*, *1080*; Large Intestine 10 (LI 10), *1080*; Large Intestine 11 (LI 11), *92*, *290*, *768*, *1080*; Large Intestine 20 (LI 20), *756*, *1080*; Liver 2 (LV 2), *112*, *832*, *1080*; Liver 3 (LV 3), *438*, *592*, *1080*; Liver 8 (LV 8), *310*, *577*, *1080*; Lung 1 (LU 1), *303*, *1081*; Lung 5 (LU 5), *297*, *1081*; Lung 7 (LU 7), *596*, *625*, *1081*; Lung 10 (LU 10), *768*, *1081*; palm pressure (Hiccup 1), *477*, *1084*; Pericardium 3 (PE 3), *480*, *1081*; Pericardium 6 (PE 6), *127*, *137*, *393*, *431*, *599*, *650*, *829*, *1081*; Shoulder Well, 99; Small Intestine 3 (SI 3), *246*, *1081*; Small Intestine 17 (SI 17), *599*, *768*, *1081*; Spleen 3 (SP 3), *112*, *1082*; Spleen 4 (SP 4), *1082*; Spleen 6 (SP 6), *127*, *191*, *480*, *592*, *650*, *697*, *1082*; Spleen 8 (SP 8), *592*, *1082*; Spleen 9 (SP 9), *1082*; Spleen 10 (SP 10), *191*, *1082*; Spleen 12 (SP 12), *1082*; Stomach 2 (ST 2), *1083*; Stomach 3 (ST 3), *438*, *1083*; Stomach 7 (ST 7), *808*, *1083*; Stomach 25 (ST 25), *519*, *1083*; Stomach 36 (ST 36), *290*, *393*, *596*, *650*, *1083*; Stomach 44 (ST 44), *650*, *1083*; TripleWarmer 3 (TW 3), *832*, *1084*; Triple Warmer 5 (TW 5), *650*, *763*, *1084*; Triple Warmer 6 (TW 6), *1084*; Triple Warmer 17 (TW 17), *445*, *832*, *1084*. *See also individual ailments*
Acupuncture, 20-21; point locations, *22-23*. *See also individual ailments*
Acute lymphocytic (lymphoblastic) leukemia (ALL), 546, 547, 548-549
Acute myelogenic leukemia (AML), 546, 547, 549
Acyclovir, 884-885
Adalat (nifedipine), 981
ADD (attention deficit disorder), 162-163
Addison's disease, 368-369
Adenocarcinomas: clear cell, 855; lung, 558, *559*
Adenoid problems, 94-95
Adenoids, 94, *95*
Adenomas: breast, 208, 211; thyroid, 824, 826
S-adenosylmethionine, 311
Adolescents, 36; acne, 90, 93; amenorrhea, 589; depression, 308; growing pains, 160, 538-539
Adrenal extract, 339
Adrenalin Chloride Solution (epinephrine), 942
Adrenaline, stress and, 597, 784
Adult-onset acne, 91
Adult-onset (Type 2) diabetes, 316, 317, 318, 319, 320, 321
Advil (ibuprofen), 961
Advil Cold and Sinus (ibuprofen, pseudoephedrine), 961, 997
Aerobic exercise, 99, 207, 455, 860
Aesculus, 117, 467
Aesculus hippocastanum (horse chestnut), 860
Aflatoxins, 528, 553
Afrin (oxymetazoline), 988
Agastache (*Agastache rugosa*), 885
Agathosma spp. (buchu), 911
Age-related macular degeneration (ARMD), 570-571
Aging: process of, 44-45. *See also* Elderly
Agoraphobia, 670, 671
Agrimony (*Agrimonia eupatoria*), 136, 434
AIDS, 96-101; treatment, 885-886
AIDS-related complex (ARC), 96
Air travel deafness, 447
Alanine, 705
Albuterol, 886
Alcohol: abuse of, 102-105, 618-619; as antiseptic, 897; and cirrhosis, 267, 268, 269; and flushed face, 380-381; and hangover, 430-431; interactions with, 884, 888, 890, 894, 895, 896, 898, 905, 906, 910, 913, 915, 917, 918, 925, 926, 933, 939, 943, 947, 956, 960, 962, 965, 978, 982, 983, 984, 985, 986, 987, 988, 992, 994, 996, 997, 999, 1012, 1022, 1024; and oral cancer, 634; for teething, danger of, 805; tinctures made with, 1025-1026
Alcoholic hepatitis, 267, 268, 469, 470
Alcoholics Anonymous (AA), 105
Alendronate, 637-638
Aletris farinosa (true unicorn root), 705

Aleve (naproxen), 980
Alexander technique, 21
Alfalfa, 886
Alfentanil: interactions with, 943
Alisma (*Alisma plantago-aquatica*), 886
Alka-Seltzer (sodium bicarbonate and citric acid), 1010
Alka-Seltzer Plus (phenylpropanolamine), 993
Alka-Seltzer Plus Cold Medicine (aspirin, chlorpheniramine), 900, 923
ALL (acute lymphocytic leukemia), 546, 547, 548-549
Allantoin, 929, 1020
Allegra-D (pseudoephedrine), 997
Allergic rhinitis, 107, 108, 432-435, 684
Allergies, 106-109, 487, 618-619; and adenoid problems, 95; and asthma, 149, 150; and CFS, 261; conjunctivitis from, 286, 287; contact dermatitis, 312, 313, 314, 315; and dandruff, 307; diaper rash as, 322, 323; and eczema, 342, 343, 344, 345; genital allergic reaction, 504-505; hay fever, 107, 108, 284-285, 432-435; hives, 482-483; insect and spider bite, 508; insect sting, 107, 109, 176-177; and laryngitis, 542-543; and pain, chronic, 653; poison ivy, oak, and sumac, 682-*683*; and sneezing, 762-763; and swallowing difficulty, *chart*, 796-797; and wheezing, 874-875
Allergy (medical specialty), 18
Allicin, 101, 261, 950
Allium cepa (homeopathic remedy), 887
Allium cepa (onion), 189, 257, 320, 480
Allium Pstulosum (scallion), 1004-1005
Allium sativum (garlic), 950; in combination, 929
Allopurinol: interactions with, 991
Aloe (*Aloe barbadensis*), 887
Aloe vera, 231, 747
Alopecia (hair loss), 422-425, *423*; androgenic, 422; involutional, 422
Alopecia areata, 422, *423*, 424
Alopecia universalis, 422
Alora (estradiol), 943
Alpha1-adrenergic blockers, 887-888; interactions with, 910
Alpha-galactosidase, 389
Alpha-tocopherol, 1036
Alprazolam, 888; interactions with, 898
ALS (amyotrophic lateral sclerosis; Lou Gehrig's disease), 554-*555*
Altace (ramipril), 999
Alternative therapies, 20-28; choice of practitioner, 29; defined, 17; homeopathic remedies, 26-27, *79*, 1027; medicine chest for, *79*; reflexology, 24, *25*. *See also* Acupressure; Herbal therapies; Yoga; *and names of individual ailments*
Althaea officinalis (marsh mallow), 974; in combinations, 911, 916, 921
Aluminum: and Alzheimer's disease, 111, 112-113; and calcium absorption, 639; interactions with, 898, 902, 906, 983, 1011
Aluminum acetate, 747
Aluminum chloride, 157, 193, 799
Aluminum hydroxide, 888; interactions with, 906, 983
Alveoli: and emphysema, 346, *347*; and pneumonia, *678*
Alzheimer's disease, 110-113
Amala, 642
Amantadine, 375, 377, 602, 661; interactions with, 937
Ambien (zolpidem), 1023
Amenorrhea (lack of period), 588-589; yoga for, *590*
American Board of Medical Specialties (ABMS), 19
American ginseng, 953
Amiloride, 888; interactions with, 891, 905, 995
Aminoglutethimide: interactions with, 996
Aminoglycosides, 191, 582; interactions with, 920, 980, 1017; neomycin, 980; tobramycin, 1016
Aminophylline: interactions with, 906, 943
Amiodarone, 450; interactions with, 938, 939
Amitriptyline, 888; interactions with, 970, 980, 988, 1016
AML (acute myelogenic leukemia), 546, 547, 549
Amlodipine, 889; interactions with, 925
Ammi visnaga, 867
Ammonium carbonicum, 348
Amomum villosum; A. xanthioides (grains-of-paradise fruit), 955; in combinations, 885, 886, 902, 922, 951
Amoxicillin, 889
Amoxicillin and clavulanate, 889
Amoxicillin-resistant bacteria, 642
Amoxil (amoxicillin), 889
Amphetamines, 163, 336, 338, 511, 630, 789; interactions with, 914, 935, 938, 953, 962, 978, 982, 997
Amphotericin, 881
Ampicillin, 274, 407, 756
Amsler grid, *571*
Amyotrophic lateral sclerosis (ALS; Lou Gehrig's disease), 554-*555*
Anabolic steroids, 91, 143-144, 337, 962
Anacardium, 391
Anacin, 900, 914
Ana-Kit (epinephrine), 942
Anal bleeding, 114-115 *chart*, 464
Anal fissure (anal ulcer), 114-115, 116-117, 200-201, 520-521
Analgesics, 889
Anal hemorrhoids, 464, *465*, 466
Anaphylactic shock (anaphylaxis), 75, 106, 108, 176, 177, 482, 508, 618-619, 796-797
Anaprox DS (naproxen), 980
Anbesol (benzocaine, phenol), 905, 992
Androgenic alopecia, 422
Androgens, 352; and acne, 90
Anemarrhena (*Anemarrhena asphodeloides*), 889; in combinations, 1009
Anemia, 118-121, 366-367, 610-611, 612-613, 1032, 1035; sickle cell, 119, 752-*753*
Anemone pulsatilla (pasqueflower), 705
Anesthesiology, 18
Anesthetics, 889-890; interactions with, 936, 1024
Anethum graveolens (dill), 273
Aneurysms, 122-*123*, 710-711; bleeding strokes from, 788, 789, 790
Angelica root (*Angelica pubescens*), 890
Angelica root, Chinese (*Angelica sinensis*; dong quai), 939-940; in combinations, 901, 922, 928, 933, 974, 995, 1002, 1019
Angina (angina pectoris), 124-127, 140-141, 248-249, 452
Angioedema, 106-107, 108, 482, 483
Angioplasty, 126, *154*, 263
Angiotensin-converting enzyme (ACE) inhibitors, 890-891; interactions with, 915, 931, 939, 995
Animal bites and rabies, 712-713
Anise and aniseed, 121, 150, 171, 216, 217, 297, 303, 348, 389, 692
Ankles: painful, *chart*, 128-129; painful, acupressure for, *650*; sprained, *771*; swollen, *chart*, 130-131
Ankylosing spondylitis, 164-165
Anorectal stricture, 114-115

Anorexia nervosa, 132-133, 218
Ansaid (flurbiprofen), 949
Antacids, 891-892; in combinations, 1008, 1010; interactions with, 893, 898, 902, 906, 914, 925, 931, 937, 938, 949, 966, 968, 969, 983, 984, 986, 994, 996, 999, 1013, 1015
Anthemis nobilis (Roman chamomile), 420
Anthocyanosides, 907
Anthralin, 707
Anthraquinones, 911, 1005
Antiacne drugs, 892
Antianxiety drugs, 892; interactions with, 896, 959, 989
Antiarrhythmic drugs, 448, 450; interactions with, 938
Antiasthmatic drugs (asthma therapy), 900
Antibiotics, 892; in combination, 1018; interactions with, 891, 895
Anticancer drugs, 892; interactions with, 925, 1013
Anticholinergic drugs, 661; interactions with, 891, 937, 966, 969, 976, 983, 987
Anticoagulant and antiplatelet drugs, 892-893; interactions with, 884, 894, 898, 902, 917, 923, 925, 935, 939, 943, 949, 968, 970, 976, 978, 984, 986, 992, 994, 996, 997, 1011, 1013, 1015, 1016, 1022
Anticonvulsant drugs, 893; interactions with, 894, 906, 913, 926, 940, 976, 984, 1011
Antidepressants, 893-894; interactions with, 918, 936, 956, 960, 965, 970, 978, 987, 997, 1012, 1016, 1022, 1024
Antidiabetic drugs, 894; interactions with, 906, 908, 910, 925, 937, 939, 970, 984, 1011, 1016
Antidiarrheal drugs, 894-895; interactions with, 937, 938, 972, 987, 990, 1011
Antidiuretic, 175
Antiemetic (antinausea) drugs, 897
Antifungal drugs, 895; in combinations, 907; interactions with, 891
Antigastroesophageal reflux drugs, 896
Antihistamines, 896; anti-itch drugs, 897; in combination, 997; interactions with, 894, 906, 913, 933, 936, 937, 953, 956, 960, 978, 987, 994, 1024
Antihyperlipidemic drugs, 923
Antihypertensive (blood pressure) drugs, 896; interactions with, 891, 905, 906, 910, 915, 935, 938, 939, 976, 987, 992, 994, 1018, 1019
Anti-insomnia drugs, 897; interactions with, 936, 960
Anti-itch drugs, 897
Antimigraine drugs, 897
Antimonium crudum, 873
Antimonium tartaricum, 297
Antimonium tartaricum, 348
Antinausea drugs, 897
Antineoplastons, 231
Antioxidants, 155, 239, 261, 455, 489, 561, 571, 977
Anti-Parkinsonism drugs, 897
Antiperspirants, 193
Antiplatelet drugs, 892-893; interactions with, 970, 1016, 1022
Antiprostaglandins, 353
Antipruritic (anti-itch) drugs, 897
Antipsychotics, 289, 517, 733, 828, 829; interactions with, 906, 960, 965, 980, 1019
Antiseptics, 897
Antispasmodic drugs, 897
Antithyroid medications, 414, 826
Antitussives (cough suppressants), 931
Antiulcer drugs, 897-898; interactions with, 914, 938, 949, 1013, 1015, 1019
Antiviral drugs, 99, 898; interactions with, 937, 949
Antrostomy, 756
Ants, fire, 508, 509
Anxiety disorders, 134-137, 364-365, 798-799, 868-869. *See also individual anxiety disorders*
Apheresis, LDL, 256
Aphthous ulcers (canker sores), 232-233, *1045*
Apis, 898-899
Apitherapy, 602
Apium graveolens (celery), 225, 411
Aplastic crises, 752
Apocrine glands, 192
ApoE (apolipoprotein E), 110-111
Apomorphine, 661
Appendectomy, 139
Appendicitis, 138-139, 200-201, 870-871
Appetite suppressants, 317
Apricot seed, 899; in combinations, 941, 970
Aqueous humor and glaucoma, 400, 401, 402
Arborvitae (biota), 907; seeds of, in combination, 1006
Arbutin, 1020
ARC (AIDS-related complex), 96
Arctium lappa (burdock), 912; in combinations, 924, 925, 958, 981
Arctostaphylos uva-ursi (uva ursi), 1020; in combinations, 911, 941
Argentum nitricum, 287, 631
Arginine, 271, 305, 395, 503, 747
ARMD (age-related macular degeneration), 570-571
Armour Thyroid (thyroid USP), 1016
Arms: injured, immobilizing, *65*; pain, *chart*, 140-141; tennis elbow, 812-815, *813*
Arnica, 899
Aromatherapy, 21. *See also individual ailments*
Arousal dysfunction, 741-742
Arrhythmias, heart, 448-451, 454, 458
Arsenicum album, 899-900
Artemisia absinthium (wormwood), 21, 201, 879
Artemisia argyi; Artemisia vulgaris (mugwort leaf), 978; in combination, 907
Arteries, *1060*; aneurysms, 122-*123*; atherosclerosis, 152-155, *153*, *154*, 453; brain, *789*; coronary, disease of, 152, *154*, 452, 453, 458-459; high blood pressure, 478-481; inflamed (arteritis), 362-363; pressure points, *48*; Raynaud's syndrome, 718-719
Arteriosclerosis (atherosclerosis), 152-155, *153*; coronary, 152, *154*, 453
Arteriovenous malformation, 789
Arthritis, 142-147, *143*; aches and pains, *chart*, 88-89; ankles, painful, *chart*, 128-129; ankles, swollen, *chart*, 130-131; arm pain, *chart*, 140-141; backache, *chart*, 164-165; dizziness, *chart*, 334-335; feet, aches and pains, *chart*, 370-371; gout, 128-129, 140-141, 370-371, 408-411, *409*, *410*, 526-527; hand and wrist pain, *chart*, 428-429; joint pain, *chart*, 526-527; knee pain, *chart*, 538-539; Lyme, 88-89, 564; neck pain, *chart*, 620-621; psoriatic, 706, 709; shoulder pain, *chart*, 750-751
Arthroscopy, 160, 807
Artificial fertilization, 503
Artificial limbs, 197
Asafetida powder, 389
Asbestos, 355
Ascariasis, 878
Asclepias syriaca (milkweed), 873
Asclepias tuberosa (pleurisy root), 681
Ascorbic acid (vitamin C), 1035
Ashwaganda, 900
Asian ginseng, 953; in combinations, 901, 925, 951, 995, 1005, 1013
Asian pennywort, 473

Asiatic cornelian cherry fruit (Asiatic dogwood; cornus), 930; in combinations, 922, 945
Asparagus racemosus (shatavari), 499
Aspartame: interactions with, 884
Aspen, 136
Aspiration (herbal formula), 311
Aspiration pneumonia, 678, 679, 680
Aspirin, 889, 900; in combinations, 914, 927, 942, 987, 988; interactions with, 884, 890, 891, 893, 898, 905, 931, 938, 983, 984, 988, 1011, 1022, 1023
Associations and organizations, 1071-1075
Asthma, 148-151, *149*
Asthma therapy, 900; interactions with, 926, 1003
Astigmatism, 862-863, 864
Aston-Patterning, 21
Astragalus (*Astragalus membranaceus*), 901; in combinations, 902, 928, 939, 1019; interactions with, 899
Astragalus Ten Formula, 260
Atarax (hydroxyzine), 960
Atenolol, 901
Atherosclerosis, 152-155, *153*; coronary, 152, *154*, 453
Athlete's foot, 156-157, 612-613, 714-715
Athletic injuries, 158-161; groin pull as, 417
Ativan (lorazepam), 972
Atopic dermatitis (eczema), 312, 313, 314, 315, 342-345, 520-521, *1044*, *1048*
Atorvastatin, 901
Atractylodes, white (*Atractylodes macrocephala*), 901-902; in combinations, 901, 922, 928, 951, 953, 955
Atrial arrhythmias, 449, 451
Atropine, 517; drugs similar to, 983, 996
Atrovent (ipratropium), 963
Attapulgite, 902; interactions with, 960
Attention deficit disorder (ADD), 162-163
Aucklandia (*Aucklandia lappa*), 902; in combinations, 922, 929, 933, 1013
Audiometry, 443-444
Augmentin (amoxicillin and clavulanate), 889
Auras, migraines with, 436
Australian fever tree (eucalyptus), 944-945
Autoimmune disorders, 486, 487; blisters from, 186; Crohn's disease as, 298; lupus, 562-563, 610-611; and thyroid problems, 824-825. *See also individual ailments*
Autonomic nervous system and arrhythmias, 449
Autumn crocus (*Colchicum*), 371, 411
Averrhoa carambola (star fruit), 537
Avita (tretinoin), 1017
Avobenzone, 795
Axid (nizatidine), 983
Aygestin (norethindrone acetate), 984
Ayurvedic medicine, 21. *See also individual ailments*
Azathioprine, 275, 299
Azithromycin, 902; interactions with, 972
Azmacort (triamcinolone), 1018
AZT (zidovudine), 99; interactions with, 884, 885, 906

B

Babies. *See* Children; Infants
Baby teeth, 804, *805*
Bach flower remedies, 136
Bacillus Calmette-Gurin (BCG) vaccine, 181
Bacitracin, 903; in combinations, 980, 995
Backache: *chart*, 164-165; in pregnancy, 688-689
Back blows for choking infants, *56*
Back problems, 166-169; backache, 164-165 *chart*, 688-689; bone spurs, 198, 199; disk problems, 164-165, 326-329, *327*, 620-621, 626-627, 672-*673*; injuries, 66, 159; pain, chronic, 651-652; pain, chronic, acupressure for, *650*; scoliosis, 736-*737*
Baclofen, 476, 555, 602; interactions with, 962
Bacterial food poisoning, 382
Bacterial infections: bladder, 182-185; blood poisoning, 190-191; boils, 191, 194-195, *772*, *773*, *774*, *775*; chlamydia, 252-253; conjunctivitis as, 286, 287; diverticulitis, 330-333, *331*; ear, 444, 445, 640-641, 642; endocarditis, 460; of eyelids, *792-793*, *1051*; gonorrhea, 406-407; impetigo, 490-491, *1045*; kidney, 534-535; laryngitis as, 542; Lyme disease, 564-565, *1049*; meningitis as, 584-585; pelvic inflammatory disease, 664-665; periodontal disease, 418-421, *419*; pneumonia as, 678, 679, 680; prostatitis, 702, 703, 704, 705; rashes from, *chart*, 714-717; and rheumatic fever, 724-725; Rocky Mountain spotted fever, 726-727; scarlet fever, 730-731; sinusitis, 754-757; sore throat from, 766, 767; staph, 772-775; strep throat, 782-783; syphilis, 802-803; tetanus, 820-821; tooth, *836*, 837; toxic shock syndrome, 838-839; tuberculosis, 844-845; and ulcers, peptic, 779, 780; vaginosis, 854, 855, 856, 857; whooping cough, 876-877
Bactericidal antibiotics: vs. bacteriostatic, 892, 942; interactions with, 943, 944
Bacteriostatic antibiotics: vs. bactericidal, 892, 942; interactions with, 920, 991
Bactrium (sulfamethoxazole and trimethoprim), 1011
Bactroban (mupirocin), 979
Bad breath, 170-171
Balanitis, 322, 504-505, 666-667, 880
Balding, 422-425, *423*
Balloon angioplasty, *154*
Balmony, 657, 879
Banana peel, 675, 873
Bandage, applying, to wound, *48*
Banding of hemorrhoids, 466
Baptisia tinctoria (wild indigo), 596
Barberry, 903; in combination, 934
Barbiturates, 107, 135, 336, 338, 512; interactions with, 884, 894, 896, 906, 913, 914, 936, 940, 944, 978, 996, 1022, 1024
Barium x-ray, 241, 289, 390, 779
Barotitis media, 447
Barotrauma, 340-341
Barrier contraception, 40
Baryta carbonica, 123
Baryta carbonica, 835
Basal cell carcinoma (BCC), 758, *759*, *760*, *1047*
Basal temperature, monitoring, 825
Basil, 310
Bayberry, 903
Bayer (aspirin), 900
BCC (basal cell carcinoma), 758, *759*, *760*, *1047*
B-complex vitamins, 1032-1035
Bead (coral) snakes, *77*; bites from, 76
Bearberry (uva ursi), 1020; in combinations, 911, 941
Beclomethasone, 903-904
Beconase AQ (beclomethasone), 903
Bedridden patients, 172-*173*
Beds for varicose vein sufferers, 861
Bedsores, 172-173
Bedwetting, 174-175
Bee pollen, 109, 631

Bees, *177*, 898-899; stings, 176-177
Bee venom therapy (BVT), 602
Behavior therapy, 133, 135, 163, 175, 219, 230, 503, 633, 659
Belladonna, 904
Benadryl (diphenhydramine), 938
Benazepril, 904-905
Ben-Gay (menthol, methyl salicylate), 974, 976
Benign multiple sclerosis, 600
Benign prostatic hyperplasia (BPH; enlarged prostate), 702-704, *703*, 705
Benzene, 355
Benzocaine, 905; in combinations, 897, 992
Benzodiazepines, 905-906; interactions with, 913, 925, 936, 937, 944, 980, 987, 1024
Benzoicum acidum, 411
Benzoin, 747
Benzoyl peroxide, 92, 93, 1018
Benztropine, 661; interactions with, 996
Berbamine, 903
Berberine, 195, 282, 903, 929
Berberis (homeopathic remedy), 705; *Berberis vulgaris*, 387
Berberis vulgaris (barberry), 903; in combination, 934
Bergamot, 195, 595, 775, 843
Beriberi, 1034
Berry aneurysms, 122, *123*
Beta-adrenergic blockers (beta blockers), 906; in combination, 887; interactions with, 888, 891, 905, 906, 910, 914, 915, 935, 944, 962, 981, 982, 984, 988, 994
Beta carotene, 1033
Betagalactosidase, 541
Beta interferon, 602
Betamethasone, 907; in combination, 927
Betapen-VK (penicillin V), 991
Betaxolol, 400, 402
Betony, wood, 440, 908
Biaxin (clarithromycin), 926
Bicarbonate of soda (sodium bicarbonate): and citric acid, 1010; interactions with, 926, 1015
Bifidobacterium, 253, 843
Bilberry, 907
Bile acid-binding resins, 923, 928
Bile and bile acids, 385, 386
Bile ducts, problems of, 268; gallstones in, 384, *385*; pancreatic cancer, blockage by, *655*
Bile salt, 386
Bilirubin in jaundice, 522, 523
Binging and purging (bulimia), 218-219
Biofeedback, 27
Bioflavonoids, 109, 155, 257, 300, 421, 571, 643, 757, 775, 853, 861, 1000, 1003; pyncogenol, 809
Biologically guided chemotherapy, 231
Biomedicine (conventional medicine): board certification in, 19; choice of practitioner, 29; defined, 17; medicine chest for, *78*; specialties, 18-20. *See also individual ailments*
Biota (*Biota orientalis*), 907; seeds of, in combination, 1006
Biotin (vitamin B_7, vitamin H), 1032
Bipolar disorder (manic-depression), 514-515, 574-577
Bipolar I vs. bipolar II, 574-575, 576
Birth control, 40-41, 42
Birth-control pills (oral contraceptives): for dysfunctional uterine bleeding, 852; for endometriosis, 352; interactions with, 906, 914, 917, 943-944, 988, 991, 994, 1011, 1013, 1015, 1019; for PMS, 695
Birthmarks, 32-33
Birth of child, 39-40; emergency, *60-61*
Bismuth drugs, 780, 781
Bismuth subsalicylate, 907-908
Bites: animal, and rabies, 712-713; insect and spider, 508-509, *1049*; snake, *76-77*
Bitter almond (apricot seed), 899; in combinations, 941, 970
Bitter orange, 757, 901, 912, 1013
Black cherry, wild, 303, 348, 680, 877
Black cohosh, 908; in combination, 1023
Black currant, 647
Black eye, 178-179
Black haw, 591
Blackheads, 90
Black-legged tick, Lyme disease caused by, 564-565
Black walnut, 908
Black widow spider, *509*; bite, 508, 509
Bladder cancer, 180-181; urinary problems from, *chart*, 846-847
Bladder incontinence, 494-497, 700, 846-847; bedwetting, 174-175
Bladder infections, 182-185; in pregnancy, 691; urinary problems from, *chart*, 846-847
Bladder retraining, 496
Bladder-stretching exercises, 175
Bladder wrack, 405, 827
Bleeding, *48*, 305; anal, 114-115 *chart*, 464; from inside ear, 58; internal, 70, 390, 391; nosebleed, 72, 692; vaginal, 848, 850, 854
Bleeding strokes, 788, 789, 790
Bleeding ulcers, 778, 780
Bleomycin: interactions with, 1013
Blepharitis, 504-505, 773
Blessed thistle, 908-909
Blindness: from cataracts, 238; diabetes and, 317
Blisters, 186-187
Blocadren (timolol), 1016
Blood: anemia, 118-121, 752-*753*, 1032, 1035; cancer of (leukemia), 546-549, *547*; cholesterol in, problems with, 254-257; coughing up, 295; dialysis, 532; Rh factor, 39; sickle cell anemia, 119, *752-753*
Blood clots, 188-189, 248-249; and hearing loss, 445; phlebitis and, 668, 669; strokes from, 788, 789, 790
Blood poisoning, 190-191
Blood pressure, 478; high, 478-481; low, 364-365
Blood pressure drugs (antihypertensives), 896; interactions with, 891, 905, 906, 910, 915, 935, 938, 939, 976, 987, 992, 994, 1018, 1019
Bloodroot, 909
Blood thinners: anticoagulant and antiplatelet drugs called, 892, 935; blood viscosity-reducing agents, 909
Blood vessels. *See* Cardiovascular system
Blood viscosity-reducing agents, 909
Blue babies, 461
Blueberry, 320
Blue chamomile, 136
Blue cohosh, 589, 647, 665, 852, 909
Blue flag, 93, 195
Board certification of specialists, 19
Body lice, 550, 551
Body mass index (BMI), 628
Body odor, 192-193
Body work, 21, 24; reflexology, 24, *25. See also individual ailments*
Body wrap, wet, 343
Boils, 191, 194-195, 556-557, 772, 773, 774, 775
Bone cancer, 196-*197*
Bone density, loss of (osteoporosis), 636-639
Bone-marrow transplantation, 549, 569
Bones, *1056-1057*
Boneset, 909-910; in combinations, 918, 961
Bone spurs, 128-129, 198-*199*, 370-371

Booster shots, tetanus, 821
Borage, 642, 647, 708
Botulism, 382, 383
Bowel movement abnormalities: *chart*, 200-201; and anal bleeding, *chart*, 114-115; constipation, 288-291, 333, 689, 691; diarrhea, 301, 324-325 *chart*; irritable bowel syndrome, 516-519
BPH (benign prostatic hyperplasia; enlarged prostate), 702-704, *703*, 705
Braces, orthopedic, for scoliosis, 736, *737*
Bradycardia, 448, 449, 450
Brain, *1064*; Alzheimer's disease, 110-113; blood vessels, *789*; cancer, 202-*203*; and dizziness, *chart*, 334-335; epilepsy, 358-359; in Parkinson's disease, 660; in rabies, 712; stroke, 788-791
Brain-wave (EEG) biofeedback, 133, 137, 163, 219, 310-311, 359, 577, 633, 687
Bran, 290-291
Branched chain amino acid (BCAA), 555
Braxton Hicks contractions, 39
Breast cancer, 204-207
Breast discomfort in pregnancy, 689
Breast examination, 38
Breast-feeding, 32, 40
Breast implants, 206
Breast lumps, 205-206, 208, 210-211, 556-557
Breast pain, 208-210
Breast problems, 208-211
Breast reconstruction, 206
Breast self-examination, 208, *210*
Breast x-rays (mammograms), 205, 208
Breath, bad, 170-171
Breathing, reestablishing: in choking victims, *54-56*; with CPR, *50-53*
Breathing exercises, 136-137, 349, 513, 633, 659, 662
Breathing problems: *chart*, 212-213; congestion, *chart*, 284-285. *See also* Respiratory problems
Breathlessness in pregnancy, 689
Breech baby, *61*
Brethaire (terbutaline), 1014
Brethine (terbutaline), 1014
Brewer's yeast, 631
Bricanyl (terbutaline), 1014
Brindall berry, 256
Broken bones (fractures), 64, *65*, 158, 160-161, 544-545; from osteoporosis, 636
Bromelain (pineapple enzyme), 155, 179, 189, 265, 305, 653, 757, 809, 811, 860, 873
Bromocriptine, 661
Brompheniramine, 910
Bronchi, lung cancer in, 558, *559*
Bronchioles, *215*; and asthma, *149*; lung cancer in, 558, *559*
Bronchitis, 212-213, 214-217, *215*, 284-285
Bronchodilators, 910; interactions with, 914, 981
Bronchopneumonia, 678
Brown recluse spider, *509*; bite, 508, 509, *1049*
Brushing of hair, 425
Bruxism, TMJ from, 807, 809
Bryonia (*Bryonia alba*), 911
Buchu, 911
Buckthorn, 911-912
Buclizine: interactions with, 937
Bufferin (aspirin), 900
Bugbane (cimicifuga), 925
Bugleweed, 415, 827
Bulimia, 218-219
Bulk-forming laxatives, 967; calcium polycarbophil, 915; psyllium hydrophilic mucilloid, 998
Bullous pemphigoid, 186
Bumblebee, *177*
Bumetanide, 912; interactions with, 988
Bumex (bumetanide), 912
Bunions, 220-*221*, 370-371
Bunolol, 400, 402
Bupleurum (*Bupleurum chinense*), 912; in combinations, 901, 925, 933
Bupropion, 310, 576, 912
Burdock, 912-913; in combinations, 924, 925, 958, 981
Burkitt's lymphoma, 567
Burns, 49, 222-223; blisters from, 186, 187; sunburn, 794-795
Bursitis, 128-129, 140-141, 224-225, 428-429, 526-527, 538-539, 750-751; with bunion, *221*
Burton, Lawrence, 231
Burzynski, Stanislav, 231
Bushmaster snake, venom of, 967
BuSpar (buspirone), 913
Buspirone, 913
Butcher's-broom, 913
B vitamins, 1032-1035
Bypass surgery, 126, 154

C

Cactus (*Cactus grandiflorus*), 126
Cadmium, 532-533
Caffeine, 889, 914; in combinations, 921; interactions with, 898, 910, 935, 953, 978, 986, 992, 994, 1024; in kola, 966
Caffeine poisoning, 829
Cajuput, 184, 642
Calamine, 251, 395, 483, 509, 579, 682, 683, 747, 795
Calan SR (verapamil), 1022
Calcarea carbonica, 914
Calcarea fluorica, 638, 652
Calcarea phosphorica, 638
Calcitonin, 637-638
Calcitriol, 707
Calcium, 1036-1037; interactions with, 902, 914, 915, 924, 938, 944, 959, 1015
Calcium absorption test, at-home, 637
Calcium carbonate, 914
Calcium channel blockers, 915; interactions with, 891, 905, 906, 925, 938
Calcium gluconate, 509, 638
Calcium pantothenate, 1034
Calcium polycarbophil, 915
Calcium sulphide, 957
Calendula (*Calendula officinalis*), 79, 139, 157, 187, 314, 344, 915-916
Calenduloside B, 915
Calluses, 292-293, *1046*
Cambridge Liquid Diet, 603
Camphor, 916; in combinations, 897, 975, 1004
Canavanine, 886
Cancer, 226-231; aging and, 45; bladder, 180-181; bone, 196-*197*; bone-marrow transplantation for, 549, 569; brain, 202-*203*; breast, 204-207; cervical, 242-243; chemotherapy for, 228, 548; colorectal, 114-115, 200-201, 276-279, *277*, 618-619; kidney, 528-*529*; leukemia, 546-549, *547*; liver, 552-553; lumps from, *chart*, 556-557; lung, 368-369, 558-561, *559*; lymphoma, 566-569; oral, 634-*635*, *1045*; ovarian, 644-*645*; pancreatic, 654-*655*; penis, 666-667; plants in treatment of, 529; prostate, 43, 698-701, *699*; quackery, 229; skin, 758-761, *759*, *1047*; stomach, 776-*777*; testicular, 816-817, 818-*819*; throat, 796-797, 822-823; thyroid, 825, 826, 827; urinary problems from, *chart*, 846-847; uterine, 848-*849*; vaginal, 854, 855, 856; and vomiting, *chart*, 870-871; warning signs, 227; as women's health issue, 41
Candidal dermatitis, 880

Candidiasis (yeast infection), 504-505, 524, 854, 855, 856, 857, 880-881, *1044, 1045*; and diaper rash, 322, 323
Candlewick plant (mullein), 979; in combinations, 929, 954
Canker sores, 232-233, *1045*
Cannabis (marijuana), 336, 337, 403, 492
Cantharis, 916
Capoten (captopril), 916
Capsaicin, 221, 527, 622, 707, 918
Capsella bursa-pastoris (shepherd's purse), 593
Capsicum frutescens (cayenne), 918; in combinations, 909, 918, 971, 1004
Capsules, herbal, 1026
Captopril, 916-917
Carafate (sucralfate), 1010
Carambola (star fruit), 537
Caraway, 121, 692
Carbacephems, 917
Carbamazepine, 917; interactions with, 898, 902, 915, 925, 940, 943, 997
Carbidopa, 661, 663, 722, 969
Carbohydrates, 1030
Carbolic acid (phenol), 992-993; in combination, 916
Carbon dichloride, 533
Carboneum sulphuratum, 833
Carbonic anhydrase inhibitors, 402
Carbon monoxide, 355, 357
Carbon tetrachloride (carbona), 533
Carbo vegetabilis, 389, 457, 877
Carbuncles, 194, 772
Carcinogens, 227, 355; and bladder cancer, 180-181; and liver cancer, 552, 553; and lung cancer, 559, 561
Carcinoid tumors, 324-325
Carcinoma: defined, 226. *See also* Cancer
Cardamom (grains-of-paradise fruit), 955; in combinations, 885, 886, 902, 922, 951
Cardiac arrest, first aid for, *50-53*
Cardiac glycosides, 463
Cardiomyopathy, 460
Cardiopulmonary resuscitation (CPR), *50-53*
Cardioselective beta blockers, 901, 976
Cardiovascular syphilis, 802
Cardiovascular system, *1060*; aging and, 44-45; aneurysms, 122-*123*; angina, 124-127, 452; and ankles, swollen, *chart*, 130-131; and arm pain, *chart*, 140-141; atherosclerosis, 152-155, *153, 154*, 453; blood clots, 188-189, 445, 668, 669; brain, blood vessels in, *789*; cholesterol problems, 254-257; circulatory problems, 262-265; and fainting, *chart*, 364-365; and fluid retention, *chart*, 378-379; heart arrhythmias, 448-451, 454, 458; heart attack, 67, 452-455; heart disease, 420, 458-463; high blood pressure, 478-481; leg pain from, *chart*, 544-545; and numbness and tingling, *chart*, 626-627; Raynaud's syndrome, 718-719; rheumatic fever, heart in, 724; stroke, 334-335, 364-365, 626-627, 788-791; vascular (migraine and cluster) headaches, 436, 437-440, 441. *See also* Blood; Veins
Cardizem (diltiazem), 938
Cardura (doxazosin), 940
Carisoprodol, 917-918
Carminative oils, 273
Carnitine, 104, 127, 257, 463, 503
Carob, 517
Carotenemia, 869
Carotenoids, 1033
Carotidynia, 620-621
Carpal tunnel syndrome (CTS), 140-141, 234-237, 428-429, 626-627
Carthamus tinctorius (safflower flower), 1002; in combination, 887
Cartilage, deterioration of, *143*
Carum carvi (caraway), 121, 692
Carvone, 1010
Cassia senna (senna), 1005-1006
Cassia (cinnamon) twigs, 926; in combinations, 902, 941, 1019
Castor-oil pack, 210, 591, 593
Cataracts, 238-*239*
Catheter ablation, 450
Catnip, 918
Caulophyllum thalictroides (blue cohosh), 589, 647, 665, 852, 909
Causticum, 175, 497, 723, 873
Cavities (tooth decay), 836, *837*
Cayenne, 918; in combinations, 909, 918, 971, 1004
Ceclor (cefaclor), 918
Cedar, yellow, 675
Cedarwood, 109, 184, 525, 707, 709
Cefaclor, 918
Cefadroxil, 918
Cefixime, 918-919
Cefoxitin, 253
Cefprozil, 919
Ceftin (cefuroxime), 919
Ceftriaxone, 407
Cefuroxime, 919
Cefzil (cefprozil), 919
Celandine, 397, 873
Celebrix (celecoxib), 919
Celecoxib, 919
Celery, 225, 411
Celiac disease, 200-201, 240-241
Cell-derived nerve growth factor, 555, 661
Cellulitis, 772
Cellulose sodium phosphate: interactions with, 891
Centella asiatica (gotu kola), 954-955
Central nervous system (CNS) depressants, 336, 338, 512; interactions with, 894, 933, 936, 956, 960, 987, 994, 1024
Central nervous system (CNS) stimulants, 919; interactions with, 890, 905, 910, 914, 935, 938, 953, 978, 981
Cephalexin, 919
Cephalosporins, 919-920; interactions with, 943, 990
Ceratonia siliqua (carob), 517
Cerclage, 247
Cerebral arteries, *789*
Cerebral atherosclerosis, 152
Cerebral hemorrhages (bleeding strokes), 788, 789, 790
Certification of specialists, 19
Cervical cancer, 242-243
Cervical caps, 839
Cervical cysts, 244-245
Cervical dysplasia, 242, 243, 245, 246, 247
Cervical eversion and cervical erosion, 244, 245, 247
Cervical incompetence, 244, 245, 247
Cervical osteoarthritis, 140-141, 334-335; as bone spurs, 198
Cervical polyps, *245*-246
Cervical problems, 244-247, *245*
Cervical stenosis, 244, 245, 247
Cervicitis, 244, 245, 246-247
Cesarean section, 39
CFS (chronic fatigue syndrome), 258-261, 366-367
Chaenomeles speciosa (Japanese quince), 607
Chalazions, 792, 793
Chamaelirium luteum (false unicorn root), 647, 665
Chamomile, 920; blue, 136; in combinations, 911, 952, 954, 989, 1020, 1023; Roman, 420
Chamomilla, 920
Charcoal, activated, 389, 411, 519
Charley horse, 159, 160, 161
Chaste tree, 921
Checkups for adults, 37; men, 42; women, 38
Chelation therapy, 112-113, 126, 155,

263, 356, 462
Chelidonium majus (celandine), 397, 873
Chelidonium majus (homeopathic remedy), 269, 387, 471
Chelone glabra (balmony), 657, 879
Chemical burns, 49
Chemical food poisoning, 382, 383
Chemical peeling, 92
Chemicals in eye, *63*
Chemotherapy, cancer, 228, 548. *See also* Cancer *for names of individual cancers*
Chenodiol: interactions with, 951
Chén pí (tangerine peel), 1013; in combinations, 902, 995
Cherry, wild, 303, 348, 680, 877
Cherry plum, 136
Chest compressions, giving, *51, 52, 53*
Chestnut, horse, 860
Chest pain: *chart*, 248-249; acupressure for, *650*
Chest thrusts for choking infant, *56*
Chi (energy), 20, 24
Chickenpox, *250*-251, 714-715, *1044*
Chicken soup as cold therapy, 283
Chickweed, 921
Chicory, 921-922
Childbirth, 39-40; emergency, *60-61*
Childhood leukemia (acute lymphocytic leukemia; ALL), 546, 547, 548-549
Children, 32-36, *1044*; adenoid problems, 94-95; athletic injuries, 158; attention deficit disorder, 162-163; bedwetting, 174-175; calluses, hereditary, 292; chickenpox, *250*-251, *1044*; choking, first aid for, *56*; colds, 280, 281; cold sores, 270, 271; colic, 272-273; CPR for, 51, *52-53*; croup, 302-303; dehydration, 301; depression, 308; diaper rash, 322-323, *1044*; eczema, 342, 345, *1044*; febrile seizures, 35, 74, 358; fever, *chart*, 372-373; German measles, 398-*399*, *1044*; glaucoma, congenital, 400, 401; growing pains (Osgood-Schlatter disease), 160, 538-539; growth charts, 34-35; hair loss, kinds of, 422, *423*; head lice, 550, 551; hearing problems, 442, 443; heart defects, congenital, 460-461; and hepatitis, 470-471; hypothyroidism, 825; immunization schedule, *chart*, 33; impetigo, 490; intussusception, 114-115; jaundice, 522, 523; lactose intolerance, 540; leukemia, 547-548; liver disorders, causes of, 267-268; measles, 578-*579, 1044*; mumps,604-605; obsessive-compulsive disorder, 632, 633; ophthalmia neonatorum, 286; otitis media, 640, 643; periodontitis, juvenile, 418, 419; posttraumatic stress disorder, 686; pulse, checking, *47, 53*; rashes, *chart*, 714-717; rheumatoid arthritis, juvenile, 142, 143; scarlet fever, 730-731; scoliosis, 736, 737; seasonal affective disorder, 738; sickle cell anemia, 752, 753; and skin cancer, 761; sore throat, 725; staph infections, 772-773; teething problems, 804-805; tonsillitis, 834-835; whooping cough, 876-877. *See also* Infants
Children's Motrin Ibuprofen Suspension (ibuprofen), 961
Chills and fever, *chart*, 372-373
Chimaphila umbellata (pipsissewa), 407, 705
Chinese angelica root (dong quai), 939-940; in combinations, 901, 922, 928, 933, 974, 995, 1002, 1019
Chinese dandelion (*Taraxacum mongolicum*), 934-935
Chinese dodder (cuscuta), 932; in combinations, 927, 945, 973, 995
Chinese foxglove root, 922; in combinations, 889, 925, 928, 929, 930, 939, 953, 973, 1002, 1005
Chinese goldthread (coptis), 929-930; in combinations, 885, 902, 925, 946, 958, 1009
Chinese herbs, 24, 26. *See also individual ailments and herbs*
Chinese medicine, traditional (TCM), 20, 22, 24
Chinese motherwort, 922
Chinese yam, 922-923; in combinations, 922, 930, 945
Chininum sulphuricum, 833
Chionanthus virginicus (fringe tree), 657
Chiropractic, 26. *See also individual ailments*
Chi yi (deep-breathing exercise), 662
Chlamydia, 252-253, 666-667
Chloasma, 692
Chloramphenicol, 274, 319, 727; interactions with, 920, 943, 991
Chlorhexidine, 923
Chloride, 1037
Chloroform, 533
Chlorophyll, 171, 193, 300
Chloroquine, 573, 706
Chlorpheniramine, 923
Chlorpromazine, 476, 733, 821; interactions with, 906, 980
Chlorpropamide, 319
Chlor-Trimeton (chlorpheniramine), 923
Chlor-Trimeton Allergy-Sinus Headache Caplets (acetaminophen), 884
Choking, *54-56*
Cholecalciferol, 1035
Cholecystectomy (gallbladder removal), 386-387
Cholesterol: and gallstones, 385, 387; problems with, 254-257
Cholesterol-reducing drugs, 923; interactions with, 891, 970, 1015, 1016
Cholestyramine, 923-924; interactions with, 970, 1015, 1016
Choline, 339, 387
Chondrosarcoma, 196
Chorea, 724
Chromium, 1037
Chromosome abnormalities, 39; in leukemia, 547
Chronic Epstein-Barr virus (CEBV), 258-261
Chronic fatigue syndrome (CFS), 258-261, 366-367
Chronic lymphocytic leukemia (CLL), *547*, 549
Chronic myelogenic leukemia (CML), 547, 549
Chronic pain, 648-653
Chronic progressive multiple sclerosis, 601
Chrysanthemum flower (*Chrysanthemum indicum*), 924
Chrysanthemum flower (*Chrysanthemum morifolium*): in combinations, 296, 924, 934, 948, 974; interactions with, 930
Chrysanthemum parthenium (feverfew), 948
Chymopapain, 328
Cibot root, 493
Cicada, 924
Cichorium intybus (chicory), 921-922
Cigarettes. *See* Smoking
Cimetidine, 924-925; interactions with, 898, 906, 914, 915, 925, 949, 968, 972, 984, 988, 994, 997, 1013, 1015, 1019
Cimicifuga (*Cimicifuga foetida; C. dahurica*), 925
Cimicifuga racemosa (black cohosh), 908; in combination, 1023
Cinnamaldehyde, 926
Cinnamates, 795
Cinnamon bark (*Cinamomum cassia*), 925-926; in combinations, 931, 1019

Cinnamon twig (*Cinnamomum cassia*), 926; in combinations, 902, 941, 1019
Cipro (ciprofloxacin), 926
Ciprofloxacin, 926; interactions with, 898, 986
Circadian rhythm sleep disorders, 511, 513
Circulatory problems, 262-265
Circulatory system, *1060. See also* Cardiovascular system
Cirrhosis, 114-115, 200-201, 266-269, 368-369, 378-379
Citric acid, 957; sodium bicarbonate and, 1010
Citronella, 509
Citrus bergamia (bergamot), 195, 595, 775, 843
Citrusel (methylcellulose), 976
Citrus reticulata (tangerine peel), 1013; in combinations, 902, 995
Cladribine, 602
Clarithromycin, 926-927; interactions with, 896, 972
Claritin; Claritin-D (loratadine; pseudoephedrine), 972, 997
Clary, 310, 493, 743
Classical (stable) angina, 124, 125
Clavulanate, amoxicillin and, 889
Clay, French, 389
Clear cell adenocarcinoma, 855
Cleavers, 93, 95, 314, 357, 596, 605, 708, 835, 913
Clemastine, 927; interactions with, 906
Climar (estradiol), 943
Climatotherapy, 707
CLL (chronic lymphocytic leukemia), *547*, 549
Clofibrate, 319, 609; interactions with, 962, 988
Clomipramine, 633
Clonazepam, 927
Clonidine, 799, 927; interactions with, 906, 1019
Clotrimazole, 927
Clot strokes, 788, 789, 790
Clove, 171, 757, 837
Clover, red, 999; in combinations, 913, 979
Clozapine, 733; interactions with, 906, 960, 980
Club moss, 973
Cluster headaches, 362-363, 436, 437, 438, 439, 440, 441
CML (chronic myelogenic leukemia), 547, 549
Cnicin, 908
Cnicus benedictus (blessed thistle), 908-909
Cnidium (*Ligusticum chuanxiong*), 890; in combinations, 931, 933, 939-940, 1002
Cnidium seeds (*Cnidium monnieri*), 927
Coal-tar preparations, 307, 313, 342, 343, 707, 709
Cobalamin (vitamin B_{12}), 1035
Cobalt, 1037
Cocaine, 336, 337, 338, 339
Cocculus, 583, 599
Coccus cacti, 877
Cochlea, *443*, *581*, *1066*; hair cells, 443
Cochlear implant, 445
Codeine, 889, 927
Codonopsis root (Codonopsis pilosula), 927-928; in combinations, 955
Coenzyme Q10 (CoQ10), 127, 230, 261, 463, 555, 603, 692
Cognitive therapy, 135, 145, 219, 659; cognitive restructuring, 652
Cohosh, black, 908; in combination, 1023
Cohosh, blue, 647, 665, 852, 909
Coix (*Coix lachryma jobi*), 928
Cola vera; Cola nitada (kola), 966; in combinations, 934, 967
Colchicine, 328, 371, 408, 409-410, 411; interactions with, 984
Colchicum, 371, 411
Cold, common, 88-89, 280-283, 284-285, 375, 684
Cold and flu preparations, 281
Cold infusion of herbal oils, 1026
Cold sores, 270-271, *1045*
Colectomy, 299-300
Colestid (colestipol), 928
Colestipol, 928
Colic, 272-273
Colitis, 84-85, 114-115, 274-275, 324-325, 526-527; pseudomembranous, 949, 972, 991, 1015
Collagen and glaucoma, 401
Collapsed lung, 248-249
Collarbone, injured, immobilizing, *65*
Collateral arteries, 453
Colocynthis, 332, 387, 518
Colon: and abdominal pains, *chart*, 84-87; cancer, 276-279, *277*; and Crohn's disease, *299*; diverticulitis, 330-333, *331*; inflammation of (colitis), 84-85, 114-115, 274-275, 324-325, 526-527; removal of, and ileostomy, 300, 301; staph infection, 773
Colonoscopy, 278
Color blindness, 862, 863
Colorectal cancer, 114-115, 200-201, 276-279, *277*, 618-619
Colostomy, 278, 279, 332
Coltsfoot, 928-929; in combinations, 961, 979; interactions with, 930
Columnar epithelium of cervix, 244
Combing of head lice, 551
Comfrey, 929
Commiphora molmol (myrrh), 979; in combinations, 916, 918, 934, 1004
Commiphora mukul (gugulipid), 155, 189, 256
Common bile duct, blockage of, 384, *385*, *655*
Common callus, 292
Common cold, 88-89, 280-283, 284-285, 375, 684
Common warts, 872, *1046*
Compartment syndrome, 748
Compazine (prochlorperazine), 996
Compound Q (tricosantin), 99
Compresses, herbal, 1026
Compulsions and obsessions, 632-633
Comtrex (acetaminophen, dextromethorphan), 884, 936
Comtrex Liqui-Gel (phenylpropanolamine), 993
Comtrex Multi-Symptom Cold Reliever (chlorpheniramine, pseudoephedrine), 923, 997
Concussion, 870-871
Conditioners, hair, 424
Conditioning, behavioral, 175
Condoms, use of, 745
Conductive hearing loss, 442-443, 444-445
Condylomata acuminata (genital warts), 396-397
Congeners and hangover, 430-431
Congenital glaucoma, 400, 401
Congenital heart disease, 460-461
Congenital lactose intolerance, 540, 541
Congestion: *chart*, 284-285; in pregnancy, 692
Congestive heart failure, 130-131, 368-369, 378-379, 458
Conium, 583
Conization, 246
Conjugated estrogen, 929
Conjunctiva, *287*
Conjunctivitis, 286-287, 504-505, *1051*
Consolida regalis (larkspur), 729
Constipation, 200-201, 288-291, 333; in pregnancy, 689, 691
Contac (acetaminophen, dextromethorphan, pseudoephedrine), 884, 936, 997
Contact dermatitis, 186, 312, 313, 314, 315, *1048*; poison ivy, oak, and sumac, 682-*683*

Contact dissolution of gallstones, 386
Contraception, 40-41, 42. *See also* Birth-control pills
Contractions, uterine, in pregnancy, 691
Convallaria majalis (lily of the valley), 463
Conventional medicine: board certification in, 19; choice of practitioner, 29; defined, 17; medicine chest for, *78*; specialties, 18-20. *See also individual ailments*
Copper, 1037-1038; inability to metabolize (Wilson's disease), 267, 268
Copperheads (snakes), *77*; bites from, 76
Coptis (*Coptis chinensis*; *C. deltoidea*), 929-930; in combinations, 885, 902, 925, 946, 958, 1009
Coral snakes, *77*; bites from, 76
Corgard (nadolol), 980
Corneal injury, 360-361
Corneal surgery, 864
Cornelian cherry fruit, Asiatic (cornus), 930; in combinations, 922, 945
Corns and calluses, 292-293, *1046*
Cornus (*Cornus officinalis*), 930; in combinations, 922, 945
Coronary artery disease (coronary heart disease), 152, 452, 453, 458-459; angioplasty for, *154*
Correctol (docusate, phenolphthalein), 939, 993
Cortaid (hydrocortisone), 960
Corticosteroids, 930-931; interactions with, 962, 966, 984, 994
Corticotropin (ACTH): interactions with, 962
Cortinelin, 1007
Cortisone, 341, 409, 424, 682, 763; deficiency (Addison's disease), 368-369; interactions with, 932, 944
Cortizone (hydrocortisone), 960
Corydalis (*Corydalis yanhusuo*), 931
Cosmetics, dermatitis from, 313
Costus root (aucklandia), 902; in combinations, 922, 929, 933, 1013
Cotrim (sulfamethoxazole and trimethoprim), 1011
Cotrimoxazole (sulfamethoxazole and trimethoprim), 1011
Cottonmouths (snakes), *77*; bites from, 76
Couch grass: in combinations, 910
Cough, 294-297; *chart*, 212-213; in bronchitis, 214, 215, 216; in emphysema, 346, 347; whooping cough, 876-877
Cough medications, 296
Cough suppressants, 931
Cough syrup, onion-honey, 297, 681
Coumadin (warfarin), 1022
Coumarin, 529; derivatives, 939
Counterstrain technique, 815
Cox-2 inhibitors, 931
CPR (cardiopulmonary resuscitation), *50-53*
Crab lice (crabs; pubic lice), 550, 551
Cradle cap, 312
Cramp bark, 136, 146, 169, 225, 440, 591, 723, 909, 1023
Cramps, menstrual, 589, 590-591; acupressure for, *592*; reflexology for, *593*
Cramps, muscle, 606-607, 608-609; in pregnancy, 691-692
Cranberry, 184, 185
Cranesbill, wild, 79, 593
Crataegus laevigata; Crataegus oxyacantha (hawthorn), 957
Creams, herbal, 1026
Crib death (sudden infant death syndrome; SIDS), 33
Crocetin, 1002
Crocus, autumn (*Colchicum*), 371, 411
Crocus sativus (saffron), 1002
Crohn's disease, 84-85, 114-115, 298-301, *299*, 324-325, 526-527, 618-619
Cromolyn, 931-932
Cromolyn sodium, 763
Croup, 302-303
Crying, prolonged, in infants, 272-273
Cryptotympana atrata (cicada), 924
CTS (carpal tunnel syndrome), 234-237, 428-429, 626-627
Cumin (*Cuminum cyminum*), 121
Cumulative trauma disorder (repetitive stress injury), 234-237
Cuprum metallicum, 477, 607
Curcuma longa (turmeric), 1019
Curcumin, 1019
Currant, black, 647
Curvature of spine, sideways (scoliosis), 736-*737*
Cuscuta (*Cuscuta chinensis*), 932; in combinations, 927, 945, 973, 995
Cutaneous horns, 758
Cuts and lacerations, 304-305
Cyanocobalamin, 1035
Cyclobenzaprine, 932-933
Cyclophosphamides, 420, 563
Cyclosporine: interactions with, 902, 915, 926, 943, 966, 984, 994, 1011
Cylindroid aneurysms, *123*
Cymbopogon citratus (lemongrass), 968
Cynanchum (*Cynanchum stautoni*), 434
Cyperus (*Cyperus rotundus*), 933
Cypress, 593, 860
Cystectomy, radical, 181
Cysteine, 675, 873
Cystic duct, 384, *385*
Cystitis (bladder infection), 182-185; in pregnancy, 691; urinary problems from, *chart*, 846-847
Cysts: acne, 90, 92; breast, 208, 210-211; cervical, 244-245; as lumps, *chart*, 556-557; ovarian, 646-647

D

Dairy products, intolerance to, 540-541
Damiana, 934; in combination, 966
Danazol, 209, 352, 592; interactions with, 962
D and C (dilation and curettage), 592
Dandelion (*Taraxacum mongolicum*), 934-935; in combination, 924
Dandelion (*Taraxacum officinale*), 934; in combination, 903
Dandruff, 306-307
Danthron: interactions with, 968
Dantrolene, 602
Darvocet-N 100 (propoxyphene), 997
Daunorubicin: interactions with, 1013
Daypro (oxaprozin), 988
DayQuil Liquid or LiquiCaps (acetaminophen, dextromethorphan, guaifenesin), 884, 936, 955
Deadly nightshade (*belladonna*), 904
Deafness and hearing impairment, 442-447
Decoctions, herbal, 1025
Decongestants, 435, 935; interactions with, 890, 905, 938
Deep-heat therapy, 225
Deep phlebitis, 544-545, 668, 669
Deep-tissue massage, 623
Deep varicose veins, 858, 859
Deer ticks, 565, *727*; Lyme disease from, 564-565
Defervescence, 798-799
Defibrillators, 450
Degenerative disk disease, disk problems known as, 327
Degenerative joint disease, osteoarthritis known as, 143
Dehydration, 610-611, 846-847, 869; diarrhea and, 301
Delirium tremens (DT), 104
Delivery, labor and, 39-40; emergency, *60-61*
Deltasone (prednisone), 996

Demulen (ethinyl estradiol, ethynodiol diacetate), 944
Dental problems: aging and, 44; bad breath as, 170-171; fluoride for preventing, 1038; gum problems, 418-421, *419*; during pregnancy, 692; teething problems, 804-805; temporomandibular joint (TMJ) syndrome, 362-363, 806-809; tooth abscess, 362-363, 372-373, 836, *837*; toothache, 836-837; tooth decay, 836, *837*
Dentinal hypersensitivity, 837
Dentistry, 18
Deodorants, 193
Depakote (valproic acid), 1021
Depigmentation of skin, 866-*867*
Depressants, central nervous system, 336, 338, 512; interactions with, 894, 933, 936, 956, 960, 987, 994, 1024
Depression, 308-311, 366-367, 514-515; manic-depression, 514-515, 574-577; seasonal affective disorder, 514-515, 738-739
Dermabrasion, 92
Dermatitis, 106, 108, 312-315, *1048*; atopic (eczema), 312, 313, 314, 315, 323, 342-345, 520-521, *1044*, *1048*; and blisters, 186; candidal, 880; as diaper rash, 322, 323; poison ivy, oak, and sumac, 682-*683*
Dermatology, 18
Dermatomyositis, 610-611
DES (diethylstilbestrol), 243, 245, 819, 855
Desensitization therapy, 671
Desipramine, 310, 576
Desmopressin, 175
Desogen (desogestrel; ethinyl estradiol), 935, 944
Desogestrel, 935
Detached retina, 862, 863, 864
Detoxification, 103-104
Devil's claw, 935-936
Dexamethasone, 415, 827
Dexatrim (phenylpropanolamine), 993
Dexbrompheniramine, 936
Dexpanthenol, 1034
Dextromethorphan, 936
Dextrothyrozine: interactions with, 962
DiaBeta (glyburide), 954
Diabetes, 316-321, 364-365, 368-369, 618-619, 798-799; hypoglycemia in, 316, 318, 484, 485
Diabetic neuropathy, 317
Diabetic retinopathy, 317
Dialysis, 531-532
Diaper rash, 322-323, 714-715, *1044*
Diaphragm: in hiatal hernia, 474, *475*; spasms of (hiccups), 476-477
Diaphragmatic breathing, 349
Diaphragms and toxic shock, 839
Diarrhea, 200-201; *chart*, 324-325; and dehydration, 301
Diastolic pressure, 478
Diathermy, 225, 814
Diazepam, 936; interactions with, 898, 980, 986, 999
Diazoxide, 485; interactions with, 988, 994
Diclofenac, 889, 936-937
Dicloxacillin, 195, 774
Dicyclomine, 937
Didanosine, 99; interactions with, 949, 966
Dideoxycytidine, 99
Diet and nutrition, 28, 1030; Food Guide Pyramid, *1031*; minerals, 1032, 1036-1041; vitamins, 1032-1036. *See also individual ailments*
Dietary Guidelines, 1030
Diethylstilbestrol (DES), 243, 245, 819, 855
Digestive problems. *See* Gastrointestinal problems
Digestive system, *1059*
Digitalis, 451
Digitalis preparations, 937; interactions with, 894, 898, 935, 939, 968, 990
Digitalis purpurea (foxglove), 450, 463
Digitate warts, 872
Digoxin, 937-938; interactions with, 891, 898, 902, 910, 913, 915, 925, 943, 990, 995, 1011, 1015
1,2-Dihydroxyethane, 533
Dihydroergotamine (D.H.E. 45), 439
Dilacor XR (diltiazem), 938
Dilantin (phenytoin), 993
Dilated pupils, *chart*, 710-711
Dilation and curettage (D and C), 592
Dill, 273
Diltiazem, 938; interactions with, 925
Dilution ratios of homeopathic remedies, 26, 1027
Dimenhydrinate, 78, 581, 598, 938
Dimetapp (brompheniramine, phenylpropanolamine), 910, 993
Dimetapp DM Elixir (dextromethorphan), 936
Dioscorea, 387
Dioscorea opposita (Chinese yam), 922-923; in combinations, 922, 930, 945
Dioscorea villosa (wild yam), 1023; in combination, 903
Diovan (valsartan), 1022
Diphenhydramine, 938; interactions with, 906
Diphenylhydantoin, phenytoin formerly known as, 993
Diphtheria, pertussis, and tetanus vaccine (DPT), 33 *chart*, 821, 877
Diplacusis, 580
Dipyridamole, 938; in combinations, 900; interactions with, 898
Discectomy, 328
Discoid lupus erythematosus (DLE), 562
Disk problems, 164-165, 326-329, *327*, 620-621, 626-627, 672-*673*
Dislocations and fractures, 64, 65, 544-545; athletic injuries, 158, 160-161
Dissecting aneurysms, 122
Disulfiram, 104; interactions with, 889, 906, 914, 991
Diuretics, 938-939; in combinations, 887; interactions with, 888, 891, 904, 905, 910, 920, 938, 962, 984, 987, 995, 996, 998
Diverticula and diverticulosis, 114-115, 330, *331*
Diverticulitis, 86-87, 324-325, 330-333, *331*
Dizziness: *chart*, 334-335; Ménière's disease, 580-583; in pregnancy, 691
DL-phenylalanine, 734
Docusate, 939
Dodder, Chinese (cuscuta), 932; in combinations, 927, 945, 973, 995
Dog tick, brown, *727*
Dogwood, Asiatic (cornus), 930; in combinations, 922, 945
Dogwood, Jamaican: in combinations, 989
Dolomite, 434
Dong quai, 939-940; in combinations, 901, 922, 928, 933, 974, 995, 1002, 1019
Dopamine, 660, 661, 897, 912, 969
Doshas, 21
Double pneumonia, 678
Douches, natural, 247, 843
Doxazosin, 940
Doxepin, 940
Doxorubicin: interactions with, 1013
Doxycycline, 940; interactions with, 917, 994
Doxylamine, 940
DPT, 33 *chart*, 821, 877
Dragon bone, 827, 985
Drainage angle in glaucoma, *401*
Drainage remedies, 535
Drixoral (acetaminophen, pseu-

doephedrine), 884, 997
Drixoral Cold and Flu; Drixoral Cold and Allergy (dexbrompheniramine), 936
Drosera, 297, 877
Drosera rotundifolia (sundew), 303, 877
Drowning or near-drowning, *57*
Drug abuse, 336-339
Drug allergies, 106, 107, 108
Drug-related hepatitis, 469, 470
Drunkenness, 102
Ductal carcinoma, 204
Dulcamara, 763
Duodenal ulcers, 778, *779*, 781
Duratuss; Duratuss G (guaifenesin; phenylpropanolamine), 955, 993
Duricef (cefadroxil), 918
Dyazide (hydrochlorothiazide, triamterene), 959, 1018
DynaCirc (isradipine), 963
Dysfunctional uterine bleeding, 850, 851, 852, 853
Dyskinesia, 829; tardive, 733
Dysmenorrhea (painful periods), 588, 590-591; acupressure for, *592*; reflexology for, *593*
Dyspareunia, 741, 742, 743
Dysplasia, cervical, 242, 243, 245, 246, 247
Dysthymia, 308, 309

E

Ear, *580-581*, *641*, *1066*
Ear, nose, and throat, 19. *See also individual ailments*
Earache, *chart*, 340-341
Eardrum, *443*; ruptured, 340-341, 444
Ear emergencies, *58*
Earwax, 340-341, 444
Eating disorders: anorexia nervosa, 132-133, 218; bulimia, 218-219
Eccrine glands, 192
Echinacea (*Echinacea* spp.), 941; in combination, 929
Echinacoside; echinacein, 941
Econazole, 856
Ecotrin (aspirin), 900
ECT (electroconvulsive therapy), 310, 576
Ecthyma, 490
Ectocervical polyps, *245*
Ectopic pregnancy, 41
Eczema, 312, 313, 314, 315, 342-345, 520-521, *1044*, *1048*; as diaper rash, 323
Eczema herpeticum, 342, 345
Edema, 378-379; in pregnancy, 691
EDTA (ethylenediaminetetraacetic acid), 112-113, 155, 263
EEG biofeedback, 133, 137, 163, 219, 310-311, 359, 577, 633, 687
E.E.S. (erythromycin), 942
Eggs (ova), 38, 646; artificial fertilization of, 503; problems of, 502
Ehrlichiosis, ticks and, 508, 509
Eicosapentaenoic acid (EPA), 344, 709
Ejaculation, problems with, 42, 741, 742
Elavil (amitriptyline), 888
Elbow, epicondylitis affecting, 158, 159, 160, 161; tennis elbow, 140-141, 812-815, *813*
Elder, 79, 109, 282, 376, 434, 596, 757, 918, 946, 961, 979
Elderly, 44-45; age-related macular degeneration, 570-571; Alzheimer's disease, 110-113; caring for, 45; cataracts, senile, 238; depression, 308-309; drug abuse, 338; hearing problems, 442; sex, 740
Elecampane, 150, 217, 348, 909
Electrical burns, 222-223
Electric shock: for arrhythmias, 450; first aid for, *59*
Electroconvulsive therapy (ECT), 310, 576
Electrolyte abnormality, 610-611
Electromyographic (EMG) biofeedback, 652
Electrophysiologic testing, 449-450
Eleutherococcus senticosus (eleuthero; Siberian ginseng), 953-954
Eleutherosides, 954
Elimination diet, 435
Elm, slippery, 1009-1010; in combination, 916
Elocon (mometasone furoate), 977
Emboli, 188
EMDR (Eye Movement Desensitization and Reprocessing), 687
Emergencies/first aid, 46-77; ABCs, checking, *47*; back injuries, 66; bleeding, *48*, *70*, *72*; burns, 49; cardiac arrest, *50-53*; chemicals, 49, *63*; childbirth, *60-61*; choking, *54-56*; diabetic, 318; dislocations, 64, *65*; drowning or near-drowning, *57*; ear, *58*; electric shock, *59*; eye, *62-63*; fractures, 64, *65*; frostbite, 69; head injuries, 66; heart attack, 67; heatstroke and heat exhaustion, 68; hypothermia, 69; internal bleeding, 70; loss of consciousness, 71; neck injuries, 66; nose, 72; poisoning, 73; Recovery Position for, *47*; respiratory arrest, *50-53*; seizures, 74; shock, 75; shock, electric, *59*; snakebites, *76-77*; supplies for, 78
EMG (electromyographic) biofeedback, 652
Emphysema, 346-349, *347*
Empyema, 676
E-Mycin (erythromycin), 942
Enalapril, 941
Encephalitis, 710-711; measles and, 578
Endocarditis, 460, 773
Endocervical polyps, *245*
Endocrine cell cancers, pancreatic, 654, 655
Endocrine problems: diabetes, 316-321, 484, 485; fatigue from, *chart*, 368-369; goiters, 404-*405*; Graves' disease, 412-415; hypoglycemia, 316, 318, 484-485; pancreatitis, 656-657; and sweating, *chart*, 798-799; thyroid, 404-*405*, 412-415, 824-827; and trembling, *chart*, 840-841
Endocrine system, *1065*
Endometrial ablation, 852, 853
Endometrial cancer (endometrial carcinoma), 848-*849*
Endometrial hyperplasia, 848
Endometriosis, *350*-353
Endoscopic examination, 385, 779
Endoscopic surgery: for kidney stones, 537; sinus, 756
Enlarged prostate (BPH), 702-704, *703*, 705
Enokidake, 488
Entex LA (guaifenesin, phenylpropanolamine), 955, 993
Environmental poisoning, 354-357, 514-515, 626-627; acute, 73, 354
Environmental Protection Agency, U.S. (EPA), 355, 356; radon policy, 561
EPA (eicosapentaenoic acid), 344, 709
Ephedra (*Ephedra sinica*), 941-942; in combinations, 890, 946, 970; interactions with, 953
Ephedrine, 942; in combination, 1015; in ephedra, 941; interactions with, 906
Epicondylitis, 158, 159, 160, 161; lateral (tennis elbow), 140-141, 812-815, *813*
Epidemiology, 18
Epidermis, development of skin cancers in, 758, *759*
Epididymitis, 816-817
Epidural injection for herniated disks, 328
Epiglottitis, 302
Epilepsy, 358-359

Epinephrine, 108, 942; interactions with, 906, 962, 970, 1016
EpiPen (epinephrine), 942
Epstein-Barr virus (EBV), 259, 567, 595, 822
Equisetum, 175
Equisetum arvense (horsetail), 959
ERCP test, 385
Erection, failure of, 42, 492-493
Ergocalciferol, 1035
Ergonomics, 237
Ergotamine, 438, 719; interactions with, 902, 943, 1012
Ery-Tab (erythromycin), 942
Erythrocin Stearate (erythromycin), 942
Erythromycin, 942-943; interactions with, 896, 901, 906, 914, 920, 938, 972, 996, 1009, 1019
Erythromycin Base (erythromycin), 942
Erythromycin estolate, 942
Erythromycins, 943; interactions with, 943, 991
Erythroplakia, 634
Esophageal thrush, 880
Esophageal ulcers, 778
Esophagus: in hiatal hernia, 474, *475*; irritation of (heartburn), 456-457
Essential oils, 21, 1026. *See also individual names*
Essential tremor, 840-841
Estrace (estradiol), 943
Estraderm (estradiol), 943
Estradiol, 943
Estrogen: and breast cancer, 205; decreased levels of, 586; in menstrual cycle, 588, 593, 921; and ovarian cancer, 644; phytoestrogens (plant estrogens), 207, 587, 639
Estrogen (hormone) replacement therapy, 112, 205, 210, 453, 496, 562, 586-587, 637, 684, 848-849
Estrogens and progestins, 943-944; conjugated estrogens, 929; interactions with estrogens, 888, 890, 905, 907, 915, 917, 962, 970, 988, 991, 1011, 1013, 1015, 1016
Estropipate, 944
Estrostep 21; Estrostep FE (norethindrone acetate), 984
Ethacrynic acid: interactions with, 962, 988
Ethambutol, 845
Ethane dioic acid, 533
Ethinyl estradiol, 944; in combination, 969, 984
Ethmoidal sinuses, 754, *755*
Ethylenediaminetetraacetic acid (EDTA), 112-113, 155, 263
Ethylene glycol (1,2-ethanediol; ethylene alcohol; ethylene dihydrate), 533
Ethynodiol diacetate, 944
Etodolac, 889, 944
Eucalyptol, 944; in combination, 897
Eucalyptus (*Eucalyptus globulus*), 944-945
Eucommia bark (*Eucommia ulmoides*), 945; in combinations, 932, 973
Eupatorium perfoliatum (boneset), 909-910; in combinations, 918, 961
Eupatorium purpureum (gravelroot), 411
Euphorbia; *Euphorbia pilulifera*, 348; interactions with, 970
Euphrasia, 763
Euphrasia officinalis (eyebright), 946
European-combination remedies, 535
Eustachian tubes, *641*; blocked, 444, 447, 640, 641
Evening primrose oil, 945
Evers Diet, 603
Evodia fruit (*Evodia rutaecarpa*), 945-946; in combination, 926
Ewing's sarcoma, 196
Excedrin Extra-Strength (acetaminophen, aspirin, caffeine), 884, 900, 914
Excedrin PM (acetaminophen, diphenhydramine), 884, 938
Excimer laser treatment of cornea, 864
Exercise tolerance (stress) test, 127
Exertional (stable) angina, 124, 125
Ex-Lax (docusate, phenolphthalein), 939, 993
Ex-Lax Gentle Natural Laxative Pills (sennosides), 1006
Exocrine cell cancers, pancreatic, 654, *655*
Exocrine insufficiency, 656, 657
Exophthalmos, *413*, 415
Expectorants, 946
Extensor carpi radialis brevis, 812, *813*
External hemorrhoids, 464, *465*, 466
Extracts, herbal, kinds of, 1025-1026
Eye, *287*, *1066*
Eyebright, 946
Eye emergencies, *62-63*
Eye exercises, 865
Eyelid glands, infected, 792-793, *1051*
Eyelid inflammation (blepharitis), 504-505, 773
Eye Movement Desensitization and Reprocessing (EMDR), 687
Eye problems: *chart*, 360-361, *1051*; aging and, 44; black eye, 178-179; cataracts, 238-*239*; chalazions, 792, 793; from cold sores, 270, 271; conjunctivitis, 286-287, *1051*; diabetic retinopathy, 317; emergencies, first aid for, *62-63*; exophthalmos, *413*, 415; glaucoma, 400-403, *401*, 710-711, 870-871; inflammation from, *chart*, 504-505; macular degeneration, 570-571; in pregnancy, 693; pupil dilation, *chart*, 710-711; sties, *772*, *773*, *774*, *775*, 792-793, *1051*; vision problems, 862-865, *863*
Eyestrain, 863, 864, 865
Eyewashes, 287

F

Facial pain: *chart*, 362-363; acupressure for, *650*
Faintness and fainting: *chart*, 364-365; in pregnancy, 691
False gout, 409
False unicorn root, 647, 665
Family planning, 40-41, 42
Family practice, 18
Famotidine, 947; interactions with, 968, 1013
Farsightedness, 862, *863*, 864
Fasts, juice and water, 489
Fat, body: excessive, 628-631; fear of, 132-133, 218-219
Fat, dietary, 1030; and breast problems, 205, 211; and gallstones, 385, 387; and prostate cancer, 699, 701
Fatigue: *chart*, 366-369; chronic fatigue syndrome, 258-261; in pregnancy, 691
Fat-soluble vitamins: vitamin A, 1033; vitamin D, 1035-1036; vitamin E, 1036; vitamin K, 1036
Fatty liver, 267, 268
Fears, phobic, 670-671
Febrile seizures, 35, 74, 358
Fecal impaction, 289
Feet: aches and pains, *chart*, 370-371; athlete's foot, 156-157, 612-613, 714-715; athletic injuries, 159; bone spurs, *199*; bunions, 220-*221*; corns and calluses, 292-293, *1046*; diabetics' care of, 321; ingrown nails, 506-*507*; nail problems, *chart*, 612-613; pain, chronic, acupressure for, *650*; plantar warts, 674-675, *1047*; psoriasis, 706; in reflexology, 24, *25*
Feldenkrais method, 21
Female condoms, 745
Female health, 38-41

Female pattern baldness, 422, *423*
Female reproductive system, 38, *855*, *1062*
Female urinary system, *1062*
Femoral hernia, 472
Fempatch (estradiol), 943
Fenfluramine: interactions with, 962, 988
Fennel, 947; in combinations, 911, 931
Fenugreek, 947-948
Ferrous gluconate, 120
Ferrous sulfate: interactions with, 949
Ferrum phosphoricum, 948
Fertility problems, 40, 42, 351, 502-503
Fetal distress, 688
Fetal-tissue implants, 661
Fever and chills: *chart*, 372-373
Fever blisters (cold sores), 270-271, *1045*
Feverfew, 948
Fever tree, Australian (eucalyptus), 944-945
Feverwort (boneset), 909-910; in combinations, 918, 961
Fiber: and colorectal cancer, reduced risk of, 279; for constipation, 290-291; for diverticulitis prevention, 333; for IBS, 519; interactions with, 938; for ulcer prevention, 781
FiberCon (calcium polycarbophil), 915
Fibrillation, ventricular, 448
Fibroadenomas, breast, 208, 211
Fibroids, 850-852, 853
Fibromyalgia, 88-89, 608-609
Fibrosis, 814
Fibrositis, 167
Field mint, 948; in combinations, 912, 924, 974
Fields, W. C., 91
Fight-or-flight response, 597, 784
Figwort: in combinations, 981
Filiform warts, 872
Filipendula ulmaria (meadowsweet), 79, 241, 383, 393, 475, 499, 735, 936, 954
Finasteride, 704
Fingernail problems: *chart*, 612-613
Finger pain: *chart*, 428-429
Fire ants, bites from, 508, 509
First aid. *See* Emergencies/first aid
First-degree burns, 222, 223
Fishhook, removing, *305*
Flag: blue, 93, 195; sweet, 475
Flammulina velutipes (enokidake), 488
Flat warts, 872, *1047*
Flavonoids, 109, 155, 257, 300, 421, 571, 643, *757*, *775*, 853, 861, 1000, 1003; pyncogenol, 809
Flax and flaxseed, 79, 290, 642, 708
Fleeceflower root (polygonum), 995
Flexeril (cyclobenzaprine), 932
Flint (silica), 1007-1008; in horsetail, 959
Floxin (ofloxacin), 986
Flu, 88-89, 284-285, 368-369, 372-373, 374-377, 526-527, 608-609, 610-611
Fluconazole, 881
Flucytosine, 881
Fluid retention: *chart*, 378-379
Fluoride, 1038
Fluorinated steroid creams, 563
Fluoroquinolones, 948-949
Fluorouracil, 760, 1013
Fluoxetine, 949; interactions with, 938
Flurbiprofen, 889, 949
Flushed face: *chart*, 380-381
Foeniculum vulgare (fennel), 947; in combinations, 911, 931, 1005
Folic acid (folacin; folate; vitamin B_9), 1032; interactions with, 924, 1011
Folium mori albae (mulberry leaf), 296; in combinations, 899, 924, 1006
Folliculitis, 772, 773, 775
Fomentations (hot compresses), 1026
Fontanels, 32
Food allergies, 106, 107, 108, 109, 653; and CFS, 261; and dandruff, 307
Food and Nutrition Board of National Research Council, 1030, 1032
Food Guide Pyramid, *1031*
Food intolerances, 107
Food poisoning, 382-383
Foot problems. *See* Feet
Foreign objects: choking on, *54-56*; in ear, *58*; in eye, *62-63*; in nose, 72
Formaldehyde, 312, 355
Formyl trichloride, 533
Fo-ti (polygonum), 995
Fourth-degree burns, 222, 223
Foxglove (*Digitalis purpurea*), 450, 463
Fractures, 64, *65*, 158, 160-161, 544-545; from osteoporosis, 636
Free radicals: and Alzheimer's disease, 111; and macular degeneration, 571
French clay, 389
Friction blisters, 186, 187
Friedman, Meyer, 454
Fringe tree, 657
Fritillaria (fritillary): in combinations, 889, 934; *Fritillaria cirrhosa* bulb, 757; interactions with, 934
Frontal sinuses, 754, *755*
Frostbite, 69
Frozen shoulder, 750-751
Fucus spp. (kelp), 965
Fucus vesiculosus (bladder wrack), 405, 827
Fungal infections: athlete's foot, 156-157; jock itch, 524-525; meningitis as, 585; rashes from, *chart*, 714-717; ringworm, *1050*; yeast, 322, 323, 504-505, 524, 854, 855, 856, 857, 880-881, *1044*, *1045*
Furosemide, 949; interactions with, 939, 962
Furuncles (boils), 191, 194-195, 556-557, 772, 773, 774, 775
Fusiform aneurysms, *123*
Fu-zheng therapy, 901

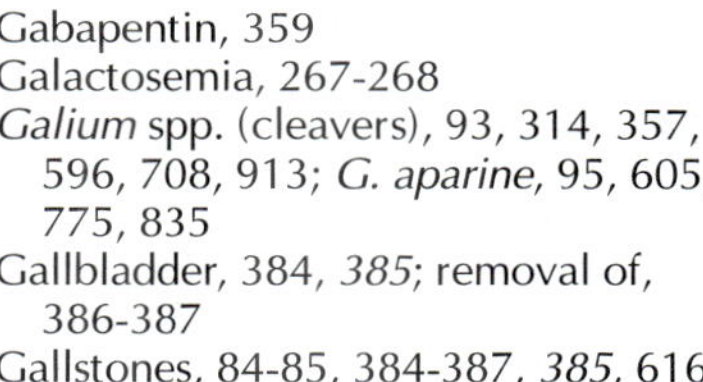

G

Gabapentin, 359
Galactosemia, 267-268
Galium spp. (cleavers), 93, 314, 357, 596, 708, 913; *G. aparine*, 95, 605, 775, 835
Gallbladder, 384, *385*; removal of, 386-387
Gallstones, 84-85, 384-387, *385*, 616-617
Gamete intrafallopian transfer (GIFT), 503
Gamma benzene hexachloride, 728, 729
Gamma globulin, 259, 487, 579
Gamma-linolenic acid (GLA), 945
Ganciclovir, 98
Gan-jian, ginger called, in China, 952
Ganoderma (*Ganoderma lucidum*), 950
Gardenia (*Gardenia jasminoides*), 749, 771, 811, 929
Gargles, homemade, 769
Garlic, 950; in combination, 929
Gas and gas pains, 388-389
Gastric cancer (gastric carcinoma; stomach cancer), *776-777*
Gastric ulcers, 778, *779*
Gastritis, 84-85, 324-325, 390-391, 616-617
Gastrodia (*Gastrodia elata*), 950-951
Gastroenteritis, 84-85, 114-115, 324-325, 392-393, 616-617, 868-869
Gastrointestinal problems, 500, 501; abdominal pains, *chart*, 84-87; anal bleeding, 114-115 *chart*, 464; anal fissure, 116-117; appendicitis, 138-139; bowel movement abnormalities, *chart*, 200-201; celiac disease,

240-241; colitis, 274-275; colorectal cancer, 276-279, *277*; constipation, 288-291, 333; Crohn's disease, 298-301, *299*; diarrhea, *chart*, 324-325; diverticulitis, 330-333, *331*; gas and gas pains, 388-389; gastritis, 390-391; gastroenteritis, 392-393; heartburn, 456-457, 474, 475; hemorrhoids, 464-467, *465*; hernia, 472-*473*; hiatal hernia, 474-*475*; indigestion, 380-381, 498-499; irritable bowel syndrome, 516-519; lactose intolerance, 540-541; nausea, *chart*, 616-619; pancreatic cancer and, *655*; in pregnancy, 689, 691; stomach cancer, 776-*777*; stomach ulcers, 778-781, *779*; vomiting, *chart*, 868-871
Gastrointestinal tract, *1059*
Gastroscopy, 779
Gathering Vitality (herbal formula), 311
Gaultheria procumbens (wintergreen), 282, 439, 651
GBE (ginkgo biloba extract), 113, 952-953
Gelsemium, 951
Gemfibrozil, 951; interactions with, 901, 996, 1009
Gene therapy for cancer, 229; brain cancer, 203; lung cancer, 560
Genetic factors: in ALS, 554; in Alzheimer's disease, 110-111; in anemia, 119; in breast cancer, 205; in cancer, 227; in cholesterol levels, 255; in cirrhosis, 267, 268; in colorectal cancer, 277, 278; in hearing loss, 443; in leukemia, 547; in lung cancer, 559; males affected by, 43; in sickle cell disease, 752
Genetics, medical, 18
Genital allergic reaction, 504-505
Genital herpes, 394-395, 666-667
Genital warts, 396-397, 666-667; cervical, 245, 246
Gentian (*Gentiana lutea*), 951
Gentiana (*Gentiana scabra*), 952
Geranium, 233, 271, 582, 593, 651, 675, 695
Geranium maculatum (wild cranesbill), 79, 593
German chamomile, 920; in combinations, 911, 952, 954, 989, 1020, 1023
German measles, 39, 398-*399*, 714-715, *1044*
GIFT (gamete intrafallopian transfer), 503
Ginger, 952; in combinations, 890, 907, 909, 929, 941, 946, 951, 971, 978, 1004, 1023
Gingerols, 952
Gingivitis, 418, 419, 420, 421
Ginkgo (*Ginkgo biloba*), 264, 952-953
Ginseng, American, 953
Ginseng, Asian, 953; in combinations, 901, 925, 951, 995, 1005, 1013
Ginseng, Siberian, 953-954
Ginsenosides, 953
GLA (gamma-linolenic acid), 945
Glands, *1065*; sweat, 192
Glandular problems: pancreatic cancer, 654-*655*. *See also* Endocrine problems
Glaucoma, 400-403, *401*, 710-711, 870-871
Glial cell-derived nerve growth factor, 661
Glioblastoma multiformes, *203*
Glipizide, 954; interactions with, 898, 999
Glomerulonephritis, 490
Glove anesthesia, 652-653
Glucagon, 485; interactions with, 962
Glucocorticoids, 637
Glucotrol (glipizide), 954
Glutamate, 791
Glutamic acid, 705
Glutamine, 781
Gluten sensitivity, 240-241
Glyburide, 954; interactions with, 999
Glycine, 305, 705
Glycolic acid, 957
Glycosides, cardiac, 463
Glycyrrhiza glabra (licorice), 970-971; in combination, 903
Glycyrrhiza uralensis (licorice), 970; in combinations, 912, 926, 941, 946, 952, 1003, 1013
Glycyrrhizic acid, 395
Glynase (glyburide), 954
GnRH (gonadotropin-releasing hormone), 852, 853
Goiters, 404-*405*
Gold, Joseph, 231
Golden chamber (herb combination), 493
Golden lock tea, 497
Goldenrod, 109, 434, 757, 946
Goldenseal, 954; in combinations, 916, 946
Gold therapy, 144-145
Goldthread, Chinese (coptis), 929-930; in combinations, 885, 902, 925, 946, 958, 1009
Gonadotropin-releasing hormone (GnRH), 852, 853
Gonorrhea, 406-407, 666-667
Gotu kola, 954-955
Gout, 128-129, 140-141, 370-371, 408-411, *409*, *410*, 428-429, 526-527
Grains-of-paradise fruit, 955; in combinations, 885, 886, 902, 922, 951
Grand mal seizures, 358, 359
Grapefruit-seed extract, 879
Grape skins, 155, 189, 257
Graphites, 117, 157, 491, 708, 801
Gravelroot, 411
Graves' disease, 412-415, 840-841
Grindelia (*Grindelia* spp.), 348
Griseofulvin, 157
Groin strain (groin pull), 416-417
Growing pains, 160, 538-539
Growth charts: female, 34; male, 35
Guaifed (guaifenesin), 955
Guaifenesin, 955
Guanabenz: interactions with, 906
Guanethidine: interactions with, 962, 976, 996
Guanfacine, 956
Gugulipid, 155, 189, 256
Guided imagery, 27
Gum problems, 418-421, *419*
Gum resin, myrrh from, 979
Gum tree (eucalyptus), 944-945
Gumweed: in combinations, 979

H

Habitrol (nicotine), 981
Hahnemann, Samuel, 26
Hair, 422; lice in, 550, 551
Hair cells of cochlea, 443
Hair follicles, 422, 423, 424; in acne, 90-91; staph infections of, 772, 773, 775
Hair loss, 422-425, *423*
Hair transplantation, 424
Halcion (triazolam), 1019
Halitosis (bad breath), 170-171
Halls Mentho-Lyptus cough drops (menthol), 974
Haloperidol, 112, 576, 733, 828; interactions with, 913, 1019
Hamamelis (homeopathic remedy), 467
Hamamelis virginiana (witch hazel), 79, 195, 251, 271, 467, 579, 683, 691, 860, 954, 979
Hamstring injury, 426-427
Hamstring stretch, *427*
Hand exercises, *146*, 237
Hand pain, *chart*, 428-429
Hands, psoriasis affecting, 706
Hangover, 430-431
Hardening of the arteries (atherosclerosis), 152-155, *153*; coronary, 152, *154*, 453
Hare's ear (bupleurum), 912; in com-

binations, 901, 925, 933
Harlequin (coral) snakes, *77*; bites from, 76
Harpagophytum procumbens (devil's claw), 935-936
Harpagoside, 935
Hashimoto's thyroiditis, 824-825
Hawthorn, 957
Hay fever, 107, 108, 284-285, 432-435
HCF (high-carbohydrate high-plant-fiber) diet, 320-321
HDL (high-density lipoprotein), 254, 255, 256, 923
Headache, 362-363, 436-441, 616-617, 868-869; in pregnancy, 691; and pupil dilation, *chart*, 710-711
Head injuries, 66, 710-711
Head lice, 550-551
Hearing, mechanics of, *443*, *1066*
Hearing aids, 445
Hearing problems, 442-447, 580
Heart, *449*, *459*
Heart and circulatory system. *See* Cardiovascular system
Heart arrhythmias, 448-451, 454, 458
Heart attack, 67, 140-141, 248-249, 452-455
Heartbeat, 448, 449; irregular, 448-451, 454, 458
Heart block, 449
Heartburn, 84-85, 248-249, 456-457, 796-797; hiatal hernia and, 474, 475; in pregnancy, 691
Heart disease, 364-365, 458-463; periodontitis and, 420. *See also individual names*
Heart murmurs, 461
Heart valve disease, 459-460, 461
Heat cramps, 606, 607
Heat rash, 714-715
Heatstroke and heat exhaustion, 68, 364-365, 372-373, 380-381
Heat therapy, 100, 147, 225
Heel spurs, *199*
Height and weight charts: adults, 37; children, 34-35
Heimlich maneuver (abdominal thrusts), *54*, *55*; infant equivalent, *56*
Hellerwork, 21
Heme vs. nonheme iron, 1038
Hemlock, Western, 705
Hemochromatosis, 120, 267, 268
Hemodialysis, 532
Hemoglobin, 118; in sickle cell anemia, 752, 753
Hemolytic anemias, 119, 120
Hemoptysis (coughing up blood), 295
Hemorrhoidectomy, 466
Hemorrhoids, 114-115, 200-201, 464-467, *465*, 520-521; in pregnancy, 691
Heparin, 957; interactions with, 898, 939
Hepar sulphuris, 957
Hepatitis, 267, 268, 269, 368-369, 468-471, 870-871
Hepatitis A, 468-469, 471
Hepatitis B, 267, 469, 470-471
Hepatitis C, 267, 469, 471
Hepatitis D, 469
Hepatitis E, 469, 471
Herbal oils: essential, 21, 1026; infused, 1026. *See also individual names*
Herbal therapies, 26; Chinese herbs, 24, 26; medicine chest, *79*; preparations, 1025-1026; safety with, 1025. *See also names of individual ailments and herbs*
Hereditary calluses, 292
Hereditary nonpolyposis colorectal cancer (HNPCC), gene for, 278
Hernias, 84-85, 472-*473*, 556-557; hiatal, 86-87, 474-*475*, 796-797, 868-869
Herniated (slipped) disks, 164-165, 326-329, *327*, 620-621, 626-627, 672-*673*
Herniorrhaphy, 473
Heroin, 337, 338, 339
Herpes, genital, 394-395, 666-667
Herpes simplex virus: cold sores from, 270-271, *1045*; eczema from, 342, 345
Herpes zoster virus: chickenpox from, *250*-251, 714-715, *1044*; shingles from, 362-363, 746-747, *1050*
Hiatal hernia, 86-87, 474-*475*, 796-797, 868-869
Hibiscus (*Hibiscus sabdariffa*), 957-958
Hiccups, 476-477
High blood pressure, 478-481
High blood pressure drugs (antihypertensives), 896; interactions with, 891, 905, 906, 910, 915, 935, 938, 939, 976, 987, 992, 994, 1018, 1019
High blood sugar (hyperglycemia), 318; and ketoacidosis, 316-317
High-carbohydrate high-plant-fiber (HCF) diet, 320-321
High-density lipoprotein (HDL), 254, 255, 256, 923
High-grade vs. low-grade lymphoma, 566-567, 568
Hip fractures, 636
Hip splinting, *65*
Histamine, 106, 482, 896, 924, 947, 983, 999; interactions with, 982
Histamine H2 blockers, 958; interactions with, 966, 968
HIV (human immunodeficiency virus), 96, 97, 98, 100, 101, 567, 885-886
Hives, 106, 107, 108, 482-483, 716-*717*, *1049*
HMG-CoA reductase inhibitors, 923, 972, 995, 1008
Hodgkin's disease, 566, 567, 568
Holistic healthcare: defined, 17; naturopathy, 28; osteopathy as, 28
Holmes-Adie syndrome, 710-711
Holmes-Rahe questionnaire, 785
Holter monitor, 449
Homeopathic remedies, 26-27, 1027; medicine chest, *79*. *See also individual ailments and remedies*
Homeostasis, goal of: in chiropractic, 26; in reflexology, 24
Homosexuals, sexual dysfunction in, 741
Homostachydrine, 886
Honey: as burn remedy, 223; scallions and, 1004
Honeybee, *177*, 602, 898-899
Honey diet, 434
Honey-onion cough syrup, 297, 681
Honeysuckle flower, 958; in combinations, 924, 934, 940, 970
Honeysuckle Forsythia Powder, 835
Honeysuc (safflower flower), 1002; in combination, 887
Hookworms, 878, 879
Hops, 958-959; in combination, 989
Hops, wild, 911
Horehound, 79, 680, 909, 929, 961, 979
Hormonal problems. *See* Endocrine problems
Hormone replacement therapy (HRT), 112, 205, 210, 453, 496, 562, 586-587, 637, 684, 848-849
Hormones, 1065; and acne, 90, 93; and breast pain, 208-209; calcitonin, 637-638; contraception based on, 40-41; for endometriosis, 352; and menstruation, 588, 592; ovaries and, 646, 647; pancreatic cancer and, 654; and PMS, 694-695; and prostate cancer, 699, 700; stress, 597, 784; and uterine problems, 851, 853. *See also* Estrogen
Hormone therapy: for cancer, 229; for hair loss, 424
Hornet, white-faced, *177*
Horse chestnut, 860
Horsetail, 959
Hot flashes, 586

Hot infusion of herbal oils, 1026
Housemaid's knee, 538-539
Huckleberry, 402-403
Human immunodeficiency virus (HIV), 96, 97, 98, 100, 101, 567
Hu ma you (sesame oil), 1006
Humibid DM (guaifenesin), 955
Humibid LA (guaifenesin), 955
Humidifiers, use of, 95, 579, 685; cool-mist, 835, 877; vs. vaporizers, 217, 349
Humulin N; Humulin R; Humulin 50/50; Humulin 70/30 (insulin), 962
Humulus lupulus (hops), 958-959; in combination, 989
Hycotuss (guaifenesin), 955
Hydantoin drugs, 993; interactions with, 1011
Hydrastis, 387
Hydrastis canadensis (goldenseal), 954; in combinations, 916, 946
Hydrazine sulfate, 231
Hydrochlorothiazide, 959; in combinations, 941, 971, 1018
Hydrocodone, 959-960
Hydrocortisone, 960; interactions with, 944; neomycin, polymyxin B, and, 980-981
Hydrocotyle rotundifolia (Asian pennywort), 473
Hydrogen peroxide, 172, 187, 233, 444, 713, 769, 897
Hydrophobia (rabies), 712-713
Hydroquinone, 867, 1020
Hydrotherapy, 27
Hydroxyapatite, microcrystalline, 161
Hydroxychloroquine, 563
Hydroxyurea, 753; interactions with, 1013
Hydroxyzine, 960
Hyoscyamus niger, 633
Hyperactivity and attention disorders, 162-163
Hyperglycemia, 318; and ketoacidosis, 316-317
Hyperhemolytic crises, 752
Hyperhidrosis, 193, 798-799
Hypericin, 100, 1003
Hypericum, 960-961
Hypericum perforatum (St.-John's-wort), 960-961, 1003
Hyperopia (farsightedness), 862, *863*, 864
Hypersensitivity, dentinal, 837
Hypertension (high blood pressure), 478-481
Hypertension, ocular, 401, 402
Hyperthermia, 100
Hyperthyroidism, 404, 405, 610-611, 798-799, 824, 825, 826, 827; Graves' disease, 412-415; and trembling, *chart*, 840-841
Hyperventilation, 137, 658, 659
Hypnotherapy, 27, 137
Hypoglycemia, 316, 318, 364-365, 484-485, 840-841
Hypoglycemics (antidiabetic drugs), oral, 987-988; interactions with, 908, 925, 939, 970, 984, 1011
Hypogonadism, 816-817
Hypopharynx, 822, *823*
Hypotension, 364-365; postural, 691
Hypothermia, 69
Hypothyroidism, 368-369, 404, 405, 415, 824-825, 827
Hyssop (*Hyssopus officinalis*), 961
Hysterectomy, 593, 849, 852; alternatives to, 851-852, 853; sex after, 740
Hytone (hydrocortisone), 960
Hytrin (terazosin), 1014

I

Ibuprofen, 889, 961; interactions with, 907
Ice rescue, *57*
Idiopathic hypertrophic subaortic stenosis, 460
Ignatia, 961
Ileostomy, 300, 301
Iletin I NPH (insulin), 962
Ileum in Crohn's disease, *299*
Ilotycin (erythromycin), 942
Imdur (isosorbide mononitrate), 963
Imipramine, 175, 219, 310, 496, 576, 659
Imitrex (sumatriptan), 1012
Immune problems, 486-489; aging and, 45; AIDS, 96-101; blisters from, 186; chronic fatigue syndrome, 258-261; Crohn's disease as, 298; Graves' disease, 412-415; lupus, 562-563, 610-611; multiple sclerosis as, 601; from stress, 597. *See also* Allergies
Immune response, 500
Immune serum globulin shots, 269, 471
Immune system, *1065*
Immunizations. *See* Vaccines
Immunization schedule: *chart*, 33
Immuno-augmentative therapy, 231
Immunoglobulin: tetanus, 821; varicella zoster, 251
Immunology, 18
Immunosuppressants: azathioprine as, 275, 299; interactions with, 901, 926, 972, 996, 1009; for lupus, 563, 611
Immunotherapy: for allergies, 108, 433; for asthma, 150; BCG, 181; for cancer, 181, 197, 207, 229, 529, 549, 560, 760, 761; passive, 98
Imodium A-D (loperamide), 971
Impaction: fecal, 289; teeth, 836
Impatiens (jewelweed), 683
Impetigo, 490-491, *1045*
Impotence, 42, 492-493
Incisional hernia, 472
Incisions and lacerations, 304-305
Inclusion conjunctivitis in infants (ophthalmia neonatorum), 286
Incompetent cervix, 244, 245, 247
Incontinence, 494-497, 846-847; bed-wetting, 174-175; after prostatectomy, 700
Indapamide, 961-962
Inderal; Inderal LA (propranolol), 997
Indian tobacco (lobelia), 971; in combination, 979
Indigestion, 84-85, 380-381, 498-499
Indomethacin, 149, 391; interactions with, 888, 890, 905, 938, 939
Industrial chemicals, environmental poisoning from, 355
Infants, 32-33; birth, *39-40, 60-61*; breast-feeding, 32, 40; choking, first aid for, *56*; CPR for, *52*; pulse, checking, *52*
Infections, 500-501; aches and pains from, *chart*, 88-89; athlete's foot, 156-157; breast, 209; and bronchitis, acute, 214, 215; cervicitis, 244, 245, 246-247; common cold, 280-283, 375; conjunctivitis as, 286, 287, *1051*; diaper rash involving, 322, 323; fatigue from, *chart*, 368-369; gastroenteritis, 392-393; immunization schedule for, *chart*, 33; inflammation from, *chart*, 504-505; of ingrown nail, 506, *507*; jock itch, 524-525; respiratory, kinds of, 720, 721; ringworm, *1050*; sickle cell anemia, 753; and stomach cancer, 776-777; swimmer's ear, 800-801; tonsil, 834-835; of wounds, 304; yeast, 524, 880-881, *1044, 1045*. *See also* Bacterial infections; Parasitic disorders; Sexually transmitted diseases (STDs); Viral infections; Warts
Infectious arthritis, 128-129, 140-141, 142, 143, 144, 145, 428-429, 526-527
Infertility, 40, 42, 351, 502-503
Inflammation. *See also names of individual ailments*: *chart*, 504-505

Influenza (flu), 88-89, 284-285, 368-369, 372-373, 374-377, 526-527, 608-609, 610-611
Infused oils, 1026
Infusions, herbal, 1025
Ingrown nail, 506-*507*, 612-613
Inguinal hernia, 84-85, 472, *473*
Injuries: athletic, 158-161; black eyes from, 178-179; childhood, 33, 34, 35; cuts, scratches, and wounds, 304-305; foot, 370-371; groin strain, 416-417; hamstring, 426-427; knee pain from, *chart*, 538-539; leg pain from, *chart*, 544-545; repetitive stress, 234-237; shin splints, 748-749; sprains and strains, 770-*771*; tennis elbow, 140-141, 812-815, *813*; and tetanus, 820, 821. *See also* Emergencies/first aid
Inner ear, 580-*581*; and dizziness, *chart*, 334-335; Ménière's disease, 580-583
Inoculations. *See* Vaccines
Inositol, 321
Insects: bee and wasp stings, 176-177; bees and wasps, *177*; bites, 508-509, *1049*; in ear, floating out, *58*; lice, 520-521, 550-551; sting allergies, 107, 109, 176-177
Insomnia, 366-367, 510-513, 514-515
Insulin, 962; interactions with, 906, 910, 937, 939, 970, 981, 984, 1015, 1016
Insulin-dependent (Type 1) diabetes mellitus (IDDM), 316, 317, 318-319, 320, 321
Insulin imbalances: diabetes, 316-321; hypoglycemia, 316, 318, 484-485
Intal (cromolyn), 931
Interferon therapy, 268, 471, 529, 549, 568, 602, 760, 761; interferon alpha (Intron A), 397
Interleukin, 549; interleukin 2, 98, 529, 761
Intermittent claudication, 262
Internal bleeding, 70, 304, 390, 391
Internal hemorrhoids, 464, *465*-466
Internal medicine, 18
Intertrigo, 880
Intervertebral disks, problems of, 164-165, 326-329, *327*, 620-621, 626-627, 672-*673*
Intestinal flu (gastroenteritis), 84-85, 324-325, 392-393, 616-617, 868-869
Intestinal problems. *See* Gastrointestinal problems
Intoxication, alcohol, 102
Intraductal papillomas, 211
Intrauterine devices (IUDs), 40; and pelvic inflammatory disease, 664, 665
Intussusception, 114-115
Inula helenium (elecampane), 150, 217, 348, 909
In vitro fertilization (IVF), 503
Involuntary movement disorders, 828-829
Involutional alopecia, 422
Iodide and thyroid, 413, 414, 825, 826; goiter, 404-405
Iodine, 1038; in combination, 897
Ipecac, 962-963
Ipratropium, 963; interactions with, 932
Iris versicolor (blue flag), 93, 195
Iron, 1038-1039; interactions with, 891, 898, 914, 925, 986, 1015; spinach and, 119
Iron deficiency anemia, 119, 120, 121
Iron excess: hemochromatosis, 120, 267, 268; iron overload, 118, 120
Iron phosphate, 948
Irritability, *chart*, 514-515
Irritable bowel syndrome (IBS), 84-85, 200-201, 324-325, 516-519
Ischemia, heart muscle, 452
Ischemic colitis, 274
Islet cell carcinomas (endocrine cell cancers), 654, 655
Ismo (isosorbide mononitrate), 963
Isocarboxazid, 963
Isoetharine, 150
Isoleucine, 555
Isolobelanine, 971
Isometheptene, 438
Isoniazid (INH), 845; interactions with, 884, 891, 906, 936, 966, 996, 1019
Isoproterenol, 149-150; interactions with, 906
Isoptin SR (verapamil), 1022
Isoquinoline alkaloids, 903
Isordil (isosorbide dinitrate), 963
Isosorbide dinitrate, 963
Isosorbide mononitrate, 963
Isotretinoin, 92
Isradipine, 963
Itching skin, *chart*, 520-521
Itraconazole: interactions with, 896, 972
IUDs (intrauterine devices), 40; and pelvic inflammatory disease, 664, 665

J

Jacksonian seizures, 358, 359
Jamaica sorrel (*Hibiscus sabdariffa*), 957-958
Jasmine, 136, 310; *Jasminum officinale*, 344, 525
Jaundice, 522-523, 868-869
Jaw: temporomandibular joint (TMJ) syndrome, 362-363, 806-809; wiring of, 630
Jet lag, 366-367, 511
Jewelry, sensitivity to, 314, 315, *1048*
Jewelweed, 683
Job's tears (coix), 928
Jock itch, 520-521, 524-525
Joint pain, *chart*, 526-527
Joint replacement, 145
Juglans nigra (black walnut), 908
Juniper (*Juniperus communis*), 964
Juniperus virginiana (cedarwood), 109, 184, 525, 707, 709
Juvenile-onset (Type 1) diabetes, 316, 317, 318-319, 320, 321
Juvenile periodontitis, 418, 419
Juvenile rheumatoid arthritis, 142, 143

K

KAI-1 (protein), 698-699
Kali bichromicum, 964
Kali iodatum, 833
Kali muriaticum, 643, 731
Kali phosphoricum, 171
Kaopectate (attapulgite, pectin), 902, 990
Kaposi's sarcoma, 758
Kava, 964-965
Kavalactones, 964
K-Dur (potassium chloride), 995
Kegel exercises, *495*, 496, 853
Kelp, 965
Keratin and acne, 90
Keratotomy, radial, 864
Ketoacidosis, 316-317, 962
Ketoconazole, 965-966; interactions with, 891, 896, 898, 906, 925, 937, 947, 972, 983, 986
Ketorolac, 889, 966
Khellin, 867
Kidney cancer, 528-*529*
Kidney disease, 368-369, 378-379, 530-533; glomerulonephritis, 490
Kidney infections, 164-165, 534-535, 868-869
Kidney stones, 86-87, 536-537; urinary problems from, *chart*, 846-847
Kidney transplant, 532
Kigelia pinnata (sausage tree), 761
Killer T cells, 760
Kissing disease, mononucleosis known as, 595
Klonopin (clonazepam), 927

Klor-Con 10 (potassium chloride), 995
Knees: athletic injuries, 159; in Osgood-Schlatter disease, 160, 538-539; pain, *chart,* 538-539
Kola, 966; in combinations, 934, 967
Kreosotum, 857
Kudzi: interactions with, 899

L

Labor and delivery, 39-40; emergency, *60-61*
Labyrinth, inner ear's, *581,* 582
Labyrinthitis, 334-335
Lacerations, 304-305
Lachesis, 967
Lactase, 389; production, lack of, 540-541
Lactobacillus acidophilus, 253, 383, 393, 518, 541, 681, 843, 857, 892, 920, 942, 949, 972, 983, 990, 1012, 1015
Lactobacillus bulgaricus, 253
Lactose intolerance, 540-541
Lactuca canadensis (wild lettuce), 877
Lactucin; lactucopicrin, 921
Lactulose, 289
Lanoxin (digoxin), 937
Laparoscopic cholecystectomy, 386
Larch, 264
Larch moss (usnea), 1020
Large cell carcinomas of lungs, 558
Large intestine. *See* Colon
Larkspur, 729
Laryngitis, 542-543
Larynx, *543;* croup, 302-303
Laser surgery: on eyes, 571, 864; on prostate, 704; for vaginal cancer, 856
Lasix Oral (furosemide), 949
Lateral epicondylitis (tennis elbow), 140-141, 812-815, *813*
Latex, aloe, 887
Lavender (*Lavandula officinalis*), 967
Law of similars, 26
Laxatives, 291, 967-968; interactions with, 893, 938, 949, 1015
L-carnitine, 127, 257, 463
L-cysteine, 675, 873
LDL (low-density lipoprotein), 153, 254, 255, 256, 923
LDL apheresis, 256
L-dopa (levodopa), 969; interactions with, 891, 905, 906, 910, 997, 1019
Lead poisoning, 355-356, 357
Lecithin, 261, 387, 603, 673
Ledebouriella divaricata (siler), 154, 344, 890, 901; interactions with, 930
Ledum, 968
Legionnaire's disease, 678, 679
Leg pain: *chart,* 544-545; in pregnancy, 691-692
Leg veins, *669;* phlebitis, 668-669; varicose, 693, 858-861
Lemon balm (melissa), 136, 273, 499, 617, 659, 747
Lemongrass, 968
Lemon oil, 376, 675, 707, 709
Lens of eye, clouding of (cataract), 238-*239*
Lentinan, 1007
Lentinus edodes (shiitake), 1007
Leonurus cardiaca (motherwort), 104, 136, 348, 415, 463, 587, 827
Leonurus heterophyllus (Chinese motherwort), 922
LES (lower esophageal sphincter), 456, 457
Lettuce, wild, 877
Leucine, 555
Leukemia, 546-549, *547*
Leukoplakia, 634
Levodopa, 969; interactions with, 891, 905, 906, 910, 997, 1019
Levonorgestrel, 969
Levothyroid (levothyroxine), 969
Levothyroxine, 969-970
Levoxine (levothyroxine), 969
Levoxyl (levothyroxine), 969
Lice, 520-521, 550-551
Licorice (*Glycyrrhiza glabra*), 970-971; in combination, 903
Licorice (*Glycyrrhiza uralensis*), 970; in combinations, 912, 926, 941, 946, 952, 1003, 1013
Lidocaine, 168, 233, 466, 499, 831
Life root, 353, 593
Ligaments, injury to, 770-*771*
Light therapy: for dermatitis, 314-315; for jaundice in infants, 523; for manic-depression, 576; for psoriasis, 707, 708; for seasonal affective disorder, 739; for vitiligo, 867
Ligusticum porterii (osha), 79
Lily of the valley, 463
Lime blossom, 512
Lincomycin, 274; interactions with, 943
Lindane (gamma benzene hexachloride), 728, 729
Linden, 121, 136, 440, 463
Ling zhi (ganoderma), 950
Linoleic acid, 603
Lipitor (atorvastatin), 901
Lipoproteins, 153, 254, 255, 256, 923
Liposuction, 630
Lisinopril, 971
Lithium, 310, 439, 575, 576, 577, 846; interactions with, 891, 894, 905, 910, 914, 915, 917, 939, 1012, 1015
Liver, 266, 368-369, 378-379; bile produced by, 385; cancer, 552-553; cirrhosis, 114-115, 200-201, 266-269; fatty, 267, 268; hepatitis, 267, 268, 269, 468-471; and jaundice, 522, 523; transplant, 268-269
Live yeast-cell derivative, 971
L-lysine, 747
Lobar pneumonia, 678
Lobelia (*Lobelia inflata*), 971; in combination, 979
Lobeline, 971
Lobular carcinoma, 204
Lockjaw (tetanus), 820-821
Lodine (etodolac), 944
Loestrin FE (ethinyl estradiol, norethindrone), 944, 984
Lonicera japonica (honeysuckle flower), 958; in combinations, 924, 934, 940, 970
Lo/Ovral (ethinyl estradiol, norgestrel), 944, 984
Loperamide, 971
Lopid (gemfibrozil), 951
Lopressor (metoprolol), 976
Lorabid (loracarbef), 972
Loracarbef, 972
Loratadine, 972
Lorazepam, 972
Lorcet Plus (hydrocodone), 959
Lortab 7.5/500 (hydrocodone), 959
Lotensin (benazepril), 904
Lotrimin AF (clotrimazole), 927
Lotrisone (betamethasone, clotrimazole), 907, 927
Lotus: in combinations, 907
Lou Gehrig's disease, 554-*555*
Lovastatin, 972; interactions with, 943, 951
Low blood pressure, 364-365
Low blood sugar (hypoglycemia), 316, 318, 364-365, 484-485
Low-density lipoprotein (LDL), 153, 254, 255, 256, 923
Lower esophageal sphincter (LES), 456, 457
Low-grade vs. high-grade lymphoma, 566-567, 568
Lozol (indapamide), 961
L-tryptophan, 261, 311
Lubrication, vaginal, inadequate, 742
Luden's cough drops (pectin), 990
Lumbar puncture, 585, 601
Lumpectomy, 206
Lumps: *chart,* 556-557; breast, 205-206, 208, 210-211, 556-557

Lung cancer, 368-369, 558-561, *559*
Lung diseases, 720, 721; abscesses, 284-285; asthma, 148-151, *149*; bronchitis, 214-217, *215*, 284-285; cancer, 368-369, 558-561, *559*; chronic obstructive, 720, 721; emphysema, 346-349, *347*; pleurisy, 676-*677*; pneumonia, 284-285, *678*-681; tuberculosis, 844-845
Lupulinic acid, 958
Lupus, 562-563, 610-611
Lycium fruit (*Lycium barbarum; L. chinense*), 973; in combination, 995
Lycopodium, 973
Lycopus spp. (bugleweed), 415, 827
Lyme arthritis, 88-89, 564
Lyme disease, 526-527, 564-565, 714-715, *1049*
Lymphadenitis, 772
Lymphatic system, 566, *567*; adenoids, 94, *95*; tonsils, 834, *835*
Lymphocytes, 566, 567; T cells, 486, 760
Lymphocytic leukemias: acute (ALL), 546, 547, 548-549; chronic (CLL), *547*, 549
Lymphoma, 556-557, 566-569
Lynch syndrome, 278
Lysine, 271, 395, 747

M

Maalox (aluminum hydroxide, magnesium hydroxide, simethicone), 888, 974, 1008
MacDougal Diet, 603
Macrobid (nitrofurantoin), 982
Macrodantin (nitrofurantoin), 982
Macronutrients, 1030
Macular degeneration, 570-571
Mad dog weed (skullcap; *Scutellaria lateriflora*), 1009; in combinations, 908, 934, 966, 967
Magnesium, 1039; interactions with, 902, 906, 949, 983, 996, 1015
Magnesium hydroxide, 974; interactions with, 983
Magnesium trisilicate, 781; interactions with, 983
Magnetic field therapy, 264
Magnolia bark (*Magnolia officinalis*), 662
Magnolia flower (*Magnolia liliflora; M. denudata*), 974
Mahonia aquifolium (Oregon grape), 499, 708
Ma huang (ephedra), 941-942; in combinations, 890, 946, 970; interactions with, 953
Major depression, 308, 309
Malabar tamarind, 256
Malabsorption, 324-325
Malaria, 572-573
Male condoms, 745
Male health, 42-43
Male reproductive system, 42, 43, *1063*
Male urinary system, *1063*
Malic acid, 261
Malignant hypertension, 478, 479
Malignant tumors. *See* Cancer
Mammograms, 205, 208
Mandarin oil, 692
Mandarin orange (tangerine) peel, 1013; in combinations, 902, 995
Manganese, 1039
Manic-depression, 514-515, 574-577
Mantoux skin test, 845
MAO (monoamine oxidase) inhibitors, 977-978; interactions with, 894, 896, 906, 907, 910, 913, 914, 915, 917, 933, 935, 936, 937, 962, 969, 976, 987, 988, 1003, 1012, 1024
Maprotiline: interactions with, 910, 944
March fractures, 159, 161
Marijuana, 336, 337, 403, 492
Marjoram, 512
Marplan (isocarboxazid), 963
Marrow transplantation, 549, 569
Marrubium vulgare (horehound), 79, 680, 909, 929, 961, 979
Marsh mallow, 974; in combinations, 911, 916, 921
Marsh tea, 968
Massage, 24
Mastectomy, 206
Mastoidectomy, 444
Mastoiditis, 340-341
Matricaria recutita (chamomile), 920; in combinations, 911, 952, 954, 989, 1020, 1023
Mattresses for bedridden patients, 173
Maxillary sinuses, 754, *755*
Maxzide-25 (hydrochlorothiazide, triamterene), 959, 1018
Mayflower, hawthorn known as, 957
Meadowsweet, 79, 241, 383, 393, 475, 499, 735, 936, 954
Measles, 578-*579*, 714-715, *1044*
Measles, mumps, and rubella vaccine (MMR), *chart* 33, 399, 579, 605
Mebendazole, 521, 879
Meckel's diverticulum, 114-115
Meclizine, 581
Medial epicondylitis, 159
Medicago sativa (alfalfa), 886
Medical genetics, 18
Medicine chest, contents of: alternative, *79*; conventional, *78*
Meditation, 27
Medorrhinum, 633
Medroxyprogesterone, 974
Mefenamic acid, 590
Mefloquine, 573
Megaloblastic anemias, kinds of, 119-120, 1032
Melaleuca spp. (tea tree oil), 1013-1014
Melanin, lack of (vitiligo), 866-*867*
Melanocytes, 758, *759*
Melanoma, 758, *759*, 760-761, *1047*
Melatonin, 367, 513
Melissa officinalis (lemon balm), 136, 273, 499, 617, 659, 747
Menadione, 1036
Ménière's disease, 334-335, 580-583, 616-617
Meningiomas, *203*
Meningitis, 372-373, 584-585, 616-617, 620-621, 710-711, 868-869, 870-871
Menopausal problems, 41, 514-515, 586-587, 798-799
Menopause, 41; uterine cancer after, 848-*849*
Menorrhagia (heavy periods), 588, 592-593
Men's health, 42-43
Men's height and weight goals, *chart* 37, 37
Menstrual problems, 38, 86-87, 588-593
Menstrual sponges and toxic shock, 839
Menstrual synchrony, 591
Menstruation, 38, 588; absence of (amenorrhea), 588-589; in adolescents, 36; and breast cancer, 205; and breast changes, 208-209; heavy (menorrhagia), 588, 592-593; myths, 589; painful (dysmenorrhea), 588, 590-591; premenstrual syndrome, 130-131, 378-379, 514-515, 694-697; retrograde, 351; and toxic shock, 838, 839
Mental disorders: alcohol abuse, 102-105; Alzheimer's disease, 110-113; anorexia nervosa, 132-133, 218; anxiety, 134-137; attention deficit disorder, 162-163; bulimia, 218-219; depression, 308-311, 514-515; drug abuse, 336-339; and fatigue, *chart*, 366-367; insomnia, 510-513, 514-515; irritability, *chart*, 514-515; in males, 43; manic-depression, 514-515, 574-577; obsessive-compulsive disorder, 632-633;

panic attacks, 626-627, 658-659; phobias, 670-671; posttraumatic stress disorder, 686-687; premenstrual syndrome, 514-515; schizophrenia, 732-733; seasonal affective disorder, 514-515, 738-739; sexual dysfunction as, 740, 741, 742, 743; stress, 459, 514-515, 597, 784-787; tics and twitches, 828-829
Mentha haplocalyx; M. arvensis (field mint), 948; in combinations, 912, 924, 974
Mentha piperita (peppermint), 992, 1005, 1020; in combination, 961; menthol from, 974-975
Mentha pulegium (pennyroyal), 991
Mentha spicata (spearmint), 1010
Menthol, 974-975; in combinations, 897, 916, 975; in peppermint, 992
Meperidine, 657; interactions with, 937
Mercurius corrosivus, 184, 300
Mercurius vivus, 975
Meridians, 20, 1076
Mestranol, 975
Metabolism, thyroid and, 412
Metacamylamine: interactions with, 891
Metamucil (psyllium hydrophilic mucilloid), 998
Metaproterenol, 150
Metastasis of breast cancer, 204
Methadone, 339, 722
Methane tetrachloride, 533
Methenamine: interactions with, 891
Methenyl chloride, 533
Methimazole, 414, 826
Methionine: interactions with, 969
Methocarbamol, 168
Methotrexate, 517; interactions with, 984, 1011, 1013
Methylcellulose, 976
Methylphenidate, 976; interactions with, 937
Methylprednisolone, 275, 415
Methyl salicylate (wintergreen oil), 889, 975-976; in combinations, 897, 916, 975; interactions with, 1022, 1023
Methysergide maleate, 439
Metoclopramide, 439, 457, 829; interactions with, 969, 987
Metoprolol, 976; interactions with, 898, 925
Metronidazole, 91, 780, 843, 856
Mevacor (lovastatin), 972
Mezereum, 491
Miconazole, 976-977
Microcrystalline hydroxyapatite, 161
Micro-K 10 (potassium chloride), 995
Micronase (glyburide), 954
Micronutrients: minerals, 1032, 1036-1041; vitamins, 1032-1036
Microwave surgery, prostate resection as, 704
Midamor (amiloride), 888
Midazolam: interactions with, 943
Middle ear infections (otitis media), 340-341, 444, 445, 640-643
Migraines, 436, 437-440, 441, 616-617, 710-711, 868-869
Milk: breast, and eczema protection, 345; heartburn and, 457; interactions with, 968, 1015; ulcers and, 781
Milk-alkali syndrome, 891
Milk thistle, 977
Milk-vetch root (astragalus), 901; in combinations, 901, 928, 939, 1019
Milkweed, 873
Mind/body medicine, 27. *See also* Yoga; *and names of individual ailments*
Minerals, 28, 1032, 1036-1041; calcium, 1036-1037; chloride, 1037; chromium, 1037; cobalt, 1037; copper, 1037-1038; fluoride, 1038; iodine, 1038; iron, 1038-1039; magnesium, 1039; manganese, 1039; molybdenum, 1039-1040; phosphorus, 1040; potassium, 1040; selenium, 1040; sodium, 1040-1041; sulfur, 1041; vanadium, 1041; zinc, 1041. *See also individual ailments*
Minitran (nitroglycerin), 983
Minor Blue Dragon Combination, 685
Minor Bupleurum Combination, 488
Minoxidil, 424; interactions with, 976, 1018
Miscarriage, 39, 688
Mistletoe, 977; mulberry, in combinations, 932, 945, 955
Mites: in house dust, 435; scabies from, 716-717, 728-729, *1050*
Mitotane: interactions with, 1013
Mitoxantrone: interactions with, 1013
Mitral valve prolapse, 459
Mixed hiatal hernias, 474, 475
MMR (measles, mumps, and rubella vaccine), 33 *chart*, 399, 579, 605
Modified radical mastectomy, 206
Mold allergies, 107
Moles, *1046*; and skin cancer, 758
Molindone: interactions with, 962
Molybdenum, 1039-1040
Mometasone furoate, 977
Moniliasis (vaginal yeast infection), 880, 881
Monistat-Derm; Monistat Dual-Pak; Monistat 7; Monistat 3 Vaginal Suppositories (miconazole), 976
Monkshood, 884
Monoamine oxidase (MAO) inhibitors, 977-978; interactions with, 894, 896, 906, 907, 910, 913, 914, 915, 917, 933, 935, 936, 937, 962, 969, 976, 987, 988, 1003, 1012, 1024
Monobenzone, 867
Monoclonal antibodies, 568
Monoket (isosorbide mononitrate), 963
Mononucleosis (mono), 368-369, 556-557, 594-597, 616-617
Morning sickness, 618-619, 688, 692, 870-871
Morphine, 229, 289, 337, 338, 454, 517, 560
Morrhuate sodium, 466
Morton's neuroma, 370-371
Mosquito-borne illness, malaria as, 572-573
Moss: club, 973; larch, 1020
Mother tinctures, homeopathic remedies from, 1027
Motherwort, 104, 136, 348, 415, 463, 587, 827; Chinese, 922
Motion sickness, 598-599, 868-869
Motivational counseling, 175
Motor neurons in ALS, 554, *555*
Motrin; Motrin IB (ibuprofen), 961
Mountain daisy, 899
Mouth guards as TMJ remedy, 809
Mouth odor, 170-171
Mouth problems, *1045*; cancer, oral, 634-*635*, *1045*; canker sores, 232-233, *1045*; oral thrush, 880, 881, 1045. *See also* Dental problems
Movement disorders, 828-829; trembling, *chart*, 840-841
Movement retraining, 21
Moxibustion, 21, 749
MS (multiple sclerosis), 600-603, *601*, 626-627, 840-841
Mucilage, 928, 947, 974, 1009
Mucin production, 781
Mucus, nasal, postnasal drip from, 684-685
Mugwort leaf, 978; in combination, 907
Mulberry leaf, 296; in combinations, 899, 924, 1006
Mullein, 979; in combinations, 929, 954
Multi-drug-resistant TB (MDR-TB), 845
Multinutrient supplements, 1030
Multiple chemical sensitivity, 354,

356
Multiple sclerosis (MS), 600-603, *601*, 626-627, 840-841
Mumps, 556-557, 604-605
Mupirocin, 979
Muriaticum acidum, 513
Muscle contraction (tension) headaches, 436, 437, 438, 439, 440, 441
Muscle cramps, 606-607, 608-609; in pregnancy, 691-692
Muscle pain, *chart*, 608-609
Muscle pulls (strains), 608-609, 770-771
Muscle relaxants, 979; interactions with, 913, 936, 956, 997, 1024
Muscle relaxation, 518-519
Muscles, *1054-1055*; in ALS, 554, *555*; herniation through, 472-*473*; in multiple sclerosis, 603; and shin splints, 748, *749*; in tennis elbow, 812, *813*; in tetanus, 820
Muscle weakness, *chart*, 610-611
Muscular dystrophy, 610-611
Muscular system, *1054-1055*
Musculoskeletal problems. *See* Arthritis; *and names of individual ailments*
Mustard poultice, 681
Myalgic encephalomyelitis (ME; chronic fatigue syndrome), 258-261
Myelin loss, 600, *601*
Myelodysplasia, 547
Myelogenic leukemias: acute (AML), 546, 547, 549; chronic (CML), 547, 549
Mylanta (aluminum hydroxide, magnesium hydroxide, simethicone), 888, 974, 1008
Mylanta Gas (simethicone), 1008
Myocardial disease, primary, 460
Myocardial infarction (heart attack), 67, 452-455
Myofascial pain dysfunction, temporomandibular joint (TMJ) syndrome known as, 806
Myofascial release therapy, 623
Myomectomy, 852, 853
Myopia (nearsightedness), 862, *863*, 864
Myotherapy, 24
Myrcene, 968
Myrica spp. (bayberry), 903
Myricitrin, 903
Myristica fragrans (nutmeg), 985
Myristicin, 985
Myrrh, 979; in combinations, 916, 918, 934, 1004
Myxedema coma, 824, 825

N

Nabothian cysts, 245
Nabumetone, 889, 980
Nadolol, 980
Naessens, Gaston, 231
Nafarelin, 352
Nail problems: *chart*, 612-613; athlete's foot as, 156, 157; infection, 504-505, 773, 775; ingrown nails, 506-*507*; psoriasis as, 706
Naltrexone, 104
Napcalen (naproxen), 980
Naprosyn (naproxen), 980
Naproxen, 889, 980
Narcolepsy, 510, 511
Narcotics: interactions with, 895, 917, 936, 960, 996, 1024; opioid analgesics as, 987
Nardil (phenelzine), 992
NARES (nonallergic rhinitis with eosinophilia syndrome), 762
Narrow-angle (acute) glaucoma, 400, *401*, 402
Nasacort (triamcinolone), 1018
Nasal cavity, *1067*
Nasal congestion, 284-285 *chart*, 692
Nasalcrom (cromolyn), 931
Nasal polyps, 614-615
Nasal sprays, 433, 643, 763; saline, 615, 685
Nasopharynx, 822, *823*
National Health and Social Life Survey, 97
National Institute of Allergy and Infectious Diseases (NIAID), work of, 98
Natrum muriaticum, 980
Natrum sulphuricum, 151, 843
Natural family planning, 40
Naturopathic medicine, 28
Nausea: *chart*, 616-619; morning sickness, 618-619, 688, 692; motion sickness, 598-599, 868-869
Nearsightedness, 862, *863*, 864
Neck injuries, 66
Neck pain, *chart*, 620-621
Needles, use of, in acupuncture, 20-21
Negative ionizers, 739
Neomycin, 980; in combinations, 903, 995; interactions with, 920
Neomycin, polymyxin B, and hydrocortisone, 980-981
Neosporin (bacitracin, neomycin, polymyxin B), 903, 980, 995
Neovascular glaucoma, 400, 403
Neovascular (wet) macular degeneration, 570, 571
Nepeta cataria (catnip), 918
Neroli oil, 450, 512
Nerve block, *747*
Nerve growth factor, cell-derived, 555, 661
Nervous system, *1064*; aging and, 45; Alzheimer's disease, 110-113; autonomic, and arrhythmias, 449; brain tumors, 202-*203*; diabetic neuropathy, 317; epilepsy, 358-359; facial pain, *chart*, 362-363; headache, 436-441; Lou Gehrig's disease, 554-*555*; multiple sclerosis, 600-603; myelin loss, 600, *601*; neuralgia, 622-*623*, *746*, *747*; and numbness and tingling, *chart*, 626-627; Parkinson's disease, 660-663; pinched nerve, 672-*673*; restless leg syndrome, 722-723; sciatica, 734-735; spinal nerves, herniated disks and, 326, *327*, 328; in tetanus, 820; tics and twitches, 828, 829; touch receptors, *1067*; and trembling, *chart*, 840-841
Nettle, 981
Neuralgia, 140-141, 362-*363*, 622-*623*; postherpetic, 622, *746*, *747*
Neural therapy, 264
Neurology, 18
Neuroma, Morton's, 370-371
Neurons in ALS, 554, *555*
Neuroscogenin, 913
Neurosyphilis, 802
Neurotherapy (EEG biofeedback), 133, 137, 163, 219, 310-311, 359, 577, 633, 687
Neutrophils, 280
Niacin, 923; interactions with, 901, 972, 996, 1009; as vitamin B3, 1032-1033
Niacinamide, 441
N'Ice cough drops (menthol), 974
Nickel, sensitivity to, 314, 315
Nicoderm (nicotine), 981
Nicorette (nicotine), 981
Nicotine, 981; interactions with, 962, 992, 997, 1024
Nicotine withdrawal, 624-625
Nicotrol; Nicotol QD (nicotine), 981
Nifedipine, 981-982
Night blindness, 862, 863, 864, 865
Nightshade, deadly, 904
Nipple adenomas, 211
Nitrates, 982; interactions with, 891, 905, 910, 982, 1008
Nitric acid, 117, 873
Nitro-Dur (nitroglycerin), 983
Nitrofurantoin, 982-983
Nitroglycerin, 983; interactions with, 915
Nitrostat (nitroglycerin), 983
Nitrous oxide, 627

Nits, 550, 551
Nizatidine, 983; interactions with, 968
Nizoral; Nizoral AD (ketoconazole), 965
Nodular goiter, 404, 405
Nodules in acne, 90
Nolvadex (tamoxifen), 1013
Nonallergic rhinitis with eosinophilia syndrome (NARES), 762
Nonheme vs. heme iron, 1038
Non-Hodgkin's lymphoma, 566-567, 568
Non-insulin-dependent (Type 2) diabetes mellitus (NIDDM), 316, 317, 318, 319, 320, 321
Nonmelanomas, 758, *759*, 760, *1047*
Nonoxynol-9, 101
Nonpotassium-sparing diuretics, 949, 959, 981, 989, 1018
Nonproductive (dry) coughs, 294, 295, 296
Nonsmall cell lung cancer, 558, *559*, 560
Nonsteroidal anti-inflammatory drugs (NSAIDs), 889, 983-984; interactions with, 884, 890, 898, 905, 907, 915, 931, 938, 939, 962, 1011
Nordette (ethinyl estradiol, levonorgestrel), 944, 969
Norepinephrine: interactions with, 982; restoration of levels of, 893, 912, 984
Norethindrone, 984; in combination, 944, 975
Norethindrone acetate, 984
Norgestimate, 984
Norgestrel, 984
Norpseudoephedrine, 941
Nortriptyline, 984
Norvasc (amlodipine), 889
Nose, *1067*
Nosebleeds, 72; in pregnancy, 692
Nose blowing, black eye and, 179
Nose drops and sprays, 433, 615, 643, 763; saline, homemade, 615, 685
Nose emergencies, 72
Notoginseng root, 985
Notopterygium root, 890
Novolin 70/30 (insulin), 962
NSAIDs (nonsteroidal anti-inflammatory drugs), 889, 983-984; interactions with, 884, 890, 898, 905, 907, 915, 931, 938, 939, 962, 1011
Nuclear medicine, 18
Nuclear sclerosis, 238
Numbness: in pregnancy, 692; and tingling, *chart*, 626-627
Nummular dermatitis, 312, 313, *1048*
Nuprin (ibuprofen), 961
Nut-grass rhizome (cyperus), 933
Nutmeg, 985
Nutritional problems: anemia as, 118-120, 121; anorexia nervosa, 132-133, 218; bulimia, 218-219; gluten sensitivity, 240-241; goiter as, 404, 405; multiple sclerosis as, 601, 603
Nutritional supplements, 1030
Nutrition and diet, 28, 1030; Food Guide Pyramid, *1031*; minerals, 1032, 1036-1041; vitamins, 1032-1036. *See also individual ailments*
Nux vomica, 985
NyQuil (acetaminophen, dextromethorphan, pseudoephedrine), 884, 936, 940, 997
Nystatin, 856, 881

O

Oak, white, 543
Oat cell cancer (small cell lung cancer), 558-559, 560
Oat preparations, 311, 315, 339, 483, 623, 625, 673, 683, 729, 747, 934, 966
Obesity, 628-631; and heart disease, 459
Obsessive-compulsive disorder (OCD), 632-633
Obstetrics and gynecology (ob-gyn), 18
Obstructive sleep apnea, 764, 765
Occupational neuritis (repetitive stress injury), 234-237
Occupation-related lung diseases, 720, 721
OCD (obsessive-compulsive disorder), 632-633
Ocular hypertension, 401, 402
Odor: body, 192-193; breath, 170-171
Oenothera biennis (evening primrose oil), 945
Ofloxacin, 986; interactions with, 898
Ogen Tablets (estropipate), 944
Oils, herbal, 1026; essential, 21, 1026; infused, 1026
Ointments, herbal, 1026
Old-man's-beard (usnea), 1020
Olfactory structures, *1067*
Omega-3 fatty acids, 101, 147, 275, 300, 563
Omeprazole, 986; interactions with, 906, 966
Onion-honey cough syrup, 297, 681
Onions: as Ayurvedic remedy, 195; as herbal therapy, 189, 320, 480, 860; red, 887; spring (scallions), 1004-1005
Open-angle (chronic) glaucoma, 400-*401*, 402
Ophthalmia neonatorum, 286
Ophthalmic antibiotics, 986
Ophthalmological examination, 863
Ophthalmology, 18
Opiates, 336, 337, 338
Opioid analgesics, 889, 987; interactions with, 891, 905, 906, 913, 915
Optic nerve in glaucoma, 401
Orajel (benzocaine), 905
Oral cancer, 634-*635*, *1045*
Oral contraceptives. *See* Birth-control pills
Oral hypoglycemics (antidiabetic drugs), 987-988; interactions with, 908, 925, 939, 984, 1011
Oral thrush, 880, 881, *1045*
Orange, bitter, 757, 901, 912, 1013
Orange flower (neroli) oil, 450, 512
Oregon grape, 499, 708
Organizations and associations, 1071-1075
Organophosphates, 356
Orgasm, problems with, 741, 742
Ornish, Dean, 154
Oropharynx, 822, *823*
Orphenadrine: interactions with, 937
Ortho-Cept (desogestrel), 935
Orthomolecular medicine, 28
Ortho-Novum (ethinyl estradiol, norethindrone), 944, 984
Ortho-Novum 1/50 (mestranol), 975
Orthopedic bracing for scoliosis, 736, 737
Ortho Tri-Cyclen; Ortho-Cyclen (norgestimate), 984
Os, cervical, 244
Osgood-Schlatter disease, 160, 538-539
Osha, 79
Osteoarthritis, 128-129, 140-141, 142, *143*-144, 145, 146-147, 164-165, 334-335, 526-527, 538-539, 620-621
Osteomyelitis, 428-429
Osteopathy, 28. *See also individual ailments*
Osteoporosis, 164-165, 636-639
Osteosarcoma, 196
Ostia, sinuses', 754, 755
Otitis externa (swimmer's ear), 340-341, 800-801
Otitis media (middle ear infection), 340-341, 444, 445, 640-643
Otolaryngology, 19
Otosclerosis, 443, 445
Outer ear infection (swimmer's ear), 340-341, 800-801

Ova (eggs), 38, 646; artificial fertilization of, 503; problems of, 502
Ovarian cancer, 644-*645*
Ovarian cysts, 646-647
Ovaries, decline in functioning of, 586
Ovary problems, 646-647
Ovcon (ethinyl estradiol, norethindrone), 944, 984
Overflow incontinence, 495
Overuse injuries, 538-539, 544-545; repetitive stress injury, 234-237; shin splints, 748-749
Overweight, 628-631
Ovulation, 38; detecting and inducing, 503; and natural family planning, 40
Oxalic acid, 533, 1007
Oxalis corniculata (wood sorrel), 473
Oxaprozin, 889, 988
Oxazepam: interactions with, 980
Oxyacanthine, 903
Oxybutynin chloride, 496
Oxycodone, 889, 988
Oxygen deprivation, 148
Oxygen starvation in anemia, 118
Oxygen therapy, 216, 441
Oxymetazoline, 988
Oxypentifylline (pentoxifylline), 991-992; interactions with, 925
Oxyphenbutazone, 319

P

PABA (para-aminobenzoic acid), 563, 761, 795
Pacemakers, 450
Paeonia lactiflora (peony), 344, 480, 719, 827
Paeonia officinalis (peony), 662
Paget's disease, 204
Pain: *chart,* 88-89; chronic, 648-653. *See also names of individual body parts*
Pain clinics, 649
Painful (vaso-occlusive) crises, 752-753
Pain management, 145
Palmar psoriasis, 706
Palmetto, saw, 1004
Palming (visualization exercise), 489
Palpitations, 448
Pamelor (nortriptyline), 984
Panax ginseng (Asian ginseng), 953; in combinations, 901, 925, 951, 995, 1005, 1013
Panax notoginseng (notoginseng root), 985
Panax pseudoginseng (pseudoginseng root; notoginseng root), 985
Panax quinquefolius (American ginseng), 953
Pancreatic cancer, 654-*655*
Pancreatitis, 86-87, 656-657
Panic attacks; panic disorder, 626-627, 658-659
Pantethine, 257
Pantothenic acid (vitamin B5), 1034
Papain, 241
Papaverine, 493; interactions with, 969
Papillomas, intraductal, 211
Pap smear, 243, 246
Para-aminobenzoic acid (PABA), 563, 761, 795
Paraesophageal hiatal hernia, 474, *475*
Parasitic disorders: itching skin from, *chart,* 520-521; lice, 550-551; malaria, 572-573; scabies, 728-729, *1050*; trichomoniasis, 842-843; worms, 878-879
Parathyroid glands, 824
Parkinson's disease, 660-663, 840-841
Parnate (tranylcypromine), 1017
Paronychia (nail infection), 504-505, 612-613, 773, 775
Parotid glands, *605*
Paroxetine, 989
Parrot fever, 680
Parsley, 989
Pasqueflower, 705
Passionflower (*Passiflora incarnata*), 989; in combinations, 908, 959
Passive immunotherapy, 98
Patchouli (agastache), 885
Patellar tendonitis, 159, 161, 538-539
Patent ductus arteriosus, 461
Pathology, 19
Pau d'arco, 990
Paxil (paroxetine), 989
PCE (erythromycin), 942
PCE (tetrachloroethylene), 533
Peak flow meter, use of, 149, 151
Pectin, 990; interactions with, 938
Pediatrics, 19
Pedicularis canadensis (wood betony), 440, 908
Pediculicides, 521, 728, 729
Pelargonium odoratissimum (geranium), 233, 271, 651, 675, 695
Pellagra, 1033
Pelvic inflammatory disease (PID), 664-665
Pelvic muscles, exercises for, *495,* 496, 853
Pemphigus, blisters from, 186, 187
Penicillins, 990-991; interactions with, 943, 1015
Penicillin V, 991
Penicillin VK (penicillin V), 991
Penile implants, 493
Penile pain, *chart,* 666-667
Pennyroyal, 991
Pennywort, Asian, 473
Pentamidine, 680
Pentoxifylline, 991-992; interactions with, 925
Peony, 344, 480, 662, 719, 827; red peony root in combinations, 922, 940, 1002; tree peony root, interactions with, 927; white peony root in combinations, 912, 933, 939
Pepcid (famotidine), 947
Pepcid AC (famotidine), 947
Peppermint, 992; in combinations, 961, 1005, 1020; menthol from, 974-975
Peptic ulcers, 84-85, 778-781, *779*
Pepto-Bismol (bismuth subsalicylate), 907
Perchloroethylene (PERC), 533
Perchloromethane, 533
Percocet (oxycodone), 988
Percodan (oxycodone), 988
Perennial hay fever, 432
Perforated and bleeding ulcers, 778, 780
Pergolide, 661
Pericardial disease, 460
Pericarditis, 460
Peridex (chlorhexidine), 923
Periodontal (gum) disease, 418-421, *419*
Periodontitis, 418-419, 420
Peripheral aneurysms, 122
Peripheral vascular disease, 544-545
Peritoneal dialysis, 532
Peritonitis, 138, 139, 330
Periungual warts, 872
Permethrin, 551, 729
Pernicious anemia, 118, 120, 1035
Personality, Type A, 43, 454, 786
Perspiration: and body odor, 192, 193; excessive, *chart,* 798-799
Pertussis (whooping cough), 876-877
Pessaries, 496, 852, 853
Pesticide poisoning, 354, 356, 357
Petit mal seizures, 358
Petroleum, 599
Petroselinum crispum (parsley), 989
Peyronie's disease, 666-667, 741
Phalen wrist flexion test, 235
Phelodendron: in combinations, 889
Phenacetin, 528
Phenazopyridine, 183
Phenelzine, 992
Phenergan (promethazine), 996
Phenobarbital, 359, 509
Phenol, 992-993; in combination, 916

Phenolphthalein, 993; in combination, 939; interactions with, 968
Phenothiazines, 829; interactions with, 891, 907, 937, 969, 1019; prochlorperazine, 996
Phenylalanine, 649, 734, 919
Phenylbutazone, 149, 319, 404; interactions with, 962, 988, 1011
Phenylephrine, 317, 433
Phenylpropanolamine, 993
Phenytoin, 993-994; interactions with, 891, 898, 902, 910, 925, 926, 936, 940, 943, 962, 966, 969, 984, 986, 988, 996, 1022
Pheromones, 591
Philadelphia chromosome, 547
Phillips' Milk of Magnesia (magnesium hydroxide), 974
Phimosis, 666-667
Phlebitis, 130-131, 668-669; and leg pain, *chart,* 544-545
Phobias, 670-671
Phosphorus, 1040
Phosphorus (homeopathic remedy), 994
Photoaging, 794
Phototherapy. *See* Light therapy
Physical medicine and rehabilitation, 19
Physical therapy: for MS, 602; for Parkinson's, 661; for TMJ, 807
Physiological jaundice, 522, 523
Physostigmine, 551
Phytate, 119
Phytoestrogens (plant estrogens), 207, 587, 639
Phytolacca, 399, 605
Phytonadione, 1036
Phytosterols, 256
Picrorhiza kurrooa, 499
PID (pelvic inflammatory disease), 664-665
Pigment loss (vitiligo), 866-*867*
Piles (hemorrhoids), 114-115, 200-201, 464-467, *465,* 520-521; in pregnancy, 691
Pilewort, 466
Pilocarpine, 402
Pimpinella anisum (anise), 121, 150, 171, 216, 217, 297, 303, 348, 389, 692, 1005
Pimples (acne), 90-93
Pinched nerve, 672-*673*
Pine, 150, 184, 216, 348, 680, 756
Pineapple enzyme (bromelain), 155, 179, 189, 265, 305, 653, 757, 809, 811, 860, 873
Pinellia (*Pinellia ternata*), 434, 885, 946, 952, 1004, 1013
Pinkeye, 286, 287, *1051*
Pinus sylvestris (pine), 150, 184, 216, 348, 680, 756
Pinworms, 520-521, 878, 879
Piper methysticum (kava), 964-965
Pipsissewa, 407, 705
Plantago major (plantain), 994
Plantago psyllium (psyllium), 997-998
Plantain, 994
Plantar calluses, 292, 293
Plantar fasciitis, 159, 160, 370-371
Plantar psoriasis, 706
Plantar warts, 370-371, 674-675, *1047*
Plant estrogens, 207, 587, 639
Plaque, arterial, *153, 154*
Plaque, dental, 418, 419, 421
Plasmodia, 572, 573
Platycodon (*Platycodon grandiflorum*), 154; in combinations, 948, 958; interactions with, 930
Pleural effusion, 676, 677
Pleural friction rub, 677
Pleurisy (pleuritis), 676-*677*
Pleurisy root, 681
Plum, cherry, 136
PMS (premenstrual syndrome), 130-131, 378-379, 514-515, 694-697
Pneumocystis pneumonia (PCP), 679, 680
Pneumonia, 88-89, 248-249, 284-285, *678*-681
Pneumothorax, 248-249
PNF stretching (Proprioceptive Neuromuscular Facilitation), 602-603
Podophyllin, 397
Podophyllum, 300, 383
Pogostemon (agastache), 885
Poisoning, 73; alcohol intoxication, 102; blood, 190-191; caffeine, 829; environmental, chronic, 354-357, 514-515, 626-627; food, 382-383
Poison ivy, 682-*683,* 1000
Poison nut, 985
Poison oak and poison sumac, 682-*683*
Poisonous snakes, bites from, *76-77*
Poisonous spiders, *509;* bites, 508, 509
Pollen extract, 435
Polycystic ovary syndrome, 647
Polygala (*Polygala tenuifolia*), 434; interactions with, 970
Polygonum (*Polygonum multiflorum*), 995
Polymox (amoxicillin), 889
Polymyalgia rheumatica, 608-609
Polymyositis, 610-611
Polymyxin B, 995; in combination, 903, 980; interactions with, 920; neomycin, hydrocortisone, and, 980-981
Polyporus (*Polyporus umbellatus*), 488
Polyps: cervical, *245*-246; colorectal, 276; nasal, 614-615
Polysaccharides, 901, 1007
Poria (*Poria cocos*), 457, 901, 922, 928
Postherpetic neuralgia, 622, 746, 747
Postnasal drip, 684-685
Postpartum depression, 40
Posttraumatic stress disorder (PTSD), 686-687
Postural dizziness, 334-335
Postural drainage, 679
Postural hypotension, 691
Posture: improvement, 21; standing and sitting, 169
Potassium, 1040; interactions with, 890, 905, 938, 939, 989, 996
Potassium bichromate, 964
Potassium chloride, 995; interactions with, 937
Potassium-sparing diuretics, 888, 939, 1018; interactions with, 890, 905, 995
Potencies (dilution ratios) of homeopathic remedies, 26, 1027
Poultices, herbal, 1026
Powders, herbal, 1026
Pranipexole, 661
Pravachol (pravastatin), 995
Pravastatin, 995-996
Prayer for stress reduction, 463
Prazosin, 704
Prednisone, 996
Preeclampsia (toxemia), 130-131, 378-379, 688
Pregnancy, 38-39; as endometriosis treatment, 352; and Graves' disease, 414
Pregnancy concerns, 39; chickenpox, 251; chlamydia, 252; German measles, 398, 399; herpes, 395; syphilis, 802
Pregnancy exercises, *689*
Pregnancy problems, 39, 130-131, 164-165, 378-379, 688-693; cervical incompetence, 244, 245, 247; morning sickness, 618-619, 688, 692, 870-871
Premarin (conjugated estrogen), 929
Premature ejaculation, 42, 741, 742
Premenstrual syndrome (PMS), 130-131, 378-379, 514-515, 694-697
Premphase (conjugated estrogen; medroxyprogesterone), 929, 974
Prempro (conjugated estrogen; medroxyprogesterone), 929, 974
Prenatal care, 39

Preparation H (live yeast-cell derivative, shark liver oil), 971, 1007
Presbycusia, 442, 443, 445
Presbyopia, 863
Preventive medicine, 20
Priapism, 666-667, 740, 741, 752
Prickly ash, 225, 421, 814, 815, 1004
Prilosec (omeprazole), 986
Primaquine, 573
Primary amenorrhea, 588, 589
Primary care physician, choosing a, 29
Primary lactose intolerance, 540-541
Primary liver cancer, 552, 553
Primary myocardial disease, 460
Primatene Dual Action Formula (ephedrine, guaifenesin, theophylline), 942, 955, 1015
Primatene Mist; Primatene Mist Suspension (epinephrine), 942
Primatene Tablets (ephedrine, theophylline), 942, 1015
Primrose, evening, 945
Prinivil (lisinopril), 971
Probenecid, 407, 410; interactions with, 906, 920, 939, 949, 972, 983, 984, 991
Procarbazine: interactions with, 1013
Procardia XL (nifedipine), 981
Prochlorperazine, 996
Proctitis, 114-115
Productive coughs, 214, 215, 216, 294, 295, 296
Professional titles, 1070
Progesterone, 209, 637, 638, 848, 849; in menstrual cycle, 588, 591, 592, 921
Progestin, 587, 852, 853
Progestins and estrogens, 943-944
Prolapsed (herniated) disks, 164-165, 326-329, *327*, 620-621, 626-627, 672-*673*
Prolapsed hemorrhoids, 464, 466
Prolapsed rectum, 114-115
Prolapsed uterus, 850, *851*, 852, 853
Promethazine, 996
Propacet 100 (propoxyphene), 997
Propantheline bromide, 496
Propoxyphene, 889, 997; interactions with, 981
Propranolol, 997; interactions with, 925, 981, 994, 996, 997
Proprioceptive Neuromuscular Facilitation (PNF stretching), 602-603
Propylthiouracil, 404, 414, 826
Prostaglandins, 353, 493, 590, 591, 592, 653, 945, 1041
Prostate cancer, 43, 698-701, *699*
Prostatectomy, 700
Prostate problems, 43, 702-705, *703*; urinary problems from, *chart*, 846-847
Prostate-specific antigen (PSA) blood test, 699-700, 701
Prostatitis, 702, 703, 704, 705
Protease inhibitors, 885
Proteins, 1030
Proventil (albuterol), 886
Provera (medroxyprogesterone), 974
Provings for homeopathic remedies, 26-27, 1027
Prozac (fluoxetine), 949, 1005
Prunella (*Prunella vulgaris*), 480, 924, 1003; in combinations, 948
Prunus armeniaca (apricot seed), 899; in combinations, 941, 970
Prunus serotina (wild black cherry), 303, 348, 680, 877
PSA (prostate-specific antigen) test, 699-700, 701
Pseudoephedrine, 997; in ephedra, 941; interactions with, 890, 905, 914, 970, 982, 1016
Pseudoginseng root (notoginseng root), 985
Pseudogout, 409
Pseudomembranous colitis, 949, 972, 991, 1015
Psittacosis, 680
Psoralen, 314, 708
Psoralen ultraviolet A (PUVA), 867
Psoriasis, 706-709, *1050*
Psoriatic arthritis, 706, 709
Psorinum, 551, 615
Psorolea fruit: in combinations, 995
Psychedelic drugs, 336
Psychiatry, 20
Psychological disorders. *See* Mental disorders
Psychoneuroimmunology, 488-489
Psychotherapy, 133, 135, 163, 219, 309, 576, 659, 687, 733, 743, 785
Psyllium, 997-998
Psyllium hydrophilic mucilloid, 998
PTSD (posttraumatic stress disorder), 686-687
Puberty, 36; delayed, 589
Pubic lice, 550, 551
Pulmonary function tests, 149
Pulmonary stenosis, 461
Pulsatilla, 998
Pulse, checking for, *47*, *50*, *52*, *53*
Puncture wounds, 304, 305
Pupil dilation, *chart*, 710-711
Purines, 410, 429
Pus in boils, 194
Pustules in acne, 90, 91
PUVA (psoralen ultraviolet A), 867
Pyelonephritis, 688
Pygeum (*Pygeum africanus*), 705
Pyrantel, 879
Pyrazinamide, 845
Pyrethrins, 551
Pyrethrum, 177, 509
Pyridoxal; pyridoxamine, 1034
Pyridoxine: interactions with, 969; as vitamin B6, 1034-1035
Pyrimethamine, 573
Pyrithione zinc, 307
Pyrrolizidine alkaloids, 910, 929
Pyrrosia (*Pyrrosia lingua*), 387, 922

Q

Qigong, 24
Quantitative computerized tomography, 637
Quercetin, 300, 861
Quercus alba (white oak), 543
Questran (cholestyramine), 923
Quicksilver, 975
Quick strep test, 783
Quinapril, 998
Quinidine, 450, 573; interactions with, 891, 937, 938
Quinine, 324, 443, 466, 555, 573, 609, 831, 938
Quinolones: fluoroquinolones, 948-949; interactions with, 891, 983

R

Rabies, 712-713
Radial keratotomy, 864
Radiation therapy for cancer, 228, 231. *See also* Cancer *for names of individual cancers*
Radical mastectomy, 206
Radioactive iodide: treatment with, 414, 826; uptake tests and scans with, 404-405, 413, 825, 826
Radiology, 20
Radon, 355; and lung cancer, 561
Raloxifine, 637-638
Ramipril, 999
Ranitidine, 888, 999; interactions with, 898, 968, 972, 988, 1013
Ranunculus ficaria (pilewort), 466
Rashes, *1044, 1048-1050. See also names of individual ailments; chart*, 714-717
Raspberry, red, 1000
Ratanhia, 117
Rattlesnakes, *77*; bites from, 76
Rauwolfia: interactions with, 938
Raynaud's disease, 718
Raynaud's phenomenon, 718-719
Raynaud's syndrome, 626-627, 718-719
Reconstructive breast surgery, 206

Recovery: from alcoholism, 104, 105; from drug addiction, 339
Recovery position, use of, *47*
Rectal and colon cancer, 276-279, *277*
Rectal examinations, 699-700
Rectal prolapse, 114-115
Rectal varicose veins (hemorrhoids), 114-115, 200-201, 464-467, *465*, 520-521; in pregnancy, 691
Red blood cells: and anemia, 118, 119, 752-*753*; and leukemia, 546, *547*; sickled, 119, 752-*753*
Red clover, 999; in combinations, 913, 979
Red onion, 887
Red raspberry, 1000
Red sage, 543, 909
Red thyme, 551
Reduction of fracture, 160-161
Reed-Sternberg cell, 566
Referred pain, testicular, 816-817
Reflexology, 24; areas, *25*. *See also individual ailments*
Refraction disorders, 862-*863*, 864
Rehabilitation after stroke, 790
Rehmannia glutinosa (Chinese foxglove root), 922; in combinations, 889, 925, 928, 929, 930, 939, 953, 973, 1002, 1005
Reishi mushroom (ganoderma), 950
Relafen (nabumetone), 980
Relapse-progressive multiple sclerosis, 600-601
Relapse-remitting multiple sclerosis, 600
Relapsing fever, ticks and, 508, 509
Relaxation response, 27
Relaxing expectorants, 297
Remodeling, bone, decrease in, 636
Renal cell carcinoma, 528, *529*
Renal failure, acute, 378-379
Repetitive stress injury (RSI), 234-237
Reproductive system: female, 38, *855*, *1062*; male, 42, 43, *1063*. *See also* Sexual problems
Rescue remedy, 136
Respiratory arrest, first aid for, *50-53*
Respiratory problems, 500, 501, 720-721. *See also individual ailments*
Respiratory system, *721*, *1061*
Restless leg syndrome, 722-723
Restoril (temazepam), 1014
Retarded ejaculation, 741, 742
Retina: diabetic retinopathy, 317; focusing images on, problems of, 862-*863*, 864; macular degeneration, 570-571; nutritional supplements for, 865
Retin-A (tretinoin), 1017
Retinal detachment, 862, 863, 864
Retinoids, 423
Retinol (retinene; retinoic acid; retinyl palmitate; vitamin A), 1033
Retrograde ejaculation, 741, 742
Retrograde menstruation, 351
Retroverted uterus, 850
Reverse prayer test, 235
Reverse transcriptase inhibitors, 885
Revici, Emanuel, 231
Reye's syndrome, 250, 251, 281, 374-375, 399, 578, 605, 618-619, 870-871
Rhamnus purshiana (buckthorn), 911
Rheumatic fever, 128-129, 428-429, 724-725
Rheumatic heart disease, 460
Rheumatoid arthritis (rheumatism), 128-129, 140-141, 142-*143*, 144, 145, 146-147, 370-371, 526-527, 538-539
Rheum palmatum (rhubarb), 387, 662
Rh factor, 39
Rhinitis, 684; hay fever, 107, 108, 284-285, 432-435; and sneezing, 762-763
Rhizotomy, 168
Rhubarb, 387, 631, 662, 901, 902
Rhus toxicodendron (*Rhus tox*), 1000
Rhythm method of natural family planning, 40
Riboflavin (vitamin B2), 1034
RICE (rest, ice, compression, elevation) treatment, 539, 545, 609, 653, 749, 770, 810-811
Rickets, 1035
Rickettsia, Rocky Mountain spotted fever from, 726-727
Rifabutin: interactions with, 926
Rifampin, 845; interactions with, 906, 915, 936, 944, 966, 988, 994, 996
Rimantadine, 375-376, 377
Ringing in ears (tinnitus), 830-833
Ringworm, 714-715, *1050*
Risperidone, 733
Ritalin (methylphenidate), 976
Robitussin-CF (dextromethorphan, guaifenesin, phenylpropanolamine), 936, 955, 993
Robitussin-DM (dextromethorphan, guaifenesin), 936, 955
Rocky Mountain spotted fever (RMSF), 716-717, 726-727
Rofecoxib, 1000
Rolaids (calcium carbonate, magnesium hydroxide), 914, 974
Rolfing (Structural Integration), 24
Roman chamomile, 420
Ropinirole, 661
Rosacea, 90, 91, 92, 380-381
Rose hip (*Rosa* spp.), 1000-1001; in combinations, 930, 958
Roselle (*Hibiscus sabdariffa*), 957-958
Rosemary, 1001; in combination, 967
Rosenman, Ray, 454
Rose oil, 310, 512, 994
Roseola, 716-717
Rosmarinus officinalis (rosemary), 1001; in combination, 967
Rotator cuff tendonitis, 158, 159
Roundworms, 878-879
Roxicet (oxycodone), 988
Roxicodone (oxycodone), 988
Royal jelly, 109
RSI (repetitive stress injury), 234-237
Rubber-band ligation of hemorrhoids, 466
Rubella (German measles), 39, 398-*399*, 714-715, *1044*
Rubus idaeus (red raspberry), 1000
Rue (rue bitterwort), 1001
Rumex acetosella (sheep sorrel), 1007
Rumex crispus (homeopathic remedy), 297
Rumex crispus (sourdock), 79, 638, 708, 803
Ruptured (herniated) disks, 164-165, 326-329, *327*, 620-621, 626-627, 672-*673*
Ruscogenin, 913
Ruscus aculeatus (butcher's-broom), 913
Ruta, 1001
Rutin, 403, 861

S

Sabadilla, 763
Sabina, 397, 852
Saccular aneurysms, *123*
SAD (seasonal affective disorder), 514-515, 738-739
Safe sex, 97; condom use, 745
Safflower flower, 1002; in combination, 887
Saffron, 1002
Safrole, 1004
Sage, 1002-1003; clary, 310, 493, 743; in combinations, 909, 961; red, 543, 909; root, interactions with, 946
St. Benedict's thistle (blessed thistle), 908-909
St. Ignatius bean, 961
St.-John's-wort, 960-961, 1003
St. Vitus's dance (chorea), 724
Salicin, 1022
Salicylates, 433, 639; interactions with, 890, 891, 905, 962, 968, 988, 996, 1022, 1023

Salicylic acid, 307, 674, 675, 707, 709, 872-873; corn remedies, 293
Salicylicum acidum, 833
Saline solution, 615, 685
Saliva and bad breath, 170
Salivary glands, parotid, *605*
Salix spp. (willow), 146, 225; *Salix alba* (white willow), 1022-1023
Salmeterol, 1003
Salmonella poisoning, 382
Salt, 980; and high blood pressure, 479
Salt plaster, 769
Salt substitutes: interactions with, 939
Salvia officinalis (sage), 1002-1003; in combinations, 909, 961; root, interactions with, 946; var. *rubia* (red), 543, 909
Sambucus nigra (elder), 79, 109, 282, 376, 434, 596, 757, 918, 946, 961, 979
Sandalwood, 184, 323, 493, 582, 692
Sang ju yin, 296
Sanguinaria canadensis (bloodroot), 909
Sanguinarine, 909
Saponins, 886, 921
Sarcomas, defined, 226
Sargassum seaweed (*Sargassum pallidum*), 1003-1004; interactions with, 970
Sarsaparilla, 803
Sassafras (*Sassafras albidum*), 1004
Saunas for cold prevention, 283
Sausage tree, 761
Saussurea (aucklandia), 902; in combinations, 922, 929, 933, 1013
Saw palmetto, 1004
Scabies, 716-717, 728-729, *1050*
Scalded skin syndrome, 772-773
Scallion, 1004-1005
Scalp massage, 441
Scalp reduction, 424
Scarlet fever, 616-617, 716-717, 730-731
SCC (squamous cell carcinoma), 758, *759*, 760, *1047*; lung, 558, *559*; oral, *1045*
Schisandra (*Schisandra chinensis*), 1005; in combination, 927
Schizophrenia, 732-733
Sciatica, 544-545, 734-735
Sciatic nerve, 734, *735*
Scoliosis, 736-*737*
Scopolamine, 581, 598-599
Scorpion stings, 508, 509
Scrapes and scratches, 304, 305
Scrophularia: in combinations, 995; interactions with, 945
Scurvy, 1035
Scutellaria baicalensis (skullcap), 1009; in combinations, 929, 934, 958; interactions with, 899
Scutellaria lateriflora (skullcap), 1009; in combinations, 908, 934, 966, 967
Seasonal affective disorder (SAD), 514-515, 738-739
Seasonal hay fever, 432
Seborrheic dermatitis, 312, 313, 315, 322, 323, *1048*
Seborrheic keratosis, *1046*
Sebum and acne, 90, 91
Secondary amenorrhea, 588-589
Secondary glaucoma, 400
Secondary hypertension, 478, 479
Secondary lactose intolerance, 540, 541
Secondary liver cancer, 552, 553
Second-degree burns, 222, 223
Sedative-hypnotic drugs, anti-insomnia drugs called, 897
Sedatives, 336, 338, 492, 512, 517; in combination, 1015; interactions with, 896, 913, 917, 918, 933, 956, 959, 960, 978, 987, 989, 994, 996, 997, 1022
Seed corns, 292
Seizures, 74; epileptic, 358-359
Selective serotonin reuptake inhibitors (SSRIs), 1005
Selegiline hydrochloride, 661
Selenium, 1040
Self-help groups for alcoholics, 105
Semicircular canals, *581*
Senecio aureus (life root), 353, 593
Senile cataracts, 238
Senna, 1005-1006
Sennosides, 1006
Sensate focus exercises, 743
Senses, *1066-1067*; aging and, 44
Sensorineural hearing loss, 442, 443, 445
Sentilla asiatica, 305
Sentinel node testing, 206
Sepia, 1006
Septal defects of heart, 461
Septicemia (blood poisoning), 190-191
Septic shock, 190, 191
Septra (sulfamethoxazole; trimethoprim), 1011
Serenoa repens (saw palmetto), 1004
Serevent (salmeterol), 1003
Serous otitis media, 641
Sertraline, 1006
Sesame oil (*Sesamum indicum*), 1006; in combinations, 950, 1019
7:1 plan (diet), 663
714X therapy, 231
Sex: condom use, 745; and contraception, 40-41, 42; during pregnancy, 690; safe, 97
Sexual dysfunction, 41, 42, 740-743; vaginismus, 741, 742, 743, 854, 855-856, 857
Sexuality, adolescent, 36
Sexually transmitted diseases (STDs), 41, 42-43, 744-745; AIDS, 96-101; and cervical cancer, 242; chlamydia, 252-253; genital herpes, 394-395; genital warts, 245, 246, 396-397; gonorrhea, 406-407; hepatitis B, 267, 469, 470-471; syphilis, 716-717, 802-803; trichomoniasis, 842-843
Sexual problems: impotence, 42, 492-493; infertility, 40, 42, 351, 502-503; penile pain, *chart*, 666-667; sexual dysfunction, 41, 42, 740-743, 854, 855-856, 857
Shaking (trembling), *chart*, 840-841
Shampoos, 424; dandruff, 306-307
Shaping technique, 652
Shark cartilage, 231
Shark liver oil, 1007
Shatavari, 499
Sheep sorrel, 1007
Shepherd's purse, 593
Shiatsu, 24
Shift-work sleep disorder, 511, 513
Shiitake, 1007
Shingles, 362-363, 520-521, 746-747, *1050*
Shin splints, 748-749
Shock, 75, 656; anaphylactic, 75, 106, 108, 176, 177, 482, 508, 618-619, 796-797; electric, first aid for, *59*; electric, for arrhythmias, 450; septic, 190, 191; in toxic shock syndrome, 838
Shoulder injuries, 158, 159; immobilizing, *65*
Shoulder pain, *chart*, 750-751
Siberian ginseng, 953-954
Sick building syndrome, 354
Sickle cell anemia, 119, 752-*753*
Sickle cell trait, 752
SIDS (sudden infant death syndrome), 33
Siegesbeckia: in combinations, 974
Sight, sense of, *1066*. *See also* Eye problems
Sildenafil, 1007-1008
Sildenafil (Viagra), 493
Silent ischemia, 452
Siler (*Ledebouriella divaricata*), 154, 344, 890, 901; interactions with, 930
Silica, 1007-1008; in horsetail, 959

Silica (homeopathic remedy), 1007-1008
Silybum marianum (milk thistle), 977
Silymarin, 104, 260, 339, 977
Simethicone, 1008
Similars, law of, 26
Simvastatin, 1008-1009
Sinemet (levodopa), 969
Sinuses, 754, *755*
Sinus headaches, 436, 437, 438, 439, 440
Sinusitis, 284-285, 362-363, 754-757
Sitz baths, 247, 465
Skeletal system, *1056-1057*
Skin, *223*; touch receptors, *1067*
Skin cancer, 758-761, *759*, *1047*
Skin-care products, dermatitis from, 313
Skin conditions, *1044-1050*. *See also* Nail problems; Warts; itching, *chart*, 520-521; rashes, *chart*, 714-717
Skin tests: for allergies, 108, 433; for tuberculosis, 845
Skipped heartbeat, 448
Skullcap (*Scutellaria baicalensis*), 1009; in combinations, 929, 934, 958; interactions with, 899
Skullcap (*Scutellaria lateriflora*), 1009; in combinations, 908, 934, 966, 967
Sleep: in PMS treatment, 697; snoring during, 764-765; TMJ prevention during, 809
Sleep apnea, 94, 366-367, 764, 765
Sleep medications, 336, 338, 512; anti-insomnia drugs, 897; interactions with, 895, 936, 960
Sleep problems, 510-513, 514-515
Sliding hiatal hernia, 474, *475*
Slings, use of, *65*, 750
Slipped (herniated) disks, 164-165, 326-329, *327*, 620-621, 626-627, 672-673
Slippery elm, 1009-1010; in combination, 916
Slo-Bid (theophylline), 1015
Slow-K (potassium chloride), 995
Small cell lung cancer, 558-559, 560
Small intestine: celiac disease, 240-241; in Crohn's disease, *299*; ileostomy, 300, 301; in inguinal hernia, *473*; lactase production, lack of, 540-541
Smell, sense of, *1067*
Smilax officinalis (sarsaparilla), 803
Smoking: and bronchitis, acute, 214; and colds, 282; and emphysema, 346, 347; and heart disease, 459; and lung cancer, 558, 559, 561; and obesity, 631; and pneumonia, 681; during pregnancy, 690; stopping, 349, 624-625; and throat cancer, 822; and ulcers, 781. *See also* Tobacco use
Smoking cessation drugs, 1010; interactions with, 997
Snakebites, *76-77*
Snakes, bushmaster, venom of, 967
Sneezing, 762-763
Snoring, 764-765
Social phobia, 670, 671
Sodium, 1040-1041
Sodium bicarbonate (bicarbonate of soda): and citric acid, 1010; interactions with, 926, 1015
Sodium chloride, 980
Sodium polystyrene sulfonate, 531; interactions with, 891
Soft corns, 292
Solidago virgaurea (goldenrod), 109, 434, 757, 946
Soma (carisoprodol), 917
Sores: bedsores, 172-173; canker sores, 232-233, *1045*; cold sores, 270-271, *1045*
Sore throats, 725, 766-769; strep throat, 782-783
Sorrel: Jamaica (*Hibiscus sabdariffa*), 957-958; sheep, 1007; wood, 473
Sourdock (*Rumex crispus*), 79, 638, 708, 803
Spanish fly, 916
Spastic colon (spastic colitis; irritable bowel syndrome), 84-85, 200-201, 324-325, 516-519
Spearmint, 1010
Specialty boards, certification by, 19
Sperm, 42; disorders of, 502
Spermatic cord, twisted, 816-817
Sphenoidal sinuses, 754, *755*
Spiders, poisonous, *509*; bites, 508, 509, *1049*
Spider venom, compounds in, as stroke remedy, 791
Spinach and iron, 119
Spinal bone spurs, 198, 199
Spinal manipulation, 168-169, 439
Spinal nerves, pinched, 672-*673*
Spinal neurons, *555*
Spinal stenosis, 164-165
Spinal tap (lumbar puncture), 585, 601
Spine, 166, *167*; backache, *chart*, 164-165; back problems, 166-169; curvature of, sideways (scoliosis), 736-*737*; disk problems, 164-165, 326-329, *327*, 620-621, 626-627, 672-*673*
Spirituality, 27
Spironolactone: interactions with, 891, 905
Spleen, *567*; and anemia, 120
Spleen pumping, 399, 579, 605
Splenic sequestration, 752
Splints for injured legs, *65*
Spondylosis, 140-141, 164-165
Spongia, 303; *S. tosta*, 543
Sporadic goiter, 404
Sports injuries, 158-161; groin pull as, 417
Sprains, 770-*771*
Spring onions (scallions), 1004-1005
Spurs, bone, 198-*199*, 370-371
Squamous cell carcinoma, 758, 759, 760, *1047*; lung, 558, *559*; oral, *1045*
Squamous cell epithelium of cervix, 244
SSRIs (selective serotonin reuptake inhibitors), 1005
Stable angina, 124, 125
Stable (Type 2) diabetes, 316, 317, 318, 319, 320, 321
Stachydrine, 886
Staging phase of cancer diagnosis, 228
Standing posture, 169
Stapedectomy, 445
Staph (*Staphylococcus aureus*) infections, 772-775; boils, 191, 194-195, 556-557, 772, 773, 774, 775
Staphysagria, 184, 305, 705
Star fruit, 537
Starvation, self-induced, 132-133
Stasis dermatitis, 312-313
STDs. *See* Sexually transmitted diseases
Steam, vaporizers for, 217, 297, 349
Steam inhalations, 282, 349, 615, 757, 769
Steere, Allen, 565
Stellaria media (chickweed), 921
Stephania: interactions with, 930
Stereotactic surgery, 661
Sterilization as contraception method, 41, 42
Steroid therapy, side effects of, 343, 708
Stiff neck, 620-621
Still, Andrew Taylor, 28
Still's disease (juvenile rheumatoid arthritis), 142, 143
Stimulant laxatives, 967, 993, 1006
Stimulants, 919; addictive, 336-337, 338; interactions with, 890, 905, 910, 914, 935, 938, 953, 978, 982
Stimulating expectorants, 297
Sting allergies, 107, 109, 176-177
Stings: bee and wasp, 176-177; scor-

pion, 508, 509
Stomach, hiatal hernia and, 474, *475*
Stomach cancer, *776-777*
Stomach flu (gastroenteritis), 84-85, 324-325, 392-393, 616-617, 868-869
Stomach inflammation (gastritis), 84-85, 324-325, 390-391
Stomach ulcers, 84-85, 616-617, 618-619, 778-781, *779*
Stools. *See* Bowel movement abnormalities
Stool-softening laxatives, 939, 967
Strabismus, 360-361
Straight-leg-raising test, 327
Strains, 608-609, 770-771; groin strain, 416-417; hamstring injury, 426-427
Strangulated hernias, 473; hiatal, 474, 475
Strawberry gingivitis, 419
Strawberry nevus, *1044*
Strep throat, 782-783; and rheumatic fever, 724-725; vs. tonsillitis, 834
Streptokinase, 189, 454
Streptozocin, 485
Stress, 364-365, 514-515, 597, 784-787; and heart disease, 459; and hypertension, coping with, 481
Stress fractures, 159, 160, 748
Stress incontinence, 494, 495, 496, 497
Stress injuries, 234-237
Stress test, 127
Stretches: for multiple sclerosis, 603; for muscle cramps, 607; for stress, 786
Stroke, 334-335, 364-365, 626-627, 788-791
Structural Integration (Rolfing), 24
Strychnine, 985
Sty, 360-361, 772, 773, 774, 775, 792-793, *1051*
Subacute thyroiditis, 824, 826-827
Subconjunctival hemorrhage, *1051*
Subluxation, 26
Sucralfate, 1010-1011; interactions with, 949, 966
Sudafed (pseudoephedrine), 997
Sudden infant death syndrome (SIDS), 33
Sulfadoxine, 573
Sulfa drugs, 107, 246
Sulfamethoxazole and trimethoprim, 1011
Sulfasalazine, 119, 299; interactions with, 938
Sulfinpyrazone, 410; interactions with, 962, 983, 1011
Sulfisoxazole, 642
Sulfites, 149, 151, 1039
Sulfonamides: in combination, 1011-1012; interactions with, 920, 959, 962, 984, 991, 994
Sulfonylureas, 1012; interactions with, 962
Sulfur, 1041
Sulphur, 1012
Sumatriptan, 1012
Sumycin (tetracycline), 1014
Sunburn, 794-795
Sundew, 303, 877
Sun exposure, skin cancers from, 758, 759, 761
Sunscreens, 795
Superficial phlebitis, 544-545, 668, 669
Superficial varicose veins, 858, 859, 860
Superoxide dismutase (SOD), lack of, 554
Support groups, 27
Supportive treatment for cancer, 228
Support stockings, 669, 859
Suprax (cefixime), 918
Surgery, 20. *See also individual ailments*
Sus-Phrine (epinephrine), 942
Swallowing difficulty, *chart*, 796-797
Swank Diet, 603
Sweating: and body odor, 192, 193; excessive, *chart*, 798-799
Sweat plant (boneset), 909-910; in combinations, 918, 961
Sweet flag, 475
Swimmer's ear, 340-341, 800-801
Symphytum, 179
Symphytum officinale (comfrey), 929
Symptoms charts. *See individual ailments*
Syndrome X, 461
Synovectomy, 145
Synovitis, rheumatoid arthritis known as, 142
Synthroid (levothyroxine), 969
Syphilinum, 803
Syphilis, 716-717, 802-803
Syrups, 1026
System-cleansing diet, 793
Systemic lupus erythematosus (SLE), 562
Systemic yeast infections, 880, 881
Systolic pressure, 478
Syzygium aromaticum (clove), 171, 757, 837

T

Tabacum, 692
Tabebuia impetiginosa (pau d'arco), 990
Tachycardia, 448, 450, 451
Tacrine hydrochloride, 112
Tagamet; Tagamet HB (cimetidine), 924
T'ai chi, 24
Tamarind, Malabar, 256
Tamoxifen, 207, 1013; interactions with, 944
Tampons, use of, 351, 353, 838, 839
Tangerine peel, 1013; in combinations, 902, 995
Tang-kuei formula, 405
Tannins, 233, 466, 615, 903, 908, 979, 1000, 1002, 1020
Tansy (*Tanacetum vulgare*), 21, 879
Tapeworms, 878, 879
Taraxacum mongolicum (dandelion), 934-935; in combination, 924
Taraxacum officinale (dandelion), 934; in combination, 903
Tardive dyskinesia (TD), 733
Tarsal tunnel syndrome, 234, 237
Taste, sense of, *1067*; changes in, during pregnancy, 693
Tavist-D (clemastine, phenylpropanolamine), 927, 993, 997
Taxol, 627, 645
TB (tuberculosis), 368-369, 844-845
TCAs (tricyclic antidepressants), 1019; interactions with, 906, 910, 913, 917, 925, 935, 937, 944, 969, 970, 976, 980, 988, 994, 1016
T cells, kinds of, 486; killer, 760
TCM (traditional Chinese medicine), 20, 22, 24
Teak tree, 499
Teas, herbal, 1025
Tea tree oil, 1013-1014
Tectona grandis (teak), 499
Teenagers. *See* Adolescents
Teeth: baby, 804, *805*. *See also* Dental problems
Teething problems, 804-805
Tegretol (carbamazepine), 917
Telogen effluvium, 422, 423
Temazepam, 1014
Temperature, basal, monitoring, 825
Temporal lobe seizures, 358
Temporomandibular joint (TMJ) syndrome, 340-341, 362-363, 806-809
Tendonitis, 128-129, 140-141, 428-429, 750-751, 810-811; athletic injuries, 158, 159, 160, 161
Tendons in tennis elbow, 812, 813
Tenex (guanfacine), 956
Tennis elbow, 140-141, 812-815, *813*
Tennis technique, proper, 815
Tenormin (atenolol), 901
TENS (transcutaneous electrical nerve

stimulator), 168, 236, 653
Tension headaches, 436, 437, 438, 439, 440, 441
Terazol (terconazole), 1014
Terazosin, 1014; interactions with, 976
Terbinafine, 157
Terbutaline, 1014
Terconazole, 1014
Teribinthina, 535
Terpenes, 915
Terpinen-4-ol, 964
Terpineol, 1013
Testicle problems, 43, 556-557; *chart*, 816-817
Testicle self-examination, 819
Testicular cancer, 816-817, 818-*819*
Testosterone, 493; and prostate cancer, 699, 700
Tetanospasmin, 820
Tetanus, 820-821
Tetrachloroethylene, 533
Tetrachloromethane, 533
Tetracycline, 1014; interactions with, 891, 898, 920, 925, 962, 968, 998
Tetracyclines, 1014-1015; interactions with, 991
Tetrahydrocannabinol (THC), 403
Thalassemia, 119, 120
Theo-Dur (theophylline), 1015
Theophylline, 1015; interactions with, 898, 902, 906, 915, 925, 926, 943, 944, 966, 972, 986, 999
TheraFlu (acetaminophen, chlorpheniramine, dextromethorphan, pseudoephedrine), 884, 923, 936, 997
Therapeutic Touch, 24, 137
Thermal biofeedback, 441
Theucrium marum, 615
Thiamine (vitamin B_1), 1033-1034
Thiazide diuretics, 408, 537; interactions with, 939, 962
Thioridazine, 112; interactions with, 906
Third-degree burns, 222, 223
Third nerve palsy, 710-711
Thistle, blessed, 908-909
Thoracic aneurysms, 122
Thorowax root (bupleurum), 912; in combinations, 901, 925, 933
Threadworms, 878, 879
Throat, 822, *823*; objects in, 54-*56*, 796-797
Throat cancer, 796-797, 822-823
Throat culture, 725, 766, 783
Thrombi, 188
Thrombophlebitis, 668-669
Thrombosed hemorrhoids, 464
Thrush, 716-717, 880, 881, *1045*; and diaper rash, 322, 323
Thuja (*Thuja occidentalis*), 21, 407, 675, 705, 843, 873
Thuja occidentalis (homeopathic remedy), 395, 397, 615
Thujone, 1003, 1023
Thyme (*Thymus vulgaris*), 193, 264, 303, 307, 344, 551, 756, 775, 803, 877
Thyroid hormones, 1015-1016; interactions with, 894, 910, 962, 997
Thyroiditis, 620-621; Hashimoto's, 824-825; subacute, 824, 826-827
Thyroid problems, 368-369, 798-799, 824-827; goiters, 404-*405*; Graves' disease, 412-415
Thyroid-stimulating hormone (TSH), 825
Thyroid USP, 1016
Thyrotoxic crisis, 412
TIAs (transient ischemic attacks), 334-335, 364-365, 626-627, 788
Tic douloureux (trigeminal neuralgia), 362-363, 622, 623
Ticks, 508, 509, *727*; Lyme disease from, 564-565, *1049*; removing, 509, 565, 727; Rocky Mountain spotted fever from, 726-727
Ticlopidine, 790
Tics and twitches, 828-829
Tilia spp. (linden), 121, 136, 440, 463
Timolol, 1016
Timoptic (timolol), 1016
Tinactin (tolnaftate), 1016
Tinctures, herbal, 1025-1026
Tinea cruris (jock itch), 520-521, 524-525
Tinel's sign test, 235
Tingling and numbness, *chart*, 626-627
Tinnitus, 830-833
TMJ (temporomandibular joint) syndrome, 340-341, 362-363, 806-809
TMP-SMZ (trimethoprim and sulfamethoxazole), 1011
Tobacco, Indian (lobelia), 971; in combination, 979
Tobacco use: interactions with, 898, 906, 925, 944, 947, 962, 983, 986, 997, 1019; and nicotine withdrawal, 624-625; and oral cancer, 634. *See also* Smoking
Tobramycin, 1016; interactions with, 920
Tobrex (tobramycin), 1016
Tocopherols, 1036
Toenail problems: *chart*, 612-613; athlete's foot as, 156, 157; ingrown nail, 506-*507*
Toes: bunions, 220-*221*; corns, 292, *1046*; gout, *409*, 410; Raynaud's syndrome, 718, 719
Tolbutamide, 319
Tolmetin, 391
Tolnaftate, 1016-1017
Tongue: cleaning, 171; taste buds, *1067*
Tonsillar abscess, 834-835
Tonsillectomy, 835
Tonsillitis, 834-835
Tonsils, 834, *835*
Tooth abscess, 362-363, 372-373, 836, *837*
Toothache, 836-837
Tooth decay, 836, *837*
Tophi, 408
Topical antibiotics, 1017
Toprol (metoprolol), 976
Toradol (ketorolac), 966
Torso, *1058*
Touch, sense of, *1067*
Touch therapy, 146
Tourette's syndrome, 828
Tourniquet, making, *76*
Toxemia (preeclampsia), 130-131, 378-379, 688
Toxic hepatitis, 469, 470
Toxic megacolon, 274
Toxic shock syndrome, 838-839
Toxins: tetanospasmin, 820. *See also* Poisoning
Toxoplasmosis, 39
t-PA (clot-dissolving drug), 454
Trabeculoplasty; trabeculectomy, 402
Traditional Chinese medicine (TCM), 20, 22, 24
Trager Psycho-physical Integration, 24
Tranquilizers, 410, 733; interactions with, 895, 917, 918, 936, 960, 996, 997, 1021, 1022, 1024
Transcutaneous electrical nerve stimulator (TENS), 168, 236, 653
Transderm-Nitro (nitroglycerin), 983
Transient insomnia, 510, 511
Transient ischemic attacks (TIAs), 334-335, 364-365, 626-627, 788
Transillumination, 755
Transitional cell carcinoma, kidney, 528
Transplants: bone marrow, 549, 569; hair, 424; kidney, 532; liver, 268-269
Transurethral resection (TUR), 181, 704
Tranylcypromine, 1017
Traumatic ulcers, 232
Traveler's diarrhea, 382
Treadmill (stress) test, 127
Trembling, *chart*, 840-841
Trench mouth (Vincent's angina), 418,

419, 420
Trental (pentoxifylline), 991
Tretinoin, 1017-1018
Triamcinolone, 1018
Triaminic DM Syrup (dextromethorphan, phenylpropanolamine), 936, 993
Triaminic Expectorant (guaifenesin, phenylpropanolamine), 955, 993
Triaminic Nite Light (chlorpheniramine, dextromethorphan, pseudoephedrine), 923, 936, 997
Triaminicol Multi-Symptom Relief (chlorpheniramine, dextromethorphan, phenylpropanolamine), 923, 936, 993
Triaminic Sore Throat Formula (acetaminophen, dextromethorphan, pseudoephedrine), 884, 936, 997
Triaminic Syrup (chlorpheniramine, phenylpropanolamine), 923, 993
Triamterene, 1018; in combination, 959; interactions with, 891, 905, 925, 962, 995
Triazolam, 1019; interactions with, 902, 943
Trichinosis, 878, 879
Trichloromethane, 533
Trichomoniasis, 842-843
Trichotillomania, 422
Tricosantin (Compound Q), 99
Tricyclic antidepressants (TCAs), 1019; interactions with, 906, 910, 913, 917, 925, 935, 937, 944, 969, 970, 976, 980, 988, 994, 1016
Trifolium pratense (red clover), 999; in combinations, 913, 979
Trigeminal neuralgia, 362-363, 622, 623
Trigonella foenum-graecum (fenugreek), 947-948
Trihexyphenidyl: interactions with, 996
Tri-Levlen (ethinyl estradiol, levonorgestrel), 944, 969
Trimethobenzamide, 392
Trimethoprim, 1019
Trimox (amoxicillin), 889
Triphasil (ethinyl estradiol, levonorgestrel), 944, 969
Triprolidine, 1019
Tritec (ranitidine), 999
Troleandomycin: in combinations, 914, 972
Tropicamide, 111
True unicorn root, 705
Trumpet (pau d'arco) tree, 990
Tryptophan, 261, 311, 513, 1033
Tuberculosis (TB), 368-369, 844-845
Tubular (cylindroid) aneurysms, *123*
Tui na, 811
Tularemia, ticks and, 508, 509
Tumor marker blood tests: KAI-1, 698-699; PSA, 699-700, 701
Tumors, 226; adenomas, 208, 211, 824, 826; brain, 202, *203*; carcinoid, 324-325; fibroids, 850-852, 853. *See also* Cancer
Tums (calcium carbonate), 914
Tums Antigas/Antacid Formula (simethicone), 1008
TUR (transurethral resection), 181, 704
Turmeric, 1019
Turnera diffusa (damiana), 934; in combination, 966
Tussilago farfara (coltsfoot), 928-929; in combinations, 961, 979; interactions with, 930
Twitches and tics, 828-829
Tylenol (acetaminophen), 884
Tylenol, with codeine, 927
Tylenol Allergy Sinus (pseudoephedrine), 997
Tylenol Cold (chlorpheniramine, dextromethorphan, pseudoephedrine), 923, 936, 997; effervescent formula (phenylpropanolamine), 993
Tylenol Cold Night Time Medication Liquid (diphenhydramine), 938
Tylenol Extra-Strength (acetaminophen), 884
Tylenol PM (diphenhydramine), 884, 938
Tylenol Sinus (pseudoephedrine), 997
Tympanostomy, 642
Type A influenza, 374, 376, 377
Type A personality, 43, 454, 786
Type B influenza, 374-375, 377
Type 1 diabetes, 316, 317, 318-319, 320, 321
Type 2 diabetes, 316, 317, 318, 319, 320, 321
Tyramine, 310, 431, 615
Tyrosine, 827

U

Ulcerated bedsores, 172
Ulcerative colitis, 84-85, 274, 275, 526-527
Ulcers: canker sores, 232-233, *1045*; ecthyma, 490; stomach, 84-85, 616-617, 618-619, 778-781, *779*
Ulmus fulva (slippery elm), 1009-1010; in combination, 916
Ultraviolet (UV) radiation: and cataracts, 238, 239; for dermatitis, 314-315; for psoriasis, 708; and skin cancer, 759; and sunburn, 794, 795; UVA, 794, 795; UVB, 238, 239, 794, 795; for vitiligo, 867
Umbilical cord, tying off, *61*
Umbilical hernia, 472, 473
Unconsciousness, 71; cardiac and respiratory arrest, *50-53*; in choking victims, 54-*55*; drowning or near-drowning, 57; fainting, *chart*, 364-365; recovery position for, *47*
Undecylenic acid, 157
Unicorn root: false, 647, 665; true, 705
Unstable angina, 124
Urea, 293, 466, 507
Urethra: and bladder infections, 182; prostate and, 702, *703*
Urge incontinence, 494-495, 496, 497
Uric acid and gout, 408, *409*, 410, 411
Urinary problems: *chart*, 846-847; bedwetting, 174-175; incontinence, 494-497, 700
Urinary system: female, *1062*; male, *1063*
Urinary tract problems: abdominal pains from, *chart*, 86-87; bladder cancer, 180-181; bladder infections, 182-185; incontinence, 494-497, 700; kidney cancer, 528-*529*; kidney disease, 368-369, 378-379, 530-533; kidney infections, 534-535; kidney stones, 536-537; in pregnancy, 691, 693; prostate cancer, 698-701, *699*; prostate problems, 702-705, *703*; urinary problems, *chart*, 846-847
Urine flow rate, measuring, 495, 704
Urology, 20
Ursodiol: interactions with, 951
Urtica dioica (nettle), 981
Urticaria (hives), 106, 107, 108, 482-483, *1049*
Urtica urens, 411, 483
Usnea (*Usnea* spp.), 1020
Usnic acid, 1020
Uterine cancer, 848-*849*
Uterine problems, 848, 850-853, *851*; cervical, 244-247, *245*; cervical cancer, 242-243
Uterine sarcoma, 848
Uva ursi, 1020; in combinations, 911, 941
Uveitis, 710-711

Vaccines, 32; *chart*, 33; AIDS, work on, 98; bacillus Calmette-Gurin (BCG), 181; chickenpox, 251; DPT

(diphtheria, pertussis, and tetanus), 821, 827; flu, 377; hepatitis, 269, 470-471; interactions with, 996; MMR (measles, mumps, and rubella), 399, 579, 605; pneumonia, 216, 680; rabies, 713
Vaccinium myrtilloides (blueberry), 320
Vaccinium myrtillus (bilberry), 907
Vagal maneuver, 451
Vaginal antifungal drugs, 1020-1021
Vaginal cancer, 854, 855, 856
Vaginal lubrication, inadequate, 742
Vaginal pain, 742
Vaginal problems, 854-857; in pregnancy, 693
Vaginal weights, 496
Vaginal yeast infections, 504-505, 524, 854, 855, 856, 857, 880, 881
Vaginismus, 741, 742, 743, 854, 855-856, 857
Vaginitis, 854-855, 856-857
Vaginosis, bacterial, 854, 855, 856, 857
Valerian (*Valeriana officinalis*), 1021; in combinations, 908, 959, 989
Valine, 555
Valium (diazepam), 936
Valproic acid, 1021-1022; interactions with, 906, 917, 994
Valsartan, 1022
Valves: heart, disorders of, 459-460, *461*; in veins, 858, *859*
Vanadium, 1041
Vancenase AQ (beclomethasone), 903
Vanceril (beclomethasone), 903
Vaporizers, use of, 217, 297, 349
VapoRub (camphor, menthol), 916, 974
Variant angina, 124
Varicella (chickenpox), *250*-251, 714-715, *1044*
Varicocele, 816-817
Varicose veins, 130-131, 378-379, 544-545, 858-861; hemorrhoidal, 464-467, *465*, 691; in pregnancy, 693
Vascular ectasia, 114-115
Vascular headaches: cluster, 436, 437, 438, 439, 440, 441; migraine, 436, 437-440, 441, 616-617, 868-869
Vasectomy, 42
Vasomotor rhinitis, 684
Vaso-occlusive (painful) crises, 752-753
Vasotec (enalapril), 941
Veal bone supplement, 638-639
Veetids (penicillin V), 991
Veins, *669*, *1060*; and ankles, swollen, *chart*, 130-131; hemorrhoidal, 464-467, *465*, 691; and leg pain, *chart*, 544-545; phlebitis, 668-669; valves, 858, *859*; varicose, 378-379, 693, 858-861
Venereal diseases. *See* Sexually transmitted diseases (STDs)
Venom, snake: lachesis, 967; sucking out, 76
Ventolin (albuterol), 886
Ventricular arrhythmias, 448
Ventricular fibrillation, 448
Verapamil, 1022; interactions with, 984
Veratrum album, 383
Verbascum thapsus (mullein), 979; in combinations, 929, 954
Verbena officinalis (vervain), 169, 339, 512, 523, 596, 659
Verelan (verapamil), 1022
Verruca vulgaris (wart), 872-873
Vertebrae, *673*
Vertebral disks, problems of, 164-165, 326-329, *327*, 620-621, 626-627, 672-*673*
Vertebral spurs, 198, 199
Vertigo (dizziness): *chart*, 334-335; Ménière's disease, 580-583; in pregnancy, 691
Vervain, 169, 339, 512, 523, 596, 659
Vestibular neurectomy, 582
Viagra (sildenafil), 493, 1007-1008
Viburnum lentago (black haw), 591
Viburnum opulus (cramp), 136, 146, 169, 225, 440, 591, 723, 909, 1023
Vicodin (hydrocordone), 959
Vicoprofen (hydrocordone), 959
Vicotuss (guaifenesin), 955
Vidarabine monohydrate, 747
Vincent's angina, 418, 419, 420
Vincristine: interactions with, 1013
Violet (*Viola yedoensis*), 195
Vioxx (rofecoxib), 1000
Viral food poisoning, 382
Viral infections, 501; AIDS, 96-101; chickenpox, *250*-251, *1044*; cold sores, 270-271, *1045*; common cold, 280-283, 375; congestion from, *chart*, 284-285; conjunctivitis as, 286, 287; croup, 302-303; eczema and, 342, 345; fever and chills from, *chart*, 372-373; flu, 374-377; genital herpes, 394-395; German measles, 39, 398-*399*, *1044*; hepatitis, 267, 268, 269, 468-471; laryngitis as, 542; lumps from, *chart*, 556-557; measles, 578-*579*, *1044*; meningitis as, 584, 585; mononucleosis, 594-597; mumps, 604-605; and otitis media, 640, 641, 643; pneumonia as, 678, 680; rabies, 712-713; rashes from, *chart*, 714-717; shingles, 362-363, 746-747, *1050*; sore throat from, 766, 767, 769. *See also* Warts
Viscum album (mistletoe), 977
Vision, *1066*
Vision problems, 862-865, *863*. *See also* Eye problems
Visualization, 489, 652, 787
Vitamin A, 1033
Vitamin B_1 (thiamine), 1033-1034
Vitamin B_2 (riboflavin), 1034
Vitamin B_3 (niacin), 1032-1033; interactions with, 972, 996, 1009
Vitamin B_5 (pantothenic acid), 1034
Vitamin B_6 (pyridoxine), 1034-1035; interactions with, 969
Vitamin B_7 (biotin, vitamin H), 1032
Vitamin B_9 (folic acid), 1032; interactions with, 924, 1011
Vitamin B_{12} (cobalamin), 1035
Vitamin B complex, 1033
Vitamin B_{12} deficiency anemia, 118, 119-120
Vitamin C (ascorbic acid), 1035
Vitamin D, 1035-1036
Vitamin E, 1036
Vitamin H (biotin, vitamin B_7), 1032
Vitamin K, 1036
Vitamins, 28, 1032-1036; interactions with, 892, 893, 923, 924, 925, 928, 944, 1010, 1011, 1022. *See also individual ailments*
Vitex, 890
Vitex agnus-castus (chaste tree), 921
Vitiligo, 866-*867*
Vivarin (caffeine), 914
Vivelle (estradiol), 943
Vocal cords, 542, *543*; problems, 796-797
Volmax (albuterol), 886
Voltaren (diclofenac), 937
Vomiting: *chart*, 868-871; self-induced, 218-219
Vulvitis, 854, 855, 856, 857

W

Walking pneumonia, 678-679
Walnut, black, 908
Warfarin, 1022; interactions with, 891, 894, 898, 923, 925, 931, 949, 966, 970, 978, 986, 999, 1011, 1013, 1016
Warts, 872-873; vs. calluses, 292; common, 872, *1046*; flat, 872, *1047*; genital, 245, 246, 396-397, 666-667; plantar, 370-371, 674-675
Wasps, *177*; stings, 176-177

Water moccasins (cottonmouths), *77*; bites from, 76
Water plantain (alisma), 886
Water rescue, *57*
Water-soluble vitamins: B vitamins, 1032-1035; vitamin C, 1035
Wax in ears, 340-341, 444
Wegener's granulomatosis, 418, 419, 420
Weight, problems with: anorexia nervosa, 132-133, 218; bulimia, 218-219; obesity, 628-631
Weight and height charts: adults, 37; children, 34-35
Weight-bearing exercises, 638
Wellbutrin (bupropion), 912
Western hemlock, 705
Wet macular degeneration, 570, 571
Wheezing, 874-875
Whiplash, 608-609, 620-621; and TMJ, 809
White atractylodes, 901-902; in combinations, 901, 922, 928, 951, 953, 955
White blood cells: in leukemia, 546, *547*, 549; in lymphatic system, 567; in lymphoma, 566; neutrophils and common cold, 280; T cells, 486, 760
White-faced hornet, *177*
Whiteheads, 90
White horehound (horehound), 79, 680, 909, 929, 961, 979
White mulberry leaf, 296, 899, 924, 1006
White oak, 543
White willow, 1022-1023
Whooping cough, 876-877
Wild black cherry, 303, 348, 680, 877
Wild chrysanthemum (*Chrysanthemum indicum*), 348, 680, 877, 924
Wild cranesbill, 79, 593
Wild hops, 911
Wild indigo, 596
Wild lettuce, 877
Wild yam, 1023; in combination, 903; Mexican, 638
Willow, 146, 225; white, 1022-1023
Wilms' tumor, 528, 529
Wilson's disease, 267, 268
Wilson's Syndrome, 825
Windflower, 998
Wintergreen, 282, 439, 651
Wintergreen oil (methyl salicylate), 889, 975-976; in combinations, 897, 916, 975; interactions with, 1022
Witch hazel, 79, 195, 251, 271, 467, 579, 683, 691, 860, 954, 979
Withania somnifera (ashwaganda), 900
Withdrawal from drugs, 338, 514-515; alcohol, 103-104, 618-619
Wolfberry (lycium fruit), 973; in combination, 995
Women's health, 38-41
Wood betony, 440, 908
Wood sorrel, 473
Wood tick, *727*
Work and tendonitis, 811
Worms, 200-201, 520-521, 878-879
Wormwood, 21, 201, 879
Wounds, 304-305; bleeding, first aid for, *48*; and tetanus, 820, 821
Wrinkles, 44
Wrist, *235*; injured, immobilizing, *65*
Wristbands, acupressure, 599
Wrist pain, *chart,* 428-429
Wymox (amoxicillin), 889

X

Xanax (alprazolam), 888
Xanthium (*Xanthium sibiricum*), 582, 757, 974

Yam, Chinese, 922-923; in combinations, 922, 930, 945
Yam, wild, 1023; in combination, 903; Mexican, 638
Yarrow, 1023; in combinations, 911, 918, 934, 941
Yeast infections, 504-505, 524, 854, 855, 856, 857, 880-881, *1044*; and diaper rash, 322, 323; oral thrush, 880, 881, *1045*
Yellow cedar, 675
Yellow jacket, *177*
Yellow jasmine, 951
Yi mu cao (Chinese motherwort), 922
Yin deficiency, 889, 955
Ylang-ylang, 493
Yoga, 27, *1085-1093*; Abdominal Massage, *518, 1085*; Boat, *352, 705, 1085*; Bow, *352, 696, 1085*; breathing exercises, 349; Bridge, *488, 1085*; C, *146, 1086*; Camel, *590, 1086*; Cat, *146, 1086*; Child, *329, 488, 774, 787, 1086*; Climbing the Wall, *205*; Cobra, 291, *696, 705, 875, 1087*; Cobra (Half), *1087*; Corpse, *256, 653, 774, 787, 1087*; Dog, 146, *1087*; Dog, Downward, *590*; Dog, Upward, *1093*; Downward Dog, *590*; Fish, *446*; Half Cobra, *1087*; Half Lotus, *774, 1089*; Half Moon, *260, 488*; Half Shoulder Stand, *446, 1091*; head movements, *833*; Head to Knee, *1088*; Hero, *1088*; Knee Down Twist, *329, 787, 1088*; Knee to Chest, 291; Locust, *352, 696, 1088*; Lotus, *774*; Lotus (Half), *774, 1089*; Mountain, *260, 1089*; Pigeon, *875, 1089*; Plow, *1089*; Posterior Stretch, *1090*; Rag Doll, *260, 329, 1090*; Seated Angle, *1090*; Shoulder Crunch, *1090*; Shoulder Stand, 415, 827, *1090*; Shoulder Stand (Half), *446, 1091*; Sphinx, *462, 577, 663, 1091*; Spider Push-Up, *146, 1091*; Spinal, *1091*; Standing Angle, *518, 1092*; Standing Yoga Mudra, *1092*; Thumb Squeezer, *146*; Tree, *1092*; Triangle, *1092*; Upward Dog, *1093*; Warrior 1, *1093*; Warrior 2, *1093*; Yoga Mudra, *1093*; Yoga Mudra, Standing, *1092*
Yohimbine, 493

Z

Zantac (ranitidine), 888, 999
Zanthoxylum americanum (prickly ash), 225, 421, 814, 815, 1004
Zefrex LA (phenylpropanolamine), 993
Zestril (lisinopril), 971
Zidovudine (AZT), 99; interactions with, 884, 885, 906, 926
Zinc, 1041; and Alzheimer's disease, 111, 113; interactions with, 949
Zinc preparations, 313, 315, 323, 345, 466, 669, 715, 795, 1041
Zingiber officinale (ginger), 952; in combinations, 890, 907, 909, 929, 941, 946, 951, 971, 978, 1004, 1023
Zithromax (azithromycin), 902
Zocor (simvastatin), 1008
Zoloft (sertraline), 1006
Zolpidem, 1023-1024
Zovirax (acyclovir), 884
Zyban (bupropion; nicotine), 912, 981

PICTURE CREDITS

All illustrations in this book were created by **Totally Incorporated.** Individual artists are listed below in alphabetical order.

Roxanna Drake, Carol Hilliard, Leslie Lien, Peter Malamas, Tipy Taylor, Patrick Wilson

---

The sources for photographs in this book are listed below. Credits from left to right are separated by semicolons; credits from top to bottom are separated by dashes.

37: Reproduced courtesy of Metropolitan Life Insurance Company.
1044: Custom Medical Stock Photo, Chicago (2); American Academy of Dermatology, Schaumburg, Ill.; NMSB/Custom Medical Stock Photo—NMSB/Custom Medical Stock Photo (2)—Keith/Custom Medical Stock Photo.
1045: © Carroll H. Weiss, 1995; Martin/Custom Medical Stock Photo—NMSB/Custom Medical Stock Photo; American Academy of Dermatology—Martin/Custom Medical Stock Photo.
1046: NMSB/Custom Medical Stock Photo (2); American Academy of Dermatology—American Academy of Dermatology; Custom Medical Stock Photo.
1047: American Academy of Dermatology; Dr. Jesse M. Kramer (2)—Nancy Wolfin, MD/ Medical Images Inc., Salisbury, Conn.; American Academy of Dermatology.
1048: American Academy of Dermatology (2)—© Carroll H. Weiss, 1995 (2).
1049: American Academy of Dermatology; Nancy Wolfin, MD/Medical Images Inc.; Custom Medical Stock Photo—© Carroll H. Weiss, 1995.
1050: English/Custom Medical Stock Photo; Leonard Morse, MD/Medical Images Inc.—American Academy of Dermatology—Biomed Comm/Custom Medical Stock Photo.
1051: SPL/Custom Medical Stock Photo—Michael English/Medical Images Inc.—SPL/Custom Medical Stock Photo.

ACKNOWLEDGMENTS

Marian Abousief, Terese Murphy Austin, Univ. of Michigan, Ann Arbor; Kathryn Bryan, Bethesda, Md.; James A. Bryant, Office of Alternative Medicine, NIH, Rockville, Md.; Karen Childs, Washington, D.C.; Jim Cirigliano, Torrance, Calif.; Anne DeBevoise, Glendale, Calif.; Alice D. Domar, PhD, Harvard Medical School, Cambridge; Kathleen Enberenz, RENFREW, Philadelphia; Mary Lee Esty, Washington, D.C.; Julia Euling, Sydbury, Mass.; Carol Fedora, Univ. of Michigan; Mitchell Fleisher, MD, Arrington, Va.; Richard Friedman, PhD, State Univ. of New York-Stony Brook, Department of Psychiatry and Behavioral Science, N.Y.; Jim Gray, PhD, The American Univ., Washington, D.C.; Judith Graykowski, Univ. of Michigan; Tracy Harnish, Univ. of Michigan; Lucy Henderson, Orinda, Calif.; Roger Jahnke, OMD, Goleta, Calif.; Wayne B. Jonas, MD, Alexandria, Va.; Joan Klyhn, New Age Health Spa, Neversink, N.Y.; Lauren LaCroix, Kline and Company, Little Falls, New Jersey; Diane Lawther, Julie J. Lea, Univ. of Michigan; Lisa Lefferts, Mothers and Others for a Livable Planet, Hyattsville, Md.; Ginger Lepre, Gary Litovitz, MD, Dominion Hospital, Falls Church, Va.; Robert McCaleb, Herb Research Foundation, Boulder, Colo.; Sarah Neises, Univ. of Michigan; G.R. Oberg, MD, The Crystal Lake Center for Allergy and Environmental Medicine, Crystal Lake, Ill.; Mary T. Panek, Josie Barnes Parker, Tammy M. Pearson, Linda P. Powers, Univ. of Michigan; Jon L. Richter, DMD, PhD, Richter Center for Treatment of Breath Disorders, Philadelphia; Jolie Martin Root, Boca Raton, Fla.; Barbara S. Schneidman, MD, MPH, American Board of Medical Specialties, Evanston, Ill.; Elaine Wu Stephenson, Univ. of Michigan; Colin M. Thomas, Washington, D.C.; Devon Thomas, Univ. of Michigan; Michael Tims, Cash Grocer, Alexandria, Va.; Jeremy Waletsky, MD, George Washington Univ., Washington, D.C.; Thomas A. Wehr, MD, NIMH, Rockville, Md.; Rita Lynn Wilson, Univ. of Michigan; William Wittman, MD, Falmouth, Mass.; Karen Beth Zamanick, MD, Northwestern Memorial Hospital, Chicago; Laura Zylstra-Garth, Washington, D.C.